Practical gastroenterology and hepatology board review toolkit

Practical gastroenterology and hepatology board review toolkit

Editor-in-Chief

Nicholas J. Talley

Section Editors

Kenneth R. DeVault
Michael B. Wallace
Bashar A. Aqel
Keith D. Lindor

Second Edition

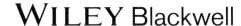

WILEY Blackwell

This edition first published 2016 © 2016 by John Wiley & Sons, Ltd

Registered office: John Wiley & Sons, Ltd, The Atrium, Southern Gate, Chichester,
West Sussex, PO19 8SQ, UK

Editorial offices: 9600 Garsington Road, Oxford, OX4 2DQ, UK
The Atrium, Southern Gate, Chichester, West Sussex, PO19 8SQ, UK
111 River Street, Hoboken, NJ 07030-5774, USA

For details of our global editorial offices, for customer services and for information about how to apply for permission to reuse the copyright material in this book please see our website at www.wiley.com/wiley-blackwell

The right of the authors to be identified as the authors of this work has been asserted in accordance with the UK Copyright, Designs and Patents Act 1988.

Library of Congress Cataloging-in-Publication Data

Names: Talley, Nicholas Joseph, editor. | Aqel, Bashar A., editor. | Lindor, Keith D., editor. | DeVault, Ken, editor. | Wallace, Michael B. (Michael Bradley), editor.
Title: Practical gastroenterology and hepatology board review toolkit / editor-in-chief, Nicholas J. Talley ; section editors, Bashar A. Aqel, Keith Lindor, Kenneth DeVault, Michael Wallace.
Description: Second edition. | Chichester, West Sussex ; Hoboken, NJ : John Wiley & Sons Inc., 2016. | Preceded by three works originally published in 2010 as individual volumes: Practical gastroenterology and hepatology. Esophagus and stomach, Practical gastroenterology and hepatology. Liver and biliary disease, and Practical gastroenterology and hepatology. Small and large intestine and pancreas. | Includes bibliographical references and index.
Identifiers: LCCN 2016000004 | ISBN 9781118829066 (pbk.) | ISBN 9781118829080 (epub) | ISBN 9781118829073 (Adobe PDF)
Subjects: | MESH: Digestive System Diseases | Diagnostic Techniques, Digestive System
Classification: LCC RC801 | NLM WI 140 | DDC 616.3/30076–dc23 LC record available at http://lccn.loc.gov/2016000004

A catalogue record for this book is available from the British Library.

Wiley also publishes its books in a variety of electronic formats. Some content that appears in print may not be available in electronic books.

Cover image: Getty/Ugreen

Set in 9/11pt MinionPro by Aptara Inc., New Delhi, India
Printed and bound in Singapore by Markono Print Media Pte Ltd

1   2016

Contents

List of contributors, ix

Foreword, xv

Preface, xvii

About the companion website, xviii

Section I: How to Ace the Boards in Gastroenterology and Hepatology

1   Introduction and Overview of the Gastroenterology Boards, 3
    Brooks Cash

Section II: Esophagus and stomach
Editors Kenneth R. DeVault and Nick J. Talley

Part 1: Pathobiology of the Esophagus and Stomach

2   Anatomy, Embryology, and Congenital Malformations of the Esophagus and Stomach, 11
    Lori A. Orlando and Roy C. Orlando

3   Esophageal and Gastric Motor Function, 15
    Kenneth R. DeVault, Ernest P. Bouras, and Nicholas J. Talley

Part 2: Other Diagnostic Modalities

4   Radiologic Approach to Diagnosis, 23
    Stephen W. Trenkner and James E. Huprich

5   Esophageal Motility Disorders, 28
    Magnus Halland and Kenneth R. DeVault

6   Gastric Motility Testing, 36
    Jan Tack

Part 3: Problem-Based Approach to Diagnosis and Differential Diagnosis

7   General Approach to History-Taking and Physical Examination of the Upper Gastrointestinal Tract, 43
    Evan S. Dellon and Eugene M. Bozymski

8   Heartburn, Regurgitation, and Chest Pain, 46
    Kenneth R. DeVault

9   Dysphagia, 52
    Dawn L. Francis

10 Miscellaneous Upper Gastrointestinal Symptoms, 56
    Mohamed Sultan and James H. Lewis

11 Dyspepsia, 70
    Nicholas J. Talley, Kate Napthali, and Kenneth McQuaid

12 Nausea and Vomiting, 74
    John K. DiBaise

13 Hematemesis, 79
    Thomas O.G. Kovacs and Dennis M. Jensen

Part 4: Diseases of the Esophagus

14 Gastroesophageal Reflux Disease, 85
    Robert T. Kavitt and Michael F. Vaezi

15 Barrett's Esophagus, 91
    Shanmugarajah Rajendra and Prateek Sharma

16 Eosinophilic Esophagitis, 98
    Jeffrey A. Alexander

17 Strictures, Rings, and Webs, 105
    Ioannis S. Papanikolaou and Peter D. Siersema

Part 5: Diseases of the Stomach

18 Peptic Ulcer Disease, 115
    Francis K.L. Chan and Nicholas J. Talley

19 *Helicobacter pylori*, 121
    Barry J. Marshall

20 Gastritis, 126
    Massimo Rugge and David Y. Graham

21 Gastroparesis, 132
    Henry P. Parkman and Nicholas J. Talley

22 Non-variceal Upper Gastrointestinal Bleeding, 138
    Thomas J. Savides

23 Other Gastric Tumors (Benign and Malignant), 145
    Sun-Chuan Dai and Michael L. Kochman

24 Eosinophilic Gastroenteritis, 152
    Magnus Halland and Nicholas J. Talley

25 Esophageal and Gastric Involvement in Systemic and Cutaneous Diseases, 156
    John M. Wo

Part 6: Functional Disease of the Esophagus and Stomach

26 Functional Esophageal Disorders, 169
    Ellionore Jarbrink-Sehgal, Kenneth R. DeVault, and Nicholas J. Talley

Section III: Intestine and Pancreas
Editor Michael Wallace

Part 1: Pathobiology of the Intestine and Pancreas

27 Clinical Anatomy, Embryology, and Congenital Anomalies, 177
    Advitya Malhotra and Joseph H. Sellin

28 Small-Intestinal Hormones and Neurotransmitters, 181
    James Reynolds

29 Mucosal Immunology of the Intestine, 187
    Maneesh Dave and William A. Faubion

30 Motor and Sensory Function, 191
Vineet S. Gudsoorkar and Eamonn M.M. Quigley

31 Neoplasia, 198
John M. Carethers

**Part 2: Problem-Based Approach to Diagnosis
and Differential Diagnosis**

32 General Approach to Relevant History-Taking and
Physical Examination, 203
Christopher L. Steele and Suzanne Rose

33 Acute Diarrhea, 213
John R. Cangemi

34 Chronic Diarrhea, 218
Lawrence R. Schiller

35 Loss of Appetite and Loss of Weight, 223
Angela Vizzini and Jaime Aranda-Michel

36 Gastrointestinal Food Allergy and Intolerance, 227
Mark T. DeMeo

37 Obesity: Presentations and Management Options, 231
*Andres Acosta, Todd A. Kellogg, and
Barham K. Abu Dayyeh*

38 Hematochezia, 237
Lisa L. Strate

39 Obscure Gastrointestinal Bleeding, 241
R. Sameer Islam and Shabana F. Pasha

40 Constipation, 246
Arnold Wald

41 Perianal Disease, 251
Leyla J. Ghazi and David A. Schwartz

42 Fecal Incontinence, 256
David Prichard and Adil E. Bharucha

43 Colorectal Cancer Screening, 261
Katherine S. Garman and Dawn Provenzale

44 Endoscopic Palliation of Malignant Obstruction, 266
Todd H. Baron

Part 3: Diseases of the Small Intestine

45 Crohn's Disease, 273
Kara M. De Felice and Sunanda V. Kane

46 Small-Bowel Tumors, 279
Nadir Arber and Menachem Moshkowitz

47 Small-Intestinal Bacterial Overgrowth, 285
Johanna Iturrino and Madhusudan Grover

48 Celiac Disease and Tropical Sprue, 291
Alberto Rubio-Tapia and Joseph A. Murray

49 Whipple's Disease, 296
Seema A. Patil and George T. Fantry

50 Short-Bowel Syndrome, 299
Alan L. Buchman

51 Protein-Losing Gastroenteropathy, 304
Lauren K. Schwartz and Carol E. Semrad

52 Acute Mesenteric Ischemia and Chronic
Mesenteric Insufficiency, 308
Timothy T. Nostrant

53 Intestinal Obstruction and Pseudo-obstruction, 313
Magnus Halland and Purna Kashyap

Part 4: Diseases of the Colon and Rectum

54 Ulcerative Colitis, 323
Sunanda V. Kane

55 *Clostridium difficile* Infection and Pseudomembranous
Colitis, 328
Byron P. Vaughn and J. Thomas Lamont

56 Colonic Ischemia, 333
Timothy T. Nostrant

57 Acute Diverticulitis, 338
Yuliya Y. Yurko and Tonia M. Young-Fadok

58 Acute Colonic Pseudo-obstruction, 343
Michael D. Saunders

59 Colonic Polyps and Colorectal Cancer, 349
John B. Kisiel, Paul J. Limburg, and Lisa A. Boardman

60 Pregnancy and Luminal Gastrointestinal Disease, 357
Sumona Saha

61 Consequences of Human Immunodeficiency
Virus Infection, 363
Vera P. Luther and P. Samuel Pegram

Part 5: Diseases of the Pancreas

62 Acute Pancreatitis and (Peri)pancreatic Fluid Collections, 371
Santhi Swaroop Vege

63 Chronic Pancreatitis and Pancreatic Pseudocysts, 378
Pierre Hindy and Scott Tenner

64 Pancreatic Cancer and Cystic Pancreatic Neoplasms, 383
William R. Brugge

**Part 6: Functional Diseases of the Small
and Large Intestine**

65 Irritable Bowel Syndrome, 391
Elizabeth J. Videlock and Lin Chang

66 Chronic Functional Constipation and Dyssynergic
Defecation, 400
Satish S.C. Rao and Yeong Yeh Lee

67 Chronic Functional Abdominal Pain, 407
Amy E. Foxx-Orenstein

68 Abdominal Bloating and Visible Distension, 412
Mark Pimentel

Part 7: Transplantation

69 Gastrointestinal Complications of Solid Organ and
Hematopoietic Cell Transplantation, 419
Natasha Chandok and Kymberly D.S. Watt

Section IV: Liver and Biliary Tract
Editors Keith Lindor and Bashar A. Aqel

Part 1: Diagnostic Approaches in Liver Disease

70 Approach to History-Taking and Physical Examination in
Liver and Biliary Disease, 429
David D. Douglas

71 Acute Liver Failure, 435
Khurram Bari and Robert J. Fontana

72 Imaging of the Liver and Bile Ducts: Radiographic and Clinical Assessment of Findings, 442
Thomas J. Byrne and Alvin C. Silva

73 Assessment of Liver Fibrosis: Liver Biopsy and Other Techniques, 450
Sumeet K. Asrani and Jayant Talwalkar

74 Endoscopic Techniques Used in the Management of Liver and Biliary Tree Disease: ERCP and EUS, 455
Toufic Kachaamy and Douglas Faigel

Part 2: Diseases of the Liver

75 Acute Viral Hepatitis: Hepatitis A, Hepatitis E, and Other Viruses, 465
Iliana Doycheva and Juan F. Gallegos-Orozco

76 Chronic Hepatitis B and D, 473
Vijayan Balan, Jorge Rakela, and Rebecca Corey

77 Hepatitis C, 480
Michael Charlton and Travis Dick

78 Bacterial and Other Non-viral Infections of the Liver, 487
Maria Teresa A. Seville, Roberto L. Patron, Ann McCullough, and Shimon Kusne

79 Alcoholic Liver Disease, 498
Moira Hilscher and Vijay Shah

80 Drug-Induced Liver Injury, 503
Einar Björnsson and Naga Chalasani

81 Autoimmune Liver Diseases, 508
Justin A. Reynolds and Elizabeth J. Carey

82 Vascular Diseases of the Liver, 513
Brenda Ernst, Pierre Noel, and Bashar A. Aqel

83 Metabolic Syndrome and Non-alcoholic Fatty Liver Disease, 522
Paul Angulo

84 Hemochromatosis, Wilson's Disease, and Alpha-1-Antitrypsin Deficiency, 530
Lisa M. Glass and Rolland C. Dickson

85 Hepatic Manifestations of Systemic Diseases, 538
Stephen Crane Hauser

86 Diseases of the Biliary Tract and Gallbladder, 543
Wajeeh Salah and M. Edwyn Harrison

87 Portal Hypertension, 554
Humberto C. Gonzalez and Patrick S. Kamath

88 TIPS, 567
Santiago Cornejo and Sailendra Naidu

89 Primary Carcinoma of the Liver, 574
Renumathy Dhanasekaran, Julie K. Heimbach, and Lewis R. Roberts

90 Pregnancy and Liver Disease, 582
J. Eileen Hay

91 Pediatric Liver Disease, 587
Tamir Miloh

Part 3: Liver Transplantation

92 Indications and Selection of Patients for Liver Transplantation, 601
Michael D. Leise and Marie A. Laryea

93 What Every Hepatologist Should Know about Liver Transplantation, 608
Peter S. Yoo and David C. Mulligan

94 Immunosuppression Used in Liver Transplantation, 617
Rebecca L. Corey and David D. Douglas

95 Medical Management of the Liver Transplant Patient, 626
William C. Palmer and Denise M. Harnois

96 Organ Allocation Policy: Practical Issues and Challenges to the Gastroenterologist, 632
Jessica Yu and Pratima Sharma

97 Endoscopic Ultrasound, 637
Thomas J. Savides

Online-Only Chapters

98 Small-Intestinal Ulcerations
Reza Y. Akhtar and Blair S. Lewis

99 Enteroscopy
G. Anton Decker, Jonathan A. Leighton, and Frank J. Lukens

100 Esophageal Dilation: An Overview
Parth J. Parekh and David A. Johnson

101 Advanced Colonoscopy, Polypectomy, and Colonoscopic Imaging
Farrah Rahmani and Douglas K. Rex

102 Physiology of Weight Regulation
Louis Chaptini and Steven Peikin

Index, 641

List of contributors

Andres Acosta, MD
Department of Gastroenterology and Hepatology
Mayo Clinic
Rochester, MN, USA

Reza Y. Akhtar, MD
Henry D. Janowitz Division of Gastroenterology
Mount Sinai School of Medicine
New York, NY, USA

Jeffrey A. Alexander, MD
Mayo Clinic
Rochester, MN, USA

Paul Angulo, MD
University of Kentucky Medical Center
Lexington, KY, USA

Bashar A. Aqel, MD
Division of Gastroenterology and Hepatology
Mayo Clinic
Scottsdale AZ, USA

Jaime Aranda-Michel
Gastroenterology, Hepatology and Liver Transplant
Swedish Health Systems
Seattle, WA, USA

Nadir Arber, MD, MSc, MHA
Tel-Aviv Sourasky Medical Center
Sackler Faculty of Medicine
Tel-Aviv University
Tel Aviv, Israel

Sumeet K. Asrani, MD
Baylor University Medical Center
Dallas, TX, USA

Vijayan Balan
Division of Gastroenterology and Hepatology
Mayo Clinic
Scottsdale, AZ, USA

Khurram Bari, MD
Department of Internal Medicine
University of Michigan Medical School
Ann Arbor, MI, USA

Todd H. Baron, MD
Division of Gastroenterology and Hepatology
Mayo Clinic
Rochester, MN, USA

Adil E. Bharucha, MBBS, MD
Division of Gastroenterology and Hepatology
Mayo Clinic
Rochester, MN, USA

Einar Björnsson, MD, PhD
Division of Gastroenterology and Hepatology
Department of Medicine
The National University Hospital of Iceland
Reykjavik, Iceland

Lisa A. Boardman, MD
Division of Gastroenterology and Hepatology
Mayo Clinic
Rochester, MN, USA

Ernest P. Bouras, MD
Division of Gastroenterology and Hepatology
Mayo Clinic
Jacksonville, FL, USA

Eugene M. Bozymski, MD
Center for Esophageal Diseases and Swallowing
Division of Gastroenterology and Hepatology
University of North Carolina School of Medicine
Chapel Hill, NC, USA

William R. Brugge, MD
Harvard Medical School and Gastrointestinal Unit
Massachusetts General Hospital
Boston, MA, USA

Alan L. Buchman, MD, MSPH
Center for Gastroenterology and Nutrition
Skokie, IL, USA

Thomas J. Byrne, MD
Division of Gastroenterology and Hepatology
Mayo Clinic
Scottsdale, AZ, USA

John R. Cangemi, MD
Division of Gastroenterology and Hepatology
Department of Internal Medicine
Mayo Clinic
Jacksonville, FL, USA

John M. Carethers, MD
Division of Gastroenterology
Department of Internal Medicine
University of Michigan
Ann Arbor, MI, USA

Elizabeth J. Carey, MD
Division of Gastroenterology and Hepatology
Mayo Clinic
Scottsdale, AZ, USA

Brooks Cash, MD
Department of Medicine
Gastroenterology Service
Walter Reed National Military Medical Center
Bethesda, MD, USA

Naga Chalasani, MD
Division of Gastroenterology and Hepatology
Department of Medicine
Indiana School of Medicine
Indianapolis, IN, USA

Francis K.L. Chan, MD
Department of Medicine and Therapeutics
The Chinese University of Hong Kong
Hong Kong, China

Natasha Chandok, MD
Division of Gastroenterology and Hepatology
University of Western Ontario
London, ON, Canada

Lin Chang, MD
Center for Neurobiology of Stress and Resilience
Division of Digestive Diseases
David Geffen School of Medicine at UCLA
Los Angeles, CA, USA

Louis Chaptini, MD
Section of Digestive Diseases
Yale University School of Medicine
New Haven, CT, USA

Michael Charlton, MD
Mayo Clinic
Rochester, MN, USA

Rebecca Corey, PharmD, BCPS
Transplant Center
Mayo Clinic Hospital
Phoenix, AZ, USA

Santiago Cornejo, MD
Department of Radiology
Mayo Clinic
Scottsdale, AZ, USA

Sun-Chuan Dai, MD
Division of Gastroenterology
University of Pennsylvania Health System
Philadelphia, PA, USA

Maneesh Dave, MD
Division of Gastroenterology and Hepatology
Mayo Clinic
Rochester, MN, USA

Barham K. Abu Dayyeh, MD
Mayo Clinic Hospital
Saint Mary's Campus
Rochester, MN, USA

G. Anton Decker, MB BCh, MRCP
Division of Gastroenterology
Mayo Clinic
Scottsdale, AZ, USA

Kara M. De Felice, MD
Division of Gastroenterology and Hepatology
Mayo Clinic
Rochester, MN, USA

Evan S. Dellon, MD, MPH
Center for Esophageal Diseases and Swallowing
Division of Gastroenterology and Hepatology
University of North Carolina School of Medicine
Chapel Hill, NC, USA

Mark T. DeMeo
Division of Gastroenterology, Hepatology and Nutrition
Department of Medicine
Rush University Medical Center
Chicago, IL, USA

Kenneth R. DeVault, MD
Division of Gastroenterology and Hepatology
Mayo Clinic
Jacksonville, FL, USA

Renumathy Dhanasekaran, MD
Division of Gastroenterology and Hepatology
Mayo Clinic
Rochester, MN, USA

John K. DiBaise, MD
Division of Gastroenterology and Hepatology
Mayo Clinic
Scottsdale, AZ, USA

Travis Dick
Intermountain Medical Center
Murray, UT, USA

Rolland C. Dickson, MD
Dartmouth Hitcock Medical Center
Lebanon, NH, USA

David D. Douglas, MD
Division of Gastroenterology and Hepatology
Mayo Clinic
Scottsdale, AZ, USA

Iliana Doycheva, MD
Division of Gastroenterology, Hepatology and Nutrition
University of Utah School of Medicine
Salt Lake City, UT, USA

Brenda Ernst, MD
Division of Hematology/Oncology
Mayo Clinic
Scottsdale, AZ, USA

Doug Faigel, MD
Division of Gastroenterology and Hepatology
Mayo Clinic
Jacksonville, FL, USA

George T. Fantry, MD
Division of Gastroenterology
University of Maryland School of Medicine
Baltimore, MD, USA

William A. Faubion, MD
Division of Gastroenterology and Hepatology
Mayo Clinic
Rochester, MN, USA

Robert J. Fontana, MD
Department of Internal Medicine
University of Michigan Medical School
Ann Arbor, MI, USA

Amy E. Foxx-Orenstein, DO
Department of Internal Medicine
Mayo Clinic
Scottsdale AZ, USA

Dawn L. Francis, MD, MHS
Division of Gastroenterology and Hepatology
Mayo Clinic
Rochester, MN, USA

Juan F. Gallegos-Orozco, MD
Division of Gastroenterology, Hepatology and Nutrition
University of Utah School of Medicine
Salt Lake City, UT, USA

Katherine S. Garman, MD
Division of Gastroenterology and Institute for Genome Sciences and Policy
Veterans Affairs Medical Center
Duke University Medical Center
Durham, NC, USA

Leyla J. Ghazi, MD
Division of Gastroenterology
Vanderbilt University
Nashville, TN, USA

Lisa M. Glass, MD
Department of Internal Medicine
Division of Gastroenterology
University of Michigan Health System
Ann Arbor, MI, USA

Humberto C. Gonzalez, MD
Division of Gastroenterology and Hepatology
Mayo Clinic
Rochester, MN, USA

David Y. Graham, MD
Baylor College of Medicine
Houston, TX, USA

Madhusudan Grover, MD
Division of Gastroenterology and Hepatology
Mayo Clinic
Rochester, MN, USA

Vineet S. Gudsoorkar, MD
Division of Gastroenterology
Department of Medicine
Houston Methodist Hospital and Weill Cornell College of Medicine
Houston, TX, USA

Magnus Halland, MD
Division of Gastroenterology and Hepatology
Mayo Clinic
Rochester, MN, USA

Denise M. Harnois, DO
Division of Transplantation
Mayo Clinic
Jacksonville, FL, USA

M. Edwyn Harrison, MD
Mayo Clinic
Scottsdale, AZ, USA

Stephen Crane Hauser, MD
Division of Gastroenterology and Hepatology
Mayo Clinic
Rochester, MN, USA

J. Eileen Hay, MD
Division of Gastroenterology and Hepatology
Mayo Clinic
Rochester, MN, USA

Julie K. Heimbach, MD
Division of Transplantation Surgery
Mayo Clinic
Rochester, MN, USA

Moira Hilscher, MD
Department of Internal Medicine
Mayo Clinic
Rochester, MN, USA

Pierre Hindy, MD
Division of Gastroenterology
Department of Medicine
State University of New York – Health Sciences Center
Brooklyn, NY, USA

James E. Huprich, MD
Division of Radiology
Mayo Clinic
Rochester, MN, USA

R. Sameer Islam, MD
Division of Gastroenterology
Mayo Clinic
Scottsdale, AZ, USA

Johanna Iturrino, MD
Division of Gastroenterology and Hepatology
Mayo Clinic
Rochester, MN, USA

Ellionore Jarbrink-Sehgal
Baylor College of Medicine
Houston, TX, USA

Dennis M. Jensen
CURE/Digestive Disease Research Center
VA Greater Los Angeles Healthcare System
Los Angeles, CA, USA

David A. Johnson, MD
Department of Internal Medicine
Gastroenterology Division
Eastern Virginia Medical School
Norfolk, VA, USA

Patrick S. Kamath, MD
Division of Gastroenterology and Hepatology
Mayo Clinic
Rochester, MN, USA

Sunanda V. Kane
Division of Gastroenterology and Hepatology
Mayo Clinic
Rochester, MN, USA

Purna Kashyap, MBBS
Department of Gastroenterology and Hepatology
Mayo Clinic
Rochester, MN, USA

Robert T. Kavitt, MD
Center for Esophageal Diseases
Section of Gastroenterology
University of Chicago
Chicago, IL, USA

Todd A. Kellogg, MD
Department of Subspeciality General Surgery
Mayo Clinic
Rochester, MN, USA

John B. Kisiel, MD
Division of Gastroenterology and Hepatology
Mayo Clinic
Rochester, MN, USA

Michael L. Kochman, MD
Division of Gastroenterology
University of Pennsylvania Health System
Philadelphia, PA, USA

Thomas O.G. Kovacs, MD
CURE/Digestive Disease Research Center
VA Greater Los Angeles Healthcare System
Los Angeles, CA, USA

Shimon Kusne, MD
Division of Infectious Diseases
Mayo Clinic
Scottsdale, AZ, USA

J. Thomas Lamont, MD
Beth Israel Deaconess Medical Center
Boston, MA, USA

Marie A. Laryea, MD
Division of Gastroenterology and Hepatology
Dalhousie University
Halifax, NS, Canada

Yeong Yeh Lee, MD
School of Medical Sciences
University of Science, Malaysia
Kubang Kerian, Kelantan, Malaysia

Jonathan A. Leighton, MD
Division of Gastroenterology
Mayo Clinic
Scottsdale, AZ, USA

Michael D. Leise, MD
William J. von Liebig Center for Transplantation and
Clinical Regeneration
Rochester, MN, USA

Blair S. Lewis, MD
Henry D. Janowitz Division of Gastroenterology
Mount Sinai School of Medicine
New York, NY, USA

James H. Lewis, MD
Division of Gastroenterology
Georgetown University Medical Center
Washington, DC, USA

Paul J. Limburg, MD, MPH
Division of Gastroenterology and Hepatology
Mayo Clinic
Rochester, MN, USA

Frank J. Lukens, MD
Department of Gastroenterology and Hepatology
Mayo Clinic
Jacksonville, FL, USA

Vera P. Luther, MD
Department of Internal Medicine
Wake Forest University School of Medicine
Winston-Salem, NC, USA

Advitya Malhotra, MD, MS
Coastal Gastroenterology Associates PA
Webster, TX, USA

Barry J. Marshall, MD
School of Biomedical, Biomolecular and Chemical
Sciences
University of Western Australia
Perth, WA, Australia

Ann McCullough, MD
Department of Laboratory Medicine and Pathology
Mayo Clinic
Scottsdale, AZ, USA

Kenneth McQuaid, MD
University of California San Francisco and San
Francisco VA Medical Center
San Francisco, CA, USA

Tamir Miloh, MD
Phoenix Children's Hospital
Phoenix, AZ, USA

Menachem Moshkowitz, MD
Tel-Aviv Sourasky Medical Center
Sackler Faculty of Medicine
Tel-Aviv University
Tel Aviv, Israel

David C. Mulligan, MD
Section of Transplantation and Immunology
Department of Surgery
Yale University School of Medicine
New Haven, CT, USA

Joseph A. Murray, MD
Division of Gastroenterology and Hepatology
Mayo Clinic
Rochester, MN, USA

Sailendra Naidu, MD
Department of Radiology
Mayo Clinic
Scottsdale AZ, USA

Kate Napthali, MD
Calvary Mater Newcastle
Waratah, NSW, Australia

Pierre Noel, MD
Division of Hematology/Oncology
Mayo Clinic
Scottsdale, AZ, USA

Timothy T. Nostrant, MD
Department of Internal Medicine
University of Michigan
Ann Arbor, MI, USA

Lori A. Orlando, MD, MHS
Division of General Internal Medicine
Duke University Medical Center
Durham, NC, USA

Roy C. Orlando, MD
Division of Gastroenterology and Hepatology
University of North Carolina School of Medicine
Chapel Hill, NC, USA

William C. Palmer
Division of Transplantation
Mayo Clinic
Jacksonville, FL, USA

Ioannis S. Papanikolaou, MD
Hepatogastroenterology Unit
2nd Department of Internal Medicine and Research
Unit
"Attikon" University General Hospital
University of Athens
Athens, Greece

Parth J. Parekh, MD
Department of Internal Medicine
Eastern Virginia Medical School
Norfolk, VA, USA

Henry P. Parkman, MD
Temple University School of Medicine
Philadelphia, PA, USA

Shabana F. Pasha, MD
Division of Gastroenterology
Mayo Clinic
Scottsdale, AZ, USA

Seema A. Patil, MD
Division of Gastroenterology
University of Maryland School of Medicine
Baltimore, MD, USA

Roberto L. Patron
Division of Infectious Diseases
Mayo Clinic
Scottsdale, AZ, USA

P. Samuel Pegram, MD
Department of Internal Medicine
Wake Forest University School of Medicine
Winston-Salem, NC, USA

Steven Peikin, MD
Division of Gastroenterology and Liver Diseases
Cooper Medical School at Rowan University
Camden, NJ, USA

Mark Pimentel, MD
Cedars-Sinai Medical Center
Los Angeles, CA, USA

David Prichard
Division of Gastroenterology and Hepatology
Mayo Clinic
Rochester, MN, USA

Dawn Provenzale, MD, MS
Veterans Affairs Medical Center
Division of Gastroenterology
Duke University Medical Center
Durham, NC, USA
VA Cooperative Studies Epidemiology Center

Eamonn M.M. Quigley, MD
Division of Gastroenterology
Department of Medicine
Houston Methodist Hospital and Weill Cornell College
of Medicine
Houston, TX, USA

Farrah Rahmani, MD
Indiana University Hospital
Indianapolis, IN, USA

Shanmugarajah Rajendra, MD
Department of Gastroenterology & Hepatology
Bankstown-Lidcombe Hospital and South Western
Sydney Clinical School
University of New South Wales
Sydney, NSW, Australia

Jorge Rakela, MD
Division of Gastroenterology and Hepatology
Mayo Clinic
Scottsdale, AZ, USA

**Satish S.C. Rao, MD, PhD, FRCP (LON),
FACG, AGAF**
Section of Gastroenterology and Hepatology
Medical College of Georgia
Georgia Regents University
Augusta, GA, USA

Douglas K. Rex, MD
Indiana University Hospital
Indianapolis, IN, USA

James Reynolds, MD
Department of Medicine
Drexel University College of Medicine
Philadelphia, PA, USA

Justin A. Reynolds
Division of Gastroenterology and Hepatology
Mayo Clinic
Scottsdale, AZ, USA

Lewis R. Roberts, MB ChB, PhD
Division of Gastroenterology and Hepatology
Mayo Clinic
Rochester, MN, USA

Suzanne Rose
Office of Academic Affairs and the Department of
Medicine
Division of Gastroenterology
University of Connecticut School of Medicine
Farmington, CT, USA

Alberto Rubio-Tapia, MD
Division of Gastroenterology and Hepatology
Mayo Clinic
Rochester, MN, USA

Massimo Rugge, MD
Baylor College of Medicine
Houston, TX, USA

Sumona Saha, MD
Division of Gastroenterology and Hepatology
University of Wisconsin School of Medicine and Public
Health
Madison, WI, USA

Wajeeh Salah, MD
Mayo Clinic Health System in Eau Claire

Michael D. Saunders, MD
Division of Gastroenterology
University of Washington Medical Center
Seattle, WA, USA

Thomas J. Savides, MD
Division of Gastroenterology
University of California
San Diego, CA, USA

Lawrence R. Schiller, MD
Division of Gastroenterology
Baylor University Medical Center
Dallas, TX, USA

David A. Schwartz, MD
Division of Gastroenterology and Hepatology
University of Maryland School of Medicine
Baltimore, MD, USA

Lauren K. Schwartz, MD
Division of Gastroenterology
Mount Sinai Hospital
New York, NY, USA

Joseph H. Sellin, MD
Division of Gastroenterology
Baylor College of Medicine
Houston, TX, USA

Carol E. Semrad, MD
Gastroenterology Section
The University of Chicago
Chicago, IL, USA

Maria Teresa A. Seville, MD
Division of Infectious Diseases
Mayo Clinic
Scottsdale, AZ, USA

Vijay Shah
Department of Internal Medicine
Mayo Clinic
Rochester, MN, USA

Prateek Sharma, MD
Division of Gastroenterology and Hepatology
Veterans Affairs Medical Center and University of
Kansas School of Medicine
Kansas City, MO, USA

Pratima Sharma, MD
Division of Gastroenterology
University of Michigan
Ann Arbor, MI, USA

Peter D. Siersema, MD, PhD
Department of Gastroenterology & Hepatology
University Medical Center Utrecht
Utrecht, The Netherlands

Alvin C. Silva, MD
Department of Radiology
Mayo Clinic
Scottsdale, AZ, USA

Christopher L. Steele, MD, MPH, MS
Resident
Osler Medical Training Program
The Johns Hopkins University School of Medicine
Baltimore, MD

Lisa L. Strate, MD, MPH
University of Washington School of Medicine
Harborview Medical Center
Seattle, WA, USA

Mohamed Sultan, MD
Division of Gastroenterology
Georgetown University Medical Center
Washington, DC, USA

Jan Tack, MD, PhD
Gastroenterology Section
University of Leuven
Leuven, Belgium

Nicholas J. Talley, MD, PhD
Faculty of Health
University of Newcastle
Newcastle, NSW, Australia

Jayant Talwalkar, MD, MPH
Division of Gastroenterology and Hepatology
Mayo Clinic
Rochester, MN, USA

Scott Tenner, MD, MPH
Division of Gastroenterology
Department of Medicine
State University of New York – Health Sciences Center
Brooklyn, NY, USA

Stephen W. Trenkner, MD
Division of Radiology
Mayo Clinic
Rochester, MN, USA

Michael F. Vaezi
Division of Gastroenterology and Hepatology
Center for Swallowing and Esophageal Disorders
Vanderbilt University Medical Center
Nashville, TN, USA

Byron P. Vaughn, MD
Beth Israel Deaconess Medical Center
Boston, MA, USA

Santhi Swaroop Vege, MD
Division of Gastroenterology and Hepatology
Mayo Clinic
Rochester, MN, USA

Elizabeth J. Videlock, MD
Center for Neurobiology of Stress and Resilience
Division of Digestive Diseases
David Geffen School of Medicine at UCLA
Los Angeles, CA, USA

Angela Vizzini, MD
Department of Dietetics
Mayo Clinic
Jacksonville, FL, USA

Arnold Wald, MD
Division of Gastroenterology and Hepatology
University of Wisconsin School of Medicine and Public Health
Madison, WI, USA

Kymberly D.S. Watt, MD
Division of Gastroenterology and Hepatology
William J. von Liebig Transplant Center
Mayo Clinic
Rochester, MN, USA

John M. Wo, MD
GI Motility and Neurogastroenterology Unit
Division of Gastroenterology & Hepatology
Indiana University School of Medicine
Indiana University Hospital
Indianapolis, IN, USA

Peter S. Yoo
Section of Transplantation and Immunology
Department of Surgery
Yale University School of Medicine
New Haven, CT, USA

Tonia M. Young-Fadok
Department of Surgery
Mayo Clinic College of Medicine
Mayo Clinic
Phoenix, AZ, USA

Jessica Yu, MD
Department of Internal Medicine
University of Michigan
Ann Arbor, MI, USA

Yuliya Y. Yurko, MD
Greenville Hospital System
Greenville, SC, USA

Foreword

I am privileged to introduce the 2nd edition of *Practical Gastroenterology and Hepatology* and the superb team of editors responsible for its development. As the knowledge base for gastroenterology and hepatology grows and evolves, a concise but comprehensive source providing the most current information and evidence is invaluable for physicians and students. Nick Talley, Ken DeVault, Michael Wallace, Bashar Aqel, and Keith Lindor, who are world-class experts in gastroenterology, endoscopy, and hepatology, have therefore worked together to produce the 2nd edition of *Practical Gastroenterology and Hepatology*, building on the success of the 1st edition. They have assembled an outstanding group of authors to produce chapters that cover all aspects of gastroenterology and hepatology. The content will be useful for physicians training or working in gastroenterology, as well as those outside the field who desire a "readable" review of key topics in digestive diseases. The 2nd edition will also be a valuable resource for those preparing for board examination, with the addition of board-style multiple choice questions and explanations of answers. Review of the list of chapters reminds us of the many areas in gastroenterology and liver with rapid evolution in knowledge base and practice – from eosinophilic esophagitis to therapies for viral hepatitis and inflammatory bowel disease to endoscopic and imaging modalities. I am therefore very pleased to have this 2nd edition available as a practical and contemporary guide to our field.

Loren Laine
Professor of Medicine
Section of Digestive Diseases
Yale School of Medicine
New Haven, CT

Preface

Welcome to the second edition of *Practical Gastroenterology and Hepatology Board Review Toolkit*, a comprehensive resource for those certifying (or recertifying) in the subspecialty and for everyone training in gastroenterology. Based on the success of the first edition, we have thoroughly revised and updated the text. Our primary goal, however, has remained unchanged: to present a fresh, modern, easy-to-read-and-digest, standalone textbook. All now presented in one slimmer, single volume, the chapters provide guidance on how to approach clinical problems (from the initial evaluation to imaging and advanced endoscopy) and how to diagnose and treat common and rare diseases every gastroenterologist must know for the boards. The emphasis is on the practical and clinically relevant, as opposed to the esoteric.

Each chapter follows a standard template structure and is written by the best of the best in the field. All focus on key knowledge, and the most important clinical facts are highlighted in an introductory summary and presented as take-home points at the end; irrelevant or unimportant information is omitted. The chapters are deliberately brief and readable; we want readers to retain the material, and immediately to be able to apply what they learn in practice.

In selected chapters, a clinical case is included, which demonstrates a common clinical situation, its approach, and its management. Simple, easy-to-follow clinical algorithms are included throughout, and the endoscopy chapters provide excellent video examples (available on the companion website: www.link.com). The book is illustrated in color, enhanced by a very pleasant layout.

An online selection of multiple-choice questions with answers and explanations has been added to aid in revision for the boards. We have guided the writing of the textbook to help ensure experienced gastroenterologists, fellows, residents, medical students, internists, primary care physicians, and surgeons will all find material of interest and practical relevance.

We thank all the authors and the publisher, who have worked very hard to create this new edition. As with the first edition, we very much hope you will enjoy reading this volume and learning its content.

Nicholas J. Talley, on behalf of the editors
2016

About the companion website

This book is accompanied by a companion website:

http://www.practicalgastrohep.com/

The website contains:
• Multiple choice questions
• Videos
Videos are listed at the end of the chapter to which they are relevant.

How to Ace the Boards in Gastroenterology and Hepatology

1 Introduction and Overview of the Gastroenterology Boards, 3
   Brooks Cash

CHAPTER 1

Introduction and Overview of the Gastroenterology Boards

Brooks Cash

Department of Medicine, Gastroenterology Service, Walter Reed National Military Medical Center, Bethesda, MD, USA

For many, taking the Gastroenterology Board Examination is a daunting experience. Uncertainty with regards to the specifics of the examination process can increase the anxiety that the boards engender. The objective of this chapter is to demystify the certification/recertification process and to delineate for the test-taker what to expect on exam day. Recent changes to the American Board of Internal Medicine (ABIM) Maintenance of Certification (MOC) program will also be discussed and explained. Hopefully, these explanations will alleviate at least some degree of test anxiety, allowing you to concentrate on learning and integrating the material that you will be tested on. A critical resource for the certification candidate is the ABIM website: www.abim.org. Through this portal, all information regarding qualifications, scheduling, payments, and test development and administration can be located. There are also numerous resources available via this website designed to prepare the candidate for the examination.

What to Expect at the Test Center

All ABIM examinations are now computer-based, and most are administered by a computer-based testing facility. You should arrive at the testing facility at least 30 minutes before the start of the examination. Late arrivals may not be allowed to sit for the examination, so it is crucial that you be familiar with the location of the testing facility and with specifics such as parking access and costs. It is highly recommended that you prepare in advance with a "dry run" trip to the testing facility well before the day of your examination. Ideally, you should do this on a weekday at the same time you plan on travelling on test day so that you have an idea of commuting requirements. You should also plan out some contingency routes in the event of significant traffic disruption on the day of the examination.

Once you arrive at the testing facility, you will be required to present your personal identification for examination security. A digital fingerprint and/or palm vein recognition scan will be performed, along with security wanding. Your signature and photograph will be taken prior to your being allowed to take the examination. Personal items are not permitted in the testing room and you will be required to leave your belongings outside in a secure storage container provided by the testing center. This includes items such as cell phones, personal digital assistants, watches, wallets, and purses. Personal earplugs, headphones, and other devices are not permitted in the test centers, though you may request earplugs

from the test administrator. While outerwear such as coats and jackets is not permitted into the examination room, sweaters are allowed, so you should plan accordingly. Prior to admission to the examination room, you will be asked to read the "ABIM Candidate Rules Checklist," agreeing to the security terms of the administration of the exam. You will be given a short orientation and then escorted to a computer workstation in the testing room to begin the examination.

The Examination

The initial certification examination consists of four 60-question tests, each administered during a 2-hour block. The entire day is scheduled to take up to 10 hours. There are 8 hours allotted for the four examinations and up to 100 minutes of optional break time that may be taken over the three intertest periods. The MOC examination differs from the initial certification examination in that only three 60-question tests are administered. The MOC test day is allotted to be approximately 8 hours, with the three 2-hour test periods and up to 80 minutes of optional break time.

A blueprint established by the Subspecialty Board of Gastroenterology, which is reviewed and updated annually in order to remain current and relevant, determines the general content of the examination. The primary content categories at the time of this writing are shown in Table 1.1, along with the percentage of the examination devoted to each broad category. The blueprint is the same for the initial certification and the MOC examinations. More specific expansion of each category is available via the ABIM website. In addition to the questions covering gastroenterology, there are also questions that are more applicable to the general practice of medicine, covering topics such as ethics and basic biostatistics. Typically, there are four to six of these general questions scattered through the tests.

The examination questions are composed of single best-answer type questions. Most describe a patient scenario that occurs in practice settings. They may include media such as radiographs, endoscopic videos, manometry tracings, or histopathology pictures to illustrate relevant findings or characteristics. The examination is designed to evaluate your knowledge, diagnostic reasoning, and judgment. Questions will adhere to a general formula aimed at testing these parameters by posing such tasks as making a diagnosis, determining a treatment plan, ordering diagnostic tests,

Practical Gastroenterology and Hepatology Board Review Toolkit, Second Edition. Edited by Nicholas J. Talley, Kenneth R. DeVault, Michael B. Wallace, Bashar A. Aqel and Keith D. Lindor.
© 2016 John Wiley & Sons, Ltd. Published 2016 by John Wiley & Sons, Ltd. Companion website: www.practicalgastrohep.com

CHAPTER 1

Table 1.1 Primary content categories for the gastroenterology certification examination.

Content category	% of exam
Esophagus	11
Stomach/duodenum	15
Liver	25
Biliary tract	10
Pancreas	11
Small intestine	10
Colon	18
Total	100

recognizing clinical features of a disease, and/or determining means of prevention, screening, staging, or follow-up.

A great deal of effort and thought goes into developing appropriate questions for the examination, and understanding this process can prepare you for what you will be expected to know as you take the examination. Most questions will begin with some text that presents the problem and provides the information required to resolve it. This is the "stem" of the question. The "lead line" is then presented, which is the question itself. This is followed by four or five possible choices, one of which is the absolutely correct answer, while the others are the "distractors." Typical lead lines will contain a task to be evaluated. Examples of lead-line tasks and specific question formats include:

1 Evaluating diagnostic inference or differential diagnosis: *Which of the following is the most likely diagnosis?*
2 Testing diagnostic knowledge: *Which of the following laboratory studies should you order next?*
3 Evaluation of the knowledge of natural history or epidemiology: *This patient is at increased risk for the development of which of the following?*
4 Testing treatment knowledge: *Which of the following drugs (or therapeutic interventions) should you now order?*
5 Evaluation of management decision-making: *Which of the following should you do next?*
6 Awareness of pathophysiology or basic science: *Which of the following is the best explanation for this patient's poor response to therapy?*
7 Testing of ability to interpret medical literature/biostatistics: *Which of the following is the best interpretation of these results?*

ABIM certification examinations are often criticized for focusing on the minutiae of specific conditions or management approaches, and a common sentiment is that whoever is writing the questions clearly must not be practicing medicine in the "real world." It is true that questions found on certification examinations often do cover some of the more esoteric aspects of a given disease or condition, perhaps especially within the subspecialty ABIM examinations. While it is easy to understand and commiserate with this sentiment, it is also important to realize that your baseline competence in recognizing and managing common conditions encountered in the practice of gastroenterology is assumed. What is being tested during a certification examination is the depth of your knowledge and understanding, which may require assessing your ability to recognize esoteric facts presented in the stems of the questions.

Maintenance of Certification Changes

An important change in the ABIM certification process occurred in 2014, when the ABIM changed its MOC program in response to increasing evidence from the public, consumer groups, and professional organizations that assessment of medical knowledge every 10 years is not sufficient for medical practice [1]. The new ABIM MOC program applies to all ABIM-certified physicians, including those who were previously "grandfathered" with indefinite certification. The hallmark of the new MOC program is exhibition of a continuous and demonstrated pattern of participation in MOC activities. Physicians who are enrolled in MOC are required to meet specific milestones every 2, 5, and 10 years. In order to continue fulfilling MOC requirements, all ABIM Board Certified physicians will be required to:

1 Earn points by completing at least one ABIM-approved MOC activity by December 31, 2015, and then every 2 years thereafter.
2 Earn 100 points, with at least 20 points in medical knowledge and 20 points in practice assessment, by December 31, 2018, and then every 5 years thereafter. A patient safety and survey requirement will also be required every 5 years.
3 Pass an MOC examination (aka, a board examination).

Diplomates with certifications that are valid indefinitely (i.e. grandfathers) will continue to be reported as "certified" by the ABIM. However, they will have to complete the aforementioned MOC milestones and pass a MOC examination by December 31, 2023 in order to be classified as "Meeting MOC Requirements." Additional information regarding these changes, as well as specific information on many unique personal situations, is available through the ABIM, and the reader is encouraged to visit http://moc2014.abim.org/whats-changing.aspx to learn more about the recent changes to the ABIM MOC program.

Specific Tips and Recommendations for the Gastroenterology Board Examination

Consider Attending a Formal Board Review Course

The Gastroenterology Board Examination is meant to test a comprehensive knowledge base, but, because it is only 180–240 questions long, there is a limit to how much content can be tested. While it is an admirable exercise in academic dedication, rereading a gastroenterology textbook that you have not opened in a meaningful way since fellowship is probably not the optimal way to prepare for the examination or to refresh your knowledge base. A more efficient use of your time would be to attend a comprehensive board review course; there are a number of very good choices available throughout the calendar year. I recommend attending one of these courses 12–18 months before you sit for the examination, to ensure that you have time to identify potential knowledge gaps, assimilate and understand any new information, and review the entire syllabus once or twice more before taking the examination. In addition to, or in lieu of, personal attendance at a board review course, it may be possible to obtain the syllabus and recorded sessions of a course for review at your leisure, though the timeframe will be compressed due to the time required to edit and package the recorded material from a course.

Review Prominent Societal Guidelines Regarding Common Disease States

Remember, the examination is meant to evaluate your knowledge, diagnostic reasoning, and judgment. Embedded in that concept is the fact that many of the questions will assess whether or not your decision-making and thought processes are within the expected standard of care for specific diseases. Review of the most recent societal guidelines for commonly encountered conditions (e.g., gastroesophageal reflux disease, colon cancer screening or surveillance, *Clostridium difficile* colitis) will underscore the standard of care for the management of these disorders and provide the evidence for this standard. While it should be obvious, it bears emphasizing that US guidelines will be the basis of ABIM-generated questions on the ABIM examination. An excellent source of compiled guidelines is the National Guideline Clearinghouse, maintained by the Agency for Healthcare Research and Quality (www.guideline.gov). While it is unlikely that the test will ask for specific societal recommendations, familiarity with the most up-to-date evidence-based guidelines will deepen your understanding of the pathophysiology, clinical associations, and management of these conditions.

Recurring Themes

There are numerous "themes" that seem to be favorites for the Gastroenterology Board Examination, which warrant additional study prior to the examination. This is by no means meant to be a comprehensive list:

- Pregnancy and gastroenterologic diseases, either pre-existing or pregnancy-induced, are favorite targets for examination questions. Questions referable to pregnancy and inflammatory bowel disease (IBD) or liver disease are prime examples.
- There will often be a manometric tracing or picture depicting at least one of the prototypical esophageal motility disorders on the examination, so familiarity with both traditional and high-resolution manometry patterns is recommended.
- There will be multiple questions related to viral hepatitis, but these questions will typically cover noncontroversial topics and established modes of therapy, rather than cutting-edge or just-approved regimens. It should be remembered that the examinations, much like textbooks and guidelines, are developed well in advance of issuance, so extremely recent information or clinical developments are unlikely to be tested.
- There will be two or three questions on ethics and simple biostatistics. The biostatistics questions may require you to calculate values such as sensitivity, specificity, number needed to treat/harm, positive/negative predictive value, or prevalence of a disease, but are unlikely to be more complicated than that, so a rudimentary working knowledge of these concepts should be sufficient.
- While rarely encountered in clinical practice, porphyria seems to be a relatively popular topic for at least one question.
- There will typically be one or two questions related to nutritional perturbations such as zinc, thiamine, or selenium deficiencies (to name a few), so memorization of the manifestations associated with nutritional disease states is recommended.
- Radiologic and histopathologic correlates will usually be "classic" examples of diseases or conditions, and you will typically be asked to recommend additional diagnostics or therapeutics based on the information derived from the radiograph or histopathology picture. Therefore, you should familiarize yourself with "classic" plain film images such as gastric or intestinal volvulus, common cholangiograms such as the "string of lakes" appearance of primary sclerosing cholangitis, and the "onion-skinning" appearance of primary sclerosing cholangitis, to mention just a few.
- Be familiar with medical eponyms and their phenotypes, especially those referable to variants of familial colorectal cancer syndromes, as these seem to be examination favorites.
- Be familiar with dermatologic manifestations of gastroenterological disease, including those associated with IBD, celiac disease, viral hepatitis, metabolic liver disease, nutritional deficiencies, and inherited colorectal cancer syndromes.

Practice Questions

Another valuable exercise to engage in well before sitting for the examination is taking mock tests or, at the very least, answering multiple sample questions and reviewing the answers. Just as there are many board review courses available, there are several good question-and-answer books that can be used to prepare for the boards. I would recommend establishing a dedicated period of time during each week beginning at least 6 months before the tests to do boluses of questions and review the answers and explanations. To avoid burnout, you should not do more than 60 at a sitting. If you, like most people, have certain areas that seem to come to you easier than others, then I would recommend that you do questions covering these topics last. While gratifying to answer correctly, you will be much better served by testing yourself on areas that you are not as comfortable with and then reviewing the rationale for the correct answers.

Hopefully, this chapter has laid the groundwork for your preparation for your certification examination and has helped to explain the processes involved in certification and MOC. With that in mind, I hope that you find the information contained in the rest of the book helpful and wish you the best of luck in your future test-taking efforts.

Reference

1 National Research Council. *Crossing the Quality Chasm: A New Health System for the 21st Century.* Committee on Quality of Health Care in America, Institute of Medicine. Washington, DC: The National Academy Press, 2001.

SECTION II

Esophagus and Stomach

Editors Kenneth R. DeVault and Nicholas J. Talley

Part 1 Pathobiology of the Esophagus and Stomach, 9

Part 2 Other Diagnostic Modalities, 21

Part 3 Problem-Based Approach to Diagnosis and Differential Diagnosis, 41

Part 4 Diseases of the Esophagus, 83

Part 5 Diseases of the Stomach, 113

Part 6 Functional Disease of the Esophagus and Stomach, 167

PART 1

Pathobiology of the Esophagus and Stomach

2 Anatomy, Embryology, and Congenital Malformations of the Esophagus and Stomach, 11
Lori A. Orlando and Roy C. Orlando

3 Esophageal and Gastric Motor Function, 15
Kenneth R. DeVault, Ernest P. Bouras, and Nicholas J. Talley

Anatomy, Embryology, and Congenital Malformations of the Esophagus and Stomach

Lori A. Orlando[1] and Roy C. Orlando[2]

[1]Division of General Internal Medicine, Duke University Medical Center, Durham, NC, USA
[2]Division of Gastroenterology and Hepatology, University of North Carolina School of Medicine, Chapel Hill, NC, USA

Summary

Understanding the anatomy and embryology of the esophagus and stomach is necessary for dealing with clinically important congenital malformations. The esophagus acts as a conduit for the transport of food from the oral cavity to the stomach, which, as a J-shaped dilation of the alimentary canal, connects with the duodenum distally. Sphincters at the upper esophagus, distal esophagus/proximal stomach, and distal stomach have strategic functions. Formation of the esophagus (primitive foregut) begins at 6 weeks, and the stomach is recognizable in the 4th week of gestation as a dilation of the distal foregut. Congenital abnormalities of the esophagus are common, while those of the stomach are rare.

Anatomy

The esophagus is a conduit for the transport of food from the oral cavity to the stomach. It is an 18–22 cm-long, hollow, muscular tube with an inner "skin-like" lining of stratified squamous epithelium. The esophagus is collapsed and airless at rest, but during swallowing it is distended by the food bolus. When the bolus is delivered to the stomach, it is stored in the gastric fundus, then mixed with acid and ground in the gastric body and antrum. Finally, it is propulsed through the pylorus and into the duodenum.

Structurally, the esophageal wall is composed of four layers: innermost mucosa, submucosa, muscularis propria, and outermost adventitia; unlike the remainder of the gastrointestinal (GI) tract, the esophagus has no serosa [1, 2]. The esophageal musculature comprises skeletal muscle in the upper third and smooth muscle in the lower two-thirds. Both skeletal and smooth muscle are innervated by the vagus nerve, with nuclei located within the central medullary swallowing center. The stomach is also innervated by the vagus nerve, which splits into two branches: the left, which innervates the dorsal wall (greater curvature), and the right, which innervates the ventral wall (lesser curvature).

Upper Esophageal Sphincter

Proximally, the esophagus begins where the inferior pharyngeal constrictor merges with the cricopharyngeus, an area of skeletal muscle known as the upper esophageal sphincter (UES). The UES is contracted at rest, creating a high-pressure zone that prevents inspired air from entering the esophagus. UES contraction is mediated by intrinsic muscle tone and vagal acetycholine release, while relaxation is mediated by inhibition of acetylcholine release [3].

Esophageal Body

The esophageal body lies within the posterior mediastinum behind the trachea and left mainstem bronchus [1]. At the T10 vertebral level, the esophageal body leaves the thorax through a hiatus within the right crus of the diaphragm. Within the hiatus, the esophageal body ends in a 2–4 cm, asymmetrically thickened, circular smooth muscle known as the lower esophageal sphincter (LES) [4]. Pain within the esophagus is mediated by stimulation of chemoreceptors in the esophageal mucosa or submucosa and mechanoreceptors in the esophageal musculature [5].

Lower Esophageal Sphincter

The LES is contracted at rest, due to intrinsic smooth muscle tone and vagal acetylcholine release. This contraction creates a high-pressure zone that prevents gastric contents from entering the esophagus. The high-pressure zone is also aided by contraction of the diaphragm and weakened in the presence of a hiatal hernia. During swallowing, LES relaxation occurs via vagal release of nitric oxide (and vasoactive intestinal peptide), enabling peristalsis to push the bolus from the esophagus into the stomach [4]. The same mechanism initiates receptive relaxation of the gastric fundus to accommodate a meal without entailing a concomitant increase in intragastric pressure.

Mucosa

On endoscopy, the esophageal stratified squamous-lined mucosa appears smooth and pink, while the stomach's simple columnar mucosa is red. Their junction is recognized by an irregular, white, "Z-shaped" line (ora serrata). Squamous cells have no secretory capacity, while gastric cells can secrete both into the lumen (acid, pepsin, and a variety of other products) and into the blood (gastrin). Below the epithelium is the lamina propria, a loose network of connective tissue with blood vessels and scattered white cells. A thin layer of smooth muscle, the muscularis mucosae, separates the lamina propria from the submucosa, a network of dense connective tissue comprising blood vessels, lymphatic channels, Meissner neuronal plexus, and, in the esophagus, submucosal glands. The

Practical Gastroenterology and Hepatology Board Review Toolkit, Second Edition. Edited by Nicholas J. Talley, Kenneth R. DeVault, Michael B. Wallace, Bashar A. Aqel and Keith D. Lindor.
© 2016 John Wiley & Sons, Ltd. Published 2016 by John Wiley & Sons, Ltd. Companion website: www.practicalgastrohep.com

esophageal glands secrete mucus and bicarbonate into collecting ducts, which deliver the fluid to the esophageal lumen. Between the inner circular and outer longitudinal layers of the muscularis propria is the Auerbach neuronal plexus.

Embryology

In the developing fetus, the GI tract and the respiratory tract develop from a common tube of endoderm. Between weeks 7 and 10, a ventral diverticulum is formed, which subsequently develops into the respiratory tract; the remaining dorsal part of the tube becomes the primitive foregut. The foregut is initially lined by ciliated columnar epithelium, but begins to transform into stratified squamous epithelium by week 16. This epithelial transition is complete by birth. At embryonic week 4, the stomach is discernable as a dilation of the distal foregut. As the stomach grows, it rotates 90° around its longitudinal axis so that the greater curvature is located dorsally and the lesser curvature ventrally.

Congenital Malformations of the Esophagus and Stomach

Congenital anomalies of the esophagus are relatively common (1 in 3000 to 1 in 4500 live births) and result from either transmission of genetic defects or intrauterine stress that impedes fetal maturation [6–8]. A clinical overview is presented in Table 2.1. In premature infants, about 50% of esophageal anomalies are also associated with anomalies at other sites; this has given rise to the term VACTERL: Vertebral, Anal, Cardiac, Tracheal, Esophageal, Renal, and Limb systems. Specific defects within this group are the patent ductus arteriosus, cardiac septal deformity, and imperforate anus.

Esophageal Atresia and Tracheoesophageal Fistula

Esophageal atresia, a failure of the primitive foregut to re-canalize, occurs as an isolated anomaly in 7% and in conjunction with a tracheoesophageal (TE) fistula in 93% of cases. In the isolated type, the upper esophagus ends in a blind pouch and the lower esophagus connects to the stomach. The condition is suspected at birth by the occurrence of choking, coughing, and regurgitation on first feeding in combination with a scaphoid gasless abdomen. The diagnosis can be confirmed by failure to pass a nasogastric tube into the stomach and air in the upper esophagus on chest radiograph following air insufflation via a nasoesophageal tube.

When esophageal atresia is associated with a TE fistula, the majority of cases are accompanied by the distal type, in which the upper esophagus ends in a blind pouch and the distal esophagus connects to the trachea. The clinical presentation of the distal type is similar to that of isolated esophageal atresia, with the addition of recurrent aspiration pneumonia and increased abdominal air. Both of these are attributed to the communication between the esophagus and trachea, permitting reflux of gastric contents into the trachea and air into the esophagus and stomach (which can be seen on plain radiographs) [7].

There are three less common types of TE fistula. The first is when both upper and lower segments of the atretic esophagus communicate with the trachea; the second is when just the upper segment communicates with the trachea; and the third or "H-type fistula" is when the esophagus is *not* atretic, but still communicates with the trachea. All TE fistula types present with recurrent aspiration pneumonia due to the communication between the esophagus and the trachea; however, they can be differentiated by other clinical features. The first two types present in infancy and are distinguished from each other by the presence or absence of bowel gas on a plain radiograph (gas present when there is an accompanying distal TE fistula). In contrast, diagnosis of the H-type TE fistula may be delayed until childhood or young adulthood [8]. The diagnosis of an H-type fistula is usually made either on bronchoscopy after ingestion of methylene blue to stain the fistula site or on esophagography.

The treatment of almost all esophageal anomalies is surgical. Success rates depend upon the type and severity of accompanying

Table 2.1 Clinical aspects of esophageal developments anomalies. Source: Long, 2002 [9]. Reproduced with permission of Elsevier.

Anomaly	Age at presentation	Predominant symptoms	Diagnosis	Treatment
Atresia alone	Newborns	Regurgitation of feedings Aspiration	Esophagogram[a] Radiograph – gasless abdomen	Surgery
Atresia + distal fistula	Newborns	Regurgitation of feedings Aspiration	Esophagogram[a] Radiograph – gasless abdomen	Surgery
H-type fistula	Infants to adults	Recurrent aspiration pneumonia Bronchiectasis	Esophagogram[a] Bronchoscopy	Surgery
Esophageal stenosis	Infants to adults	Dysphagia Food impaction	Esophagogram[a] Endoscopy[b]	Bougienage[c] Surgery[d]
Duplication cysts	Infants to adults	Dyspnea, stridor, cough (infants) Dysphagia, chest pain (adults)	EUS[a] MRI/CT[b] Esophagogram	Surgery
Vascular anomalies	Infants to adults	Dyspnea, stridor, cough (infants) Dysphagia (adults)	Esophagogram[a] Angiography[b] MRI/CT/EUS	Diet modification[c] Surgery[d]
Esophageal rings	Children to adults	Dysphagia Food impaction	Esophagogram[a] Endoscopy[b]	Bougienage
Esophageal webs	Children to adults	Dysphagia	Esophagogram[a] Endoscopy[b]	Bougienage

[a]Diagnostic test of choice.
[b]Confirmatory test.
[c]Primary therapeutic approach.
[d]Secondary therapeutic approach.
EUS; endoscopic ultrasonography; MRI, magnetic resonance imaging; CT, computed tomography.

genetic abnormalities. For isolated atresias, surgical success is about 90%; however, there is an increased risk of gastroesophageal reflux disease after correction due to abnormalities of both esophageal motility and luminal acid clearance.

Congenital Stenosis

Esophageal stenosis, which varies in length from 2 to 20 cm, is rare and typically occurs in males [10]. The precise cause is unknown, and most cases present with solid-food dysphagia and regurgitation in infancy or childhood. Diagnosis is made by either esophagography or endoscopy. Treatment is by endoscopic-guided bougienage, which has variable efficacy according to the length and the complexity of the stricture. It is possible that some – perhaps many – of the cases once considered congenital stenosis are actually involved with eosinophilic esophagitis (see Chapter 16).

Esophageal Duplications

Congenital duplications of the esophagus are rare and arise as epithelial-lined outpouchings off the primitive foregut. There are two types: cystic and tubular. Cysts account for 80% of the duplications and are usually single, fluid-filled structures. They do not communicate with the lumen and, when large, are often associated with compression of the adjacent tracheobronchial tree, resulting in cough, stridor, wheezing, cyanosis, or chest pain. When asymptomatic, they may be detected as mediastinal masses on chest radiography or submucosal lesions on esophagogram. The diagnosis is confirmed by computed tomography (CT), magnetic resonance imaging (MRI) or endoscopic ultrasonography (EUS). Surgical excision is usually required to exclude a cystic neoplasm [11].

Tubular esophageal duplications are less common and, unlike the cystic type, *do* communicate with the true lumen [11]. They usually cause chest pain, dysphagia, or regurgitation in infancy, and the diagnosis is established by esophagography or endoscopy. Reconstructive surgery is indicated for those patients who are symptomatic [11–13].

Vascular Anomalies

Intrathoracic vascular anomalies are present in 2–3% of the population. Most are asymptomatic, but some may develop symptoms via esophageal compression (dysphagia and regurgitation) in childhood or adulthood. Dysphagia lusoria, the most common vascular compression of the esophagus, is due to an aberrant right subclavian artery, arising off the left side of the aortic arch [14]. Diagnosis is made by a pencil-like extrinsic esophageal compression at the level of the third to fourth thoracic vertebrae on barium esophagogram [14]. Confirmation is made by CT, MRI, or EUS [14, 15]. Initial treatment is dietary modification (mechanical soft diet) for symptom control, with surgery reserved for refractory cases.

Esophageal Rings

The distal esophagus may contain up to two "rings": the muscular A ring and the mucosal B or Schatzki ring. The A ring is 4–5 mm thick and represents an enlargement of the upper end of the LES [16, 17]. It is both uncommon and rarely symptomatic. The B ring, which is 2 mm thick, represents the squamocolumnar junction [16, 17]. It is common and usually asymptomatic, unless the lumen size is compressed to less than 15 mm, at which point intermittent solid-food dysphagia or acute impaction may occur [16, 17].

Esophageal Webs

Esophageal webs are thin mucosal protrusions extending from the anterior wall of the esophagus in the cervical region. They are thus best visualized on a lateral view of an esophagram. Unlike rings, webs rarely encircle the lumen [18]. Nonetheless, cervical webs can cause solid-food dysphagia. The triad of cervical webs, dysphagia, and iron-deficiency anemia is referred to as the Plummer–Vinson or Paterson–Brown-Kelly syndrome [18]. The syndrome is significant as it increases the risk of squamous cell carcinoma of the pharynx and esophagus and may also be associated with celiac sprue [18,19]. Treatment with iron has been reported to not only correct the iron deficiency but also induce resolution of the web. Isolated cervical webs are treated by esophageal bougienage.

Heterotopic Gastric Mucosa

Heterotopic gastric mucosa is also known as the "inlet patch." It is seen on 10% of endoscopies as a small, red island of mucosa just below the UES. Typically, inlet patches are asymptomatic, though rarely they secrete acid and cause strictures or ulcers [20], and even more rarely they evolve into adenocarcinoma [21].

Congenital Malformations of the Stomach

Congenital malformations of the stomach are very uncommon. They include gastric atresia, microgastria, gastric volvulus, gastric diverticulum, and gastric duplications. When symptomatic, these lesions typically present with epigastric pain, nausea, and vomiting, reflecting the degree of gastric outlet obstruction. Gastric atresia may be associated with both Down syndrome and epidermolysis bullosa. Unlike esophageal duplications, gastric duplications rarely communicate with the lumen, and therefore develop into masses within the stomach wall. Congenital laxity of ligaments attaching stomach to duodenum, spleen, liver, and diaphragm are contributing causes of gastric volvulus, and are either mesenteroaxial or organoaxial in type based on the axis of rotation. Mesenteroaxial gastric volvulus may be asymptomatic or symptomatic with chronic, intermittent, upper gastrointestinal (GI) symptoms [22]. Organoaxial gastric volvulus is typically acute, presenting with abdominal pain, retching, and inability to pass a nasogastric tube (Borchardt triad). It is commonly associated with a diaphragmatic hernia, and a gas-filled viscus in the thorax may be seen on chest radiography. Diagnosis is confirmed by upper GI series (UGI).

Take Home Points

- Dysphagia lusoria is due to an aberrant right subclavian artery. Diagnosis is made by a pencil-like extrinsic esophageal compression at the level of the third to fourth thoracic vertebrae.
- The triad of cervical webs, dysphagia, and iron-deficiency anemia is referred to as the Plummer–Vinson or Paterson–Brown-Kelly syndrome. The syndrome is significant as it increases the risk of squamous cell carcinoma of the pharynx and esophagus and may be associated with celiac sprue.
- As the "inlet patch" seen on 10% of endoscopies, heterotopic gastric mucosa rarely secrete acid and cause strictures or ulcers, and even more rarely evolve into adenocarcinoma.
- Organoaxial gastric volvulus is typically acute, presenting with abdominal pain, retching, and inability to pass a nasogastric tube (Borchardt triad).

CHAPTER 2

Videos of interest to readers of this chapter can be found by visiting the companion website at:

http://www.practicalgastrohep.com/

2.1 Endoscopic case presentation.

2.2 The role of endoscopy in caustic ingestion.

2.3 Transit of an esophageal capsule from the mouth to the stomach.

2.4 Unsedated transnasal endoscopy.

2.5 Esophagogastroduodenoscopy of a Type III paraesophageal hernia.

2.6 Dynamic computed tomography scan video of a large Type III hiatal hernia.

References

1 Skandalakis JE, Ellis H. Embryologic and anatomic basis of esophageal surgery. *Surg Clin North Am* 2000; **80**: 85–155.

2 Ergun GA, Kahrilas PJ. Esophageal muscular anatomy and physiology. In: *Atlas of Esophageal Diseases*, 2nd edn. Philadelphia, PA: Current Medicine, 2002: 2–18.

3 Mittal RK, Balaban DH. The esophagogastric junction. *N Engl J Med* 1997; **336**: 924–32.

4 Hornby PJ, Abrahams TP. Central control of lower esophageal sphincter relaxation. *Am J Med* 2000; **108** (Supp. 4A): 90S.

5 Orlando RC. Esophageal perception and noncardiac chest pain. *Gastroenterol Clin N Am* 2004; **33**: 25–33.

6 Spitz L, Kiely EM, Morecroft JA, *et al.* Oesophageal atresia: at-risk groups for the 1990s. *J Pediatr Surg* 1994; **29**: 723–5.

7 Deurloo JA, Ekkelkamp S, Schoorl M, *et al.* Esophageal atresia: historical evolution of management and results in 371 patients. *Ann Thorac Surg* 2002; **73**: 267–72.

8 Danton MHD, McMahon J, McGiugan J, *et al.* Congenital oesophageal respiratory tract fistula presenting in adult life. *Eur Respir J* 1993; **6**: 1412.

9 Long JD, Orlando RC. Anatomy, histology, embryology, and developmental anomalies of the esophagus. In: Feldman M, Friedman LS, Brandt LJ, eds. *Sleisenger and Fordtran's Gastrointestinal and Liver Disease, Vol 1: Pathophysiology/Diagnosis/Management*, 7th edn. Philadelphia, PA: Elsevier, 2002.

10 Amae S, Nio M, Kamiyama T, *et al.* Clinical characteristics and management of congenital esophageal stenosis: a report of 14 cases. *J Pediatr Surg* 2003; **38**: 565–70.

11 Geller A, Wang KK, DiMagno EP. Diagnosis of foregut duplication cysts by endoscopic ultrasonography. *Gastroenterology* 1995; **109**: 838–42.

12 Cioffi U, Bonavina L, De Simone M, *et al.* Presentation and surgical management of bronchogenic and esophageal duplication cysts in adults. *Chest* 1998; **113**: 1492–6.

13 Ratan ML, Anand R, Mittal SK, *et al.* Communicating oesophageal duplication: a report of two cases. *Gut* 1988; **29**: 254–6.

14 Janssen M, Baggen MGA, Veen HF, *et al.* Dysphagia lusoria: clinical aspects, manometric findings, diagnosis, and therapy. *Am J Gastroenterol* 2000; **95**: 1411–16.

15 De Luca L, Bergman JGHM, Tytgat GNJ, *et al.* EUS imaging of the arteria lusoria: case series and review. *Gastrointest Endosc* 2000; **52**: 670–3.

16 Tobin RW. Esophageal rings, webs, and diverticula. *J Clin Gastroenterol* 1998; **27**: 285–95.

17 Hirano I, Gilliam J, Goyal RK. Clinical and manometric features of the lower esophageal muscular ring. *Am J Gastroenterol* 2000; **95**: 43–9.

18 Dickey W, McConnell B. Celiac disease presenting as the Paterson–Brown-Kelly (Plummer–Vinson) syndrome. *Am J Gastroenterol* 1999; **94**: 527–9.

19 Jessner W, Vogelsang H, Puspok A, *et al.* Plummer–Vinson syndrome associated with celiac disease and complicated by postcricoid carcinoma and carcinoma of the tongue. *Am J Gastroenterol* 2003; **98**: 1208–9.

20 Von Rahden BHA, Stein HJ, Becker K, *et al.* Heterotopic gastric mucosa of the esophagus: literature-review and proposal of a clinicopathologic classification. *Am J Gastroenterol* 2004; **99**: 543–51.

21 Galan AR, Katzka DA, Castell DO. Acid secretion from an esophageal inlet patch demonstrated by ambulatory pH monitoring. *Gastroenterology* 1998; **115**: 1574–6.

22 Godshall D, Mossallam U, Rosenbaum R. Gastric volvulus: case report and review of the literature. *J Emerg Med* 1999; **17**: 837–40.

CHAPTER 2

CHAPTER 3

Esophageal and Gastric Motor Function

Kenneth R. DeVault,[1] Ernest P. Bouras,[1] and Nicholas J. Talley[2]

[1] Division of Gastroenterology and Hepatology, Mayo Clinic, Jacksonville, FL, USA
[2] Faculty of Health, University of Newcastle, Newcastle, NSW, Australia

Summary

The esophagus and stomach have specific motor functions that propel ingested material through the upper gastrointestinal (GI) tract, while the stomach also helps to grind the food into a more digestible form. The proximal, striated muscle portion of the esophagus quickly moves the bolus into the distal esophagus, where smooth muscle contractions propel it through the lower esophageal sphincter (LES) into the stomach. In addition to allowing the bolus to pass, the LES is tonically contracted in its resting state, which prevents gastroesophageal reflux. The proximal stomach receptively relaxes to accommodate the swallowed bolus, while the distal stomach has functions to grind the food into smaller sizes to facilitate digestion. The antrum and pylorus have an additional function as a "sieve" to prevent emptying of particles until they have been reduced to an appropriate size. The stomach has a specific region that coordinates the motor activity of the stomach and to a degree the entire upper GI tract (pacemaker region). This region initiates the periodic contraction profile that pushes both digested and undigested material through the GI tract (phase III of the migrating motor complex). This complicated physiology is affected by both hormones and extrinsic innervation, but the pacemaker resides in the specialized nervous system of the GI tract, most likely in the interstitial Cajal cells.

Esophageal Motor Function

The esophagus is a tubular structure of approximately 18–25 cm length (somewhat dependent on body height) with two major functions: propulsion of swallowed material to the stomach and prevention of the reflux gastric content back toward the mouth. At rest, the smooth muscle of the esophagus is relaxed, with the exception of the sphincters located on either end: the striated-muscle upper esophageal sphincter (UES) and the smooth-muscle LES. These sphincters are very important, since the pressure of the thoracic cavity is lower than that of either the external environment or the stomach (without the sphincters, air and gastric content would be pulled into the esophagus).

Innervation of Esophageal Muscle

The proximal portion of the esophagus is composed of striated muscle that is not under voluntary control, but is directly innervated by cholinergic nerves that have their cell bodies in the brainstem (predominantly the nucleus ambiguous). Vagal nerves going to the smooth muscle have their cell bodies in the dorsal motor complex and do not directly synapse on the muscle, but instead synapse on myenteric neurons. Cholinergic innervation excites both the longitudinal and circular muscle, while the non-adrenergic, non-cholinergic transmitter mainly inhibits activity in the circular muscle [1]. The final mediator of this relaxation is most likely nitric oxide (NO) or a similar compound [2]. Peristalsis can occur in a deinnervated esophagus through intramural enteric neurological activity.

Esophageal motor activity and much of the motor activity of the GI tract in general seems to be localized in specialized neurons within the myenteric plexus in the wall of the organ, which are labeled the interstitial Cajal cells (ICCs) [3]. These cells are found between most nerves and smooth muscle and are major moderators of the nerve–smooth muscle interaction. They may have a role in modulating muscle activity independent of central stimulation, have been shown to play a key role in the relaxation of the LES [4], and are abnormal in diseases such as achalasia [5].

Oral, Pharyngeal, and Upper Esophageal Sphincter Function

Coordinated activity in the mouth and pharynx is required in order to process a bolus, to avoid aspiration of that bolus, and to transfer the bolus to the esophagus in order to initiate peristalsis. Chewing and swallowing is a complicated process under control of multiple cranial nerves. The process begins with mastication of the bolus, which is under voluntary control and involves the brainstem and cranial nerves (CN) V, VII, and XII. Once the decision to initiate the swallow is made, a very rapid process (involving CN V, X, XI, and XII) begins, but quickly (in less than 0.5 seconds) becomes automatic, involving those nerves and brainstem coordination. The phase begins with the tongue preparing the bolus then forcing it posteriorly and continues with the palate and posterior pharynx closing to prevent nasal regurgitation. The next event is protection of the airway, as the pharynx is lifted proximally and anteriorly, which results in the closure of the airway by the epiglottis. Sequential contractions of pharyngeal muscle then move the bolus toward the entrance to the esophagus.

The upper esophageal "sphincter" (UES) is not a true smooth-muscle sphincter, but is, in fact, a functional closure between the pharynx and the esophagus comprising several different muscles

Practical Gastroenterology and Hepatology Board Review Toolkit, Second Edition. Edited by Nicholas J. Talley, Kenneth R. DeVault, Michael B. Wallace, Bashar A. Aqel and Keith D. Lindor.

and is slit-like rather than round (unlike the other GI-tract sphincters). At rest, UES muscle is tonically contracted and closed due to neural excitation. Within 0.3 seconds after a swallow begins, neural stimulation to the UES ceases and the thyrohyoid and other muscles contract, which pulls the larynx upward and forward to open the sphincter [6]. This entire process takes 0.5–1.0 second in most individuals. Assuming the pharynx contracts as the UES opens, the bolus is cleared into the esophageal body by post-relaxation contractions of muscles in the UES region. The UES is also affected by what occurs more distally, in that fluid or acid in the esophagus tends to result in an increase in UES pressure, presumptively to prevent the aspiration of refluxed material. In addition, the UES relaxes to allow air to escape during a belch. The mechanism that distinguishes between air and fluid is not clear (just as the same mechanism is not clear on the other end of the GI tract!).

Motor Function of the Esophageal Body

Once a bolus enters the esophagus, it quickly transits the striated-muscle portion (which varies from a minimal segment to up to one-third of the length of the esophagus, with a segment of "transition" or mixed muscle). Upon reaching the smooth muscle, the process becomes automated and essentially outside conscious control. The esophageal smooth muscle consists of two layers: an outer longitudinal layer and an inner circular layer. It appears that contraction of the longitudinal muscle allows the circular muscle to have a firmer substrate upon which to act. It has been suggested that the circular-muscle contraction would have to increase by up to 90% without longitudinal muscle contraction [7].

The circular muscle distal to the bolus relaxes (receptive relaxation) and the muscle proximal to the bolus contracts. Both receptive relaxation and esophageal contraction are at least partially controlled by the vagus nerve, with relaxation moderated by vasoactive intestinal polypeptide (VIP) and NO, and contraction by cholinergic innervation. The smooth muscle of the esophagus actually relaxes, and remains relaxed until the bolus arrives, and, interestingly, if multiple swallows occur (as in gulping water), the esophagus remains relaxed until the last swallow, when peristalsis moves down the organ. This response is termed "deglutitive inhibition" and can result in abnormal motility testing in normal patients who repetitively swallow during esophageal manometry [8]. It takes between 6 and 8 seconds for a bolus to move from the mouth to the stomach, with a velocity of 3–4 cm/second. Normal esophageal contraction should last less than 7 seconds and have a bolus pressure between 35 and 180 mmHg [9]. Although air (with belching) and gastric content (with vomiting or regurgitation) can move retrograde through the esophagus, this is due to gastric contraction, and normal esophageal muscle cannot produce coordinated retrograde activity. In fact, when isolated muscle from the distal and proximal smooth muscle is electrically stimulated contraction occurs at different rates, suggesting that peristalsis is programmed into the smooth muscle itself.

The process of transfer of a swallowed bolus through the esophagus is often termed "primary peristalsis." Peristalsis can also be initiated independent of swallowing, usually after esophageal distension; this has been termed "secondary peristalsis." This response is independent of central nervous system control and is preserved in an isolated organ preparation. Secondary peristalsis is important in the clearance of material left behind after primary peristalsis and material refluxed from the stomach. In addition to primary and secondary contractions, the esophagus at times may activate and produce peristalsis independent of swallowing or intraluminal distension (tertiary peristalsis). This must be distinguished from uncoordinated contractions, which radiologists often observe with barium testing and describe as "tertiary" contractions, as well as from the simultaneous contractions seen at manometry that define esophageal spasm [10].

Lower Esophageal Sphincter

The muscle of the LES is different from the smooth muscle of the non-sphincteric portions of the GI tract in that it is contracted in the resting state and relaxes with stimulation. In a resting state, the majority of the LES pressure is provided by the tonic contraction of smooth muscle, but some additional "pressure" is provided by diaphragmatic contraction. The resting pressure of this sphincter needs to be more than 10 mmHg in order to prevent the spontaneous reflux of gastric material into the esophagus and must relax in order to allow the bolus to pass. Interestingly, the LES relaxes within 1–2 seconds of swallowing and remains relaxed until the bolus arrives and passes (6–8 seconds). This relaxation occurs even with "dry" swallows, and the LES can remain relaxed for very long periods of time during repetitive swallowing. Central control appears to enter well proximal to the LES, since surgical vagotomy in the lower esophagus has minimal to no effect on LES pressure or relaxation [11]. LES tone is dependent on the influx of extracellular calcium and can be attenuated with calcium channel blockers [12]. NO plays an important role in LES relaxation. Nitrates and phosphodiesterase inhibitors such as sildenafil also lower LES pressure in health and disease [13].

Gastroesophageal reflux is common when the resting LES pressure is very low, especially in the presence of a hiatal hernia, but the more common reflux-associated event at the LES is what has been termed "transient LES relaxation" (TLESR) [14]. TLESR is evoked by gastric distension and by stimulation of gastric vagal afferent neurons. It is also increased by cholecystokinin, acetylcholine, and NO, and is decreased by gamma aminobutyric acid (GABA-B receptor) and opioids [15]. Preventing TLESR is a major target for several ongoing research programs and may eventually represent a more physiologic way of treating some patients with gastroesophageal reflux disease (GERD).

Figure 3.1 illustrates typical esophageal peristalsis, as demonstrated with high-resolution manometry.

Gastric Motor Function

Motor activity has several major functions in the stomach. In response to eating, the proximal stomach normally relaxes (accommodation). The distal stomach contracts in a coordinated fashion to begin to mix (trituration) and eventually empty. In addition, emptying of the stomach helps to coordinate the motility of the rest of the upper GI tract.

Electrophysiology of Gastric Motility

Much of the motor activity of the stomach is controlled by an innate, cyclical electrical activity. This activity is felt to originate at a site along the greater curvature of the stomach that has been described as a "gastric pacemaker" [16]. From this point, electrical activity is transmitted throughout the stomach in the form of an activity occurring at a frequency of about three cycles per minute (CPM) that is known as the "slow wave" [17]. When this activity is occurring at a low level, no motor activity occurs, but when the amplitude of the cycles is sufficient, calcium channels open, spikes of activity produce action potentials, and motor activity ensues. This electrical activity has different effects on different areas of the stomach, due to innate difference in the excitability of muscles in those areas [18].

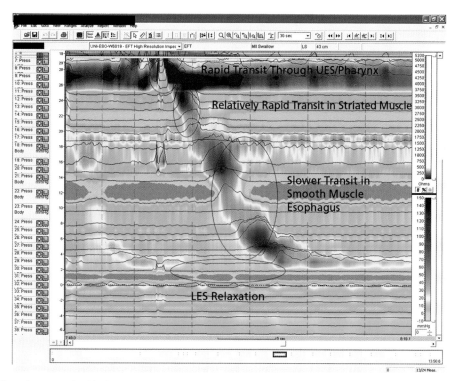

Figure 3.1 Esophageal motility: example of high-resolution motility tracing to demonstrate the progression of a bolus through the esophagus. With swallowing, there is rapid transit through the UES/pharyngeal region. The bolus continues to move relatively rapidly through the striated muscle and then transitions into slower transit in the smooth muscle. The LES actually relaxes with the initiation of swallowing and remains relaxed until the bolus passes into the stomach.

It is important to understand that the frequency of gastric contractions cannot exceed 3 CPM.

ICCs play a key role in the stomach, just as in the esophagus [19]. The ICCs are directly coupled to smooth-muscle cells (SMCs) and result in their excitation when 3 CPM activity reaches threshold amplitude. In fact, the slow wave itself is most likely a function of the ICCs [20]. In contrast to the small bowel and colon, it appears that almost all gastric ICCs receive direct vagal innervation [21]. The ICCs play a role in the relaxation of the pylorus and appear to be lost in infantile pyloric stenosis [22].

The stomach, unlike the esophagus, receives innervation from both the vagus nerve (cell bodies in the dorsal motor nucleus) and the splanchnic nerves (cell bodies in the prevertebral celiac ganglia). While these nerves certainly affect motility, they contain a predominance of efferent, sensory fibers.

Proximal Stomach

The muscle in the proximal stomach has a degree of tonic contraction at rest and does not usually exhibit 3 CPM activity. With a meal, it relaxes to allow the stomach to distend (up to threefold) and provide a reservoir for the swallowed material. The muscle then contracts and pushes the bolus toward the distal stomach. In the past, this was thought to be due to an overall pressure gradient, but modern studies have found that the activity of even the proximal stomach is pulsatile and under the control of the gastric pacemaker. This relaxation is under vagal control, is diminished or lost with vagotomy or significant vagal neuropathy, and appears to be mediated by NO- and VIP-releasing nerves [23]. Poor gastric accommodation has also been suggested to play a role in some patients with dyspepsia and may cause early satiation (inability to finish a normal-sized meal) [24]. Other factors that decrease fundic tone (and increase

accommodation) include: antral distension (a full stomach) [25], duodenal acidification and distension [26], and intraluminal fat or protein and nutrients in the ileum [27]. The fundus also relaxes with swallowing [28] and during nausea and vomiting. Surgical fundoplication obliterates part of the fundus and seems to impair relaxation, usually through a mechanical means, though some patients also undoubtedly suffer vagus nerve damage during their surgery [29].

Distal Stomach

The muscle from the distal stomach initially contracts at 3 CPM to mix the bolus with secreted acid and enzymes in order to break the food down into smaller particles prior to emptying. When food is sufficiently digested, peristaltic contractions (again at 3 CPM) force the bolus toward the pylorus [30]. The pylorus is the sphincter between the stomach and duodenum; it has greater muscular bulk than the remainder of the stomach and has unique myogenic activity. During trituration, the pylorus is contracted and closed, which keeps the bolus in the stomach or allows only the better-digested (i.e., smaller) portions of the gastric content to empty. Later, when the bolus is more completely digested, the pylorus relaxes in coordination with antral contractions to allow more of the bolus to exit the stomach. In fact, ultrasound-based studies suggest that most flow through the pylorus occurs during relatively prolonged periods of opening, when the gastric antrum and duodenal bulb become essentially a common cavity [31].

Gastric emptying of solids classically occurs in two phases. The first (lag phase) is characterized by minimal solid emptying and may last up to 60 minutes. The majority of emptying occurs during the second (linear) phase [32], which is felt to begin after the meal has been triturated into particles of 1 mm or less in diameter. Emptying of fats presents an additional challenge in that fats are liquid at

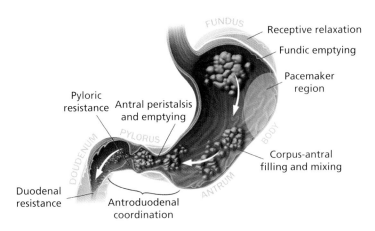

Figure 3.2 Gastric motility. See text for details, but in brief gastric function can be divided into what happens in the proximal stomach (receptive relaxation and fundic empting) and what happens in the corpus and distal stomach (mixing, peristalsis, and emptying). In addition, there is a gastric pacemaker that helps to coordinate not only gastric motility, but the motility of the upper small intestine. The pylorus provides resistance to emptying, which aids mixing, and opens to allow the bolus to pass into the duodenum.

body temperature, do not mix well with the aqueous solutions in the stomach, and tend to float on the top of the liquid layer, all of which results in slow emptying of this food component [33].

During fasting, there are periodic "housekeeper contractions," which are also known as phase III of the migrating motor complex. Particles that were not broken down sufficiently during tituration are emptied by these phase III contractions. This event appears to be initiated in the duodenum, but also affects gastric muscle [34]. When a phase III is initiated, the LES contracts, tone increases in the proximal stomach, and 1 CPM-high amplitude waves develop in the body of the stomach. The 3 CPM contractions in the antrum become more pronounced, and as the activity reaches the distal stomach, the pylorus relaxes, allowing material to move into the duodenum. In the GI tract distal to the stomach, phase III activity is peristaltic, while in the stomach it tends to occur in all areas relatively simultaneously. Motilin is a peptide hormone that appears to induce this activity and offers a therapeutic target for patients with disturbed gastric motility [35].

Gastric Emptying: A Coordinated Activity?

Given the previously described physiology, how does the stomach process and transport an ingested meal? There is no one answer to this question. The stomach (assuming it is intact, with intact innervation) handles low- or no-calorie liquids in a very simple fashion: it distends, liquids are distributed throughout it, and the liquids then empty at a steady rate until most have exited it. If there are substantial calories or even osmols in the liquid, emptying is slowed, most likely due to feedback from receptors in the duodenum [36] (Table 3.1). Solids are handled differently, depending initially on the

size of particles in the ingested material and later on the size of those in the digested meals. Digestible solids (defined in general as particles that can be broken down to 1 mm or smaller by the stomach) empty more like liquids (after they are digested to that size), while indigestible solids remain in the stomach longer, some not being emptied until phase III of the migrating motor complex. The complicated nature of this activity is compounded by the fact that most ingested meals are a combination of liquids and both digestible and indigestible solids, as is illustrated in Figure 3.2.

Take Home Points

- The esophagus and stomach have innate muscle activity, with an intramural "nervous" system. This activity is affected and, in some cases, controlled by extrinsic nervous input (primarily via the vagus nerve).
- The esophagus has striated muscle in the proximal portion, smooth muscle in the distal portion, and a sphincter at either end (upper and lower esophageal sphincters (UES and LES)).
- After swallowing, the bolus enters the esophagus and is passed to the stomach in 5–10 seconds.
- The LES is tonically closed (to prevent reflux) and opens with the initiation of swallowing, then closes when the bolus passes into the stomach.
- With eating, the proximal stomach relaxes (receptive relaxation), allowing the bolus to be easily accommodated. This function is under control of the vagus nerve.
- The distal stomach and pylorus are involved in the grinding of food into small pieces and in the control of gastric emptying.
- The stomach has an intramural "pacemaker region" that controls specific aspects of both gastric and small-bowel motility.

Table 3.1 Factors that slow gastric emptying.

Meal factors	Volume
	Acidity
	Osmolarity
	Nutrient density
	Carbonation
	Certain amino acids
	l-tryptophan
Medications	Narcotics
	Anticholinergics
	Calcium channel blockers
Other factors	Rectal or colonic distension
	Pregnancy
	Female sex
	Blood glucose
	Circular motion
	Cold-induced pain

References

1 Crist J, Gidda JS, Goyal RK. Intramural mechanism of esophageal peristalsis: roles of cholinergic and noncholinergic nerves. *Proc Natl Acad Sci USA* 1984; **81**: 3595–9.

2 Yamato S, Spechler SJ, Goyal RK. Role of nitric oxide in esophageal peristalsis in the opossum. *Gastroenterology* 1992; **103**: 197–204.

3 Daniel EE, Posey-Daniel V. Neuromuscular structures in opossum esophagus: role of interstitial cells of Cajal. *Am J Physiol* 1984; **246**: G305–15.

4 Morris G, Reese L, Wang X-Y, Sanders KM. Interstitial cells of Cajal mediate enteric inhibitory neurotransmission in the lower esophageal and pyloric sphincters. *Gastroenterology* 1998; **115**: 314–29.

5 Mearin F, Mourelle M, Guarner F, *et al.* Patients with achalasia lack nitric oxide synthase in the gastro-oesophageal junction. *Eur J Clin Invest* 1993; **23**: 724–8.

6 Jacob P, Kahrilas PJ, Logemann JA, *et al.* Upper esophageal sphincter opening and modulation during swallowing. *Gastroenterology* 1989; **97**: 1469–78.

7 Brasseur JG, Nicosia MA, Pal A, Miller LS. Function of longitudinal vs circular muscle fibers in esophageal peristalsis, deduced with mathematical modeling. *World J Gastroenterol* 2007; **13**: 1335–46.

8 Meyer GW, Gerhardt DC, Castell DO. Human esophageal response to rapid swallowing: muscle refractory period or neural inhibition? *Am J Physiol* 1981; **241**: G129–36.

9 Richter JE, Wu WC, Johns DN, *et al.* Esophageal manometry in 95 healthy adult volunteers. Variability of pressures with age and frequency of "abnormal" contractions. *Dig Dis Sci* 1987; **32**: 583–92.

10 Meyer GW, Castell DO. Anatomy and physiology of the esophageal body. In: Castell DO, Johnson LF, eds. *Esophageal Function in Health and Disease.* New York: Elsevier Biomedical, 1983: 1–29.

11 Higgs RH, Castell DO. The effect of truncal vagotomy on lower esophageal sphincter pressure and response to cholinergic stimulation. *Proc Soc Exp Biol Med* 1976; **153**: 379–82.

12 Biancani P, Hillemeier C, Bitar KN, Makhlouf GM. Contraction mediated by Ca^{2+} influx in esophageal muscle and by Ca^{2+} release in the LES. *Am J Physiol* 1987; **253**: G760–6.

13 Lee JI, Park H, Kim JH, *et al.* The effect of sildenafil on oesophageal motor function in healthy subjects and patients with nutcracker oesophagus. *Neurogastroenterol Motil* 2003; **15**: 617–23.

14 Dodds WJ, Dent J, Hogan WJ, *et al.* Mechanisms of gastro-esophageal reflux in patients with reflux esophagitis. *N Engl J Med* 1982; **307**: 1547–52.

15 Hirsch DP, Tytgat GN, Boeckxstaens GE. Transient lower oesophageal sphincter relaxations – a pharmacological target for gastro-oesophageal reflux disease? *Aliment Pharmacol Ther* 2002; **16**: 17–26.

16 Szurszewski JH. Electrophysiological basis of gastrointestinal motility. In: Johnson LR, ed. *Physiology of the Gastrointestinal Tract*, 2nd edn. New York: Raven Press, 1986: 383–42.

17 Wilson P, Perdikis G, Redmond EJ, *et al.* Prolonged ambulatory antroduodenal manometry in humans. *Am J Gastroenterol* 1994; **89**: 1489–95.

18 Hinder RA, Kelly KA. Human gastric pacesetter potential. Site of origin, spread, and response to gastric transection and proximal gastric vagotomy. *Am J Surg* 1977; **133**: 29–33.

19 Horowitz B, Ward SM, Sanders KM. Cellular and molecular basis for electrical rhythmicity in gastrointestinal muscles. *Annu Rev Physiol* 1999; **61**: 19–43.

20 Huizinga JD. Physiology and pathophysiology of the intestinal cell of Cajal: from bench to bedside. II. Gastric motility: lessons from mutant mice on slow waves and innervation. *Am J Physiol* 2001; **281**: G1129–34.

21 Powley T. Vagal input to the enteric nervous system. *Gut* 2000; **47** (Suppl. 4): iv30–32.

22 Vanderwinden J-M, Liu H, De Laet M-H, Vanderhaegen J-J. Study of the interstitial cells of Cajal in infantile hypertrophic pyloric stenosis. *Gastroenterology* 1996; **111**: 279–88.

23 Jansson G. Extrinsic nervous control of gastric motility. An experimental study in the cat. *Acta Physiol Scand* 1969; **326**: 1–42.

24 Tack J, Piessevaux H, Coulie B, *et al.* Role of impaired gastric accommodation to a meal in functional dyspepsia. *Gastroenterology* 1998; **115**: 1346–52.

25 De Ponti F, Azpiroz F. Malagelada JR. Reflex gastric relaxation in response to distention of the duodenum. *Am J Physiol* 1987; **252**: G595–601.

26 Kelly KA, Code CF. Effect of transthoracic vagotomy on canine gastric electrical activity. *Gastroenterology* 1969; **57**: 51–8.

27 Azpiroz F, Malagelada JR. Physiological variations in canine gastric tone measured by an electronic barostat. *Am J Physiol* 185; **248**: G229–37.

28 Jansson G. Extrinsic nervous control of gastric motility: an experimental study in the cat. *Acta Physiol Scand* 1969; **326** (Suppl.): 1–42.

29 DeVault KR, Swain JM, Wentling GK, *et al.* Evaluation of vagus nerve function before and after antireflux surgery. *J Gastrointest Surg* 2004; **8**: 883–8; disc. 888–9.

30 Ehrlein HJ, Heisinger E. Computer analysis of mechanical activity of gastroduodenal junction in unanesthetized dogs. *Q J Exp Phyisol* 1982; **67**: 17–29.

31 Pallotta N, Cicala M, Frandina C, Corazziara E. Antro-pyloric contractile patterns and transpyloric flow after meal ingestion in humans. *Am J Gastroenterol* 1998; **93**: 2513–22.

32 Siegel JA, Urbain JL, Adler LP, *et al.* Biphasic nature of gastric emptying. *Gut* 1988; **29**: 85–9.

33 Meyer JH, Mayer EA, Jehn D, *et al.* Gastric processing and emptying of fat. *Gastroenterology* 1986; **90**: 1176–87.

34 Kellow JE, Borody TJ, Phillips SF, *et al.* Human interdigestive motility: variations in patterns from esophagus to colon. *Gastroenterology* 1986; **91**: 386–95.

35 Peeters T, Matthijs G, Depoortere I, *et al.* Erythromycin is a motilin receptor agonist. *Am J Physiol* 1989; **257**: G470–4.

36 Hunt JN, Spurrell WR. The pattern of emptying of the human stomach. *J Physiol (Lond)* 1951; **115**: 157–68.

CHAPTER 3

PART 2

Other Diagnostic Modalities

4 Radiologic Approach to Diagnosis, 23
Stephen W. Trenkner and James E. Huprich

5 Esophageal Motility Disorders, 28
Magnus Halland and Kenneth R. DeVault

6 Gastric Motility Testing, 36
Jan Tack

Radiologic Approach to Diagnosis

Stephen W. Trenkner and James E. Huprich

Division of Radiology, Mayo Clinic, Rochester, MN, USA

Esophagus

Techniques

The primary imaging study of the esophagus is the barium esophagram [1]. It is performed with the patient standing (double contrast) or lying down (single contrast). It evaluates the structure of the esophagus and cardia, and to some extent swallowing, esophageal peristalsis, and gastroesophageal reflux. Occasionally, the patient is given a 13 mm barium tablet to evaluate the diameter of strictures. Swallowing marshmallows is rarely helpful.

When the swallowing mechanism is of primary concern, the esophagram should be performed in conjunction with a modified barium swallow [2]. The modified barium swallow is done with the assistance of a speech pathologist or occupational therapist. The swallow is evaluated with both liquids and solids. When an abnormality is detected, the therapists are invaluable in retraining the patient to swallow safely.

The esophagram is excellent for evaluating perforations and postoperative anatomy. In these cases, water-soluble contrast is used, followed by barium if the initial study is negative for perforation.

Computed tomography (CT) plays a limited role in the evaluation of the esophagus. It can be used to stage esophageal cancer and to evaluate abnormalities extrinsic to the esophagus. In the case of an esophageal lipoma, CT is diagnostic.

Dysphagia

Dysphagia is the feeling of difficulty in passing liquids or solids from the mouth to the stomach [1]. The abnormality may be structural or functional and may involve anywhere between the mouth and the gastric cardia. When ordering studies, it is important to remember that patients are not always able to localize the level of obstruction [3]. An obstructing lesion in the distal esophagus or cardia may be perceived in the neck. Conversely, a proximal obstructing lesion is rarely referred distally. Therefore, patients with symptoms in the neck require an evaluation of swallowing, often followed by an esophagram. If the symptoms are perceived in the chest, usually only an esophageal evaluation is needed.

While endoscopy is superior for evaluating reflux esophagitis, and provides the opportunity for biopsies, barium studies provide an excellent overview of swallowing and the esophagus. The esophagram is also excellent for defining the size and type of hiatal hernia (sliding, paraesophageal, or mixed). The esophagram is also superior to endoscopy for detecting Schatzki rings (mucosal rings)

(Figure 4.1), which are a common cause of dysphagia [4]. Other advantages of the esophagram include the detection of cervical esophageal webs and assessment of esophageal size – both too narrow and too wide (Figure 4.2).

Imaging after Antireflux Surgery

In the past decade, there has been an 8 to 10-fold increase in the number of laparoscopic antireflux procedures performed. Approximately 50% of patients have persistent or new symptoms within 3 months following surgery and 2–17% will eventually have objective evidence of failed antireflux surgery. Managing such patients has occupied a significant portion of the gastroenterologist's practice. Barium studies play an important role in the evaluation of these challenging patients. Familiarity with their techniques is important to a successful patient outcome.

The purpose of antireflux surgery is to restore the function of the lower esophageal sphincter (LES) and return the gastroesophageal junction (GEJ) to an intra-abdominal location. Fundoplication types can be divided into (i) complete (Nissen) and (ii) partial fundoplications (e.g., Belsey, Toupet, Dor). Partial fundoplications can further be divided into anterior and posterior types, depending upon the location of the plication. The choice of fundoplication type depends upon many factors. In general, complete wraps (e.g., Nissen) provide better protection against reflux but have a higher incidence of dysphagia, especially in patients with poor esophageal function.

The successful radiographic evaluation of patients with fundoplications depends upon the use of proper technique and possession of a thorough knowledge of the surgical anatomy. The radiologist must be familiar with double-contrast upper gastrointestinal series (UGI) techniques for the proper evaluation of these patients.

Complete and partial fundoplications each have characteristic radiographic appearances. In both types, a soft-tissue density representing the wrap is seen in the gastric fundus (Figure 4.3). The fundic soft-tissue density appears larger in the case of a complete versus a partial wrap. In both cases, the esophageal lumen appears narrowed as it passes through the wrap. Since the wrap completely surrounds the esophagus in a complete fundoplication, the esophageal lumen appears centered within the wrap. In partial fundoplications, the lumen is eccentrically located within the wrap, either anteriorly (in posterior fundoplications) or posteriorly (in anterior fundoplications). In all cases, the wrap should be located below the diaphragm, indicating an intra-abdominal location. One

Practical Gastroenterology and Hepatology Board Review Toolkit, Second Edition. Edited by Nicholas J. Talley, Kenneth R. DeVault, Michael B. Wallace, Bashar A. Aqel and Keith D. Lindor.

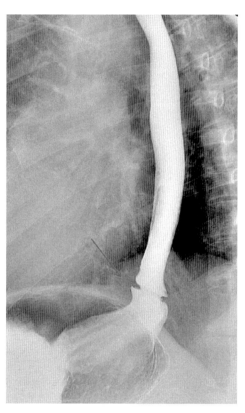

Figure 4.1 Schatzki ring (arrow).

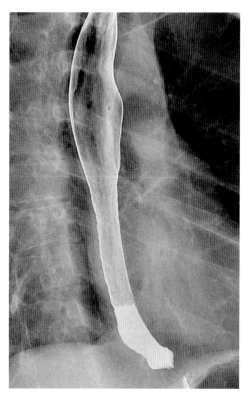

Figure 4.2 Narrowing of the distal third of the esophagus and subtle rings resulting from eosinophilic esophagitis.

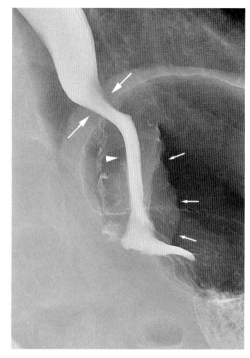

Figure 4.3 Normal Nissen fundoplication. The barium-filled esophageal lumen (arrowhead) is slightly narrowed as it passes through the wrap, represented by the soft-tissue density in the gastric fundus (small arrows). Note that the wrap is located entirely below the diaphragmatic hiatus (large arrows) and no hiatal hernia or any portion of the gastric fundus is seen above the wrap.

other very important radiographic sign of an intact fundoplication is the absence of any portion of the stomach or hiatal hernia above the wrap. The radiographic features of an intact fundoplication are stated in Table 4.1.

Radiographic changes during the first 3 months following antireflux surgery may cause concern if one is not aware of their temporary nature. In the early postoperative period, there is delayed emptying of barium from the esophagus as a result of swelling. The soft-tissue density in the gastric fundus may appear quite large initially – approximately the size of an apricot. The soft-tissue density shrinks over the following months to less than half the original size. During the first few days after surgery, the stomach may be somewhat dilated, reflecting temporary delayed gastric emptying. Recognition of these normal transient changes can be reassuring to the patient.

The diagnosis of failed antireflux surgery is based upon persistent or new symptoms associated with an anatomical or physiological abnormality. Various classifications of types of anatomical failure, based upon barium studies, have been published [5–7]. However, if one adheres to the simple criteria listed in Table 4.1, most cases of anatomical failure can be recognized.

Table 4.1 Signs of intact fundoplication on barium swallows.

1. Soft-tissue density (wrap) within the gastric fundus
2. Wrap located below the diaphragm
3. Slightly narrowed esophageal lumen passes centrally (in complete fundoplications) or eccentrically (partial fundoplication) within the soft-tissue density
4. No stomach (or hiatal hernia) above the wrap

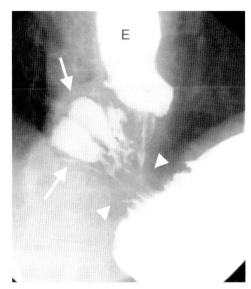

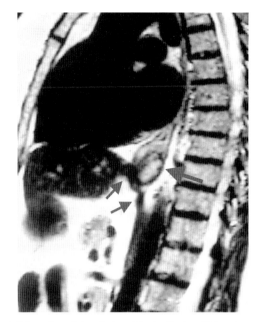

Figure 4.4 Disrupted Nissen fundoplication. Barium filling a bizarrely shaped paraesophageal hernia (arrows) located above the diaphragmatic hiatus (arrowheads) adjacent to the esophagus (E). Note the absence of the normal soft-tissue density in the gastric fundus, indicating herniation of the disrupted wrap through the hiatus into the chest.

Dysphagia persisting more than 6 months after a fundoplication may be caused by a wrap that is too tight. Diagnosis is usually difficult. However, findings of delayed emptying of the esophagus in the upright position and an excessively long luminal narrowing may provide clues to the diagnosis.

The most common finding of fundoplication failure is the appearance or reappearance of a hiatal hernia. In most cases, portions of

Figure 4.5 Intrathoracic herniation of fundoplication. This patient experienced severe dysphagia several months after laparoscopic Nissen fundoplication. Endoscopy and barium studies showed an intact wrap. This sagittal MR image through the diaphragmatic hiatus demonstrates the fundoplication (large arrow) to be located above the diaphragm (small arrows). Source: Lord *et al.*, 2000 [8].

the wrap remain intact, causing an asymmetrical, sometimes bizarre appearance (Figure 4.4). With complete disruption of the wrap and failure of the hiatal closure, a larger hiatal hernia may result. Herniation of an intact wrap above the diaphragm is less common but

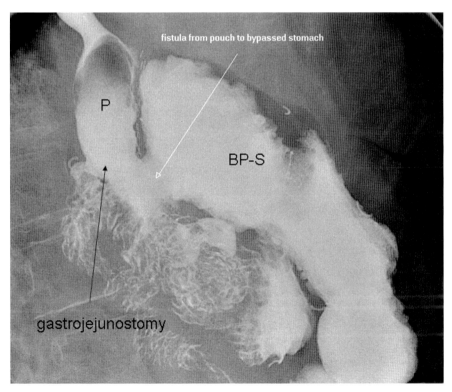

Figure 4.6 RYGBP with a large area of breakdown in the staple line between the gastric pouch (P) and the bypassed portion of the stomach (BP-S).

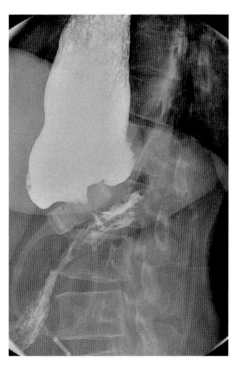

Figure 4.7 This band is too tight, causing gross esophageal dilation.

may be more difficult to diagnose, especially if there is no associated hiatal hernia. In these cases, CT or magnetic resonance imaging (MRI) may be of value in demonstrating the supradiaphragmatic location of the wrap (Figure 4.5).

Stomach

Techniques

The major imaging study of the stomach is the UGI, an evaluation of the area from the mouth to the duodenal/jejunal junction. The UGI therefore incorporates the esophageal evaluation discussed previously, but also includes an evaluation of the stomach and duodenum. Like the esophagram, it is a biphasic technique, including both double and single contrast [9]. When perforation is suspected, water-soluble contrast is used.

CT plays a secondary role in gastric imaging. It can be used to stage gastric malignancies and is helpful in defining intramural tumors, such as gastrointestinal stromal tumors (GISTs) and extrinsic abnormalities.

Major Indications

Barium evaluation of the stomach is less clinically relevant than the esophagram. The UGI is often ordered when an esophagram is all that is needed. Endoscopy has largely replaced the UGI for evaluation of the gastric mucosa.

Probably the current leading indication for a UGI is to evaluate the postoperative stomach. With the decline in partial gastrectomies for ulcers, we are now mainly evaluating morbid obesity procedures. The two main procedures are the Roux-en-Y gastric bypass (RYGBP) and laparoscopic adjustable gastric banding (LAGB) [10].

The RYGBP consists of a small gastric pouch that is attached to the Roux limb. Further down, the Roux limb is anastomosed to the jejunum. The UGI is excellent for evaluating the major complications, including obstructions and fistulas, between the gastric pouch and bypassed stomach (Figure 4.6).

The LAGB is an inflatable silicone band that is surgically placed around the proximal stomach. The band is connected to a subcutaneous port, allowing its inflation and deflation. Inflating the band narrows the proximal stomach, restricting food intake. Adverse symptoms occur when the band is too tight (Figure 4.7) or there is slippage of the stomach above the band (Figure 4.8). Both problems are easily assessed with a UGI. The band may also erode through the gastric wall, which can be detected by UGI or endoscopy.

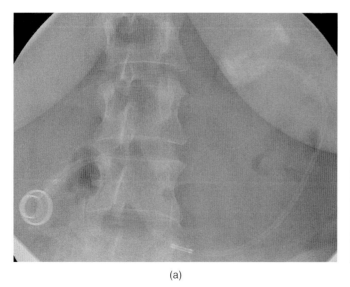

(a)

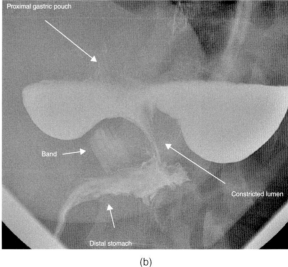

(b)

Figure 4.8 (a) LAGB on plain film. (b) Slipped LAGB. Almost no stomach is seen above the band in normal cases.

Take Home Points

- When the swallowing mechanism is of primary concern, the esophagram should be performed in conjunction with a modified barium swallow.
- Patients with symptoms in the neck need an evaluation of swallowing.
- Esophagram is superior to endoscopy for detecting Schatzki rings (mucosal rings).
- Radiographic changes during the first 3 months following antireflux surgery are often temporary.
- Dysphagia persisting more than 6 months after a fundoplication may be caused by a wrap that is too tight.
- The current leading indication for a UGI is evaluation of the postoperative stomach.

References

1 Levine MS, Rubesin SE. Radiologic investigation of dysphagia. *AJR* 1990; **154**: 1157–63.

2 Logemann JA. Role of the modified barium swallow in management of patients with dysphagia. *Otolaryngol Head Neck Surg* 1997; **116**: 335–8.

3 Wilcox CM, Alexander LN, Clark WS. Localization of an obstructing esophageal lesion: is the patient accurate? *Digestive Diseases and Sciences* 1995; **40**: 2192–6.

4 Ott DJ, Chen YM, Wu WC, *et al.* Radiographic and endoscopic sensitivity in detecting lower esophageal mucosal ring. *AJR* 1986; **147**: 261–5.

5 Horgan S, Pohl D, Bogetti D, *et al.* Failed antireflux surgery: what have we learned from reoperations? *Arch Surg* 1999; **134**: 809–17.

6 Saik R, Peskin G. The study of fundoplication disruption and deformity. *Am J Surg* 1977; **134**: 19–22.

7 Thoeni R, Moss A. The radiographic appearance of complications following Nissen fundoplication. *Radiology* 1979; **131**: 17–21.

8 Lord R, Huprich J, Katkhouda N. Gastrointestinal: complications of fundoplication. *JGH* 2000; **15**(10): 1221.

9 Levine MS, Rubesin SE, Herlinger H, Laufer I. Double-contrast upper gastrointestinal examination: technique and interpretation. *Radiology* 1988; **168**: 593–602.

10 Trenkner SW. Imaging of morbid obesity procedures and their complications. *Abdom Imaging* 2009; **34**(3): 335–44.

CHAPTER 4

Esophageal Motility Disorders

Magnus Halland[1] and Kenneth R. DeVault[2]

[1] Division of Gastroenterology and Hepatology, Mayo Clinic, Rochester, MN, USA
[2] Division of Gastroenterology and Hepatology, Mayo Clinic, Jacksonville, FL, USA

Summary

Achalasia is the most important esophageal motility disorder to recognize and treat. Despite the unknown etiology of this disease, many therapeutic options exist – once the presence of achalasia mimics, including cancer have been carefully excluded. Per-oral endoscopic myotomy (POEM) is emerging as a minimally invasive therapeutic option. The pathophysiological understanding of achalasia and non-achalasia motility disorders has been improved by the development of high-resolution esophageal manometry. Many centers now use the "Chicago classification" to describe abnormal manometric patterns.

Case

An 85-year-old man presents with heartburn and increasing dysphagia to solids and liquids. His symptoms have gradually increased over the past 4 years. He has lost 7 kg of weight in the last 18 months. He can no longer belch, refuses to eat at restaurants for fear of regurgitation, and has experienced awakening at night with fluid in his mouth. A trial of a proton pump inhibitor (PPI) has only been partially effective. A recent endoscopy was essentially unremarkable, apart from some fluid and candidiases noted in the distal esophagus. A computed tomography (CT) scan of the chest is negative, but a dilated esophagus is noted.

Introduction

The normal physiology associated with esophageal peristalsis is described in Chapter 3. This physiology can become disordered in several ways. There can be a loss of coordination or development of high-pressure contractions, which may produce dysphagia, chest pain, or both (spastic dysmotility). There can also be disorders with weak or ineffective peristalsis. This dysfunction may be either primary (idiopathic) or secondary to many different systemic diseases.

This chapter discusses the pathophysiology, diagnosis, and therapy of common esophageal motor disorders.

Esophageal Diagnostics

Historically, the assessment of esophageal motility was made on barium esophagraphy, which was supplemented by development water-perfused esophageal manometry. More recently, the advent of high-resolution solid-state catheters with an increased number of sensors has provided much more detailed information about esophageal pathophysiology. In particular, the development of esophageal pressure topography (EPT) has advanced the understanding of normal and abnormal esophageal motor patterns and simplified the interpretation of esophageal tracings. Many centers now use the "Chicago classification" to characterize and diagnose esophageal motility disorders. This classification provides a "hierarchy" of esophageal motor disorders in order of clinical significance and serves as a diagnostic algorithm. It utilizes a number of key metrics to assess esophageal function:

- Integrated relaxation pressure (IRP): measures the mean esophagogastric junction (EGJ) pressure after a swallow.
- Distal contractile integral (DCI): measures the duration and amplitude of the distal esophageal contraction.
- Contractile deceleration point (CDP), contractile front velocity (CVI), distal latency (DL): used to determine the velocity and timing of the swallow.

The findings of an esophageal manometry must always be interpreted in the clinical context of the patient's symptoms, coexisting illnesses, medication use, and prior surgery. Correlation with barium esophagography remains important, particularly in cases of suspected achalasia.

Normal esophageal peristalsis requires a balance of excitatory neurologic input (usually cholinergic) and inhibitory input (non-adrenergic, non-cholinergic – NANC) [1]. When these forces become imbalanced, the esophageal peristaltic sequence may become disordered and produce symptoms. Achalasia is the best-described esophageal motility disorder; the clinical implications of many of the other observable abnormal manometric patterns are less certain [2].

Achalasia

Achalasia is an uncommon disorder with an estimated incidence of 1 in 100 000 annually. Classically, achalasia has been defined by a combination of two cardinal features:

- A lower esophageal sphincter (LES) that fails to relax with swallows.
- Aperistalsis of the esophageal body.

It is important to note that achalasia can be present with a normal or elevated esophageal sphincter pressure that fails to relax. The

Practical Gastroenterology and Hepatology Board Review Toolkit, Second Edition. Edited by Nicholas J. Talley, Kenneth R. DeVault, Michael B. Wallace, Bashar A. Aqel and Keith D. Lindor.

etiology remains elusive, but it is hypothesized that viral infections or autoimmune processes may produce the phenotype in genetically susceptible individuals. It appears that loss of the inhibitory NANC nerves (especially those containing vasoactive intestinal polypeptide (VIP) and nitric oxide (NO)) in the lower esophagus brings about this disorder [3].

Clinical Presentation

Patients with achalasia typically present with several months to many years of dysphagia. Achalasia may occur in any age group, including children. It is often progressive, starting as intermittent dysphagia to solids and progressing to dysphagia to liquids and solids. Patients often learn to stand up and move about when dysphagia occurs, which may force the bolus into the stomach. Frank regurgitation, nocturnal aspiration, and pulmonary compromise complicate advanced cases. Chest pain is another common symptom of achalasia, and may be the only symptom in some cases. These symptoms can occasionally be confused with heartburn, and many achalasia patients are mistakenly given trials of acid blockers at some point in the course of their illness. Weight loss often occurs later in the course and is frequently the reason for a more detailed evaluation leading to the diagnosis.

Clinical suspicion, barium testing, manometry, and endoscopy combine to make this diagnosis, which may be delayed for years when clinical suspicion is insufficient. Barium testing almost always suggests the diagnosis. The typical finding is a dilated esophagus with a smoothly tapered, narrowed lower portion, which has been described as a "bird-beak" appearance (Figure 5.1). Advanced cases may develop large epiphrenic diverticula. When the esophagus becomes so dilated that a portion extends inferior to the LES, treatment becomes very difficult and esophagectomy is often required.

Manometry is required to confirm achalasia. The classic finding is an elevated IRP and an aperistaltic esophageal body (Figure 5.2).

With the advent of high-resolution manometry (HRM), it is now clear that three subtypes of achalasia exist:
- Type 1: elevated IRP and absent peristalsis.
- Type 2: elevated IRP with panesophageal pressurization.
- Type 3: elevated IRP and peristaltic fragments or spastic contraction.

Endoscopy is neither sensitive nor specific as a diagnostic tool in achalasia, but is still important, as tumors at the EGJ may produce a radiographic and manometric appearance identical to that of idiopathic achalasia. Endoscopy, with a careful retroflexed view of the EGJ, can usually (but not always) exclude a mucosal lesion, producing secondary achalasia. The mucosa of the esophagus is frequently thickened due to chronic stasis, but achalasia may be complicated by *Candida albicans* infection in some cases. If the clinical suspicion for a malignant cause is high, endoscopic ultrasonography (EUS) can be performed to rule out a submucosal process.

Importantly, a number of disorders can mimic achalasia:
- Tumors in the area of the LES:
  - esophageal malignancies:
    - adenocarcinoma;
    - squamous cell carcinoma;
    - lymphoma.
  - other malignancies:
    - liver;
    - gastric;
    - lung;
    - peritoneal;
    - kidney.
- Benign stromal tumors (e.g., gastrointestinal (GI) stromal tumor).
- Postoperative status after fundoplication or bariatric surgery.

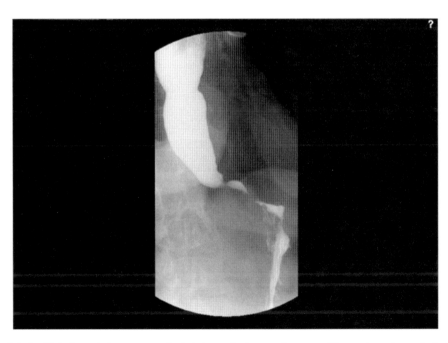

Figure 5.1 Barium of achalasia: this is the typical appearance of achalasia on a barium esophagogram. The esophagus is usually (but not always) dilated, with a smooth tapering into what has been described as a "bird-beak" appearance. Secondary achalasia due to a malignancy at the esophagogastric junction may have an appearance identical to that of idiopathic achalasia and must be excluded with endoscopic visualization.

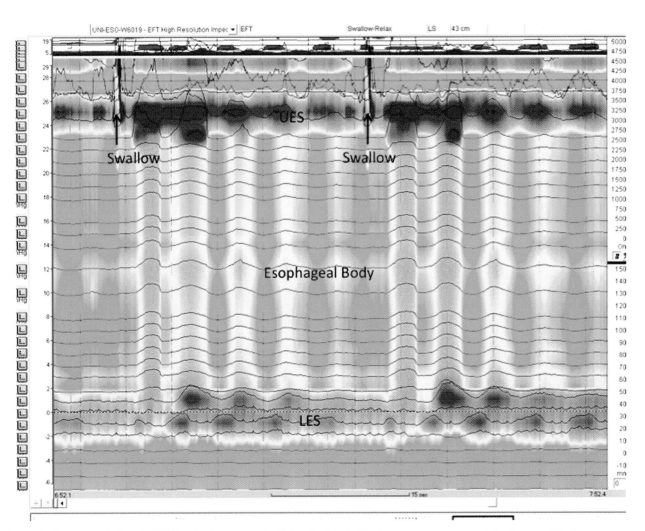

Figure 5.2 Manometry of achalasia: HRM tracing from a patient with type 2 achalasia. The two swallows can be seen to begin normally in the upper esophageal sphincter area, but the esophageal body has only simultaneous, repetitive, low-pressure contractions and there is minimal evidence of relaxation of the LES.

Chagas Disease

Chagas disease is a multisystem infectious disease caused by the protozoan *Trypanosoma cruzi*, which is endemic in certain Central and South American countries. It has a similar esophageal presentation to achalasia, but, unlike achalasia, affects other organs, including the small bowel, colon, rectum, and heart [4]. Reference laboratories now have antibody tests for this disease, which should be considered in an achalasia patient presenting from an endemic area.

- Paraneoplastic phenomena: usually due to small-cell lung cancer – a paraneoplastic panel that includes antibiodies to Hu may be diagnostic.
- Sarcoidosis.
- Amyloidosis.
- Sphingolipidosis (Anderson–Fabry disease).
- Neurofibromatosis.

Remember: malignancy can produce achalasia by three potential mechanisms: direct obstruction at the EGJ from the tumor itself; infiltration of the myenteric plexus, producing a more typical "neurogenic" achalasia; and production of autoantibodies by a distant malignancy, such as a small-cell carcinoma [5]. In patients with advanced age, smoking history, or severe weight loss, cross-sectional imaging is recommended, and positron emission tomography (PET) may also be helpful.

Therapy

Current achalasia therapies focus on relieving the obstruction at the EGJ and hence allowing the still aperistaltic esophagus to essentially empty through a combination of gravity and the force generated by the proximal striated muscle components. The main therapeutic options are:

- heller myotomy (laparoscopic, in many cases);
- pneumatic dilatation;
- per-oral endoscopic myotomy (POEM).

Injection of botulinum toxin A is often effective but not durable, and thus is usually reserved for cases where advanced age or comorbidities make other therapies unattractive. Botulinium toxin injection can be used in cases of diagnostic uncertainty, but due to concerns about subsequent fibrosis at the EGJ, which may make definitive therapy more difficult, this approach is rarely employed. Medical therapies with calcium channel blockers or sildenafil are generally not effective but may be trialed if no other option is viable.

Mechanical disruption of the LES has been the traditional treatment for achalasia and can be accomplished in one of three ways:

forceful pneumatic dilation, surgical myotomy, or POEM. Traditional (20 mm or less) dilation provides no significant benefit in patients with achalasia. Forceful, pneumatic dilation with 30–40 mm balloons is more effective. These balloons do not fit through the endoscope, so they are placed under fluoroscopic control after endoscopic localization of the LES. The exact method of pneumatic dilation varies among experts, but modern studies suggest starting with a smaller balloon (30 mm) and working up to a larger one if symptoms persist. A contrast study may be obtained immediately after the dilation if there are concerns about a possible perforation, which has been reported in up to 3% of cases. Late perforation is possible, so patients should be observed closely for up to 24 hours. Interestingly, some (perhaps most) limited perforations can be managed conservatively with antibiotics and nil-by-mouth status. If surgery is required for a perforation, a simultaneous myotomy should be performed, if technically possible. Some authors advocate a timed barium study after dilation as a way to determine whether the dilation was sufficient [13]. They then advocate an additional dilation with a larger balloon when emptying remains poor independent of symptom response. Interestingly, younger patients do not seem to respond as well to pneumatic dilation [14].

The most common surgical approach to achalasia is the so-called "modified Heller myotomy," which has been performed since the early part of the 20th century. This procedure divides the muscle fibers of the distal esophagus and proximal stomach down to the level of the mucosa, which reliably produces a drop in LES pressure into the normal or even hypotensive range [15].

Traditionally, Heller procedures were performed through an open thoracotomy, with all of the perioperative risk and discomfort associated with that procedure. The surgery can now be performed via either a laparoscopic or a thoracoscopic approach in most cases [16]. Most centers favor the laparoscopic approach, where a very loose, partial (Toupet) fundoplication is performed after the myotomy, with results comparable to the older, open approach [17]. Although most patients respond to this surgery, some do not. Postoperative dysphagia may result from an incomplete myotomy, scarring at the myotomy site, obstruction from the fundoplication, paraesophageal hernias, diverticula, or massive esophageal dilation. If it appears that the problem is an incomplete myotomy or fundoplication, pneumatic dilation may be attempted, but some patients will need a surgical revision to either loosen the fundoplication or extend the myotomy, or both. In refractory cases, and in those with a massively dilated esophagus, esophagectomy may be the only option for symptomatic improvement, especially in patients experiencing pulmonary or nutritional compromise [18].

POEM is emerging as a possible less invasive alternative to laparoscopic Heller myotomy. During this procedure, a submucosal tunnel is created with a standard endoscope in the proximal esophagus. This tunnel is then extended down to the LES and proximal gastric cardia. A myotomy is performed using electrocautery and the submucosal tunnel is subsequently closed. Currently, some centers perform POEM as a pure endoscopic procedure, while others combine it with a laparoscopic antireflux procedure to minimize the potential impact of post-POEM reflux. Short-term outcomes have been comparable with Heller myotomy, but long-term results are pending.

Prognosis

Regardless of the therapeutic approach, achalasia is not considered a "curable" illness. There have been reports of a return of peristalsis after treatment, but this is probably the exception rather than the rule [7]. Although therapeutic decisions are generally not made based on achalasia subtyping, the various forms appear to predict response to therapy. Specifically, type 1 achalasia is thought to represent a more advanced form of the disease, while patients with type 2 achalasia appear to have improved chances of symptom resolution. A diagnosis of type 3 achalasia carries the worst prognosis in terms of post-intervention dysphagia and pain, most likely due to the failure to address the spastic pathophysiology in the esophageal body by current LES-directed therapies such as Heller myotomy and pneumatic dilatation. It is possible that the longer myotomy allowed by POEM may be a better alternative in type 3 achalasia.

EGJ

Outflow Obstruction

This disorder is defined as an IRP equal to or greater than the upper limit of normal and, in some cases, weak peristalsis. This pattern can be observed in patients who have an anatomical anomaly in the region of the LES (e.g., fundoplication, hiatal hernia, tumor) and may also represent evolving achalasia. Treatment is currently individualized based on symptoms, if an anatomical target can be identified. Some experts believe EGJ obstruction to represent "early achalasia" but this remains to be proven.

Non-Achalasia Esophageal Motility Disorders

Distal Esophageal Spasm

Distal esophageal spasm (DES) is a rare esophageal motility disorder in which LES relaxation is normal, but abnormal esophageal body contractions produce chest pain and dysphagia. The manometric observation of rapid or simultaneous contractions used to be thought of as a diagnostic feature, but the advent of HRM has significantly impacted on the understanding of esophageal spasm. In a large study of 2000 patient studies with EPT, the finding of a rapid contractile velocity was very non-specific. However, by assessing the distal latency on swallows, a patient group with significant dysphagia and chest pain can be identified. A considerable overlap between type 3 achalasia and spasm exists, and thus only a few patients truly fulfill criteria for DES based on the Chicago classification.

As with achalasia, the underlying etiology of the disorder is poorly understood, but it is likely related to loss of inhibitory innervation of the esophagus.

Patients with DES usually present with chest pain, dysphagia, or both, but up to 20% will have heartburn as their primary complaint [21]. Findings on barium studies that had previously been though to represent spasm are poorly associated with significant abnormalities on HRM (Figure 5.3). The treatment of DES is medical. Nitrates, calcium channel blockers, and sildenafil/vardenafil have all been used with moderate success. Cold liquids seem to be more likely to produce symptoms, and warm water swallows have been used as therapy in DES [24]. In patients with pain and less dysphagia, a trial of a low-dose antidepressant may be reasonable (trazodone 50–150 mg at bedtime [25] and imipramine 50 mg at bedtime [26] have been best studied). Botox injection at the LES has been used in an open-label trial with promising results but has not been subjected to an adequately controlled trial [27]. Others will try to inject botox into the parts of the esophagus with more of a "spastic" appearance, but this has not been well studied. Pneumatic dilation [28] and even long myotomy [29] are options in refractory cases.

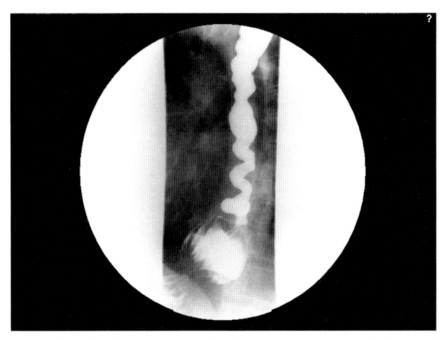

Figure 5.3 Distal esophageal spasm (DES): this is the classic appearance of esophageal spasm on barium testing. The diagnosis of DES cannot be made on barium alone and must be confirmed with manometry, showing a mixture of 20% or more simultaneous contractions with some normally propagated contractions.

Gastroesophageal reflux disease (GERD) can coexist with DES, and a trial of acid suppression or an ambulatory reflux test is also reasonable. Clinial and manometric monitoring for development of achalasia is important.

Hypercontractile Esophagus

The widespread use of manometry for patients with chest pain and dysphagia in the 1980s led to the observation that there is a group of patients (particularly chest-pain patients) that has a higher than expected pressure in an otherwise normally peristaltic esophagus. This group was initially described as "super squeezers," but the term "nutcracker esophagus" was later coined and became the standard label [30] (Figure 5.4). There is some controversy over the clinical significance as a number of health controls also exhibit this pattern on HRM. HRM utilizes the DCI as a measure of the vigor of the contraction. By using data from normal controls, nutcracker esophagus is now defined as a DCI > 5000 mmHg/s/cm; when a DCI > 8000 is observed, the term "jackhammer esophagus" is used. A great number of patients who previously would have been defined as having spasm now fall into this diagnostic category. Although the full clinical spectrum of these patients is not fully understood, the DCI appears to correlate with symptoms of chest pain and dysphagia. Hypercontractile (jackhammer) esophagus is not observed in health. Current therapeutic approaches include trials of pain modulators such as tricyclic antidepressant and more traditional antispasm therapy (calcium channel blockers, sildenafil). Long surgical myotomy and POEM of the esophageal body have been trialed on a case by case basis.

Disorders with Absent, Weak, or Frequent Failed Peristalsis

The classic disorder associated with severe loss of peristalsis is scleroderma or systemic sclerosis. Patients with these disorders are found to have an aperistaltic (or nearly so) esophagus and, in contrast to achalasia, a very low-pressure LES, as evidenced by a low IRP. Patients often present with dysphagia and severe GERD, and usually have other symptoms and findings, which makes the diagnosis evident. The absence of peristalsis and LES pressure predisposes to particularly severe gastroesophageal reflux, and patients frequently develop strictures and Barrett's esophagus. In recent years, it has been suggested that some of the lung disease associated with scleroderma may in fact be due to reflux and aspiration [33]. Patients are occasionally diagnosed in error with achalasia when they have a distal stricture or tumor that makes their esophagus appear more consistent with that diagnosis. Esophageal involvement may be the only GI manifestation of disease, but other patients will have small-bowel and colon symptoms, and the most severe cases will lose the ability to maintain oral nutrition.

Although scleroderma is the classic disorder, peristaltic dysfunction has been associated with almost all of the connective-tissue disorders. The potential etiologies of hypotensive esophageal dysmotility include:

- GERD.
- Rheumatologic disease:
  ○ scleroderma;
  ○ mixed connective-tissue disease;
  ○ rheumatoid arthritis (RA);
  ○ systemic lupus erythematosus (SLE).
- Endocrine disease:
  ○ diabetes;
  ○ hypothyroidism.
- Miscellaneous:
  ○ alcoholism;
  ○ amyloidosis;
  ○ intestinal pseudo-obstruction;
  ○ steroid myopathy;
  ○ multiple sclerosis.

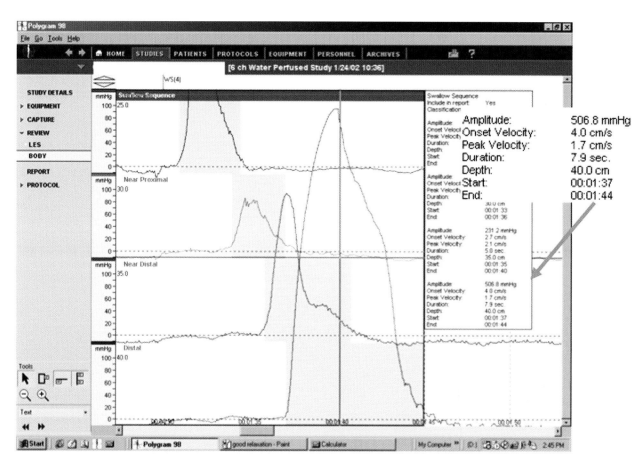

Figure 5.4 Nutcracker esophagus is defined as a statistically determined increase in peristaltic pressures in the distal esophagus (>180 mmHg). Many feel this "diagnosis" to be more a marker of anxiety than anything else, but an occasional patient has very high pressures that seem to be a marker of underlying neuropathy. This example shows a distal pressure of >500 mmHg in a patient with severe chest pain with swallowing.

CHAPTER 5

• Drugs:
  ◦ opiates;
  ◦ anticholinergics.
• Idiopathic.

Diagnosis relies on the examiner having sufficient clinical suspicion based on the patient's underlying non-esophageal conditions; for example, patients with scleroderma are diagnosed based on their cutaneous findings, while patients with diabetes are diagnosed based on their history or on simple blood tests. Generally, a barium swallow will suggest an esophageal disorder, but confirmation is obtained with manometry. In difficult cases, the LES pressure (or lack thereof) is the deciding factor between achalasia and a scleroderma-like condition. An esophagogastroduodenoscopy (EGD) is important in screening for Barrett's esophagus and in dilating strictures, if present; both are common in scleroderma and similar disorders.

There is no specific treatment for severe hypotensive esophageal dysmotility, but patients may have severe acid reflux, and most benefit from PPI therapy. Furthermore, non-pharmacologic management of GERD becomes very important, and all patients should be advised to eat small meals, avoid eating several hours prior to bedtime, and consider bed head elevation. Reflux may be particularly difficult to treat and require dosing more than once daily. Although somewhat controversial, severe reflux cases, particularly if there is fear of aspiration, may benefit from a carefully performed, very loose, partial fundoplication [36]. If there is associated gastric

dysmotility, promotility agents may be of benefit. Rarely, patients will develop enough nutritional compromise that tube-based enteral nutrition will be needed.

The finding of other minor perstaltic disorders, including weak peristalsis and frequent failed peristalsis, is often of uncertain clinical significance. In particular, such observations are made in patients with GERD and in aging patients. The widespread availability of motility testing and the increase in reflux surgery brought about by the laparoscopic technique have led to more patients with GERD undergoing manometry. Studies have revealed that GERD patients commonly have a variety of motility issues, ranging from mild, non-specific changes to aperistalsis that is identical to that seen with scleroderma. The vast majority of GERD patients do not require motility testing, nor is there a clinical indication to search for a motility disorder. On the other hand, patients with dysphagia and GERD who do not have a stricture and those being considered for reflux surgery should be studied. There is controversy over whether these disorders improve with medical or surgical therapy [37]. Most surgeons continue to "tailor" their surgery based on motility, and limit the fundoplication to a partial repair in patients with severe dysmotility, though modern data seem to refute the assumption that this approach decreases postoperative dysphagia [38]. Nevertheless, preoperative manometry remains a reasonable option to exclude the occasional achalasia patient presenting with GERD-like symptoms (somewhere between 1 and 3% of patients referred for reflux surgery may have achalasia). Dysphagia in patients with severe hypomotility who have undergone fundoplication is particularly difficult to diagnose and treat. Dysphagia may require pneumatic dilation or takedown of the fundoplication in some patients who do not respond to traditional dilation (up to 20 mm) [39].

A decrease in esophageal amplitude pressures has been reported in the eighth and ninth decades of life [40]. This has resulted in the identification of a group of older patients who have aperistalsis but whose manometry and radiographic studies do not support the diagnosis of either achalasia or "scleroderma" esophagus. These disorders appear to be more than a simple manometric curiosity, because radiological studies have demonstrated poor bolus clearance from the esophagus in older patients [41].

Case Continued

The patient undergoes a barium swallow that demonstrates a dilated esophagus with a smoothly tapered narrowing at the esophagogastric junction. Achalasia is confirmed manometrically. Laparoscopic myotomy, pneumatic dilation, and POEM are all discussed with the patient, who chooses pneumatic dilation. A 30 mm pneumatic dilator is confirmed to be across the LES fluoroscopically and then inflated to 12 lb/in² for 15 seconds. There is a moderate amount of blood on the dilator. A water-soluble contrast swallow is performed, and no perforation is noted. At 6-week follow-up, the patient is swallowing much better and has gained back 2 kg of the weight lost.

Take Home Points

- Achalasia is the prototypical esophageal motility disorder, characterized by aperistalsis of the esophageal body and a poorly relaxing LES with an elevated IRP on HRM using the Chicago classification.
- Achalasia is treated by improving LES relaxation with surgery, pneumatic dilation, or POEM.
- Distal esophageal spasm is a very rare disorder. The predominant symptom is dysphagia.
- Scleroderma (systemic sclerosis) produces an aperistaltic esophagus with a very weak LES and predisposes to severe reflux complications.
- Most patients with a weak esophagus actually do not have scleroderma; they may have other rheumatologic conditions or, perhaps most commonly, severe GERD.
- Non-specific dysmotility may occur with other systemic illnesses such as diabetes, as well as in aging.

References

1 Devault KR, Rattan S. Physiological role of neuropeptides in the gastrointestinal smooth muscle sphincters: neuropeptide and VIP-oxide interactions. In: Walsh J, Dockray G, eds. *Gut Peptides: Biochemistry and Physiology*. New York: Raven Press, 1994: 715–48.

2 Spechler SJ, Castell DO. Non-achalasia esophageal motility abnormalities. In: Castell DO, Richter HE, eds. *The Esophagus*, 4th edn. Philadelphia, PA: Lippincott, Williams & Wilkins, 2004: 262–74.

3 Csendes A, Smok G, Braghetto I, *et al.* Gastroesophageal sphincter pressure and histological changes in distal esophagus in patients with achalasia of the esophagus. *Dig Dis Sci* 1985; **30**: 941–5.

4 Oliveira RB, Filho FJ, Dantas RO, *et al.* The spectrum of esophageal motor disorders in Chagas' disease. *Am J Gastroenterol* 1995; **90**: 119–24.

5 Liu W, Fackler W, Rice TW, *et al.* The pathogenesis of pseudoachalasia: a clinicopathologic study of 13 cases of a rare entity. *Am J Surg Pathol* 2002; **26**: 784–8.

6 Dunaway PM, Wong RKH. Risk and surveillance intervals for squamous cell carcinoma in achalasia. *Gastrointest Endosc Clin North Am* 2001; **11**: 425–34.

7 Bianco A, Cagossi M, Scrimieri D, Greco AV. Appearance of esophageal peristalsis in treated idiopathic achalasia. *Dig Dis Sci* 1986; **31**: 40–8.

8 Bortolotti M, Mari C, Lopilator C, *et al.* Effects of sildenafil on esophageal motility of patients with idiopathic achalasia. *Gastroenterology* 2000; **118**: 253–7.

9 Pasricha PJ, Ravich WJ, Hendrix TR, *et al.* Intrasphincteric botulinum toxin for the treatment of achalasia. *N Engl J Med* 1995; **322**: 774–8.

10 Vaezi MF, Richter JE, Wilcox CM, *et al.* Botulinum toxin versus pneumatic dilation in the treatment of achalasia: a randomized trial. *Gut* 1999; **44**: 231–9.

11 Horgan S, Hudda K, Eubanks T, *et al.* Does botulinum toxin injection make esophagomyotomy a more difficult operation? *Surg Endosc* 1999; **13**: 576–9.

12 Gideon RM, Castell DO, Yarze J. Prospective randomized comparison of pneumatic dilatation technique in patients with idiopathic achalasia. *Dig Dis Sci* 1999; **44**: 1853–7.

13 Vaezi MF, Baker ME, Richter JE. Assessment of esophageal emptying postpneumatic dilation: use of the timed barium esophagram. *Am J Gastroenterol* 1999; **94**: 1802–7.

14 Clouse RE, Abramson BK, Todorczuk JR. Achalasia in the elderly: effects of aging on clinical presentation and outcome. *Dig Dis Sci* 1991; **36**: 225–8.

15 Csendes A, Velasco N, Braghetto I, Henriquez A. A prospective randomized study comparing forceful dilatation and esophagomyotomy in patients with achalasia of the esophagus. *Gastroenterology* 1981; **80**: 789–95.

16 Pellegrini C, Wetter LA, Patti M, *et al.* Thoracoscopic esophagomyotomy: initial experience with a new approach for the treatment of achalasia. *Ann Surg* 1992; **216**: 291–6.

17 Zaninotto G, Costantini M, Molena D, *et al.* Treatment of esophageal achalasia with laparoscopic Heller myotomy and Dor partial anterior fundoplication: prospective evaluation of 100 consecutive patients. *J Gastrointest Surg* 2000; **4**: 282–9.

18 Banbury MK, Rice TW, Goldblum JR, *et al.* Esophagectomy with gastric reconstruction for achalasia. *J Thorac Cardiovasc Surg* 1999; **117**: 1077–84.

19 Vantrappen G, Janssens J, Hellemans J, Coremans G. Achalasia, diffuse esophageal spasm, and related motility disorders. *Gastroenterology* 1979; **76**: 450–7.

20 Pehlivanov N, Liu J, Kassab GS, *et al.* Relationship between esophageal muscle thickness and intraluminal pressure in patients with esophageal spasm. *Am J Physiol Gastrointest Liver Physiol* 2002; **282**: G1016–23.

21 Reidel WL, Clouse RE. Variations in clinical presentation of patients with esophageal contraction abnormalities. *Dig Dis Sci* 1985; **30**: 1065–71.

22 Pandolfino JE, Kahrilas PJ. American Gastroenterological Association medical position statement: clinical use of esophageal manometry. *Gastroenterology* 2005; **128**: 207–8.

23 Song CW, Lee SJ, Jeen YT, *et al.* Inconsistent association of esophageal symptoms, psychometric abnormalities and dysmotility. *Am J Gastroenterol* 2001; **96**: 2312–16.

24 Triadafilopoulos G, Tsang HP, Segall GM. Hot water swallows improve symptoms and accelerate esophageal clearance in esophageal motility disorders. *J Clin Gastroenterol* 1998; **26**: 239–44.

25 Clouse RE, Lustman PJ, Eckert TC, *et al.* Low-dose trazodone for symptomatic patients with esophageal contraction abnormalities: a double-blind, placebo-controlled trial. *Gastroenterology* 1987; **92**: 1027–36.

26 Cannon RO, Quyyumi AA, Mincemoyer R, *et al.* Imipramine in patients with chest pain despite normal coronary angiograms. *N Engl J Med* 1994; **330**: 1411–17.

27 Storr M, Allescher HD, Rosch T, *et al.* Treatment of symptomatic diffuse esophageal spasm by endoscopic injections of botulinum toxin: a prospective study with long term follow up. *Gastrointest Endosc* 2001; **54**: 754–9.

28 Ebert EC, Ouyang A, Wright SH, *et al.* Pneumatic dilatation in patients with symptomatic diffuse esophageal spasm and lower esophageal sphincter dysfunction. *Dig Dis Sci* 1983; **28**: 481–5.

29 Ellis FH Jr. Long esophagomyotomy for diffuse esophageal spasm and related disorders: an historical overview. *Dis Esophagus* 1998; **11**: 210–14.

30 Benjamin SB, Gerhardt DC, Castell DO. High amplitude, peristaltic esophageal contractions associated with chest pain and/or dysphagia. *Gastroenterology* 1979; **77**: 478–83.

31 Anderson KO, Dalton CB, Bradley LA, Richer JE. Stress induces alterations of esophageal pressures in healthy volunteers and non-cardiac chest pain patients. *Dig Dis Sci* 1989; **34**: 83–91.

32 Cohen S, Fisher R, Lipshutz W, *et al.* The pathogenesis of esophageal dysfunction in scleroderma and Raynaud's disease. *J Clin Invest* 1972; **51**: 2663–8.

33 Ebert EC. Esophageal disease in scleroderma. *J Clin Gastroenterol* 2006; **40**: 769–75.

34 Schneider HA, Yonker RA, Longley S, *et al.* Scleroderma esophagus: a nonspecific entity. *Ann Intern Med* 1984; **100**: 848–50.

35 Clouse RE, Lustman PJ, Reidel WL. Correlation of esophageal motility abnormalities with neuropsychiatric status in diabetics. *Gastroenterology* 1986; **90**: 1146–54.

36 Orringer MB. Surgical management of scleroderma reflux esophagitis. *Surg Clin North Am* 1983; **63**: 859–67.

37 Hunter JG, Trus TL, Branum GD, *et al.* A physiologic approach to laparoscopic fundoplication for gastro-esophageal reflux disease. *Ann Surg* 1996; **223**: 673–85.

38 Varin O, Velstra B, DeSutter S, Ceelen W. Total vs partial fundoplication in the treatment of gastroesophageal reflux: a meta-analysis. *Arch Surg* 2009; **144**: 273–8.

39 Hui JM, Hunt DR, de Carle DJ, *et al.* Esophageal pneumatic dilation for postfundoplication dysphagia: safety, efficacy, and predictors of outcome. *Am J Gastroenterol* 2002; **97**: 2986–91.

40 Bloem BR, Lagaay AM, van Beek W, *et al.* Prevalence of subjective dysphagia in community residents aged over 87. *BMJ* 1990; **300**: 721–2.

41 Aviv JE, Martin JH, Jones ME, *et al.* Age-related changes in pharyngeal and supraglottic sensation. *Ann Otol Rhinol Laryngol* 1994; **103**: 749–52.

42 Eckhardt VF, LeCompte PM. Esophageal ganglia and smooth muscle in the elderly. *Am J Dig Dis* 1978; **23**: 443.

43 Adams CW, Brain RH, Trounce JR. Ganglion cells in achalasia of the cardia. *Virchows Arch A Pathol Anat Histol* 1976; **372**: 75–9.

44 Leite LP, Johnston BT, Barrett J, *et al.* Ineffective esophageal motility (IEM). The primary finding in patients with nonspecific esophageal motility disorder. *Dig Dis Sci* 1997; **42**: 1859–65.

CHAPTER 5

Gastric Motility Testing

Jan Tack

Gastroenterology Section, University of Leuven, Leuven, Belgium

Summary

Tests of gastric motor function include gastric emptying tests, antro-duodenal manometry, electrogastrograpy, and tests to study gastric accommodation. Tests of gastric motor function have limited diagnostic specificity, and their impact on management is hampered by the lack of therapeutic alternatives for patients with gastric motor disorders. Gastric emptying tests are most frequently applied clinically, and they may be useful when invasive or experimental therapies for gastroparesis are considered. Antroduodenal manometry is mostly useful in cases of severe, potentially generalized motor disorders. Electrogastrography and tests of gastric accommodation have mainly research applications.

Introduction

In patients presenting with gastrointestinal (GI) symptoms, conventional diagnostic approaches such as endoscopy with biopsies and radiological or biochemical examinations may identify an underlying abnormality that explains the patient's symptoms. When no such underlying disease can be found, it is often assumed that disorders of GI motor or sensory function underlie symptom generation [1].

Symptoms related to feeding may include epigastric pain and burning, early satiation, postprandial fullness, anorexia, belching, nausea, and vomiting. These symptoms, in the absence of organic causes, may suggest a disturbance of gastric function, and a number of tests have been developed to study the motor (and sensory) function of the stomach.

Gastric motor disorders can be either primary (i.e., no apparent underlying cause is present) or secondary (i.e., they are related to another medical condition). The primary and secondary gastric motor disorders are listed in Table 6.1. Tests are especially useful if they have diagnostic specificity (i.e., the outcome of the test may yield a clear diagnosis) and if they are able to explain the patient's symptoms. Diagnostic tests may also determine the choice of therapy, help to predict response to therapy, and predict the long-term prognosis of the underlying condition.

Gastric Motility Testing

Assessment of gastric motor function is generally pursued after the exclusion of structural disease, using esophagogastroduodenoscopy (EGD), radiology, and laboratory testing. The most common tests are measurement of gastric emptying rate, electrogastrography, GI manometry, and gastric accommodation testing.

Gastric Emptying Testing

Measurement of Gastric Emptying Rate

Several techniques are available to quantify gastric emptying of solid or liquid meals, but solid emptying rate is considered clinically most relevant. When evaluating suspected dumping syndrome, assessment of liquid emptying may also be considered. Radionuclide gastric emptying measurement is considered the standard method by which to assess gastric emptying rate. Depending on the label used, solid and liquid emptying can be assessed separately or simultaneously. The solid and/or liquid meals are labeled with (different) radioisotopes. A gamma camera measures the number of counts in an investigator-determined region of interest (total, proximal, or distal stomach, small intestine) for a certain time after ingestion of a meal. Mathematical processing involves corrections for distance to the camera and isotope decay and curve-fitting, which allows calculation of the half-emptying time, the lag phase (period of delay after meal ingestion before emptying starts), and the percentage labeled meal retention at different time points (Figure 6.1). Although not routinely applied, the technique also has the ability to provide information on distribution within the stomach. Disadvantages include the use of radioactive substances, the considerable costs, and the poor level of standardization of meal compositions and measuring times among different laboratories. In a recent consensus document, supported by the American Neurogastroenterology and Motility Society (ANMS) and the American Society of Nuclear Medicine (ASNC), a single standardized protocol for gastric emptying scintigraphy was proposed [2]. One potential weakness of this proposal is the use of an egg replacement meal, which lacks lipids. As it is not uncommon for patients to report symptom aggravation after lipid-rich meals, it is unclear whether lack of lipids compromises the ability of the meal to detect abnormalities in certain patient groups.

Breath tests can also be used to measure gastric emptying rates. The solid or liquid phase of a meal is labeled with a ^{13}C-containing substrate (octanoic acid, acetic acid, glycin, or spirulina) [3]. As soon as the substrate enters the small bowel, it is metabolized with generation of $^{13}CO_2$, which appears in the breath. Breath sampling at regular intervals and mathematical processing of the $^{13}CO_2$ content over time allows calculation of a gastric emptying curve. The advantages of this test are the use of non-radioactive materials and

---

Practical Gastroenterology and Hepatology Board Review Toolkit, Second Edition. Edited by Nicholas J. Talley, Kenneth R. DeVault, Michael B. Wallace, Bashar A. Aqel and Keith D. Lindor.

Table 6.1 Primary and secondary disorders of gastric motor and sensory function.

Primary disorders	FD – postprandial distress syndrome
	FD – epigastric pain syndrome
	Idiopathic gastroparesis
	Chronic idiopathic nausea
	Functional vomiting
	Cyclic vomiting syndrome
	Aerophagia
	Rumination syndrome
Secondary disorders	Metabolic disorders (diabetes, thyroid dysfunction)
	Postsurgical
	Drug-induced gastric motor disorders
	Central nervous system disorders
	Extrinsic neuropathy
	Intestinal neuropathy
	Intestinal myopathy

FD, functional dyspepsia.

the ability to perform it outside a hospital setting. Disadvantages are the absence of standardization of meal and substrate. The test is well accepted in Europe, but has not gained clinical application in the United States.

Real-time ultrasonography has also been applied to the measurement of gastric emptying [4]. The method is based on serial measurements of the cross-sectional area of the gastric antrum. Despite some attractive features, such as its non-invasive character, the absence of radiation burden, and the widespread availability of the equipment, ultrasonographic determination of gastric emptying rate has the disadvantages of being time-consuming and unsuitable for use with solid meals. Moreover, antral volume is determined not only by gastric emptying rate, but also by redistribution of the meal inside the stomach, such as in cases of impaired accommodation.

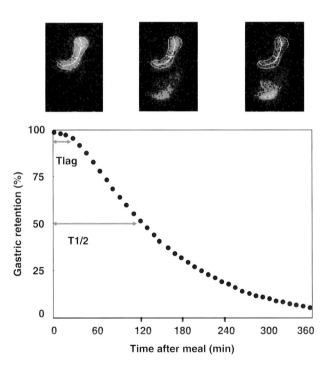

Figure 6.1 Scintigraphic assessment of gastric emptying rate. The presence of the radiolabeled meal is quantified in a region of interest, representing the stomach (upper panels). The presence of the label in the stomach region of interest over time is plotted, allowing quantification of the gastric half-emptying time and lag phase.

The Smartpill (SmartPill Corporation, Buffalo, NY) is a nondigestible capsule that records luminal pH, temperature, and pressure during transit through the GI tract, transmitting the data to an ambulatory data recorder [5]. The device therefore provides a measure of gastric emptying time, small-bowel transit time, and whole-gut transit time. Simultaneous manometry studies have demonstrated that the return of gastric phase 3 activity is the principal mechanism underlying emptying of the capsule from the stomach after a meal [6]. However, in a US multicenter study, gastric emptying times determined by the Smartpill capsule correlated acceptably well with scintigraphy results and were able to distinguish between health and gastroparesis with good diagnostic accuracy [7]. Furthermore, the Smartpill also provides information on the amplitude of contractions, which is of uncertain clinical relevance, and on intestinal and colonic transit times as the capsule traverses the rest of the GI tract.

Impact of Gastric Emptying Testing

Gastric emptying tests do not have a high diagnostic specificity. Delayed gastric emptying, for instance, can be found in the majority of patients with anorexia nervosa, and several common drugs and coexisting neurological and endocrine disorders can affect gastric emptying rate. Similarly, one can find rapid gastric emptying, especially of liquids, in patients with dumping syndrome, but a diagnosis of dumping syndrome cannot be made on the basis of rapid emptying alone, but requires specific additional tests or observations [8].

The relationship between gastric emptying rate and symptom pattern is also a matter of controversy. Studies in functional dyspepsia (FD) patients have found associations between delayed gastric emptying and the presence and severity of symptoms of postprandial fullness, nausea, and vomiting. However, the correlation of delayed emptying with the presence or severity of specific symptoms is weak, limiting its use in providing an explanation of symptoms. The impact of establishing abnormalities in gastric emptying on the therapeutic approach is also limited. The limited treatment options for patients with gastric motility disorders eliminate the need for a test to guide choices. Moreover, most studies find no correlation between the severity of delayed emptying and the response to prokinetic therapy [9].

Routine gastric emptying testing in patients with symptoms suggestive of impaired gastric motility therefore cannot be recommended, but it can be applied in patients who fail to respond to initial empiric treatment approaches, especially when more invasive or experimental treatment modalities, such as jejunal tube feeding or gastric electrical stimulation, are considered.

Electrogastrography

Measurement of Gastric Electrical Rhythm

Cutaneous electrodes placed over the stomach region allow the measurement of gastric electrical activity. This electrogastrogram (EGG) provides information on the frequency and regularity of gastric pacemaker activity, as well as on changes in the power of the signal after meal ingestion [10].

Impact of Gastric Electrical Rhythm Testing

The EGG has been advocated to distinguish between patients with normal and delayed emptying, and to explain intractable nausea. However, EGG abnormalities can also be induced through central mechanisms (e.g., vertigo-induced nausea). Furthermore, as EGG

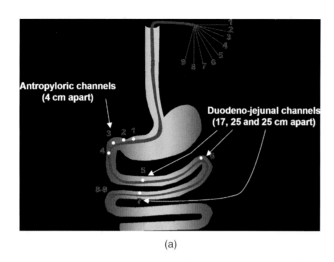

(a)

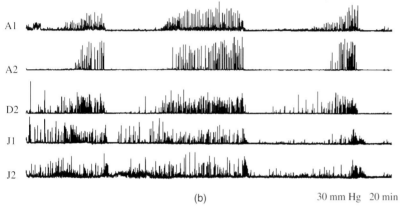

(b)   30 mm Hg   20 min

Figure 6.2 (a) The principle of antroduodenojejunal manometry, which uses a catheter with manometry ports in the stomach and different parts of the small intestine. (b) Example of interdigestive motility as recorded via catheter in the antrum (A channels), duodenum (D channel), and jejunum (J channels).

findings are unlikely to alter clinical management, EGG remains mainly a research tool.

Gastrointestinal Manometry

Antroduodenal Manometry

Antroduodenal manometry quantifies contractility in regions that determine interdigestive motility and gastric emptying [11]. The technique is only available at a small number of specialized centers, and is mainly used in the evaluation of patients with potentially generalized motility disorders, such as chronic idiopathic intestinal pseudo-obstruction syndromes. The key features that are evaluated on antroduodenal manometry are the number and amplitude of contractions and their pattern in the interdigestive and in the postprandial state (Figure 6.2). So-called "clustered contractions" may be indicative of mechanical obstruction.

Impact of Antroduodenal Manometry

Antral hypomotility is a non-specific finding, often associated with delayed gastric emptying. In patients with pseudo-obstruction syndrome and in radiation enteropathy, aberrant configuration and migration of intestinal phase 3 are indicators of a major motor disorder. Adequate assessment of interdigestive motility requires a prolonged measurement in the fasting state; some centers use 24-hour antroduodenojejal manometry, which provides a long nocturnal period for optimal evaluation of interdigestive motility. After a standard meal, up to 10 hours may be required before return to normal interdigestive motility occurs.

With its ability to diagnose patterns suggestive of intestinal neuropathy (normal contractile strength but abnormal patterns), intestinal myopathy (decreased contractile strength), retrogradely propagated phase 3 activity, and patterns suggestive of mechanical subobstruction, intestinal manometry has the potential to provide diagnostic specificity and to impact on management choices. This is a highly technical and often challenging procedure that justifies referral to a specialized center.

Gastric Accommodation Testing

Methods for the Measurement of Accommodation

The gastric barostat measures changes in tone and sensitivity to distension of the proximal stomach [12]. The procedure is invasive, as it requires positioning of a double lumen polyvinyl tube with an adherent plastic bag through the mouth into the stomach. The barostat is the gold standard for measurement of gastric accommodation (meal-induced relaxation of the proximal stomach), which may be impaired in FD, but also in diabetic gastropathy and rumination syndrome and after antireflux surgery. The gastric barostat can also be used to quantify sensitivity to gastric distension.

A number of other means of assessing gastric accommodation have been proposed, including tolerance of an oral water or nutrient load, and gastric volume imaging by means of scintigraphy, ultrasound, single positron emission computed tomography (SPECT), or magnetic resonance imaging (MRI). Recently, manometric recording of the intragastric pressure drop in response to a meal was proposed as an easier way of estimating gastric accommodation [13].

These methods require further validation and additional studies before they can be applied clinically.

Impact of Accommodation Testing

Although impaired accommodation has been associated with early satiation and weight loss, accommodation measurements are also influenced by emotions, such as anxiety. In the absence of an established therapy for impaired accommodation, measuring accommodation does not influence the choice and outcome of therapy, and remains a research tool. The same is true for gastric hypersensitivity, which can also be measured with the barostat.

Take Home Points

- The most frequently applied tests of gastric motor function are measurement of gastric emptying rate (scintigraphy or breath test), GI manometry, and electrogastrography.
- Gastric emptying testing can be applied to help explain symptoms, but the impact on management is limited.
- In rare or refractory cases, small-bowel manometry may lead to specific diagnoses.
- The main limit to a greater clinical usefulness of gastric motility testing is the lack of therapeutic alternatives.

References

1 Tack J, Talley NJ, Camilleri M, *et al*. Functional gastroduodenal disorders. *Gastroenterology* 2006; **130**: 1466–79.

2 McCallum RW, Nowak T, Nusynowitz ML, *et al*; American Neurogastroenterology and Motility Society and the Society of Nuclear Medicine. Consensus recommendations for gastric emptying scintigraphy: a joint report of the American Neurogastroenterology and Motility Society and the Society of Nuclear Medicine. *Am J Gastroenterol* 2008; **103**: 753–63.

3 Sanaka M, Yamamoto T, Kuyama Y. Retention, fixation and loss of the [13C] label: a review for the understanding of gastric emptying breath tests. *Dig Dis Sci* 2008; **53**: 1747–56.

4 Gentilcore D, Hausken T, Horowitz M, Jones KL. Measurements of gastric emptying of low- and high-nutrient liquids using 3D ultrasonography and scintigraphy in healthy subjects. *Neurogastroenterol Motil* 2006; **18**: 1062–8.

5 Kuo B, McCallum RW, Koch KL, *et al*. Comparison of gastric emptying of a nondigestible capsule to a radio-labelled meal in healthy and gastroparetic subjects. *Aliment Pharmacol Ther* 2008; **27**: 186–96.

6 Cassilly D, Kantor S, Knight LC, *et al*. Gastric emptying of a non-digestible solid: assessment with simultaneous SmartPill pH and pressure capsule, antroduodenal manometry, gastric emptying scintigraphy. *Neurogastroenterol Motil* 2008; **20**: 311–19.

7 Rao SS, Kuo B, McCallum RW, *et al*. Investigation of colonic and whole-gut transit with wireless motility capsule and radiopaque markers in constipation. *Clin Gastroenterol Hepatol* 2009; **7**: 537–44.

8 Tack J, Arts J, Caenepeel P, *et al*. Pathophysiology, diagnosis and management of postoperative dumping syndrome. *Nat Rev Gastroenterol Hepatol* 2009; **6**(10): 583–90.

9 Janssen P, Harris MS, Jones M, *et al*. The relation between symptom improvement and gastric emptying in the treatment of diabetic and idiopathic gastroparesis. *Am J Gastroenterol* 2013; **108**(9): 1382–91.

10 Huizinga JD. Physiology and pathophysiology of the interstitial cell of Cajal: from bench to bedside II. Gastric motility: lessons from mutant mice on slow waves and innervation. *Am J Physiol* 2001; **281**: G1119–34.

11 Camilleri M, Bharucha AE, di Lorenzo C, *et al*. American Neurogastroenterology and Motility Society consensus statement on intraluminal measurement of gastrointestinal and colonic motility in clinical practice. *Neurogastroenterol Motil* 2008; **20**: 1269–82.

12 Sarnelli G, Vos R, Cuomo R, *et al*. Reproducibility of gastric barostat studies in healthy controls and in dyspeptic patients. *Am J Gastroenterol* 2001; **96**: 1047–53.

13 Janssen P, Verschueren S, Giao Ly H, *et al*. Intragastric pressure during food intake: a physiological and minimally invasive method to assess gastric accommodation. *Neurogastroenterol Motil* 2011; **23**(4): 316–22, e153–4.

PART 3

Problem-Based Approach to Diagnosis and Differential Diagnosis

7 General Approach to History-Taking and Physical Examination of the Upper Gastrointestinal Tract, 43
Evan S. Dellon and Eugene M. Bozymski

8 Heartburn, Regurgitation, and Chest Pain, 46
Kenneth R. DeVault

9 Dysphagia, 52
Dawn L. Francis

10 Miscellaneous Upper Gastrointestinal Symptoms, 56
Mohamed Sultan and James H. Lewis

11 Dyspepsia, 70
Nicholas J. Talley, Kate Napthali, and Kenneth McQuaid

12 Nausea and Vomiting, 74
John K. DiBaise

13 Hematemesis, 79
Thomas O.G. Kovacs and Dennis M. Jensen

General Approach to History-Taking and Physical Examination of the Upper Gastrointestinal Tract

Evan S. Dellon and Eugene M. Bozymski

Center for Esophageal Diseases and Swallowing, Division of Gastroenterology and Hepatology, University of North Carolina School of Medicine, Chapel Hill, NC, USA

Summary

The history and physical exam (H&P) remains the cornerstone of the doctor–patient relationship, forming the basis of clinical information-gathering and medical decision-making. With the wide adoption of electronic medical records, direct interactions between doctors and patients may be threatened. Moreover, in the current age of rapidly evolving technologies, it may seem expedient to proceed directly to testing after a cursory history, but this is a trap that must be avoided. A thorough yet targeted H&P is the only way to construct an appropriate differential diagnosis (DDx), which guides judicious use of the numerous testing modalities available. This chapter will discuss an approach to the H&P that emphasizes developing a physician–patient rapport and a complete DDx.

Setting the Stage

A good visit starts with introducing yourself to the patient by making eye contact and shaking their hand. If there is a sink in the room, it is good practice to wash your hands in the patient's view prior to shaking hands. Then, take a seat at the same level as the patient, preferably without any barriers (such as a desk) between you. Even if data capture is required on a computer, it is strongly preferable to face the patient directly, interact with them, and not type or look directly into a computer monitor or other handheld screen. The first question is the most important and should be sufficiently open-ended to allow the patient to fully describe their concerns. Possible options include: "What can I help you with?", "What brings you into the office today?", and "I see Dr. So-and-So referred you. I've reviewed your records, but I wanted to hear what's been going on from your perspective." It is less advisable to start with a directed or yes/no question because it immediately limits what the patient might tell you. Open-ended questions will certainly allow the patient to provide you with more information about their visit.

It is also important to allow the patient to speak without interruption. Data indicate that on average, physicians interrupt patients after only 18 seconds [1]. This temptation to ask questions immediately should be suppressed. In most cases, if the patient talks for enough time and you listen carefully, they will tell you what is wrong with them. After a certain amount of time, directed questions or redirection will be appropriate. Experienced clinicians have learned

how to redirect without appearing to interrupt the patient: "These symptoms seem to have affected your life greatly. Let's go back to the beginning. Can you tell me where exactly the pain was located the very first time it occurred?"

A final general point is that if there are records to review from prior evaluation, it is best to do this before seeing the patient rather than shuffle though pages while the patient is talking. Any prior information should certainly play into the overall diagnostic picture, but keeping an open mind is key during the early phase of the H&P, particularly during consults for second opinions. Symptoms should then be explored in depth, with special focus on onset, exacerbating and relieving factors, progression, and other associated factors. A thorough medication history, including over-the-counter drugs and supplements, is imperative given the number of agents available with myriad potential side effects. The remainder of this chapter will review the approach to the H&P for common symptoms of upper gastrointestinal (GI) tract diseases.

Heartburn

Heartburn – pyrosis – a substernal burning sensation that radiates orad, is the cardinal symptom of gastroesophageal reflux disease (GERD). When approaching a patient with this complaint, the symptom must be elicited accurately. Because heartburn is experienced frequently but perhaps imprecisely, when patients say they have "heartburn" or "reflux," what they may really be describing could be dysphagia, chest pain, shortness of breath, dyspepsia, or even abdominal pain [2, 3]. When discussing this complaint, focused questioning should be used to clarify exactly what is meant by the term the patient is using. Questioning should also attempt to exclude other conditions that might present with central chest pain mimicking heartburn from reflux. For example, when does the symptom occur? If it is postprandial, nocturnal, or exacerbated by lying supine or bending over, then it is more consistent with GERD. If it is exertional, then heart disease should be considered. Since symptom overlap may make differentiation difficult, cardiac evaluation will often be necessary. It is not uncommon for gastroenterologists to detect unstable angina masquerading as "GERD" [4]. The physical exam is generally normal in patients with heartburn from GERD, but clues pointing to severe acid exposure (e.g., tooth enamel loss) may be detected.

Practical Gastroenterology and Hepatology Board Review Toolkit, Second Edition. Edited by Nicholas J. Talley, Kenneth R. DeVault, Michael B. Wallace, Bashar A. Aqel and Keith D. Lindor.
© 2016 John Wiley & Sons, Ltd. Published 2016 by John Wiley & Sons, Ltd. Companion website: www.practicalgastrohep.com

Dysphagia

When a patient presents with a chief complaint of difficulty swallowing, the H&P should be used to distinguish between oropharyngeal (or transfer) dysphagia and esophageal dysphagia, whether the symptoms most likely represent a structural or motor disease, and what the most appropriate first-line test might be [5]. Dysphagia can be sought by asking the patient whether food "sticks," is "hung-up," or "slows down" after swallowing. Symptoms of difficulty passing the bolus to the back of the mouth or initiating swallowing, regurgitation of food or liquid through the nose, coughing during swallows, and frank aspiration are all suggestive of oropharyngeal dysphagia [6]. If these are elicited, physical exam should search for focal or global neurologic deficits that might suggest an underlying etiology.

Classically, dysphagia to solid foods alone or dysphagia for solids that progresses to solid and liquid dysphagia has been associated with structural disease. In contrast, dysphagia for liquids alone or for a combination of liquids and solids is indicative of a motor disorder. History should construct a careful timeline of the symptoms, paying attention to specific foods (e.g., meat vs. rice vs. bread), consistencies (e.g., dry vs. soft vs. liquid), and temperature triggers. It is also important to determine whether dysphagia is not "progressing" because the patient has adapted by eating smaller bites or softer foods, avoiding certain items altogether, or chewing thoroughly. Loss of weight and behaviors related to eating can also help quantify the severity of dysphagia for patients who might be minimizing symptoms with dietary modification. Risk factors for malignancy (smoking, alcohol, GERD, family history) and systemic signs and symptoms associated with connective tissue diseases should be examined. With the increasing recognition of eosinophilic esophagitis, it is important to inquire specifically about atopic diseases, longstanding dysphagia, episodes of food bolus or foreign body impaction, and dietary modification [7, 8]. While patients often point to a substernal area where they feel food "hanging-up," there can be poor correlation between this localization and a potentially causative structural lesion, particularly for proximal locations [9]. Physical examination is typically unrevealing in patients with esophageal dysphagia, except for the finding of tylosis palmaris (hyperkeratosis of the palmar surface of the hands rarely seen with esophageal cancer), but if a motor disorder is suggested on history, a thorough exam for signs of scleroderma (e.g., sclerodactyly, periungual telangiectasias, shiny skin), arthritis, CREST syndrome, or other connective tissue diseases is mandated.

Nausea/Vomiting

The patient complaining of nausea and/or vomiting presents a challenge to the gastroenterologist because these symptoms are nonspecific, the potential causes are legion, and evaluation may range from minimal to extensive. As with heartburn, the history for nausea and vomiting should initially focus on asking the patient to explicitly describe what they are experiencing [10]. Nausea is defined as a sensation of impending emesis, while the act of emesis is the expulsion of gastric contents. These should be distinguished from reflux, regurgitation, rumination, indigestion, abdominal pain, early satiety, and sitophobia.

Next, the H&P should focus on determining whether these symptoms represent a primary or secondary process, whether they are structural or functional, and whether they might be a side effect of a medication or supplement. For example, the patient who complains of constant and longstanding nausea alone, with no emesis or associated symptoms, almost certainly has a functional GI disorder. In contrast, worsening postprandial nausea and vomiting associated with abdominal distension that develops in a patient with known Crohn's disease may represent obstructive symptoms from a critical intestinal stenosis. The presence of a succussion splash remote from eating on physical exam raises the issue of gastric outlet obstruction or gastroparesis. Extra-GI or central nervous system etiologies, while rare, should be kept in the differential.

Abdominal Pain

Abdominal pain is the most frequent presenting symptom the gastroenterologist encounters [11], and it should always be evaluated systematically. A complete history includes eliciting information about the acuity of onset, triggering events, location, radiation, quality, progression, and exacerbating and relieving factors. Location and chronicity can help narrow the DDx to structures in that specific area. The quality of the pain is most useful for characterizing colic, a paroxysmal cramping sensation typical of an intermittently obstructed hollow viscus. Biliary colic is typically localized to the right-upper quadrant or the epigastrium. Pancreatic pain is frequently severe and bores into the mid-back from the epigastric region and may be eased by sitting and leaning forward.

On physical exam, the severity of the patient's symptoms can be correlated with the presence or absence of signs that might require urgent surgical intervention (e.g., guarding or rebound). Another useful finding is that of Carnett's sign, a worsening of discomfort with tightening of abdominal musculature [12], which can indicate a musculoskeletal etiology. When functional abdominal pain is a possibility, examination with distraction – the application of abdominal pressure with the stethoscope while "listening" or conducting a conversation with the patient – is invaluable. Pain related to mesenteric vascular insufficiency generally is postprandial and periumbilical, is said to present with abdominal pain out of proportion to the findings on exam, and can be difficult to diagnose in the early stages. A high level of suspicion for this condition is required, particularly in patients with vascular disease. Finally, it is important to consider non-GI causes of abdominal pain, especially those that can be life–threatening, such as an aortic dissection or aneurysm, but also those which might cause referred pain, such as neurologic or musculoskeletal disorders.

Diarrhea

While many patients who present with diarrhea have a lower-GI source, it is important to keep upper-GI causes of diarrhea on the DDx in the appropriate clinical context. Nocturnal diarrhea is not often related to a functional problem. Malabsorptive diarrhea, either from pancreatic insufficiency, bacterial overgrowth, or celiac disease, can be characterized by steatorrhea. Because many patients do not see frank fat, oil, or grease mixed with their stools, or because they do not actually look at each stool in detail, this sign is often difficult to elicit on history [13]. Instead, asking about "peanut butter" consistency and the color of the stool may provide a more "real-world" prompt for the patient. In addition, small-bowel sources of diarrhea, such as infectious (Giardia, Whipple's disease), autoimmune (celiac disease), infiltrative (amyloid), or malignant (lymphoma) causes, should be kept on the differential, and upper endoscopy with biopsies should be pursued when indicated. Diarrhea may be related to a wide variety of medications, making a good medication history imperative. A timely example is antibiotic use facilitating the development of C. *Difficile* pseudomembranous colitis.

Finishing the Visit

After the initial H&P has been conducted, it is important to describe your thought processes to the patient, outlining the DDx and options for further diagnosis and treatment, before making recommendations. This allows patient preferences and concerns to be discussed and addressed. It is equally important to summarize the plan going forward and to ask the patient to repeat their understanding of the next steps required. With the utilization of electronic records and meaningful-use requirements, more and more clinicians are providing written summaries to patients. This and so-called "open access" medical records may help with adherence to the prescribed therapies [14]. It is also very useful to ask, "Is there anything else you'd like to mention today?" in order to avoid a "doorknob" moment [15]. A good visit ends with a follow-up appointment being made, when possible, and with the understanding that the initial H&P is just the first step in the therapeutic doctor–patient relationship.

• At the end of the visit, summarize the DDx and evaluation or treatment plan. It is useful to have the patient repeat their understanding of the plan, since no matter how skilled the physician at eliciting information on the H&P, the patient must act to carry this plan forward.

• *Lavabo manus meus* ("I wash my hands") is a precept that we should always follow, and one that we should practice before and between patient encounters.

Take Home Points

• Listening to and talking with the patient are the most important initial diagnostic tests available.

• Ask an open-ended question to allow the patient to describe their symptoms and chief complaints without interruption.

• Ask directed questions to clarify exactly what is meant by each symptom. For example, ensure a patient's "heartburn" means pyrosis and not angina.

• Qualify each symptom by learning about the acuity of onset, triggering events, quality, progression, and exacerbating and relieving factors.

• When discussing difficult topics or relating bad news, it is acceptable to show empathy or emotion. Providing tissues to a tearful patient or touching them on the shoulder can be reassuring in the right setting.

• After the H&P, the tempo of the planned evaluation should match the relative acuity and severity of the patient's symptoms. For example, progressive dysphagia and weight loss over a month requires expedited evaluation, while longstanding chronic abdominal pain may be worked up less rapidly.

References

1 Beckman HB, Frankel RM. The effect of physician behavior on the collection of data. *Ann Intern Med* 1984; **101**(5): 692–6.

2 Kahrilas PJ, Shaheen NJ, Vaezi MF. American Gastroenterological Association Institute technical review on the management of gastroesophageal reflux disease. *Gastroenterology* 2008; **135**(4): 1392–413.e1–5.

3 Katz PO, Gerson LB, Vela MF. Guidelines for the diagnosis and management of gastroesophageal reflux disease. *Am J Gastroenterol* 2013; **108**(3): 308–28, quiz 329.

4 Ruigomez A, Garcia Rodriguez LA, Wallander MA, *et al.* Natural history of gastro-oesophageal reflux disease diagnosed in general practice. *Aliment Pharmacol Ther* 2004; **20**(7):751–60.

5 Pasha SF, Acosta RD, Chandrasekhara V, *et al.* The role of endoscopy in the evaluation and management of dysphagia. *Gastrointest Endosc* 2014; **79**(2): 191–201.

6 Cook IJ. Diagnostic evaluation of dysphagia. *Nat Clin Pract Gastroenterol Hepatol* 2008; **5**(7): 393–403.

7 Liacouras CA, Furuta GT, Hirano I, *et al.* Eosinophilic esophagitis: updated consensus recommendations for children and adults. *J Allergy Clin Immunol* 2011; **128**: 3–20.e6.

8 Dellon ES, Gonsalves N, Hirano I, *et al.* ACG Clinical Guideline: evidence based approach to the diagnosis and management of esophageal eosinophilia and eosinophilic esophagitis. *Am J Gastroenterol* 2013; **108**: 679–92.

9 Roeder BE, Murray JA, Dierkhising RA. Patient localization of esophageal dysphagia. *Dig Dis Sci* 2004; **49**(4): 697–701.

10 Quigley EM, Hasler WL, Parkman HP. AGA technical review on nausea and vomiting. *Gastroenterology* 2001; **120**(1): 263–86.

11 Peery AF, Dellon ES, Lund J, *et al.* Burden of gastrointestinal disease in the United States: 2012 update. *Gastroenterology* 2012; **143**(5): 1179–87.e1–3.

12 Anon. Abdominal wall tenderness test: could Carnett cut costs? *Lancet* 1991; **337**(8750): 1134.

13 Fine KD, Schiller LR. AGA technical review on the evaluation and management of chronic diarrhea. *Gastroenterology* 1999; **116**(6): 1464–86.

14 Walker J, Darer JD, Elmore JG, Delbanco T. The road toward fully transparent medical records. *N Engl J Med* 2014; **370**(1): 6–8.

15 Jackson G. "Oh…by the way…": doorknob syndrome. *Int J Clin Pract* 2005; **59**(8): 869.

CHAPTER 7

Heartburn, Regurgitation, and Chest Pain

Kenneth R. DeVault

Division of Gastroenterology and Hepatology, Mayo Clinic, Jacksonville, FL, USA

Heartburn and regurgitation are the cardinal symptoms of gastroesophageal reflux disease (GERD). Chest pain is another common symptom, and the esophagus should be considered once cardiac causes have been excluded.

Heartburn and Regurgitation

Heartburn is probably the most common gastrointestinal (GI) complaint in the Western world. One systematic review [1] identified 31 articles, reporting 78 000 patients, that assessed the period prevalence of heartburn in the community. In these Western populations, 25% of people reported heartburn at least once a month, 12% at least once a week, and 5% daily. However, most people do not consider heartburn a major medical problem and seldom report this complaint to their physicians. For example, a large population survey from Olmsted County, Minnesota [2] found that only 5.4% of people had seen a physician for their heartburn in the last year, despite describing their symptoms as moderately severe in intensity and having a duration of 5 years or more.

"Heartburn" is a commonly used but frequently misunderstood word. It has many synonyms, including "indigestion," "acid regurgitation," "sour stomach," and "bitter belching." Heartburn is usually best described as burning discomfort experienced behind the breastbone. The terms "burning," "hot," and "acidic" are typically used by patients unless the symptom becomes so intense that pain is experienced. In those situations, the patient commonly complains of both heartburn and pain. Heartburn typically radiates toward the neck, throat, and, occasionally, the back. Heartburn is particularly aggravated by foods: it is frequently noted within 1 hour of eating, and usually after the largest meal of the day. Foods high in fats, sugars, chocolate, onions, and carminatives may aggravate heartburn, usually by reducing lower esophageal sphincter (LES) pressure [3]. Other foods commonly associated with heartburn, including citrus products, tomato-based foods, and spicy foods, do not affect LES pressure but are direct irritants to the esophageal mucosa [4]. This mechanism is independent of pH and is probably related to high osmolarity.

The supine position frequently aggravates heartburn, especially if subjects eat late in the evening or have bedtime snacks. This sensation occurs within 1–2 hours of reclining [5] and, in contrast to peptic ulcer disease, does not awaken the subject in the early morning. Some patients say their heartburn is more pronounced while lying on the right side [6]. Nighttime heartburn may affect quality of life in some patients, causing sleep difficulties and impaired next-day function [7]. Maneuvers that increase intra-abdominal pressure may aggravate heartburn, including bending over, lifting heavy objects, and undertaking isometric exercises. Recent studies suggest that sleep deprivation and psychological or auditory stress may exacerbate heartburn by lowering the threshold for symptom perception rather than by actually increasing the amount of acid reflux [8–10].

Heartburn is frequently accompanied by regurgitation, defined as the perception of flow of refluxed gastric content into the mouth or hypopharnyx [11]. The fluid has a bitter, acidic taste, is common after meals, and is worsened by stooping or the supine position. Among patients with daily regurgitation, LES pressure is usually low; some have associated gastroparesis and esophagitis is common, making this symptom more difficulty to treat medically than heartburn. It is important to distinguish regurgitation from "vomiting" and "waterbrash." The absence of nausea, retching, and abdominal contractions should suggest that regurgitation, and not vomiting, is present. Waterbrash is an uncommon symptom that involves the sudden filling of the mouth with clear, slightly salty fluid. This fluid is not regurgitated material but rather secretions from the salivary glands as part of the protective vagally mediated reflex from the distal esophagus [12]. Rumination is another commonly overlooked condition that can mimic reflux, both symptomatically and on pH testing [13].

Heartburn Symptoms as Predictors of GERD

The accuracy of heartburn and regurgitation in the diagnosis of GERD is difficult to define. A recent systematic review [14] identified seven studies that assessed the accuracy of reflux symptoms in the diagnosis of esophagitis. A total of 5134 patients were included, with 894 (17%) having esophagitis. The sensitivity of reflux symptoms was generally disappointing, with a range of 30–76% (pooled sensitivity 55%: 95% CI 45–68%), while the specificity was between 62 and 96%. These results are similar to those of the much-cited study by Klauser *et al.* [15], where the presence of heartburn had a sensitivity of 78% and a specificity of 60% in a highly selected population referred for esophageal pH monitoring. Finally, *post hoc* analysis of five esophagitis studies involving nearly 12 000 patients found the severity of heartburn was an unreliable indicator of the severity of erosive disease. This was particularly true in elderly patients (over 70 years of age) [16].

Practical Gastroenterology and Hepatology Board Review Toolkit, Second Edition. Edited by Nicholas J. Talley, Kenneth R. DeVault, Michael B. Wallace, Bashar A. Aqel and Keith D. Lindor.
© 2016 John Wiley & Sons, Ltd. Published 2016 by John Wiley & Sons, Ltd. Companion website: www.practicalgastrohep.com

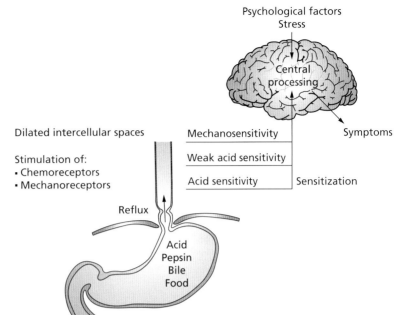

Figure 8.1 Schematic representation of the mechanisms involved in the generation of heartburn. These mechanisms and pathways include activation of chemoreceptors by acid, weak acid, and bile refluxates and mechanoreceptors. Dilated intercellular spaces (DISs) may facilitate the activation of these receptors. Afferent signaling and perception can be enhanced by sensitization of affluent sensory neurons, central brain processing, psychological factors, and stress. Source: Ang 2008. Reproduced with permission of the Nature Publishing Group.

Mechanisms of Heartburn

The underlying mechanisms of heartburn symptoms are only partially understood. The etiology appears multifactorial, potentially arising from chemostimulation, mechanostimulation, or hyperalgesia (Figure 8.1) [17].

Role of Acid Reflux

Acid reflux is critical, but it is not the sole cause of heartburn, as demonstrated by an esophageal acid perfusion study conducted by Smith *et al.* [18]. In this double-blind study, 25 patients with heartburn were randomly perfused with eight solutions of different pH (1.0–6.0). An overall positive correlation (R = 0.77) was demonstrated between the time of onset of pain and the pH of the infused solution. Solutions of pH 1.0 and 1.5 induced heartburn in all patients, but even the pH 6.0 solution produced heartburn in more than 40% of patients. Ambulatory pH monitoring consistently finds that only a small proportion of acid reflux episodes evoke heartburn.

Nerve endings and acid-sensitive ion channels are found in the deepest layer of the esophageal mucosa, which are normally shielded from luminal influences by anatomical barriers. The presence of dilated intercellular spaces (DISs) within the stratified squamous epithelium is now recognized as the earliest lesion in the damaged esophagus. DISs are present in animal models of GERD and in GERD patients – even those with visually normal mucosa [19]. This defect decreases mucosal resistance, allowing the diffusion of acid and luminal contents into the intercellular spaces. Activation of chemosensitive nociceptors occurs with signals transmitted to the brain, which generate the perception of heartburn [20]. Some researchers propose that resolution of DISs after proton pump inhibitor (PPI) therapy is the key to heartburn relief [21].

Role of Weakly Acid Reflux

With combined impedance/pH monitoring, esophageal refluxate can be further characterized as acidic (nadir pH < 4), weakly acidic (nadir pH 4–7), or non-acidic (nadir pH > 7) [22]. Off PPIs, heartburn is most commonly associated with acid reflux, but up to 15% of episodes occur with weakly acidic reflux [23]. A high proximal extent of the esophageal refluxate, a low nadir pH, and a large pH drop, as well as a large reflux volume and prolonged acid clearance times, are more likely associated with heartburn symptoms. On twice-daily PPI therapy, the relationship is modified, with studies finding that 17–37% of patients have symptom production with non-acid, usually weakly acidic reflux [24, 25]. Cough and regurgitation are the most common non-acid-associated symptoms.

Role of Bile Reflux

Esophageal infusion of bile acids can generate heartburn symptoms, but not with the rapidity and intensity of acid infusion [26]. The likely mechanism is the release of intracellular mediators via damage to lipid membranes [27]. Combined 24-hour pH and bilirubin absorbance monitoring (indirect measure of bile) finds that acid and bile reflux occur simultaneously during most reflux episodes, being found in 100% of patients with complicated Barrett's esophagus, 89% of patients with simple Barrett's esophagus, 79% of patients with esophagitis, and 50% of patients without esophagitis [28]. Off PPI therapy, Koek *et al.* [29] observed that less than 10% of symptoms were related to bile reflux alone, but the majority of symptoms on BID PPIs were related to bile reflux as compared to acid reflux.

Role of Esophageal Mechanical Stimulation

The concept that mechanical stimulation of the esophagus may have a role in heartburn symptoms has attracted increasing support. Esophageal balloon distension, especially in the proximal esophagus, can produce the symptom of heartburn [30]. Researchers postulate that the proximal esophagus has a larger number of mechanoreceptors than the distal esophagus, contributing to the generation of symptoms during reflux events. Acid exposure might also reduce the threshold for mechanoreceptor stimulation [31]. Sustained esophageal contractions represent prolonged contractions of the longitudinal esophageal smooth muscle (identified by high-frequency intraluminal ultrasound) and may produce chest pain. Balaban *et al.* [32] demonstrated a strong correlation between spontaneous chest pain or chest pain induced by edrophanium chloride and sustained contractions. These contractions did not occlude the esophageal lumen and were not associated with changes in intraluminal esophageal pressure, indicating that the circular muscles are not involved.

Role of Esophageal Hypersensitivity

Esophageal hypersensitivity contributes to heartburn complaints, especially in the subgroup of GERD patients with normal acid exposure, but a close relationship exists between reflux events and heartburn perception [33, 34]. These patients are also hypersensitive to mechanical distension, as shown by balloon studies. The proposed mechanisms are complex, but studies suggest altered brain processing (central sensitization), rather than abnormal esophageal wall receptors, is key to the development of visceral hypersensitivity [35]. Anxiety and stress contribute to this increased perception of heartburn via both central mechanisms, and possibly peripherally by DISs in the esophageal mucosa [36].

Chest Pain

While heartburn and regurgitation are almost always esophageal symptoms, the differential diagnosis of chest pain can be very challenging. Cardiac and pulmonary disease should be excluded prior to implicating the esophagus, though these etiologies can certainly coexist with esophageal disease. Traditionally, assessment of patients is based on the description of the pain, the overall clinical picture, electrocardiogram (ECG), and cardiac enzymes, including troponin levels. However, due to extensive overlap between cardiac and non-cardiac causes of chest pain, reliance on history alone does not provide optimal exclusion of cardiac or non-cardiac causes [37]. There are several potential esophageal mechanisms for the production of chest pain, which will be discussed in subsequent sections. A potential approach to patients with chest pain is presented in Figure 8.2.

Gastroesophageal reflux related chest pain

GERD is the most common esophageal cause of non-cardiac chest pain (NCCP) [38]. There are currently only a few useful diagnostic tests available by which to assess GERD in patients with NCCP; these include upper endoscopy, esophageal pH monitoring, esophageal impedance and pH, and the PPI test.

Upper endoscopy

Alarm symptoms such as recent weight loss, dysphagia or odynophagia, decreased appetite, hematemesis, and anemia are important indications for upper endoscopy in individuals with NCCP. Upper endoscopy is ideal for detecting erosive esophagitis, esophageal stricture, ulcers, and Barrett's esophagus. However, the diagnostic yield of upper endoscopy among individuals with NCCP is variable. Hsia *et al.* [39], in their endoscopic assessment of 100 consecutive NCCP patients, found that 24% had esophagitis. A recent study of 3688 consecutive NCCP patients who had an upper endoscopy reported that 44.1% had normal findings, 28.3% had hiatal hernia, 19.4% erosive esophagitis, 4.4% Barrett's esophagus, and 3.6% stricture or stenosis [40]. Therefore, the current literature suggests that there may be only limited utility in using upper endoscopy in assessing NCCP patients.

The PPI Test

This is a cost-effective method of quickly diagnosing and treating simultaneously GERD-related NCCP [41] Importantly, this simple and non-invasive method is available to all physicians and specialists, and those in primary care. The dose can range from 1 to 3 PPIs per day and the trial length is usually 7 days to 4 weeks, depending on the frequency of the chest pain symptoms.

There have been two meta-analyses that have assessed the role of PPI therapy in the diagnosis of NCCP. The first aimed to determine the efficacy of short-term PPIs among those with NCCP, as well as how useful PPIs are in diagnosing reflux-related NCCP. The analysis contained eight randomized controlled trials (RCTs) with either a parallel or crossover design comparing PPI therapy with placebo. The results showed that NCCP patients taking PPIs have reduced episodes of chest pain (RR = 0.54; 95% CI: 0.41–0.71). The number needed to treat was 3 (95% CI: 2–4). Moreover, the pooled sensitivity, specificity, and diagnostic odds ratios (ORs) for the PPI test compared to 24-hour pH monitoring and endoscopy were 80%,

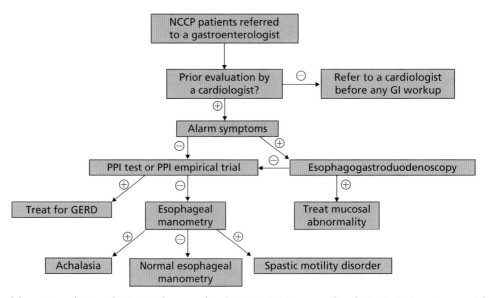

Figure 8.2 Proposed diagnostic evaluation of patients with non-cardiac chest pain. NCCP, non-cardiac chest pain; PPI, proton pump inhibitor; GERD, gastroesophageal reflux disease.

74%, and 13.83 (95% CI: 5.48–34.91), respectively [42]. The second analysis included eight randomized, placebo-controlled studies. It revealed that the PPI test had a much higher sensitivity (80%; 95% CI: 71–87%) and specificity (74%; 95% CI: 64–83%) compared with the placebo group (sensitivity 19% (95% CI: 12–29%), specificity 77% (95% CI: 62–87%)). Overall, the PPI test had greater discriminatory power, with a summary diagnostic OR of 19.35 (95% CI: 8.54–43.84), compared with 0.61 (95% CI: 0.20–1.86) in the placebo group [43].

Esophageal pH Monitoring

This includes both the standard catheter-based ambulatory 24-hour esophageal pH monitoring and the wireless "catheterless" Bravo pH monitoring systems, which are used in correlation with symptoms [44]. Just over half of all NCCP patients are found to have abnormal esophageal acid exposure or a positive symptom index alone. It must be remembered that abnormal distal esophageal acid exposure during pH testing does not necessarily mean that the chest pain experienced by the patient is due to GERD. This test has numerous disadvantages, which include cost and availability for physicians and inconvenience for patients. Currently, most experts reserve esophageal pH monitoring for NCCP patients who fail PPI therapy, though for the test to be optimally diagnostic, the patient should be taken off PPI prior to testing.

Multichannel Intraluminal Esophageal Impedance and pH Sensor

The combination of an impedance catheter and a pH probe provides a unique opportunity to study physiologic and pathologic events within the esophagus and their relationship to symptoms. In addition, the recording assembly can disclose the characteristics of the gastric refluxate (acidic, weakly acidic, alkaline, gas, liquid, and mixed gas and liquid). The specific value of the multichannel intraluminal impedance plus pH sensor and the documentation of weakly acidic reflux in patients with NCCP remains to be elucidated.

Motility Disorders

In patients with non-GERD-related NCCP, esophageal dysmotility is relatively uncommon. Studies have consistently demonstrated that approximately 70% of patients with non-GERD–related NCCP have normal esophageal motility during esophageal manometry [45, 46]. Overall, the relationship between non-GERD-related NCCP and esophageal dysmotility remains an area of controversy. This is primarily because of the common documentation of esophageal dysmotility in NCCP patients undergoing esophageal manometry without concomitant reports of chest pain symptoms.

Esophageal Manometry

At present, esophageal manometry is the optimal method for assessing motility disorders of the esophagus [48]. The exact role of abnormal motility in NCCP patients and chest pain remains controversial. DiMarino et al. [50] suggested that esophageal dysmotility may not be the cause of patients' chest pain, but instead a proxy marker of an underlying motor disorder.

Other Tests Not Routinely Used

A barium swallow (esophagram) is not useful in the diagnosis of GERD, but should be considered in NCCP cases with dysphagia. An assortment of provocative tests (the edrophonium test (Tensilon test) and the Bernstein test) have been used to evaluate patients with NCCP. Enthusiasm about their diagnostic role has been tempered by a low sensitivity. Presently, few motility laboratories are using these tests on a routine basis. The balloon distension test is currently used primarily for research purposes to determine perception thresholds for pain in patients with functional chest pain of presumed esophageal origin, though a few labs continue to use this clinically.

Differentiating Esophageal from Non-esophageal Causes of NCCP

There can be overlap of esophageal and non-esophageal causes of chest pain. Patients with documented coronary artery disease are likely to have concomitant chest pain of esophageal origin [49]. Although there are a number of esophageal disorders reported in patients with coronary artery disease, the most common is gastroesophageal reflux [50, 51]. Research suggests that cardiac manipulation (e.g., coronary angioplasty) can induce esophageal motility abnormalities but not gastroesophageal reflux [52]. In one study, anti-anginal treatment became partially ineffective in patients with coronary artery disease who also demonstrated esophageal abnormalities [50]. Recently, a small case series found that patients reported a reduction in symptoms related to atrial fibrillation after treatment of GERD symptoms with PPI therapy; this was verified by combined 24-hour pH and ambulatory Holter monitoring [53]. In addition, Lux et al. [54] have shown a statistically significant association between ST-segment abnormalities and gastroesophageal reflux or esophageal dysmotility Thus, the interaction between the heart and esophagus in causing chest pain is a complex one, and patients with chest pain should therefore first undergo a thorough diagnostic assessment by a cardiologist, and only if negative should they be referred to a gastroenterologist for further evaluation.

Functional Chest Pain

Functional chest pain is one of the functional GI disorders (FGIDs). Very little is known about functional chest pain, and the underlying pathophysiology remains poorly understood. Diagnosis is usually based on symptoms and exclusion of organic disease. It can be an extremely debilitating condition that impacts greatly on quality of life, with frequent physician consultations, diagnostic tests, and use of medications (over-the-counter and prescription). Guidelines as to the classification of functional chest pain have been developed by the Rome Foundation [55]. Functional chest pain (NCCP) is defined as "episodes of unexplained chest pain that usually are midline in location and of visceral quality, and therefore potentially of esophageal origin. The pain is easily confused with cardiac angina and pain from other esophageal disorders, including achalasia and gastroesophageal reflux disease (GERD)." The Rome Committee developed the following diagnostic criteria for functional chest pain of presumed esophageal origin, which must include *all* of the following: (i) midline chest pain or discomfort that is not of burning quality; (ii) absence of evidence that gastroesophageal reflux is the cause of the symptom; and (iii) absence of histopathology-based esophageal motility disorders. In addition, these criteria must be fulfilled for the last 3 months, with symptom onset at least 6 months before diagnosis. There may be benefit in using the Rome III criteria in clinical practice to define functional chest pain; however, these criteria have not been assessed in any clinical studies. There are advantages and disadvantages to using these criteria [56], but they are not, unfortunately, widely used clinically for chest pain, perhaps due to the specificity of the diagnostic criteria. Studies have found that other functional GI disorders, such as irritable bowel syndrome

(IBS) and functional dyspepsia (FD), overlap with functional chest pain [56].

Psychological Evaluation

This is an important part of chest pain assessment, as many chest pain patients with either a cardiac or a non-cardiac cause suffer from a psychological disorder (depression, anxiety, neuroticism). Psychogenic chest pain hurts just as much as pain of organic origin, but it can be difficult if not impossible to determine which came first: the chest pain or the psychological state. Other studies have found higher rates of psychological disorders (up to 80%) among chest pain patients. Use of a screening questionnaire would be optimal, as a structured psychiatric interview is time-consuming and requires a specialized assessor for maximum efficacy.

Psychologically active medications have been used in NCCP. Studied agents include paroxetine, sertraline, imipramine, venlafaxine, and trazodone. Some but not all of them have proven efficacy in randomized trials

---

Take Home Points

- Heartburn and regurgitation are the cardinal symptoms of gastroesophageal reflux disease (GERD).
- These complaints usually occur after consuming "refluxogenic" foods and can be aggravated by exercise or the supine position.
- Recent studies have found the sensitivity of reflux symptoms to be relatively disappointing for GERD (30–76%) and an unreliable indicator of the severity of erosive esophagitis. This should perhaps not be surprising, as acid reflux is not the sole mechanism of heartburn symptoms.
- Other factors include the reflux of bile and weak acid, mechanical stimulation of the esophagus, esophageal hyperalgesia, and psychological comorbidity.
- Chest pain is a more confusing symptom, but the esophagus should be considered as a possible etiology for pain, once cardiac disease has been ruled out.
- Esophageal and cardiac pain can occur in the same patient, producing confusion for both the patient and providers.

References

1 Moayyedi P, Axon ATR. Gastro–oesophageal reflux disease: the extent of the problem. *Aliment Pharmacol Ther* 2005; **22**(Suppl. 1): 11–19.

2 Locke GM, Talley NJ, Fett SL, *et al.* Prevalence and clinical spectrum of gastroesophageal reflux: a population–based study in Olmsted County, Minnesota. *Gastroenterology* 1997; **112**: 1448–53.

3 Price SF, Smithson KW, Castell DO. Food sensitivity in reflux esophagitis. *Gastroenterology* 1978; **75**: 240–6.

4 Feldman M, Barnett C. Relationship between the acidity and osmolality of popular beverages and reported postprandial heartburn. *Gastroenterology* 1995; **108**: 125–31.

5 Fujiwara Y, Machida A, Watanabe Y, *et al.* Association between dinner-to-bedtime and gastroesophageal reflux disease. *Am J Gastroenterol* 2005; **100**: 2633–6.

6 Katz LC, Just R, Castell DO. Body position affects recumbent postprandial reflux. *J Clin Gastroenterol* 1994; **18**: 280–3.

7 Shaker R, Castell DO, Schoenfeld PS, Spechler SJ. Nighttime heartburn is an underappreciated clinical problem that impacts sleep and daytime function: the results of a Gallup survey conducted on behalf of the American Gastroenterological Association. *Am J Gastroenterol* 2003; **98**: 1487–92.

8 Schey R, Dickman R, Parthasarthy S, *et al.* Sleep deprivation is hyperalgesic in patients with gastroesophageal reflux disease. *Gastroenterology* 2007; **133**: 1787–95.

9 Wright CE, Ebrecht M, Mitchell R, *et al.* The effect of psychological stress on symptom severity and perception in patients with gastroesophageal reflux disease. *J Psychosom Res* 2005; **59**: 415–24.

10 Fass R, Naliboff BD, Fass SS, *et al.* The effect of auditory stress on perception of intraesophageal acid in patients with gastroesophageal reflux disease. *Gastroenterology* 2008; **134**: 696–705.

11 Wong WM, Wong BCY. Definition and diagnosis of gastroesophageal reflux disease. *J Gastroenterol Hepatol* 2004; **19**(Suppl. 3): S26–32.

12 Helms JF, Dodds WJ, Hogan WJ. Salivary response to esophageal acid in normal and patients with reflux esophagitis. *Gastroenterology* 1987; **93**: 1393–9.

13 Saleh CM, Bredenoord AJ. Utilization of esophageal function testing for the diagnosis of the rumination syndrome and belching disorders. *Gastrointest Endosc Clin N Am* 2014; **24**: 633–42.

14 Moayyedi P, Talley NJ, Fennerty MB, Vakil N. Can the clinical history distinguish between organic and functional dyspepsia? *JAMA* 2006; **295**: 1566–76.

15 Klauser AG, Schindlbeck NE, Muller-Lissner SA. Symptoms in gastro-oesophageal reflux disease. *Lancet* 1990; **335**: 205–8.

16 Johnson DA, Fennerty MB. Heartburn severity underestimates erosive esophagitis in elderly patients with gastroesophageal reflux disease. *Gastroenterology* 2004; **126**: 660–8.

17 Ang D, Sifrim D, Tack J. Mechanisms of heartburn. *Nat Clin Prac Gastroenterol Hepatol* 2008; **5**: 383–92.

18 Smith JL, Opekun AR, Larkai E, *et al.* Sensitivity of the esophageal mucosa to pH in gastroesophageal reflux disease. *Gastroenterology* 1989; **96**: 683–9.

19 Malenstein HV, Farre R, Sifrim D. Esophageal dilated intercellular spaces (DIS) and nonerosive reflux disease. *Am J Gastroenterol* 2008; **103**: 1021–8.

20 Barlow WJ, Orlando RC. The pathogenesis of heartburn in nonerosive reflux disaease: a unifying hypothesis. *Gastroenterology* 2005; **128**: 771–8.

21 Calabrese C, Bortolotti M, Fabbri A, *et al.* Reversibility of GERD ultrastructural alteration and relief of symptoms after omeprazole treatment. *Am J Gastroenterol* 2005; **100**: 537–42.

22 Sifrim D, Castell DO, Dent J, *et al.* Gastro–oesophageal reflux monitoring: review and consensus report on detection and definitions of acid, non-acid, and gas reflux. *Gut* 2004; **53**: 1024–31.

23 Bredenoord AJ, Weusten BLAM, Curvers WL, *et al.* Determinants of perception of heartburn and regurgitation. *Gut* 2006; **55**: 313–18.

24 Zerbib F, Roman S, Ropert A, *et al.* Esophageal pH impedance monitoring and symptom analysis in GERD: a study in patients off and on therapy. *Am J Gastroenterol* 2006; **101**: 1956–63.

25 Maine I, Tutuian R, Shay S, *et al.* Acid and non- acid reflux in patients with persistent symptoms despite acid suppressive therapy: a multicentre study using combined ambulatory impedance-pH monitoring. *Gut* 2006; **55**: 1398–402.

26 Siddiqui A, Rodriguez-Stanley S, Zubaidi S, *et al.* Esophageal visceral sensitivity to bile salts in patients with functional heartburn and in healthy control subjects. *Dig Dis Sci* 2005; **50**: 81–5.

27 Tack J. Review article: The role of bile and pepsin in the pathophysiology and treatment of gastroesophageal reflux disease. *Aliment Pharmacol Ther* 2006; **24**(Suppl): 10–16.

28 Vaezi MF, Richter JE. Role of acid and duodenogastroesophageal reflux in GERD. *Gastroenterology* 1006; **111**: 1992–9.

29 Koek GH. The role of acid and duodenal gastroesophageal reflux in symptomatic GERD. *Am J Gastroenterol* 2001; **96**: 2033–40.

30 Patel S, Rao S. Biomechanical and sensory parameters of the human esophagus at four levels. *Am J Physiol Gastrointest Liver Physiol* 1998; **275**: G187–91.

31 Peghini P, Johnston BT, Leite LP, *et al.* Mucosal acid exposure sensitizes a subset of normal subjects to intra-oesophageal balloon distension. *Eur J Gastroenterol Hepatol* 1996; **8**: 978–83.

32 Balaban DH, Yamamoto Y, Liu J, *et al.* Sustained esophageal contraction: a marker of esophageal chest pain identified by intraluminal ultrasonography. *Gastroenterology* 1999; **116**: 29–37.

33 Trimble KC, Pryde A, Heading RC. Lowered esophageal sensory thresholds in patients with symptomatic but not excess gastro-oesophageal reflux: evidence for a spectrum of visceral sensitivity in GORD. *Gut* 1995; **37**: 7–12.

34 Rao SC, Gregersen H, Hayek B, *et al.* Unexplained chest pain: the hypersensitive, hyperactive and poorly compliant esophagus. *Ann Intern Med* 1996; **124**: 950–8.

35 Sarkar S, Hobson AR, Furlong PL, *et al.* Central neural mechanisms mediating human visceral hypersensitivity. *Am J Physiol Gastroentest Liver Physiol* 2001; **881**: G1196–202.

36 Naliboff BD, Mayer M, Fass R, *et al.* The effect of life stress on symptoms of heartburn. *Psych Med* 2004; **66**: 426–34.

37 Eslick GD, Talley NJ. Natural history and predictors of outcome for non-cardiac chest pain: a prospective 4-year cohort study. *Neurogastroenterol Motil* 2008; **20**: 989–97.

38 Bortolotti M, Marzocchi A, Bacchelli S, *et al.* The esophagus as a possible cause of chest pain in patients with and without angina pectoris. *Hepatogastroenterology* 1990; **37**: 316–18.

39 Hsia PC, Maher KA, Lewis JH, *et al.* Utility of upper endoscopy in the evaluation of noncardiac chest pain. *Gastrointest Endosc* 1991; **37**: 22–6.

40 Dickman R, Mattek N, Holub J, *et al.* Prevalence of upper gastrointestinal tract findings in patients with noncardiac chest pain versus those with gastroesophageal reflux disease (GERD)-related symptoms: results from a national endoscopic database. *Am J Gastroenterol* 2007; **102**: 1173–9.

41 Fass R, Fennerty MB, Ofman JJ, *et al.* The clinical and economic value of a short course of omeprazole patients with noncardiac chest pain. *Gastroenterology* 1998; **115**: 42–9.

42 Wang W, Huang J, Zheng G, *et al.* Is proton pump inhibitor testing an effective approach to diagnose gastroesophageal reflux disease in patients with noncardiac chest pain? *Arch Intern Med* 2005; **165**: 1222–8.

43 Cremonini F, Wise J, Moayyedi P, *et al.* Diagnostic and therapeutic use of proton pump inhibitors in non-cardiac chest pain: a meta-analysis. *Am J Gastroenterol* 2005; **100**: 1226–32.

44 Prakash C, Clouse RE. Wireless pH monitoring in patients with non-cardiac chest pain. *Am J Gastroenterol* 2006; **101**: 446–52.

45 Dekel R, Pearson T, Wendel C, *et al.* Assessment of oesophageal motor function in patients with dysphagia or chest pain – the Clinical Outcomes Research Initiative experience. *Aliment Pharmacol Ther* 2003; **18**: 1083–9.

46 Katz PO, Dalton CB, Richter JE, *et al.* Esophageal testing of patients with noncardiac chest pain or dysphagia. Results of three years' experience with 1161 patients. *Ann Intern Med* 1987; **106**: 593–7.

47 Knippig C, Fass R, Malfertheiner P. Tests for the evaluation of functional gastrointestinal disorders. *Dig Dis* 2001; **19**: 232–9.

48 DiMarino AJ Jr., Allen ML, Lynn RB, Zamani S. Clinical value of esophageal motility testing. *Dig Dis* 1998; **16**: 198–204.

49 Ghillebert G, Janssens J. Oesophageal pain in coronary artery disease. *Gut* 1998; **42**: 312–19.

50 Bortolotti M, Marzocchi A, Bacchelli S, *et al.* The esophagus as a possible cause of chest pain in patients with and without angina pectoris. *Hepatogastroenterology* 1990; **37**: 316–18.

51 Schofield PM, Whorwell PJ, Brooks NH, *et al.* Oesophageal function in patients with angina pectoris: a comparison of patients with normal coronary angiograms and patients with coronary artery disease. *Digestion* 1989; **42**: 70–8.

52 Makk LJ, Leesar M, Joseph A, *et al.* Cardioesophageal reflexes: an invasive human study. *Dig Dis Sci* 2000; **45**: 2451–4.

53 Gerson LB, Friday K, Triadafilopoulos G. Potential relationship between gastroesophageal reflux disease and atrial arrhythmias. *J Clin Gastroenterol* 2006; **40**: 828–32.

54 Lux G, Van Els J, The GS, *et al.* Ambulatory oesophageal pressure, pH and ECG recording in patients with normal and pathological coronary angiography and intermittent chest pain. *Neurogastroenterol Motil* 1995; **7**: 23–30.

55 Galmiche JP, Clouse RE, Bálint A, *et al.* Functional esophageal disorders. *Gastroenterology* 2006; **130**: 1459–65.

56 Dipalli RS, Remes-Troche JM, Andersen L, Rao SSC. Functional chest pain – esophageal or overlapping functional disorder. *J Clin Gastroenterol* 2007; **41**: 264–9.

CHAPTER 8

Dysphagia

Dawn L. Francis
Division of Gastroenterology and Hepatology, Mayo Clinic, Rochester, MN, USA

Summary

"Dysphagia" refers to the subjective sensation of difficulty in swallowing. Dysphagia is a distinct symptom from other swallowing-related complaints such as odynophagia, which refers to painful swallowing, and globus sensation, the sensation of a lump in the throat.

Dysphagia is a common complaint that can occur in any age group, but it is more common in the elderly population. As many as 10% of people over the age of 50 complain of dysphagia [1]. No matter the age, dysphagia is considered an alarm symptom and should prompt a diagnostic evaluation to define its etiology. A thorough patient history suggests the correct etiology in as many as 85% of patients [2]. Table 9.1 lists the questions to use to elicit the salient points of the patient's history. The differential diagnosis of dysphagia is broad and includes anatomic abnormalities, motility disorders, and infiltrative disorders.

Pathophysiology

There are a number of potential physiologic problems that can lead to the symptom of dysphagia or odynophagia. These can be broadly categorized as infections, mucosal abnormalities, anatomic abnormalities, and functional problems of the oropharynx and esophagus.

Infections

Odynophagia is often caused by infection of the oropharynx with fungal organisms or viruses. Dysphagia without odynophagia can also be caused by infection. The infections that cause the symptoms of odynophagia and dysphagia are usually opportunistic and occur in immunosuppressed or elderly patients, such as those with candida, herpes simplex virus (HSV), or cytomegalovirus (CMV).

Mucosal Abnormalities

There are a number of mucosal abnormalities that can cause odynophagia, dysphagia, or both. Those associated with odynophagia are usually caused by radiation injury or head and neck cancer. Those most commonly associated with dysphagia are peptic esophagitis, esophageal carcinoma, eosinophilic esophagitis, and pill esophagitis.

Anatomic Abnormalities

Anatomic abnormalities that may cause dysphagia include cricopharyngeal bar, Zenker's diverticulum, esophageal webs, peptic stricture, distal esophageal rings, vascular compression of the esophagus, and compression of the esophagus by cervical osteophytes.

Functional Abnormalities

Odynophagia or oropharyngeal dysphagia may be caused by weakness of the oropharynx, cricopharyngeal hypertrophy, or several different neuromuscular disorders. Esophageal dysphagia may be caused by ineffective esophageal motility, aperistalsis, hypertensive lower esophageal sphincter (LES), nutcracker esophagus, diffuse esophageal spasm (DES), or achalasia

Clinical Features

The most important function of the patient history is to define the patient's dysphagia as oropharyngeal or "transfer" dysphagia versus esophageal dysphagia. Oropharyngeal dysphagia is often characterized by the complaint of difficulty initiating a swallow, difficulty transitioning a food bolus or liquid into the esophagus, meal-induced coughing or "choking," or food "getting stuck" immediately after swallowing. The patient will often localize the sensation to the cervical esophagus above the suprasternal notch.

The timing of the onset and worsening of symptoms of dysphagia is also important. Progressive dysphagia is often associated with an esophageal carcinoma, peptic stricture, or achalasia, whereas intermittent dysphagia may indicate the presence of a lower esophageal ring. Patients with esophageal motility disorders may have either progressive or intermittent symptoms.

An important part of the medical history is characterizing the types of food that produce symptoms; that is, solids, liquids, or both. For example, dysphagia for both solids and liquids often indicates an underlying esophageal motility disorder, whereas dysphagia for solids alone usually represents an anatomic obstruction.

Oropharyngeal Dysphagia

There are many disorders that cause oropharyngeal dysphagia (Table 9.2). Generally, these include neuromuscular diseases, systemic diseases, and mechanical obstruction. When neuromuscular diseases cause oropharyngeal dysphagia, other neurological or muscular symptoms may be present, including recurrent bouts of aspiration pneumonia due to inadequate airway protection, hoarseness, dysarthria, and pharyngonasal regurgitation.

Mechanical and anatomic causes of oropharyngeal dysphagia include cervical osteophytes, thyromegaly, pharyngeal tonsillar

Practical Gastroenterology and Hepatology Board Review Toolkit, Second Edition. Edited by Nicholas J. Talley, Kenneth R. DeVault, Michael B. Wallace, Bashar A. Aqel and Keith D. Lindor.
© 2016 John Wiley & Sons, Ltd. Published 2016 by John Wiley & Sons, Ltd. Companion website: www.practicalgastrohep.com

Table 9.1 Focused questions for patients with dysphagia.

Question	Comments
How long have you had trouble swallowing? Have your symptoms worsened with time? Is your swallowing difficulty continuous or intermittent?	Progressive dysphagia is often associated with an esophageal carcinoma, peptic stricture or achalasia. Intermittent dysphagia may indicate the presence of a lower esophageal ring. Patients with motility disorders may have either progressive or intermittent symptoms, depending on the disorder.
Do you have trouble initiating a swallow or do you feel food getting "stuck" or "hanging up" a few seconds after swallowing?	Oropharyngeal dysphagia is often characterized by difficulty initiating a swallow and esophageal dysphagia by the onset of symptoms several seconds after the initiation of a swallow.
Do you have problems swallowing solids, liquids, or both?	Dysphagia for both solids and liquids often indicates an underlying esophageal motility disorder, whereas dysphagia for solids alone usually represents an anatomic obstruction.
Do you cough or choke after swallowing?	Coughing or choking after swallowing is often caused by oropharyngeal dysphagia or a Zenker's diverticulum.
Have you had unintentional weight loss?	Weight loss may be present with dysphagia of any type but is most often associated with esophageal carcinoma or achalasia.

Table 9.3 Causes of esophageal dysphagia.

Extraesophageal	Cervical osteophytes
	Enlarged left atrium
	Enlarged aorta
	Enlarged or aberrant subclavian artery (dysphagia lusoria)
	Mediastinal mass
Intraesophageal	Benign tumors or lesions
	Esophageal carcinoma
	Caustic esophagitis
	Dermatologic conditions (lichen planus, pemphigoid/pemphigus)
	Diverticula
	Eosinophilic esophagitis
	Infection
	Radiation injury
	Rings or webs
	Stricture (benign or malignant)
	Scarring from surgery
Motility disorders	Achalasia
	Aperistalsis
	Diffuse esophageal spasm
	Hypertensive LES
	Ineffective motility
	Nutcracker esophagus

LES, lower esophageal sphincter.

CHAPTER 9

enlargement, a cricopharyngeal bar (also known as hypertensive upper esophageal sphincter (UES)), and Zenker's diverticulum.

Esophageal Dysphagia

Patients with esophageal dysphagia describe the onset of symptoms several seconds after the initiation of a swallow. They can sense that the food or liquid bolus has traversed the oral cavity and has entered the esophagus. They complain of food feeling "stuck" or "hung up" in transition to the stomach. They usually feel symptoms in the retrosternal area, but may also feel the problem near the suprasternal notch. Retrosternal dysphagia usually corresponds to the location of the lesion, while suprasternal dysphagia may represent a proximal obstruction or be referred from below. Occasionally, patients will describe their dysphagia as regurgitation of liquid occurring during or just after a meal. This can be misdiagnosed as gastroesophageal reflux, especially in patients with achalasia.

Esophageal dysphagia can be caused by a number of diseases (see Table 9.3), but is most often the result of a mechanical obstruction or one of a small number of motility disorders. Esophageal dysphagia that is caused by a motility disorder is commonly characterized by dysphagia to both solids and liquids. Dysphagia that is associated with only solid foods is more likely due to a mechanical

Table 9.2 Causes of oropharyngeal dysphagia.

Mechanical obstruction	Cervical osteophyte
	Cricopharyngeal bar
	Thyromegaly
	Zenker's diverticulum
Neuromuscular	Amyotrophic lateral sclerosis
	Brainstem tumors
	Cerebrovascular accident
	Multiple sclerosis
	Parkinson's disease
	Peripheral neuropathy
Skeletal muscle disorders	Myasthenia gravis
	Muscular dystrophies
	Polymyosisits

obstruction, though mechanical obstructions may progress to the extent that there is dysphagia for both solids and liquids.

If there is episodic and non-progressive dysphagia without weight loss, then the obstruction is likely secondary to an esophageal web or a distal esophageal ring. If solid food dysphagia is progressive, then the problem may be an esophageal stricture, carcinoma of the esophagus, or achalasia. When weight loss is present with solid food dysphagia, concern for an esophageal carcinoma comes to the forefront.

Diagnosis

There are a limited number of tests that can be performed to evaluate dysphagia. These include videofluoroscopic swallowing evaluation, barium esophagram, esophageal manometry, and upper intestinal endoscopy for esophageal dysphagia. All barium tests should include a solid bolus unless the liquid phase is clearly abnormal. The goal of testing is to identify structural abnormalities that can be treated endoscopically or surgically, detect treatable underlying systemic disease, and define functional disorders.

The choice of initial test is based on the clinical presentation and available expertise. If the patient has symptoms and history that are consistent with oropharyngeal dysphagia, one may elect to start the diagnostic workup with videofluoroscopy that can identify the presence of aspiration and help in directing swallowing rehabilitation. Alternatively, if the patient has complaints that are more consistent with an esophageal anatomic abnormality, a barium esophagram or upper endoscopy may be the best first step. For those who have an initial barium esophagram that suggests achalasia, esophageal manometry would be an appropriate next step. Many experts recommend that esophageal biopsies be obtained for patients with esophageal dysphagia if there is no endoscopic evidence of anatomic narrowing to rule out eosinophilic esophagitis.

Therapeutics

The aims of treatment for dysphagia are to improve the mechanics of food bolus transfer, to ameliorate the sensation of dysphagia,

Table 9.4 Treatment of oropharyngeal dysphagia.

Neuromuscular disorders	Swallowing rehabilitation Medical treatment targeted at the underlying disease: • Myasthenia gravis • Parkinson's disease • Multiple sclerosis
Zenker's diverticulum	Botulinum toxin injection of UES Cricopharyngeal myotomy with diverticulectomy
Hypertensive UES/ cricopharyngeal bar	Bougie dilation UES botulinum toxin injection Cricopharyngeal myotomy

UES, upper esophageal sphincter.

to prevent esophageal food bolus impaction, and to prevent aspiration and its complications. The treatment strategy requires correct identification of the etiology of the patient's dysphagia for targeted interventions (Tables 9.4 and 9.5).

Oropharyngeal dysphagia

Swallowing rehabilitation by a swallowing professional (in most cases, a speech pathologist) is the mainstay of treatment for patients with oropharyngeal dysphagia caused by neuromuscular dysfunction and benefits most patients in this category [3, 4]. Any patient with oropharyngeal dysphagia should be cautioned to chew food thoroughly and slowly and to avoid alcohol during meals. Consuming food quickly and without focused attention can lead to aspiration.

There are a number of maneuvers one can make during swallowing that may reduce oropharyngeal dysphagia, and these can be tailored to the specific defect leading to the dysphagia. Some authors believe that swallowing rehabilitation can improve oropharyngeal dysphagia even when it is caused by an anatomic abnormality. This has been demonstrated in patients with defects brought about by surgical resection of oropharyngeal tissue [5] or by caustic injury [6].

Specific pharmacologic intervention may be available for patients with oropharyngeal dysphagia caused by an underlying neurologic disease that has a medical treatment, such as myasthenia gravis or Parkinson's disease. However, many patients with oropharyngeal dysphagia have an underlying disease that is progressive and does

Table 9.5 Treatment of esophageal dysphagia.

Mucosal disease	
Infection	Antifungals Antivirals
Eosinophilic esophagitis	Topical or systemic corticosteroids Allergy testing/avoidance of allergens
Peptic esophagitis	PPIs
Motility disorders	
DES, nutcracker esophagus	Nitrates, calcium channel blockers Sildenafil Trazadone/impramine Esophageal dilation Botulinum toxin in distal esophagus LES myotomy
Achalasia	LES myotomy for surgical candidates Botulinum toxin injection to LES Pneumatic dilations
Benign strictures, webs, and rings	Esophageal dilation Intralesional injection of corticosteroids Temporary self-expanding plastic stents Surgery

PPI, proton pump inhibitor; DES, distal esophageal spasm; LES, lower esophageal sphincter.

not have good treatment options. For these patients, swallowing rehabilitation may prolong the amount of time in which they can meet their nutritional needs orally, but ultimately many require non-oral feeding to prevent aspiration, such as with a percutaneous gastrostomy tube.

Patients who have oropharyngeal dysphagia due to an anatomic abnormality such as a Zenker's diverticulum or cricopharyngeal bar typically require an endoscopic or surgical intervention. Bougie dilation has been used successfully with oropharyngeal dysphagia caused by a hypertensive UES [7] or primary cricopharyngeal dysfunction [8]. Botulinum toxin injection at the UES has also been effective for hypertensive UES and Zenker's diverticulum [9].

Patients with inadequate pharyngeal contraction or lack of coordination between the hypopharynx and the UES, a hypertensive UES, or Zenker's diverticulum may be candidates for a cricopharyngeal myotomy. The success of this surgical intervention depends on the patient having an intact neurologic system, adequate propulsive force generated by the tongue and pharyngeal constrictors, intact initiation of swallowing, videofluorographic demonstration of obstruction to bolus flow at the level of the cricopharyngeus muscle, and manometeric evidence of relatively elevated UES pressure in comparison to the pharynx [10].

Esophageal Dysphagia

Mucosal Disease

Esophageal dysphagia caused by mucosal disease such as infection, eosinophilic esophagitis, or peptic esophagitis can be treated with targeted medical therapy. Candida esophagitis is typically treated with fluconazole for 10–14 days. Viral esophagitis often requires 6 weeks of treatment with the appropriate antiviral. Eosinophilic esophagitis is often treated with swallowed topical corticosteroids, such as fluticasone delivered in a metered-dose inhaler for 6–8 weeks. Patients with gastroesophageal reflux disease (GERD)-related strictures or motility disorders benefit from aggressive acid suppression. This is typically accomplished with proton pump inhibitors (PPIs) or H2 receptor antagonists [11, 12]. PPI therapy has been shown to decrease the recurrence of esophageal strictures.

Anatomic Narrowing from Benign Disease

Esophageal narrowing caused by esophageal webs, rings, or benign strictures is typically treated with esophageal dilation by either solid dilators (e.g., Savary, Maloney, or American) or balloon dilators. Patients with esophageal strictures that require repeated dilation may benefit from intralesional corticosteroids [13], which can be performed with standard endoscopy. In severe cases, placement of a temporary self-expanding plastic esophageal stent can be helpful. Patients with refractory and severe benign esophageal strictures may require surgical resection.

Anatomic Narrowing from Malignant Disease

The reason dysphagia is an alarm symptom is because of the possibility of malignancy. Nearly 50% of patients with esophageal cancer present with disease that is already metastatic. For such patients, placement of an esophageal stent will improve their dysphagia symptoms. For those that have resectable disease, surgery is the definitive treatment.

Motility Disorders

It is known that cold foods or liquids can make some esophageal motility problems worse, so these should be avoided in patients with such disorders – especially those of the hypertensive category, such as nutcracker esophagus and DES.

There are medications available for some esophageal hypertensive motility disorders (e.g., DES, nutcracker esophagus, hypertensive LES). Nitrates and calcium channel blockers have been used with some effect. Sildenafil inactivates nitric oxide-stimulated cyclic guanosine monophosphate, and, as a result, can relax the LES. Several investigators have studied the effect of 50 mg sildenafil on the LES. It has been found to be associated with symptom relief in a group of 11 patients with nutcracker esophagus or DES [14]. Trazadone and imipramine have been shown to be effective in relieving chest pain in patients with esophageal motility disorders. They likely work by modifying visceral sensation.

Certain motility disorders may be improved with dilation, most notably achalasia and perhaps nutcracker esophagus. Pneumatic dilation with large-diameter balloons (30–40 mm) has been used with some success in patients with achalasia, but the perforation risk is significant, and many clinicians have thus moved away from dilation as a first-line treatment for achalasia.

Botulinum toxin has been used with variable success in patients with achalasia. The effect is shorter-lasting than of myotomy, but it appears to be a safe alternative to pneumatic dilation for patients who are not surgical candidates [15]. Botulinum toxin has been reported to be effective in DES and other non-specific motility disorders in small, uncontrolled studies.

LES myotomy is primarily used for achalasia and, in severe cases, DES. The modified Heller approach is the most common. The Heller myotomy relieves symptoms associated with achalasia in up to 90% of patients, with a mortality rate similar to that of pneumatic dilation (0.3%). The response seems to be more durable than that of pneumatic dilation [16]. As laparoscopic myotomy becomes more common, it is increasingly used to treat achalasia in patients who are surgical candidates. Finally, an endoscopic approach to myotomy (per-oral endoscopic myotomy, POEM) has been introduced in several centers. This may be an appropriate alternative to laparoscopic myotomy and pneumatic dilation.

Prognosis

Most patients with esophageal dysphagia do well with treatment focused on the underlying etiology. Patients with oropharyngeal dysphagia fare less well, as the cause of the oropharyngeal dysphagia is usually a progressive and untreatable neuromuscular disease. Though swallowing rehabilitation can help, patients may ultimately require non-oral feeding to prevent aspiration.

Take Home Points

- Odynophagia is often caused by infection of the oropharynx with fungal organisms or viruses.
- Oropharyngeal dysphagia is often characterized by the complaint of difficulty initiating a swallow and of a sensation above the suprasternal notch.
- Progressive dysphagia can be caused by an esophageal carcinoma, peptic stricture, or achalasia.
- Dysphagia for both solids and liquids often indicates an underlying esophageal motility disorder.
- If solid-food dysphagia is progressive, then the problem may be an esophageal stricture, carcinoma of the esophagus, or achalasia.
- Swallowing rehabilitation by a swallowing professional is the mainstay of treatment for patients with oropharyngeal dysphagia caused by neuromuscular dysfunction.

- Oropharyngeal dysphagia due to an anatomic abnormality such as a Zenker's diverticulum or cricopharyngeal bar typically requires an endoscopic or surgical intervention.
- Esophageal strictures that require repeated dilation may benefit from intralesional corticosteroids.

Videos of interest to readers of this chapter can be found by visiting the companion website at:

http://www.practicalgastrohep.com/

9.1 Distal esophageal food bolus impaction.
9.2 Endoscopic investigation of a periduodenal mass.

References

1 Lindgren S, Janzon L. Prevalence of swallowing complaints and clinical findings among 50–79-year-old men and women in an urban population. *Dysphagia* 1991; **6**: 187–92.

2 Edwards DA. Discriminative information in the diagnosis of dysphagia. *J R Coll Physicians Lond* 1975; **9**(3): 257–63.

3 Neuman S. Swallowing therapy with neurologic patients: results of direct and indirect therapy methods in 66 patients suffering from neurological disorders. *Dysphagia* 1993; **8**(2): 150–3.

4 Huckabee ML, Cannito MP. Outcomes of swallowing rehabilitation in chronic brainstem dsyphagia: a retrospective evaluation. *Dysphagia* 1999; **14**: 93–109.

5 Zuydam AC, Rogers SN, Brown JS, et al. Swallowing rehabilitation after oropharyngeal resection for squamous cell carcinoma. *Br J Oral Maxillofac Surg* 2000; **38**(5): 513–18.

6 Shikowitz MJ, Levy J, Villano D, et al. Speech and swallowing rehabilitation following devastating caustic ingestion: techniques and indicators for success. *Laryngoscope* 1996; **106**(2; Suppl. 78): 1–12.

7 Hatlebakk J, Castell J, Spiegel J, et al. Dilatation therapy for dysphagia in patients with upper esophageal sphincter dysfunction – manometric and symptomatic response. *Dis Esophagus* 1998; **11**(4): 254–9.

8 Solt J, Bajor J, Moizs M, et al. Primary cricopharyngeal dysfunction: treatment with balloon catheter dilatation. *Gastrointest Endosc* 2001; **54**(6): 767–71.

9 Yokoyama T, Asai M, Kumada M, et al. Botulinum toxin injection into the cricopharyngeal muscle for dysphagia: report of 2 successful cases. *J Oto-Rhino-Laryngol Soc Jap* 2003; **106**(7): 754–7.

10 Buchholz DW. Cricopharyngeal myotomy may be effective treatment for selected patients with neurogenic oropharyngeal dysphagia. *Dysphagia* 1995; **10**: 255.

11 Stal JM, Gregor JC, Preiksaitis HG, et al. A cost-utility analysis comparing omeprazole with ranitidine in the maintenance therapy of peptic esophageal stricture. *Can J Gastroenterol* 1998; **12**(1): 43–9.

12 Marks RD, Richter JE, Rizzo J, et al. Omeprazole versus H2-receptor antagonists in treating patients with peptic stricture and esophagitis. *Gastroenterology* 1994; **106**(4): 907–15.

13 Kochhar R, Makharia G. Usefulness of intralesional triamcinolone in treatment of benign esophageal strictures. *Gastrointest Endosc* 2002; **56**(6): 829–34.

14 Eherer AJ, Schwetz I, Hammer HF, et al. Effect of sildenafil on oesophageal motor function in healthy subjects and patients with oesophageal motor disorders. *Gut* 2002; **50**: 758.

15 Pasricha PJ, Ravich WJ, Hendrix TR, et al. Intrasphincteric botulinum toxin for the treatment of achalasia. *NEJM* 1995; **332**(12): 774–8.

16 Vela MF, Richter JE, Khandwala F, et al. The long-term efficacy of pneumatic dilation and Heller myotomy for the treatment of achalasia. *Clin Gastroenterol Hepatol* 2006; **4**(5): 580–7.

CHAPTER 9

Miscellaneous Upper Gastrointestinal Symptoms

Mohamed Sultan and James H. Lewis

Division of Gastroenterology, Georgetown University Medical Center, Washington, DC, USA

Belching (Eructation) and Aerophagia

Summary

Eructation (belching) is the escape of air from the esophagus or stomach into the pharynx, accompanied by the characteristic belching sound [1]. Belching can be physiologic or pathologic. Excessive belching may be associated with reflux and functional dyspepsia (FD), but extreme belching may be a manifestation of an anxiety or stress. Aerophagia is a behavioral disorder in which patients swallow copious amounts of air, often leading to significant abdominal distention and bloating. It has also been associated with continuous positive airway pressure (CPAP) therapy. In our experience, belching and aerophagia may be confused by some patients as being hiccups. Physicians should be aware of these conditions, their potentially different etiologies, and approaches to their management.

Case

A 38-year-old male with long-standing anxiety is referred by his primary care physician with persistent belching for the past year. He was initially diagnosed by his physician as having gastroesophageal reflux disease (GERD) and was treated empirically with a proton pump inhibitor (PPI), without benefit. He does not report classic heartburn, dysphagia, or abdominal pain. He presents to your office seeking symptom relief, as he finds his condition socially embarrassing and states it interferes with his work, since coworkers are constantly bothered by the loud sounds he emits. You observe that he burps repetitively up to 20 times per minute, noting that he does not burp when speaking to you or when he is distracted.

Definition and Epidemiology

In some cultures (e.g., India, Turkey, some Middle Eastern countries, and parts of China), belching after a meal is considered a sign of appreciation to the host, indicating satiety and contentment. In patients, it may be related to underlying GERD, FD, anxiety, or another stress-related condition [2, 3]. Two types of belch have been recognized: gastric belch and supragastric belch [1, 3]. Gastric belch is a normal physiologic phenomenon. It occurs up to 25 times per day and can be seen in patients with reflux and other dyspeptic disorders. It is associated with transient lower esophageal sphincter (LES) relaxation (TLESR) resulting from proximal gastric

distention, which allows venting of air out of the stomach [1, 2, 4]. Supragastric belching originates in the esophagus [1, 3, 5], where ingested air is immediately brought back out – often voluntarily, but never during sleep [6]. It is usually not associated with other gastrointestinal (GI) symptoms. Some patients report that supragastric belching initially began as a means to relieve bloating or abdominal discomfort and simply became uncontrollable [1]. It may have a psychological basis [7]. Gastric belches are relatively uncommon compared to supragastric belches [8].

Aerophagia can be distinguished from excessive supragastric belching in that the former involves true air-swallowing, in which peristaltic contractions of the esophagus transport the air into the stomach [1, 9]. Patients can swallow a large quantity of air (up to 4 L per minute), which accumulates in the GI tract, causing abdominal distention and bloating. It is associated most often with behavioral or psychiatric disorders, but certain lifestyle choices (such as smoking cigarettes, drinking carbonated beverages, chewing gum, and eating too fast, in some cases associated with high CPAP pressures used to treat sleep apnea disorders) are also recognized causes [10–12]. Among patients on CPAP found to have aerophagia, GERD symptoms (especially at night) were more than twice as prevalent as in those without aerophagia [10]; these patients were also more likely to be on acid-suppressive medications (45.5 vs. 18.2%, $p < 0.05$) than were the controls [11].

Pathophysiology

Gastric belch occurs when swallowed air escapes from the stomach into the esophagus as a result of vagally mediated TLESR from proximal gastric distention [1, 4]. Subsequent relaxation of the upper esophageal sphincter (UES) as the air is vented into the esophagus allows it to be expelled into the pharynx [1, 4, 8]. This is considered a physiologic reflex. In contrast, supragastric belching occurs when air is rapidly swallowed into the esophagus and immediately expelled, with little or no air entering the stomach [1, 9]. This is generally under the voluntary control of the patient. Often, the process of supragastric belching is triggered by emotional stress or by dyspeptic symptoms that the patient misinterprets as being caused by excessive gas or other related symptoms stemming from the GI tract [3].

In a study utilizing concurrent high-resolution manometry and impedance monitoring in patients with severe, frequent burping, it was found that most exhibited supragastric belches [8]. These were characterized by a downward (aboral) movement of the diaphragm

Practical Gastroenterology and Hepatology Board Review Toolkit, Second Edition. Edited by Nicholas J. Talley, Kenneth R. DeVault, Michael B. Wallace, Bashar A. Aqel and Keith D. Lindor.
© 2016 John Wiley & Sons, Ltd. Published 2016 by John Wiley & Sons, Ltd. Companion website: www.practicalgastrohep.com

Table 10.1 Chain of events in supragastric belching (after Kessing *et al.* 2012 [8]).

1. Concurrent contraction of the esophagogastric junction (EGJ) and aboral displacement of the diaphragm
2. Decrease in pressure in the esophageal body
3. Relaxation of the upper esophageal sphincter (UES)
4. Sucking of air into the esophagus
5. Forcing out of air from the esophagus in a retrograde direction

Table 10.2 Causes of belching (eructation).

GI causes (most common)	Extra-GI causes (less common)
• GERD • FD • Esophagitis • Esophageal dysmotility • Gastritis • Gallbladder disease • Pancreatitis • IBS • Gastroparesis • Hiatal hernia • SIBO • Peptic ulcer disease • Gastritis • Celiac disease • Lactose intolerance	• Cardiovascular (unstable angina, MI, and heart failure) • Pulmonary (PNA, pleural effusion, pneumothorax) • CNS (stroke, meningitis, encephalitis, subarachnoid hemorrhage) • Miscellaneous (smoking cigarettes, drinking carbonated beverages)

GI, gastrointestinal; GERD, gastroesophageal reflux disease; FD, functional dyspepsia; IBS, irritable bowel syndrome; SIBO, small-intestine bacterial overgrowth; MI, myocardial infarction; PNA, pulmonary nodular amyloidosis; CNS, central nervous system.

with an increase in esophagogastric junction (EGJ) pressure, a decrease in luminal esophageal pressure, and subsequent relaxation of the UES. The negative intrathoracic pressure created allows for antegrade airflow into the esophagus. However, almost immediately (within 1 second), an increase in esophageal and gastric pressure expels the air out of the esophagus in the retrograde direction (Table 10.1, Figure 10.1). In contrast, the manometry of a gastric belch is defined by a decrease in LES pressure (which is significantly lower than that seen during supragastric belching) and a simultaneous increase in esophageal pressure, creating a "common cavity" phenomenon. This precedes the venting of air into the esophagus, followed by UES relaxation, which allows the air to escape into the pharynx and oral cavity. Gastric belches are not felt to be under voluntary control [1, 2, 4, 8].

Patients with aerophagia and excessive intestinal gas can be shown to exhibit excessive air-swallowing by impedance monitoring [13]. They belch to a much lesser degree than those with classic eructation [9]. Watson [11] has suggested a relationship between GERD, LES pathophysiology, and the development of aerophagia in patients using CPAP [11]. Patients with aerophagia on CPAP can be shown to have greater degrees of nocturnal reflux compared to those without CPAP-associated aerophagia [12].

Clinical Features

Supragastric belching is a voluntary, behavioral act (think of the impromptu burping contests that are frequently held in college ratskellers). However, this form of eructation may also be a presenting feature of underlying psychiatric disorders and certain medical conditions, such as encephalitis (Table 10.2) [1,2,7]. Sufferers belch repetitively, but not while asleep or speaking, or when they are distracted [1,7]. Both gastric and supragastric belching can be a manifestation of GERD [3, 14, 15], and eructation can be a significant factor in reducing health-related quality of life [16].

In a study describing the initial presentation of patients with aerophagia seeking medical attention at the Mayo Clinic (Rochester, MN) between 1996 and 2003, the most common symptoms reported were belching (56% of cases), abdominal pain (19%), bloating (27%), and abdominal distension (19%). Patients with FD had a higher prevalence of nausea, vomiting, early satiety, weight loss, and abdominal pain than did the aerophagia patients. In contrast, significantly more individuals with aerophagia had anxiety (19%) compared to those with FD (6%) [17]. Adult and pediatric patients with primary aerophagia often present with excessive intestinal gas and bloating rather than eructation [10], and complications such as ileus, volvulus, and intestinal perforation have been reported in extreme cases [18]. In studies of aerophagia among school-aged children, air-swallowing was associated with sleeping difficulties, chronic diarrhea, photophobia, headaches, and limb pain [19, 20]. Causes of aerophagia are given in Table 10.3.

Diagnostic Testing

The diagnosis of supragastric belching can usually be made by simply observing the subject in the office. Repetitive belching up to 20 times a minute may be seen, although the burping stops when the patient is talking or when distracted. Some patients confuse eructation with singultus (hiccups), but the astute clinician should

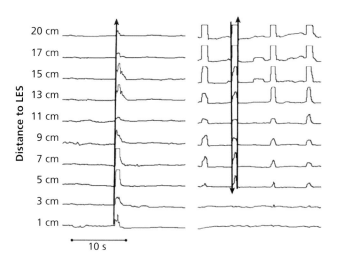

Figure 10.1 Manometric differences between gastric (left) and supragastric (right) belching. During the gastric belch, air moves in a proximal direction. During the supragastric belch, air enters the esophagus from a proximal direction and is immediately expelled in a retrograde direction. Source: Bredenoord 2007 [2]. Reproduced with permission of Elsevier.

Table 10.3 Causes of aerophagia.

Anxiety/behavioral disorders
Emotional/physical stress
Continuous positive airway pressure (CPAP)
Tourette's syndrome
Cognitive impairment, mental retardation
Laryngectomy
Huntington's disease
Rett's syndrome and other neurodevelopment disorders
Tricyclic antidepressants (and other drugs causing dry mouth)

be able to distinguish the two quite easily, both by the sound that is made and by whether the diaphragm is contracting (in hiccups). Conventional manometry for belching has largely been supplanted by the use of high-resolution manometry and impedance monitoring. While this is usually reserved for research studies, it can be of use in differentiating between the variants in difficult cases and helping to guide therapy [1]. Interestingly, the size of the gastric air bubble is not different among patients with gastric and supragastric belching [5]. If there are associated alarm symptoms such as heartburn, dysphagia, weight loss, GI bleeding, vomiting, bloating, or diarrhea, then it is recommended that a further workup with upper endoscopy and biopsy, or other testing modalities, be considered, depending on the suspected underlying disorder (e.g., breath testing for small-intestine bacterial overgrowth (SIBO), lactose intolerance, or *H. pylori* gastritis; celiac disease serology; gastric emptying scintigraphy; esophageal pH testing).

For aerophagia, excessive GI air will be present on abdominal radiographs in patients observed to have excessive air-swallowing [10]. Abdominal distention, tympany, signs of ileus, and so on may be present on physical exam. Esophageal impedance has also been used in this setting to help differentiate patients from those with supragastric belching [1, 5]. Rarely will massive abdominal distention, ileus, volvulus, or bowel perforation occur [18].

Therapeutic Approach

Gastric belching is a benign physiologic condition that requires no specific treatment. On the other hand, supragastric belching can impair quality of life [16], and therapy for this voluntary, behavioral disorder should be aimed at the underlying cause. Bredenoord advises that the patient should be made to understand the mechanism of his or her belching, and that efforts should be made to uncover the principal cause(s) [1]. Treating underlying esophageal reflux and other recognized GI disorders has been effective [3]. Speech, behavioral, and psychotherapy may be useful when no underlying cause is found [1, 21]. Katzka has described his method of controlling belching using a breathing approach. He instructs the patient to breathe slowly though an open mouth while lying supine and then while in a sitting position. Wide mouth opening is taught as a rescue measure. Following this protocol, four out of five patients were able to control their belching successfully [23]. With respect to drug therapy, baclofen, a gamma aminobutyric acid (GABA) receptor agonist used as an antispasmodic in conditions such as multiple sclerosis (MS), was demonstrated to significantly reduce the number of supragastric belches when given in a dose of 10 mg thrice daily [24].

For aerophagia, minimization of air-swallowing can be achieved by refraining from sucking on hard candies, chewing gum, eating too rapidly, and drinking carbonated beverages, and by drinking through a straw [1, 10]. The empiric use of simethicone-containing anti-gas products may also be helpful [1]. Treating underlying conditions leading to excessive gas and flatus, such as reflux disease, celiac disease, lactose intolerance, and SIBO may also help to control symptoms. As many instances appear to stem from a psychological condition, speech therapy may be helpful, along with behavioral and psychiatric approaches [1, 3]. Baclofen has also been used to control aerophagia [24]. In instances where extreme aerophagia causes massive bowel distention – placing the patient at risk of life-threatening complications, such as perforation, volvulus, and severe ileus (seen predominantly in patients with severe neurological or

cognitive impairment disorders) – surgical intervention has been utilized [18, 25].

Take Home Points

- Gastric belching is a physiologic reflex, whereas supragastric belching is a behavioral disorder.
- "Aerophagia" refers to excessive air-swallowing leading to accumulation of gas in the GI tract.
- Supragastric eructation can be distinguished from gastric belches and aerophagia manometrically.
- Diagnosing and treating underlying conditions (such as GERD) may help control belching.
- Consider psychological assessment and behavioral therapies for patients with associated anxiety or other psychological disorders where belching or aerophagia may impair quality of life.
- Anti-gas measures such as avoiding carbonated beverages, drinking through a straw, and eating slowly may help decrease aerophagia.
- Use of baclofen and simethicone-containing products may be of benefit in eructation and aerophagia.
- Surgical intervention has been required in cases of life-threatening massive abdominal distention or perforation due to extreme aerophagia.

Halitosis

Summary

The majority of cases of halitosis originate from the oral cavity. Less commonly, halitosis can be caused by a systemic (e.g., liver failure), esophageal, or gastric disease. Initial evaluation may lead to an oral source, such as poor dentition, periodontal disease, or a dental or tonsillar abscess. Mouthwash can reduce oral bacteria and neutralize odors. On rare occasions, gas chromatography is useful to distinguish the offending gas. Since the tongue may be a source, tongue cleaning is warranted.

Case

A 48-year-old female comes to the physician stating that the last two social relationships in which she was involved ended with the man saying he didn't enjoy kissing her because she had bad breath. She has gone to the dentist, who told her that she had no dental or periodontal problems. She has tried six different mouthwashes that she saw advertised on TV, but they didn't work for her like they did for the ladies in the commercials, who smiled and kissed their husbands with relief. She says she has read in a magazine that there is some stomach infection that can cause halitosis and she wants to be tested for that. She also has symptoms of reflux, but taking antacids and over-the-counter acid suppressants hasn't made a difference.

The gastroenterologist reluctantly schedules her for an endoscopy, which is normal except for a small hiatal hernia. Biopsies from the antrum and body are taken and both reveal *H. pylori*. The patient is placed on a 14-day course of PPI and two antibiotics, and reports that her breath has improved. A urea breath test for *H. pylori* 3 months later shows no evidence of infection. She contacts one of the men who had been offended by her breath and they have a few more dates, but eventually he breaks up with her saying he doesn't like her personality. She meets another man 6 months later over the Internet and they are eventually married in Aruba.

Definition and Epidemiology

"Halitosis" describes an unpleasant or offensive odor in the breath. This condition has been associated with psychosocial embarrassment and may impact personal relationships [26]. It is quite common, affecting people of all ages, with a prevalence based on a few population studies from various countries ranging from 15 to 30% [27–29].

Bad breath is worse upon awakening; this is termed "morning halitosis" [26]. This usually has no clinical consequence, resulting from increased microbial metabolic activity during sleep and decreased salivary flow [30]. More than three-quarters of patients complaining of chronic halitosis have a cause that stems from the oral cavity, such as poor dental hygiene, periodontal disease, ill-fitting dentures that trap food, tongue coatings, tonsilliths, or pharyngeal infections [31–33]

Halitophobics are individuals who fear they have bad breath, when in fact they do not. They wrongly interpret the actions of others as an indication of their having offensive breath and often become fixated with teeth-cleaning, gum-chewing, and using mouthwash [26]. Such patients constitute up to 25% of those seeking professional counseling for bad breath [34].

Etiology and Pathophysiology

Halitosis originates from either the oral cavity, the nasal passages, or the tonsils, with systemic or respiratory causes being less common (Table 10.4) [31–33,35]; 80–90% of all cases originate from the oral cavity [31–33, 36]. The tongue is the major source of halitosis, and periodontal disease represents a relatively small fraction of the overall problem [31,37–39]. The oral malodor arises from microbial degradation of organic substrates present in saliva, oral soft tissues, and retained debris. Microbial degradation products are volatile sulfur-containing compounds (VSCs) [40]. Many Gram-positive and -negative bacteria have been implicated; these are most likely to accumulate when food debris collects in between teeth, in the gingival crevices, and at the posterior portion of the tongue. The dorsal aspect of the tongue may retain large amounts of desquamated cells, leukocytes, and microorganisms [26,41]. Oral pathology, such as advanced gingivitis and periodontal disease, also contributes to halitosis [37]. Other dental problems and poor oral hygiene have been associated with halitosis, including peri-implant disease, deep carious lesions, exposed necrotic tooth pulp, oral wounds, imperfect dental restorations, and unclean dentures [42]. Xerostomia due to disease or medications also has potential to cause or enhance malodor.

The nasal passages are the second most common cause of halitosis [36]. Nasal malodour is "cheesy," which differs from other forms of bad breath [43]. Causes include sinusitis, nasal polyps affecting airflow, and a history of cleft palate or other craniofacial anomalies. Foreign bodies placed in nostrils are a common cause of halitosis in children [44]. The tonsils are a minor but important cause of halitosis; the odor is created from tonsilloliths that form in the crypts of the tonsils [45]. Because tonsil stones contain mouth debris primarily made up of active bacteria, they emit large amounts of sulfur, which causes bad breath. These anaerobic bacteria thrive in conditions that are lacking in oxygen but rich in food particles and postnasal mucus. As a result, tonsil stones emit odorous sulfur compounds, resembling the smell of rotting eggs. This kind of halitosis is especially noticeable when someone with tonsil stones accidentally bites down on one that has become dislodged from a tonsil crevice.

Other causes of halitosis include respiratory, bronchial, and lung infections, which may result in nasal or sinus secretions passing into the oropharynx [31]. Some systemic causes of bad breath include kidney failure, liver failure, various carcinomas, medications, metabolic dysfunction, and biochemical disorders [46]. Classically, acetone breath has been associated with uncontrolled diabetes, but this is not very common. Interestingly, no differences in malodor measurements are seen between diabetics and non-diabetics [47]. Carcinomas in the oral cavity, pharynx, tonsils, base of the tongue, and nasopharynx are other potential causes of halitosis in a patient with the appropriate risk factors [30,31]. Halitosis has been reported in several patients who have suffered a stroke [48].

Trimethylaminuria ("fish-odor syndrome") is a rare disorder characterized by oral and body malodor. This genetic disorder involves the inability to break down trimethylamine-N-oxide, resulting in excess trimethylamine, which produces a pungent ammoniacal odor, similar to that of rotten fish. Management includes reducing or eliminating precursors of trimethylamine in the diet, such as rapeseed oil, carnitine, certain legumes, and sulfur-containing foods, including eggs [49].

Halitosis is rarely associated with diseases of the esophagus, stomach, and intestines and is generally not an indication for endoscopy. Recently, an association has been described between halitosis and GERD, but this is still somewhat speculative [50]. In contrast, *H. pylori* has been shown to produce sulfur compounds, and has been considered as a possible cause of halitosis [51].

Some halitosis results purely from lifestyle choices. Certain habits, such as cigarette-smoking and alcohol consumption, are common causes of bad breath. The ingestion of certain foods, such as garlic, onions, spices, cabbage, cauliflower, and radishes, is classically associated with halitosis [30]. So-called "garlic breath" may persist for several hours or days despite meticulous oral hygiene, as the organosulfides are absorbed into systemic circulation and excreted through the lungs for hours after ingestion in the form of a gas (allyl methyl sulfide) [52].

Diagnosis

Before halitosis can be managed effectively, an accurate diagnosis must be achieved. A detailed history, including medical and dental history, diet, and a detailed oral and periodontal exam, is a necessary part of the evaluation. However, it is difficult for a patient to self-assess the extent of their disorder and it is recommended that they bring a confidant to the visit to provide more accurate data [53].

Table 10.4 Causes of halitosis.

Oral disease	Tongue, food particles, gingivitis, peridontitis, pericoronitis, xerostomia, oral ulceration, oral malignancy, peri-implant disease, deep carious lesions, exposed necrotic tooth pulp, oral wounds, imperfect dental restorations, unclean dentures
Nasal passages	Sinusitis, nasal polyps, history of cleft palate or craniofacial anomalies, foreign bodies
Oropharynx/ respiratory	Tonsilliths, foreign body, bronchial or lung infections, xerostomia
Systemic	Liver failure, chronic kidney disease, various carcinomas (oral cavity, pharynx, tonsils, tongue, nasopharynx), medications, metabolic dysfunction (diabetes), biochemical disorders (trimethylaminuria), stroke
Gastrointestinal	*H. pylori*, gastroesophageal reflux disease (GERD)
Lifestyle	Cigarette-smoking, alcohol, garlic, onions, spices, cabbage, cauliflower, radish

Physical exam includes a detailed oral and periodontal examination, preferably by a dentist, periodontist, otolaryngologist, or other expert in oral hygiene [33]. The ultimate assessment is made by smelling the exhaled air of the mouth and of the nose and comparing the two [54]. Odor from the mouth but not the nose is likely to have an oral source. Odor from the nose alone is likely to be coming from the nares or sinuses [55]. If the odors from the nose and mouth are similar, then the halitosis likely has a systemic cause. The Finkelstein tonsil-smelling test involves massaging the tonsils and smelling the squeezed discharge, which has a distinctive fetid odor when there is chronic infection [45]. More objective measurements of halitosis are available, but they are generally not used clinically because of their expense and due to time constraints. Instruments used to detect VSCs generally cannot detect other classes of volatile compound and are therefore insensitive [30]. Gas chromatography is the method of choice for distinguishing the gas mixture of bad breath, and less cumbersome, less expensive gas chromatographs are being developed [30].

Therapeutics

Management of halitosis depends largely on the identified cause. The majority of patients have an oral source, and management will focus on managing oral halitosis (Figure 10.2). Treatment is aimed at educating the patient as to the common causes of halitosis and the tools available to prevent it, which include good oral hygiene, with brushing and flossing. Avoiding smoking, drugs, and food that may contribute to halitosis is often recommended. In addition, chewing gum or sucking on breath mints or fennel seeds may mask the bad breath. Treatment is also directed at reducing accumulation of food debris and malodor-producing bacteria. This requires treating oral/dental diseases, making sure dentures or prosthetics are well-fitting, improving oral hygiene, and reducing tongue coating.

Oral hygiene involves regular tooth-brushing, flossing, and tongue-scraping. Rinsing and gargling with mouthwash have been used to reduce oral bacteria and neutralize exhaled odoriferous compounds [56]. Mouthwashes containing chlorhexidine gluconate, cetylpyridinium chloride, or triclosan have shown some benefit [57, 58]. A recent Cochrane review pooled five randomized controlled trials (RCTs) and concluded that mouth rinses may play an effective role in reducing halitosis, but some of the trials had incomplete data [59].

If oral hygiene is already good, the tongue is the likely source of halitosis, and hence tongue-cleaning is indicated. The aim is to dislodge trapped food, cells, and bacteria from between the filiform papillae in order to decrease the concentration of VSCs. Tongue-cleaning may be done with a tongue scraper or toothbrush. Studies have shown a limited benefit of prolonged tongue-scraping, but many still recommend this be done regularly [41, 60]. A combination of brushing and tongue-scraping may provide more benefit than either method alone [61]. Tonsilliths causing halitosis have been treated successfully with laser cryptolysis [45, 62].

Antibiotics aimed at eliminating mouth flora have been used by multiple physicians, but they often result in only a transient relief of halitosis and their use is not advisable. Treatment of *H. pylori* with triple therapy in patients with FD resulted in resolution of halitosis in one study [63]. Dental referral for patients with persistent halitosis is reasonable, when odor is deemed to be originating from an oral source. If the cause of halitosis is identified (e.g., periodontal disease, gingivitis, postnasal drip, systemic illness), treatment is to resolve the patient's underlying condition. Vaccines targeting fusobacteria nucleatum, which are a major cause of plaque biofilm, will offer a unique approach to combating halitosis in the future [64].

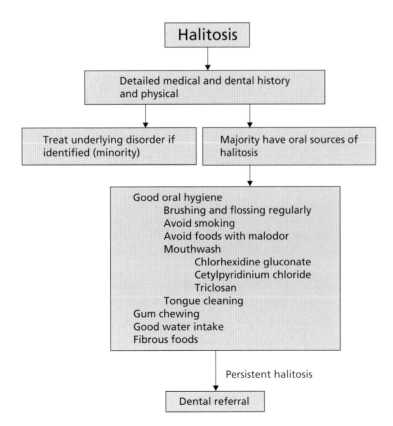

Figure 10.2 Treatment algorithm for halitosis.

CHAPTER 10

Take Home Points

Diagnosis:

- 80–90% of cases of halitosis originate from the oral cavity, with the tongue and periodontal disease being the major sources.
- Tonsilliths are a minor but important cause of halitosis.
- Halitosis is rarely associated with diseases of the esophagus, stomach, or intestines and is generally not an indication for endoscopy.
- A detailed history, including medical and dental history, diet, and a detailed oral and periodontal exam, is an important part of the evaluation.
- Therapy:
- Treatment focuses on educating the patient as to the common causes of halitosis and what tools are available to prevent it; these include good oral hygiene, with brushing and flossing, and the avoidance of smoking and certain foods.
- Mouthwash can reduce oral bacteria and neutralize odoriferous compounds.
- Studies have shown a limited benefit of prolonged tongue-scraping, but this is still recommended in patients with halitosis.
- Dental referral for patients with persistent halitosis is reasonable.
- Effective halitosis vaccines appear to be in development.

Hiccups

Summary

Most instances of transient hiccups are of little clinical significance. If hiccups last for more than 48 hours, that often implies an underlying structural, physical, or neoplastic disorder, which necessitates an evaluation for a cause. The afferent limb of the hiccup arc is via the vagus and phrenic nerves, and the efferent limb is via the phrenic nerve. More than 100 conditions have been associated with hiccups. Men are more likely to have an underlying cause discovered than women. Hiccups are commonly seen with medications used for endoscopy, but the explanation is not clear. Among the GI causes of hiccups are GERD, infectious esophagitis, achalasia, and carcinomatosis. Chlorpromazine is the only Food and Drug Administration (FDA)-approved drug for hiccups. Baclofen has emerged as the most successful pharmacologic treatment.

Case

A 54-year-old male is hospitalized for persistent vomiting, dehydration, abdominal pain, and hiccups of 1 week's duration. He had been receiving outpatient external beam radiation therapy for retroperitoneal sarcoma that was initially treated with local resection 10 months earlier, but was admitted from the radiation oncology clinic after a recent abdominal computed tomography (CT) scan revealed progression of his disease with studding of the peritoneum consistent with carcinomatosis and dilated small-bowel loops with air/fluid levels consistent with obstruction. The stomach is also found to be dilated, but his abdomen is only minimally distended. He refuses nasogastric decompression, preferring to be made nothing by mouth (nil per os, NPO) and given intravenous fluids. His hiccups have increased in frequency to about 12 times per minute and are now occurring around the clock and interfering with his ability to sleep.

Chlorpromazine is administered at a dose of 25 mg IV every 8 hours, but this produces unwanted somnolence and hypotension and is discontinued in favor of metoclopramide 10 mg IV every 6 hours. However, the hiccups still fail to respond after another 72 hours and the patient is evaluated by the gastroenterology service,

which recommendeds a percutaneous endoscopic gastrostomy (PEG) for decompression, since he is adamant that he does not want a nasogastric tube; however, the PEG is also refused. It is recommended that baclofen 10 mg every 6 hours be tried. Over the course of the next 48 hours, the hiccups decrease in frequency, and they disappear 2 days later. The patient is able to tolerate small amounts of liquids and is discharged on baclofen.

Definition and Epidemiology

Hiccups have long been considered a medical curiosity. Although most hiccups occur as brief, self-limited episodes lasting up to a few minutes, persistent hiccups that last longer than 48 hours or recur at frequent intervals often imply an underlying physical, structural, metabolic, neoplastic, or infectious cause. Occasionally, hiccups are intractable, occurring continuously for months or years, and can result in significant morbidity [65]. Intractable hiccups are responsible for approximately 4000 hospitalizations per year in the United States [66]. Interestingly, hiccups affect men more than women [67].

The term "hiccup" refers to the onomatopeic attempt to vocalize the sound produced by the abrupt closure of the glottis after the sudden contraction of the inspiratory muscles [68]. "Hiccough" was used in the older literature and likely represented the previously held belief that hiccups occur as a result of abnormal respiratory reflex. The medical term for hiccups, "singultus," is derived from the Latin root *singult*, meaning the act of catching one's breath during sobbing [65].

Pathophysiology/Clinical Features

Hiccups do not appear to serve any particularly useful or protective function. However, because they may occur during fetal and neonatal life and are seen in other mammals, they may represent a primitive or vestigial reflex whose functional or behavioral significance has been lost [69, 70]. One theory speculates that intrauterine hiccups permit training of the diaphragm without aspiration of amniotic fluid [71].

A relationship between hiccups and the phrenic nerve was recognized by an Edinburgh physician in 1833 [72]. Current theories, developed further by Bailey and colleagues, describe the concept of a hiccup reflex arc [73, 74]. In current theory, the afferent limb of hiccup reflex is composed of the vagus and phrenic nerves and the sympathetic chain arising from T6–T12, with a hiccup center located in the upper spinal cord (C3–C5). The efferent limb remains primarily the phrenic nerve, although nerves to the glottis and accessory muscles of the respiration are also involved, as patients are reported to continue to hiccup even after transection of both phrenic nerves [65, 75]. This reflex pathway is similar to those that produce coughing, sneezing, swallowing, and vomiting [68] (Figure 10.3).

More than 100 conditions have been associated with hiccups, including a variety of structural, metabolic, inflammatory, neoplastic, infectious, and drug-related causes (Table 10.5). For many, a relationship with one or more limbs of the reflex arc can be demonstrated, whereas for others, the association is more obscure [65].

Benign Transient Causes

Transient hiccups are benign and occur in nearly all individuals from time to time. Such hiccups are often caused by overdistension of the stomach, commonly due to overeating, drinking carbonated beverages, aerophagia, drinking alcohol, and sudden excitement or emotional stress [65]. The mechanism is presumed to be gastric

Inhalation   Exhalation

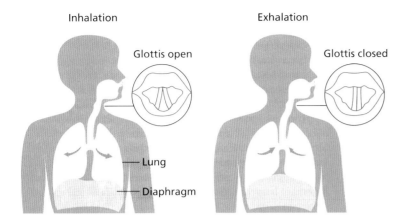

Figure 10.3 Anatomic representation of the diaphragm, lungs, and glottis in inhalation and exhalation during hiccups.

distension, stimulating gastric branches of vagus nerve, or direct irritation of the diaphragm by an overinflated stomach [65, 68]. Alcohol-induced hiccups are also likely to result from gastric distension and/or the central effects of alcohol on the cerebral cortex, which remove inhibitions normally serving to dampen the hiccup reflex [76]. Sudden excitement, emotional stress, smoking, and changes in food/body temperature have also been associated with temporary hiccups [68].

Table 10.5 Causes of persistent hiccups. Source: Lewis 1995.

Central nervous system
Structural lesions: intracranial neoplasms, hydrocephalus, MS, brainstem tumors, syringomyelia, ventriculi–peritoneal shunt, glaucoma, Parkinson's disease
Vascular lesions: vascular insufficiency, arteriovenous malformation, intracranial hemorrhage, temporal arteritis
Trauma: skull fracture, epilepsy
Infectious: meningitis, encephalitis, neurosyphilis, brain abscess
Toxic–metabolic
Chronic kidney disease, diabetes mellitus, alcohol, gout, hyponatremia, hypokalemia, hypocalcemia, hypocarbia, fever, insulin shock therapy
Diaphragmatic irritation
Diaphragmatic tumors, eventration, myocardial infarction, pericarditis, hiatus hernia, splenomegaly, hepatomegaly, subphrenic abscess, perihepatitis, esophageal cancer, aberrant cardiac pacemaker electrode
Vagus nerve irritation
Meningeal branches: meningitis
Pharyngeal branches pharyngitis, laryngitis
Auricular branches: hair, insect, foreign body
Recurrent laryngeal nerve: goiter, neck cyst, tumors, scrofula
Thoracic branches: pneumonia, empyema, bronchitis, asthma, pleuritis, achalasia, sarcoidosis, esophageal obstruction, esophagitis, thoracic aortic aneurysm, tuberculosis, myocardial infarction, pericarditis, mediastinitis, cor pulmonale, herpes zoster, lung cancer, mediastinal hematoma
Abdominal branches: gastric distension, gastric cancer, gastritis, peptic ulcer, gastric ulcer, pancreatic cancer, pancreatitis, pseudocyst, intra-abdominal abscess, bowel obstruction, cholelithiasis, cholecystitis, abdominal aortic aneurysm, ulcerative colitis, Crohn disease, GI hemorrhage, prostatic disorders, parasitic infestation, appendicitis, hepatitis
Drugs
Methyldopa, short-acting barbiturates, dexamethasone, methylprednisolone, diazepam, chlordiazepoxide
General anesthesia
Inadequate ventilation, suppression of normal inhibitory influences, intubation, recovery period, traction of viscera, hyperextension of neck, gastric distension or ileus
Postoperative
Manipulation of diaphragm, prostatic and urinary tract surgery, craniotomy, thoracotomy, laparotomy
Infectious
Meningitis, encephalitis, typhoid fever, cholera, *Candida* esophagitis, malaria, herpes zoster, acute rheumatic fever, influenza, tuberculosis
Psychogenic
Hysterical neurosis, conversion reaction, sudden shock, grief reaction, malingering, personality disorders, anorexia nervosa, enuresis

Intraoperative hiccups may occur for a number of reasons, including extension of the neck with stretching of the roots of the phrenic nerve, use of short-acting barbiturates, inadequate ventilation during anesthesia, gastric distension, or ileus. A light plane of anesthesia may suppress inhibitory influences that normally function to prevent hiccups. Postoperative hiccups account for as much as 25% of hiccups in men, usually appearing within 4 days of surgery. A majority of these episodes follow intra-abdominal surgery, with the remainder resulting from urinary tract, central nervous system (CNS), and chest surgery procedures [68]. Hiccups are also commonly seen during endoscopy, either from the use of opioids or midazolam used for sedation, or from gastric distension from air insufflation.

Persistent Hiccups
The longer the duration of a hiccup bout, the more likely an organic cause exists. The etiopathogenic causes of persistent and intractable hiccups can be broadly categorized as CNS disorders, toxic–metabolic causes, diseases affecting the diaphragm or vagus nerve, drugs, general anesthesia, postoperative causes, and inflammatory, neoplastic, and infectious causes (Table 10.5). All these causes stimulate one or more limbs of the hiccup reflex arc.

Of particular interest to gastroenterologists are the GI and hepatic causes of hiccups. Conditions such as GERD, infectious esophagitis, esophageal obstruction (stricture, cancer, rings), achalasia, abdominal carcinomatosis, and widespread surgical adhesions have been associated with hiccups [68]. Significant morbidity has been associated with intractable hiccups. Inability to eat, significant weight loss, exhaustion, insomnia, cardiac arrhythmias, and even death have all been associated with persistent hiccups [65].

Evaluation
Brief hiccup bouts are common and do not require medical intervention. However, persistent and intractable hiccups necessitate a thorough evaluation in order to find the underlying etiology and guide successful treatment. The extent of the workup should reflect the degree of morbidity. An underlying organic cause is discovered in 90% of men with persistent hiccups, whereas women are less likely to have a specific cause identified [65]. A complete history, including the duration of the hiccups, alcohol and drug use, and medications, should be sought. Physical examination should be focused on eliciting structural or neurological abnormalities, mass lesions, tenderness, or inflammation. Hiccups have been attributed to foreign bodies in the ear canal, prompting a thorough aural exam.

Initial laboratory tests should include a complete blood count (CBC), chemistry panel, urinanalysis, and chest X-ray. Liver-associated enzymes, thyroid tests, electrocardiogram (ECG), and imaging of the abdomen, pelvis, thorax, and head are often performed routinely. In cases where the likely cause of hiccups remains obscure, additional testing can be pursued, including lumbar puncture, panendoscopy, esophageal manometry, pulmonary function tests, bronchoscopy, and electroencephalogram (EEG). Exploratory laparotomy or other surgery is occasionally required.

Therapeutics

Numerous therapies have been proposed for the control or elimination of hiccups [77]. However, most of these are based on a small number of isolated case reports and many of the better-known hiccup "cures" are mostly anecdotal. Whenever possible, treatment should be directed at the specific illness causing the hiccups (Figure 10.4).

Non-pharmalogic Therapy

Many of the original "hiccup cures" can be traced back hundreds or thousands of years. Plato is credited with being the first to recommend a sudden slap on the back as a means of scaring away hiccups. This probably worked by inducing a sudden gasp in the person being struck, thereby breaking the hiccup cycle, and giving rise to other therapies aimed at disrupting the respiratory rhythm [65,78]. These included breath-holding, gargling with water, and tickling the nose to induce sneezing [79, 80]. Other physical and mechanical cures attempt to disrupt the diaphragmatic contractions that occur during hiccupping. Pulling the knees up to the chest or leaning forward to compress the diaphragm [65] may increase positive airway pressure and hyperinflate the lungs, which stimulates the Hering–Breuer reflex and disrupts the abnormal hiccup pattern [81]. Performing a Valsalva maneuver, hyperventilating, inducing involuntary gasping using smelling salts, and inhaling 5% carbon dioxide have also been described [68]. Counterstimulating the vagal branches of the

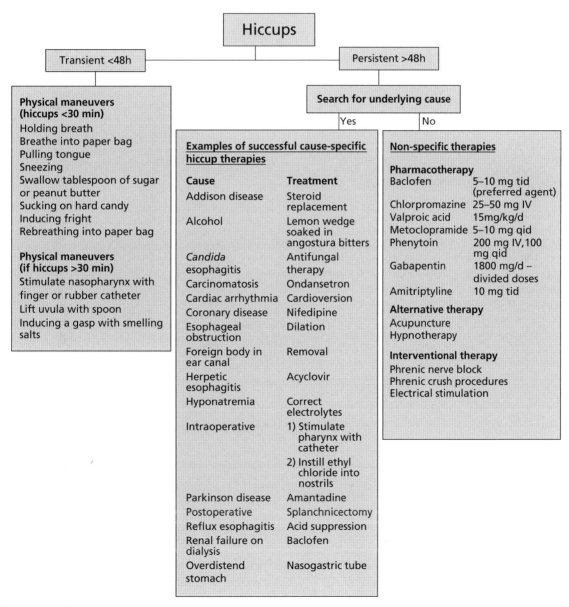

Figure 10.4 Algorithm for treating hiccups.

pharynx has been accomplished by swallowing a teaspoon of sugar in a single "gulp."

Relief of gastric distension with emetics, gastric lavage, or nasogastric aspiration may be an effective way of relieving hiccups when the stomach is overdistended with air, food, or liquid. Stimulation of the oropharynx is often cited as a way of terminating hiccups. This can be achieved by placing traction on the tongue, lifting the uvula with a spoon, manipulating the pharynx with a rubber tube or cotton swab, or swallowing granulated sugar, honey, or peanut butter. Each method has anecdotal success, suggesting that irritation of the soft palate or pharynx may inhibit afferent impulses transmitted by the vagus nerve [68].

Hypnotherapy and acupuncture have reportedly been used to cure hiccups arising from a number of different causes [80]. While acupuncture for hiccups has traditionally been practiced in East Asia, it is becoming a more commonplace therapy in Western centers as well, especially when no specific cause of hiccups can be identified. However, recent systematic reviews of hiccup treatments found insufficient evidence to guide therapy with acupuncture or other non-pharmacological or drug interventions [81, 82].

Pharmacotherapy

Several pharmacologic agents have been used for the treatment of persistent or intractable hiccups, although there are few controlled trials to confirm what is largely anecdotal evidence of their success [65, 68, 81]. The following agents have been the most frequently employed for hiccups of various causes. Doses and routes of administration are provided in Figure 10.4.

- **Baclofen:** An analog of the inhibitory neurotransmitter GABA, baclofen has emerged as the most successful general hiccup therapy, with multiple studies showing successful treatment of hiccups [83–87]. Baclofen is believed to reduce excitability and depress reflex hiccup activity, as demonstrated in animal studies. It has also found utility in the treatment of rumination and supragastric belching [88]. Baclofen is relatively fast-acting, with a half-life of 3–4 hours, and is cleared by the kidneys. Side effects include drowsiness, insomnia, weakness, ataxia, dizziness, and confusion, and may be poorly tolerated by elderly patients. The drug should be used cautiously in patients with renal failure [89, 90].
- **Chlorpromazine**: A phenothiazine antipsychotic, chlorpromazine is the only medication specifically approved by the FDA for the treatment of hiccups. Its use was first described in the 1950s, with an 80% success rate [91]. Intravenous administration is considered to be most effective, although the drug must be infused slowly to prevent hypotension. Oral doses (25–50 mg three times per day) have been used successfully as an alternative therapy for the treatment of hiccups [66]. Chlorpromazine tends to be more poorly tolerated in the elderly, causing dizziness and orthostatic hypotension.
- **Metoclopramide**: A dopamine antagonist and gastric motility agent, metoclopramide is often used in the treatment of hiccups, although it is not as effective as chloropromazine [92]. It has terminated hiccups in patients with gastric distension caused by diabetic gastroparesis.
- **Anticonvulsants**: Anticonvulsants such as phenytoin, valproic acid, carbamazepine, gabapentin, and the benzodiazepenes have had limited success in terminating hiccups [93–96].

Gabapentin has been shown to treat hiccups in patients with cancer and CNS disorders (Guillain–Barré and stroke) [66, 97–99]. A systematic review of case series and case reports demonstrates it is well tolerated, but is probably only useful as a second-line agent in stroke patients or those in palliative care settings [100].

Anesthesia-related hiccups have been stopped with methylphenidate, ethyl chloride spray, ephedrine, and catheter stimulation of the pharynx [101–103]. Postoperative hiccups have been cured with amphetamine and ketamine [104–106]. Marijuana has even been used in patients with acquired immunodeficiency syndrome (AIDS) [107]. Amantadine, a dopaminergic agonist, has had anecdotal success in treating hiccups in patients with Parkinson's disease [68]. Chronic hiccups associated with esophageal disorders (e.g., GERD, achalasia, esophagitis) have been relieved with appropriate treatment of the specific underlying condition [65, 68].

Conclusion

While the majority of hiccups are either socially amusing, embarrassing, or annoying, they are self-limited and rarely require treatment other than simple physical maneuvers such as holding the breath, pulling on the tongue, sneezing, sucking on hard candy, or swallowing some sugar or peanut butter. Persistent or intractable hiccups can be associated with significant morbidity and often require an extensive evaluation to find the cause. If an underlying condition cannot be treated specifically or effectively (e.g., carcinomatosis), pharmacologic therapy may be tried. If this proves unsuccessful, alternative therapeutic approaches, including acupuncture and hypnosis, can be attempted [80, 82].

Surgical approaches, including phrenic nerve-crushing and transection, or the use of phrenic nerve block with a local anesthetic, are reserved for refractory cases. Unfortunately, results have been variable, and such procedures may result in impaired respiratory function [68]. Electrical stimulation of the phrenic nerve has seen limited use in treating refractory hiccups [108].

Take Home Points

Evaluation:
- Transient hiccups are benign, last seconds to minutes, and do not require evaluation.
- Bouts lasting more than 48 hours often imply an underlying physical, infectious, structural, neoplastic, or metabolic disorder.
- Persistent hiccups necessitate a thorough evaluation in order to find the underlying etiology and guide successful treatment.
- The extent of the workup should reflect the degree of morbidity of the hiccups; even an extensive evaluation may at times fail to uncover a specific or readily treatable cause.

Treatment:
- Treatment begins with various physical and mechanical maneuvers for transient hiccups.
- Treat the specific underlying cause, when one is identified (e.g., GERD).
- Baclofen remains the only pharmacologic therapy with proven efficacy in the controlled clinical trial setting.
- Acupuncture, hypnosis, and surgical therapies to crush or transect phrenic nerves have been used in refractory cases.

Rumination

Summary

Rumination syndrome is a functional gastroduodenal disorder of unknown etiology characterized by repetitive, effortless regurgitation of recently ingested food into the mouth followed by remastication and reswallowing or expectoration [109–111]. It can be confused with bulimia, gastroesophageal reflux, functional vomiting, and gastroparesis, and the diagnosis is often delayed. However, recognizing the rumination syndrome is essential to avoiding inappropriate tests and offering unnecessary or ineffective treatments. For most cases, reassurance and behavioral therapy to regulate postprandial breathing are effective in managing the condition.

> ## Case
>
> An 18-year-old female presents with daily regurgitation with meals for 1 year. This occurs only when she is eating or shortly after eating. She has made a habit of rechewing and reswallowing the regurgitated food, but will spit it out when the regurgitant is bitter or sour. Persistent symptoms have led to reduced oral intake and 9 kg (20 lb) weight loss. She is given a diagnosis of GERD and told to start daily PPI. This fails to help her, and she returns for a further opinion.

Epidemiology

In contrast to the rumination seen in animals, the regurgitant is recognizable as recently consumed food [112]. While originally described in mentally challenged infants, the syndrome has been described in individuals of all ages and cognitive abilities [113–116]. There is almost an equal prevalence among disabled infants (6–10%) [113, 114] and institutionalized adults (8–10%) [115]. The syndrome is now recognized as a cause of postprandial regurgitation in children, adolescents, and adults with normal development [110, 111, 116, 117], although the prevalence of rumination in the normal development group is largely unknown. In part, this is due to the secretive nature of the condition in many patients and a lack of awareness among physicians [116]. The syndrome may remain misdiagnosed or undiagnosed for years [110], as it is frequently confused with anorexia nervosa, bulimia, GERD, and other motility disorders, such as gastroparesis and functional vomiting [112]. While some patients may have GERD or gastroparesis, these disorders are considered secondary to rumination and not the primary cause [109]. Criteria proposed by Chial *et al.* [111] (Table 10.6) are considered more accurate in children and adolescents than were the Rome II criteria at the time [109], but these have been supplanted by Rome III consensus criteria in the various age groups [112,118–120] (Table 10.7).

Clinical Features

Repetitive regurgitation usually begins within minutes of starting a meal and may persist for more than 60 minutes after completing it. A sensation of belching may precede regurgitation, and the regurgitated contents often consist of recognizable food [109,110].

Table 10.6 Modified clinical criteria for rumination syndrome in children and adolescents, proposed by Chial *et al.* in 2003 [111]. Source: Chial 2003. Reproduced with permission of the American Academy of Pediatrics.

At least 6 weeks, which may not be consecutive, in the previous 12 months of recurrent regurgitation of recently ingested food which:

1. Begins within 30 min of meal ingestion.
2. Is associated with either reswallowing or expulsion of food.
3. Stops within 90 min of onset or when regurgitant becomes acidic.
4. Is not associated with mechanical obstruction.
5. Does not respond to standard treatment for gastroesophageal reflux disease (i.e., medical therapy or lifestyle medication measures).
6. Is not associated with nocturnal symptoms.

Table 10.7 Rome III consensus criteria for rumination syndrome. Source: Adapted from [112, 118–120].

Neonate/toddler
Must include all of the following for at least 3 months:
1. Repetitive contractions of the abdominal muscles, diaphragm, and tongue.
2. Regurgitation of gastric content into the mouth, which is either expectorated or rechewed and reswallowed.
3. Three or more of the following:
   a. onset between 3 and 8 months;
   b. does not respond to management for GERD or to anticholinergic drugs, hand restraints, formula changes, or gavage or gastrostomy feedings;
   c. unaccompanied by signs of nausea or distress;
   d. does not occur during sleep or when the infant is interacting with individuals in the environment.

Child/adolescent
Must include all of the following:
1. Repeated painless regurgitation and rechewing or expulsion of food that:
   a. begin soon after ingestion of a meal;
   b. do not occur during sleep;
   c. do not respond to standard treatment for gastroesophageal reflux.
2. No retching.
3. No evidence of an inflammatory, anatomic, metabolic, or neoplastic process that explains the subject's symptoms.

Adult
Must include both of the following:
1. Persistent or recurrent regurgitation of recently ingested food into the mouth, with subsequent spitting or remastication and swallowing.
2. Regurgitation not preceded by retching.

Supportive criteria:
1. Regurgitation events usually not preceded by nausea.
2. Cessation of the process when the regurgitated material becomes acidic.
3. Regurgitant containing recognizable food, with a pleasant taste.

The patient makes a conscious decision to reswallow or expectorate the regurgitant [110]. Symptoms often cease when the remasticated food becomes acidic or bitter to the taste [110,111]. Weight loss may be considerable, and is not uncommon in female adolescents. Many individuals describe their regurgitation as vomiting, but close questioning can distinguish between the two.

In a series of 147 children and adolescents studied at the Mayo Clinic, Chial *et al.* [111] found that two-thirds were female, with a mean age of 15 years, and that they required more than 2 years of evaluation prior to having the diagnosis made. Only 16% had a psychiatric illness recorded. In a series of 38 adults and adolescents also followed at the Mayo Clinic, O'Brien *et al.* [110] noted that the patients saw an average of five physicians over 2.75 years prior to being given the diagnosis of rumination. No obvious triggering events were uncovered as a cause for the rumination in this group. Women outnumbered men by a ratio of three to one, but the authors noted that this was a lower F : M ratio than seen in bulimia.

Among 21 adults without a psychiatric history at a Korean tertiary referral center [109], no patient had a parent or sibling with rumination. Three patients (14.3%) had concurrent diabetes mellitus, and five (23.8%) had a history of abdominal surgery prior to the diagnosis of rumination syndrome. Three (14.3%) had a history of alcoholism and four (19.1%) smoked.

Pathophysiology and Diagnosis

While the etiology and pathophysiology of rumination remain unclear, it involves a rise in intragastric pressure generated by a voluntary contraction of the abdominal musculature at a time of low pressure in the LES, resulting in retrograde movement of gastric contents into the esophagus in the early postprandial period [112].

Normally, in health, LES pressure increases with increased intra-abdominal pressure. In contrast, in rumination, transient LES

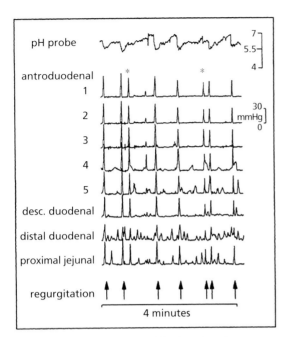

Figure 10.5 GI manometric tracing and distal esophageal pH in a rumination patient. Note the concurrence of regurgitation (arrows) with decreases in pH and R or simultaneous waves, consistent with increased intra-abdominal pressure. * Two R waves that are not associated with regurgitation or a decrease in intraesophageal pH. Source: O'Brien 1995. Reproduced with permission of Elsevier.

relaxations occur during these abdominal straining events. With the increase in gastric pressure that overcomes the LES pressure in rumination, allowing gastric contents to move into the esophagus, relaxation of the UES occurs and the contents can move orad into the pharynx and mouth. In addition, a forward extension of the head is thought to assist in opening the UES at the same moment [121].

Gastroduodenal manometry demonstrates brief, simultaneous increases in gastric and small-bowel pressure known as rumination or "R" waves, which are seen in all abdominal recording ports during the postprandial period [110] (Figure 10.5). While these R waves are characteristic of rumination, they are not present in up to 60% of patients and may not correlate with regurgitation events [110], which limits the usefulness of this diagnostic test. In contrast, high-resolution manometry and pH impedance measurement studies have revealed a typical motor pattern during rumination, defined as a reflux event extending into the proximal esophagus associated with an abdominal pressure increase of >30 mmHg and an esophageal pressure increase on combined pressure–impedance monitoring [122].

Three manometric variants of rumination are recognized [122] (Figure 10.6). Primary rumination is characterized by increased abdominal pressures preceding the retrograde flow of gastric contents. This primary rumination pattern is seen in 100% of individuals with the syndrome and is the predominant mechanism in two-thirds of patients. Secondary rumination is similar to the primary event, but the increase in abdominal pressure occurs after the onset of a reflux event, with the increased abdominal pressure considered secondary to reflux. This pattern occurs in approximately 45% of individuals, but is the predominant mechanism in only a minority. A third variant is known as supragastric belch-associated rumination, which is characterized by an aboral movement of the diaphragm that

creates a negative pressure in the body of the esophagus and concurrent relaxation of the UES. This allows inflow of air into the esophagus, followed by the immediate expulsion of the air. Abdominal pressure increases during the supragastric belch, allowing rumination to occur as the abdominal pressure increase occurs during the expulsion of air. This variant occurrs in 36% of patients and is the predominant mechanism in 25% [122].

Differential Diagnosis

Patients with rumination often have additional symptoms, such as nausea, heartburn, abdominal discomfort, diarrhea, constipation, and weight loss. As a result, the syndrome is frequently confused with other disorders, such as anorexia nervosa, bulimia, gastroparesis, and functional vomiting, and not surprisingly, many individuals undergo extensive testing before a diagnosis of rumination is finally made [110–112].

For those who undergo pH testing for possible GERD, impedance monitoring may actually be suggestive of acid reflux, but the tracings classically show a high number of repetitive events in the first postprandial hour and an erratic pattern of back-and-forth movement of regurgitation and reswallowing. In addition, there is an absence of nocturnal regurgitation events [112]. Gastric-emptying studies may be difficult to perform in these patients, as the potential for expectoration is high and so such studies are often incomplete. In contrast to the relatively rapid postprandial regurgitation seen with rumination, postprandial vomiting from gastroparesis is often delayed for many hours [110], after which the food is no longer recognizable as such by taste [112]. Moreover, while vomiting may be intermittent or dependent on the meal in gastroparesis, rumination invariably occurs with every meal, and often also after ingestion of only liquids [112].

While a lack of awareness of the clinical features, the female predominance, and the considerable weight loss on presentation often contributes to the misdiagnosis or underdiagnosis of the rumination syndrome, a thorough history and clinical observation are usually sufficient to confirm its presence, without the need for manometry [110].

Treatment

Treatment of rumination is best accomplished with behavioral modification and biofeedback therapy administered in a formal eating-regulation program. The behavioral approach focuses on diaphragmatic breathing as a means to create a competing behavior and break the cycle of food regurgitation [109, 111, 112, 123–125]. Chitkara et al. [124] have described a technique whereby the patient is taught to place a hand on the chest and one on the abdomen, and is instructed that only the hand on the abdomen should move with breathing. This helps teach patients to relax their abdominal muscles during and after eating, which directly competes with the urge to regurgitate. The success of this and others maneuvers is reported to be good, with 30–66% of patients having rumination disappear, and an additional 20–55% experiencing improvement [112]. Among 21 adults treated with prokinetic agents and psychotherapy over a 6-month period, abnormal esophageal manometric measurements improved in 8, remained unchanged in 10, and worsened in 3 [109]. Overall, the use of oral medications, such as antidepressants, antiemetics, PPIs, prokinetics, and anticholinergics, has been disappointing [110,112]. However, baclofen in a dose of 10 mg thrice daily has been shown to reduce rumination based on high-resolution manometry and impedance recordings [126] and may be considered as an adjunct to behavioral therapy. Similarly,

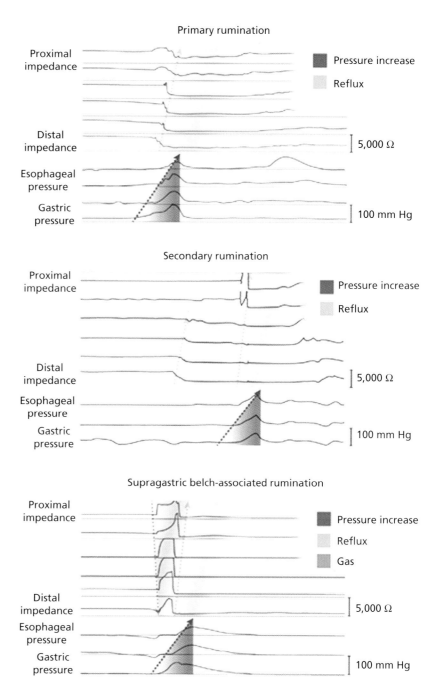

Figure 10.6 Three manometric variants of rumination, as measured by combined ambulatory manometry and pH impedance monitoring. Source: Boudewijn 2014 [14]. Reproduced with permission of Macmillan Publishers.

chewing gum has been suggested as an alternative for children and adolescents [112]. While surgical intervention (e.g., Nissen fundoplication, gastric pacing) has been performed, it is generally not recommended, and in fact may worsen rumination symptoms due to the patient's loss of ability to engage in this behavior in the absence of an effective psychological intervention [112].

Take Home Points

- Rumination can be recognized in children, adolescents, and adults, and must be distinguished from bulimia, GERD, and vomiting syndromes.

- A clinical history and observation are usually adequate to make the diagnosis, but manometry has a role in more difficult cases.
- Weight loss is not uncommon and may be considerable, leading to a misdiagnosis of bulimia or anorexia nervosa.
- Gastroduodenal manometry with characteristic "rumination" waves is not necessary to make the diagnosis; R waves are absent in up to 60% of cases.
- Timely diagnosis, reassurance, and behavioral therapy are crucial to avoiding continued deterioration, inappropriate tests, and unnecessary treatments.
- Behavioral modification therapy aimed at teaching diaphragmatic breathing is the mainstay of rumination treatment.

CHAPTER 10

References

1 Bredenoord AJ. Management of belching, hiccups, and aerophagia. *Clin Gastroenterol Hepatol* 2013; **11**(1): 6–12.

2 Bredenoord AJ, Smout AJ. Physiologic and pathologic belching. *Clin Gastroenterol Hepatol* 2007; **5**(7): 772–5.

3 Hemmink GJ, Bredenoord AJ, Weusten BL, *et al.* Supragastric belching in patients with reflux symptoms. *Am J Gastroenterol* 2009; **104**(8): 1992–7.

4 Kessing BF, Conchillo JM, Bredenoord AJ, *et al.* Review article: the clinical relevance of transient lower esophageal sphincter relaxations in gastro-oesophageal reflux disease. *Aliment Pharmacol Ther* 2011; **33**: 650–61.

5 Bredenoord AJ, Weusten BL, Sifrim D, *et al.* Aerophagia, gastric, and supragastric belching: a study using intraluminal electrical impedance monitoring. *Gut* 2004; **53**(11): 1561–5.

6 Karamanolis G, Triantafyllou K, Tsiamoulos Z, *et al.* Effect of sleep on excessive belching; a 24-hour impedance-pH study. *J Clin Gastroenterol* 2011; **44**: 332–4.

7 Bredenoord AJ, Weusten BL, Timmer R, Smout AJ. Psychological factors affect the frequency of belching in patients with aerophagia. *Am J Gastroenterol* 2006; **101**(12): 2777–81.

8 Kessing BF, Bredenoord AJ, Smout AJ. Mechanisms of gastric and supragastric belching: a study using concurrent high-resolution manometry and impedance monitoring. *Neurogastroenterol Motil* 2012; **24**(12): e573–9.

9 Bredenoord AJ. Excessive belching and aerophagia: two different disorders. *Dis Esophagus* 2010; **23**(4): 347–52.

10 Loening-Baucke V, Swidsinski A. Observational study of children with aerophagia. *Clin Pediatr (Phila)* 2008; **47**(7): 664–9.

11 Watson NF. Aerophagia and gastroesophageal reflux disease in patients using continuous positive airway pressure: a preliminary observation. *J Clin Sleep Med* 2008; **4**(5): 434–8.

12 Shepherd K, Hillman D, Esatwood P. Symptoms of aerophagia are common in patients on continuous positive airway pressure therapy and are related to the presence of nighttime gastroesophageal reflux. *J Clin Sleep Med* 2013; **9**(1): 13–17.

13 Hemmink GJ, Weusten BL, Bredenoord AJ, *et al.* Aerophagia: excessive air swallowing demonstrated by esophageal impedance monitoring. *Clin Gastroenterol Hepatol* 2009; **7**: 1127–9.

14 Yi CH, Liu TT, Chen CL. Atypical symptoms in patients with gastroesophageal reflux disease. *J Neurogastroenterol Motil* 2012; **18**(3): 278–83.

15 Li J, Xiao Y, Peng S, *et al.* Characteristics of belching, swallowing, and gastroesophageal reflux in belching patients based on Rome III criteria. *J Gastroenterol Hepatol* 2013; **28**(8): 1282–7.

16 Bredenoord AJ, Smout AJ. Impaired health-related quality of life in patients with excessive supragastric belching. *Eur J Gastroenterol Hepatol* 2010; **22**(12): 1420–3.

17 Chitkara DK Bredenoord AJ, Rucker MJ, Talley NJ. Aerophagia in adults: a comparison with functional dyspepsia. *Aliment Pharmacol Ther* 2005; **22**(9): 855–8.

18 Basaran UN, Inan M, Aksu B, Ceylan T. Colon perforation due to pathologic aerophagia in an intellectually disabled child. *J Pediatr Child Health* 2007; **43**(10): 710–12.

19 Devanarayana NM, Rajindrajith S. Aerophagia among Sri Lankan schoolchildren: epidemiological patterns and symptom characteristics. *J Pediatr Gastroenterol Nutr* 2012; **54**(4): 516–20.

20 Hwang JB, Choi WJ, Kim JS, *et al.* Clinical features of pathologic childhood aerophagia: early recognition and essential diagnostic criteria. *J Pediatr Gastroenterol Nutr* 2005; **41**(5): 612–16.

21 Hemmink GJ, Ten Cate L, Bredenoord AJ, *et al.* Speech therapy in patients with excessive supragastric belching – a pilot study. *Neurogastroenterol Motil* 2010; **22**: 24–8, e2–3.

22 Cigrang JA, Hunter CM, Peterson AL. Behavioral treatment of chronic belching due to aerophagia in a normal adult. *Behav Modif* 2006; **30**(3): 341–51.

23 Katzka DA. Simple office-based behavioral approach to patients with chronic belching. *Dis Esophagus* 2013; **26**(6): 570–3.

24 Blondeau K, Boecxstaens V, Rommel N, *et al.* Baclofen improves symptoms and reduces postprandial flow events in patients with rumination and supragastric belching. *Clin Gastroenterol Hepatol* 2012; **10**(4): 379–84.

25 Fukuzawa H, Urushihara N, Fukumoto K, *et al.* Esophagogastric separation and abdominal esophagostomy via jejunal interposition: a new operation for extreme forms of pathologic aerophagia. *J Pediatr Surg* 2011; **46**(10): 2035–7.

26 Porter SR, Scully C. Oral malodour (halitosis). *BMJ* 2006; **333**: 632–5.

27 Rosenberg M, Knaan T, Cohen D. Association among bad breath, body mass index, and alcohol intake. *J Dent Res* 2007; **86**: 997–1000.

28 Liu XN, Shinada K, Chen XC, *et al.* Oral malodor-related parameters in the Chinese general population. *J Clin Periodontol* 2006; **33**: 31–6.

29 Nadanovsky P, Carvalho LB, Ponce de Leon A. Oral malodour and its association with age and sex in a general population in Brazil. *Oral Dis* 2007; **13**: 105–9.

30 Scully C, Greenman J. Halitosis (breath odor). *Periodontol 2000* 2008; **48**: 66–75.

31 Quirynen M, Dadamio J, Van den Velde S, *et al.* Characteristics of 2000 patients who visited a halitosis clinic. *J Clin Peridontol* 2009; **36**(11): 970–5.

32 Aylikci BU, Colak H. Halitosis: from diagnosis to management. *J Nat Sci Biol Med* 2013; **4**(1): 14–23.

33 Bollen CM, Beikler T. Halitosis: the multidisciplinary approach. *Int J Oral Sci* 2012; **4**(2): 55–63.

34 Seemann R, Bizhang M, Djamchidi C, *et al.* The proportion of pseudo-halitosis patients in a multidisciplinary breath malodour consultation. *Int Dent J* 2006; **56**: 77–81.

35 Tangerman A. Halitosis in medicine: a review. *Int Dent J* 2002; **52**(Suppl. 3): 201–6.

36 Delanghe G, Ghyselen J, van Steenberghe D, Feenstra L. Multidisciplinary breath-odour clinic. *Lancet* 1997; **350**: 187.

37 John M, Vandana KL. Detection and measurement of oral malodour in periodontitis patients. *Indian J Dent Res* 2006; **17**(1): 2–6.

38 Bosy A, Kulkarni GV, Rosenberg M, McCulloch CA. Relationship of oral malodor to periodontitis: evidence of independence in discrete subpopulations. *J Periodontol* 1994; **65**: 37–46.

39 Rosenberg M. Bad breath and periodontal disease: how related are they? *J Clin Periodontol* 2006; **33**: 29–30.

40 Ademovski SE, Persson GR, Winkel E, *et al.* The short-term treatment effects on the microbiota at the dorsum of the tongue in intra-oral halitosis patients – a randomized clinical trial. *Clin Oral Investig* 2013; **17**(2): 463–73.

41 Outhouse TL, Al-Alawi R, Fedorowicz Z, Keenan JV. Tongue scraping for treating halitosis. *Cochrane Database Syst Rev* 2006(2):CD005519.

42 van den Broek AM, Feenstra L, de Baat C. A review of the current literature on aetiology and measurement methods of halitosis. *J Dent* 2007; **35**: 627–35.

43 Rosenberg M. Clinical assessment of bad breath: current concepts. *J Am Dent Assoc* 1996; **127**: 475–82.

44 Katz HP, Katz JR, Bernstein M, Marcin J. Unusual presentation of nasal foreign bodies in children. *JAMA* 1979; **241**: 1496.

45 Finkelstein Y, Talmi YP, Ophir D, Berger G. Laser cryptolysis for the treatment of halitosis. *Otolaryngol Head Neck Surg* 2004; **131**(4): 372–7.

46 Durham TM, Malloy T, Hodges ED. Halitosis: knowing when "bad breath" signals systemic disease. *Geriatrics* 1993; **48**: 55–9.

47 Kamaraj DR, Bhushan KS, Laxman VK, Mathew J. Detection of odoriferous subgingival and tongue microbiota in diabetic and nondiabetic patients with oral malodor using polymerase chain reaction. *Indian J Dent Res* 2011; **22**(2): 260–5.

48 Tseng WS. Halitosis: could it be a predictor of stroke? *Med Hypotheses* 2014; **82**(3): 335–7.

49 Li M, Al-Sarraf A, Sinclair G, Frohlich J. Fish odour syndrome. *Can Med Assoc J* 2011; **183**(8): 929–31.

50 Struch F, Schwahn C, Wallaschofski H, *et al.* Self-reported halitosis and gastroesophageal reflux disease in the general population. *J Gen Intern Med* 2008; **23**: 260–6.

51 Lee H, Kho HS, Chung JW, *et al.* Volatile sulfur compounds produced by *Helicobacter pylori.* *J Clin Gastroenterol* 2006; **40**: 421–6.

52 Suarez F, Springfield J, Furne J, Levitt M. Differentiation of mouth versus gut as site of origin of odoriferous breath gases after garlic ingestion. *Am J Physiol* 1999; **276**. G425–30.

53 Rosenberg M, Kozlovsky A, Gelernter I, *et al.* Self-estimation of oral malodor. *J Dent Res* 1995; **74**: 1577–82.

54 Donaldson AC, Riggio MP, Rolph HJ, *et al.* Clinical examination of subjects with halitosis. *Oral Dis* 2007; **13**: 63–70.

55 Rosenberg M, McCulloch CA. Measurement of oral malodor: current methods and future prospects. *J Periodontol* 1992; **63**: 776–82.

56 Porter SR, Scully C. Oral malodour (halitosis). *BMJ* 2006; **333**: 632–5.

57 Roldan S, Herrera D, O'Connor A, *et al.* A combined therapeutic approach to manage oral halitosis: a 3-month prospective case series. *J Periodontol* 2005; **76**: 1025–33.

58 Roldan S, Winkel EG, Herrera D, *et al.* The effects of a new mouthrinse containing chlorhexidine, cetylpyridinium chloride and zinc lactate on the microflora of oral halitosis patients: a dual-centre, double-blind placebo-controlled study. *J Clin Periodontol* 2003; **30**: 427–34.

59 Fedorowicz Z, Aljufairi H, Nasser M, *et al.* Mouthrinses for the treatment of halitosis. *Cochrane Database Syst Rev* 2008(4):CD006701.

60 Erovic Ademovski S, Lingstrom P, Winkel E, *et al.* Comparison of different treatment modalities for oral halitosis. *Acta Odontol Scand* 2012; **70**(3): 224–33.

61 Kuo YW, Yen M, Fetzer S, Lee JD. Toothbrushing versus toothbrushing plus tongue cleaning in reducing halitosis and tongue coating: a systematic review and meta-analysis. *Nurs Res* 2013; **62**(6): 422–9.

62 Ata N, Ovet G, Alatas N. Effectiveness of radiofrequency cryptolysis for the treatment to caseums. *Am J Otolaryngol* 2014; **35**(2): 93–8.

63 Katsinelos P, Tziomalos K, Chatzimavroudis G, *et al.* Eradication therapy in *Helicobacter pylori*-positive patients with halitosis: long-term outcome. *Med Princ Pract* 2007; **16**: 119–23.

64 Liu PF, Huang IF, Shu CW, Huang CM. Halitosis vaccines targeting FomA, a biofilm-bridging protein of fusobacterium nucleatum. *Curr Mol Med* 2013; **13**(8): 1358–67.

65 Lewis JH. Hiccups: causes and cures. *J Clin Gastroenterol* 1985; **7**: 539–52.

66 Schuchmann JA, Browne BA. Persistent hiccups during rehabilitation hospitalization: three case reports and review of the literature. *Am J Phys Med Rehabil* 2007; **86**: 1013–18.

67 Fisher CM. Protracted hiccup – a male malady. *Trans Am Neurol Assoc* 1967; **92**: 231–3.

68 Lewis JH. Hiccups: reasons and remedies. In: Lewis JH, ed. *A Pharmalogic Approach to Gastrointestinal Disorders*. Baltimore, MD: Williams & Wilkins, 1995: 209–27.

69 Dunn PM. Fetal hiccups. *Lancet* 1977; **2**: 505.

70 Miller FC, Gonzales F, Mueller E, McCart D. Fetal hiccups: an associated fetal heart rate pattern. *Obstet Gynecol* 1983; **62**: 253–5.

71 Fuller GN. Hiccups and human purpose. *Nature* 1990; **343**: 420.

72 Shortt T. Hiccup, its causes and cure. *Med Surg J (Edinburgh)* 1833; **39**: 305.

73 Samuels L. Hiccup; a ten year review of anatomy, etiology, and treatment. *Can Med Assoc J* 1952; **67**: 315–22.

74 Bailey H. Persistent hiccup. *Practitioner* 1943; **150**: 173–7.

75 Salem MR. An effective method for the treatment of hiccups during anesthesia. *Anesthesiology* 1967; **28**: 463–4.

76 Hulbert NG. Hiccoughing (hiccup or singultus). *Practitioner* 1951; **167**: 286–9.

77 Friedman NL. Hiccups: a treatment review. *Pharmacotherapy* 1996; **16**: 986–95.

78 Obis P Jr. Remedies for hiccups. *Nursing* 1974; **4**: 88.

79 Engleman EG, Lankton J, Lankton B. Granulated sugar as treatment for hiccups in conscious patients. *N Engl J Med* 1971; **285**: 1489.

80 Bendersky G, Baren M. Hypnosis in the termination of hiccups unresponsive to conventional treatment. *Arch Intern Med* 1959; **104**: 417–20.

81 Moretto EN, Wee B, Wiffen PJ, Murchison AG. Interventions for treating persistent and intractable hiccups in adults. *Cochrane Database Syst Rev* 2013(1):CD008768.

82 Choi TY, Lee MS, Ernst E. Acupuncture for cancer patients suffering from hiccups: a systematic review and meta-analysis. *Complement Ther Med* 2012; **20**(6): 447–55.

83 Ramirez FC, Graham DY. Treatment of intractable hiccup with baclofen: results of a double-blind randomized, controlled, cross-over study. *Am J Gastroenterol* 1992; **87**: 1789–91.

84 Guelaud C, Similowski T, Bizec JL, *et al.* Baclofen therapy for chronic hiccup. *Eur Respir J* 1995; **8**: 235–7.

85 Burke AM, White AB, Brill N. Baclofen for intractable hiccups. *N Engl J Med* 1988; **319**: 1354.

86 Turkyilmaz A, Eroglu A. Use of baclofen in the treatment of esophageal stent-related hiccups. *Ann Thorac Surg* 2008; **85**: 328–30.

87 Mirijello A, Addolorato G, D'Angelo C, *et al.* Baclofen in the treatment of persistent hiccup: a case series. *Int J Clin Pract* 2013; **67**(9): 918–21.

88 Blondeau K, Boecxstaerns V, Rommel N, *et al.* Baclofen improves symptoms and reduces postprandial flow events in patients with rumination and supragastric belching. *Clin Gastroenterol Hepatol* 2012; **10**(4): 379–84.

89 Chou CL, Chen CA, Lin SH, Huang HH. Baclofen-induced neurotoxicity in chronic renal failure patients with intractable hiccups. *South Med J* 2006; **99**: 1308–9.

90 Lee J, Shin HS, Jung YS, Rim H. Two cases of baclofen-induced encephalopathy in hemodialysis and peritoneal dialysis patients. *Ren Fail* 2013; **35**(6): 860–2.

91 Friedgood CE, Ripstein CB. Chlorpromazine (thorazine) in the treatment of intractable hiccups. *J Am Med Assoc* 1955; **157**: 309–10.

92 Madanagopolan N. Metoclopramide in hiccup. *Curr Med Res Opin* 1975; **3**: 371–4.

93 Petroski D, Patel AN. Letter: Diphenylhydantoin for intractable hiccups. *Lancet* 1974; **1**: 739.

94 Jacobson PL, Messenheimer JA, Farmer TW. Treatment of intractable hiccups with valproic acid. *Neurology* 1981; **31**: 1458–60.

95 McFarling DA, Susac JO. Letter: Carbamazepine for hiccoughs. *JAMA* 1974; **230**: 962.

96 Fariello RG, Mutani R. Letter: Treatment of hiccup. *Lancet* 1974; **2**: 1201.

97 Hernandez JL, Pajaron M, Garcia-Regata O, *et al.* Gabapentin for intractable hiccup. *Am J Med* 2004; **117**: 279–81.

98 Porzio G, Aielli F, Narducci F, *et al.* Hiccup in patients with advanced cancer successfully treated with gabapentin: report of three cases. *N Z Med J* 2003; **116**: U605.

99 Tegeler ML, Baumrucker SJ. Gabapentin for intractable hiccups in palliative care. *Am J Hosp Palliat Care* 2008; **25**: 52–4.

100 Thompson DF, Brooks KG. Gabapentin therapy of hiccups. *Ann Pharmacother* 2013; **47**(6): 897–903.

101 Macris SG, Gregory GA, Way WL. Methylphenidate for hiccups. *Anesthesiology* 1971; **34**: 200–1.

102 Vasiloff N, Cohen DD, Dillon JB. Effective treatment of hiccup with intravenous methylphenidate. *Can Anaesth Soc J* 1965; **12**: 306–10.

103 Sohn YZ, Conrad LJ, Katz RL. Hiccup and ephedrine. *Can Anaesth Soc J* 1978; **25**: 431–2.

104 Shantha TR. Ketamine for the treatment of hiccups during and following anesthesia: a preliminary report. *Anesth Analg* 1973; **52**: 822–4.

105 Tavakoli M, Corssen G. Control of hiccups by ketamine: a preliminary report. *ALA J Med Sci* 1974; **11**: 229–30.

106 Teodorowicz J, Zimny M. The effect of ketamine in patients with refractory hiccup in the postoperative period. Preliminary report. *Anaesth Resusc Intensive Ther* 1975; **3**: 271–2.

107 Gilson I, Busalacchi M. Marijuana for intractable hiccups. *Lancet* 1998; **351**: 267.

108 Okuda Y, Kitajima T, Asai T. Use of a nerve stimulator for phrenic nerve block in treatment of hiccups. *Anesthesiology* 1998; **88**: 525–7.

109 Lee H, Rhee PL, Park EH, *et al.* Clinical outcome of rumination syndrome in adults without psychiatric illness: a prospective study. *J Gastroenterol Hepatol* 2007; **22**(11): 1741–7.

110 O'Brien M, Bruce BK, Camilleri M. The rumination syndrome: clinical features rather than manometric diagnosis. *Gastroenterology* 1995; **108**: 1024–9.

111 Chial HJ, Camilleri M, Williams DE. Rumination syndrome in children and adolescents: diagnosis, treatment, and prognosis. *Pediatrics* 2003; **111**: 158–62.

112 Tack J, Blondeau K, Boecxstaerns V, Rommel N. Review article: The pathophysiology, differential diagnosis and management of rumination syndrome. *Aliment Pharmacol Ther* 2011; **33**(7): 782–8.

113 Chatoor J, Dickson L, Einhorn A. Rumination: etiology and treatment. *Pediatr Ann* 1984; **13**: 924–9.

114 Winton A, Singh NN. Rumination in pediatric populations: a behavioral analysis. *J Am Acad Child Adolesc Psychiatry* 1983; **22**: 269–75.

115 Rogers B, Stratton P, Victor J, *et al.* Chronic regurgitation among persons with mental retardation: a need for combined medical and interdisciplinary strategies. *Am J Ment Retard* 1992; **96**: 522–7.

116 Malcolm A, Thumshirn MB, Camilleri M, Williams DE. Rumination syndrome. *Mayo Clin Proc* 1997; **72**(7): 646–52.

117 Amarnath R, Abell TL, Malagelada JR. The rumination syndrome in adults. *Ann Intern Med* 1986; **105**, 513–18.

118 Hyman PE, Milla PJ, Benninga MA. Childhood functional gastrointestinal disorders: neonate/toddler. *Gastroenterology* 2006; **130**: 1519–26.

119 Rasquin A, Di Lorenzo C, Forbes D. Childhood functional gastrointestinal disorders: child/adolescent. *Gastroenterology* 2006; **130**: 1527–37.

120 Tack J, Talley NJ, Camilleri M. Functional gastroduodenal disorders. *Gastroenterology* 2006; **130**: 1466–79.

121 Khan S, Hyman PE, Cocjin J, *et al.* Rumination syndrome in adolescents. *J Pediatr* 2000; **136**: 528–31.

122 Kessing BF, Bredenoord AJ, Smout AJPM. Objective manometric criteria for the rumination syndrome. *Am J Gastroenterol* 2014; **109**(1): 52–9.

123 Wagaman JR, Williams DE, Camilleri M. Behavioral intervention for the treatment of rumination. *J Pediatr Gastroenterol Nutr* 1998; **27**: 596–8.

124 Chitkara DK, Van Tilburg M, Whitehead WE, Talley NJ. Teaching diaphragmatic breathing for rumination syndrome. *Am J Gastroenterology* 2006; **101**: 2449–52.

125 Tucker E, Knowles K, Wright J, Fox MR. Rumination variations:aetiology and classification of abnormal behavioural responses to digestive symptoms based on high-resolution manometry studies. *Aliment Pharmacol Ther* 2013; **37**(2): 263–74.

126 Blondeau K, Boecxstaerns V, Rommel N, *et al.* Baclofen improves symptoms and reduces postprandial flow events in patients with rumination and supragastric belching. *Clin Gastroenterol Hepatol* 2012; **10**(4): 379–84.

CHAPTER 11

Dyspepsia

Nicholas J. Talley,[1] Kate Napthali,[2] and Kenneth McQuaid[3]

[1] Faculty of Health, University of Newcastle, Newcastle, NSW, Australia
[2] Calvary Mater Newcastle, Waratah, NSW, Australia
[3] University of California San Francisco and San Francisco VA Medical Center, San Francisco, CA, USA

Summary

Dyspepsia is a symptom consisting of postprandial distress, early satiation, or epigastric pain or discomfort. It is described by patients using a variety of terms, including "indigestion." The etiology is suspected by the clinician to arise from the upper gastrointestinal (GI) tract, but other etiologies must also be considered. Most patients with these symptoms have functional dyspepsia (FD). The most common organic etiologies include peptic ulcer, gastroesophageal reflux disease (GERD), and medication side effect. In patients less than 55 years of age who have no alarm features, the most cost-effective approach is an initial test-and-treat strategy for *H. pylori*, followed by empiric proton pump inhibitor (PPI) therapy and, ultimately, esophagogastroduodenoscopy (EGD), if symptoms persist.

Case

A 57-year-old man with a 1-year history of gout, hypertension, diabetes, and previous alcohol abuse presents with the complaint of "indigestion," describing frequent "fullness" after meals. He denies heartburn, epigastric burning or pain, nausea, vomiting, and weight loss. The primary care physician obtained an *H. pylori* serology, which is negative, and prescribed once-daily PPI without benefit. What is the differential diagnosis? What is the next step in management?

Introduction

Dyspepsia is a common symptom in practice [1], and an evidence-based approach to management is key [2–4]. Dyspepsia is not associated with a shortening of survival [5]. The majority of patients presenting with chronic dyspepsia have no structural findings at EGD and are labeled as having FD. A subset of patients with FD (25%) has slow gastric emptying [2]. This overlaps with a rare and more severe motility disorder, gastroparesis, sometimes causing confusion. In gastroparesis, vomiting is usual and weight loss more frequent.

Functional gastrointestinal disorders (FGIDs) categorize patients who present with chronic GI symptoms but have no definitive abnormalities on structural evaluation that can explain them. "Chronic" refers to a 6-month history of symptoms or longer. FGIDs are not a major emphasis on the Board exams but represent very common presentations in clinical practice, so questions will be included. Management is facilitated by making a positive clinical diagnosis (do not wait until every known test is negative), reassuring the patient, and individualizing care based on the symptoms and comorbidities. The absence of obvious GI pathology does not mean the syndrome is psychiatric. Learning a few key facts emphasized in this chapter will ensure you answer Board questions correctly every time!

Dyspepsia

Definitions

"Dyspepsia" is best considered a label for a symptom complex [6]. It is *not* a diagnosis itself and patients often do not know the word (they may say they have "indigestion," "bloating," "gas," "pain," "discomfort," or "fullness," not "dyspepsia"). Some authorities insist on including reflux symptoms (most notably heartburn) under the umbrella term "dyspepsia," but this is confusing and best avoided [6].

Dyspepsia, according to the Rome classification, is restricted to specifically mean only epigastric pain or epigastric burning, fullness after eating (postprandial fullness), or an inability to finish a normal-sized meal (early satiety) [2]. Other upper GI symptoms may be present, but these are not classified as dyspepsia. This restricted definition will be applied here. Dyspepsia affects up to 40% of adults, but most do not seek care [1].

Differential Diagnosis

Dyspepsia may be organic or functional. Most sufferers have FD (Table 11.1).

Think about an organic explanation if there are alarm features (although the positive predictive value (PPV) of alarm features is low, the negative predictive value (NPV) is high; that is, many with alarm features do not have malignancy) [7].

Alarm features suggesting the need to search for an organic cause of chronic dyspepsia (especially malignancy) include:

- age ≥ 55 years at onset in the United States;
- family history of GI malignancy;
- dysphagia;
- weight loss;

Practical Gastroenterology and Hepatology Board Review Toolkit, Second Edition. Edited by Nicholas J. Talley, Kenneth R. DeVault, Michael B. Wallace, Bashar A. Aqel and Keith D. Lindor.

Table 11.1 Causes of dyspepsia.

Most common	FD
	Peptic ulcer disease (usually secondary to *H. pylori* and/or NSAIDs)
	Gastroesophageal reflux disease
	Medication side effect
Less common	Carbohydrate malabsorption (e.g., lactose intolerance, sorbitol in "sugar-free" foods)
	Malignancy: stomach, esophagus, pancreas, hepatobiliary
	IBS
	Gastroparesis (diabetes, vagotomy)
	Small-bowel bacterial overgrowth (consider diabetes, prior surgery)
	Biliary pain (cholelithiasis, cholecholithiasis)
	Chronic pancreatitis (especially if there is a history of alcohol abuse)
	Chronic mesenteric ischemia
	Infection: viral, parasitic (*Giardia*, *Strongyloides*, *Anisakiasis*), bacterial (syphilis)
	Crohn's disease
	Infiltrative disease (e.g., sarcoidosis)
	Metabolic disturbances (e.g., thyroid disease, hyperparathyroidism)
	Pregnancy

FD, functional dyspepsia; NSAID, non-steroidal anti-inflammatory drug; IBS, irritable bowel syndrome.

- GI bleeding;
- anemia;
- persistent vomiting.

Organic causes of dyspepsia include peptic ulcer disease (consider *H. pylori* infection, non-steroidal anti-inflammatory drugs (NSAIDs), and, rarely, Zollinger Ellison syndrome), malignancy (often in the setting of such alarm symptoms as weight loss), and GERD (presenting with predominant dyspepsia rather than typical reflux symptoms) [8]. Think about chronic pancreatitis, an uncommon cause, if there are risk factors (e.g., heavy alcohol use); pain may radiate through to the back. Medications can cause dyspepsia, which will resolve when they are ceased [2] (Table 11.2).

Biliary pain from gallstones is usually distinguishable from other causes of epigastric pain by its severity, unpredicatability, radiation, and course (lasting hours); it is not usually colicky. A fear of eating

Table 11.2 Common culprit drugs.

NSAIDs
Anti-inflammatory/immunomodulators: prednisone, azathioprine, methotrexate
Minerals: potassium, iron
Oral antibiotics: penicillins, cephalosporins, macrolides
HIV protease inhibitors
Digoxin
Nitrates
Loop diuretics
Antihypertensive medications: ACE inhibitors, ARBs
Cholesterol-lowering agents: niacin, fibric acid derivatives (gemfibrozil, fenofibrate)
Narcotics
Colchicine
Estrogens: oral contraceptives, hormonal replacement
Parkinson drugs: levodopa, dopamine agonists, MAO B inhibitors
Diabetes medications: metformin, acarbose, exenatide
Neuropsychiatric medications: cholinesterase inhibitors (donepezil, rivastigmine); SSRIs (e.g., fluoxetine, sertraline); serotonin-norepinephrine reuptake inhibitors (e.g., venlafaxine, duloxetine)

NSAID, non-steroidal anti-inflammatory drug; HIV, human immunodeficiency virus; ACE, angiotensin-converting enzyme; ARB, angiotensin receptor blocker; MAO, monoamine oxidase; SSRI, selective serotonin reuptake inhibitor.

and weight loss should prompt investigations for mesenteric angina in the right clinical setting (vasculopath).

Celiac disease is the great mimic in gastroenterology and may present with dyspepsia in a small number of cases.

Gastroparesis is slow gastric emptying and upper GI symptoms in the absence of mechanical obstruction; it can be idiopathic or occur in diabetes mellitus. Suspect this severe motility disorder if there is persistent vomiting.

Rare cases of dyspepsia include gastric infiltrative disease (e.g., Crohn's, sarcoid), biochemical disorders (e.g., hypercalcemia, heavy metal poisoning), and arterial compression (e.g., celiac artery compression syndrome). Liver disease (e.g., hepatoma) may cause pain confused with dyspepsia.

Management of Dyspepsia

Your clinical evaluation determines next steps. If the patient has chronic dyspepsia with no obvious explanation (e.g., a recent drug was commenced), alarm features should be reviewed. If the patient is older than 55 or has other alarm features, do a prompt EGD to look especially for malignancy and peptic ulcer disease [2,4]. Most often, EGD will be negative (you then need to go down the FD management pathway).

If there are no alarm features, you have two evidence-based alternatives [3,7]:

1 Test and treat *H. pylori*. Stop acid suppression, if already taken for at least a week (to avoid false-negative testing), and then undertake a urea breath or stool antigen test for *H. pylori* (serology cannot distinguish current from past infection). If positive, treat the infection. If negative, prescribe a trial of PPI for 4–8 weeks. If therapy fails, conduct an EGD.

2 Trial acid suppression without testing for *H. pylori* (and only if the background prevalence of *H. pylori* in the local setting is low; e.g., less than 10%). If this fails, do an EGD.

We recommend the first option, which is cost-effective in most settings.

Treatment of chronic dyspepsia after a negative EGD depends on the diagnosis. Most patients do not need a further workup, but do think about celiac disease (consider a tissue transglutaminase (tTG), and remember this will be negative if IgA-deficient). If there are risk factors, consider pancreaticobiliary disease (a routine ultrasound is *not* recommended). Most will have FD.

Functional Dyspepsia

FD affects 10% of Americans [1]. Most do not consult, but of those that do, many are misdiagnosed as GERD (and when PPIs fail, PPI-resistant GERD). FD commonly overlaps with irritable bowel syndrome (IBS) and GERD (more than expected by chance), suggesting shared pathogenic factors.

Classification

FD is subdivided [2] into:
- Epigastric pain syndrome (EPS, characterized by epigastric pain or epigastric burning).
- Postprandial distress syndrome (PDS, characterized by postprandial fullness or early satiety).

See the Rome criteria for exact diagnostic criteria (www.rome.org). In clinical practice, patients often have both PDS and EPS, but in epidemiological studies these syndromes are distinct.

Pathophysiology

Classically, the focus has been on gastric dysfunction – a subset have slow gastric emptying (25%) [9]. The gastric fundus fails to relax in a subset, leading to early satiety. Others have gastric or duodenal hypersensitivity [2]. Duodenal abnormalities have generated much interest in recent years. Pathophysiologically, PDS has been linked to a subtle excess of eosinophils in the duodenum [10]. It is conceivable that pathology in the duodenum could alter, through reflex pathways, stomach function.

Gastric emptying testing is unhelpful in terms of guiding diagnosis or therapy in most cases [2].

H. pylori can cause chronic dyspepsia [11]. However, many with this infection have no symptoms. In other words, it is possible to have *H. pylori* and FD but for them not to be linked.

> ### Case Continued
>
> A careful medication and dietary history is obtained. The patient has been taking metformin for 1 year and recently started exenatide. He also consumes many "sugar-free" products containing sorbitol. Despite the absence of alarm features, EGD is performed because of the patient's age. The EGD is normal.

Management Approach to FD

The first step is to determine whether or not *H. pylori* infection is present. If it is present, it is reasonable to offer eradication therapy. Only a minority of patients will respond to eradication treatment (i.e., only some who are infected have true *H. pylori*-related dyspepsia; number needed to treat = 17) [11]. However, responders are likely to have long-term relief. Further, eradication of *H. pylori* reduces the risk of missing a peptic ulcer disease that is the real cause of the dyspepsia, and may reduce the long-term risk of gastric adenocarcinoma, assuming gastric atrophy is absent.

The next consideration is acid suppression [12]. Both PPIs and histamine type 2 receptor antagonists (H2RAs) improve symptoms in a minority, but they are better than placebo. Those with epigastric pain are more likely to respond. If one class of drug fails, you can consider switching to the alternative, but this is not evidence-based.

A prokinetic can be considered for FD, especially in those with PDS [11]. Prokinetic therapy appears to be efficacious whether or not gastric emptying is slowed, so assessing gastric emptying is not routinely recommended. Metoclopramide should usually be avoided because of its side effects, especially in the elderly (tardive dyskinesia). Domperidone helps some patients but is not Food and Drug Administration (FDA)-approved (and can cause QT prolongation). Acotiamide, available in Japan, relaxes the gastric fundus and reduces PDS (including early satiety) [13]. Other drugs that relax the gastric fundus and may help some patients include the antianxiety agent buspirone and the antimigraine drug sumatriptan, but this remains experimental.

Antidepressants are of limited value [13]. Tricyclic antidepressant therapy in low dose may help some patients. Mirtazepine may improve appetite and dyspepsia. Selective serotonin reuptake inhibitors (SSRIs) are no better than placebo. Psychological treatment helps some patients, but evidence is limited, as is therapist availability [13]. Combination therapies can benefit some patients [14].

Other Gastroduodenal Disorders

There are other distinct gastroduodenal syndromes that you must also be able to recognize:

- Chronic nausea and vomiting disorders: most notably cyclic vomiting syndrome (CVS). This is a clinical diagnosis and is characterized by very discreet episodes of nausea and vomiting, with symptom-free intervals in between. Patients may have abdominal pain in between attacks. Tricyclic antidepressant therapy can reduce CVS attacks. Cannabis use can cause CVS (cannabinoid hyperemesis); a clinical clue is relief with hot baths or showers. Cannabis is often taken to help nausea, but actually causes the vomiting. Stopping cannabis can be curative.

- Chronic belching: may occur from extraesophageal belching (a learned habit of swallowing air that only travels into the esophagus and is then belched up – you may see the glottis moving as the patient swallows and belches) or gastric belching (from excess air in the stomach due to air-swallowing). Esophageal pH impedance is diagnostic but usually unnecessary. Belching may respond to behavioral therapy or possibly baclofen.

- Rumination: often mislabeled "vomiting" by the patient, this is actually effortless regurgitation of stomach contents. These often taste nice and may be spat out or reswallowed (Board clue: When were you last able to retain vomitus in your mouth voluntarily? You can't! This is how you tell it is rumination, not vomiting). Rumination may respond to diaphragmatic rebreathing training during meals, which abolishes the events; if severe, fundoplication may help.

> ### Take Home Points
>
> - Dyspepsia is a symptom of postprandial distress, early satiation, or epigastric burning or pain that is referred to by patients by various terms, including "indigestion."
> - The majority of patients with these symptoms have functional dyspepsia (FD).
> - The most common organic etiologies include peptic ulcer (*H. pylori*- or NSAID-related), GERD, *H. pylori*-related gastritis, and medication side effect.
> - A prompt diagnostic EGD is warranted in patients ≥ 55 years or with alarm features.
> - In young patients (<55 years) without alarm features, the most cost-effective approach is a test-and-treat strategy for *H. pylori*, followed by empiric PPI therapy, if needed. Patients with persistent symptoms after 4–8 weeks of empirical treatment should undergo EGD. Further workup is not advised in most patients with presumed FD.
> - FD includes two entities: postprandial distress syndrome (PDS), with predominant meal-related symptoms, and the epigastric pain syndrome (EPS).
> - Defined abnormalities of stomach function are only present in a proportion of patients and may not be associated with the severity of symptoms.
> - The diagnosis of FD does *not* require evidence of disordered stomach function (e.g., delayed gastric emptying).
> - The initial management of FD should involve acknowledgement and validation of symptoms, followed by reassurance.
> - The efficacy of medical therapy for FD is limited. Acid suppression is a safe first-line measure.

References

1 El-Serag HB, Talley NJ. Systemic review: the prevalence and clinical course of functional dyspepsia. *Aliment Pharmacol Ther* 2004; **19**(6): 643–54.

2 Tack J, Talley NJ, Camilleri M, *et al.* Functional gastroduodenal disorders. *Gastroenterology* 2006; **130**(5): 1466–79.

3 Talley NJ, Vakil NB, Moayyedi P. American gastroenterological association technical review on the evaluation of dyspepsia. *Gastroenterology* 2005; **129**(5): 1756–80.

4 Talley NJ, Vakil N; Practice Parameters Committee of the American College of Gastroenterology. Guidelines for the management of dyspepsia. *Am J Gastroenterol* 2005; **100**(10): 2324–37.

5 Ford AC, Forman D, Bailey AG, *et al.* Effect of dyspepsia on survival: a longitudinal 10-year follow-up study. *Am J Gastroenterol* 2012; **107**(6): 912–21.

6 Bytzer P, Talley NJ. Dyspepsia. *Ann Intern Med* 2001; **134**(9 Pt. 2): 815–22.

7 Vakil N, Moayyedi P, Fennerty MB, Talley NJ. Limited value of alarm features in the diagnosis of upper gastrointestinal malignancy: systematic review and meta-analysis. *Gastroenterology* 2006; **131**(2): 390–401; quiz 659–60.

8 Ford AC, Marwaha A, Lim A, Moayyedi P. What is the prevalence of clinically significant endoscopic findings in subjects with dyspepsia? Systematic review and meta-analysis. *Clin Gastroenterol Hepatol* 2010; **8**(10): 830–7.e1–2.

9 Haag S, Talley NJ, Holtmann G. Symptom patterns in functional dyspepsia and irritable bowel syndrome: relationship to disturbances in gastric emptying and response to a nutrient challenge in consulters and non-consulters. *Gut* 2004; **53**(10): 1445–51.

10 Talley NJ, Walker MM, Aro P, *et al.* Non-ulcer dyspepsia and duodenal eosinophilia: an adult endoscopic population-based case-control study. *Clin Gastroenterol Hepatol* 2007; **5**(10): 1175–83.

11 Moayyedi P, Soo S, Deeks J, *et al.* Pharmacological interventions for non-ulcer dyspepsia. *Cochrane Database Syst Rev* 2006(4):CD001960.

12 Moayyedi P, Delaney BC, Vakil N, *et al.* The efficacy of proton pump inhibitors in nonulcer dyspepsia: a systematic review and economic analysis. *Gastroenterology* 2004; **127**(5): 1329–37.

13 Talley, NJ, Ford A. Functional dyspepsia. *N Engl J Med* 2015; **373**: 1853–63.

14 Haag S, Senf W, Tagay S, *et al.* Is there a benefit from intensified medical and psychological interventions in patients with functional dyspepsia not responding to conventional therapy? *Aliment Pharmacol Ther* 2007; **25**(8): 973–86.

CHAPTER 11

Nausea and Vomiting

John K. DiBaise

Division of Gastroenterology and Hepatology, Mayo Clinic, Scottsdale, AZ, USA

Case

A 27-year-old man presents for evaluation of gastroparesis. He was healthy until approximately 3 months ago, when he developed an insidious onset of nausea and vomiting. His evaluation elsewhere, consisting of routine laboratory studies, abdominal ultrasound, and cholecystokinin-cholescintigraphy, was normal, leading to the eventual performance of a gastric emptying test that demonstrated delayed emptying of a solid meal. A trial of metoclopramide and promethazine did not result in improvement of his symptoms. Presently, he has constant nausea, feels full upon eating small portions, and about every other day will vomit items he had eaten several hours previously. He denies abdominal pain, but has noticed a decrease in appetite, frequent pyrosis, and a slight increase in frequency of his bowel movements. He has lost about 15 kg. Physical examination reveals an overweight young man but is otherwise unremarkable.

On the basis of his lack of previous medical problems and the diversity of his gastrointestinal (GI) symptoms, celiac disease is suspected, and, indeed, IgA tissue transglutaminase antibodies are highly positive, as are anti-endomysial antibodies. Subsequent upper endoscopy confirms the diagnosis, demonstrating scalloping of the duodenal folds with marked villous atrophy histologically. Los Angeles classification grade B esophagitis is also noted.

Treatment with a gluten-free diet and daily proton pump inhibitor (PPI) is initiated, and leads to a near-complete resolution of his symptoms and an improvement in his weight when seen in follow-up.

Definition and Epidemiology

Nausea and vomiting are common, frequently distressing, and occasionally disabling symptoms that can occur due to a variety of causes. *Nausea* is the painless, unpleasant, subjective feeling of an impending need to vomit. In contrast, *vomiting* is the rapid, forceful expulsion of upper GI contents from the mouth. Nausea is frequently not followed by vomiting; however, vomiting is usually preceded by nausea. *Retching* refers to the repetitive contractions of the abdominal musculature and labored, rhythmic respirations that usually precede vomiting but may also occur without subsequent vomiting (i.e., "dry heaves"). Vomiting must be differentiated from *regurgitation*, which describes the effortless flow of gastroesophageal contents into the mouth, and *rumination*, whereby an effortless regurgitation of recently ingested food into the mouth occurs, followed by rechewing and reswallowing or spitting out.

Both regurgitation and rumination are usually not preceded by nausea or, by definition, retching.

While it is difficult to accurately assess the economic burden related to nausea and vomiting, when considering only the more common causes of acute nausea and vomiting, such as acute gastroenteritis, postoperative effects, pregnancy, and chemotherapy, it is apparent that the socioeconomic burden to affected patients and society (i.e., employers, health care industry) is significant, at least in part due to restricted activities and social functioning, lost work productivity, increased length of hospitalization, and home nursing support [1].

Pathophysiology

Much is known about the pathophysiology of vomiting, due to its stereotypical behavior and relative ease of study using experimental models. In contrast, much less is known about nausea, as it cannot be readily studied in animals. During the retching phase of vomiting, diaphragmatic, respiratory, and abdominal muscles simultaneously contract or relax and the glottis closes. With expulsion, prolonged contraction of several groups of muscles, including the abdominal, intercostal, and laryngeal and pharyngeal muscles occurs in the absence of diaphragmatic contraction and the glottis opens. Heart and respiratory rates increase, sweating occurs, giant retrograde contractions develop in the small bowel, and both the gastric fundus and lower esophageal sphincter (LES) relax. Thus, it is important to realize that expulsion results not from a primary change in gut function but instead because of changes in intra-abdominal and intrathoracic pressure generated by the muscles of respiration.

Coordination of this combination of events takes place at the level of the medulla oblongata [2]. The major components of this neural circuitry include the area postrema in the floor of the fourth ventricle, which lies outside the blood–brain barrier (BBB) and contains a "chemoreceptor trigger zone" that detects emetic agents in the blood and cerebrospinal fluid (CSF) and transmits this information to the nucleus tractus solitarius (NTS). Vagal afferent nerves from the gut that detect noxious luminal contents and changes in tone also terminate in the NTS. Neurons from the NTS project to a central pattern generator, which then coordinates the previously described behaviors by projecting information to the various nuclei involved. The neurotransmitters involved in these processes are incompletely understood. Importantly, this central pattern generator is not a discrete site (i.e., "vomiting center") but instead

Practical Gastroenterology and Hepatology Board Review Toolkit, Second Edition. Edited by Nicholas J. Talley, Kenneth R. DeVault, Michael B. Wallace, Bashar A. Aqel and Keith D. Lindor.
© 2016 John Wiley & Sons, Ltd. Published 2016 by John Wiley & Sons, Ltd. Companion website: www.practicalgastrohep.com

consists of groups of loosely organized neurons throughout the medulla that must be activated in the appropriate sequence.

Clinical Features

A thorough history detailing the temporal features of the nausea and vomiting, the presence of associated symptoms, and the characteristics of the emesis, along with a careful physical examination, are crucial elements in determining the cause and consequences of nausea and vomiting [3]. Determining whether the symptoms are acute or chronic is the first step. Most episodes of acute nausea and vomiting have a recognized primary cause and resolve spontaneously or can be readily resolved. In contrast, chronic nausea and vomiting, defined as the persistence of nausea and vomiting for over a month, frequently presents more of a clinical challenge, because of an inability to identify the underlying cause or adequately control the symptoms. Table 12.1 lists some clinical features that may help in the identification of the diagnosis.

Findings on physical examination that may both aid in the diagnosis and assess the consequences of nausea and vomiting include resting tachycardia, orthostasis, poor skin turgor, and dry mucus membranes, which suggest the presence of significant dehydration. A general examination may detect changes associated with systemic conditions like scleroderma, Addison's disease, and hypo- or hyperthyroid disease. Lanugo-like hair, parotid gland enlargement, loss of dental enamel, and calluses on the dorsal aspect of the hand are associated with eating disorders. The presence of generalized lymphadenopathy, occult blood in the stool, and cachexia raises the possibility of an underlying neoplasm. Jaundice, conjunctival icterus, and/or hepatomegaly suggest the presence of benign or malignant hepatic disease. Focal neurologic signs, papilledema, nystagmus, nuchal rigidity, altered mentation, abnormal deep tendon reflexes, and the presence of asterixis suggest central, labyrinthine, infectious, or metabolic origins of nausea and vomiting. The abdominal examination is of particular importance in the evaluation of nausea and vomiting. Hypo- and hyperactive bowel sounds suggest the presence of an ileus and a bowel obstruction, respectively. Abdominal distension also raises the possibility of bowel obstruction. A succussion splash may be present in gastric outlet obstruction or

gastroparesis. Abdominal tenderness or peritoneal signs suggest the presence of an intraabdominal inflammatory or infectious process. An abdominal mass may reflect either a benign or a malignant process.

Diagnosis

Although a diagnosis is possible after completing a thorough history and examination in most cases of acute nausea and vomiting, for those whose symptoms persist or are chronic and the diagnosis remains uncertain, further testing guided by the clinical presentation is generally indicated. Additional testing may include laboratory studies, radiologic and endoscopic imaging studies, and, occasionally, an assessment of GI motor activity. Unfortunately, no controlled trials exist to guide this diagnostic evaluation; therefore, recommendations are typically based upon expert consensus and opinion [3]. Importantly, correction of the clinical consequences of vomiting, such as dehydration, electrolyte abnormalities, and malnutrition, and suppression of symptoms using empiric antiemetic and/or prokinetic treatment, should be initiated either before or concurrently with the diagnostic evaluation.

Laboratory Testing

As most cases of acute nausea and vomiting are self-limited, testing may not be needed. In cases where the symptoms are more significant or particularly concerning signs and symptoms or potential complications are present, initial laboratory studies may include electrolytes, renal function, glucose, hemogram, liver tests, and pancreatic enzymes. Pregnancy testing should be performed in women of childbearing potential when symptoms persist or imaging studies are being considered. When the symptoms are more persistent or become chronic, additional blood tests to consider include thyroid studies, cortisol level, C-reactive protein, erythrocyte sedimentation rate, and celiac disease antibodies. Serum drug levels should be considered in individuals taking drugs such as digoxin and theophylline. Additional serologic testing may be indicated when the initial tests are abnormal or the history is suggestive.

Radiologic and Endoscopic Imaging

When the diagnosis remains unclear, an evaluation of the GI tract by radiologic and endoscopic means should be considered. While recognizing that they are imperfect in terms of both sensitivity and specificity due to their ease and cost, supine and upright plain films of the abdomen should be considered initially to exclude intestinal obstruction. If inconclusive for small-bowel obstruction and clinical suspicion persists, further evaluation using barium-contrast small-bowel series or a more detailed enteroclysis should be considered, although in the present day, computed tomography (CT) enterography seems to be replacing barium studies as the modality of choice [4]. CT enterography has the advantage of not only providing images of the small-bowel lumen but also imaging the small bowel wall and other structures within the abdomen and retroperitoneum, as well as allowing for a determination of the patency of the mesenteric vessels. Magnetic resonance enterography has similar capabilities and has the advantage of not including radiation exposure, but is more costly than CT and oftentimes provides a claustrophobic experience for the patient [5]. Ultrasonography is another method by which to image the gallbladder and hepatobiliary system without the need for radiation, but tends to be less useful for

Table 12.1 Clinical features that may aid in the diagnosis of nausea and vomiting.

Clinical feature	Examples
Associated symptom(s)	
Abdominal pain	Pancreatitis, intestinal obstruction
Altered menses	Pregnancy
Chest pain	Myocardial infarction
Depression, anxiety	Psychiatric cause
Diarrhea, fever	Gastroenteritis
Headache, neck stiffness, altered mental status, focal neurological signs	Brain tumor, meningitis
Tinnitus, vertigo	Meniere's disease
Weight loss	Neoplasm
Characteristics of the emesis	
Bloody or coffee-ground	Ulcer, Mallory–Weiss tear
Bilious	Obstruction distal to major papilla
Continuous	Conversion disorder
Episodic	Cyclic vomiting syndrome (CVS)
Feculent	Intestinal obstruction
Food eaten >1 hour previously	Gastroparesis
Food eaten <1 hour previously	Bulimia/rumination
Morning vomiting	Pregnancy
Projectile	Gastric outlet obstruction

visualizing the pancreas and is more operator-dependent. CT or magnetic resonance imaging (MRI) of the brain may be indicated in those with severe, unexplained nausea and vomiting, but is generally most useful when a headache or neurologic signs are present. Although more costly and involving increased risk, esophagogastroduodenoscopy (EGD) is more useful than a barium-contrast study of the upper gut for detecting mucosal lesions and allows for mucosal biopsies to be taken and gastric outlet obstruction to be treated, when present. If colonic obstruction is suspected, a contrast enema (typically using gastrograffin) or CT imaging should be performed before colonoscopy is considered.

Gastrointestinal Motility Testing

Routine laboratory testing and radiologic and endoscopic imaging studies are often normal in individuals with chronic nausea and vomiting. In this setting, testing of GI motility may be appropriate. The most common test used to screen for gastric motor dysfunction measures the rate of gastric emptying following the ingestion of a standardized meal. In the United States, this is most commonly accomplished clinically using a meal labeled with a radionuclide; however, gastric emptying can also be measured using ultrasonography, MRI, and a stable-isotope breath test, which, while benefiting from a lack of need for radiation, suffer from limitations related to availability, operator-dependence, meal content, and cost [6]. Unfortunately, regardless of the method used, inconsistencies in test methodologies and generally poor correlation between the test results and the clinical response to prokinetic medications have led to frustration over the clinical utility of this test. Furthermore, an abnormal test does not prove that the symptoms are caused by abnormal gastric emptying. As a consequence, empiric treatment with a course of a prokinetic and/or an antiemetic may be worthwhile before ordering a test of gastric emptying. If a gastric emptying test is ordered, it must include 4-hour imaging, as studies that interpolate emptying from 1–2-hour imaging are unreliable.

Other tests that have been advocated as alternatives or complements to the gastric emptying test include electrogastrography (EGG) and gastroduodenal or small-bowel manometry. EGG uses cutaneous electrodes to record the gastric slow-wave activity, while manometry involves the direct recording of intraluminal pressure activity via a catheter, incorporating pressure sensors positioned in the distal stomach, duodenum, and/or jejunum. Unfortunately, similar problems exist regarding the clinical relevance of the test results, and they are further limited by a general lack of availability and expertise in their interpretation [6]. Therefore, the place of these tests in the evaluation of the individual with chronic unexplained nausea and vomiting remains poorly defined [3].

Psychological Assessment

An evaluation of psychological causes should be considered in those individuals with chronic unexplained nausea and vomiting after common organic causes and gut dysmotility have been excluded. Obtaining a history of a prior or active eating disorder can be important and should lead to appropriate referral.

Differential Diagnosis

A diverse array of disorders can produce acute or chronic nausea with or without vomiting (Table 12.2). In the acute setting, these symptoms most often arise in order to protect the individual from toxic insults. A pathophysiological explanation is usually less clear in the setting of chronic nausea and vomiting, but it most certainly depends upon the underlying etiology.

Therapeutics

The standard approach to the management of nausea and vomiting is threefold [3] (Figure 12.1): (i) correction of fluid, electrolyte, and nutritional deficiencies; (ii) treatment of the underlying cause, if known; and (iii) suppression of the symptoms using dietary, pharmacological, and, sometimes, surgical interventions.

In the acute setting, once medical and surgical emergencies have been excluded and the individual has been assessed for complications of nausea and vomiting (e.g., dehydration, malnutrition), a decision needs to be made about whether hospitalization is necessary. Fortunately, most cases are self-limited and not severe enough to require hospitalization; however, hospitalization should be considered in cases of severe dehydration or electrolyte abnormalities, when age or medical comorbidities increase the likelihood of complications, and when outpatient management has failed. Rehydration with oral fluids is generally sufficient for most cases of acute nausea and vomiting, along with short-term antiemetic therapy (generally administered orally or rectally) and plans for follow-up if symptoms worsen or do not improve.

Dietary Modification

The treatment of chronic nausea and vomiting, while similar, tends to be more challenging, particularly when a specific cause has not been identified – an all too common situation. Furthermore,

Table 12.2 Acute and chronic causes of nausea and vomiting.

Medications	Antiarrhythmics, antibiotics, anticonvulsants, antiparkinsonian drugs, cancer chemotherapy, digoxin, exenatide, hypervitaminosis A, lubiprostone, metformin, narcotics, nicotine patch, nonsteroidal anti-inflammatory drugs (NSAIDs), sulfasalazine, theophylline
Drugs	Alcohol, marijuana (cannabinoid-hyperemesis syndrome), opiates
Toxin exposures	Arsenic poisoning, food poisoning, heavy metals
Radiation therapy	
Infections	Gastrointestinal, non-gastrointestinal
Organic GI conditions	Celiac disease, cholecystitis, cholelithiasis, Crohn's disease, eosinophilic gastroenteritis, food allergy, gastroesophageal reflux disease (GERD), hepatitis, hepatic failure, mechanical bowel obstruction, mesenteric ischemia, pancreatic cancer, pancreatitis, peptic ulcer disease, postoperative effects
Functional GI conditions	Chronic intestinal pseudo-obstruction, cyclic vomiting syndrome (CVS), functional dyspepsia, chronic idiopathic nausea, functional vomiting, gastroparesis
Non-GI conditions	Addison's disease, angioedema, acute intermittent porphyria, brain tumor, congestive heart failure, diabetic ketoacidosis, hypercalcemia, hyper/hypothyroidism, increased intracranial pressure, Meniere's disease, migraine, motion sickness, myocardial infarction, nephrolithiasis, occult malignancy, pregnancy, severe pain, uremia
Psychiatric conditions	Anxiety, conversion disorder, depression, eating disorder, panic disorder

GI, gastrointestinal.

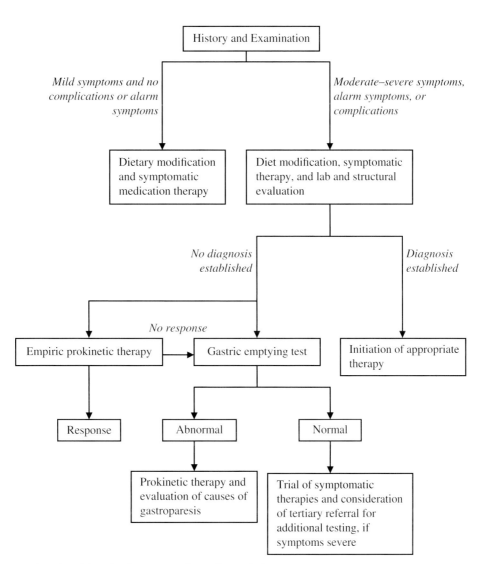

Figure 12.1 Management algorithm. Adapted with permission from reference [13].

nutritional problems tend to be more of an issue than in the acute setting. Because of the limitations of pharmacological therapies in this situation, dietary modification tends to play a more important role in terms not only of nutritional replenishment but also of symptom relief. Ingestion of a liquid diet when symptoms are most severe, with gradual advancement to a more solid diet when symptoms lessen, is generally recommended [7]. Other commonly utilized strategies include the ingestion of small-portion meals and a restriction of fat and fiber intake. The use of oral nutritional supplements is often recommended, and when nutrition is severely compromised and symptoms are persistent, enteral or parenteral nutrition support may be needed.

Pharmacological Options

Acute and chronic nausea and vomiting are often relieved, at least partially, with the use of antiemetic and prokinetic medications; however, there are no controlled trials of therapies outside the setting of surgery, chemotherapy, and radiation therapy to support any specific medical therapy, and the issue of which drug is preferable in which patients remains poorly defined. Antiemetics suppress nausea and vomiting through actions primarily within the

central nervous system (CNS), although newer agents appear to work at least in part to block receptors in the peripheral endings of vagal afferents [2]. Prokinetics act peripherally to alter GI motor function primarily via cholinergic agonism, motilin agonism, and/or dopamine antagonism [7]. There are a number of classes of antiemetic agent (Table 12.3), and side effects tend to vary based on the class. Antiemetics are available in a variety of formulations (e.g., oral, rectal, parenteral) and may be used in combination.

Table 12.3 Classes of antiemetic agent.

Class	Examples
Anticholinergic	Scopolamine
Antihistamine	Meclizine, hydroxyzine
Phenothiazine	Prochlorperazine, promethazine
Benzamide	Trimethobenzamide, metoclopramide
Butyrophenone	Droperidol
Serotonin (5-HT$_3$) antagonist	Ondansetron, granisetron
Neurokinin-1 antagonist	Aprepitant
Corticosteroid	Dexamethasone
Benzodiazepine	Lorazepam, diazepam
Cannabinoid	Dronabinol

Prokinetic agents are typically used when GI dysmotility is suspected or proven. Unfortunately, the few agents that are currently readily available in the United States (e.g., metoclopramide, erythromycin) are limited by side effects, a modest efficacy, and tolerance to long-term use. Combination antiemetic and prokinetic therapy is often used with variable success to manage chronic nausea and vomiting related to gut dysmotility syndromes.

Low-dose tricyclic antidepressants (e.g., amitriptyline, nortriptyline, doxepin) at a median dose of about 50 mg/day for 3–6 months appear to be used fairly commonly in clinical practice to treat chronic nausea and vomiting, usually of a functional etiology based mostly on small, uncontrolled trials [8]. Antimigraine drugs, including tricyclic antidepressants, are commonly used to prevent attacks of cyclic vomiting syndrome (CVS), while antiseizure medications have recently also been suggested to be useful [9].

Surgical Options

While infrequently utilized, surgical treatments may be helpful and/or necessary in both acute and chronic nausea and vomiting. Those with chronic severe nausea and vomiting, particularly those with severe gastroparesis, may benefit from a gastrostomy and/or jejunostomy tube for the purpose of supplementing oral nutrition, decompressing the gut, or both [10]. Completion gastrectomy may be worthwhile in the patient with severe postsurgical gastroparesis [11]. High-frequency gastric electrical stimulation via serosally implanted electrodes is a new therapeutic approach for patients with medically refractory gastroparesis, and a recent report suggests it may be effective in treating chronic severe nausea and vomiting, regardless of whether gastric emptying is delayed or not [7,12].

Psychological, Behavioral, and Integrative Options

Integrative management approaches such as ginger, pyridoxine, hypnotherapy, and acupuncture/acupressure have been suggested to be useful. Psychological therapies, biofeedback therapy, and relaxation techniques may also be of benefit to some individuals.

- For those whose symptoms are severe, associated with complications, or chronic and the diagnosis remains uncertain, further testing guided by the clinical presentation is generally indicated to enable a diagnosis and allow targeted treatment. Additional testing might include laboratory studies, a structural evaluation of the GI tract, and, occasionally, an assessment of GI motor activity.
- Correction of the clinical consequences of vomiting, such as dehydration, electrolyte abnormalities and malnutrition, and suppression of symptoms using empiric antiemetic and/or prokinetic treatment, should generally be initiated either before or concurrently with the diagnostic evaluation.
- Hospitalization should be considered when severe dehydration, electrolyte abnormalities, or malnutrition are present, when age or medical comorbidities increase the likelihood of complications, and when outpatient management has failed.
- The standard approach to managing nausea and vomiting includes correction of fluid, electrolyte, and nutritional deficiencies, treatment of the underlying cause, if known, and suppression of the symptoms using dietary, pharmacological, and, sometimes, surgical interventions.

References

1 Sandler RS, Everhart JE, Donowitz M, *et al.* The burden of selected digestive diseases in the United States. *Gastroenterology* 2002; **122**: 1500–11.

2 Hornby PJ. Central neurocircuitry associated with emesis. *Am J Med* 2001; **111**: 106S–12S.

3 Quigley EMM, Hasler WL, Parkman HP. AGA technical review on nausea and vomiting. *Gastroenterology* 2001; **120**: 263–86.

4 Fletcher JG, Huprich J, Loftus Jr EV, *et al.* Computerized tomography enterography and its role in small-bowel imaging. *Clin Gastroenterol Hepatol* 2008; **6**: 283–9.

5 Gonçalves Neto JA, Elazzazzi M, Altun E, Semelka RC. When should abdominal magnetic resonance imaging be used? *Clin Gastroenterol Hepatol* 2008; **6**: 610–15.

6 Camilleri M, Hasler WL, Parkman HP, *et al.* Measurement of gastroduodenal motility in the GI laboratory. *Gastroenterology* 1998; **115**: 747–62.

7 Abell TL, Bernstein RK, Cutts T, *et al.* Treatment of gastroparesis: a multidisciplinary clinical review. *Neurogastroenterol Motil* 2006; **18**: 263–83.

8 Prakash C, Lustman PJ, Freedland KE, Clouse RE. Tricyclic antidepressants for functional nausea and vomiting: clinical outcome in 37 patients. *Dig Dis Sci* 1998; **43**: 1951–6.

9 Clouse RE, Sayuk GS, Lustman PJ, Prakash C. Zonisamide or levetiracetam for adults with cyclic vomiting syndrome: a case series. *Clin Gastroenterol Hepatol* 2007; **5**: 44–8.

10 DiBaise JK, Decker GA. Enteral access options and management in the patient with intestinal failure. *J Clin Gastroenterol* 2007; **41**: 647–56.

11 Jones MP, Maganti K. A systematic review of surgical therapy for gastroparesis. *Am J Gastroenterol* 2003; **98**: 2122–9.

12 Gourcerol G, Leblanc I, Leroi AM, *et al.* Gastric electrical stimulation in medically refractory nausea and vomiting. *Eur J Gastroenterol Hepatol* 2007; **19**: 29–35.

13 Hasler WL, Chey WD. Nausea and vomiting. *Gastroenterology* 2003; **125**: 1860–7.

Take Home Points

- A wide variety of disorders can produce acute or chronic nausea with or without vomiting. Most cases of nausea and vomiting are self-limited, with infectious gastroenteritis and food poisoning accounting for the majority.
- In most cases of nausea and vomiting, a diagnosis is possible following the completion of a thorough history and a careful physical examination, and additional testing is not needed. Pregnancy should always be considered in women of childbearing age.

CHAPTER 12

Hematemesis

Thomas O.G. Kovacs and Dennis M. Jensen

CURE/Digestive Disease Research Center, VA Greater Los Angeles Healthcare System, Los Angeles, CA, USA

Summary

Upper gastrointestinal (GI) bleeding, which is defined as hemorrhage proximal to the ligament of Treitz, occurs frequently and is a common cause of hospitalization or inpatient bleeding, resulting in substantial patient morbidity, mortality, and medical care expense [1–4]. Hematemesis, which consists of vomiting either bright red blood (suggestive of recent and/or continued hemorrhage) or darker, "coffee-ground" liquid (suggestive of older or quiescent bleeding), is one of the most common manifestations of acute upper GI hemorrhage. About 40–50% of upper GI bleeding cases are caused by peptic ulcer disease (duodenal, gastric, and marginal) [3]. Variceal hemorrhage occurs in 14–20% [3]. Other, less common but still important potential etiologies are listed in Table 13.1.

Initial Approach to the Patient

The initial approach to the patient with upper GI bleeding includes evaluation of the severity of the hemorrhage, patient resuscitation, a medical history and physical examination, and consideration of possible interventions. The initial clinical assessment should focus on the patient's hemodynamic state, which has a higher initial priority than other considerations, including localization of the bleeding source. Patient resuscitation should begin early. Important determinants of resuscitation include adequate intravenous (IV) access, accurate assessment of blood loss, and appropriate fluid and blood product infusion [1]. The initial aim of therapy is to restore blood volume through fluid replacement, in order to ensure that tissue perfusion and oxygen delivery are not compromised.

Large-bore (14–18 gauge) IV catheters are recommended for infusion of normal saline and to maintain systolic blood pressure > 100 mmHg and pulse < 100 bpm. Packed red blood cell transfusions are given to maintain the hemocrit greater than 24–30%, depending on the patient's age and comorbidities. Supplemental oxygen provides adequate oxygen-carrying capacity in the elderly and in those with associated cardiopulmonary conditions.

Airway protection is also important, especially with severe upper GI hemorrhage. Endotracheal intubation should be strongly considered in patients with ongoing hematemesis or altered mental status, to prevent aspiration and to prepare for emergency endoscopy. Aspiration is a common cause of endoscopy-associated hypoxia and a leading cause of the morbidity and mortality related to severe upper GI bleeding, especially in cirrhotics. For example, in a non-randomized study, respiratory complications occurred in 22% of patients with severe acute upper GI bleeding. Risk factors for respiratory complications included advanced liver disease, esophageal bleeding, and age > 70 years. Patients with respiratory complications had a much higher mortality than patients without (70 versus 4%) [3].

If present, an associated coagulopathy should be corrected with fresh frozen plasma (FFP) infusion to lower prolonged prothrombin time to <15 seconds (or to reduce an elevated International Normalized Ratio (INR) to <1.5), and with platelet transfusion, to provide a platelet count >50 000/mm3.

History

In a patient with acute upper GI bleeding, the initial history should be brief and focused on determining the symptoms of severity and the potential etiologies of the hemorrhage. Recurrent or ongoing hematemesis, melena or hematochezia, syncope, dizziness, and chest pain are all markers of severity and acuity. Essential history includes prior episodes of upper GI bleeding and their cause, past history of chronic liver disease or peptic ulcer, and use of aspirin, non-steroidal anti-inflammatory drugs (NSAIDs), or anticoagulants such as warfarin or clopidogrel. The presence of symptoms of gastroesophageal reflux disease (GERD), prior vomiting or retching, past upper GI surgery, and past abdominal aortic aneurysm repair should also be quickly determined.

Physical Examination

In a patient with acute upper GI bleeding, the patient's pulse, blood pressure, and orthostatic changes may help determine the degree of hypovolemia and guide resuscitation. Resting tachycardia (pulse ≥ 100 bpm) suggests mild to moderate hypovolemia, while hypotension (systolic blood pressure < 100 mmHg) represents an approximate 40% loss of blood volume. Orthostatic hypotension (pulse increase of ≥ 20 bpm or decrease in systolic pressure ≥ 20 mmHg on standing) suggests a ≥15% loss of blood volume [5]. Other important physical findings include abdominal surgical scars, tenderness or a mass, and features of chronic liver disease, especially those associated with portal hypertension, such as ascites, splenomegaly, and ecchymoses or petechiae.

Laboratory Studies

Important laboratory studies should include complete blood count (CBC) with platelet count, coagulation profiles, and serum

Practical Gastroenterology and Hepatology Board Review Toolkit, Second Edition. Edited by Nicholas J. Talley, Kenneth R. DeVault, Michael B. Wallace, Bashar A. Aqel and Keith D. Lindor.

Table 13.1 Causes of hematemesis and prevalence of causes of upper GI hemorrhage.

	CURE data	Others [11]
Peptic ulcer disease	45%	35–50%
Varices (esophageal or gastric)	15%	10–15%
Gastric or duodenal erosions	10%	5–15%
Angioectasias (including gastric antral vascular ectasia – watermelon stomach)	7%	5–10%
Mallory–Weiss tear	7%	5–10%
Esophagitis	5%	3–7%
Upper GI tumor	5%	2–5%
Portal hypertension Gastropathy	2%	1–3%
Large giatal gernia – Cameron lesions	2%	1–2%
Dieulafoy's lesion	2%	0.5–1.0%
Aortoenteric fistula	<1%	<1%

chemistry, especially blood urea nitrogen (BUN), creatinine, and liver function tests (LFTs). Patients with acute upper GI bleeding will usually have an elevated BUN level secondary to an increased intestinal absorption of degraded blood urea and hypovolemia leading to prerenal azothemia. An elevated BUN/creatinine ratio greater than 20: 1 suggests an upper GI rather than lower GI source for the bleed. Blood should also be sent for type and cross-match for packed red blood cells and other blood products (platelets or FFP), if these are low.

Nasogastric Aspiration

Nasogastric or orogastric tube placement for aspiration and lavage may be useful in detecting the presence of intragastric blood (either large-volume red blood or coffee grounds), in emptying the stomach prior to endoscopy, and in lessening the likelihood of aspiration. The finding of a bloody nasogastric aspirate predicted high-risk endoscopic stigmata in a study of patients with acute upper GI bleeding [6]. However, in this same study, the nasogastric aspirate was most useful in hemodynamically stable patients without hematemesis, but with either melena or hematochezia. High-risk endoscopic findings occurred in about 15% of patients without coffee grounds or blood in their nasogastric aspirates [6].

A bilious non-bloody nasogastric aspirate in a patient with GI bleeding implies that the bleeding is distal to the ligament of Treitz or has stopped several hours previously. There is no role for guaiac-testing nasogastric tube aspirates for the presence of occult blood, since nasogastric tube insertion is likely to produce trauma with minor bleeding and a false-positive result. Patients with witnessed hematemesis do not need nasogastric tube placement for diagnostic evaluation. Further, there is no therapeutic value to iced saline lavage. If lavage is performed, lukewarm water is just as effective as and cheaper than saline. However, a randomized trial of gastric lavage prior to endoscopy showed only an improvement in endoscopic visualization of the gastric fundus, without any additional beneficial outcome [7].

IV erythromycin (a motilin receptor agonist that stimulates GI motility) may improve the quality of endoscopic examination in patients with upper GI hemorrhage by promoting the emptying of intragastric blood. A recent cost-effectiveness study confirmed that giving IV erythromycin before endoscopy for upper GI bleeding resulted in cost savings and an increase in quality-adjusted life years [8]. Because of these benefits, IV erythromycin 250 mg or IV metoclopramide 10 mg, 30–60 minutes prior to endoscopy, is recommended for selected patients with severe upper GI hemorrhage, in order to potentially improve upper GI visualization.

Triage

Patients with severe upper GI hemorrhage should be hospitalized. If they are hemodynamically unstable, have active ongoing hematemesis or large-volume bright blood per nasogastric tube or rectum (e.g. hematochezia), and have associated medical comorbidities that may be aggravated by the bleeding, they should be admitted to an intensive care unit (ICU) for continuous monitoring [1]. Selected patients with self-limited upper GI bleeding, stable vital signs, and absence of liver disease or coagulopathy, and who are dependable and have help at home, can be considered for outpatient management rather than hospitalization [9].

Clinical and laboratory parameters have been used to guide risk-stratification of patients with upper GI bleeding. Both the Blatchford score and the clinical Rockall score have been used prior to upper endoscopy in patients with acute upper GI bleeding to predict those at high versus low risk. In a recent study, patients with a low-risk clinical score had a decreased chance of having high-risk endoscopic stigmata and a very low risk of adverse outcomes, suggesting that this clinical scoring system may be applied in the future to reduce the need for urgent endoscopy [9].

Medical Therapy

After initial resuscitation and evaluation, medical therapy should be started. Several studies and meta-analyses of proton pump inhibitor (PPI) use in peptic ulcer bleeding have confirmed that PPIs reduce rebleeding, surgery, transfusion requirements, and duration of hospitalization, without decreasing mortality [10, 11]. These reports suggest that IV PPI infusion is most beneficial after endoscopic hemostasis of high-risk ulcer stigmata, but not as a standalone therapy. These stigmata of ulcer hemorrhage include active bleeding, non-bleeding visible vessel, and adherent clot, but not oozing bleeding (without other stigmata), clean ulcer base, or flat spots [11]. The recommended dose of PPIs for these high-risk ulcer stigmata, based on published randomized trials, is the equivalent of omeprazole 80 mg by IV bolus, followed by an 8 mg/h infusion for 72 hours [1,11]. However, PPIs are not approved by the US Food and Drug Administration (FDA) for such medical therapy of either upper GI or peptic ulcer bleeding. Early, pre-endoscopy IV PPI bolus and infusion in patients with upper GI hemorrhage is controversial. In one report, such pre-endoscopy PPI infusion decreased the need for endoscopic therapy, the number of actively bleeding peptic ulcers, and the duration of hospitalization, but did not change other clinical outcomes [12]. Other studies have not shown any significant benefit in important clinical outcomes such as mortality, rebleeding, and surgery [13], or in cost-effectiveness in North America [14]. In patients with upper GI hemorrhage presumed to be from ulcers, IV PPI therapy in some dosage schedule before endoscopy appears reasonable in view of its potential benefits and negligible risks [1,11].

In patients with upper GI bleeding and associated liver disease, pharmacological therapy with octreotide should be started as soon as variceal hemorrhage is suspected and should be continued for 3–5 days after the diagnosis is confirmed [11,15]. Octreotide is safe and can be given continuously for 5 days or longer. Octreotide should be administered as an initial IV bolus of 50 µg, followed by a continuous infusion of 50 µg/h. Clinical trials suggest that octreotide is particularly useful as an adjunct to endoscopic therapy. Additionally, patients with cirrhosis and GI hemorrhage should receive short-term (7 days maximum) antibiotic prophylaxis. Oral norfloxacin (400 mg BID) or IV ciprofloxacin, if oral administration is not possible, is recommended, except in patients with advanced cirrhosis in whom IV ceftriaxone (1 g/day) may be preferable [11,15].

After the patient has been stabilized and medical treatment instituted, urgent endoscopy is recommended for diagnosis and therapy, because of its high accuracy and low complication rate [11, 16]. Endoscopy using large single-channel or double-channel therapeutic endoscopes is diagnostic in about 95% of upper GI hemorrhage patients [11]. Endoscopy may also reveal stigmata of hemorrhage on ulcers or varices with important prognostic value, assisting in the triage of patients into high or low risk [11, 16]. (These specific findings will be discussed further in Chapter 22.)

The timing of endoscopy may depend on several variables, including available resources, but patients with active bleeding should be endoscoped soon after resuscitation [11]. Urgent endoscopy (within 6 hours) should be considered, particularly in patients with cirrhosis or recurrent in-patient bleeding, or in the rare patient with suspected aortoenteric fistula. For other hemodynamically stable upper GI-bleed patients, urgent endoscopy should be performed within 12 hours.

Acknowledgements

Dr. Jensen's research in GI bleeding is supported by NIH-NIDDK.K24 DK02650 and NIH-NIDDK.AM 41301 CURE CORE Grant (Human Studies Core).

Take Home Points

For upper GI bleed presenting as hematemesis:
- Assess pulse, blood pressure, orthostasis.
- Take focused GI and drug history.
- Obtain lab studies.
- Start resuscitation.
- Admit to ICU versus monitored bed.
- Perform endotracheal intubation if hematemesis persists or if there is altered mental status.
- Start IV PPI.
- Start IV octreotide infusion and antibiotics, if cirrhotic.
- Consider IV erythromycin or metoclopramide.
- Consider nasogastric tube insertion if hematemesis is not witnessed.
- Perform upper endoscopy for diagnosis and therapy within 12 hours.

References

1 Kovacs TOG. Management of upper gastrointestinal bleeding. *Curr Gastroenterol Rep* 2008; **10**: 535–42.

2 Kovacs TOG, Jensen DM. The short-term medical management of non-variceal upper gastrointestinal bleeding. *Drugs* 2008; **68**: 2105–11.

3 Kovacs TOG, Jensen DM. Recent advances in the endoscopic diagnosis and therapy of upper gastrointestinal, small intestinal, and colonic bleeding. *Med Clin N Am* 2002; **86**: 1319–56.

4 Gralnek IM, Barkun AN, Bardou M. Management of acute bleeding from a peptic ulcer. *N Engl J Med* 2008; **359**: 928–37.

5 Kupfer Y, Cappell MS, Tessler S. Acute gastrointestinal bleeding in the intensive care unit. The internist's perspective. *Gastroenterol Clin N Am* 2000; **29**: 275–307.

6 Aljebreen AM, Fallone CA, Barkun AN. Nasogastric aspirate predicts high-risk endoscopic lesions in patients with acute upper-GI bleeding. *Gastrointest Endosc* 2004; **59**: 172–8.

7 Lee SD, Kearney DJ. A randomized, controlled trial of gastric lavage prior to endoscopy for acute upper gastrointestinal bleeding. *J Clin Gastroenterol* 2004; **38**: 861–5.

8 Winstead NS, Wilcox CM. Erythromycin prior to endoscopy for acute upper gastrointestinal hemorrhage: a cost-effectiveness analysis. *Aliment Pharmacol Ther* 2007; **26**: 1371–7.

9 Romagnuolo J, Barkun AN, Armstrong D, et al. Simple clinical predictors may obviate urgent endoscopy in selected patients with non-variceal upper gastrointestinal tract bleeding. *Arch Intern Med* 2007; **167**: 265–70.

10 Bardou M, Toubouti Y, Benhaberou-Brun D, et al. Meta-analysis: proton-pump inhibition in high-risk patients with peptic ulcer bleeding. *Aliment Pharmacol Ther* 2005; **21**: 677–86.

11 Savides TS, Jensen DM. GI bleeding. In: Feldman M, Friedman LS, Brandt LJ, eds. *Slessenger and Fordtran's Gastrointestinal and Liver Disease Pathophsiology/Diagnosis/Management*, 8th edn. Philadelphia, PA: Saunders/Elsevier, 2009.

12 Lau JY, Leung WK, Wu JCY, et al. Omeprazole before endoscopy in patients with gastrointestinal bleeding. *N Engl J Med* 2007; **356**: 1631–40.

13 Dorward S, Sreedharan A, Leontiadis GI, et al. Proton pump inhibitor treatment initiated prior to endoscopic diagnosis in upper gastrointestinal bleeding. *Cochrane Database Syst Rev* 2006(18):CD005415.

14 Al-Sobah S, Burkun AN, Herba K, et al. Cost-effectiveness of proton-pump inhibition before endoscopy in upper gastrointestinal bleeding. *Clin Gastroenterol Hepatol* 2008; **6**: 418–25.

15 Garcia-Tsao G, Sanyal AJ, Grace ND, et al. Prevention and management of gastroesophageal varices and variceal hemorrhage in cirrhosis. *Hepatology* 2007; **46**: 922–38.

16 Kovacs TOG, Jensen DM. Endoscopic treatment of peptic ulcer bleeding. *Curr Treat Opt Gastroenterol* 2007; **10**: 143–8.

PART 4

Diseases of the Esophagus

14 Gastroesophageal Reflux Disease, 85
Robert T. Kavitt and Michael F. Vaezi

15 Barrett's Esophagus, 91
Shanmugarajah Rajendra and Prateek Sharma

16 Eosinophilic Esophagitis, 98
Jeffrey A. Alexander

17 Strictures, Rings, and Webs, 105
Ioannis S. Papanikolaou and Peter D. Siersema

Gastroesophageal Reflux Disease

Robert T. Kavitt[1] and Michael F. Vaezi[2]

[1]Center for Esophageal Diseases, Section of Gastroenterology, University of Chicago, Chicago, IL, USA

[2]Division of Gastroenterology and Hepatology, Center for Swallowing and Esophageal Disorders, Vanderbilt University Medical Center, Nashville, TN, USA

Summary

Gastroesophageal reflux disease (GERD) is a disorder commonly seen by primary care physicians and gastroenterologists. The pathophysiology of GERD is primarily related to failure of the antireflux mechanism of the lower esophageal sphincter (LES), among other etiologies. Most patients have non-erosive reflux disease (NERD), while a minority may exhibit erosive esophagitis. GERD commonly presents with heartburn and regurgitation. However, due to unknown mechanisms, some patients with GERD present with extraesophageal symptoms such as dental erosions, laryngitis, asthma, cough, and non-cardiac chest pain. Therapeutic trials with acid-suppressive medications and ambulatory reflux monitoring are often used in patients with suspected GERD. Acid suppression is the mainstay of GERD therapy, while antireflux surgery is an option for selected patients.

Case

A 46-year-old female presents in referral from her ear, nose, and throat (ENT) physician for evaluation and treatment of her throat-clearing and chronic cough. She has a history of asthma and postnasal drip from seasonal allergies and has been treated aggressively by her pulmonary and allergy physician for the past 3 years. She has undergone laryngoscopy by her ENT physician, which showed laryngeal irritation that suggested GERD. The patient is on once-daily proton pump inhibitor (PPI) intermittently, which has only minimally helped her symptoms. She does have heartburn and occasional regurgitation, especially at night when in the supine position.

Definition and Epidemiology

GERD is defined as chronic symptoms or mucosal damage secondary to the abnormal reflux of gastric contents into the esophagus [1]. GERD is a common medical condition with a prevalence of 10–20% in the Western world [2]. "Reflux esophagitis" refers to a disorder in a subgroup of patients with GERD consisting of histopathologically demonstrated characteristic changes in the esophageal mucosa. NERD is the presence of typical GERD symptoms in a patient without endoscopic findings of esophageal erosion. Classic symptoms include heartburn and regurgitation.

The 2006 Montreal consensus group recognized extraesophageal syndromes with "established" associations, including those with GERD and chronic cough syndrome, reflux laryngitis syndrome, reflux asthma syndrome, and reflux dental erosion syndrome [3]. Less well established symptoms include pharyngitis, sinusitis, idiopathic pulmonary fibrosis, and recurrent otitis media. Figure 14.1 illustrates potential esophageal and extraesophageal manifestations of GERD. The exact prevalence of the various extraesophageal manifestations is unknown. Estimates vary due to differences in definitions and in the methods used to establish the diagnosis. However, the prevalence of GERD may vary depending on each extraesophageal manifestation (Table 14.1).

Key Terms

- **Microaspiration**: Non-overt entrance of gastroduodenal contents into the larynx or airways due to a problem with protective mechanisms.
- **Regurgitation**: The perception of flow of refluxed gastric content into the mouth or hypopharynx.
- **Globus sensation**: A feeling of choking or a lump in the throat that is more prominent between meals and generally disappears at night.
- **Non-cardiac chest pain**: Crushing chest pain identical to angina, where after a thorough workup no evidence of ischemia is found.
- **Dysphagia**: A perceived impassage of food from the mouth into the stomach.

Pathophysiology

GERD occurs when the normal antireflux barrier between the stomach and the esophagus is impaired, either transiently or permanently. Therefore, defects in the esophagogastric barrier, such as LES incompetence, transient LES relaxations (TLESRs), and hiatal hernia are the primary factors involved in the development of GERD [4]. TLESRs are short relaxations of the LES that do not occur in response to swallowing. Studies have demonstrated that TLESRs are the primary mechanism for gastroesophageal reflux in normal individuals and in patients with mild GERD. Conversely, those with severe GERD and complications are more likely to have a permanent structural alteration, such as low LES pressure or a large hiatal hernia [5]. Delayed gastric emptying can also be a contributing factor

Practical Gastroenterology and Hepatology Board Review Toolkit, Second Edition. Edited by Nicholas J. Talley, Kenneth R. DeVault, Michael B. Wallace, Bashar A. Aqel and Keith D. Lindor.

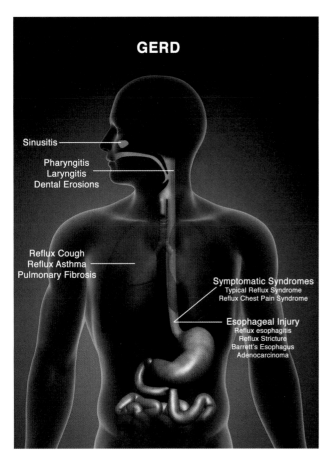

Figure 14.1 Esophageal and extraesophageal manifestations of GERD. Esophageal syndromes include typical and atypical chest pain syndromes and reflux esophagitis, stricture, Barrett's esophagus, and adenocarcinoma. Extraesophageal syndromes include pharyngitis, laryngitis, dental erosions, cough, asthma, and pulmonary fibrosis. Source: Patel 2013 [23]. Reproduced with permission of Elsevier.

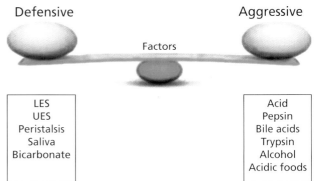

Figure 14.2 Pathophysiology of GERD: aggressive and defensive factors.

luminal layers of this epithelium are exposed to the highest concentrations of acid and protect the deeper layers. The junctions between cells are "tight" and limit the diffusion of hydrogen ions. Postepithelial defense is provided by factors derived from the blood supply to the esophageal mucosa. This blood flow both carries nutrients to the esophageal lining and carries away and neutralizes harmful factors.

Two mechanisms have been proposed to explain extraesophageal symptoms of GERD: microaspiration (reflux) and vagal stimulation (reflex) (Table 14.2) [6]. Microaspiration involves the entrance of gastroduodenal contents into the larynx or airways due to a failure of normal protective mechanisms. These chemicals can include acid, pepsin, bile, and pancreatic enzymes. Chronic irritation causes laryngitis, chronic cough, or asthma. In the second mechanism, the presence of acid within the distal esophagus causes stimulation of acid-sensitive receptors innervated by the vagus nerve. As the esophagus and bronchial tree share innervation by the vagal nerve, this stimulation may result in non-cardiac chest pain, cough, or asthma.

Clinical Features

Classic symptoms of GERD are heartburn, defined as a retrosternal burning discomfort, and acid regurgitation. Symptoms often occur after meals and may increase when a patient is recumbent. Other ancillary symptoms seen in typical reflux are dysphagia, odynophagia, and belching.

When acid refluxes into the esophagus, in sufficient amounts for a sufficient duration, the mucosa begins to break down, resulting in the most specific sign of GERD: erosive esophagitis. This can vary from mild erosions to severe circumferential ulcerations. Symptom severity in GERD patients is not highly predictive of the presence or absence of esophagitis, and esophagitis can only be diagnosed with endoscopy. Severe esophagitis may lead to stricture formation.

to the development of GERD. Symptoms develop when the offensive factors in the gastroduodenal contents, such as acid, pepsin, bile acids, and trypsin, overcome several lines of esophageal defense, including esophageal acid clearance and mucosal resistance. As more components of esophageal defense break down, the severity of reflux increases (Figure 14.2).

The distal esophagus is exposed to acid for up to 5% of a 24-hour period in normal controls. It may take at least twice this exposure to result in esophagitis. Unlike the stomach, the esophagus does not have a well-developed pre-epithelial defense, and the majority of resistance comes from the epithelium itself. The lining of the esophagus is composed of a stratified squamous epithelium. The more

Table 14.1 Prevalence of various conditions in patients with GERD and the general population. Source: Garcia-Compean 2000 [22]. Reproduced with permission of Karger Publishers

	GERD (%)	General population (%)
Chest pain	69	31
Chronic cough	75	25
Asthma	45–80	10
Dental erosions	20–55	2 19

Table 14.2 Extraesophageal manifestations of GERD and their proposed mechanisms.

Symptom	Mechanism
Chest pain	Visceral hypersensitivity, vagal stimulation
Chronic cough	Microaspiration, vagal stimulation
Asthma	Microaspiration, vagal stimulation
Laryngitis	Laryngopharyngeal reflux, chronic cough
Otitis media	Reflux into middle ear cavity
Obstructive sleep apnea	May cause GERD through negative intrathoracic pressure and traction on phrenoesophageal ligament
Dental erosions	Chemical erosion

Patients with typical reflux symptoms who lack evidence of Barrett's esophagus or erosive esophagitis are described as having NERD. Patients with GERD may present with evidence of laryngopharyngeal reflux, asthma, chronic cough, non-cardiac chest pain, or dental erosions.

Laryngopharyngeal Reflux

Symptoms of laryngopharyngeal reflux may include hoarseness, throat-clearing, cough, sore or burning throat, dysphagia, and globus sensation. Chronic laryngitis and difficult-to-treat sore throat are associated with acid reflux in as many as 60% of patients [7]. Failure to diagnose early symptoms of laryngopharyngeal reflux may result in progression to the more serious complications of contact ulcers, granuloma, subglottic stenosis, and lower-airway disease [8]. However, prospective controlled data in this area are lacking.

Symptoms of laryngopharyngeal reflux may be caused by smoking, toxic inhalants, allergies, postnasal drip, alcohol, chronic cough and infections, vocal cord dysfunction, or muscle tension dysphonia in those with hoarseness. In patients with structural laryngeal pathology, it is important that an otolaryngologist with experience continues with patient follow-up as individual causes are explored and treated.

Asthma

Asthma has a strong correlation with GERD. The relationship is complicated by the fact that each condition seems to induce the other. GERD can induce asthma by vagally mediated or microaspiration mechanisms. Asthma can induce GERD by several mechanisms: first, an asthma exacerbation results in negative intrathoracic pressure, which may overcome the tension in the LES and cause reflux; second, medications used to treat asthma (theophylline, beta-agonists, steroids) can affect the protective mechanisms against GERD.

Patients with asthma whose symptoms are worse after meals or who do not respond to traditional asthma medications should be suspected of having GERD. Additionally, patients who experience heartburn and regurgitation before the onset of asthma symptoms may have GERD as a potential cause for worsening asthma symptoms. Patients often present with adult-onset symptoms that are only partially responsive to aggressive asthma therapies. Most will report the presence of heartburn and, occasionally, regurgitation. Aggressive therapy of *both* GERD and asthma is indicated in this group, in order to provide symptomatic relief for these difficult-to-treat patients.

Chronic Cough

GERD is one of the three most common causes of chronic cough (asthma and postnasal drip being the other two) [9, 10]. GERD-related chronic cough typically occurs during the day, in the upright position, and is non-productive. GERD should be suspected in patients with cough whose symptoms have been chronic, who are not smokers, who are not on any cough-inducing medications (such as angiotensin-converting enzyme (ACE) inhibitors), who have normal chest X-ray, and in whom there is no evidence of asthma or postnasal drip.

Non-cardiac Chest Pain

In approximately one-third of patients with angina-type symptoms, ischemia is excluded and no etiology for the pain is found; 25–50%

Table 14.3 Differential diagnosis of GERD.

Eosinophilic esophagitis
Esophageal motility disorder
Coronary artery disease
Pill or infectious esophagitis
Peptic ulcer disease or non-ulcer dyspepsia
Diseases of the biliary tract

of these patients will have abnormal reflux events on pH monitoring, suggesting that GERD may have a role in causing the chest pain. Direct contact of the esophageal mucosa with gastroduodenal agents such as acid and pepsin, leading to vagal stimulation, is the most likely cause of these symptoms [11]. Other gastrointestinal (GI) etiologies may include esophageal motility disorders such as nutcracker esophagus or diffuse esophageal spasm.

GERD-related chest pain may be indistinguishable from angina. Other causes of chest pain can include esophageal motility disorders, gastritis, peptic ulcer disease, or chronic pancreatitis. Because of the difficulty in distinguishing GERD-related chest pain and angina and the implications of making the incorrect diagnosis, cardiac chest pain should always be ruled out before diagnosing GERD or embarking on a search for GI causes for chest pain.

Diagnosis of GERD and Extraesophageal Reflux

There is no diagnostic gold standard for the detection of GERD (Table 14.3). Classic symptoms of acid regurgitation and heartburn are specific but not sensitive for the diagnosis of GERD, as determined by abnormal 24-hour pH monitoring. Therefore, it is reasonable to consider an initial empiric trial of antisecretory therapy in a patient with classic GERD symptoms in the absence of alarm signs, such as dysphagia, odynophagia, weight loss, chest pain, and choking. Further diagnostic testing should be considered if there is no response to an empiric course of antisecretory therapy or if alarm symptoms are present.

Endoscopy

Endoscopy is the technique of choice for evaluation of the mucosa in patients with symptoms of GERD. Reflux esophagitis is present when erosions or ulcerations are present at the squamocolumnar junction. There are many grading systems that can be used to characterize the severity of esophagitis, the most common of which is the Los Angeles (LA) classification [12] (Figure 14.3). The presence of esophagitis and the finding of Barrett's esophagus are diagnostic of GERD. Upper endoscopy is indicated primarily to evaluate alarm symptoms and to evaluate those thought to be at risk for Barrett's esophagus. Risk factors for Barrett's esophagus include age over 50, symptoms for over 5–10 years, obesity, and male sex [13].

Esophagitis is uncommonly seen in extraesophageal GERD patients. Therefore, it is neither a sensitive nor a specific tool for diagnosing extraesophageal GERD. However, if a patient has warning signs or is considering surgery, endoscopy is indicated. In most patients presenting with continued symptoms, endoscopy is performed not to rule in GERD but to rule out other upper GI structural causes for the patient's symptoms.

pH Monitoring

Ambulatory 24-hour pH testing can be a useful way of quantitating esophageal acid exposure and allows for the correlation of

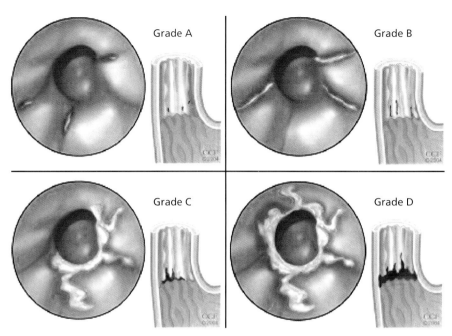

Figure 14.3 Various grades of esophagitis, according to the modified LA classification. Source: Nayar 2004 [24]. Reproduced with permission of Elsevier.

symptoms to reflux events. Transnasal catheter-based testing can monitor pH and impedance, while wireless capsule-based testing monitors pH. The electrode of an ambulatory pH probe is positioned 5 cm above the upper border of the LES. Wireless testing involves the use of a radiotelemetry pH recording capsule that attaches to the esophageal mucosa 6 cm above the squamocolumnar junction using endoscopy or 5 cm above the proximal LES border using manometry. Testing on therapy can help determine whether acid suppression is effective, while testing off therapy can determine the level of acid reflux occurring at baseline.

The utility of 24-hour pH monitoring is hampered by poor sensitivity (70–80%) and frequent false negatives (20–50%). Studies are conflicting as to the usefulness of pH monitoring in diagnosing extraesophageal GERD. There may be several reasons for this, including variable probe position, the definition of abnormal reflux, day-to-day variability of reflux events, and the intermittent nature of reflux events. The presence of acid in the upper esophagus and hypopharynx may be seen in up to 10% of asymptomatic volunteers. Therefore, 24-hour pH monitoring can neither definitively diagnose nor exclude extraesophageal reflux as the cause of a patient's symptoms. Wireless pH monitoring may increase the sensitivity of pH monitoring by capturing rare events during prolonged monitoring. Impedance/pH monitoring increases the sensitivity of the traditional ambulatory pH testing by detecting non-acid liquid (decreased impedance) or gas reflux (increased impedance). The most recent American Gastroenterological Association (AGA) guidelines suggest empiric therapy followed by pH monitoring for those unresponsive [14].

Laryngoscopy

Patients with laryngeal symptoms are often referred to ENT for laryngoscopy. Findings on laryngoscopy do not necessarily implicate gastric contents as the causative irritants. The initial endoscopic lesions associated with GERD were erosions and lesions such as vocal cord ulcerations. However, erythema and edema are

now considered by many in the ENT community to suggest GERD [15]. The identifying findings in reflux laryngitis include erythematous arytenoids and a gray appearance of the interarytenoid region. Additionally, patients with GERD may exhibit abnormalities such as erythema and edema of the posterior larynx, vocal cord polyps, granuloma, subglottic stenosis, ulcerations, vocal cord nodules, leukoplakia, and cancer. These findings are not specific for GERD; other causes may include smoking, alcohol, postnasal drip, viral illness, voice overuse, and environmental allergens. Laryngoscopy in patients with throat symptoms is not to rule in GERD but to rule out cancer and causes other than GERD.

Therapeutic Approach

GERD

The goals of treatment in GERD are to relieve symptoms, heal esophagitis, prevent recurrence of symptoms, and prevent complications. A variety of lifestyle modifications are recommended in the treatment of GERD. These include avoidance of precipitating foods, avoidance of recumbency for 3 hours postprandially, elevation of the head of the bed, smoking cessation, and weight loss [16]. However, although these measures make sense physiologically, few data are available in the literature to support them. Additionally, with the availability of potent acid-suppressive agents, dietary modification as the primary therapy for GERD is no longer overly emphasized.

Antacids and alginic acid can provide temporary relief of episodic heartburn. Despite the wide use of these over-the-counter products, surprisingly few data are available as to their utility for healing reflux esophagitis or for the long-term management of GERD symptoms.

The cornerstone of GERD therapy is the administration of agents that decrease gastric acid secretion, thereby reducing esophageal acid exposure. Histamine receptor antagonists (H_2 blockers) in standard divided doses achieve complete symptom relief in approximately 60% of patients and heal esophagitis in about 50%. The H$_2$ blockers are most useful for patients with GERD of mild to moderate severity, in whom the highest rates of healing can be anticipated. However, healing rates with these agents are poor in patients who have severe reflux esophagitis. Few data document the long-term efficacy of H$_2$ blockers used in any dosage, and tolerance to the antisecretory effects of these agents develops in many patients. For patients with severe GERD, most authorities prescribe PPIs rather than high-dose H$_2$-blocker therapy.

PPIs are superior to H$_2$ blockers in both healing erosive esophagitis and relieving symptoms, with healing rates approaching 90% [17]. For most patients, GERD is a chronic relapsing disease with almost universal recurrence of symptoms after treatment withdrawal; thus, it requires maintenance therapy in many patients. Long-term therapy with PPIs, which maintains remission in 80% of patients, is superior to that with H$_2$ blockers, which achieve a remission rate of 50% [18].

Prokinetic drugs are typically not effective as monotherapy for GERD, and their side-effect profiles often limit their use. Metoclopramide may increase LES pressure, improve gastric emptying, and enhance peristalsis of the esophagus. Side effects include tardive dyskinesia, drowsiness, agitation, and dystonic reactions, among others. The 2013 American College of Gastroenterology Guidelines for the Diagnosis and Management of Gastroesophageal Reflux Disease conclude that in the absence of gastroparesis, there is no clear role for the use of metoclopramide in the management of GERD [13].

Antireflux surgery, performed primarily by the laparoscopic approach, remains an option for carefully selected patients with well-documented GERD [19]. The ideal candidate is the patient with typical symptoms that respond completely to antisecretory therapy. The patients who opt for surgery typically have concerns about the cost or potential adverse effects associated with long-term PPI therapy. Patients with large hiatal hernias and predominant regurgitation symptoms are also good candidates. However, in some patients, GERD is refractory to acid suppression with high-dose PPI therapy; any consideration of surgery in such patients must be guarded, and the clinician should document continued evidence of ongoing esophageal acid exposure or damage during therapy. At this time, surgery is not advised in patients with GERD unresponsive to PPIs who have no evidence of esophageal acid exposure or non-acid regurgitation.

Extraesophageal Reflux

Given the non-specific nature of extraesophageal symptoms and the poor sensitivity and specificity of diagnostic tests such as pH monitoring, laryngoscopy, and endoscopy in establishing a GERD etiology, empiric therapy with PPIs has become common practice. Most therapeutic trials of these syndromes have used twice-daily dosing of PPIs for treatment periods of 2–4 months. The rationale for this dosing comes from pH-monitoring data demonstrating that the likelihood of normalizing esophageal acid exposure with twice-daily PPIs in GERD patients is 93–99%; the logic is then that lesser dosing does not exclude the possibility of a poor response due to inadequate acid suppression. Patients are difficult to treat and may not respond to traditional therapy, perhaps because of the overdiagnosis of extraesophageal GERD. Figure 14.4 highlights a suggested algorithm for the evaluation and treatment of suspected GERD and suspected gastroesophageal reflux laryngitis.

The fact that placebo-controlled trials in patients with extraesophageal symptoms show limited or no benefit from PPIs

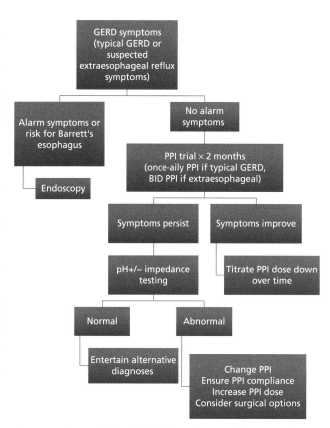

Figure 14.4 Suggested algorithm for the evaluation and treatment of suspected GERD and suspected gastroesophageal reflux laryngitis.

compared to placebo probably has several causes: (i) an overlap in extraesophageal symptoms and signs between GERD and other causes, which leads to overdiagnosis of GERD; (ii) the multifactorial nature of the presenting extraesophageal symptoms, with GERD as only one of the causes; and (iii) the possibility of weakly acidic or non-acid reflux as the etiology for persistent symptoms in some patients who are unresponsive to PPI therapy.

Initial therapy with twice-daily PPI dosing should be limited with an endpoint of titration to the lowest dose of acid suppression with controlled symptoms or to no acid suppression if symptoms do not improve after 2 months of therapy. pH/impedance monitoring on therapy might be considered to help identify that small subgroup that continues to have abnormal esophageal acid or non-acid exposure. However, in most non-responders, a search for other potential etiologies should be conducted.

Allen & Anvari [20] studied the surgical treatment of GERD in chronic cough. In their 42 patients, 51% had resolution of cough and 31% had improvement. They later determined that response to PPI predicted surgical outcome. A retrospective cohort study found that among 27 patients presenting with extraesophageal reflux symptoms and evidence of GERD, 59% noted at least partial improvement in their presenting symptom after fundoplication. Both heartburn with or without regurgitation and esophageal pH <4 for more than 12% of a 24-hr period predicted symptom resolution after surgery [21]. At this point, surgical fundoplication cannot be recommended to those unresponsive to PPI therapy unless symptoms such as regurgitation are accompanied by endoscopic findings of hiatal hernia and baseline abnormal acid reflux parameters.

Case Continued

The patient has no warning signs that necessitate endoscopy. She has not had an adequate trial of PPI therapy, since she has only been intermittently on a once-daily PPI. Therefore, she is initiated on a 2-month trial of twice-daily PPI without any further testing. She has complete resolution of her heartburn, and her throat-clearing and cough improve. She does not notice a difference in her asthma symptoms. Impedance pH monitoring on therapy suggests control of acid and non-acid reflux. pH monitoring off therapy suggests only mild reflux at baseline in the upright position, and the PPI dose is reduced to once-daily, to be taken before breakfast. The patient continues to show symptomatic improvement of her heartburn and throat-clearing.

Take Home Points

- Empiric therapy (usually with a PPI) is indicated in the majority of patients with suspected GERD.
- Endoscopy is indicated in patients with alarm symptoms or at increased risk of Barrett's esophagus.
- Ambulatory reflux testing is indicated in patients who do not respond to empiric therapy and in whom GERD is still a concern, and to confirm the disease prior to endoscopic or surgical therapy.
- Surgical therapy, performed by an experienced surgeon, is a maintenance option for the patient with typical symptoms of heartburn and regurgitation and with well-documented GERD.
- Extraesophageal reflux disease is an increasingly recognized complication of reflux of gastric contents presenting with different symptomatic manifestations.
- Reflux into the larynx can cause laryngeal irritation, which can lead to voice symptoms.
- Dual impedance/pH monitoring may improve the sensitivity and specificity of diagnostic testing; however, outcome data are needed if we are to better understand its role in this group of patients.

Videos of interest to readers of this chapter can be found by visiting the companion website at:

http://www.practicalgastrohep.com/

14.1 Endoscopic appearance of fundoplication.

References

1 DeVault KR, Castell DO. Updated guidelines for the diagnosis and treatment of gastroesophageal reflux disease. *Am J Gastroenterol* 2005; **100**(1): 190–200.

2 Dent J, El-Serag HB, Wallander MA, Johansson S. Epidemiology of gastro-oesophageal reflux disease: a systematic review. *Gut* 2005; **54**(5): 710–17.

3 Vakil N, van Zanten SV, Kahrilas P, *et al.* The Montreal definition and classification of gastroesophageal reflux disease: a global evidence-based consensus. *Am J Gastroenterol* 2006; **101**(8): 1900–20, quiz 43.

4 Orlando RC. Pathogenesis of gastroesophageal reflux disease. *Gastroenterol Clin N Am* 2002; **31**(4 Suppl.): S35–44.

5 Mittal RK, Holloway RH, Penagini R, *et al.* Transient lower esophageal sphincter relaxation. *Gastroenterology* 1995; **109**(2): 601–10.

6 Vakil N. The frontiers of reflux disease. *Dig Dis Sci* 2006; **51**(11): 1887–95.

7 Vaezi MF, Hicks DM, Abelson TI, Richter JE. Laryngeal signs and symptoms and gastroesophageal reflux disease (GERD): a critical assessment of cause and effect association. *Clin Gastroenterol Hepatol* 2003; **1**(5): 333–44.

8 El-Serag HB, Hepworth EJ, Lee P, Sonnenberg A. Gastroesophageal reflux disease is a risk factor for laryngeal and pharyngeal cancer. *Am J Gastroenterol* 2001; **96**(7): 2013–18.

9 Irwin RS, Richter JE. Gastroesophageal reflux and chronic cough. *Am J Gastroenterol* 2000; **95**(8 Suppl.): S9–14.

10 Irwin RS, Curley FJ, French CL. Chronic cough. The spectrum and frequency of causes, key components of the diagnostic evaluation, and outcome of specific therapy. *Am Rev Respir Dis* 1990; **141**(3): 640–7.

11 Richter J. Chest pain and gastroesophageal reflux disease. *J Clin Gastroenterol* 2000; **30**: S39–41.

12 Lundell LR, Dent J, Bennett JR, *et al.* Endoscopic assessment of oesophagitis: clinical and functional correlates and further validation of the Los Angeles classification. *Gut* 1999; **45**(2): 172–80.

13 Katz PO, Gerson LB, Vela MF. Guidelines for the diagnosis and management of gastroesophageal reflux disease. *Am J Gastroenterol* 2013; **108**(3): 308–28, quiz 29.

14 Kahrilas PJ, Shaheen NJ, Vaezi MF, *et al.* American Gastroenterological Association Medical Position Statement on the management of gastroesophageal reflux disease. *Gastroenterology* 2008; **135**(4): 1383–91, e1–5.

15 Ahmed TF, Khandwala F, Abelson TI, *et al.* Chronic laryngitis associated with gastroesophageal reflux: prospective assessment of differences in practice patterns between gastroenterologists and ENT physicians. *Am J Gastroenterol* 2006; **101**(3): 470–8.

16 Meining A, Classen M. The role of diet and lifestyle measures in the pathogenesis and treatment of gastroesophageal reflux disease. *Am J Gastroenterol* 2000; **95**(10): 2692–7.

17 Chiba N, De Gara CJ, Wilkinson JM, Hunt RH. Speed of healing and symptom relief in grade II to IV gastroesophageal reflux disease: a meta-analysis. *Gastroenterology* 1997; **112**(6): 1798–810.

18 Vigneri S, Termini R, Leandro G, *et al.* A comparison of five maintenance therapies for reflux esophagitis. *N Engl J Med* 1995; **333**(17): 1106–10.

19 Rice TW. Why antireflux surgery fails. *Dig Dis* 2000; **18**(1): 43–7.

20 Allen CJ, Anvari M. Gastro-oesophageal reflux related cough and its response to laparoscopic fundoplication. *Thorax* 1998; **53**(11): 963–8.

21 Francis DG, Slaughter JC, Garrett CG, *et al.* Traditional reflux parameters and not impedance monitoring predict outcome post fundoplication in extraesophageal reflux. *Laryngoscope* 2011; **121**(9): 1902–9.

22 Garcia-Compean D, Gonzalez MV, Galindo G, *et al.* Prevalence of gastroesophageal reflux disease in patients with extraesophageal symptoms referred from otolaryngology, allergy, and cardiology practices: a prospective study. *Dig Dis* 2000; **18**(3): 178–82.

23 Patel D, Vaezi MF. Normal esophageal physiology and laryngopharyngeal reflux. *Otolaryngol Clin N Am* 2013; **46**(6): 1023–41.

24 Nayar DS, Vaezi MF. Classifications of esophagitis: who needs them? *Gastrointest Endosc* 2004; **60**(2): 253–7.

CHAPTER 15

Barrett's Esophagus

Shanmugarajah Rajendra[1] and Prateek Sharma[2]

[1]Department of Gastroenterology & Hepatology, Bankstown-Lidcombe Hospital and South Western Sydney Clinical School, University of New South Wales, Sydney, NSW, Australia

[2]Division of Gastroenterology and Hepatology, Veterans Affairs Medical Center and University of Kansas School of Medicine, Kansas City, MO, USA

Summary

Barrett's esophagus is the most important and recognizable precursor lesion for esophageal adenocarcinoma (EAC), which is one of the fastest-growing cancers in the Western world. Paradoxically, the cancer risk in Barrett's esophagus has been progressively downgraded, which raises fundamental questions about our understanding of the known and unknown risk factors and molecular aberrations that are involved in the Barrett's metaplasia–dysplasia–carcinoma sequence. Future research has to be directed at these areas in order to fine tune our screening and surveillance programs and so identify more accurately the high-risk group of progressors to esophageal adenocarcinoma that would benefit most from endoscopic therapy.

Case

A 48-year-old white male with trivial heartburn on occasional antacids is referred to you by a surgical colleague for further management of long-segment Barrett's esophagus diagnosed endoscopically (C13 M14). Four quadrant biopsies obtained every alternate centimeter reveal intestinal metaplasia with goblet cells without dysplasia. He is well read on the malignant potential of Barrett's esophagus and wonders if further molecular testing of the biopsies would aid in-fine tuning his risk of progression to esophageal adenocarcinoma. In addition, he would like to know if endoscopic surveillance would be beneficial, and if so, how frequently.

Definition

Barrett's esophagus is suspected on endoscopy as salmon-colored mucosa in the distal third of the esophagus and is defined as a condition in which any extent of metaplastic columnar replaces the stratified squamous epithelium that normally lines the distal esophagus. Intestinal metaplasia is required for the diagnosis, as it is thought to be the only type of esophageal epithelium that predisposes to malignancy [1]. Nevertheless, a large study involving 8522 patients with Barrett's esophagus has shown that there is still a risk of malignant progression in patients without intestinal metaplasia (0.07% per year) as compared to those with intestinal metaplasia (0.38% per year) on index biopsy [2]. The British Society of Gastroenterology (BSG) omits goblet cell metaplasia in its definition of Barrett's esophagus [3] as sampling errors at index endoscopy may miss areas of intestinal metaplasia, which may preclude patients from entering endoscopic surveillance programs.

Gastroesophageal reflux disease (GERD) and Barrett's esophagus are the most important known risk factors for EAC. The incidence of EAC increased 600% in the United States between 1975 and 2001 (from 4 to 23 cases per million) [4], with similar increase in other Western countries, including the United Kingdom, Australia, and the Netherlands. Reasons include the increasing prevalence of GERD possibly related to abdominal adiposity, widespread eradication of *Helicobacter pylori* infection, and increased ingestion of refined food, with a concomitant reduction in consumption of fruit and vegetables.

Paradoxically, there has been a reduction in the risk estimate of cancer in Barrett's esophagus over time [2,5]. The recent discovery of a strong association of transcriptionally active high-risk human papillomavirus (hr-HPV) with Barrett's dysplasia and EAC but not Barrett's esophagus may shed some light on this anomaly (Figure 15.1) [6]. Viral integration into the host genome was found to be an early event, and both increasing viral load and integration were significantly associated with disease severity in the Barrett's metaplasia–dysplasia–adenocarcinoma pathway [7]. Thus, hr-HPV may be another plausible explanation for the significant rise of EAC, as has been the case with head and neck tumors [6,8].

Epidemiology, Genetics, Environmental Influence, and Natural History

Barrett's esophagus affects predominantly white and South Asian (Indian) males, smokers, and those with age > 50, chronic GERD, hiatal hernia, and abdominal adiposity [1,9] (Table 15.1). It is estimated to affect 1.6% of the adult Swedish population at the low end [10] and 6.8% of Americans at the high [11]. The prevalence of Barrett's esophagus in Asians is also increasing, as evidenced by hospital studies from Malaysia, South Korea, Japan, China, and India [9]. Ethnic differences in the prevalence of heartburn, esophagitis, and Barrett's esophagus are well documented in multiracial Asian patients [12–14] (Table 15.2). These racial differences, as well as familial aggregation of GERD symptoms, Barrett's esophagus/adenocarcinoma, and twin studies, suggest the possibility of a genetic component to GERD and Barrett's esophagus [15]. Environmental factors (e.g., *H. pylori* infection) may be protective for Barrett's esophagus in both Asians and Caucasians [16,17].

Practical Gastroenterology and Hepatology Board Review Toolkit, Second Edition. Edited by Nicholas J. Talley, Kenneth R. DeVault, Michael B. Wallace, Bashar A. Aqel and Keith D. Lindor.
© 2016 John Wiley & Sons, Ltd. Published 2016 by John Wiley & Sons, Ltd. Companion website: www.practicalgastrohep.com

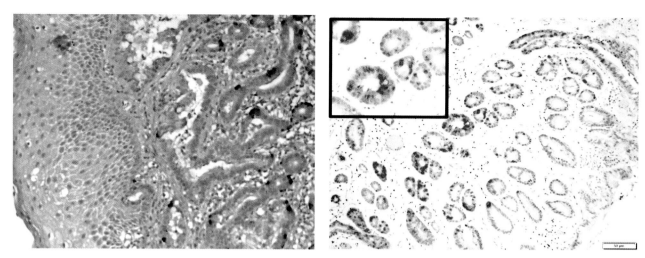

Figure 15.1 The left-hand panel reveals the *in situ* hybridization image of the hr-HPV genome in Barrett's esophagus, Barrett's dysplasia, and EAC cells but not the squamous epithelium, raising the concept of viral tropism for esophageal glandular tissue. The panel on the right demonstrates a novel RNA *in situ* hybridization targeting hr-HPV 16 and 18 E6/E7 messenger RNA transcripts in esophageal dysplastic/adenocarcinoma cells. Source: Courtesy Professor S. Rajendra & Dr. B. Wang.

In those patients with chronic GERD, the prevalence of Barrett's esophagus is 10–15% [18]. A large proportion of patients with Barrett's esophagus are asymptomatic, and >90% do not progress to cancer [19]. No prior diagnosis of Barrett's esophagus was found in 95% of patients with EAC, and 80% of esophageal cancer patients had no prior diagnosis of GERD [20]. Two large population-based studies published in 2011 from Northern Ireland and Denmark

Table 15.1 Positive and negative associations with Barrett's esophagus/EAC.

Positive association	Negative association
GERD (heartburn)	Non-steroidal anti-inflammatory drugs (NSAIDs)
Male sex	Statins
Age	*H. pylori*
Caucasians, including South Asians	Diet rich in fruits and vegetables
Familial	
Genetic: single-nucleotide polymorphisms (SNPs)	
Rs9936833 on chromosome 16q24, close to FOXF1	
Rs9257809 on chromosome 6p21, within the major histocompatibility complex (MHC)	
(? HLA-B07 in Asians with Barrett's esophagus)	
Hiatus hernia	
Smoking	
Abdominal adiposity	
Transcriptionally active hr-HPV (16/18)	

Table 15.2 Prevalence of Barrett's esophagus in patients of different racial groups examined in the same endoscopy units. Source: Sharma 2006 [14]. Reproduced with permission of Wiley.

Authors	Country	Race	n	(n)
Hirota 1999	USA	White	611	40
		Black	200	0
Rajendra 2004	Malaysia	Malays	502	7
		Chinese	824	10
		Indians	659	15
Ford 2004	UK	White	15 063	690
		Asian	5297	45

have reduced the risk estimate of cancer in non-dysplastic Barrett's esophagus (NDBE) to 0.13% (1 case per 769 patient years) and 0.12% (1 case per 860 patient years), respectively [2,5]. Moreover, the cancer risk in Barrett's esophagus remains relatively constant over time [2].

The malignancy potential in Barrett's low-grade dysplasia (LGD) is poorly defined [1], due to poor interobserver correlation (reactive changes secondary to esophagitis versus LGD), biopsy sampling error, and regression of LGD as a result of immunosurveillance. A large multicenter study revealed that the incidence of EAC among patients with Barrett's LGD was 0.6% per year [21]. More recently, it was reported that the incidence rate of EAC amongst 621 Danish patients with LGD was 0.5% per annum [5]. In the Northern Ireland Barrett's Esophagus Register study, subgroup analysis of 374 patients with LGD followed up for a mean of 7 years revealed the risk for developing high-grade dysplasia (HGD) or cancer was 1.4% per year [2].

In a meta-analysis involving four studies that included patients with HGD, the incidence of EAC was estimated to be between 5.6 and 6.6% per annum [22].

Predictors of Progression

Dysplasia is considered the best histopathological marker of cancer risk in Barrett's esophagus, though given its shortcomings, other biomarkers have been proposed for the risk of cancer progression. Chromosome instability is strongly associated with progression from Barrett's esophagus to EAC [20], and a biomarker panel detecting the presence of 9p LOH (inactivation of p16), 17p LOH (inactivation of p53), and aneuploidy/tetraploidy (DNA content abnormalities) may be superior to histology alone for risk-stratifying patients with Barrett's metaplasia, indefinite dysplasia, or LGD [1]. P53 immunohistochemistry is another good clinical molecular marker for predicting disease progression in Barrett's dysplasia, and as such has been recommended as an adjunct to routine clinical diagnosis [3]. It is the authors' opinion that significant negative staining for p53 in Barrett's dysplasia (10–50%) (thought to be due to silencing mutations of this gene) remains a major hurdle to widespread routine clinical use as a sole molecular marker.

Biomarkers relating to the transcriptional activity of hr-HPV in relation to identifying the high-risk group of progressors to malignancy should be investigated, given recent publications linking this virus with Barrett's dysplasia and EAC [6, 7]. Genome-wide association studies (GWASs) have found an association between Barrett's esophagus and two variants on chromosome 6p21 (major histocompatibility complex, MHC) and 16q24 as compared with controls [23]. The association of these variants with EAC was validated in another case–control study [24]. Interestingly, in a small prospective study involving multiethnic South East Asian patients, a strong association between HLA-B7 (0702/0706) (MHC class I) and Barrett's esophagus in Indians (who have a Caucasian genetic makeup), as compared with South Asian controls, has been demonstrated [25]. Furthermore, loss of MHC class I and gain of class II were observed to be early events in Barrett's esophagus [26].

Screening

Screening the general population with GERD for Barrett's esophagus is not currently recommended. Patients at risk of EAC (i.e., age ≥50 years, Caucasian, male, chronic GERD, hiatal hernia, abdominal adiposity, elevated body mass index (BMI)) should be screened, though this is not a universal recommendation across gastroenterology societies [1]. The ingestible esophageal sampling device (Cytosponge), together with immunocytochemistry for trefoil factor 3, may make screening for Barrett's esophagus more attractive [27]. It is pertinent to note that there are no randomized controlled trials (RCTs) demonstrating benefit in terms of decreasing the incidence or mortality of EAC or cost-effectiveness in screening for Barrett's esophagus.

Endoscopic Surveillance

The current recommendations for surveillance in Barrett's esophagus are to perform two endoscopies with biopsy within a year and then endoscopy every 3–5 years [1,28]. Absence of dysplasia on the first two endoscopies does not preclude NDBE from progressing to HGD or EAC [21]. Patients with LGD should undergo endoscopic surveillance at intervals of 6–12 months and those with HGD in the absence of eradication therapy, 3-monthly. The American Gastroenterological Association (AGA) recommends endoscopic eradication therapy rather than surveillance for treatment of patients with HGD and the most recent American College of Gastroenterology guidelines suggest eradication of both low and high grade dysplasia. Central reporting of histopathology by experienced gastrointestinal (GI) pathologists should be undertaken. Patients with dysplasia should be on proton pump inhibitor (PPI) therapy to reduce inflammatory changes, which could make histopathological interpretation difficult. A large retrospective case–control study involving 8272 individuals with Barrett's esophagus found that endoscopic surveillance for this condition was not associated with a significant reduced risk of death from EAC [29].

Evaluation

During endoscopy, with minimal air insufflation and quiet respiration (and in the absence of a hiatus hernia), the squamocolumnar junction (SCJ) is located at and coincides with the gastroesophageal junction (GEJ). The SCJ is the transformation zone where stratified squamous epithelium transitions to columnar lining. Assessment for Barrett's esophagus is done if the SCJ is located above the GEJ. Barrett's esophagus is measured from the proximal (top) end of the longitudinal gastric folds at the GEJ to the area of columnar

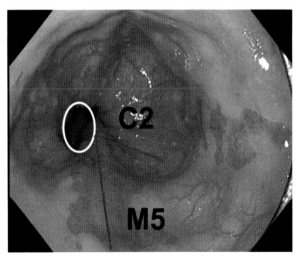

Figure 15.2 Endoscopic Barrett's esophagus: Prague C&M criteria. Patient with 5 cm-long Barrett's, distal 2 cm-circumferential and proximal 3 cm in the form of a tongue: Barrett's: C2M5. Source: Courtesy Professor P. Sharma.

epithelium that terminates at the site of the squamocolumnar demarcation. Barrett's esophagus was initially categorized as long-segment (>3 cm) versus short-segment (≤3 cm). The risk of cancer varies with the length of esophageal intestinal metaplasia (0.57% in long-segment Barrett's esophagus versus 0.26% in short-segment Barrett's esophagus) [30,31], although this is not a universal finding [32]. The Prague C and M criteria identify both the circumferential extent (C) and the maximum extent (M) of Barrett's metaplasia and have been demonstrated to have excellent interobserver agreement among endoscopists (Figure 15.2) [32]. This is so for columnar epithelium extending at least 1 cm above the GEJ. Endoscopic evaluation of the columnar lined esophagus should be carefully performed using high-resolution white-light endoscopy. Four-quadrant biopsy specimens should be obtained every 1–2 cm, as well as targeted biopsies of apparent lesions from patients with Barrett's esophagus. In patients with known or suspected Barrett's dysplasia, four-quadrant biopsy specimens should be obtained every 1 cm [1]. Specific biopsy specimens of any mucosal irregularity should be sent separately to the pathologist for evaluation. Endoscopists using high-definition white-light imaging to assess patients with Barrett's esophagus should spend approximately 1 minute per centimeter of columnar lining prior to obtaining biopsies [33]. A recent meta-analysis revealed that electronic and dye chromoendoscopy led to a 33% increase in the detection of dysplasia/cancer [34]. Moreover, narrow-band imaging (electronic chromoendoscopy) targeted biopsies have a similar intestinal metaplasia detection rate as high-definition white-light endoscopy with the Seattle protocol, while requiring fewer samples [35].

Management

The three main objectives in managing Barrett's esophagus are:
- Treatment of GERD, both by antisecretory therapy and with surgery.
- Cancer prevention.
- Removal of diseased epithelium in appropriate patient subgroups, using endotherapy.

Managing Underlying GERD

Lifestyle modification should be undertaken. This includes losing weight, eating small frequent meals, avoiding acidic and spicy foods, and raising the head of the bed by 6 inches [36].

PPIs are the mainstay of treatment, but addition of H_2-receptor antagonists may be required to combat nocturnal acid break-through. Pro-kinetic therapy may be of use if volume regurgitation is a problem.

An antireflux operation can be considered (most commonly, a Nissen fundoplication) in patients with significant volume regurgitation or those responding to medical therapy who want a surgical alternative. It is important to note that neither surgery nor medical therapy has been shown to prevent EAC.

Cancer Prevention

Indirect evidence exists to support the use of PPIs as chemoprophylaxis in Barrett's esophagus, though there are no prospective clinical studies as yet demonstrating that this class of antisecretory therapy prevents the development of dysplasia or cancer [37, 38]. The yet-to-be-reported Aspirin Esomeprazole Chemoprevention Trial (ASPECT) may clarify this issue.

Meta-analyses have shown that non-steroidal anti-inflammatory drugs (NSAIDs) and aspirin reduce the risk of EAC by 43 and 50%, respectively [39,40]. Currently, it is appropriate to consider prescription of low-dose aspirin for Barrett's esophagus subjects (who are already on a PPI) with concomitant risk factors for cardiovascular disease (CVD). Interestingly, the BSG does not recommend the use of aspirin/NSAIDs as chemopreventitive agents in patients with Barrett's esophagus, perhaps due to the unfavorable risk/benefit ratio (GI bleeding and hemorrhagic stroke) [3].

Statin use may also be associated with a lower risk of cancer in patients with Barrett's esophagus. A meta-analysis has revealed a 41% reduction in the risk of EAC in 2125 patients with Barrett's esophagus (NNT = 389) [41].

Endotherapy

Elimination of metaplastic/dysplastic cells involves ablation, endoscopic mucosal resection (EMR), and esophagectomy. Ablation can take the form of heat injury (multipolar electrocautery (MPEC), argon plasma coagulation (APC), laser), neodymium-doped yttrium aluminum garnet (Nd-YAG), radio-frequency ablation (RFA), cold injury (cryotherapy), and photochemical injury (photodynamic therapy, PDT). Post ablation/EMR, antisecretory therapy in the form of PPIs is prescribed, so the esophageal mucosa heals with the growth of new squamous epithelium (neosquamous epithelium).

Non-dysplastic Barrett's Esophagus

The use of invasive ablative therapies in NDBE is difficult to justify given the low risk for malignancy in Barrett's metaplasia, especially after multiple negative biopsies, the inadequately understood natural history of this condition (which has so far precluded identification of the high-risk population of progressors to EAC), and the potential for complications with endotherapy. A recent study revealed that RFA for NDBE was not cost-effective when compared with endoscopic surveillance and ablation if HGD developed [42].

Though endoscopic surveillance is currently recommended by most gastroenterology societies worldwide, there are no discernible data to suggest that it reduces mortality from EAC. The standard surveillance protocol in the United States and United Kingdom recommends 2–5-yearly surveillance endoscopies. The recent guidelines from the United Kingdom have advocated endoscopic surveillance only in Barrett's esophagus patients with biopsies showing intestinal metaplasia: 3–5-yearly in those with short-segment Barrett's esophagus and 2–3-yearly in those with long-segment [3].

Barrett's Low-Grade Dysplasia

The definition of dysplasia is fraught with difficulties, and without a well-defined uniform natural history (and with widely varying risk estimates for progression to cancer) it is difficult to be definite about ablative therapy in this group. It can certainly be considered as a therapeutic option in the future if the high-risk population of progressors can be better characterized [43].

If surveillance is undertaken, the next endoscopy should be within 6 months after the index examination with a diagnosis of LGD. If no progression of dysplasia is detected, annual endoscopy until there is no dysplasia for 2 consecutive years, followed by the non-dysplastic surveillance protocol, can be adopted.

RFA therapy (consisting of a balloon-based bipolar radiofrequency ablation catheter, sizing catheters, and a radiofrequency energy generator that delivers radiofrequency energy to the esophageal epithelium) eradicated dysplasia in 83–98% of subjects with LGD. It is a durable and relatively safe procedure [44, 45]. Intestinal metaplasia was eradicated in 98% of patients after 2 years, and 90% of patients with LGD remained free of dysplasia at a mean follow-up of more than 3 years. These trials have demonstrated short-term benefit in eliminating LGD, but there are no long-term data to show cancer prevention.

However, a recent multicenter trial involving 136 patients with LGD subjected to either RFA or surveillance (1 : 1 ratio) revealed that ablation reduced the risk of progression to HGD or adenocarcinoma from 26.5 to 1.5% (absolute risk reduction of 25%) over a 3-year follow-up, suggesting an early interventional approach is more appropriate [46] and was supported in the most recent guidelines from the American College of Gastroenterology.

Barrett's High-Grade Dysplasia and Intramucosal Adenocarcinoma

The combination of EMR and ablative therapy, particularly RFA, has replaced esophagectomy as the standard of care in the management of HGD and esophageal intramucosal cancer (that has not breached the muscularis mucosae). Nevertheless, all such patients should be discussed at a multidisciplinary meeting involving the GI pathologist, interventional endoscopist, upper GI surgeon, and medical oncologist/radiotherapist. Endoscopic ablative therapy should be undertaken in centers of excellence where ablative skills, patient volume, and specialized care are optimal. Endoscopic ultrasound (EUS) utilizing the TNM classification is useful in deciding whether patients with adenocarcinoma are offered endoscopic therapy or esophagectomy [43]. Prior to EMR being performed, gross tumor morphology should be assessed using the Paris classification (Table 15.3).

Table 15.3 Paris classification of the endoscopic appearance of superficial neoplastic lesions of the digestive tract mucosa.

Type I	Protruding
Type IIa	Slightly elevated
Type IIb	Completely flat
Type IIc	Slightly depressed
Type III	Excavated

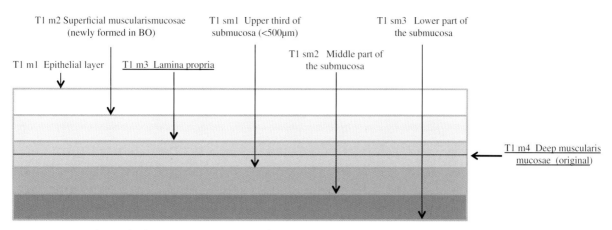

Figure 15.3 Intramucosal Barrett's adenocarcinoma (T1) subclassification. Lymph node metastasis in intramucosal cancer is 1–2%, and that involving the upper third of the submucosa is between 0 and 20%.

All visible lesions should undergo EMR (histological assessment of the whole lesion, permitting definition of lateral extent plus depth). EUS has its limitations in differentiating HGD from a T1m or a T1sm lesion (see Figure 15.3). Complications include stricture formation, hemorrhage, and perforation. Mucosally confined esophageal carcinoma has a very low risk of metastatic lymphadenopathy (1–2%), which makes endoscopic resection feasible [47]. RFA is currently the first choice of ablative therapy for flat dysplastic/neoplastic epithelium. In the AIM dysplasia trial (HGD = 63), complete eradication of HGD occurred in 81% of those in the ablation group, as compared with 19% in the control group. In the HGD group, complete eradication of dysplasia was achieved in 95% at 2 years and in 96% at 3 years [44, 45]. All patients should be on high-dose PPI therapy twice daily during and after treatment, and should continue to have lifelong endoscopic surveillance. If the neoplasia has breached the muscularis mucosae, then by definition the submucosa is involved and lymph node metastases are in the order of 10–20%, and esophagectomy (distal or subtotal) is indicated [48]. Nevertheless, some investigators have reported that the upper third of the submucosa (sm1) has a very low risk of lymph node metastasis [49, 50]. Others have reported a risk of lymph node involvement of between 0 and 8% in sm1 EAC [51], though one study from the Mayo Clinic has found that up to 12.9% of cancers confined to the first third of the submucosa have lymph node metastasis [52]. Thus, the jury is still out as to whether sm1 cancers might be eligible for endoscopic resection with a curative intent.

It is important that esophagectomies are performed by an experienced surgeon in a high-volume center in order to minimize morbidity and mortality (4.9% at a centre performing more than 50 esophagectomies) [53]. The 5-year survival rate in patients post-esophagectomy is between 90 and 95%. Significant morbidity occurs in approximately 40–50%, including pulmonary complications, anastomotic leak, dysphagia, loss of appetite, early satiety, fatigue, and loss of functional esophagus. Surveillance is still required postsurgery.

Take Home Points
- Barrett's esophagus is suspected on endoscopy as salmon-colored mucosa in the distal third of the esophagus and is defined as a condition in which any extent of metaplastic columnar replaces the stratified squamous epithelium that normally lines the distal

esophagus. Traditionally, intestinal metaplasia has been required for the diagnosis, as it is thought to be the only type of esophageal epithelium that predisposes to malignancy, though recent data suggest that columnar lining without goblet cells also carries a cancer risk of 0.07% per annum.
- Currently, endoscopic surveillance is recommended by most gastroenterology societies worldwide, though there is a lack of data to back this practice in relation to reducing mortality from EAC.
- NDBE should not be subjected to ablative therapy. It is difficult to be definite about ablative therapy in patients with LGD. Treatment could be considered as part of a clinical trial or if the high-risk group of progressors to EAC could be identified in the future.
- The combination of EMR and ablative therapy, particularly RFA, has replaced esophagectomy as the standard of care in the management of HGD and esophageal intramucosal cancer. RFA appears to be a safe and durable procedure and results in complete eradication of dysplasia in 95% of patients with HGD at 2 years post-treatment. The question as to whether Sm1 cancers might be eligible for endoscopic resection with a curative intent is yet to be resolved.
- It is imperative that we identify the high-risk group of progressors to EAC. Apart from p53 immunohistochemistry, which is probably the best current clinical molecular marker for predicting disease progression in Barrett's dysplasia, we must think outside the box and cast the net wide in search of additional biomarkers (e.g., high-risk human papilloma virus, hr-HPV). In future, genome-wide technology may provide molecular signatures to aid diagnosis and risk stratification in Barrett's esophagus.

Videos of interest to readers of this chapter can be found by visiting the companion website at:

http://www.practicalgastrohep.com/

15.1 Chromoendoscopy of Barrett esophagus using methylene blue staining.

15.2 Examination of Barrett esophagus: high magnification and acetic acid.

15.3 Examination of Barrett esophagus: white light endoscopy and narrow-band imaging.

15.4 Examination of Barrett esophagus: high magnification and narrow-band imaging.

15.5 Examination of Barrett esophagus: cap-assisted endoscopy.

References

1 Spechler SJ, Sharma P, Souza RF, et al. American Gastroenterological Association medical position statement on the management of Barrett's esophagus. *Gastroenterology* 2011; **140**: 1084–91.

2 Bhat S, Coleman HG, Yousef F, et al. Risk of malignant progression in Barrett's esophagus patients: results from a large population-based study. *J Natl Cancer Inst* 2011; **103**: 1049–57.

3 Fitzgerald RC, di Pietro M, Ragunath K, et al. British Society of Gastroenterology guidelines on the diagnosis and management of Barrett's oesophagus. *Gut* 2014; **63**: 7–42.

4 Pohl H, Welch HG. The role of overdiagnosis and reclassification in the marked increase of esophageal adenocarcinoma incidence. *J Natl Cancer Inst* 2005; **97**: 142–6.

5 Hvid-Jensen F, Pedersen L, Drewes AM, et al. Incidence of adenocarcinoma among patients with Barrett's esophagus. *N Engl J Med* 2011; **365**: 1375–83.

6 Rajendra S, Wang B, Snow ET, et al. Transcriptionally active human papillomavirus is strongly associated with Barrett's dysplasia and esophageal adenocarcinoma. *Am J Gastroenterol* 2013; **108**: 1082–93.

7 Wang B, Rajendra S, Pavey D, et al. Viral load and integration status of high-risk human papillomaviruses in the Barrett's metaplasia-dysplasia-adenocarcinoma sequence. *Am J Gastroenterol* 2013; **108**: 1814–16.

8 Marur S, D'Souza G, Westra WH, et al. HPV-associated head and neck cancer: a virus-related cancer epidemic. *Lancet Oncol* 2013; **11**: 781–9.

9 Rajendra S. Barrett's oesophagus in Asians – are ethnic differences due to genes or the environment? *J Intern Med* 2011; **270**: 421–7.

10 Ronkainen J, Aro P, Storskrubb T, et al. Prevalence of Barrett's esophagus in the general population: an endoscopic study. *Gastroenterology* 2005; **129**: 1825–31.

11 Rex DK, Cummings OW, Shaw M, et al. Screening for Barrett's esophagus in colonoscopy patients with and without heartburn. *Gastroenterology* 2003; **125**: 1670–7.

12 Rajendra S, Alahuddin S. Racial differences in the prevalence of heartburn. *Aliment Pharmacol Ther* 2004; **19**: 375–6.

13 Rajendra S, Kutty K, Karim N. Ethnic differences in the prevalence of endoscopic esophagitis and Barrett's esophagus: the long and short of it all. *Dig Dis Sci* 2004; **49**: 237–42.

14 Cameron A. Molecular biology of Barrett's esophagus. In: Sharma P, Sampliner R, eds. *Barrett's Esophagus and Esophageal Adenocarcinoma*. Malden, MA: Blackwell Publishing, 2006: 82–91.

15 Chak A, Lee T, Kinnard MF, et al. Familial aggregation of Barrett's oesophagus, oesophageal adenocarcinoma, and oesophagogastric junctional adenocarcinoma in Caucasian adults. *Gut* 2002; **51**: 323–8.

16 Rajendra S, Ackroyd R, Robertson IK, et al. Helicobacter pylori, ethnicity, and the gastroesophageal reflux disease spectrum: a study from the East. *Helicobacter* 2007; **12**: 177–83.

17 Corley DA, Kubo A, Levin TR, et al. Helicobacter pylori infection and the risk of Barrett's oesophagus: a community-based study. *Gut* 2008; **57**: 727–33.

18 Sharma P. Clinical practice. Barrett's esophagus. *N Engl J Med* 2009; **361**: 2548–56.

19 Reid BJ, Blount PL, Feng Z, et al. Optimizing endoscopic biopsy detection of early cancers in Barrett's high-grade dysplasia. *Am J Gastroenterol* 2000; **95**: 3089–96.

20 Reid BJ, Li X, Galipeau PC, et al. Barrett's oesophagus and oesophageal adenocarcinoma: time for a new synthesis. *Nat Rev Cancer* 2010; **10**: 87–101.

21 Sharma P, Falk GW, Weston AP, et al. Dysplasia and cancer in a large multicenter cohort of patients with Barrett's esophagus. *Clin Gastroenterol Hepatol* 2006; **4**: 566–72.

22 Rastogi A, Puli S, El-Serag HB, et al. Incidence of esophageal adenocarcinoma in patients with Barrett's esophagus and high-grade dysplasia: a meta-analysis. *Gastrointest Endosc* 2008; **67**: 394–8.

23 Su Z, Gay LJ, Strange A, et al. Common variants at the MHC locus and at chromosome 16q24.1 predispose to Barrett's esophagus. *Nat Genet* 2012; **44**: 1131–6.

24 Dura P, van Veen EM, Salomon J, et al. Barrett associated MHC and FOXF1 variants also increase esophageal carcinoma risk. *Int J Cancer* 2013; **133**: 1751–5.

25 Rajendra S, Ackroyd R, Murad S, et al. Human leucocyte antigen determinants of susceptibility to Barrett's oesophagus in Asians – a preliminary study. *Aliment Pharmacol Ther* 2005; **21**: 1377–83.

26 Rajendra S, Ackroyd R, Karim N, et al. Loss of human leucocyte antigen class I and gain of class II expression are early events in carcinogenesis: clues from a study of Barrett's oesophagus. *J Clin Pathol* 2006; **59**: 952–7.

27 Kadri SR, Lao-Sirieix P, O'Donovan M, et al. Acceptability and accuracy of a non-endoscopic screening test for Barrett's oesophagus in primary care: cohort study. *BMJ* 2010; **341**: c4372.

28 Wang KK, Sampliner RE. Updated guidelines 2008 for the diagnosis, surveillance and therapy of Barrett's esophagus. *Am J Gastroenterol* 2008; **103**: 788–97.

29 Corley DA, Mehtani K, Quesenberry C, et al. Impact of endoscopic surveillance on mortality from Barrett's esophagus-associated esophageal adenocarcinomas. *Gastroenterology* 2013; **145**: 312–19.

30 Sharma P, Morales TG, Sampliner RE. Short segment Barrett's esophagus – the need for standardization of the definition and of endoscopic criteria. *Am J Gastroenterol* 1998; **93**: 1033–6.

31 Yousef F, Cardwell C, Cantwell MM, et al. The incidence of esophageal cancer and high-grade dysplasia in Barrett's esophagus: a systematic review and meta-analysis. *Am J Epidemiol* 2008; **168**: 237–49.

32 Sharma P, Dent J, Armstrong D, et al. The development and validation of an endoscopic grading system for Barrett's esophagus: the Prague C & M criteria. *Gastroenterology* 2006; **131**: 1392–9.

33 Gupta N, Gaddam S, Wani SB, et al. Longer inspection time is associated with increased detection of high-grade dysplasia and esophageal adenocarcinoma in Barrett's esophagus. *Gastrointest Endosc* 2012; **76**: 531–8.

34 Qumseya BJ, Wang H, Badie N, et al. Advanced imaging technologies increase detection of dysplasia and neoplasia in patients with Barrett's esophagus: a meta-analysis and systematic review. *Clin Gastroenterol Hepatol* 2013; **11**: 1562–70.

35 Sharma P, Hawes RH, Bansal A, et al. Standard endoscopy with random biopsies versus narrow band imaging targeted biopsies in Barrett's oesophagus: a prospective, international, randomised controlled trial. *Gut* 2013; **62**: 15–21.

36 Harvey RF, Gordon PC, Hadley N, et al. Effects of sleeping with the bed-head raised and of ranitidine in patients with severe peptic oesophagitis. *Lancet* 1987; **2**: 1200–3.

37 Nguyen DM, El-Serag HB, Henderson L, et al. Medication usage and the risk of neoplasia in patients with Barrett's esophagus. *Clin Gastroenterol Hepatol* 2009, 7: 1299–304.

38 Cooper BT, Chapman W, Neumann CS, et al. Continuous treatment of Barrett's oesophagus patients with proton pump inhibitors up to 13 years: observations on regression and cancer incidence. *Aliment Pharmacol Ther* 2006; **23**: 727–33.

39 Liao LM, Vaughan TL, Corley DA, et al. Nonsteroidal anti-inflammatory drug use reduces risk of adenocarcinomas of the esophagus and esophagogastric junction in a pooled analysis. *Gastroenterology* 2012; **142**: 442–52.

40 Corley DA, Kerlikowske K, Verma R, et al. Protective association of aspirin/NSAIDs and esophageal cancer: a systematic review and meta-analysis. *Gastroenterology* 2003; **124**: 47–56.

41 Singh S, Singh AG, Singh PP, et al. Statins are associated with reduced risk of esophageal cancer, particularly in patients with Barrett's esophagus: a systematic review and meta-analysis. *Clin Gastroenterol Hepatol* 2013; **11**: 620–9.

42 Hur C, Choi SE, Rubenstein JH, et al. The cost effectiveness of radiofrequency ablation for Barrett's esophagus. *Gastroenterology* 2012; **143**: 567–75.

43 Rajendra S, Sharma P. Management of Barrett's oesophagus and intramucosal oesophageal cancer: a review of recent development. *Therap Adv Gastroenterol* 2012; **5**: 285–99.

44 Shaheen NJ, Sharma P, Overholt BF, et al. Radiofrequency ablation in Barrett's esophagus with dysplasia. *N Engl J Med* 2009; **360**: 2277–88.

45 Shaheen NJ, Overholt BF, Sampliner RE, et al. Durability of radiofrequency ablation in Barrett's esophagus with dysplasia. *Gastroenterology* 2011; **141**: 460–8.

46 Phoa KN, van Vilsteren FG, Weusten BL, et al. Radiofrequency ablation vs endoscopic surveillance for patients with Barrett esophagus and low-grade dysplasia: a randomized clinical trial. *JAMA* 2014; **311**: 1209–17.

47 Dunbar KB, Spechler SJ. The risk of lymph-node metastases in patients with high-grade dysplasia or intramucosal carcinoma in Barrett's esophagus: a systematic review. *Am J Gastroenterol* 2012; **107**: 850–62.

48 Leers JM, DeMeester SR, Oezcelik A, et al. The prevalence of lymph node metastases in patients with T1 esophageal adenocarcinoma a retrospective review of esophagectomy specimens. *Ann Surg* 2011; **253**: 271–8.

49 Stein HJ, Feith M, Bruecher BL, *et al.* Early esophageal cancer: pattern of lymphatic spread and prognostic factors for long-term survival after surgical resection. *Ann Surg* 2005; **242**: 566–73.

50 Buskens CJ, Westerterp M, Lagarde SM, *et al.* Prediction of appropriateness of local endoscopic treatment for high-grade dysplasia and early adenocarcinoma by EUS and histopathologic features. *Gastrointest Endosc* 2004; **60**: 703–10.

51 Liu L, Hofstetter WL, Rashid A, *et al.* Significance of the depth of tumor invasion and lymph node metastasis in superficially invasive (T1) esophageal adenocarcinoma. *Am J Surg Pathol* 2005; **29**: 1079–85.

52 Badreddine RJ, Prasad GA, Lewis JT, *et al.* Depth of submucosal invasion does not predict lymph node metastasis and survival of patients with esophageal carcinoma. *Clin Gastroenterol Hepatol* 2010; **8**: 248–53.

53 van Lanschot JJ, Hulscher JB, Buskens CJ, *et al.* Hospital volume and hospital mortality for esophagectomy. *Cancer* 2001; **91**: 1574–8.

CHAPTER 16

Eosinophilic Esophagitis

Jeffrey A. Alexander

Mayo Clinic, Rochester, MN, USA

Case

A 38-year-old male presents with 8 years of solid-food dysphagia. He eats slowly, chews well, and takes liquid with each swallow. He particularly has trouble with dry meats and bread. Once a week, he has food stick for several minutes before passing. He had a meat impaction removed endoscopically 6 years ago. He has heartburn once a week and takes antacids about once a month. He has a history of seasonal allergies and mild asthma.

His physical exam is normal, showing good dentition and moist mucus membranes.

Definition and Epidemiology

The first case of eosinophilic esophagitis (EoE) was described by Landres in 1978 [1]. EoE is defined by a consensus group as a chronic, immune/antigen-mediated esophageal disease characterized clinically by symptoms related to esophageal dysfunction and histologically by eosinophil-predominant inflammation [2]. A diagnosis of EoE requires several conditions: (i) esophageal symptoms; (ii) 15 or more eosinophils/hpf on esophageal biopsy; (iii) eosinophilia limited to the esophagus; and (iv) exclusion of other causes of esophageal eosinophilia, including gastroesophageal reflux disease (GERD) and proton pump inhibitor (PPI)-responsive esophageal eosinophilia (PPI-REE) (Table 16.1). The disease should remit with treatments of dietary exclusion and topical steroids [2].

EoE behaves somewhat differently in adults versus children. The primary symptom in adults is solid-food dysphagia and food impaction, while in children a variety of symptoms, including nausea and failure to thrive, are common. This chapter will focus on adult EoE, commenting on pediatric EoE where appropriate.

About 70% of EoE patients are males, and this disease has been reported worldwide [3]. EoE may be more common in cold, arid climates and in rural communities [4, 5]. To date, there has been no proven ethnic or socioeconomic predilection for EoE, but details are minimal. However, the majority of reports have come from Westernized developed countries, raising the possibility of predisposing geographic or socioeconomic factors. Some studies have suggested a seasonal variation in EoE, with more activity during the higher aeroallergen seasons [6–8], but this has not been a universal finding [9–11].

Population studies have shown an increasing prevalence of EoE over time, with reported prevalence rates from 8.9 to 57.0/100 000 people; the most recent studies show a rate of 43–57/100 000 [12–16]. The incidence of EoE has also been increasing over time according to three population-based studies, with a current estimated annual incidence of 2.5–15.9/100 000 [13, 15, 17]. It remains uncertain whether this represents a true increased incidence or merely increased recognition; it's likely to be a little of both. Physicians have dilated the normal-appearing esophagus without biopsies in patients with solid-food dysphagia with success for years; it is likely many of these patients had unrecognized EoE. It is highly likely as well that this disease has truly been increasing in incidence, as have other allergic diseases over the last several decades.

EoE is not rare; the incidence appears similar to that of Crohn's disease, which has an annual incidence of 7.9/100 000 in Olmsted County, Minnesota [18]. Eosinophilic esophageal infiltration (EEI) is seen in 5–7% of those undergoing esophagogastroduodenoscopy (EGD) for any reason and 12–15% of those undergoing EGD for dysphagia [19–22]. Interestingly, ≥15 eosinophils/hpf were found histologically in 1.1% of 1000 randomly selected people in northern Sweden [23]. This is over 20 times the prevalence of EoE we have recognized clinically, suggesting that the majority of patients with esophageal eosinophilia may well be minimally symptomatic.

Pathophysiology

Our understanding of this newly recognized disease is only in its infancy; the pathophysiology of EoE is only beginning to be unraveled. The leading hypothesis suggests that antigenic exposure to a food or aeroallergen, in a genetically predisposed host, leads to esophageal eosinophilia. This process involves a Th2 cytokine response and is mediated by interleukins (IL)-4, -5, and -13.

The role of food allergens is supported by the dramatic response of esophageal eosinophilia and symptoms to elemental diets [24,25]. Moreover, there are reports of the clustering of new cases during the aeroallergen season, suggesting an allergic mechanism [7,13,26,27].

Familial clustering of EoE has been reported [12, 28, 29]. A positive family history of EoE in a first-degree relative is seen in about 5–10% of pediatric EoE patients, suggesting a genetic predisposition to the disease [12, 24]. Furthermore, the estimated sibling recurrence risk with EoE is higher than that in many other atopic diseases with familial inheritance patterns [30].

Genetic studies have demonstrated dysregulation of 1% of the human genome in children with EoE [31]. This genetic footprint is clearly different than that in GERD patients, and can resolve with dietary and corticosteroid therapy [32, 33]. Interestingly, in these

Practical Gastroenterology and Hepatology Board Review Toolkit, Second Edition. Edited by Nicholas J. Talley, Kenneth R. DeVault, Michael B. Wallace, Bashar A. Aqel and Keith D. Lindor.
© 2016 John Wiley & Sons, Ltd. Published 2016 by John Wiley & Sons, Ltd. Companion website: www.practicalgastrohep.com

Table 16.1 EoE definition.

1 Esophageal symptoms	Adults: dysphagia, food impaction, heartburn, regurgitation, chest pain
	Children: dysphagia, food impaction, feeding disorder, vomiting abdominal pain, heartburn, regurgitation, diarrhea
2 Histology	≥15 eosinophils/hpf on any one biopsy specimen
	Eosinophilia limited to the esophageal mucosa
3 Exclusion of other diseases associated with esophageal eosinophilia, including GERD and PPI-REE	

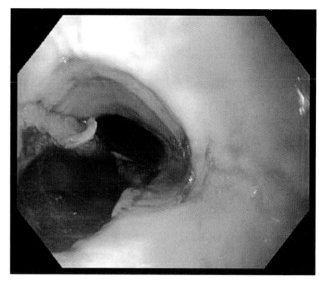

Figure 16.1 Mucosal tear post-dilation in EoE.

studies the gene encoding the eotaxin-3 gene was increased 53-fold. Eotaxin 3 is primarily produced by esophageal epithelium in response to IL-13, which is presumed to be secreted in response to inhaled or absorbed antigens [31, 34]. This process involves a complex association of eosinophils and mast cells and is only beginning to be unraveled. The proinflammatory stimulus transforming growth factor (TGF)-β is expressed by eosinophils and mast cells. This and other mediators likely play a role in remodeling at the cellular level. This process involves angiogenesis and leads to subepithelial fibrosis [35]. The pathogenesis of dysphagia in EoE can result from stricture formation and loss of wall compliance related to this fibrosis [36]. However, the rapid response to topical steroid therapy suggests there is likely a non-fibrotic mechanism delaying the transport of solid food as well, which is not well understood at this time. The mechanism of the multiple symptoms in children is poorly understood, though some of the symptoms may be related to underappreciated food impaction.

GERD can cause esophageal eosinophilia, and the frequency of GERD in patients with esophageal eosinophilia and dysphagia is 19–58% [37–39]. It is postulated that acid esophageal injury may damage cellular tight junctions, leading to greater antigen exposure [40, 41]. PPI-responsive esophageal eosinophilia is now a well recognized entity [2]. PPI treatment may improve esophageal eosinophilia not only by blocking acid, but also through direct anti-inflammatory effects of esophageal mucosa [42, 43]. It is likely GERD and EoE are interrelated diseases, but the actual mechanism of this relationship needs to be further elucidated.

Clinical Features

EoE in adults presents with the primary symptom of solid-food dysphagia and food impaction, beginning in early adulthood. Commonly, symptoms of dysphagia will have been present for years before the diagnosis is made. EoE has been reported to be present in 30–50% of patients presenting with food impaction [44–47]. The symptoms of EoE in children can be considerably different than those in adults. As children, dysphagia becomes more prominent, but at a very young age, the presentation can vary considerably [12]. Young children may present with symptoms of heartburn and regurgitation, emesis, vomiting, failure to thrive, abdominal pain, chest pain, or diarrhea. It is uncertain what roles dysphagia and food impaction play in these symptoms in young children, who may have a difficult time expressing their symptomatology.

EoE is frequently associated with other atopic diseases, including allergic rhinitis, asthma, and atopic dermatitis. One of these is present in up to 80% of children and slightly less than 50% of adults with EoE [48]. About 30% of adults and 50% of children have elevated blood eosinophilia counts, but generally less than twice normal [3]. Serum IgE levels have been reported elevated in about 70% of EoE patients [3].

The endoscopic findings of EoE are suggestive but not specific for the disease. The most common endoscopic findings are horizontal circular rings and linear vertical furrows. Loss of vasculature or edema and white spots, felt to represent eosinophilic abscesses, are seen slightly less frequently [49]. Strictures may be present throughout the esophagus with EoE but are most common in the proximal and midesophagus. The mucosal fragility or "crepe paper esophagus" can lead to linear mucosal shearing after passing an endoscope or dilator (Figure 16.1). Notably, a normal-appearing esophagus can be present in up to 40% of EoE patients [20, 22, 49]. EoE is present in 12–15% of adult patients undergoing EGD for dysphagia [20, 22].

Esophageal manometry has been abnormal in the minority of adult EoE patients studied [50]. Various abnormalities have been reported, but hypocontractility is the most common finding. Endoscopic ultrasound generally shows thickening of the mucosa, submucosa, and muscularis propria in EoE [51, 52].

Esophageal intraepithelial eosinophils are the hallmark of EoE. There are no specific histopathologic findings that clearly separate EoE from other etiologies of esophageal eosinophilia. However, certain features have been found to be suggestive of EoE: superficial layering of eosinophils, eosinophilic abscesses (a cluster of four or more eosinophils), basal-zone hyperplasia and papillary lengthening, spongiosis, lamina propria fibrosis, and an increase in mast cells [2].

Diagnosis

The diagnosis of EoE is made by the typical history, endoscopy with biopsy, and the exclusion of other diseases that can cause esophageal eosinophilia, including PPI-REE. As previously mentioned, the typical endoscopic findings support but are not required for the diagnosis. Eosinophilic infiltration may vary significantly throughout the esophagus; however, eosinophilia is usually detectable at all levels of the esophagus [53–55]. At least six specimens should be obtained, including samples from the distal and more proximal esophagus [53, 56].

Case Continued

The primary differential diagnosis of non-progressive solid-food dysphagia in a young adult is EoE, esophageal ring, extrinsic vascular esophageal compression, achalasia, and GERD with a peptic stricture. The history of food impaction, mild GERD symptoms, and atopy brings EoE, peptic stricture, or a ring to the top of the list. A barium swallow is always a reasonable first test for the evaluation of dysphagia. However, with no history to suggest oropharyngeal dysphagia and no liquid dysphagia, we choose to start the evaluation with a complete blood count (CBC) and upper endoscopy with esophageal biopsy.

The patient's CBC is only remarkable for an absolute eosinophil count of 320. His upper endoscopy shows concentric rings and furrows in the upper two-thirds of the esophagus. Midesophageal biopsies show hyperplastic squamous mucosa with up to 60 eosinophils/hpf.

These findings are felt to be consistent with EoE, but diagnostic treatment trial of twice-daily PPI therapy is required to exclude PPI-REE and confirm the EoE diagnosis.

Differential Diagnosis

The differential diagnosis of solid-food dysphagia is shown in Table 16.2. Eosinophils in esophageal mucosa are a non-specific finding. Esophageal eosinophilia has been seen in many conditions, including GERD and PPI-REE, Crohn's disease, vasculitis, celiac disease pemphigus, graft-versus-host disease, achalasia, connective-tissue disease, drug hypersensitivity reactions, infection, and the eosinophilic diseases of hypereosinophilic syndrome, eosinophilic gastroenteritis, and primary EoE. Eosinophilic gastroenteritis can have mucosal, submucosal, or serosal eosinophilic infiltration, can involve any area of the gastrointestinal (GI) tract, and can present with a multitude of GI symptoms. In EoE, the esophageal infiltration is limited to the esophageal mucosa.

Esophageal eosinophilia can be seen not uncommonly in GERD. Increased esophageal 24-hour acid exposure is seen in 19–58% of patients with symptomatic EEI [37–39]. Resolution of esophageal symptoms and marked histologic esophageal eosinophilia has been well documented with PPI therapy (PPI-REE) [2,19,48,57]. Resolution of EEI has been reported in 33–74% of patients treated with PPI medication [14,19,37,38]. PPI medications will treat acid-induced increased permeability of the esophageal mucosa, but it has been suggested that PPI treatment may decrease eosinophilia by a direct anti-inflammatory effect as well [42,43]. The relationship between GERD and EoE, as well as the terminology of PPI-REE, will likely evolve further with time [48].

Therapeutics

Treatment of Active Disease

Steroids

Swallowed topical steroid therapy is well established in the treatment of EoE, having been used to treat it for over 15 years. Currently, there are two open-label, two placebo-controlled, four comparator, and one maintenance trial of steroid therapy in the treatment of EoE [58]. There is at present no commercially available preparation designed to deliver the steroid to the esophagus. Current regimens consist of swallowing steroid preparations designed for inhalation treatment for asthma. It appears that a viscous liquid preparation is more effective than an aerosolized preparation [59]. When used in proper dose, steroids lead to complete histologic responses in the range of 60–70% of patients and at least a partial histologic response in over 90% of patients [37–39, 59–63]. Symptom response rates appear to be somewhat less than histologic rates, with at least a partial symptomatic response of only 60–75%. Acute treatment should be for 2–4 weeks with fluticasone 880 µg bid or budesonide 1–2 mg bid in adults and fluticasone 440–880 µg bid or budesonide 0.5–1.0 mg bid in children. Maintenance therapy seems promising in one trial, but likely needs a higher dose than the 0.25 mg budesonide bid that trial uses [51]. In the short term, steroids are associated with about a 20–25% incidence of asymptomatic esophageal candidiasis, but otherwise appear to be well tolerated.

Systemic steroid therapy has shown to be effective in EoE in doses up to 60 mg, or 1–2 mg/kg in children [64]. Due to their toxicity, and given the availability of other therapies, systemic steroids are rarely used in the treatment of EoE.

Dietary Therapy

Elemental diets have been dramatically successful in children and adults with EoE [24, 25]. Liacoros has found a 97% histologic and clinical response in 164 children treated with an elemental diet, with average time to response of 8.5 days [24]. These diets are expensive and unpalatable, requiring nasal gastric tube placement in 80% of patients. A six- or eight-food-elimination diet, avoiding cow's milk, eggs, soy, nuts, wheat, fish ± legumes, and cereals has led to a clinical and histologic response in about 70% of children and adults with EoE [65–67]. Wheat and milk are the most common allergens. This process requires a motivated, compliant patient and may take five or more EGDs over several months' time. Skin prick testing in adult trials was not predictive of food challenge results [66, 67]. Patients require histologic sampling to assess response to restriction and food reintroduction [66, 67]. Pilot studies suggest that potentially, the esophageal mucosa could be sampled without the need for endoscopy in the future [68, 69]. Long-term data are lacking, but the response appears to be sustained for at least 3 years in adults [67].

Table 16.2 Differential diagnosis of solid-food dysphagia.

Condition	Comment
Esophageal rings/webs	Some Schatzki rings are EoE-related
Peptic stricture	GERD symptoms may or may not be present
Achalasia	Progresses to solid and liquid dysphagia over time
GERD	Likely overlap with EoE
Pill-induced stricture	Odynophagia common, more acute onset
Extrinsic vascular compression	Aorta, subclavian artery, thoracic aneurysm
Extrinsic malignant compression	Shorter duration and progressive symptoms
Esophageal malignancy	Shorter duration and progressive symptoms
Infection	Shorter-duration symptoms. Candida, HSV, CMV, HIV. Odynophagia often present
Distal esophageal spasm	Liquid dysphagia and pain unassociated with food impaction more common
Connective-tissue diseases	Often solid and liquid dysphagia
Neuromuscular diseases	Primarily oropharyngeal symptoms with transfer and liquid dysphagia with aspiration
Cricopharyngeal narrowing ± Zenkers diverticulum	Primarily oropharyngeal symptoms

EoE, eosinophilic esophagitis; GERD, gastroesophageal reflux disease; HSV, herpes simplex virus; CMV, cytomegalovirus; HIV, human immunodeficiency virus.

Dietary therapy directed by allergy testing in children has had mixed results. The largest study showed a 77% response rate to a food-elimination diet directed by skin prick testing (immediate hypersensitivity) and skin patch testing (delayed hypersensitivity) [70]. Milk allergy testing has a low negative predictive value (NPV), and most pediatric allergists will restrict cow's milk regardless of allergy testing [70]. Patch testing has a small incremental yield over skin prick testing alone.

In motivated patients, food-elimination diets should be attempted. Vitamin and micronutrient deficiencies can develop and patients should be followed by a dietician with expertise in this area. Elemental diets should be reserved for refractory patients.

Other Agents

The leukotriene receptor antagonist montelukast used in high dose (up to 100 mg/day) has been shown to lead to symptomatic remission and maintenance of remission in a small open-label experience in eight patients, which has not been confirmed in two smaller studies at 10 mg/day [71–73]. Oral cromolyn sodium did not seem to be effective in 14 pediatric patients treated [24]. Antihistamines (H1 blockers) and allergy immunotherapy have not been formally studied but may be of theoretic benefit.

Monoclonal antibodies to IL-5 have shown some histologic benefit, but not a statistically significant symptomatic benefit [74–76]. A small study of a selective CHRTH2 antagonist, which blocks the effects of prostaglandin D2 on eosinophils and Th2 lymphocytes, has shown a significant decrease in esophageal eosinophilia [77]. Anti-immunoglobulin E (IgE) antibodies and Infliximab have not been effective for relief of symptoms or improvement in histology [75,78].

Esophageal Dilation

Esophageal dilation is an effective therapy for EoE and is the primary therapy for fibrotic stricturing disease. Dysphagia is significantly improved in 83–93% of patients, and over 40% of patients will have a response for more than 2 years [79–81] However, esophageal perforation has been reported in EoE associated with food impaction, as well as with mere passage of an endoscope [82–85]. Esophageal dilation in EoE is frequently associated with esophageal mucosal tears (Figure 16.1) and pain, as well as anecdotal reports of perforation [84, 86]. Pain is common post-dilation and is present in up to 74% of patients, typically resolving over several days [79]. Esophageal perforation was reported in 8% of 38 patients dilated in one series, causing significant concern [87]. However, in the hands of experienced physicians, dilation can be reasonably safely performed: the four largest series found a 0.3% perforation rate in 887 dilations [79, 81, 88, 89]. One should take caution in dilating EoE, however: following the rule of only using three sequential dilators after feeling resistance seems reasonable.

Esophageal dilation as the initial therapy for EoE is supported by some, but it is our feeling, in light of the potential risk and lack of effect on eosiniophilic inflammation, that dilation should be reserved for adults who have persistent symptoms after medical or dietary therapy, or in conjunction with these if the minimal esophageal diameter is less than 10 mm at presentation. Dilation is often needed to treat esophageal fibrosis, but does not turn off the inflammation that originally induced this fibrosis.

Maintenance Therapy

Recurrence of symptoms post-therapy is extremely common, and recurrence of histologic inflammation is nearly universal post-steroid treatment of EoE [51, 90, 91]. This esophageal eosinophilia can lead to wall fibrosis, resulting in a loss of compliance, esophageal stricture, and recurrent food impaction [36,90,92–95]. Patients presenting for evaluation after more than 20 years of untreated EoE symptoms have a >70% chance of having a significant esophageal stricture [94]. There are many who advocate long-term maintenance therapy in all patients with EoE, but others suggest it should only be used in those with frequent recurrent symptoms and/or those with significant esophageal fibrosis leading to small-caliber esophagus [94,96]. In the only trial of maintenance steroid therapy in EoE, a dose of 0.25 mg budesonide bid had a modest benefit on symptoms and histology and was very well tolerated [51]. It is highly likely that topical steroid in a higher dose will be an effective maintenance agent in EoE. Moreover, dietary treatment appears effective as maintenance therapy out to at least 3 years [66,67]. The role of selective or universal maintenance therapy will be resolved with time; however, treatment long-term with topical steroids, potentially other drug therapy, or dietary restriction is clearly needed in many patients with EoE.

Therapeutic End Point

The end point of therapy in adults is controversial: should we aim for symptomatic response or histologic remission? In adult patients, symptoms resulting from inflammation tend to correlate with histology, but symptoms as a result of fibrosis leading to stricturing disease and loss of compliance may persist despite histologic remission [36, 97]. With the growing awareness of stricturing disease, loss of compliance, and food impactions resulting from untreated inflammation, the pendulum is swinging to histologic healing to prevent long-term esophageal sequele [96]. Those who have incomplete histologic responses to dietary or steroid therapy can be offered the alternative treatment option: higher dose of steroid, or potentially even combination therapy. However, we really don't have prospective long-term studies on the frequency of fibrotic sequela in all patients. Therefore, it remains unclear if further therapy is beneficial in the asymptomatic patient. Further long-term studies in adult patients will be needed before we can clearly define whether the appropriate end point of treatment is symptomatic or histologic. In children, symptoms may be very difficult to evaluate, and histologic remission is needed.

From the limited data currently available, it is not possible to make definite evidence-based recommendations for many aspects of the management of EoE; a proposed management algorithm is displayed in Figure 16.2.

Case Continued

The patient is treated for 3 weeks with omeprazole 20 mg bid. His heartburn resolves, but there is no response of his dysphagia. Repeat EGD shows persistent esophageal eosinophilia. He is treated with swallowed budesonide 1.5 mg bid for 6 weeks, with complete resolution of his dysphagia after 1 week of therapy.

His symptoms recur 6 months later and he responds again to topical steroid therapy. He is currently on maintenance therapy with 1.5 mg budesonide daily and is considering an endoscopy-directed six-food elimination trial.

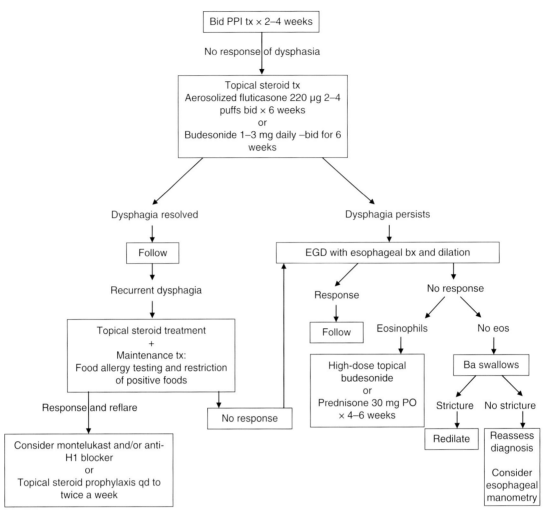

Figure 16.2 Management algorithm for adults with EoE.

Prognosis

In retrospective trials, we found symptomatic recurrence in 91% of our adult patients within 13 months of stopping steroid therapy; Liacouras reported almost universal recurrence in 381 pediatric patients after dietary or steroid therapy [24, 90]. In prospective controlled trials, histologic recurrence was universal, and symptomatic recurrence post-treatment occurred in 35% of patients at 6 months and 64% patients at 1 year [51, 91].

Straumann *et al.* [21] have followed 30 adult patients for a mean follow-up of 7.2 years. The disease course was variable, but only resolved in 10% of patients. The disease did cause dysphagia, requiring eating and dietary adjustment, but did not significantly affect quality of life or longevity. Interestingly, six of the seven patients from whom subepithelial tissue was available had evidence of fibrosis present. The same group looked at patients with untreated disease and found the prevalence of endoscopically evident esophageal stricture to be related to time of disease activity; a stricture rate of over 70% was seen in those with 20 years of untreated disease [94].

Therefore, it appears that histologic recurrence post-steroid therapy is nearly universal, symptomatic recurrence post-treatment is very high, and longstanding disease can be associated with esophageal stricture. This highlights the need for maintenance therapy in the majority of (if not all) EoE patients.

Take Home Points

- Eosinophilic esophagitis (EoE) in adult patients presents with solid-food dysphagia and food impaction.
- One-half of patients have a history of seasonal allergies, asthma, or allergic dermatitis.
- Typical endoscopic findings of concentric rings, furrows, white spots, or mucosal fragility are present in the majority of patients.
- The diagnosis is made by 15 or more eosinophils/hpf on esophageal biopsy and the exclusion of other causes of esophageal eosinophilia.
- All patients with solid-food dysphagia require esophageal biopsy.
- All patients should be treated with high-dose proton pump inhibitor (PPI) therapy to exclude PPI-responsive esophageal eosinophilia (PPI-REE).
- Most patients respond to topical steroid therapy, but recurrent dysphagia after stopping therapy is extremely common.
- Response rates to food-elimination diets are high.
- Esophageal dilation can be performed and is effective, but it may be associated with slightly increased risk of perforation.
- We are still very early in our understanding of the pathophysiology, treatment, and potential prevention of EoE.
- We have numerous questions to answer regarding the etiology and pathogenesis, natural history, and treatment of EoE, including the end points of therapy, maintenance therapy, and the role of treatment in the asymptomatic patient.

Videos of interest to readers of this chapter can be found by visiting the companion website at:

http://www.practicalgastrohep.com/

16.1 Typical rings and furrows of eosinophilic esophagitis.
16.2 Typical rings and subtle furrows of eosinophilic esophagitis with distal food impaction.

References

1 Landres RT, Kuster GG, Strum WB. Eosinophilic esophagitis in a patient with vigorous achalasia. *Gastroenterology* 1978; **74**: 1298–301.

2 Liacouras CA, Furuta GT, Hirano I, *et al.* Eosinophilic esophagitis: updated consensus recommendations for children and adults. *J Allergy Clin Immunol* 2011; **128**(1): 3–20.e6.

3 Furuta GT, Liacouras CA, Collins MH, *et al.* Eosinophilic esophagitis in children and adults: a systematic review and consensus recommendations for diagnosis and treatment. *Gastroenterology* 2007; **133**: 1342–63.

4 Hurrell JM, Genta RM, Dellon ES. Prevalence of esophageal eosinophilia varies by climate zone in the United States. *Am J Gastroenterol* 2012; **107**: 698–706.

5 Jensen ET, Hoffman K, Shaheen NJ, *et al.* Esophageal eosinophilia is increased in rural areas with low population density: results from a national pathology database. *Am J Gastroenterol* 2014; **109**: 668–75.

6 Prasad GA, Alexander JA, Schleck CD, *et al.* Epidemiology of eosinophilic esophagitis over three decades in Olmsted County, Minnesota. *Clin Gastroenterol Hepatol* 2009; **7**: 1055–61.

7 Wang FY, Gupta SK, Fitzgerald JF. Is there a seasonal variation in the incidence or intensity of allergic eosinophilic esophagitis in newly diagnosed children? *J Clin Gastroenterol* 2007; **41**: 451–3.

8 Almansa C, Krishna M, Buchner AM, *et al.* Seasonal distribution in newly diagnosed cases of eosinophilic esophagitis in adults. *Am J Gastroenterol* 2009; **104**: 828–33.

9 Elitsur Y, Aswani R, Lund V, Dementieva Y. Seasonal distribution and eosinophilic esophagitis: the experience in children living in rural communities. *J Clin Gastroenterol* 2013; **47**: 287–8.

10 Sorser SA, Barawi M, Hagglund K, *et al.* Eosinophilic esophagitis in children and adolescents: epidemiology, clinical presentation and seasonal variation. *J Gastroenterol* 2013; **48**: 81–5.

11 van Rhijn BD, Verheij J, Smout AJ, Bredenoord AJ. Rapidly increasing incidence of eosinophilic esophagitis in a large cohort. *Neurogastroenterol Motil* 2013; **25**: 47–52, e45.

12 Noel RJ, Putnam PE, Rothenberg ME. Eosinophilic esophagitis. *N Engl J Med* 2004; **351**: 940–1.

13 Prasad GA, Alexander JA, Schleck CD, *et al.* Epidemiology of eosinophilic esophagitis over three decades in Olmsted County, Minnesota. *Clin Gastroenterol Hepatol* 2009; **7**: 1055–61.

14 Dellon ES, Jensen ET, Martin CF, *et al.* Prevalence of eosinophilic esophagitis in the United States. *Clin Gastroenterol Hepatol* 2014; **12**(4): 589–96.e1.

15 Hruz P, Straumann A, Bussmann C, *et al.* Escalating incidence of eosinophilic esophagitis: a 20-year prospective, population-based study in Olten County, Switzerland. *J Allergy Clin Immunol* 2011; **128**: 1349–50, e1345.

16 Straumann A, Simon HU. Eosinophilic esophagitis: escalating epidemiology? *J Allergy Clin Immunol* 2005; **115**: 418–19.

17 Noel RJ, Putnam PE, Rothenberg ME. Eosinophilic esophagitis. *N Engl J Med* 2004; **351**: 940–1.

18 Loftus CG, Loftus EV Jr, Harmsen WS, *et al.* Update on the incidence and prevalence of Crohn's disease and ulcerative colitis in Olmsted County, Minnesota, 1940–2000. *Inflamm Bowel Dis* 2007; **13**: 254–61.

19 Molina-Infante J, Ferrando-Lamana L, Ripoll C, *et al.* Esophageal eosinophilic infiltration responds to proton pump inhibition in most adults. *Clin Gastroenterol Hepatol* 2011; **9**: 110–17.

20 Prasad GA, Talley NJ, Romero Y, *et al.* Prevalence and predictive factors of eosinophilic esophagitis in patients presenting with dysphagia: a prospective study. *Am J Gastroenterol* 2007; **102**: 2627–32.

21 Veerappan GR, Perry JL, Duncan TJ, *et al.* Prevalence of eosinophilic esophagitis in an adult population undergoing upper endoscopy: a prospective study. *Clin Gastroenterol Hepatol* 2009; **7**: 420–6, 426, e421–2.

22 Mackenzie SH, Go M, Chadwick B, *et al.* Eosinophilic oesophagitis in patients presenting with dysphagia – a prospective analysis. *Aliment Pharmacol Ther* 2008; **28**: 1140–6.

23 Ronkainen J, Talley NJ, Aro P, *et al.* Prevalence of oesophageal eosinophils and eosinophilic oesophagitis in adults: the population-based Kalixanda study. *Gut* 2007; **56**: 615–20.

24 Liacouras CA, Spergel JM, Ruchelli E, *et al.* Eosinophilic esophagitis: a 10-year experience in 381 children. *Clin Gastroenterol Hepatol* 2005; **3**: 1198–206.

25 Peterson KA, Byrne KR, Vinson LA, *et al.* Elemental diet induces histologic response in adult eosinophilic esophagitis. *Am J Gastroenterol* 2013; **108**: 759–66.

26 Onbasi K, Sin AZ, Doganavsargil B, *et al.* Eosinophil infiltration of the oesophageal mucosa in patients with pollen allergy during the season. *Clin Exp Allergy* 2005; **35**: 1423–31.

27 Fogg MI, Ruchelli E, Spergel JM. Pollen and eosinophilic esophagitis. *J Allergy Clin Immunol* 2003; **112**: 796–97.

28 Patel SM, Falchuk KR. Three brothers with dysphagia caused by eosinophilic esophagitis. *Gastrointest Endosc* 2005; **61**: 165–7.

29 Zink DA, Amin M, Gebara S, Desai TK. Familial dysphagia and eosinophilia. *Gastrointest Endosc* 2007; **65**: 330–4.

30 Blanchard C, Wang N, Rothenberg ME. Eosinophilic esophagitis: pathogenesis, genetics, and therapy. *J Allergy Clin Immunol* 2006; **118**: 1054–9.

31 Blanchard C, Wang N, Stringer KF, *et al.* Eotaxin-3 and a uniquely conserved gene-expression profile in eosinophilic esophagitis. *J Clin Invest* 2006; **116**: 536–47.

32 Sherrill JD, Rothenberg ME. Genetic dissection of eosinophilic esophagitis provides insight into disease pathogenesis and treatment strategies. *J Allergy Clin Immunol.* 2011; **128**: 23–32, quiz 33–4.

33 Wen T, Stucke EM, Grotjan TM, *et al.* Molecular diagnosis of eosinophilic esophagitis by gene expression profiling. *Gastroenterology* 2013; **145**: 1289–99.

34 Rothenberg ME. Biology and treatment of eosinophilic esophagitis. *Gastroenterology* 2009; **137**: 1238–49.

35 Aceves SS, Newbury RO, Dohil R, *et al.* Esophageal remodeling in pediatric eosinophilic esophagitis. *J Allergy Clin Immunol* 2007; **119**: 206–12.

36 Kwiatek MA, Hirano I, Kahrilas PJ, *et al.* Mechanical properties of the esophagus in eosinophilic esophagitis. *Gastroenterology* 2011; **140**: 82–90.

37 Moawad FJ, Veerappan GR, Dias JA, *et al.* Randomized controlled trial comparing aerosolized swallowed fluticasone to esomeprazole for esophageal eosinophilia. *Am J Gastroenterol* 2013; **108**: 366–72.

38 Peterson KA, Thomas KL, Hilden K, *et al.* Comparison of esomeprazole to aerosolized, swallowed fluticasone for eosinophilic esophagitis. *Dig Dis Sci* 2010; **55**(5): 1313–19.

39 Remedios M, Campbell C, Jones DM, Kerlin P. Eosinophilic esophagitis in adults: clinical, endoscopic, histologic findings, and response to treatment with fluticasone propionate. *Gastrointest Endosc* 2006; **63**: 3–12.

40 Tobey NA, Carson JL, Alkiek RA, Orlando RC. Dilated intercellular spaces: a morphological feature of acid reflux – damaged human esophageal epithelium. *Gastroenterology* 1996; **111**: 1200–5.

41 Spechler SJ, Genta RM, Souza RF. Thoughts on the complex relationship between gastroesophageal reflux disease and eosinophilic esophagitis. *Am J Gastroenterol* 2007; **102**: 1301–6.

42 Zhang X, Cheng E, Huo X, *et al.* Omeprazole blocks STAT6 binding to the eotaxin-3 promoter in eosinophilic esophagitis cells. *PLoS One* 2012; **7**: e50037.

43 Cheng E, Zhang X, Huo X, *et al.* Omeprazole blocks eotaxin-3 expression by oesophageal squamous cells from patients with eosinophilic oesophagitis and GORD. *Gut* 2013; **62**: 824–32.

44 Desai TK, Stecevic V, Chang CH, *et al.* Association of eosinophilic inflammation with esophageal food impaction in adults. *Gastrointest Endosc* 2005; **61**: 795–801.

45 Prasad GA, Reddy JG, Boyd-Enders FT, *et al.* Predictors of recurrent esophageal food impaction: a case-control study. *J Clin Gastroenterol* 2008; **42**: 771–5.

46 Kerlin P, Jones D, Remedios M, Campbell C. Prevalence of eosinophilic esophagitis in adults with food bolus obstruction of the esophagus. *J Clin Gastroenterol* 2007; **41**: 356–61.

47 Sperry SL, Crockett SD, Miller CB, *et al.* Esophageal foreign-body impactions: epidemiology, time trends, and the impact of the increasing prevalence of eosinophilic esophagitis. *Gastrointest Endosc* 2011; **74**: 985–91.

48 Dellon ES. Diagnosis and management of eosinophilic esophagitis. *Clin Gastroenterol Hepatol* 2012; **10**: 1066–78.

49 Kim HP, Vance RB, Shaheen NJ, Dellon ES. The prevalence and diagnostic utility of endoscopic features of eosinophilic esophagitis: a meta-analysis. *Clin Gastroenterol Hepatol* 2012; **10**: 988–96, e985.

50 Roman S, Hirano I, Kwiatek MA, *et al.* Manometric features of eosinophilic esophagitis in esophageal pressure topography. *Neurogastroenterol Motil* 2011; **23**: 208–14, e111.

51 Straumann A, Conus S, Degen L, *et al.* Long-term budesonide maintenance treatment is partially effective for patients with eosinophilic esophagitis. *Clin Gastroenterol Hepatol* 2011; **9**: 400–9, e401.

52 Fox VL. Eosinophilic esophagitis: endoscopic findings. *Gastrointest Endosc Clin N Am* 2008; **18**: 45–57, viii.

53 Gonsalves N, Policarpio-Nicolas M, Zhang Q, *et al.* Histopathologic variability and endoscopic correlates in adults with eosinophilic esophagitis. *Gastrointest Endosc* 2006; **64**: 313–19.

54 Konikoff MR, Noel RJ, Blanchard C, *et al.* A randomized, double-blind, placebo-controlled trial of fluticasone propionate for pediatric eosinophilic esophagitis. *Gastroenterology* 2006; **131**: 1381–91.

55 Saffari H, Peterson KA, Fang JC, *et al.* Patchy eosinophil distributions in an esophagectomy specimen from a patient with eosinophilic esophagitis: implications for endoscopic biopsy. *J Allergy Clin Immunol* 2012; **130**: 798–800.

56 Nielsen JA, Lager DJ, Lewin M, *et al.* The optimal number of biopsy fragments to establish a morphologic diagnosis of eosinophilic esophagitis. *Am J Gastroenterol* 2014; **109**: 515–20.

57 Ngo P, Furuta GT, Antonioli DA, Fox VL. Eosinophils in the esophagus – peptic or allergic eosinophilic esophagitis? Case series of three patients with esophageal eosinophilia. *Am J Gastroenterol* 2006; **101**: 1666–70.

58 Alexander JA. Steroid treatment of eosinophilic esophagitis in adults. *Gastroenterol Clin N Am* 2014; **43**: 357–73.

59 Dellon ES, Sheikh A, Speck O, *et al.* Viscous topical is more effective than nebulized steroid therapy for patients with eosinophilic esophagitis. *Gastroenterology* 2012; **143**: 321–4, e321.

60 Arora AS, Perrault J, Smyrk TC. Topical corticosteroid treatment of dysphagia due to eosinophilic esophagitis in adults. *Mayo Clin Proc* 2003; **78**: 830–5.

61 Straumann A, Conus S, Degen L, *et al.* Budesonide is effective in adolescent and adult patients with active eosinophilic esophagitis. *Gastroenterology* 2010; **139**: 1526–37.

62 Alexander JA, Jung KW, Arora AS, *et al.* Swallowed fluticasone improves histologic but not symptomatic response of adults with eosinophilic esophagitis. *Clin Gastroenterol Hepatol* 2012; **10**: 742–9, e741.

63 Francis DL, Foxx-Orenstein A, Arora AS, *et al.* Results of ambulatory pH monitoring do not reliably predict response to therapy in patients with eosinophilic oesophagitis. *Aliment Pharmacol Ther* 2012; **35**: 300–7.

64 Liacouras CA, Wenner WJ, Brown K, Ruchelli E. Primary eosinophilic esophagitis in children: successful treatment with oral corticosteroids. *J Pediatr Gastroenterol Nutr* 1998; **26**: 380–5.

65 Kagalwalla AF, Sentongo TA, Ritz S, *et al.* Effect of six-food elimination diet on clinical and histologic outcomes in eosinophilic esophagitis. *Clin Gastroenterol Hepatol* 2006; **4**: 1097–102.

66 Gonsalves N, Yang GY, Doerfler B, *et al.* Elimination diet effectively treats eosinophilic esophagitis in adults; food reintroduction identifies causative factors. *Gastroenterology* 2012; **142**: 1451–9, e1451, quiz e1414–55.

67 Lucendo AJ, Arias A, Gonzalez-Cervera J, *et al.* Empiric 6-food elimination diet induced and maintained prolonged remission in patients with adult eosinophilic esophagitis: a prospective study on the food cause of the disease. *J Allergy Clin Immunol* 2013; **131**: 797–804.

68 Furuta GT, Kagalwalla AF, Lee JJ, *et al.* The oesophageal string test: a novel, minimally invasive method measures mucosal inflammation in eosinophilic oesophagitis. *Gut* 2013; **62**: 1395–405.

69 Katzka D, Fitzgerald R, Alexander J, Geno D. 56 cytosponge evalutation of eosiniophilic esophagitis in comparison to endoscopy: accuracy, safety, and tolerability. *Gastroenterology* 2014; **146**(5): S16.

70 Spergel JM, Brown-Whitehorn T, Beausoleil JL, *et al.* Predictive values for skin prick test and atopy patch test for eosinophilic esophagitis. *J Allergy Clin Immunol* 2007; **119**: 509–11.

71 Attwood SE, Lewis CJ, Bronder CS, *et al.* Eosinophilic oesophagitis: a novel treatment using Montelukast. *Gut* 2003; **52**: 181–5.

72 Stumphy J, Al-Zubeidi D, Guerin L, *et al.* Observations on use of montelukast in pediatric eosinophilic esophagitis: insights for the future. *Dis Esophagus* 2011; **24**: 229–34.

73 Lucendo AJ, De Rezende LC, Jimenez-Contreras S, *et al.* Montelukast was inefficient in maintaining steroid-induced remission in adult eosinophilic esophagitis. *Dig Dis Sci* 2011; **56**: 3551–8.

74 Spergel JM, Rothenberg ME, Collins MH, *et al.* Reslizumab in children and adolescents with eosinophilic esophagitis: results of a double-blind, randomized, placebo-controlled trial. *J Allergy Clin Immunol* 2012; **129**: 456–63, 463. e451–3.

75 Straumann A, Bussmann C, Conus S, *et al.* Anti-TNF-alpha (infliximab) therapy for severe adult eosinophilic esophagitis. *J Allergy Clin Immunol* 2008; **122**: 425–7.

76 Assa'ad AH, Gupta SK, Collins MH, *et al.* An antibody against IL-5 reduces numbers of esophageal intraepithelial eosinophils in children with eosinophilic esophagitis. *Gastroenterology* 2011; **141**: 1593–604.

77 Straumann A, Hoesli S, Bussmann C, *et al.* Anti-eosinophil activity and clinical efficacy of the CRTH2 antagonist OC000459 in eosinophilic esophagitis. *Allergy* 2013; **68**: 375–85.

78 Fang JC HK, Gleich GJ, *et al.* A pilot study of the treatment of eosinophilic esophagitis with omalizumab. *Gastroenterology* 2011; **140**: S506.

79 Schoepfer AM, Gonsalves N, Bussmann C, *et al.* Esophageal dilation in eosinophilic esophagitis: effectiveness, safety, and impact on the underlying inflammation. *Am J Gastroenterol* 2010; **105**: 1062–70.

80 Bohm M, Richter JE, Kelsen S, Thomas R. Esophageal dilation: simple and effective treatment for adults with eosinophilic esophagitis and esophageal rings and narrowing. *Dis Esophagus* 2010; **23**: 377–85.

81 Dellon ES, Gibbs WB, Rubinas TC, *et al.* Esophageal dilation in eosinophilic esophagitis: safety and predictors of clinical response and complications. *Gastrointest Endosc* 2010; **71**: 706–12.

82 Cohen MS, Kaufman A, DiMarino AJ Jr, Cohen S. Eosinophilic esophagitis presenting as spontaneous esophageal rupture (Boerhaave's syndrome). *Clin Gastroenterol Hepatol* 2007; **5**: A24.

83 Riou PJ, Nicholson AG, Pastorino U. Esophageal rupture in a patient with idiopathic eosinophilic esophagitis. *Ann Thorac Surg* 1996; **62**: 1854–6.

84 Kaplan M, Mutlu EA, Jakate S, *et al.* Endoscopy in eosinophilic esophagitis: "feline" esophagus and perforation risk. *Clin Gastroenterol Hepatol* 2003; **1**: 433–7.

85 Straumann A, Rossi L, Simon HU, *et al.* Fragility of the esophageal mucosa: a pathognomonic endoscopic sign of primary eosinophilic esophagitis? *Gastrointest Endosc* 2003; **57**: 407–12.

86 Croese J, Fairley SK, Masson JW, *et al.* Clinical and endoscopic features of eosinophilic esophagitis in adults. *Gastrointest Endosc* 2003; **58**: 516–22.

87 Cohen MS, Kaufman AB, Palazzo JP, *et al.* An audit of endoscopic complications in adult eosinophilic esophagitis. *Clin Gastroenterol Hepatol* 2007; **5**: 1149–53.

88 Jung KW, Gundersen N, Kopacova J, *et al.* Occurrence of and risk factors for complications after endoscopic dilation in eosinophilic esophagitis. *Gastrointest Endosc* 2011; **73**: 15–21.

89 Ally MR, Dias J, Veerappan GR, *et al.* Safety of dilation in adults with eosinophilic esophagitis. *Dis Esophagus* 2013; **26**: 241–5.

90 Helou EF, Simonson J, Arora AS. 3-yr-follow-up of topical corticosteroid treatment for eosinophilic esophagitis in adults. *Am J Gastroenterol* 2008; **103**: 2194–9.

91 Schaefer ET, Fitzgerald JF, Molleston JP, *et al.* Comparison of oral prednisone and topical fluticasone in the treatment of eosinophilic esophagitis: a randomized trial in children. *Clin Gastroenterol Hepatol* 2008; **6**: 165–73.

92 Straumann A, Spichtin HP, Grize L, *et al.* Natural history of primary eosinophilic esophagitis: a follow-up of 30 adult patients for up to 11.5 years. *Gastroenterology* 2003; **125**: 1660–9.

93 Chehade M, Sampson HA, Morotti RA, Magid MS. Esophageal subepithelial fibrosis in children with eosinophilic esophagitis. *J Pediatr Gastroenterol Nutr* 2007; **45**: 319–28.

94 Schoepfer AM, Safroneeva E, Bussmann C, *et al.* Delay in diagnosis of eosinophilic esophagitis increases risk for stricture formation in a time-dependent manner. *Gastroenterology* 2013; **145**: 1230–6, e1232.

95 Nicodeme F, Hirano I, Chen J, *et al.* Esophageal distensibility as a measure of disease severity in patients with eosinophilic esophagitis. *Clin Gastroenterol Hepatol* 2013; **11**: 1101–7, e1101.

96 Katzka DA. The skinny on eosinophilic esophagitis. *Gastroenterology* 2013; **145**: 1186–8.

97 Gentile N, Ravi K, Trenkner S, *et al.* The sensitivity and specificity of esophagogastroduodenoscopy (EGD) for the small caliber esophagus in esophageal eosinophilic infiltration (EEI). *Am J Gastroenterol* 2012; **107**: S17.

CHAPTER 17

Strictures, Rings, and Webs

Ioannis S. Papanikolaou[1] and Peter D. Siersema[2]

[1] Hepatogastroenterology Unit, 2nd Department of Internal Medicine and Research Unit, "Attikon" University General Hospital, University of Athens, Athens, Greece
[2] Department of Gastroenterology & Hepatology, University Medical Center Utrecht, Utrecht, The Netherlands

Case

A 55-year-old white man presents with a 10-month history of worsening dysphagia to solids. In the past 5 years, he had frequent symptoms of heartburn and regurgitation, particularly when bending forward and during the night while in bed. These symptoms have quite suddenly resolved, and he has noticed dysphagia. His body weight has gradually increased over the past few years, while his appetite has not changed. An esophagogastroduodenoscopy (EGD) is performed, which shows a regular, smooth, 1–2 cm-long stricture in the distal esophagus, just above the gastroesophageal junction (GEJ). The stricture can be passed only with a small-caliber (5.9 mm) endoscope. Biopsies are taken, but only show a moderate inflammatory reaction and fibrous tissue, with no evidence of malignancy. He is diagnosed with a peptic stricture, and the stricture is dilated using various diameter Savary–Gilliard dilators up to 18 mm. He is then placed on proton pump inhibitors (PPIs). After dilation, the symptoms do not recur and he is able to resume a normal diet.

Definition and Epidemiology

Benign esophageal strictures, rings, and webs result from numerous etiologies and pathophysiologic mechanisms (Table 17.1) and manifest as dysphagia of variable severity [1]. In addition, benign esophageal strictures, rings, and webs can be classified according to complexity, which is associated with the type and number of therapeutic procedures needed. In this setting, strictures that are short, focal straight, and allow passage of an endoscope are considered simple strictures (e.g., peptic strictures, webs, and rings). On the other hand, strictures that are longer (>2 cm), angulated, irregular, and lead to a markedly narrowed lumen are defined as complex. The former require usually one to three dilations to relieve dysphagia, and only one-quarter need additional treatment. The latter are commonly refractory to initial treatment and tend to recur. Refractoriness is defined as the inability to successfully remediate the anatomic problem to a diameter of at least 14 mm over five sessions at 2-week intervals. On the other hand, the term "recurrent stricture" refers to the inability to maintain a satisfactory luminal diameter for 4 weeks once the target diameter of 14 mm has been achieved [1].

Though dysphagia is a common condition, occurring in 5–8% of the general population over 50 years [2], it is difficult to obtain detailed information on incidence and prevalence rates, due to the various etiologies (Table 17.1) [3]. An estimated 40–50% of benign esophageal strictures are peptic in origin and result from gastroesophageal reflux disease (GERD). The prevalence of strictures among GERD patients undergoing endoscopy used to be 4–20%, but this has diminished due to the widespread use of PPIs. Approximately 50–60% of cases of benign esophageal strictures are attributed to causes other than gastroesophageal reflux. Examples include strictures secondary to chest radiation, caustic ingestions, surgical anastomosis following esophageal resection, and strictures due to external compression of the esophagus. In addition, eosinophilic esophagitis (EoE) represents an increasingly recognized cause of esophageal strictures, occurring particularly in young men. Its diagnosis is important, since effective medical management can be offered. However, in the case of stenosis that does not respond to conservative measures, endoscopic dilation is indicated. Notably, dilation of stenosis in the background of EoE carries a risk of mucosal tearing and perforation [4].

An esophageal web represents a thin mucosal fold that protrudes into the lumen and is covered by squamous epithelium. They most commonly occur anteriorly in the cervical esophagus, but their prevalence is difficult to assess, since they are often missed during endoscopy. Webs have been associated with iron deficiency, and the triad of iron-deficiency anemia, dysphagia, and a cervical esophageal web is known as Plummer–Vinson or Paterson–Brown-Kelly syndrome. Recognition of this syndrome is important, since it is related to esophageal squamous carcinoma. Esophageal webs have also been associated with Zenker's diverticulum and can be seen as extracutaneous manifestations of various dermatologic and immunologic diseases [5].

Schatzki rings are the most common type of esophageal ring normally located at the distal esophagus. There are two types of Schatzki ring: A and B. The former is a muscular ring just proximal to the esophagogastric junction (EGJ), corresponding to the lower esophageal sphincter (LES). A rings are rare and are usually seen in children. B rings are mucosal structures that are found precisely at the squamocolumnar junction (SCJ) and are covered with squamous mucosa proximally and columnar epithelium distally. Schatzki rings are usually associated with GERD; however, their exact pathogenesis remains uncertain. Moreover, Schatzki rings are almost always associated with hiatal hernias.

Practical Gastroenterology and Hepatology Board Review Toolkit, Second Edition. Edited by Nicholas J. Talley, Kenneth R. DeVault, Michael B. Wallace, Bashar A. Aqel and Keith D. Lindor.
© 2016 John Wiley & Sons, Ltd. Published 2016 by John Wiley & Sons, Ltd. Companion website: www.practicalgastrohep.com

Table 17.1 Differential diagnosis of esophageal dysphagia. Source: Kochman 2005 [1]. Reproduced with permission of Elsevier.

Inflammatory and/or fibrotic strictures	Peptic Caustic Pill-induced Radiation-induced
Mucosal rings and webs	Schatzki ring EoE
Cancer	Primary (squamous carcinoma, adenocarcinoma) Secondary (e.g., lung, breast, melanoma)
Intramural lesions	Leiomyoma Granular cell tumor
Extramural lesions	Aberrant right subclavian artery (dysphagia lusoria) Mediastinal masses Lung cancer
Anatomical abnormalities	Hiatus hernia Esophageal diverticulum
Motility disorders	Achalasia and achalasia-like disorders Pseudoachalasia Hypomotility secondary to systemic disease (e.g., scleroderma, amyloid, diabetes)

Pathophysiology

Benign esophageal strictures result from esophageal injury. The volume, dwell time, concentration, and depth of the injury produced by the underlying causative etiology determine the severity and recurrence risk after treatment of the stricture [6]. The pathologic processes in benign esophageal strictures can be quite diverse. An inflammatory component is found in almost all benign strictures, but not to the same degree or for the same period of time. For example, the initial inflammatory reaction in peptic and caustic strictures can be severe, but this will ultimately resolve with a satisfactory outcome for the stricture. On the other hand, transmural (ischemic) insults to the esophagus, such as are seen in postoperative anastomotic and postradiation strictures, may be more difficult and need more time to resolve, and sometimes require prolonged treatment. Any treatment in these situations is a temporizing maneuver, allowing the inflammatory reaction to resolve over time. In particular, if there is ongoing or repeated injury to the esophageal mucosa, the resulting acute inflammation and healing reaction with fibrosis may maintain the stricture.

Clinical Features

Patients with a benign stricture, web, or ring all have symptoms in common, but they may have some discriminating symptoms depending on the underlying disease. Obtaining a careful history is mandatory before deciding which diagnostic algorithm should be used (Table 17.2).

Dysphagia is the primary symptom of any type of esophageal obstruction, though it is often a late symptom. Typically, the patient will describe food "sticking" or "holding up," but at times the presenting symptoms may be atypical. Atypical symptoms of dysphagia include meal-related regurgitation (often reported as vomiting), a sense of fullness or filling up retrosternally, and hiccups during meals. There should be two aims when taking a dysphagia history: to establish whether or not dysphagia is actually present (i.e., to distinguish true dysphagia from globus sensation or a difficulty in swallowing); and to determine whether the site of the problem is pharyngeal or esophageal. Importantly, subjective localization of the lesion by the patient correlates poorly with the true site of stenosis. The progressive or intermittent presentation of dysphagia should also be

clarified. Finally, the physician must seek for possible unintentional weight loss, which is an alarm symptom for malignancy.

The type of food that produces the symptom of dysphagia is suggestive of the underlying disease. Dysphagia to both solids and liquids from the onset of symptoms is probably caused by a motility disorder of the esophagus. In contrast, dysphagia for solids that later involves liquids is more likely to reflect mechanical obstruction.

If dysphagia is present, it usually starts with difficulty passing larger solid food challenges, typically meat, down the esophagus, followed by dysphagia for all solids. Solid food obstruction becomes permanent when the esophageal lumen is reduced to approximately 12 mm (which equals 50% of normal). Patients often ignore the early symptoms of dysphagia for some time. They compensate for this by eating softer or minced food, eating slowly, or using variable amounts of fluid to facilitate the passage of food down the esophagus. Suddenly, complete obstruction for all food – and later for fluids – occurs during a meal. This is a challenging problem to endoscopists, because it usually occurs during the nighttime following dinner and necessitates immediate intervention. Regurgitation during meals, as well as spontaneous regurgitation between meals or at night, is easily separated from vomiting because it is not associated with nausea. Unlike regurgitation that is related to GERD, the regurgitated fluid and/or food in patients with an esophageal stricture is generally not noxious to taste and is composed primarily of indigested material and saliva.

Odynophagia is not always present, but can develop with erosive or ulcerative esophageal disease, or with increased intraesophageal pressure and distension. Examples of the former include benign esophageal strictures with an ongoing inflammatory component (as is seen in GERD), caustic injury, and postradiation esophagitis.

It is important to take a thorough previous medical history, which should take into account the previous application of radiation therapy on the chest (postradiation stricture), the use of medication (e.g., non-steroidal anti-inflammatory drugs (NSAIDs), potassium chloride, and alendronate – pill-induced stricture), the accidental or intentional use of caustic fluids (caustic stricture), the performance of a surgical procedure in the esophagus or stomach (anastomotic stricture), and a history of chronic heartburn. Additionally, known allergies and atopic conditions should be revealed, since they are common in patients with EoE (Tables 17.1 and 17.2).

Table 17.2 Clinical features in patients with benign strictures, rings, or webs.

Symptom	Comment
Dysphagia	Starting with large solids, followed by all solids, then liquids, and finally no food or drinks
Regurgitation	Mostly in advanced cases
Odynophagia	In cases with erosions or ulceration (reflux esophagitis, radiation injury, caustic injury)
Previous medical history	Radiation therapy on chest, esophageal or gastric resection
History of esophageal injury	GERD, caustic, radiation therapy, pills
Other symptoms	Heartburn (GERD), systemic disease (scleroderma)
Sialorrhea	Related to severity of obstruction
Weight loss	Uncommon with benign stricture, rings, or webs (more common with malignancy)
History of smoking and alcohol abuse	Malignant disorder (esophageal cancer, lung cancer)

GERD, gastroesophageal reflux disease.

Table 17.3 Diagnostic modalities in benign strictures, rings, and webs.

Method	Comment
EGD	Allows inspection of localization of the stricture
	Allows biopsies to be obtained and endoscopic treatment to be performed
Radiography	A barium swallow detects small strictures, rings, or webs and identifies coexisting perforations, leaks, and fistulae
	A CT scan detects extramural lesions and small tumors around the GEJ
Esophageal manometry	Detects motility disorders

EGD, esophagogastroduodenoscopy; CT, computed tomography; GEJ, gastroesophageal junction.

Diagnosis

Diagnostic testing to identify the etiology of esophageal dysphagia should be based on the patient history. Available modalities include endoscopy, imaging, and esophageal manomentry [7–9] (Table 17.3).

Esophagogastroduodenoscopy

Patients with esophageal dysphagia should be referred for upper endoscopy. Endoscopy can reveal the responsible lesion and offers the opportunity for tissue sampling and therapeutic intervention (e.g., dilation). During endoscopy, peptic strictures and Schatzki rings are always found in the distal esophagus. Moreover, endoscopy will identify anastomotic, postradiation, and pill-induced strictures (e.g., from tetracyclines, bisphosphonates), as well as caustic ones, which are commonly multifocal. Infective esophagitis (e.g., that caused by herpes simplex virus (HSV), cytomegalovirus (CMV), or Candida) has typical appearances. The presence of food, fluid, or salivary residue within a dilated esophagus is highly suggestive of a dysmotility disorder, particularly achalasia, and the patient should be referred for manometry.

Numerous endoscopic findings have been associated with EoE, including circular rings, strictures, linear furrows, white papules, and a small-caliber esophagus. The diagnosis is established by distal and proximal esophageal biopsies, which demonstrate an increased number of eosinophils (>15 per high power field). If no clear structural abnormality is seen, esophageal biopsies should also be obtained (to rule out EoE) in any case of unexplained dysphagia or food impaction.

Barium Swallow

Barium esophagogram may be helpful as an initial test in cases of a suspected proximal esophageal lesion (e.g., Zenker's diverticulum), known complex stricture (to determine an endoscopic intervention), or suspected achalasia, or as a second test following a negative upper endoscopy, since lesions such as rings and extrinsic esophageal compression can be missed initially. This technique is also able to detect a perforation, leak, or fistula, in combination with a stricture. If a structural disorder is still suspected, it is important to determine whether the barium swallow study included prone views and a marshmallow or pill swallow. Mucosal rings and webs, in particular, are frequently overlooked unless adequate and deliberate distension of the esophagus is achieved by evaluating the esophageal contours in the prone position, preferably while the patient performs the Valsalva.

Motility Testing

Esophageal manometry should be offered to patients with dysphagia in whom upper endoscopy is not diagnostic and/or an esophageal motility disorder is suspected. Up to 50% of patients with non-structural dysphagia are diagnosed by manometry as suffering from achalasia or a non-specific motility disorder.

Differential Diagnosis

The amount of time for which the dysphagia has been present and whether it is intermittent and/or progressive will help to define the likely cause. Slowly progressive, long-standing dysphagia, particularly against a background of reflux, is suggestive of a peptic stricture. However, the physician should remember that the severity of heartburn correlates poorly with esophageal mucosal damage. Patients who have mucosal changes, including strictures and Barrett's esophagus, could have had minimal or no heartburn in the immediate past. On the other hand, a short history of dysphagia, particularly with rapid progression (weeks or months) and associated weight loss, is highly suggestive of esophageal cancer.

Long-standing, intermittent, non-progressive dysphagia purely for solids is indicative of a fixed structural lesion, such as a distal esophageal ring or proximal esophageal mucosal web. The latter in association with iron deficiency comprises the Plummer–Vinson or Paterson–Brown-Kelly syndrome, in which anemia, koilonychia, glossitis, cheilitis, and other symptoms/signs of iron deficiency may be present. Intermittent dysphagia to solids and/or history of food impaction in a middle-aged male patient with a history of allergies should raise concern in the direction of EoE. Finally, it is important to emphasize that the (previous) medical history will also allow a diagnosis to be made, as in the setting of irradiation to the chest, upper gastrointestinal (GI) surgical procedures, and caustic agent ingestion.

Treatment

Treatment of an esophageal stricture depends on the characteristics of the stricture, the endoscopist's experience, and the available equipment. The majority of simple strictures can be treated successfully with mechanical dilators (bougie) or balloon dilators. Common etiologies include peptic injury, (Schatzki) rings, and webs. One to three dilations are usually sufficient to relieve symptoms related to simple strictures. Complex esophageal strictures are more difficult to treat. The most common causes include caustic ingestion, radiation injury, and postsurgical anastomotic strictures. These strictures often require at least three dilation sessions, and are associated with high recurrence rates. When this is the case, they are considered to be refractory and other treatment modalities will be required. Dilatation in EoE should be used only as an adjunctive therapy when medical measures (i.e., swallowed fluticasone or budenoside) fail. It should be performed carefully, since it has been linked to an increased risk of esophageal tearing and perforation. Both mechanical and balloon dilators and balloons have been proven efficacious (Table 17.4).

It is important to treat esophageal strictures in a stepwise fashion, starting with the least invasive treatment modality (Table 17.5). If this is not sufficient to relieve the dysphagia, the next treatment modality in the algorithm should be applied. In this section, the various treatments for strictures are discussed. At the end of the section, an algorithm for the treatment of refractory strictures is proposed.

Table 17.4 Treatment modalities in benign strictures, rings, and webs.

Dilation therapy	Bougie
	Balloon
	Combined antegrade and retrograde dilation (CARD)
Dilation with intralesion steroid injection	
Incisional therapy	Needle knife
	Argon plasma coagulation (APC)
Stent placement	Self-expanding metal stent (SEMS)
	Self-expanding plastic stent (SEPS)
	Self-expanding biodegradable stent
Self-bougienage	

Dilation Therapy

Treatment of benign esophageal strictures aims to relieve symptoms of dysphagia, while avoiding complications and preventing of recurrences. Dilation is the first-line treatment option for benign esophageal strictures. Dilators can be categorized into mechanical (bougie) and balloon dilators. Mechanical dilators are further subdivided into bougies that are used with or without a guidewire and fluoroscopy. The most commonly used guidewire-assisted bougie is the polyvinyl Savary–Gilliard dilator, which has a tapered tip and is available in multiple sizes. The American dilators are similar products that are impregnated with barium and are thus easier to see fluoroscopically. Balloon dilators can be passed through the scope and are also available with or without a guidewire.

Bougie dilators dilate a stenotic segment by using gradually increasing dilator diameters, resulting in both a longitudina and a radial force on the stricture. Balloon dilation can be performed under direct vision. In contrast to bougies, balloon dilators deliver only a radial force, resulting in a simultaneously applied dilating force across the entire length of the stricture. Despite these mechanistic differences, no clear advantage of either balloon or bougie dilation has been demonstrated in terms of efficacy and safety [10]. An advantage of bougie dilators is that they are more cost-effective because they are reusable, whereas balloon dilators are intended for a single use only.I Importantly, PPIs should be prescribed following esophageal dilation to promote mucosal healing and reduce the risk of stricture recurrence.

The most frequently reported complications of esophageal dilation are perforation, hemorrhage, and bacteremia. Perforation rates varying between 0.1 and 0.4% have been reported. In general, it is accepted that the risk of perforation is minimal only when the "rule of three" is applied, meaning that no more than three dilators of progressively increasing diameter should be passed in a single session, corresponding with a total 3 mm increase in diameter [11]. Though this "rule" is easily applicable as a clinical guideline, no studies have demonstrated that it indeed improves safety and efficacy. It is commonly advised to limit initial dilation to 33–39 Fr (about

Table 17.5 Treatment algorithm for benign esophageal strictures, rings, and webs.

Step	Action
1	Dilation (Savary–Gilliard or balloon) to 16–18 mm (up to five sessions)
2	Dilation combined with intralesional four-quadrant triamcinolone acetate injections (max. three sessions)
	Incisional therapy (max. three sessions) for Schatzki rings and anastomotic strictures
3	Stent placement
4	Self-bougienage
5	Surgery

11–13 mm). Nevertheless, there is no evidence that this prevents development of complications. As already noted, dilation of strictures due to EoE carries a greater risk of perforation, a matter of which patients should be aware [12].

The efficacy and safety of endoscopic dilation without fluoroscopy have been shown. However, it is generally advocated that fluoroscopic guidance be used to enhance safety during dilation of complex strictures.

Most patients are instructed to avoid antiplatelet agents and anticoagulants for 5–7 days prior to the procedure, to minimize bleeding risk. Guidelines issued by the American Heart Association (AHA) and the American Society of Gastrointestinal Endoscopy (ASGE) no longer recommend antibiotic prophylaxis for esophageal dilations, even in high-risk groups [9].

Combined Antegrade and Retrograde Dilation

Most complex strictures can be endoscopically passed with a guidewire, followed by dilation. Occasionally, it can be difficult to identify the true lumen of a stenotic esophagus (e.g., in postradiation strictures in the cervical esophagus). In these circumstances, the passing of a guidewire for dilation through antegrade endoscopy is unsuccessful. In order to reduce the potential risk of perforation, the combined antegrade and retrograde dilation (CARD) technique can be applied [13]. The principle of the CARD technique is double endoscopic access to the proximal and distal ends of the stricture, resulting in better control during dilation.

Dilation and Intralesional Steroid Injection Therapy

In the 1960s, the efficacy of intralesional corticosteroid injections into benign esophageal strictures of dogs and children was demonstrated. Over the last decade, this treatment has increasingly been employed in the treatment of refractory benign esophageal strictures. The mechanism of action is suggested to be the local inhibition of the inflammatory response, resulting in a reduction in collagen formation.

It has been demonstrated that there is an increase in intervals between dilations and a reduction in the frequency of dilations when dilation is combined with intralesional injections with triamcinolone acetonide [14]. There is no certainty about the optimal technique of intralesional steroid injection (i.e., the optimal dose is per session is (varying between 40 and 80 mg), the number of injections per session (four to eight), the injection site (upper margin or inside stricture), the interval between treatment sessions, and the maximum number of treatment sessions). Only a few complications (perforation ($n = 2$) and *Candida albicans* infections ($n = 2$)) have been reported. However, recent studies question the efficacy of intralesional steroid injection at least in anastomotic strictures [15].

Incisional Therapy

Strictures at the esophagogastric anastomosis following esophageal resection have been reported in up to 30% of patients. Postoperative complications, such as anastomotic leakage, fistula formation, and ischemia of the proximal gastric tube, contribute to anastomotic stricture formation. The success rate of dilation of anastomotic strictures ranges from 70 to 90%, with up to 40% of patients requiring more than three dilation sessions to achieve an adequate result [16]. An alternative treatment option for refractory benign anastomotic strictures is to use incisional therapy [17], which can be performed with needle-knife electrocautery or argon plasma coagulation (APC). The author incises the stricture in four quadrants and,

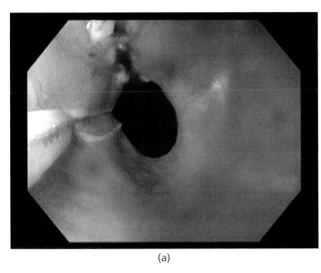

(a)

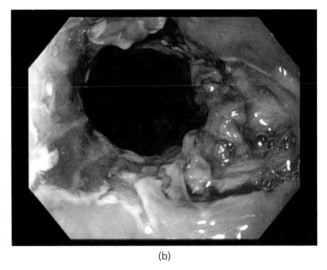

(b)

Figure 17.1 (a) Anastomotic stricture after esophageal resection with gastric tube interposition, treated with incisional therapy with needle-knife electrocautery. (b) Wide-open anastomosis following incisional therapy.

in addition, coagulates the bridging (fibrous) tissue in between the incisions in order to establish a maximally wide luminal diameter (Figure 17.1).

In short anastomotic strictures (≤10 mm), a single treatment session is usually effective, but longer strictures (>10 mm) require more electrocautery procedures. Incisional therapy can also be considered in refractory Schatzki rings. Only limited experience but no complications have been reported. More studies are needed to confirm the initial results and define the patients most amenable to this treatment.

Stents

Placement of a self-expanding metal stent (SEMS) is frequently used for the palliation of dysphagia from esophageal or gastric cardia cancer. Over the last few years, stents have become increasingly important in various clinical applications, such as sealing benign esophageal leaks or perforations and dilating refractory benign esophageal strictures. In these strictures, the idea is that dilation for a prolonged period of time will ultimately reduce the risk of recurrent stricture formation. The introduction of self-expanding plastic stents (SEPS) has given a further boost to the use of stents for these indications. Very recently, self-expanding biodegradable stents have been developed and used in esophageal strictures of benign origin.

Self-Expanding Metal Stents

To date, numerous patients have been reported with a SEMS placed for a benign esophageal stricture [18]. In most patients, strictures were resistant to (repeat) dilation. Indications for SEMS placement included achalasia, caustic strictures, postradiation strictures, anastomotic strictures, peptic strictures, and some other causes. Uncovered SEMS were chiefly used in initial studies, but these were associated with a very high incidence of complications. Currently, only fully covered SEMS are used for benign esophageal obstruction. Their removability is of great importance; however, stent migration rates remain high.

As already indicated, a limitation of uncovered and partially covered SEMS is the occurrence of hyperplastic tissue ingrowth through the uncovered stent meshes. Tissue ingrowth has been considered to result from a combination of factors, particularly the

type of metal used (stainless steel or nitinol), the size and radial force of the stent, and the duration of stenting. The risk of tissue ingrowth increases with stenting time, but it can already be observed 2–6 weeks after stent placement [19]. This tissue reaction causes the uncovered stent parts to embed in the esophageal wall, which precludes easy removal. An obvious advantage of this anchoring is that migration of uncovered or partially covered SEMS is rare, though migration is more frequent with fully covered SEMS. Hyperplastic tissue overgrowth at both ends of a fully covered SEMS can also be observed. Tissue in- or overgrowth is the cause of recurrent dysphagia in 15–20% of patients treated with a SEMS for a benign esophageal stricture, whereas stent migration is seen in 10–15% of patients. SEMS are otherwise relatively safe, with major complication (i.e., retrosternal pain, reflux with or without esophagitis) seen in 10–20% of patients, and (rarely) perforation [18].

Due to high rates of complications related to uncovered or partially covered SEMS, only fully covered ones are used nowadays in refractory or recurring benign esophageal stenoses. They demonstrate significant rates of dysphagia relief, though they are associated with migration in about one-quarter to one-third of cases. Notably, stent migration rates seem to be lower with flared, fully covered SEMS.

In published series, SEMS were not removed in all patients. This is likely due to patient-related factors, such as old age and comorbidity. In addition, it can be imagined that physicians were sometimes reluctant to remove an imbedded SEMS. Limited reports have shown that approximately 40–50% of patients had no clinical evidence of a recurrent stricture after stent removal.

Self-Expanding Plastic Stents

SEPS are the other stent type used for this indication. The Polyflex stent is the only SEPS currently available (Figure 17.2). It is a silicone device with an encapsulated monofilament braid made of polyester. Several studies have evaluated the use of SEPS in benign esophageal strictures. Indications for stent placement in these series included anastomotic strictures, followed by peptic strictures, caustic strictures, postradiation strictures, and some other causes.

Though initial studies with Polyflex stents showed promising results, more recent studies have been less favorable, with high stent

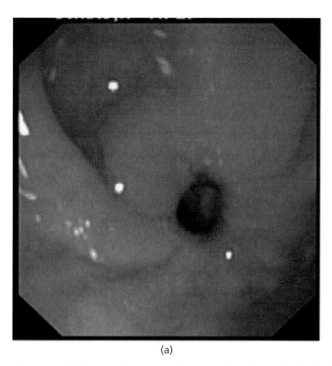
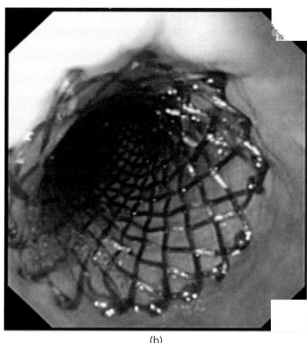

(a)   (b)

Figure 17.2 (a) Anastomotic stricture in the proximal esophagus, for which a (b) self-expanding biodegradable stent was placed.

migration rates and recurrent strictures after stent removal reported in up to 90% of patients. An advantage of Polyflex stents is that they are easily removable, and hyperplastic tissue overgrowth is less likely after Polyflex stent placement for benign esophageal strictures, probably due to the non-metal material used, the fully covered design, and the relatively low radial force at the stent ends. On the other hand, migration rates are high after Polyflex stent placement, occurring in almost 50% of patients [20, 21]. This high migration rate is likely the result of the fully covered stent design, the smooth outer surface of the stent, and the insufficient anchoring support provided by the stricture. Major complications are seen in less than 10% of patients and consist of perforations, fistulas, bleeding, reflux esophagitis, and pain. A systematic review of SEPS placement in recurrent and/or refractory benign esophageal strictures demonstrated a beneficial risk/benefit ratio and suggested the use of SEPS as an alternative to dilation and before definite surgery [22].

In various studies, Polyflex stents were removed in all patients after stenting times varying between 4 weeks and 18 months. Long-term improvement of dysphagia was seen in only 40% of patients.

Self-Expanding Biodegradable Stents

Recently, a self-expanding biodegradable stent has been developed, which is currently only available outside the United States. It is believed that biodegradable stents will be introduced in the Unities States within 1–2 years.

A biodegradable stent is uncovered, with no antireflux valve. The stent degrades in approximately 2–4 months, depending on whether PPIs are prescribed. Biodegradable stents have been used in malignant obstruction during neoadjuvant therapy, and to a larger extent also in benign refractory strictures. A comparison study between temporary placement of either SEPS or biodegradable stents in benign esophageal strictures revealed prolonged relief of dysphagia in 30 and 33%, respectively; however, the latter type of stent required fewer interventions [23].

Management of Refractory Benign Esophageal Strictures

It is important to treat esophageal strictures in a stepwise fashion, starting with the least invasive treatment modality (Table 17.5). If this is not sufficient to relieve dysphagia, the next treatment modality in the algorithm should be applied.

Step 1

The first step in managing a benign esophageal stricture is balloon or Savary–Gilliard bougie dilation, preferably to 16–18 mm. It is recommended to perform at least five dilations to the maximum diameter before deciding whether to switch to an alternate treatment. In the author's institution, dilations are performed once a week or twice weekly in order to reach the maximum diameter in a relatively short period of time.

If a stricture is considered to be refractory, the treatment plan should first be discussed with the patient, because in some refractory benign esophageal strictures, many endoscopy sessions are indicated (Figure 17.1). It is important to have the patient's cooperation and to make sure that they know the treatment options and what can be expected. Some patients will not be willing to undergo a multitude of endoscopy sessions and will prefer, after just one or two dilation sessions, to have a stent placed (step 3) or even to opt for a surgical solution (step 4).

Step 2

After maximum dilation, the next step is to combine dilation with intralesional steroid injections. In the author's institution, triamcinolone acetate 20 mg/mL is used for intralesional injection, which is injected in four aliquots of 1.0 mL at the proximal margin of the stricture, followed by dilation. There is, however, no evidence to substantiate this protocol. It is suggested that dilation plus intralesional steroid injection be limited to a maximum of three sessions, because, in the author's experience, more treatment sessions are rarely effective.

In refractory Schatzki rings and anastomotic strictures, refractory strictures can also be treated with incisional therapy using needle-knife electrocautery or APC. Again, it is suggested that a maximum of three treatment sessions be performed, mainly due to a lack of further effect after this point.

Step 3

Stent placement can be considered when an adequate luminal diameter has not been established with previous treatment modalities or when the stricture still recurs within a short time interval. The preferred stent in patients with a long stricture in the mid-esophagus (2–4 cm) (e.g., due to caustic injury or radiation therapy) is a fully covered SEMS, SEPS, or self-expanding biodegradable stent. As Polyflex stents are associated with considerable side effects, they are no longer used in the author's institution. The same stent types can also be considered in patients with an anastomotic stricture in the proximal or distal esophagus (e.g., a peptic stricture).

It is not clear how long a stent should be left in the esophagus, though a period of 4–8 weeks, and 8–16 weeks in highly refractory strictures, is required to allow scar tissue remodeling. Factors that influence stenting time include the underlying cause, the time since injury to the esophagus, and the length of the stricture. The protocol for stent placement in refractory benign esophageal strictures that is followed in the author's institution is shown in Table 17.6.

When stent placement is not successful and the stricture still persists, one should consider continuing stenting for a longer period and, depending on the time to occurrence of hyperplastic tissue in- and overgrowth in a particular patient, replacing the stent at intervals determined by this fibrous tissue growth. As discussed, it is likely that the inflammatory reaction underlying the stricture will finally subside and the luminal diameter achieved at that time will remain.

Step 4

An alternative treatment option is to teach the patient self-bougienage using Maloney dilators. This is not a common practice, but it is safe and effective when patients have learned the technique. In the author's experience, self-bougienage is most successful with a favorable anatomy (e.g., proximal stricture of caustic or anastomotic origin without significant diverticulum formation).

There is a subgroup of patients in whom all efforts to dilate a refractory benign esophageal stricture are unsuccessful. On the other hand, there are also patients who are unable to tolerate stent placement, or who just do not have enough patience to let the stricture resolve. In these patients, a surgical procedure can be considered.

Table 17.6 Guidelines for the use of stents with benign esophageal strictures, rings, and webs.

1	Strictures that are caused by ischemic injury, present within 6–12 months of the injury, and/or longer than 5 cm are stented for 8–16 weeks
2	In all other cases, stents are inserted for a shorter period, usually 4–8 weeks
3	When symptoms recur after stent removal, a second stent is placed
4	Fully covered SEMS or SEPS carry a risk of hyperplastic tissue overgrowth, and periodic endoscopy at 6-week intervals is recommended
5	Self-expanding biodegradable stents can be considered as alternative to fully covered stents, as stent removal is not required

SEMS, self-expanding metal stent; SEPS, self-expanding plastic stent.

Take Home Points

Diagnosis:
- Benign esophageal strictures, rings, and webs can be subdivided according to underlying pathologic mechanisms (inflammatory disorder, anatomic disorder, intra- or extramural lesions, motility disorder).
- Benign esophageal disorders, rings, and webs can also be classified according to treatment response as simple or complex, with the latter frequently requiring repeated and prolonged treatment.
- Patients with a benign stricture, web, or ring all have several symptoms in common (dysphagia, regurgitation, and odynophagia), but may have some discriminating symptoms, depending on the type of injury to the esophageal wall.
- A careful assessment of a patient's history can provide information of mandatory importance and direct the diagnostic and therapeutic manipulations.
- The most valuable investigation in patients with esophageal dysphagia is esophagogastroduodenoscopy (EGD), followed by radiography (barium swallow or computed tomography (CT) of the chest) and esophageal manometry.

Therapy:
- Most strictures can be treated with bougie or balloon dilation. Refractory strictures need an alternative treatment, such as intralesional steroid injection, incisional therapy, stent placement, self-bougienage, or surgery.
- It is important to treat esophageal strictures in a stepwise fashion, starting with the least invasive treatment. If this is not sufficient to relieve dysphagia, the next treatment modality in the algorithm should be applied.
- An alternative to repeat dilation in anastomotic strictures is to use incisional therapy with needle-knife electrocautery or argon plasma coagulation (APC).
- The idea behind dilation for a prolonged period using self-expanding metal stents (SEMS), self-expanding plastic stents (SEPS), or self-expanding biodegradable stents is that it will reduce the risk of recurrent stricture formation.
- If the various treatment modalities are not effective in relieving dysphagia, a patient can be taught to apply self-bougienage, or, ultimately, surgery can be performed.

References

1 Kochman ML, McClave SA, Boyce HW. The refractory and the recurrent esophageal stricture: a definition. *Gastrointest Endosc* 2005; **62**: 474–5.

2 Lindgren MD, Janzon L. Prevalence of swallowing complaints and clinical findings among 50–70 year old men and women in an urban population. *Dysphagia* 1991; **6**: 187–92.

3 Spechler SJ. AGA technical review on treatment of patients with dysphagia caused by benign disorders of the distal esophagus. *Gastroenterology* 1999; **117**: 233–54.

4 Kidambi T, Toto E, Ho N, *et al.* Temporal trends in the relative pre valence of dysphagia etiologies from 1999–2009. *World J Gastroenterol* 2012; **18**: 4335–41.

5 Hoffman RM, Jaffe PE. Plummer-Vinson syndrome: a case report and literature review. *Arch Intern Med* 1995; **155**: 2008–11.

6 Siersema PD, Hirdes MM. What is the optimal duration of stent placement for refractory, benign esophageal strictures? *Nat Clin Pract Gastroenterol Hepatol* 2009; **6**: 146–7.

7 Cook IJ. Diagnostic evaluation of dysphagia. *Nat Clin Pract Gastroenterol Hepatol* 2008; **5**: 393–403.

8 Ferguson DD. Evaluation and management of benign esophageal strictures. *Dis Esophagus* 2005; **18**: 359–64.

9 ASGE Standard of Practice Committee, Pasha SF, Acosta RD, *et al.* The role of endoscopy in the evaluation and management of dysphagia. *Gastrointest Endosc* 2014; **79**: 191–201.

10 Saeed ZA, Winchester CB, Ferro PS, *et al.* Prospective randomized comparison of polyvinyl bougies and through-the-scope balloons for dilation of peptic strictures of the esophagus. *Gastrointest Endosc* 1995; **41**: 189–95.

CHAPTER 17

11 Lew RJ, Kochman ML. A review of endoscopic methods of esophageal dilatation. *J Clin Gastroenterol* 2002; **35**: 117–26.b12.

12 Richter JE. Esophageal dilation in eosinophilic esophagitis. *Best Pract Res Clin Gastroenterol* 2015; **29**: 815–28.

13 Bueno R, Swanson SJ, Jaklitsch MT, *et al.* Combined antegrade and retrograde dilation: a new endoscopic technique in the management of complex esophageal obstruction. *Gastrointest Endosc* 2001; **54**: 368–72.

14 Ramage JI Jr, Rumalla A, Baron TH, *et al.* A prospective, randomized, double-blind, placebo-controlled trial of endoscopic steroid injection therapy for recalcitrant esophageal peptic strictures. *Am J Gastroenterol* 2005; **100**: 2419–25.

15 Hirdes MM, van Hooft JE, Koornstra JJ, *et al.* Endoscopic corticosteroid injections do not reduce dysphagia after endoscopic dilation therapy in patients with benign esophagogastric anastomotic strictures. *Clin Gastroenterol Hepatol* 2013; **11**: 795–801.

16 Honkoop P, Siersema PD, Tilanus HW, *et al.* Benign anastomotic strictures after transhiatal esophagectomy and cervical esophagogastrostomy: risk factors and management. *J Thorac Cardiovasc Surg* 1996; **111**: 1141–6.

17 Hordijk ML, Siersema PD, Tilanus HW, *et al.* Electrocautery therapy for refractory anastomotic strictures of the esophagus. *Gastrointest Endosc* 2006; **63**: 157–63.

18 Siersema PD. Stenting for benign esophageal strictures. *Endoscopy* 2009; **41**: 363–73.

19 Cwikiel W, Willén R, Stridbeck H, *et al.* Self-expanding stent in the treatment of benign esophageal strictures: experimental study in pigs and presentation of clinical cases. *Radiology* 1993; **187**: 667–71.

20 Holm AN, de la Mora Levy JG, Gostout CJ, *et al.* Self-expanding plastic stents in treatment of benign esophageal conditions. *Gastrointest Endosc* 2008; **67**: 20–5.

21 Dua KS, Vleggaar FP, Santharam R, *et al.* Removable self-expanding plastic esophageal stent as a continuous, non-permanent dilator in treating refractory benign esophageal strictures: a prospective two-center study. *Am J Gastroenterol* 2008; **103**: 2988–94.

22 Repici A, Hassan C, Sharma P, *et al.* Systematic review: the role of self-expanding plastic stents for benign oesophageal strictures. *Aliment Pharmacol Ther* 2010; **31**: 1268–75.

23 van Boeckel PG, Vleggaar FP, Siersema PD. A comparison of temporary self-expanding plastic and biodegradable stents for refractory benign esophageal strictures. *Clin Gastroenterol Hepatol* 2011; **9**(8): 653–9.

PART 5

Diseases of the Stomach

18 Peptic Ulcer Disease, 115
Francis K.L. Chan and Nicholas J. Talley

19 *Helicobacter pylori*, 121
Barry J. Marshall

20 Gastritis, 126
Massimo Rugge and David Y. Graham

21 Gastroparesis, 132
Henry P. Parkman and Nicholas J. Talley

22 Non-variceal Upper Gastrointestinal Bleeding, 138
Thomas J. Savides

23 Other Gastric Tumors (Benign and Malignant), 145
Sun-Chuan Dai and Michael L. Kochman

24 Eosinophilic Gastroenteritis, 152
Magnus Halland and Nicholas J. Talley

25 Esophageal and Gastric Involvement in Systemic and Cutaneous Diseases, 156
John M. Wo

Peptic Ulcer Disease

Francis K.L. Chan[1] and Nicholas J. Talley[2]

[1] Department of Medicine and Therapeutics, The Chinese University of Hong Kong, Hong Kong, China
[2] Faculty of Health, University of Newcastle, Newcastle, NSW, Australia

Summary

Unlike many chronic medical conditions, peptic ulcer disease is a potentially curable or avoidable condition because *Helicobacter pylori* infection and the use of non-steroidal anti-inflammatory drugs (NSAIDs) account for the vast majority of cases. The key to successful management rests on choosing appropriate *H. pylori* diagnostic tests according to specific clinical settings (e.g., avoid using urease tests in the presence of proton pump inhibitor (PPI) therapy), obtaining a careful drug history so as to identify NSAID exposure (e.g., over-the-counter NSAIDs), and assessing both the gastrointestinal (GI) and the cardiovascular risks of individual patients before prescribing NSAIDs. With the declining prevalence of *H. pylori* infection, ulcers not associated with *H. pylori* or NSAID use are increasingly recognized. In patients presenting with peptic ulcer bleeding, endoscopic therapy is highly effective in achieving hemostasis. However, early rebleeding is common and causes significant morbidity and mortality. The use of a PPI before and after endoscopic diagnosis of peptic ulcer bleeding has significantly improved clinical outcomes but has failed to reduce mortality.

Case

An 85-year-old female presents with weakness and an occasional episode of dizziness. She has noticed no other symptoms, but does report that her stools are darker than the past. Her medical history is significant for osteoarthritis and a possible transient ischemic attack (TIA) several years ago. Medications include propranolol, daily 81 mg aspirin, and two or three 200 mg ibuprofen most days. On physical examination, she is pale and her pulse is 120 bpm. She had mild epigastric tenderness and her rectal exam shows dark, but not black stool that is heme-positive on testing. Initial laboratory testing is significant for an Hgb of 7.8 with microcytic indices. A colonoscopy 1 year ago was normal.

She is started on omeprazole 20 mg daily, is told to stop ibuprofen, and is transfused with 2 units of packed red blood cells (RBCs). The next day, she feels much better and undergoes an esophagogastroduodenoscopy (EGD). This demonstrates a normal esophagus and a 2.5 cm bland-appearing ulcer in the antrum. The duodenum is normal. Biopsy from the ulcer is benign, but shows moderate numbers of *H. pylori* organisms. Her omeprazole is increased to twice daily, and she is given 10 days of amoxicillin and clarithromycin. At the conclusion of the 10 days, her omeprazole is decreased to once daily. A follow-up endoscopy 6 weeks later shows

the ulcer to be healed, and biopsies do not show *Helicobacter*. At 1 year, she remains on daily omeprazole and has returned to the occasional use of ibuprofen without additional episodes of bleeding.

Background and Epidemiology

Peptic ulcer disease and its complications are leading causes of morbidity and mortality worldwide. Peptic ulcer disease is the most common cause of acute upper GI bleeding. The incidence of acute upper GI bleeding ranges from 36 to 172 per 100 000 population. Despite major improvements in clinical care, the mortality rate after an episode of acute upper GI bleeding remains high at 5–14% [1]. In contrast, due to advances in endoscopic treatment, operations for peptic ulcer complications have fallen by 80% in the last 3 decades.

Etiologies

The most common causes of peptic ulcer disease are *H. pylori* infection and the use of NSAIDs, including low-dose aspirin. As the prevalence of *H. pylori* infection is declining, ulcers associated with the use of NSAIDs and low-dose aspirin have become increasingly important in the elderly. Interestingly, the incidence of ulcers not associated with *H. pylori* or NSAID use is also rising [2].

Helicobacter pylori

The discovery of *H. pylori* by Marshall and Warren revolutionized our understanding of upper GI disorders. *H. pylori* infection is associated with gastritis, peptic ulcers, mucosa-associated lymphoid tissue lymphomas, and gastric cancer.

Aspirin and Non-steroidal Anti-inflammatory Drugs

NSAIDs, including low-dose aspirin, are the most commonly used drugs worldwide. It has been estimated that about 70% of people aged 65 years and older use NSAIDs at least once a week. Around 40–50% of bleeding peptic ulcers are etiologically linked to aspirin or NSAIDs. The proportion is expected to rise in aging populations.

Topical injury is not an important mechanism of NSAID-induced gastric ulceration. There is good evidence that NSAIDs damage the stomach by suppressing gastric prostaglandin synthesis. The discovery of two isoforms of cyclo-oxygenase (COX-1 and COX-2) has led to the development of COX-2-selective NSAIDs as

Practical Gastroenterology and Hepatology Board Review Toolkit, Second Edition. Edited by Nicholas J. Talley, Kenneth R. DeVault, Michael B. Wallace, Bashar A. Aqel and Keith D. Lindor.

gastric-sparing anti-inflammatory analgesics. Current evidence indicates that COX-2-selective NSAIDs induce fewer ulcers than do non-selective NSAIDs.

A history of peptic ulcer bleeding is the most important factor predicting recurrent ulcer complications associated with aspirin and NSAID use. Other risk factors include old age (>75), comorbid illnesses, coexisting *H. pylori* infection, and concomitant use of aspirin, corticosteroids, or anticoagulants. Though corticosteroids and anticoagulants are not ulcerogenic themselves, they markedly increase the risk of GI bleeding if used together with aspirin or NSAIDs [3].

Non-NSAID, Non-*H. pylori* Idiopathic Ulcers

As the prevalence of *H. pylori* infection is declining, the proportion of ulcers not associated with *H. pylori* or NSAID use is increasing. Previously, it was thought that the relative proportion of idiopathic ulcers increased only as a consequence of the declining prevalence of *H. pylori*-related ulcers. Current evidence, however, indicates that there is a genuine rise in the absolute incidence of non-NSAID, non-*H. pylori* idiopathic ulcers [2]. The pathogenesis of idiopathic ulcer remains uncertain, but several studies suggest that this condition probably accounts for up to 20% of all peptic ulcer disease [2,4]. Compared to patients with *H. pylori*-related bleeding ulcers, those with non-NSAID, non-*H. pylori* idiopathic bleeding ulcers are older, suffer from more severe illnesses, and have a higher risk of recurrent ulcer bleeding [2].

Before making a diagnosis of idiopathic ulcers, however, one should carefully scrutinize the patient's drug history to exclude any surreptitious use of NSAIDs. In addition, recent use of acid suppressants or antibiotics and blood in the stomach are important causes of false-negative tests for *H. pylori*. One study showed that some patients with idiopathic ulcers actually had *H. pylori* detected in duodenal metaplasia [5]. Repeating diagnostic tests for *H. pylori* is advisable. Finally, uncommon but well-recognized conditions such as Crohn's disease, cytomegalovirus (CMV) disease, and Zollinger–Ellison syndrome should also be considered.

Clinical Features

Patients with peptic ulcers often complain of dyspepsia. However, dyspepsia is a poor predictor of peptic ulcers, because this non-specific symptom is common in other upper GI conditions. On the other hand, up to 80% of patients receiving NSAIDs develop ulcer complications without any warning symptoms. Among patients with a history of ulcer who receive a COX-2 inhibitor or a combination of a PPI and a non-selective NSAID, it has been shown that those who develop breakthrough dyspepsia have a significantly higher likelihood of developing recurrent ulcers than their asymptomatic counterparts [6]. In patients presenting with upper GI bleeding, fresh blood hematemesis, hypotension, anemia, and comorbid illnesses are predictors of poor clinical outcome such as death. The presence of chronic liver stigmata, however, may indicate variceal bleeding. Chronic pyloric and duodenal ulcers may result in gastric outlet obstruction. Patients present with epigastric distension and repeated vomiting. On physical examination, epigastric distension and succussion splash may be found.

Perforated peptic ulcer is a surgical emergency. Abdominal tenderness, rebound tenderness, guarding, and reduced bowel sounds may be found. It is important to note that some perforated peptic ulcers may seal off spontaneously, and peritonism may not be

apparent. If this possibility is not considered and endoscopy is arranged, unsealing of the perforation may occur.

Diagnosis

Peptic ulcer can be diagnosed EGD. All patients with peptic ulcer should be tested for *H. pylori* infection regardless of any history of NSAID use. It is important to biopsy gastric ulcers in order to exclude dysplasia or carcinoma. In addition, physicians should obtain a detailed drug history in order to identify any recent use of prescription or over-the-counter NSAIDs.

H. pylori testing should be routine. It is important to note that both the rapid urease test and histology have low sensitivity during acute bleeding and in the presence of acid-suppressive therapy [7]. Thus, patients with bleeding peptic ulcers should be tested for *H. pylori* after the acute bleeding episode has subsided and at least 1 week after stopping acid-suppressive therapy. Alternatively, a serology test can be performed at the time of acute bleeding (a positive serology indicates current or past infection).

In patients with gastric outlet obstruction, a plain radiograph may show dilated gastric shadow with displaced transverse colon and small-bowel loops. The stomach should be decompressed with a sump drain or nasogastric tube before endoscopy to reduce the risk of aspiration.

In *H. pylori*-negative, NSAID-negative ulcer, consider missed infection (test off PPI, antibiotics by mouth), surreptitious NSAID use, neoplasia or infiltrative diseases, ischemia (e.g., crack cocaine), and Zollinger–Ellison syndrome (test serum gastrin off PPI).

In patients suspected to have perforated peptic ulcer, a plain chest radiograph may show free gas under the diaphragm. If the plain film is non-diagnostic, a contrast computed tomography (CT) scan may show free peritoneal gas, fluid in the peritoneum, or inflammatory changes at the site of perforation.

Therapeutics

H. pylori Ulcers

There is good evidence from meta-analyses of randomized trials that eradication of *H. pylori* alone is sufficient to heal symptomatic and bleeding peptic ulcers, such that additional acid-suppressive therapy is not required [8]. Therefore, the treatment of *H. pylori*-related peptic ulcer is intended to ensure successful eradication of the bacterium. This goal can be achieved in 70% of cases using 7–14 days of PPI-based triple therapies.

In patients with duodenal ulcer, confirmation of *H. pylori* eradication by non-invasive methods (e.g., ^{13}C-urea breath test or *H. pylori* stool antigen test) is a validated surrogate marker for healing of the duodenal ulcer. Eradication of *H. pylori* also effectively heals gastric ulcers. For patients with large (>1.5 cm) gastric ulcers, however, adding a PPI to *H. pylori* eradication therapy is recommended to promote ulcer healing.

Unlike duodenal ulcers, gastric ulcers must be adequately biopsied at diagnosis (×6); then healing needs to be confirmed endoscopically. Biopsy is mandatory to exclude malignancy.

In patients with *H. pylori*-related bleeding peptic ulcers, an additional course of PPI therapy is advisable to prevent early rebleeding, though there are data showing that eradication of *H. pylori* alone is sufficient to heal bleeding peptic ulcers [9]. After ulcer healing and successful eradication of *H. pylori*, maintenance acid-suppressive therapy is not required because recurrent ulcer or ulcer bleeding is very uncommon unless NSAID use coexists [10].

NSAID Ulcers

Treatment of Active Ulcers

Patients should stop taking NSAIDs in the presence of active ulcers. If continuous NSAID therapy is required, standard doses of histamine type 2 receptor antagonists (H2RAs) effectively heal duodenal ulcers, but not gastric ulcers. Current evidence indicates that PPIs are superior to standard-dose H2RA therapy and full-dose misoprostol in healing ulcers [11]. Since *H. pylori*-related ulcers cannot be differentiated from NSAID-induced ulcers and *H. pylori* infection is a risk factor for peptic ulcers associated with NSAID use, all patients should be tested for *H. pylori*, and if it is present, the infection should be eradicated [12]. Eradication of *H. pylori* does not impair ulcer healing [13].

Prevention of Ulcers

Aspirin- and NSAID-induced ulcer is an avoidable, iatrogenic condition. Before prescribing these drugs, physicians should review whether the benefits will outweigh their risks. Simple analgesics (e.g., acetaminophen) should be the first-line therapy for pain relief in degenerative arthritis. When NSAIDs are deemed necessary, the least ulcerogenic should be used at the lowest effective dose and for the shortest duration. Test-and-treating *H. pylori* infection before the prescription of NSAIDs has been shown to reduce the risk of peptic ulcers [14]. All patients with a history of peptic ulcer should be tested for *H. pylori* infection.

Patients who require NSAIDs can be stratified according to their level of GI risk, namely: low (absence of risk factors), moderate (presence of one or two risk factors), and high (history of ulcer complications, multiple risk factors, or concomitant use of corticosteroids or anticoagulant therapy). Low-risk patients should receive the least ulcerogenic NSAIDs (e.g., ibuprofen) at their lowest effective doses. Moderate-risk patients should receive prophylaxis with a PPI or misoprostol. There is evidence from randomized trials that a COX-2-selective NSAID alone is comparable to a non-selective NSAID plus a PPI in terms of the risk of ulcer bleeding [15]. High-risk patients should avoid taking NSAIDs if possible, because neither a COX-2 inhibitor alone nor a non-selective NSAID plus a PPI can eliminate the ulcer risk [6]. Short-term corticosteroid therapy can be considered for acute, self-limiting arthritis (e.g., gout). If long-term NSAID therapy is required, the combination of a COX-2-selective NSAID and a PPI or misoprostol provides the best protection [16,17].

NSAID Users with High Cardiovascular Risk

Patients with a history of coronary artery disease or multiple cardiovascular risk factors should receive low-dose aspirin. Current evidence suggests that COX-2-selective NSAIDs and some non-selective NSAIDs such as diclofenac and ibuprofen increase the risk

of myocardial infarction. In addition, concomitant use of ibuprofen and low-dose aspirin should be avoided, because ibuprofen has been shown to attenuate the cardioprotective effect of aspirin. Meta-analyses of randomized trials [18] indicate that full-dose naproxen (500 mg twice daily) does not increase the risk of myocardial infarction, and this is thus the preferred NSAID in patients with increased cardiovascular risk. However, naproxen is very ulcerogenic and concomitant use of low-dose aspirin will markedly increase the risk of ulcer complications, such that prophylaxis with a PPI or misoprostol is recommended [19] (Table 18.1).

Antiplatelet Therapy in Patients with High Ulcer Risk

For many years, the American Heart Association (AHA) and the American College of Cardiology (ACC) have strongly recommended the use of clopidogrel in patients with major GI intolerance to aspirin. This recommendation was largely based on *post hoc* secondary analysis of safety data from clinical trials that were not designed to evaluate the GI safety of clopidogrel, however [20]. In a double-blind, randomized comparison of clopidogrel with aspirin plus a PPI in patients with prior peptic ulcer bleeding, the recurrent ulcer bleeding rate in 1 year was significantly lower in the aspirin-plus-PPI group (0.7%) than in the clopidogrel group (8.6%) [21]. In an updated expert consensus report, aspirin plus a PPI is recommended in patients requiring antiplatelet therapy with high GI risk [22]. However, PPI cotherapy may increase the risk of recurrent myocardial infarction in patients receiving clopidogrel [23,24].

Non-NSAID, Non-*H. pylori* Idiopathic Ulcers

The optimal management of patients with non-NSAID, non-*H. pylori* ulcers remain uncertain, since the pathogenesis and natural history of this condition is poorly understood [25]. One should be careful not to incorrectly diagnose it due to a false-negative *H. pylori* test or a failure to obtain a detailed drug history. There is evidence that the risk of recurrent ulcer bleeding is high among patients with a history of non-NSAID, non-*H. pylori* ulcer bleeding [2]. Long-term prophylaxis with a PPI is therefore advisable.

Peptic Ulcer Bleeding

Peptic ulcer bleeding is a serious complication of peptic ulcers. Advances in endoscopic and pharmacological treatment have improved the outcomes of this condition. Surgical treatment is rarely performed nowadays. Despite interobserver variability, the Forrest classification is still commonly used to predict the risk of recurrent bleeding based on the presence of stigmata of recent hemorrhage (Table 18.2). A number of risk-stratification schemes are also available to aid clinicians in determining the prognosis and the risk of rebleeding, such as the Rockall score and the Glasgow–Blatchford bleeding score (GBS) (Table 18.3).

Table 18.1 Recommendations for the use of NSAIDs according to GI and cardiovascular risk.

Cardiovascular risk	GI risk[a]		
	Low	Moderate	High
Low	NSAID	NSAID + PPI/misoprostol or COX-2 inhibitor	COX-2 inhibitor + PPI
High[b]	Naproxen + PPI/misoprostol	Naproxen + PPI/misoprostol	Avoid NSAIDs and COX-2 inhibitors

[a] GI risk is defined as low (no risk factors), moderate (presence of one or two risk factors), or high (multiple risk factors, previous ulcer complications, or concomitant use of corticosteroids or anticoagulants). All patients with a history of ulcers who require NSAIDs should be tested for *H. pylori*, and if the infection is present, eradication therapy should be given.

[b] High cardiovascular risk is defined as the requirement for low-dose aspirin in order to prevent myocardial infarction.

NSAID, non-steroidal anti-inflammatory drug; PPI, proton pump inhibitor; COX, cyclo-oxygenase.

Table 18.2 Forrest classification of peptic ulcers.

Forrest class	Description	Risk of rebleeding if untreated (%)
IA	Arterial spurting	100
IB	Arterial oozing	55
IIA	Non-bleeding visible vessel	43
IIB	Adherent blood clot	22
IIC	Pigmented spot	10
III	Clean base	5

A prospective cohort study compared the GBS score with the Rockall score in patients admitted to general hospitals with upper GI bleeding [26]. It was found that the GBS score was superior to the Rockall score for prediction of need for intervention or death. In addition, patients who were classified as low-risk (GBS score of 0) were managed safely as outpatients without adverse events [26].

Endoscopic Hemostasis

Endoscopic hemostasis can be achieved using injection therapy, thermal devices, and mechanical devices. Diluted epinephrine (1 : 10000) injection around bleeding ulcers is commonly performed because of its efficacy and simplicity of use. The heater probe is a thermal device that compresses the walls of the bleeding vessel together and seals them off using thermal energy – a condition called "coaptive coagulation." The success of heater probe treatment requires the application of firm pressure over the bleeding point. This can be technically demanding in difficult locations such as the posterior duodenal wall. The hemoclip is a mechanical device that controls bleeding by obliterating the feeding vessel. Its deployment can be difficult if the ulcer base is fibrotic or the location of ulcer only allows tangential application.

A meta-analysis of randomized trials indicates that dual endoscopic therapy (epinephrine injection plus a thermal or mechanical device) reduces early rebleeding and the need for surgical intervention compared to epinephrine injection alone. In contrast, dual endoscopic therapy has not been shown to be superior

Table 18.3 Glasgow–Blatchford score (GBS). Source: Glasgow–Blatchford, https://en.wikipedia.org/wiki/Glasgow-Blatchford_score#cite_note-5. Used under CC-BY-SA 3.0, http://creativecommons.org/licenses/by-sa/3.0/.

Admission risk marker	Score component value
Blood urea (mmol/L)[5]	
6.5–8.0	2
8.0–10.0	3
10.0–25.0	4
>25	6
Hemoglobin (g/L) for men	
12.0–12.9	1
10.0–11.9	3
<10.0	6
Hemoglobin (g/L) for women	
10.0–11.9	1
<10.0	6
Systolic blood pressure (mmHg)	
100–109	1
90–99	2
<90	3
Other markers	
Pulse ≥100 (per minute)	1
Presentation with melena	1
Presentation with syncope	2
Hepatic disease	2
Cardiac failure	2

In the validation group, scores of 6 or more were associated with a >50% risk of needing an intervention.

to monotherapy using a thermal or mechanical device. Though epinephrine injection alone is inferior to other mono- or dual-therapies, none of the endoscopic hemostatic strategies can improve survival when compared to epinephrine injection alone [27, 28].

Acid-Suppressive Therapy

Platelets function optimally at neutral pH. This explains why acute upper GI bleeding can be torrential and lethal. Potent suppression of gastric acid leads to clot stabilization and is expected to reduce the risk of bleeding. A systematic review of randomized trials has shown that both oral and intravenous PPI initiated after endoscopic diagnosis of peptic ulcer bleeding reduce the risk of rebleeding and surgical requirement, but fail to reduce mortality [29]. The optimal dose and route of administration of adjuvant PPI therapy remain controversial. To date, the use of intravenous high-dose PPI (e.g., 80 mg of omeprazole bolus injection followed by 8 mg/h infusion for 72 hours) after endoscopic hemostatic therapy is the most studied method, but high-dose oral PPI may be an alternative [30].

Should PPI therapy be initiated before endoscopy in patients presenting with hematemesis or melena? In a double-blind randomized trial of high-dose PPI infusion before endoscopy the following morning, patients receiving preemptive PPI required significantly less endoscopic treatment than the placebo group [31]. A systematic review found that both oral and intravenous PPI given before endoscopy reduced the need for endoscopic therapy when compared to placebo or H2RA [32]. It follows that preemptive PPI is particularly useful in hospitals where 24-hour emergency endoscopy is not readily available. However, clinicians should not have the misconception that preemptive PPI can substitute timely endoscopic treatment, because the former does not reduce rebleeding, surgical requirement, and mortality [32].

Rebleeding

Close monitoring is required after endoscopic therapy for peptic ulcer bleeding. Repeating endoscopy and surgery are both effective in controlling recurrent ulcer bleeding. The mortality does not differ using either approach [33]. Endoscopy results in fewer complications, but is more likely to fail if the patient develops hypotension during rebleeding or the ulcer is more than 2 cm in size. Scheduled second-look endoscopy after initial hemostasis may reduce the risk of rebleeding but has no effect on the duration of hospitalization or mortality [34]. Emerging evidence suggests that angiographic embolization is also effective in managing refractory bleeding [35]. Avoid blood transfusion unless the hemoglobin falls below 7.0 g/dL as outcomes are better [36]. Figure 18.1 shows an algorithm for the management of peptic ulcer bleeding.

Take Home Points

- *Helicobacter pylori* infection and the use of non-steroidal anti-inflammatory drugs (NSAIDs), including low-dose aspirin, are the two most common causes of peptic ulcer disease.
- Eradication of *H. pylori* infection alone heals peptic ulcer and prevents ulcer relapse.
- In cases of gastric ulcer, standard teaching is to confirm healing after 6 weeks of therapy and to biopsy if the ulcer is still present (but if adequately biopsied at baseline, this may not be necessary). Uncomplicated duodenal ulcers do not need follow up endoscopy unless they are symptomatic.
- NSAID-induced ulcer complications are potentially avoidable. Risk factors include history of ulcer, old age, the use of high-dose or

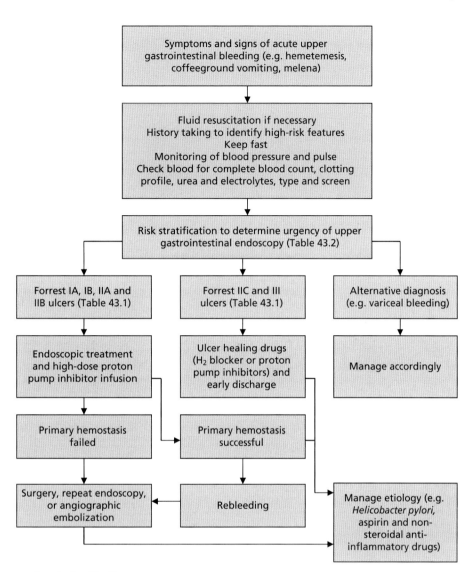

Figure 18.1 Management of peptic ulcer bleeding.

multiple NSAIDs, concomitant use of aspirin, anticoagulants, or corticosteroids, and *H. pylori* infection.
- Combination of a non-selective NSAID and a gastroprotective agent (PPI or misoprostol) or substitution for a cyclo-oxygenase (COX)-2 selective NSAID reduces the risk of ulcer complications.
- COX-2-selective and some non-selective NSAIDs increase the risk of myocardial infarction.
- Physicians should assess patients' gastrointestinal (GI) and cardiovascular risks before prescribing NSAIDs. Patients with low cardiovascular risk can be managed according to the number and type of GI risk factors. Naproxen is preferred in patients with high cardiovascular risk.
- Patients with high GI risk who require aspirin should receive PPI prophylaxis.
- Clopidogrel is not an alternative to aspirin in patients with high GI risk.
- Endoscopic therapy using epinephrine injection plus a thermal or mechanical device is superior to epinephrine injection alone and reduces early rebleeding and surgical requirement.
- Infusion of high-dose PPI after endoscopy for bleeding peptic ulcers reduces early rebleeding, transfusion, surgical requirement, and duration of hospital stay but has no effect on mortality.

References

1 Rockall TA, Logan RF, Devlin HB, Northfield TC. Incidence of and mortality from acute upper gastrointestinal haemorrhage in the United Kingdom. Steering Committee and members of the National Audit of Acute Upper Gastrointestinal Haemorrhage. *BMJ* 1995; **311**(6999): 222–6.

2 Hung LC, Ching JY, Sung JJ, *et al.* Long-term outcome of *Helicobacter pylori*-negative idiopathic bleeding ulcers: a prospective cohort study. *Gastroenterology* 2005; **128**(7): 1845–50.

3 Chan FK. Primer: managing NSAID-induced ulcer complications – balancing gastrointestinal and cardiovascular risks. *Nat Clin Pract Gastroenterol Hepatol* 2006; **3**(10): 563–73.

4 Laine L, Hopkins RJ, Girardi LS. Has the impact of *Helicobacter pylori* therapy on ulcer recurrence in the United States been overstated? A meta-analysis of rigorously designed trials. *Am J Gastroenterol* 1998; **93**(9): 1409–15.

5 Pietroiusti A, Forlini A, Magrini A, *et al.* Isolated *H. pylori* duodenal colonization and idiopathic duodenal ulcers. *Am J Gastroenterol* 2008; **103**(1): 55–61.

6 Chan FK, Hung LC, Suen BY, *et al.* Celecoxib versus diclofenac plus omeprazole in high-risk arthritis patients: results of a randomized double-blind trial. *Gastroenterology* 2004; **127**(4): 1038–43.

7 Gisbert JP, Abraira V. Accuracy of *Helicobacter pylori* diagnostic tests in patients with bleeding peptic ulcer: a systematic review and meta-analysis. *Am J Gastroenterol* 2006; **101**(4): 848–63.

8 Ford AC, Delaney BC, Forman D, Moayyedi P. Eradication therapy in *Helicobacter pylori* positive peptic ulcer disease: systematic review and economic analysis. *Am J Gastroenterol* 2004; **99**(9): 1833–55.

9 Sung JJ, Leung WK, Suen R, *et al*. One-week antibiotics versus maintenance acid suppression therapy for Helicobacter pylori-associated peptic ulcer bleeding. *Dig Dis Sci* 1997; **42**(12): 2524–8.

10 Gisbert JP, Calvet X, Feu F, *et al*. Eradication of Helicobacter pylori for the prevention of peptic ulcer rebleeding. *Helicobacter* 2007; **12**(4): 279–86.

11 Hawkey CJ, Karrasch JA, Szczepanski L, *et al*. Omeprazole compared with misoprostol for ulcers associated with nonsteroidal antiinflammatory drugs. Omeprazole versus Misoprostol for NSAID-induced Ulcer Management (OMNIUM) Study Group. *N Engl J Med* 1998; **338**(11): 727–34.

12 Venerito M, Malfertheiner P. Interaction of *Helicobacter pylori* infection and nonsteroidal anti-inflammatory drugs in gastric and duodenal ulcers. *Helicobacter* 2010; **15**(4): 239–50.

13 Chan FK, Sung JJ, Suen R, *et al*. Does eradication of Helicobacter pylori impair healing of nonsteroidal anti-inflammatory drug associated bleeding peptic ulcers? A prospective randomized study. *Aliment Pharmacol Ther* 1998; **12**(12): 1201–5.

14 Chan FK, To KF, Wu JC, *et al*. Eradication of *Helicobacter pylori* and risk of peptic ulcers in patients starting long-term treatment with non-steroidal anti-inflammatory drugs: a randomised trial. *Lancet* 2002; **359**(9300): 9–13.

15 Chan FK, Hung LC, Suen BY, *et al*. Celecoxib versus diclofenac and omeprazole in reducing the risk of recurrent ulcer bleeding in patients with arthritis. *N Engl J Med* 2002; **347**(26): 2104–10.

16 Chan FK, Wong VW, Suen BY, *et al*. Combination of a cyclo-oxygenase-2 inhibitor and a proton-pump inhibitor for prevention of recurrent ulcer bleeding in patients at very high risk: a double-blind, randomised trial. *Lancet* 2007; **369**(9573): 1621–6.

17 Targownik LE, Metge CJ, Leung S, Chateau DG. The relative efficacies of gastroprotective strategies in chronic users of nonsteroidal anti-inflammatory drugs. *Gastroenterology* 2008; **134**(4): 937–44.

18 Kearney PM, Baigent C, Godwin J, *et al*. Do selective cyclo-oxygenase-2 inhibitors and traditional non-steroidal anti-inflammatory drugs increase the risk of atherothrombosis? Meta-analysis of randomised trials. *BMJ* 2006; **332**(7553): 1302–8.

19 McGettigan P, Henry D. Cardiovascular risk and inhibition of cyclooxygenase: a systematic review of the observational studies of selective and nonselective inhibitors of cyclooxygenase 2. *JAMA* 2006; **296**(13): 1633–44.

20 Braunwald E, Antman EM, Beasley JW, *et al*. ACC/AHA guideline update for the management of patients with unstable angina and non-ST-segment elevation myocardial infarction – 2002: summary article: a report of the American College of Cardiology/American Heart Association Task Force on Practice Guidelines (Committee on the Management of Patients With Unstable Angina). *Circulation* 2002; **106**(14): 1893–900.

21 Chan FK, Ching JY, Hung LC, *et al*. Clopidogrel versus aspirin and esomeprazole to prevent recurrent ulcer bleeding. *N Engl J Med* 2005; **352**(3): 238–44.

22 Bhatt DL, Scheiman J, Abraham NS, *et al*. ACCF/ACG/AHA 2008 expert consensus document on reducing the gastrointestinal risks of antiplatelet therapy and NSAID use: a report of the American College of Cardiology Foundation Task Force on Clinical Expert Consensus Documents. *Circulation* 2008; **118**(18): 1894–909.

23 Ho PM, Maddox TM, Wang L, *et al*. Risk of adverse outcomes associated with concomitant use of clopidogrel and proton pump inhibitors following acute coronary syndrome. *JAMA* 2009; **301**(9): 937–44.

24 Juurlink DN, Gomes T, Ko DT, *et al*. A population-based study of the drug interaction between proton pump inhibitors and clopidogrel. *CMAJ* 2009; **180**(7): 713–18.

25 Charpignon C, Lesgourgues B, Pariente A, *et al*. Peptic ulcer disease: one in five is related to neither Helicobacter pylori nor aspirin/NSAID intake. *Aliment Pharmacol Ther* 2013; **38**(8): 946–54.

26 Stanley AJ, Ashley D, Dalton HR, *et al*. Outpatient management of patients with low-risk upper-gastrointestinal haemorrhage: multicentre validation and prospective evaluation. *Lancet* 2009; **373**(9657): 42–7.

27 Marmo R, Rotondano G, Piscopo R, *et al*. Dual therapy versus monotherapy in the endoscopic treatment of high-risk bleeding ulcers: a meta-analysis of controlled trials. *Am J Gastroenterol* 2007; **102**(2): 279–89, quiz 469.

28 Vergara M, Bennett C, Calvet X, Gisbert JP. Epinephrine injection versus epinephrine injection and a second endoscopic method in high-risk bleeding ulcers. Cochrane Database Syst Rev 2014(10):CD005584.

29 Leontiadis GI, Sreedharan A, Dorward S, *et al*. Systematic reviews of the clinical effectiveness and cost-effectiveness of proton pump inhibitors in acute upper gastrointestinal bleeding. *Health Technol Assess* 2007; **11**(51): iii–iv, 1–164.

30 Sung JJ, Suen BY, Wu JC, *et al*. Effects of intravenous and oral esomeprazole in the prevention of recurrent bleeding from peptic ulcers after endoscopic therapy. *Am J Gastroenterol* 2014; **109**(7): 1005–10.

31 Lau JY, Leung WK, Wu JC, *et al*. Omeprazole before endoscopy in patients with gastrointestinal bleeding. *N Engl J Med* 2007; **356**(16): 1631–40.

32 Dorward S, Sreedharan A, Leontiadis GI, *et al*. Proton pump inhibitor treatment initiated prior to endoscopic diagnosis in upper gastrointestinal bleeding. *Cochrane Database Syst Rev* 2006(4):CD005415.

33 Lau JY, Sung JJ, Lam YH, *et al*. Endoscopic retreatment compared with surgery in patients with recurrent bleeding after initial endoscopic control of bleeding ulcers. *N Engl J Med* 1999; **340**(10): 751–6.

34 Marmo R, Rotondano G, Bianco MA, *et al*. Outcome of endoscopic treatment for peptic ulcer bleeding: Is a second look necessary? A meta-analysis. *Gastrointest Endosc* 2003; **57**(1): 62–7.

35 Cheung FK, Lau JY. Management of massive peptic ulcer bleeding. *Gastroenterol Clin N Am* 2009; **38**(2): 231–43.

36 Villanueva C, Colomo A, Bosch A, *et al*. Transfusion strategies for acute upper gastrointestinal bleeding. *N Engl J Med* 2013; **368**: 11–21.

CHAPTER 18

Helicobacter pylori

Barry J. Marshall

School of Biomedical, Biomolecular and Chemical Sciences, University of Western Australia, Perth, WA, Australia

Summary

Helicobacter pylori infection of the stomach is the most important cause of peptic ulcer disease. Half the world's population is infected by *H. pylori*, including about 20% of those in developed countries and the majority in developing countries. It is usually acquired in early childhood and is permanent unless specifically treated. Decades after the acute *H. pylori* infection, 20% of cases develop peptic ulcer disease. The remainder are asymptomatic but carry a 1–5% risk of stomach cancer in later life.

Diagnosis is via serology, urea breath test (UBT), and stool antigen test, or else via urease test or histology of gastric biopsies. Therapy cures 70% using an acid pump blocker concurrently with two antibiotics for 7–10 days. Cure of peptic ulcer, remission of lymphoma, and decreased cancer risk follow the bacteriologic cure. Reinfection is uncommon.

Case

A 38-year-old female patient presents with upper abdominal discomfort. This symptom has been present for the past 2 years. It is made worse with meals, particularly large and fatty meals. She has no real heartburn, dysphagia, or other esophageal symptoms. There is some nausea, no vomiting, and she has gained 5 kg over the past year. Her bowel movements are normal. There is no fever, chills, or other associated symptoms. Her internist orders an upper abdominal ultrasound and upper gastrointestinal (GI) X-ray, both of which are normal. On further questioning, it is found that she is somewhat concerned because her father (in her home country of Paraguay) died of gastric cancer and she has heard that this tends to run in families. Her physical exam and general screening laboratories are both normal.

Bacteriology

H. pylori is a Gram-negative, spiral-shaped organism measuring approximately 0.5 µm in diameter and 3–5 µm in length. It has two to six polar-sheathed flagella, which allow the bacterium to move in the viscous environment of the gastric mucus.

Prior to the first isolation and characterization of this organism in 1982 [1], it was assumed that the human stomach was sterile because bacteria are usually killed by acid at pH <3.0. Upon its discovery, a new genus, *Helicobacter*, was created; since then at least 30 new species have been added, mainly isolated from the stomach and GI tracts of mammals.

The genome of *H. pylori* was sequenced in 1997 [2]. It has a single circular chromosome of 1.7 Mb with 1500 genes, of which only 1000 are present in all strains. The small size of the *H. pylori* genome confirms that it has fewer regulatory genes than other bacteria, supporting the hypothesis that *H. pylori* lives only in the human stomach, as it does not possess the enzymatic pathways necessary to survive in other environments.

H. pylori is nutritionally fastidious and can be cultivated in the laboratory from gastric biopsies on agar plates containing blood or serum, under microaerobic conditions, or in the presence of air enriched with 10% CO_2. Optimum growth is obtained at 37 °C after 4–5 days for primary culture or 2 days for subsequent subculture. The growth of small, translucent, water droplet-like colonies that are urease-, catalase-, and oxidase-positive and which show the characteristic spiral morphology is usually adequate for the identification of *H. pylori*. Large amounts of urease are produced, which are used to break down urea to ammonia and bicarbonate, allowing the organism to survive in acid. Diagnosis by culture is usually reserved for cases in which bacterial susceptibility data are required or for use in research studies.

Epidemiology and Transmission

H. pylori infects more than half the people on earth, particularly in developing countries, where the majority of the population may be infected. In Western countries and in countries emerging from a developing to a Western economy, the prevalence of *H. pylori* in the community is decreasing, due to improved standards of hygiene, smaller families, and increasing awareness of the infection. In the United States, for example, *Helicobacter* infected about 60% of the population in 1965 but currently infects only about 20%; immigrants are infected in proportion to the prevalence rate in their home country [3, 4].

The transmission of *H. pylori* is not totally understood, because it can rarely be cultured from environmental samples. It has occasionally been cultured from feces, saliva, and dental plaque, but, for the most part, it lives only in the stomach; saliva transfer is thus thought to be a likely means of transmission, particularly between mother and child. In support of this, *H. pylori* does seem to run in families, and children are more likely to have exactly the same strain as their mother. The major mode of transmission

Practical Gastroenterology and Hepatology Board Review Toolkit, Second Edition. Edited by Nicholas J. Talley, Kenneth R. DeVault, Michael B. Wallace, Bashar A. Aqel and Keith D. Lindor.
© 2016 John Wiley & Sons, Ltd. Published 2016 by John Wiley & Sons, Ltd. Companion website: www.practicalgastrohep.com

of *H. pylori* in developing countries is probably via contaminated water [5].

Emphasizing the possible transmission of *H. pylori* via feces or gastric secretions, some papers show that medical staff, nursing staff, and, especially, gastroenterologists are likely to be infected by *H. pylori*. Similarly, those who experience a vomiting illness are likely to spread the infection within their family [6].

Reinfection after treatment is uncommon in Western countries (1%) but common in countries with a high prevalence. However, our poor understanding of the transmission of *H. pylori* is reflected in data such as those from Malaysia, an emerging economy, where the reinfection rate is only about 2% despite a high prevalence [7]. In Malaysia, the prevalence varies greatly between racial groups [7].

Pathogenesis and Disease Associations

Upon entering the stomach, *H. pylori* colonizes the mucus layer above the secreting gastric epithelial cells. Adherent *H. pylori* organisms can inject a toxin, called cag A, into the epithelial cells, which release interleukin 8 (IL-8) and so attract polymorphonuclear leukocytes and components of the innate immune system. This acute inflammatory reaction produces IL-1B, which serves to inhibit acid secretion. Thus, in the first few days of the acute infection, acid secretion falls to near zero and the syndrome of "acute gastritis with hypochlorhydria" develops, probably as a mild illness that is largely unnoticed in young children. This status of low acidity may continue for months, years, or possibly even a lifetime. Subsequently, acute inflammation settles and chronic inflammation sets in. Immunoglobulin M (IgM) antibodies develop, followed by antibodies to IgG and IgA, as *H. pylori* colonization reaches a stable form. In this mid stage, lasting most of the infected person's lifetime, acid secretion returns, but there are often no symptoms.

In some people, gastritis impairs normal secretion of somatostatin, thereby permitting increased secretion of gastrin [8]. People with duodenal ulcer thus tend to have a raised fasting basal acid secretion. After decades of infection, the chronic inflammation can lead to intestinal metaplasia in the gastric mucosa, with atrophy of the acid-secreting tissue and the return of a low-acid state.

When *Helicobacter* is eradicated, the inflammation largely resolves and a mild infiltrate of lymphocytes and plasma cells remains. Intestinal metaplasia does not resolve and the presence of associated atrophy marks a continuing cancer risk even after the eradication of *H. pylori*.

Duodenal and Gastric Ulcers

In duodenal ulcer, the *H. pylori* infection causes chronic gastritis of the antrum, but acid secretion is normal or high because the upper 75% of the stomach is mostly spared. Duodenal ulcers are associated with infected islands of gastric metaplasia (a normal anatomical variant) in the duodenal bulb. Duodenal and gastric ulcers form a continuum through the pylorus. Duodenal ulcers are not associated with gastric cancer, but gastric ulcers do carry a risk of malignancy and therefore must be adequately biopsied. In duodenal ulcer, the gastric mucosa returns to near normality after the *Helicobacter* has been eradicated. After *H. pylori* eradication, 80–90% of patients may experience a total ulcer cure. Gastric ulcers are more likely to be associated with non-steroidal anti-inflammatory drugs (NSAIDs) than are duodenal ulcers. The *H. pylori* contribution to peptic ulcer has decreased in Western countries as a result of widespread treatment and decreased prevalence. As a result, NSAIDs now account for about 50% of "peptic ulcers."

Gastric MALT Lymphoma

Lymphoma of the mucosa-associated lymphoid tissue (MALT) is the most common lymphoma of the GI tract. This indolent B-cell gastric tumor is strongly associated with *H. pylori*; 75% of people undergo clinical remission of the disease when *H. pylori* is eradicated [9]. Those with undifferentiated MALT lymphoma of the stomach or associated MALT lymphoma outside the stomach are not cured, though occasional exceptions occur, so the bacterium should always be eliminated. Histological studies of patients in clinical remission still reveal a clonal population of lymphocytes in the gastric epithelium. Thus, follow-up to prove continuing absence of *H. pylori* (with a combination of tests such as UBT plus serology) is essential for long-term care.

Gastric cancer is associated with chronic gastritis. In Japan, where gastric cancer was until recently the most common malignancy, almost everyone with gastric cancer has evidence of current or past *H. pylori* infection, as indicated by specific antibodies, atrophy of the gastric acid secreting glands, and intestinal metaplasia. However, some countries with a high prevalence of *H. pylori* do not have a correspondingly high incidence of gastric cancer (e.g., Thailand, countries in the Middle East) [10]. Bacterial factors (cagA toxin activity), as well as dietary (high-salt diet) and cultural factors, may also affect cancer risk.

Persons with intestinal metaplasia and widespread gastric atrophy carry a cancer risk, which continues after eradication of *H. pylori* but possibly reduces in time [11]. In those who do not have these changes in the gastric mucosa, eradication of *H. pylori* reduces the risk of gastric cancer.

Other Conditions Associated with *H. pylori*

Numerous other conditions have been associated with *H. pylori* infections. Many of these are rare and anecdotal, but a few warrant brief mention.

The syndrome of functional dyspepsia refers to the presence of epigastric pain or discomfort in the absence of peptic ulcer disease. In prospective double-blind studies where *H. pylori* has been eradicated, complete symptomatic cures have been noted in about 15% of cases [12].

Iron deficiency associated with *H. pylori* infection presumably results from slight chronic gastric mucosal iron loss. In prospective studies in Japan, iron levels increased after eradication of *H. pylori*. The effect of treatment is small, but in a population with low iron intake, some people probably do develop iron-deficiency anemia related to *H. pylori*. Therefore, in all those with iron-deficiency anemia who do not have a serious source identified, eradication of *H. pylori* is justified.

Idiopathic thrombocytopenic purpura (ITP) has been reported to be associated with *H. pylori*. Since other treatments for ITP are hazardous, a course of antibiotics to eradicate *H. pylori* is an excellent first choice, with a cure rate of 30–59% in some studies. Therefore, always test and treat *H. pylori* in patients with ITP [13].

Some of these recorded associations with *H. pylori* are listed in Table 19.1.

Diagnosis

Accurate diagnosis of *H. pylori* is essential for good treatment compliance by the patient and enthusiastic participation by the physician. Diagnostic tests can be characterized as non-invasive versus invasive, and also as tests for active disease versus past disease. Serology for specific IgG antibodies against *H. pylori* is highly sensitive,

Table 19.1 Non-gastric conditions associated with *H. pylori*.

Studies/reports	Diseases	
Substantial evidence from several studies	Iron deficiency	Proven association; possible clinical relevance when nutrition is poor [14]
	Idiopathic thrombocytopenic purpura (ITP)	Several reports, but prospective data are weak [14]
	Chronic urticaria	A systematic review concluded that bacterial eradication is associated with remission [15]

so *H. pylori* infection can be virtually excluded if the test is negative. The IgG level may stay in the positive range for years after eradication of *H. pylori*.

The UBT is based on the ability of *H. pylori* to secrete a large amount of urease enzyme, which splits urea into CO_2 and ammonia. Therefore, if the patient is given a small dose of urea labeled with ^{13}C or ^{14}C, the CO_2 they breathe out will likewise be labeled. Breath tests are highly specific and can be used for initial diagnosis of *H. pylori* in a similar way to serology. However, they are essential for non-invasive follow-up testing of *H. pylori*, since they test for the actual live *H. pylori* organisms in the gastric mucosa. Wait 4 weeks or longer to test after antibiotic treatment. During breath–testing, it is important that the patient not be taking any medications that inhibit *H. pylori*. Acid pump blockers should be ceased for at least 7 days before performing the UBT.

An alternative test for active disease is the *Helicobacter* fecal antigen test. Organisms shed from the stomach are passed into the intestine and appear in the feces [16].

At endoscopy, accurate diagnosis of *H. pylori* is made by studying biopsy samples of the gastric mucosa (Figure 19.1). These tests may be negative when the patient is taking an inhibitory compound in the days before endoscopy. Acute GI bleeding can also lead to a false-negative test. In persons with active *H. pylori* disease, at least two biopsies should be taken for histology from opposite sides of the gastric antrum and examined with hematoxylin stain, eosin stain, and either a Giemsa, toluidine blue, or silver stain for *H. pylori* organisms. Immunohistochemical stains can be used to prove the organisms are *H. pylori*. *H. pylori* is usually less abundant in the corpus, but corpus biopsies are useful to see the extent of the gastritis.

A useful addition to diagnosis is the rapid urease test. An antral biopsy is taken from the prepyloric lesser curve and placed into a medium that contains urea. In the presence of *H. pylori*, the urea is split into CO_2 and ammonia, which raises the pH and so produces a color change in the indicator dye after about 10 minutes. This allows the gastroenterologist to make a diagnosis in the endoscopy room.

Gastric biopsies may also be cultured in order to determine the antibiotic sensitivities of the organism. This is not routine, but may be considered in patients who have failed multiple (more than three) previous therapies. *H. pylori* is almost universally sensitive to penicillin and tetracycline, and most strains are initially sensitive to clarithromycin and metronidazole, but after being exposed to these latter two the organism usually becomes resistant. Antibiotic resistance develops in *H. pylori* because of its high spontaneous mutation rate.

Treatment

Successful eradication rates have fallen. Compliance with treatment increases the success rate, but at least 30 % will still fail first-line optimal therapy.

There are three groups of medications that are used in a successful *H. pylori* eradication therapy:

1 Drugs that can be used repeatedly, as *H. pylori* remains susceptible.
2 Drugs that can only be used once, as *H. pylori* becomes resistant.
3 Drugs that decrease acid secretion and assist antibiotic action.

The drugs that can be used repeatedly are amoxicillin, tetracycline, and bismuth (Pepto-Bismol – bismuth subsalicylate in the United States or bismuth subcitrate elsewhere). These are usually given in a 7–14-day course, which leads to widespread suppression of the organism. Given alone, they only rarely cure the infection, so a second antibiotic drug is given concurrently. In this group are metronidazole, clarithromycin, the quinolones, and the rifamycins, such as rifabutin. These must always be given with a suppressive agent from the first group. If treatment needs to be repeated, a different drug from this group should be used. Finally, in order for antibiotics to work effectively in the gastric mucosa, acid secretion must be inhibited. This is done with high-dose proton pump inhibitors (PPIs).

The most widely used therapy in the United States is a 10-day course of a PPI twice daily, amoxicillin 1 g twice daily, and clarithromycin 500 mg twice daily. In Australia and Europe, this "triple-therapy" treatment is given only for 7 days. Extending these 7 days to 14 increases the rate of eradication by about 5%. In penicillin-allergic patients, switch metronidazole (500 mg daily) for amoxicillin.

Quadruple therapy comprises bismuth, a PPI, metronidazole, and tetracycline for 14 days and is equivalent to triple therapy [17]. Prescribe quadruple therapy if initial triple-therapy treatment failed or if clarithromycin resistance is known to be high (>15% of the population). A capsule containing bismuth subcitrate (140 mg), metronidazole (125 mg), and tetracycline (125 mg) is available and is Food and Drug Administration (FDA) approved. The dosing is three capsules four times daily, plus a PPI twice daily.

The concept of "sequential therapy" has been promoted because it can give an improved cure rate compared to triple therapy, with decreased side effects. Typical sequential therapy consists of a total 10-day treatment of high-dose PPI, with amoxicillin added in the first 5 days, to be replaced by clarithromycin and metronidazole for the next 5 days [18]. Simplified treatment packs of sequential therapy are presently unavailable, so they are less convenient to prescribe than triple therapy.

In practice, patients are given the standard treatment with PPI, amoxicillin, and clarithromycin. If the treatment has failed, consider trying quadruple therapy. If this fails too, consider a PPI, amoxicillin, and levofloxcian (250 mg) twice daily. Rescue-therapy combinations can otherwise include a PPI, amoxicillin, rifabutin, and ciprofloxiacin [19]. Probiotics (e.g., saccharomryces boulardii) may slightly increase eradication rates but are not routine.

Controversies in Management

Who to Diagnose and Who to Treat

Anyone with persistent dyspepsia might reasonably be tested for *H. pylori* and treated if it is found to be present. In those who come from a country where gastric cancer is common, endoscopic diagnosis is preferred as it allows malignancy to be excluded and *H. pylori* diagnosed at the same time (e.g., Hong Kong). In Western countries, where gastric cancer is relatively uncommon, those below the age of 50 with simple dyspepsia without alarm symptoms (e.g., weight loss, GI bleeding, etc.) may reasonably be subjected to

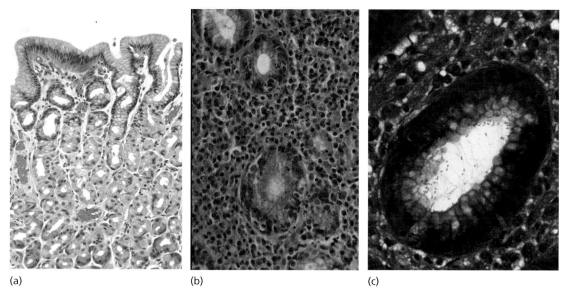

(a)   (b)   (c)

Figure 19.1 Histology of *H. pylori* infection: (a) normal mucosa (H&E 100×); (b) active gastritis with HP (H&E 250×); (c) numerous HP bacilli (Toludene blue stain 500×).

"test-and-treat" strategies, whereby the physician performs a convenient diagnostic test for *H. pylori*, prescribes treatment to eradicate it (if the test is positive), then follows up 1 month later with a test of active infection (e.g., UBT) to confirm eradication. If treatment fails, the physician may choose to treat the patient again. If symptoms persist, consider endoscopy.

Well-known indications for *H. pylori* eradication are any history of peptic ulcer, gastric cancer in the patient's family, and gastric MALT lymphoma. It is not cost-effective to screen and treat *H. pylori* in asymptomatic people, except in populations at high risk of gastric cancer, such as Japanese Americans [20].

Pregnancy
Usually, treatment is deferred until delivery. Avoid bismuth and tetracycline in pregnancy. *H. pylori* may be linked to hyperemesis gravidarum.

Cancer Prevention
First-degree relatives of those with gastric adenocarcinoma have an increased risk of cancer caused by their *H. pylori* infection [21]. However, it is controversial to screen asymptomatic family members of gastric cancer patients. Prospective treatment studies have shown some protection from gastric cancer; that is, there are fewer new cancer cases in those from whom *H. pylori* has been eradicated. However, some cancers still occur in the stomach after *H. pylori* has been cured [22]. The presence of atrophic gastritis and intestinal metaplasia serve to prolong the risk of gastric adenocarcinoma for several years after *H. pylori* eradication.

After eradication of *H. pylori*, hypochlorhydric patients with widespread asymptomatic gastritis may increase their acid secretion, thereby unmasking an incompetent lower esophageal sphincter (LES). A link between *H. pylori* disappearance and obesity has also been observed [23]. On a population basis, it is inevitable that gastroesophageal reflux disease (GERD) would increase if the whole asymptomatic population were treated for *H. pylori*. On the other hand, the risk of a continuing low-acid state due to atrophic gastritis is known to confer at least a sixfold increased rate of gastric adenocarcinoma in individuals with persistent *H. pylori*. The practical response to this controversy is to test and treat any patients who have *H. pylori* but to be on the lookout for new GERD symptoms. The physician should discuss the pros and cons of *H. pylori* therapy with the patient. Most patients are concerned about the small cancer risk of *H. pylori*, the potential for transmitting the organism to family members, and the possibility that eradication of chronic inflammation of the gastric mucosa might lead to symptom relief.

Case Continued
Given the presentation of ulcer-negative dyspepsia in an emigrant from a country with a high prevalence of *H. pylori*, a test-and-treat strategy is considered, though the number needed to treat in order to achieve a cure of these symptoms may be quite high (since significant ulcer disease has been excluded by the barium test). On the other hand, given this patient's family history and concerns, an esophagogastroduodenoscopy (EGD) may be justified. She undergoes an EGD, which demonstrates diffuse erythema of the stomach. Biopsy confirms *H. pylori* infection, but there are no areas of histological concern. Eradication therapy produces a partial improvement in her upper GI symptoms, and follow-up breath-testing confirms eradication.

Take Home Points
- *Helicobacter pylori* is a bacterial pathogen that causes gastritis, peptic ulcers, and gastric cancer (both adenocarcinoma and mucosa-associated lymphoid tissue (MALT) lymphoma).
- Disease outcome is dependent upon bacterial and host factors.
- Diagnosis may be made by endoscopic biopsy, breath-testing, stool tests, and serology (but serology does not distinguish current from past infection).
- Eradication is by combination antibiotic therapy.

References

1 Marshall B, Royce H, Annear D. Original isolation of *Campylobacter pyloridis* from human gastric mucosa. *Microbios Lett* 1984; **25**(25): 83–8.

2 Tomb JF, White O, Kerlavage AR, *et al.* The complete genome sequence of the gastric pathogen *Helicobacter pylori*. *Nature* 1997; **388**(6642): 539–47.

3 Parsonnet J, Friedman GD, Vandersteen DP, *et al. Helicobacter pylori* infection and the risk of gastric carcinoma. *N Engl J Med* 1991; **325**(16): 1127–31.

4 Perez-Perez GI, Olivares AZ, Foo FY, *et al.* Seroprevalence of *Helicobacter pylori* in New York City populations originating in East Asia. *J Urban Health* 2005; **82**(3): 510–16.

5 Ahmed KS, Khan AA, Ahmed I, *et al.* Impact of household hygiene and water source on the prevalence and transmission of *Helicobacter pylori*: a South Indian perspective. *Singapore Med J* 2007; **48**(6): 543–9.

6 Perry S, de la Luz Sanchez M, Yang S, *et al.* Gastroenteritis and transmission of *Helicobacter pylori* infection in households. *Emerg Infect Dis* 2006; **12**(11): 1701–8.

7 Goh KL, Parasakthi N. The racial cohort phenomenon: seroepidemiology of *Helicobacter pylori* infection in a multiracial South-East Asian country. *Eur J Gastroenterol Hepatol* 2001; **13**(2): 177–83.

8 El-Omar EM, Oien K, El-Nujumi A, *et al. Helicobacter pylori* infection and chronic gastric acid hyposecretion. *Gastroenterology* 1997; **113**(1): 15–24.

9 Bayerdorffer E, Neubauer A, Rudolph B, *et al.* Regression of primary gastric lymphoma of mucosa-associated lymphoid tissue type after cure of *Helicobacter pylori* infection. *MALT Lymphoma Study Group. Lancet* 1995; **345**(8965): 1591–4.

10 Yamaoka Y, Kato M, Asaka M. Geographic differences in gastric cancer incidence can be explained by differences between *Helicobacter pylori* strains. *Intern Med* 2008; **47**(12): 1077–83.

11 Asaka M, Sugiyama T, Nobuta A, *et al.* Atrophic gastritis and intestinal metaplasia in Japan: results of a large multicenter study. *Helicobacter* 2001; **6**(4): 294–9.

12 Moayyedi P, Soo S, Deeks J, *et al.* Eradication of *Helicobacter pylori* for non-ulcer dyspepsia. *Cochrane Database Syst Rev* 2006(2):CD002096.

13 Stasi R, Sarpatwari A, Segal JB, *et al.* Effects of eradication of *Helicobacter pylori* infection in patients with immune thrombocytopenic purpura: a systematic review. *Blood* 2009; **113**(6): 1231–40.

14 Suzuki H, Marshall BJ, Hibi T. Overview: *Helicobacter pylori* and extragastric disease. *Int J Hematol* 2006; **84**(4): 291–300.

15 Federman DG, Kirsner RS, Moriarty JP, Concato J. The effect of antibiotic therapy for patients infected with *Helicobacter pylori* who have chronic urticaria. *J Am Acad Dermatol* 2003; **49**(5): 861–4.

16 Gisbert JP, de la Morena F, Abraira V. Accuracy of monoclonal stool antigen test for the diagnosis of *H. pylori* infection: a systematic review and meta-analysis. *Am J Gastroenterol* 2006; **101**(8): 1921–30.

17 Delchier JC, Malfertheiner P, Thieroff-Ekerdt R. Use of a combination formulation of bismuth, metronidazole and tetracycline with omeprazole as a rescue therapy for eradication of *Helicobacter pylori*. *Aliment Pharmacol Ther* 2014; **40**(2): 171–7.

18 Vaira D, Zullo A, Vakil N, *et al.* Sequential therapy versus standard triple-drug therapy for *Helicobacter pylori* eradication: a randomized trial. *Ann Intern Med* 2007; **146**(8): 556–63.

19 Tay CY, Windsor HM, Thirriot F, *et al. Helicobacter pylori* eradication in Western Australia using novel quadruple therapy combinations. *Aliment Pharmacol Ther* 2012; **36**(11–12): 1076–83.

20 Talley NJ, Fock KM, Moayyedi P. Gastric Cancer Consensus conference recommends *Helicobacter pylori* screening and treatment in asymptomatic persons from high-risk populations to prevent gastric cancer. *Am J Gastroenterol* 2008; **103**(3): 510–14.

21 Motta CR, Cunha MP, Queiroz DM, *et al.* Gastric precancerous lesions and *Helicobacter pylori* infection in relatives of gastric cancer patients from Northeastern Brazil. *Digestion* 2008; **78**(1): 3–8.

22 Fock KM. Review article: The epidemiology and prevention of gastric cancer. *Aliment Pharmacol Ther* 2014; **40**(3): 250–60.

23 Lender N, Talley NJ, Enck P, *et al.* Review article: Associations between *Helicobacter pylori* and obesity – an ecological study. *Aliment Pharmacol Ther* 2014; **40**(1): 24–31.

CHAPTER 19

Gastritis

Massimo Rugge and David Y. Graham

Baylor College of Medicine, Houston, TX, USA

Summary

Gastritis is defined as inflammation of stomach mucosa and classified on the basis of etiology [1–5]. The most common forms of gastritis are infectious (*Helicobacter pylori*), chemical, and autoimmune. Diagnostic tools includes clinical evaluation, serology (pepsinogens and antibodies against infectious agents and/or autoantigens), endoscopy (standardized biopsy protocols should be applied), and histology. Histology distinguishes non-atrophic from atrophic gastritis (atrophy = loss of appropriate glands). Most of the gastric cancers arise in atrophic mucosa. Atrophic-intestinalized glands may de-differentiate in an advanced precancerous lesion defined as intraepithelial neoplasia (IEN). IEN can progress in invasive gastric carcinoma (intestinal type). The histology report should be clinically informative. Histology can also be used for cancer risk stratification, using the OLGA or OLGIM staging systems, and can provide a clinicopathological rationale for identification of those who would benefit from clinical/endoscopic follow-up.

Definitions

"Gastritis" is a widely misused term, as it is often used to denote endoscopic findings such as redness or symptoms such as those experienced after eating spicy foods. Clinically, gastric abnormalities associated with clinical or endoscopic findings are divided into inflammatory conditions and non-inflammatory or focally inflammatory conditions, called gastropathies [6]. While this distinction is theoretically appropriate, histologically they almost always reveal an inflammatory component, such as that associated with non-steroidal anti-inflammatory drug (NSAID)-induced erosions or duodenogastric bile reflux [7].

Assessment

The approach to gastritis is both clinical (including serology) and histological. Clinical features assist in interpretation of both the endoscopic and the histological findings. For example, interpretation of endoscopic findings of multiple, small, antral erosions would be advanced by knowing that the patient took aspirin the morning of the procedure. Similarly, the finding of antral and corpus atrophy in a patient with vitamin B_{12} deficiency (pernicious anemia) would point toward the process being the end result of a chronic *H. pylori* infection rather than an autoimmune phenomenon. In contrast, primary autoimmune gastritis involves only the gastric corpus.

A diagnosis of gastritis implies that one has histologically examined the gastric mucosa. Most often, the tissue specimens are obtained at endoscopy. Standardized biopsy protocols should be used, and many different biopsy sampling protocols have been proposed [4, 8]. The most recent is the Sydney system and its modifications, in which mucosa from the oxyntic, antral, and incisura angularis areas are sampled (Figure 20.1), in addition to specimens from any focal lesions seen [9]. Because the histology assessment may be conditioned by the location of the biopsy samples, antral specimens (including the incisura) and corpus biopsies can be combined, but in separate bottles. Biopsy samples obtained from focal lesions (if any) should also be placed in separate bottles. If more extensive sampling of the corpus is done (e.g., two lesser-curve and two greater-curve specimens), three bottles should be used to separate the lesser- and greater-curve corpus specimens. This is based on the notion that atrophy extends proximally more quickly along the lesser curve than the greater curve.

Biopsy samples should be handled as little as possible, and after fixation should be embedded on edge. The basic stain is H&E. When *H. pylori* is suspected, a special stain such as a modified Giemsa, a triple stain such as the Genta or El-Zimaity, or immunohistochemical staining should be used [10, 11]. The widespread use of proton pump inhibitors (PPIs) may be associated with an increased presence of non-*H. pylori* organisms, and in our experience, less-experienced pathologists often overdiagnose the infection based on the presence of a few silver-stained particles in otherwise non-inflamed tissue. In such instances, it is prudent to confirm the infection using immunohistochemical staining. Extensive gastric mucosa intestinalization may limit the accuracy of histology in *H. pylori* histological assessment.

The histology report should be clinically informative and the terminology should be suggested by the Sydney system or, more recently, by an international group of gastroenterologists and pathologists known as the OLGA staging system [12]. The OLGA system categorizes gastritis in five stages according to the progressively increasing extension of atrophy (histologically assessed in both antral and oxyntic compartments: OLGA-staging system Stages I–IV) (Table 20.1). OLGA staging is particularly useful in regions where gastric cancer is still prevalent, as it provides information about the cancer risk and includes assessment of the etiology of gastritis (*H. pylori*, autoimmune, etc.). More recently, another staging system has been proposed (OLGIM) based on the semiquantitative histology score of intestinal metaplasia. The rationale

Practical Gastroenterology and Hepatology Board Review Toolkit, Second Edition. Edited by Nicholas J. Talley, Kenneth R. DeVault, Michael B. Wallace, Bashar A. Aqel and Keith D. Lindor.

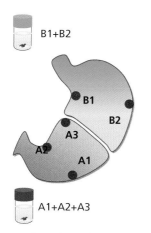

B1+B2

B1

B2

A3

A2

A1

A1+A2+A3

Figure 20.1 Biopsy protocol sampling in the routine assessment of gastritis. Biopsy samples from antral (A1, A2), oxyntic (B1, B2), and incisura angularis (A3) mucosa should be obtained. Antral specimens (including incisura angularis) can be placed in one vial and the corpus biopsies in another.

behind this system is equivalent to that of the OLGA staging: both support the priority of moving from a descriptive histology report to a more consistent (less equivocal) assessment of the gastritis-associated cancer risk.

Non-invasive tests can also provide important information that can complement or supplant histologic mapping studies. For example, pepsinogens levels: Pepsinogen I (PgI) is present in fundic chief cells, whereas PgII is present in the antrum and corpus [13, 14]. Pepsinogen testing is especially useful in excluding extensive atrophy and as a non-invasive test to identify those likely to benefit from histologic examination. The negative predictive value (NPV) of normal PgI and of the PgI : PgII ratio is very high, whereas the presence of a PgI < 70 and a PgI : PgII ratio < 3.0 suggest extensive atrophic gastritis [15].

Gastrin 17 levels provide evidence of acid secretion (high gastrin 17 = low acid secretion; low gastrin 17 typically = high acid secretion). Antiparietal cell antibodies assist in the diagnosis of autoimmune gastritis.

Basic Morphology

Inflammatory Infiltrate: Mononuclear Cells

The inflammatory infiltrate mainly consists of lymphocytes, plasmocytes, histiocytes, and granulocytes within the lamina propria, and may also infiltrate single glands units. Lymphocytes may be dispersed or organized in follicular (or nodular) structures.

The term "lymphocytic gastritis" is applied to those conditions in which single lymphocytes are detected within the columnar epithelia of the majority of the glandular structures and suggests, but is not diagnostic of, an immune-mediated pathogenesis [16]. A more severe (nodular) lymphocyte intraglandular infiltrate may destroy the continuity of the glandular epithelia; such a "lymphoepithelial lesion" is considered almost pathognomonic of primary gastric (almost always *H. pylori*-associated) lymphomas [17].

Inflammatory Infiltrate: Polymorphs (Neutrophils and Eosinophils)

When neutrophils are detected within the lamina propria and/or the glandular lumen, the patient has an "active gastritis." The presence of a predominant eosinophil population is assessed as eosinophilic gastritis [18].

Fibrosis of the Lamina Propria and Smooth-Muscle Hyperplasia

Irrespective of its etiology, the expansion of the collagen tissue of the lamina propria (fibrosis) couples with loss of glandular units and the lesion is assessed as mucosa atrophy. Fibrosis of the lamina propria may also be focal (i.e., scar of peptic ulcer).

Hyperplasia of the muscularis mucosae may result from long-term PPI therapy; smooth-muscle fascicles may push apart the glandular coils, causing a pseudoatrophic pattern. Muscularis mucosae hyperplasia (most often coexisting with foveolar hyperplasia; see next section) is frequently encountered as part of the so-called "reactive gastropathy." The low-level inflammatory tract of this histological lesion does not properly allow its categorization among "gastritis"; it generally results from duodenogastric reflux, and its associated cancer risk is considered negligible.

Hyperplasia of Glandular Elements

All inflammatory conditions of the gastric mucosa are associated with some degree of regenerative epithelial modification, and this is typically seen adjacent to peptic ulcers and erosions (regenerative hyperplasia). Expansion of the proliferative compartment of the gastric glands (neck region) results in foveolar hyperplasia. Chemical (biliary reflux into the stomach or NSAID use) and infectious stimuli increasing the cellular turnover result in hyperplastic foveolae. Atypical regeneration of the glandular neck and/or expansion of the glandular proliferative compartment may cause difficulty in differentiating regenerative from dysplastic lesions (see lesions indefinite for IEN).

Changes occurring in the oxyntic epithelia as result of PPIs in response to the inhibition of the acid secretion are sometimes considered hyperplastic changes but may simply represent a remodeling of the epithelial structure due to cytoskeletal rearrangements. Similar cytologic alteration have been described in association with *H. pylori* infection.

Table 20.1 OLGA system for gastritis staging [9]. The gastritis stage results from the combination of the atrophy scores detected at the antral mucosa and at the corpus mucosa. Source: Correa 2008 [9]. Reproduced with permission of Elsevier.

Atrophy score		Corpus			
		No atrophy (score 0)	Mild atrophy (score 1)	Moderate atrophy (score 2)	Severe atrophy (score 3)
Antrum	No atrophy (score 0) (including incisura angularis)	Stage 0	Stage I	Stage II	Stage II
	Mild atrophy (score 1) (including incisura angularis)	Stage I	Stage I	Stage II	Stage III
	Moderate atrophy (score 2) (including incisura angularis)	Stage II	Stage II	Stage III	Stage IV
	Severe atrophy (score 3) (including incisura angularis)	Stage III	Stage III	Stage IV	Stage IV

Table 20.2 Atrophy in gastric mucosa.

Atrophy	Histological type	Location and key lesions		Grading
		Antrum	Corpus	
0 Absent (= score 0) 1 Indefinite (no score is applicable) 2 Present	2.1 Non-metaplastic	Glands: shrinking/vanishing Lamina propria: fibrosis	Glands: shrinking/vanishing Lamina propria: fibrosis	2.1.1 Mild = G1 (1–30%) 2.1.2 Moderate = G2 (31–60%) 2.1.3 Severe = G3 (>60%)
	2.2 Metaplastic	Intestinal metaplasia	Intestinal metaplasia Pseudopyloric metaplasia	2.2.1 Mild = G1 (1–30%) 2.2.2 Moderate = G2 (31–60%) 2.2.3 Severe = G3 (>60%)

Glandular Atrophy

Atrophy is defined as the loss of appropriate gastric glands. Different phenotypes of atrophic transformation may be present (Table 20.2), including: (i) vanishing or evident shrinkage of glandular units replaced by fibrosis ("scaring") of the lamina propria (such a situation results in a reduced glandular mass, but does not imply any modification of the original (mucosecreting or oxyntic) cell phenotype); and (ii) metaplastic replacement of the native glands by glands featuring a new cellular commitment (= intestinal and/or pseudopyloric metaplasia). The number of glands is not necessarily lower, but the metaplastic replacement of the original glandular units decreases the population of the native glands (which are "appropriate" for the compartment considered). A formal classification of atrophic changes has been proposed (Table 20.2).

Metaplasia Phenotypes

By definition, metaplasia is a transformation of the native commitment of a cell. Within the stomach, the metaplastic transformation always implies loss of appropriate (native) glands (i.e., atrophy). Two main histotypes of gastric gland metaplasia are described. Pseudopyloric metaplasia (also know as SPAM (spasmolytic polypeptide-expressing metaplasia)) of native corpus epithelia is characterized histologically as antral-appearing mucosa obtained from what was anatomically corpus mucosa [19]. It is particularly important for the endoscopist to identify the location of the biopsy specimens, otherwise they will likely miss the fact that the antral-appearing mucosa is a metaplastic epithelia. The original commitment of a pseudopyloric-metaplastic epithelium can be revealed by positive immunostain for PgI, which is only found in the corpus (oxyntic) mucosa.

The most easily identified variant of metaplasia is the intestinal type. Intestinal metaplasia may arise in native mucosecreting (antral) epithelia or in previously antralized oxyntic glands (i.e., from pseudopyloric metaplasia). Different subtypes of intestinal metaplasia have been proposed based on whether the metaplastic epithelium phenotype resembles large-bowel epithelia (colonic-type intestinal metaplasia, also known as Type II–III intestinal metaplasia) or small intestinal mucosa (also known as Type I intestinal metaplasia) [20].

Particularly in the cardia region, a third type of metaplastic transformation can occasionally be faced (pseudopancreatic metaplasia). The clinical relevance of this metaplasia is negligible.

Endocrine Cells Hyperplasia

Normally, endocrine cell hyperplasia is secondary to gastric achlorhydria, usually associated with corpus atrophy. In such a condition, the hyperplasia of the endocrine enterochromaffin-like (ECL) cells may be micronodular or diffuse. Less frequently, (neuro)endocrine (nodular) tumors (well-differentiated endocrine tumors; i.e., Type I carcinoids) may develop. Such tumors almost never metastasize, and when indicated, they should be simply resected. They often regress following removal of the source of gastrin (i.e., antral resection).

Intraepithelial Neoplasia (Synonym: Non-invasive Neoplasia; Formerly Defined as Dysplasia)

In longstanding (atrophic) gastritis, mainly due to *H. pylori* infection, the glands may undergo neoplastic transformation confined within the basal membrane, formerly defined as "gastric dysplasia." Because molecular studies have detected a number of the genotypic alterations common to both gastric dysplasia and gastric cancer, both are recognized as neoplastic. Dysplasia has therefore been redefined as an intraepithelial or non-invasive neoplasia (i.e., confined by the dysplastic glands' basal membrane) [21, 22]. The continuity/integrity of the dysplastic glands' basal membrane separates the dysplastic epithelia from the stroma (i.e., lamina propria), excluding the potential for invasion required for any metastatic implant. It was previously thought that cancer often arose from intestinal metaplastic cells, but more recent studies have challenged that hypothesis, and currently the cell of origin is considered unknown.

Classification

Current classifications are based on etiology. Table 20.3 summarizes the etiological classification of gastritis.

Main Forms of Gastritis

Helicobacter pylori Gastritis

H. pylori gastritis is by far the most frequent and important form of gastritis. In never-treated, infected patients, *H. pylori* is usually easily detectable within the mucous gel layer covering gastric mucosa. It is more abundant in the antrum and cardia than in oxyntic mucosa and, while it can be detected with the H&E stain, randomized controlled trials (RCTs) have shown that accuracy is best with special stains. In cases with extensive gastric intestinalization and in patients treated with PPIs, diagnosis may be difficult even with special stains; as already noted, less-experienced pathologists tend to overdiagnose the infection based on the presence of a few silver-stained particles in otherwise non-inflamed tissue.

The presence of the infection is suggested by both mononuclear and neutrophil (i.e., "active") inflammation (neutrophils may fill the foveolar lumen, producing pit microabscesses). Lymphoid follicles are also frequently detected. After successful eradication

Table 20.3 Etiological classification of gastritis.

Etiological category	Agents	Specific etiology	Clinical presentation	Notes (Prevalence: high***, low**, very low*)
Transmissible agents	Viruses	CMV	Acute	Non-atrophic**
		HSV	Acute	Non-atrophic**
	Bacteria	*Helicobacter pylori*	Acute or chronic	Non-atrophic and atrophic; Type B***
		Mycobacterium tuberculosis	? Acute	Non-atrophic*
		Mycobacterium avium complex	? Acute	Non-atrophic*
		Mycobacterium diphtheriae	Acute	Non-atrophic*
		Actinomyces	Acute	Non-atrophic*
		Spirochaeta	Acute	Non-atrophic*
	Fungi	*Candida*	Acute	Non-atrophic**
		Histoplasma	Acute	Non-atrophic*
		Phycomycosis	Acute	Non-atrophic*
	Parasites	*Cryptosporidium*	Acute	Non-atrophic*
		Strongyloides	Acute	Non-atrophic*
		Anisakis	Acute	Non-atrophic*
		Ascaris lumbricoides	Acute	Non-atrophic*
Chemical agents (most frequently gastropathies)	Environment (dietary and drug-related)	Dietary factors	Chronic	Non-atrophic and atrophic***
		Drugs: NSAIDs, ticlopidine	Acute	Non-atrophic; Type C***
		Alcohol	Acute	Non-atrophic; Type C**
		Cocaine	Acute	Non-atrophic; Type C*
		Bile (reflux)	Acute or chronic	Non-atrophic; Type C***
Physical agents	Radiations		Acute or chronic	Non-atrophic and atrophic+
Immunomediated	Different pathogenesis	Autoimmune	Chronic	Atrophic (corpus); Type A**
		Drugs (ticlopidine)	Acute	
		? Gluten	Chronic	Lymphocytic gastritis**
		Food sensitivity	Acute or chronic	Eosinophilic gastritis**
		H. pylori (autoimmune) component	Chronic	Non-atrophic and atrophic
		GVHD	Acute or chronic	Non-atrophic and atrophic+
		Idiopathic	Acute or chronic	
Idiopathic		Crohn disease	? Chronic	Non-atrophic/focal atrophy**
		Sarcoidosis	? Chronic	Non-atrophic or focal atrophy*
		Wegener granulomatosis	? Chronic	Non-atrophic or focal atrophy*
		Collagenous gastritis	Acute	Non-atrophic*

CMV, cytomegalovirus; HSV, herpes simplex virus; NSAID, non-steroidal anti-inflammatory drug; GVHD, graft-versus-host disease.

therapy, neutrophils quickly disappear, whereas the mononuclear component remains detectable for many weeks to months. However, the persistence of neutrophils and/or mononuclear infiltrate should suggest the possibility of therapeutic failure, even if organisms are not seen. This is especially a problem when PPI therapy is continued.

H. pylori infection is the major cause of gastric atrophy. Atrophic changes (metaplastic and non-metaplastic) detected in a biopsy sample obtained from both angularis incisura and antral mucosa should be primarily considered as part of an *H. pylori* gastritis. In long-standing infection (i.e., elderly subjects) or in young infected patients with concomitant risk factors, atrophic changes also occur in oxyntic mucosa, typically as pseudopyloric metaplasia often coexisting with multifocal (antral and corpus) intestinal metaplasia. Such patients are at increased risk of gastric cancer [23].

H. pylori gastritis is also strongly suggested endoscopically by the presence of follicular gastritis, which represents the endoscopic visualization of the multiple lymphoid follicles in the antrum. Experienced endoscopists are often able to correctly assess atrophy/intestinal metaplasia, which should feature an irregular surface, often with patchy pink and pale areas, using standard white-light endoscopy (Figure 20.2).

Chemical Gastritis/Gastropathies

The exposure of gastric mucosa to bile reflux (due either to partial gastrectomy or to dysmotility), to aspirin or other NSAIDs, or

to other chemical injuries (possibly alcohol, etc.) may result in a wide spectrum of mucosal changes [24]. The histological lesions range from minimal to severe (also hemorrhagic) mucosal damage. Based on their trivial inflammatory trait, these conditions have

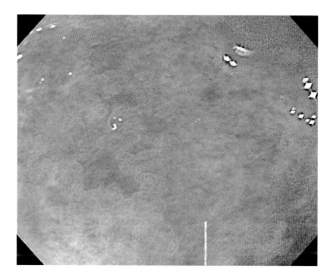

Figure 20.2 Extensive intestinal metaplasia, seen endoscopically. The pattern of irregular pink patches within a white, often velvety background is typical of intestinal metaplasia. When extensive, both the white and the pink mucosa typically show intestinal metaplasia histologically.

been defined as "chemical gastropathies." The pathogenesis of such abnormalities is not completely understood, and it differs slightly according to the different etiologies.

Postgastrectomy gastric reflux of bile salts and pancreaticoduodenal secretions alters the mucus barrier and allows increased back-diffusion of hydrogen ions. The exposure of gastric mucosa to this noxious chemical environment accelerates the turnover of the gastric epithelium; the overproliferation of the epithelial compartment may result in polypoid lesions. Concomitant histamine-mediated vascular response and the release of other proinflammatory cytokines produces vascular ectasia, edema, muscularis mucosa hyperplasia, and variable mucosal fibrosis. It is not clear whether there is any relation between the histological findings and symptoms. Most chemical gastropathies are asymptomatic and non-atrophic. In intact stomachs, the reflux of duodenal content may also result in similar abnormalities.

In 10–50% of long-term NSAID users, endoscopy and/or histology document variable gastric mucosa alterations. NSAIDs reduce the synthesis of prostaglandins, resulting in inefficient protection of the superficial epithelial layer (decreased secretion of both mucus and bicarbonate). The variable unbalance of the cytoprotection and the characteristics of the chemical agent are thought to be the main determinants of the severity of the mucosal damage. Mucosa lesions range from minimal alterations (only detectable at histology: low-grade interfoveolar edema, foveolar hyperplasia, vascular ectasia) to multiple erosions/ulcers with bleeding. Concomitant *H. pylori* infection is a risk factor for more severe gastric lesions; it is likely responsible for an inflammatory component, which is usually undetectable in "pure" chemical forms.

Autoimmune Gastritis

Autoimmune gastritis is a corpus-restricted inflammation caused by selective autoimmune damage of parietal cells (antiparietal cell and anti-intrinsic-factor antibodies). The clinical manifestations of the full-blown disease include hypoachlorhydria, hypergastrinemia, a low PgI : PgII ratio (which parallels the loss of oxyntic gland population), and vitamin B_{12}-deficient macrocytic anemia. The disease may coexist with immunomediated diseases (Hashimoto thyroditis, insulin-dependent diabetes, vitiligo).

In the early stage, oxyntic mucosa shows rich, full-thickness lymphocyte infiltrate, which is even organized in follicular structures (non-atrophic stage). In advanced cases, the corpus-restricted gastritis is characteristically atrophic. The native oxyntic glands are replaced by metaplastic glandular units (pseudopyloric metaplasia comes first; gland intestinalization represents a more advanced stage). Autoimmune gastritis may coexist with *H. pylori* infection, and a previous history of bacterial infection may be recorded in patients with autoimmune gastritis. In such patients, the corpus-based autoimmune disease may be combined with the antral lesions resulting from the bacterial etiology. These situations can result in extensive (antrum and corpus) atrophic gastritis, potentially harboring a high risk of cancer progression [25, 26].

Hypoachlorhydria triggers gastrin hypersecretion (hyperplasia of gastrin secreting cells in antral mucosa), which stimulates the ECL cells of the oxyntic compartment. Such a situation may result in ECL-cell hyperplasia (linear and micronodular). Micronodular ECL-cell hyperplasia can evolve into well-differentiated endocrine tumors (type I carcinoid). It is important to note that such tumors are typically only locally invasive [27, 28].

Take Home Points

- Gastritis is defined as inflammation of the gastric mucosa.
- Histological assessment of gastritis is bases on validated protocols of biopsy sampling.
- Worldwide, *Helicobacter pylori* infection is the most prevalent etiology.
- Atrophic pangastritis is the major risk factor for gastric cancer.
- Reporting gastritis in terms of staging (OLGA or OLGIM staging systems: Stages 0–IV) provides an estimate of gastritis-associated cancer risk.
- Gastritis staging (particularly in the setting of *H. pylori* infection) may represent the rationale for differentiated protocols of follow-up of atrophic gastritis.
- Non-invasive testing may complement or supplant more expensive invasive procedures. The most informative tests are: the urea breath test (UBT) and the stool antigen test for *H. pylori* infection; serum levels of pepsinogen I and II (PgI and PgII) for atrophy; and serum gastrin 17 and antiparietal cell antibody levels for autoimmune gastritis.
- Chemical gastritis is mostly non-atrophic (low cancer risk).
- Autoimmune atrophic gastritis is associated with an increased risk of neuroendocrine well-differentiated tumors (Type I), and possibly also of gastric adenocarcinoma.

References

1 Owen DA. Gastritis and carditis. *Mod Pathol* 2003; **16**: 325–41.

2 Correa P. Chronic gastritis: a clinico-pathological classification. *Am J Gastroenterol* 1988; **83**: 504–9.

3 Price AB. The Sydney System: histological division. *J Gastroenterol Hepatol* 1991; **6**: 209–22.

4 Dixon MF, Genta RM, Yardley JH, *et al.* Classification and grading of gastritis. The updated Sydney System. International Workshop on the Histopathology of Gastritis, Houston 1994. *Am J Surg Pathol* 1996; **20**: 1161–81.

5 Whitehead R. The classification of chronic gastritis: current status. *J Clin Gastroenterol* 1995; **21** (Suppl. 1): S131–4.

6 Srivastava A, Lauwers GY. Pathology of non-infective gastritis. *Histopathology* 2007; **50**: 15–29.

7 Sepulveda AR, Patil M. Practical approach to the pathologic diagnosis of gastritis. *Arch Pathol Lab Med* 2008; **132**: 1586–93.

8 Sipponen P, Stolte M. Clinical impact of routine biopsies of the gastric antrum and body. *Endoscopy* 1997; **29**: 671–8.

9 Rugge M, Correa P, Di Mario F, *et al.* OLGA staging for gastritis: a tutorial. *Dig Liver Dis* 2008; **40**: 650–8.

10 Genta RM, Robason GO, Graham DY. Simultaneous visualization of *Helicobacter pylori* and gastric morphology: a new stain. *Hum Pathol* 1994; **25**: 221–6.

11 el-Zimaity HM, Wu J, Graham DY. Modified Genta triple stain for identifying *Helicobacter pylori*. *J Clin Pathol* 1999; **52**: 693–4.

12 Rugge M, Genta RM. Staging gastritis: an international proposal. *Gastroenterology* 2005; **129**: 1807–8.

13 Pasechnikov VD, Chukov SZ, Kotelevets SM, *et al.* Invasive and non-invasive diagnosis of *Helicobacter pylori*-associated atrophic gastritis: a comparative study. *Scand J Gastroenterol* 2005; **40**: 297–301.

14 Sipponen P, Graham DY. Importance of atrophic gastritis in diagnostics and prevention of gastric cancer: application of plasma biomarkers. *Scand J Gastroenterol* 2007; **42**: 2–10.

15 Dinis-Ribeiro M, Yamaki G, Miki K, *et al.* Meta-analysis on the validity of pepsinogen test for gastric carcinoma, dysplasia or chronic atrophic gastritis screening. *J Med Screen* 2004; **11**: 141–7.

16 Haot J, Hamichi L, Wallez L, *et al.* Lymphocytic gastritis: a newly described entity: a retrospective endoscopic and histological study. *Gut* 1988; **29**: 1258–64.

17 Rugge M, Correa P, Dixon MF, *et al.* Gastric mucosal atrophy: interobserver consistency using new criteria for classification and grading. *Aliment Pharmacol Ther* 2002; **16**: 1249–59.

18 Lwin T, Melton SD, Genta RM. Eosinophilic gastritis: histopathological characterization and quantification of the normal gastric eosinophil content. *Mod Pathol* 2011; **24**: 556–63.

19 Weis VG, Goldenring JR. Current understanding of SPEM and its standing in the preneoplastic process. *Gastric Cancer* 2009; **12**: 189–97

20 Filipe MI, Munoz N, Matko I, *et al.* Intestinal metaplasia types and the risk of gastric cancer: a cohort study in Slovenia. *Int J Cancer* 1994; **57**: 324–9.

21 Rugge M, Correa P, Dixon MF, *et al.* Gastric dysplasia: the Padova international classification. *Am J Surg Pathol* 2000; **24**: 167–76.

22 Rugge M, Cassaro M, Di Mario F, *et al.* The long term outcome of gastric non-invasive neoplasia. *Gut* 2003; **52**: 1111–16.

23 Uemura N, Okamoto S, Yamamoto S, *et al. Helicobacter pylori* infection and the development of gastric cancer. *N Engl J Med* 2001; **345**: 784–9.

24 De Nardi FG, Riddell RH. Reactive (chemical) gastropathy and gastritis. In: Graham DY, Genta RM, Dixon MF, eds. *Gastritis*. Philadelphia, PA: Lippincott Williams & Wilkins, 1999: 125–46.

25 Neumann WL, Coss E, Rugge M, *et al.* Autoimmune atrophic gastritis-pathogenesis, pathology and management. *Nat Rev Gastroenterol Hepatol* 2013; **10**: 529–41.

26 Rugge M, Fassan M, Pizzi M, *et al.* Autoimmune gastritis: histology phenotype and OLGA staging. *Aliment Pharmacol Ther* 2012; **35**: 1460–6.

27 Rindi G, Kloppel G, Alhman H, *et al.* TNM staging of foregut (neuro)endocrine tumors: a consensus proposal including a grading system. *Virchows Arch* 2006; **449**: 395–401.

28 Rindi G, Kloppel G. Endocrine tumors of the gut and pancreas tumor biology and classification. *Neuroendocrinology* 2004; **80** (Suppl. 1): 12–15.

CHAPTER 20

Gastroparesis

Henry P. Parkman[1] and Nicholas J. Talley[2]

[1] Temple University School of Medicine, Philadelphia, PA, USA
[2] Faculty of Health, University of Newcastle, Newcastle, NSW, Australia

Summary

Gastroparesis is a disorder characterized by symptoms of, and evidence for, gastric retention in the absence of mechanical obstruction. Gastroparesis can occur in many clinical settings, with varied symptoms and symptom severity, but it is uncommon [1–3]. The most frequently reported symptoms include nausea, vomiting, early satiety, and postprandial fullness. Abdominal pain, weight loss, malnutrition, and dehydration may be prominent in severe cases. In diabetics, gastroparesis may adversely affect glycemic control. Diagnostic evaluation in patients with symptoms suggestive of gastroparesis generally consists of esophagogastroduodenoscopy (EGD) and a gastric emptying test. Management of this condition can be particularly challenging.

Case

A 19-year-old female presents with nausea and vomiting. Approximately 1 year ago, she became ill while on a cruise ship in the Caribbean. Several other passengers also became ill, but no clear etiology was ever determined. Her acute illness resolved, but she remained nauseated. She began 3 months ago to experience episodic vomiting. Initially, this occurred on a weekly basis, but it has progressed to several episodes of vomiting every day. She is usually well in the morning, but as she begins to eat, she gets more and more nauseated, and she normally begins to vomit in the early afternoon. She feels distended and uncomfortable all the time, has limited her diet to mostly liquids, and has lost weight, from 70 to 55 kg. She is fatigued, but otherwise has no other symptoms, and she has no other significant past medical, social, or family history.

Upper endoscopy demonstrates a moderate amount of retained gastric content despite a 12-hour fast. The underlying mucosa of the esophagus, stomach, and duodenum are normal. A small-bowel X-ray is also negative, with a normal-appearing terminal ileum. Nuclear medicine gastric emptying testing demonstrates delayed gastric emptying at 2 hours (65% retention; normal <60%) and 4 hours (25% retention; normal <10%). A trial of metoclopramide is not tolerated due to severe worsening in her fatigue. Erythromycin actually increases her nausea. Domperidone of 20 mg four times daily is started; she is able to tolerate a low-residue diet and has stabilized her weight.

Etiology

Most cases of gastroparesis are idiopathic [2]. It was initially described as an infrequent complication of long-standing diabetes, especially in association with other complications of diabetes, such as neuropathy. Diabetes mellitus is the most common systemic disease associated with gastroparesis. Postsurgical gastroparesis, often with vagotomy or damage to the vagus nerve, represents the third most common etiology. Delayed gastric emptying can also be seen in patients with gastroesophageal reflux disease (GERD), where reflux symptoms may predominate, and in patients with functional dyspepsia. In a series of 146 patients with gastroparesis [4], the three major categories were idiopathic (36%), diabetic (29%), and postsurgical (13%). Whatever the cause, gastroparesis has a major impact on quality of life. It affects women more than men.

Diabetic Gastroparesis

Gastroparesis is a well-recognized complication of diabetes mellitus. Classically, gastroparesis occurs in patients with long-standing type 1 diabetes mellitus who have other associated complications of diabetes, such as retinopathy, nephropathy, and peripheral neuropathy. Many affected patients may have other signs of autonomic dysfunction, including postural hypotension. Gastroparesis can also occur in patients with type 2 diabetes. The prevalence of gastroparesis in patients with either type 1 or type 2 diabetes has been reported from academic centers to range from 25 to 50%, though the magnitude of gastric delay is modest in many cases. Patients who have had diabetes for a relatively short time may have accelerated emptying from impairment of fundic relaxation caused by vagal dysfunction.

In diabetic patients, delayed gastric emptying contributes to erratic glycemic control because of unpredictable delivery of food into the duodenum. Delayed gastric emptying of nutrients in conjunction with insulin administration may produce hypoglycemia. Conversely, acceleration of the emptying of nutrients with prokinetic agents has been reported to cause early postprandial hyperglycemia. Difficulty in the control of blood glucose levels may be an early indication that a diabetic patient is developing gastric motor dysfunction.

Hyperglycemia itself can reversibly interfere with gastric motility in several ways: by decreasing antral contractility, decreasing the occurance of phase III of the migrating motor complex, increasing pyloric contractions, causing disturbances in gastric myoelectric activity, delaying gastric emptying, or modulating fundic relaxation.

Practical Gastroenterology and Hepatology Board Review Toolkit, Second Edition. Edited by Nicholas J. Talley, Kenneth R. DeVault, Michael B. Wallace, Bashar A. Aqel and Keith D. Lindor.
© 2016 John Wiley & Sons, Ltd. Published 2016 by John Wiley & Sons, Ltd. Companion website: www.practicalgastrohep.com

Postsurgical Gastroparesis

Gastroparesis may occur as a complication of a number of abdominal surgical procedures. In the past, most cases resulted from vagotomy performed in combination with gastric drainage to correct medically refractory or complicated peptic ulcer disease. Since the advent of laparoscopic techniques for the treatment of GERD, gastroparesis has become a recognized complication of fundoplication (possibly from vagal injury during the surgery).

Approximately 5% of patients undergoing vagotomy with antrectomy and gastrojejunostomy (Billroth I procedure) develop severe postsurgical gastroparesis. In these patients, the antrum is not present to triturate solids, and the proximal stomach is unable to generate sufficient pressure to empty solid food residue. The combination of vagotomy, distal gastric resection, and Roux-en-Y gastrojejunostomy predisposes to severe gastric stasis, resulting from slow emptying from the gastric remnant and delayed small-bowel transit in the denervated Roux efferent limb. The Roux-en-Y stasis syndrome – characterized by postprandial abdominal pain, bloating, nausea, and vomiting – is particularly difficult to manage.

Idiopathic Gastroparesis

"Idiopathic gastroparesis" refers to a symptomatic patient with no detectable primary underlying abnormality to explain their delayed gastric emptying. Most patients with idiopathic gastroparesis are women, typically young or middle-aged. Symptoms of idiopathic gastroparesis overlap with those of functional dyspepsia, and in some patients it may be difficult to provide a definitive distinction between the two. Upper abdominal pain/discomfort and postprandial fullness/early satiety are typically the predominant symptoms in functional dyspepsia, whereas nausea, vomiting, and bloating predominate in idiopathic gastroparesis.

A subset of patients with idiopathic gastroparesis report sudden onset of symptoms after a viral prodrome, suggesting a potential viral etiology [3, 4]. Previously healthy subjects develop the sudden onset of nausea, vomiting, diarrhea, fever, and cramps suggestive of a systemic viral infection. However, instead of experiencing resolution of symptoms, these individuals have persistent nausea, vomiting, and early satiety. Viruses that have been implicated in these cases include cytomegalovirus, Epstein–Barr virus (EBV), and varicella zoster. These patients may have slow resolution of their symptoms over several years.

Some patients have cyclic or episodic vomiting episodes, suggesting cyclic vomiting syndrome (CVS). Over time, some of these patients may develop more frequent symptom episodes, termed "coalescent CVS." Delayed gastric emptying is uncommon in CVS; most cases have rapid gastric emptying.

Sometimes, rumination syndrome is confused with vomiting, and patients may be investigated for gastroparesis (but gastric emptying is normal).

Clinical Presentation

Symptoms of gastroparesis are variable; they include early satiety, nausea, vomiting, bloating, and upper abdominal pain. In one series of 146 patients with gastroparesis, nausea was present in 92%, vomiting in 84%, abdominal bloating in 75%, and early satiety in 60% [4]. Complications of gastroparesis include esophagitis, Mallory–Weiss tear, and vegetable-laden bezoars.

Symptoms of gastroparesis may simulate symptoms related to other structural disorders of the stomach and proximal gastrointestinal (GI) tract, such as peptic ulcer disease, partial gastric or small-bowel obstruction, gastric cancer, and pancreaticobiliary disorders.

Though it has been a common assumption that the GI symptoms can be attributed to delay in gastric emptying, most investigations have observed only weak correlations between symptom severity and the degree of gastric stasis. In patients with diabetes, abdominal fullness and bloating have been found to be associated with delayed gastric emptying. In individuals with symptoms of gastroparesis who have normal rates of gastric emptying, other motor, myoelectric, or sensory abnormalities may be responsible for the symptoms.

Abdominal discomfort or pain is present in 46–89% of patients with gastroparesis but is usually not the predominant symptom. Nevertheless, treatment of abdominal pain in gastroparesis can be challenging. In diabetic patients with dyspeptic symptoms, gastric distension elicits exaggerated nausea, bloating, and abdominal discomfort, suggesting that sensory nerve dysfunction may participate in symptom genesis in some patients with gastroparesis.

Evaluation of Patients with Suspected Gastroparesis

A careful history and careful physical examination are important parts of patient evaluation. Symptom onset and progression of the disease, with understanding of the periods of exacerbation, are particularly important. History should include reviewing the patient's medications to help identify and eliminate drugs that can aggravate symptoms. Physical examination may reveal signs of dehydration or malnutrition. The presence of a succussion splash, detected by auscultation over the epigastrium while moving the patient side to side or rapidly palpating the epigastrium, indicates excessive fluid in the stomach from gastroparesis or mechanical gastric outlet obstruction.

Laboratory studies should be performed to identify electrolyte abnormalities such as hypokalemia and metabolic alkalosis, renal insufficiency, anemia, pancreatitis, or thyroid dysfunction. In females with the recent onset of symptoms, a pregnancy test should be obtained. An abdominal obstruction series can be performed to evaluate for mechanical gastric outlet or small-bowel obstruction. Most patients will need an EGD to exclude mechanical obstruction or ulcer disease. The presence of retained food in the stomach after overnight fasting without evidence of mechanical obstruction is suggestive of gastroparesis. Bezoars may be found in severe cases.

The diagnosis of gastroparesis is made when a delay in gastric emptying is present and laboratory studies rule out metabolic causes of symptoms and endoscopic and/or radiographic testing exclude luminal blockage. The classic test for measurement of gastric emptying is scintigraphy [5]. Other methods include a wireless motility capsule capable of recording pH and pressure (SmartPill, Buffalo, NY), which can assess gastric emptying using the acidic gastric residence time of the capsule, and a ^{13}C-ocanoate breath test (OBT), which has been shown to correlate well with gastric emptying for solids by scintigraphy. These tests are discussed in this section.

Scintigraphy

Gastric-emptying scintigraphy of a solid-phase meal is considered the standard for diagnosis of gastroparesis as it quantifies the emptying of a physiologic caloric meal. Measurement of gastric emptying of solids is more sensitive for detection of gastroparesis, as liquid emptying may remain normal even in the presence of advanced disease.

For solid-phase testing, most centers use a ^{99m}Tc sulfur colloid-labeled egg sandwich as the test meal, with standard imaging at 0, 1, 2, and 4 hours. The radiolabel should be cooked into the meal to ensure radioisotope binding to the solid phase. Scintigraphic assessment of emptying should be extended to at least 2 hours after meal ingestion. Even with extension of the scintigraphic study to this length, there may be significant day-to-day variability (up to 20%) in rates of gastric emptying. For shorter durations, the test is less reliable, due to larger variations in normal gastric emptying. Extending scintigraphy to 4 hours improves accuracy in determining the presence of delayed gastric emptying. A 4-hour gastric-emptying scintigraphy test using a radiolabeled EggBeaters meal with jam, toast, and water is advocated by the Society of Nuclear Medicine and Molecular Imaging (SNMMI) and the American Neurogastroenterology and Motility Society (ANMS) [6, 7].

Emptying of solids typically exhibits a lag phase, followed by a prolonged linear emptying phase. A variety of parameters can be calculated from the emptying profile of a radiolabeled meal, such as half emptying time and duration of lag phase. The simplest approach to interpreting a gastric-emptying study is to report the percentage retention at defined times after meal ingestion: usually 2 and 4 hours, with normal being less than 60% remaining in the stomach at 2 hours and less than 10% remaining at 4 hours [7].

Patients should discontinue medications that may affect gastric emptying. For most medications, this will be at 48–72 hours. Opiate analgesics and anticholinergic agents delay gastric emptying. Other medications can slow gastric emptying, including tricyclic antidepressants, calcium channel blockers, and cyclosporine (not tacrolimus). Prokinetic agents that accelerate emptying may give a falsely normal gastric-emptying result. Serotonin receptor antagonists such as ondansetron, which have little effect on gastric emptying, may be given for severe symptoms before performance of gastric scintigraphy. Hyperglycemia (glucose level >270 mg/dL) delays gastric emptying in diabetic patients. It is not unreasonable to defer gastric-emptying testing until relative euglycemia is achieved, in order to obtain a reliable determination of emptying parameters in the absence of acute metabolic derangement.

Dual labeling of solids with ^{99m}technetium and liquids with ^{111}indium allows for assessment of gastric emptying of solids and liquids, which may be useful in assessing the differential handling of the postsurgical stomach. This will help determine whether symptoms result from delayed solid emptying or rapid liquid emptying. Continued imaging of ^{111}indium may be used to assess small-bowel transit.

Wireless Motility Capsule

The SmartPill wireless motility capsule is an ingestible capsule that measures pH, pressure, and temperature using miniaturized wireless sensor technology. The wireless motility capsule is swallowed by the patient and information is recorded as it travels through the GI tract. Gastric emptying is determined from the time at which the wireless motility capsule is swallowed until there is a rapid increase in the pH recorded by the wireless motility capsule, indicating emptying from the acidic stomach to the alkaline duodenum. In addition, the wireless motility capsule characterizes pressure patterns and provides motility indices for the stomach, small intestine, and colon. The gastric residence time of the wireless motility capsule has a high correlation (85%) with the T-90 of gastric-emptying scintigraphy, suggesting that the gastric residence time of the wireless motility capsule represents a time near the end of the emptying of a solid meal [8]. A 5-hour cut-off value for the SmartPill gastric

residence time has been found to be best in identifying subjects with delayed or normal gastric emptying based on scintigraphy on the day of the test, with a sensitivity of 83% and a specificity of 83%. The SmartPill GI Monitoring System is approved by the US Food and Drug Administration (FDA) for the assessment of gastric pH, gastric emptying, and total GI transit time.

Breath-Testing

Breath tests using the non-radioactive isotope ^{13}C bound to a digestible substance have been validated for the measurement of gastric emptying [9]. Most commonly, ^{13}C-labeled octanoate, a medium-chain triglyceride, is bound into a solid meal such as a muffin. Other studies have bound ^{13}C to acetate or to proteinaceous algae (*Spirulina*). After ingestion and stomach emptying, ^{13}C-octanoate is absorbed in the small intestine and metabolized to $^{13}CO_2$, which is then expelled from the lungs during respiration. The rate-limiting step is the rate of solid gastric emptying. Thus, ^{13}C-octanoate breath-testing provides a measure of solid-phase emptying. The octanoate breath test provides reproducible results that correlate with findings on gastric-emptying scintigraphy. ^{13}C breath tests do not use ionizing radiation and can be used to test patients in the community or even at the bedside, where gamma camera facilities are not readily available. Breath samples can be preserved and shipped to a laboratory for analysis.

Treatment

The general principles for treating symptomatic gastroparesis are: (i) to correct and prevent fluid, electrolyte, and nutritional deficiencies; (ii) to control symptoms; and (iii) to identify and rectify the underlying cause of gastroparesis, if possible [3,10].

Management of this condition can be particularly challenging. Care of patients generally relies on dietary modification, medications that stimulate gastric motor activity (Table 21.1), and antiemetic drug therapy (Table 21.2) [10,11]. Though in most cases rigorous investigations have not assessed therapeutic responses as a function of symptom severity, a number of basic recommendations can be made (Table 21.3) [10].

For mild symptoms, dietary modifications should be tried. When possible, patients should avoid the use of medications that delay gastric emptying. Low doses of antiemetic or prokinetic medications can be taken on an as-needed basis. Diabetic patients should strive for optimal glycemic control, to minimize the effects of hyperglycemia on gastric function.

For individuals with compensated gastroparesis, treatment recommendations commonly involve a combination of antiemetic and

Table 21.1 Prokinetic medication classes for the treatment of gastroparesis.

Class	Presently available agents	Agents available under special circumstances
Dopamine D_2 receptor antagonists	Metoclopramide	Domperidone
Motilin receptor agonists	Erythromycin Clarithromycin Azithromycin	
Muscarinic receptor agonists	Bethanechol	
Acetylcholinesterase inhibitors	Physostigmine Neostigmine	

Table 21.2 Antiemetic therapy for gastroparesis.

Prokinetic agents with antiemetic properties (antagonize dopamine receptors)	Metoclopramide Domperidone
Phenothiazine derivatives (antagonize dopamine receptors in area postrema)	Prochlorperazine Trimethobenzamide
Antihistamines (H1 receptor antagonists)	Diphenhydramine Promethazine Meclizine
Anticholinergic agents	Scopolamine
Antiserotoninergic (5-HT-3 receptor antagonists)	Ondansetron Granisetron Dolasetron Palonosetron
Substance P/neurokinin-1 receptor antagonists	Aprepitant

prokinetic medications given at regularly scheduled intervals to relieve more chronic symptoms of nausea, vomiting, fullness, and bloating. Unfortunately, these agents frequently have no effect on the pain and discomfort that may be associated with gastroparesis. In such patients, measures need to be directed at pain control, but these should be measures that do not exacerbate other symptoms of gastroparesis.

For patients with severe gastroparesis, care may include enteral nutritional support through a jejunostomy tube and/or other surgical intervention, such as gastric electric stimulation.

Dietary Treatment

The liquid nutrient component of ingested meals should be increased, because liquid emptying is often preserved. Fats and fiber tend to decrease gastric emptying; thus, their intake should be minimized. Indigestible fiber and roughage may predispose to bezoar formation. Foods that cannot be reliably chewed into smaller constituency should be avoided. Six frequent but small meals are often recommended to limit the calorie intake with each meal while still achieving adequate total calories over a day [12].

Metabolic Control

Diabetic patients with gastroparesis frequently exhibit labile blood glucose concentrations with prolonged periods of significant hyperglycemia. Hyperglycemia itself can delay gastric emptying. Hyperglycemia can also counteract the accelerating effects of prokinetic agents on gastric emptying. Improvement of glucose control increases antral contractility, corrects gastric dysrhythmias, and accelerates emptying. To date, there have been no long-term studies confirming the beneficial effects of maintenance of near euglycemia on gastroparetic symptoms. Nevertheless, the consistent findings of physiologic studies in healthy volunteers and diabetic patients provide a compelling argument to strive for near-normal blood glucose levels in affected diabetic patients [13].

Prokinetic Agents

Current prokinetic agents for treatment include the oral agents metoclopramide and erythromycin (Table 21.1).

Metoclopramide

Metoclopramide, a substituted benzamide that is structurally related to procainamide, exhibits both prokinetic and antiemetic actions. The drug serves as a dopamine receptor antagonist both in the central nervous system (CNS) and in the stomach. The prokinetic properties of metoclopramide are limited to the proximal gut. Metoclopramide, with its antinausea and prokinetic actions, is widely used for the treatment of gastroparesis. Metoclopramide provides symptomatic relief and accelerates gastric emptying of solids and liquids in patients with idiopathic, diabetic, and postvagotomy gastroparesis. Metoclopramide is effective for the short-term treatment of gastroparesis for up to several weeks; however, symptomatic improvement does not necessarily accompany improvement in gastric emptying. The long-term utility of metoclopramide has not been proven. Metoclopramide is approved for the treatment of diabetic gastroparesis and for the prevention of postoperative and chemotherapy-induced nausea and vomiting. The usual dosage is 5–10 mg four times a day (but start at a low dose). In some patients, rather than the pill form, liquid metoclopramide is used, which may be better tolerated. Metoclopramide is also available for parenteral use (intravenous or intramuscular).

Unfortunately, side effects are relatively common with metoclopramide; it can cause both acute and chronic CNS side effects in some patients. Acute side effects include dystonic reactions, resulting from an idiosyncratic reaction. Longer treatment can produce depression or anxiety. QT prolongation and hyperprolactinemia can occur. Rare cases of tardive dyskinesia (often irreversible) have been reported with long-term treatment, and the FDA has issued a "black box" warning, which has markedly decreased the use of this agent. If used, the health-care provider should discuss and document these potential risks.

Table 21.3 ANMS consensus recommendations for the treatment of gastroparesis. A top-down vertical stepped-care approach, dependent on the severity of gastroparesis, is recommended. Treatments from different categories (columns) are often used in combination. Source: Abell 2006 [10]. Reproduced with permission of Wiley.

Psychological measures	Glycemic control	Nutritional care	Prokinetic medications	Antiemetic therapies	Pain control
Empathy and education	Twice-daily long-acting insulin plus periprandial short-acting insulin	Small, frequent meals, low in fat and fiber	Metoclopramide or erythromycin PRN	Phenothiazine or dopamine receptor antagonist PRN	Acetaminophen or non-steroidal agents
Patient support groups	Insulin pump	Primarily liquid diet Liquid nutrient supplements	Metoclopramide or erythromycin scheduled dosing	Muscarinic receptor antagonist or 5-HT-3 antagonist	Tramadol or propoxyphene
Behavioral or relaxation therapy	Pancreas transplant	Enteral feedings Central or peripheral parenteral nutrition, short-term	Domperidone	Tetrahydrocannabinol, lorazepam, or alternative therapies Gastric electrical stimulation	Newer antidepressants, SNRIs Fentanyl patch or methadone Referral for pain specialist Nerve block

PRN, as needed; TCA, tricyclic antidepressant; SNRI, serotonin-norepinephrine reuptake inhibitor.

Erythromycin

The macrolide antibiotic erythromycin exerts prokinetic effects via action on gastroduodenal receptors for motilin, an endogenous peptide responsible for initiation of the phase III migrating motor complex in the upper gut. Clinically, erythromycin has been shown to stimulate gastric emptying in diabetic gastroparesis, idiopathic gastroparesis, and postvagotomy gastroparesis. Erythromycin may be most potent when used intravenously. Limited data exist concerning the clinical efficacy of erythromycin in reducing symptoms of gastroparesis. In studies on oral erythromycin with symptom assessment as a clinical end point, improvement was noted in 43% of patients [10]. The benefit wanes because of tachyphylaxis, so a 4-week treatment followed by a drug holiday can be helpful.

Oral administration of erythromycin should be initiated at low doses (e.g., 125 mg three or four times daily). Liquid-suspension erythromycin may be preferred because it is rapidly and more reliably absorbed. Intravenous erythromycin (100 mg every 8 hours) is used for inpatients hospitalized for severe refractory gastroparesis.

Side effects of erythromycin at higher doses include nausea, vomiting, and abdominal pain. Because these symptoms may mimic those of gastroparesis, erythromycin can have a narrow therapeutic window in some patients. Erythromycin may be associated with higher mortality from cardiac disease, especially when combined with agents that inhibit cytochrome P-450, such as calcium channel blockers.

Azithromycin also has a risk of long QT and sudden death, and is not generally recommended as treatment for gastroparesis.

Domperidone

The effects of domperidone on the upper gut are similar to those of metoclopramide, including stimulation of antral contractions and promotion of antroduodenal coordination. Domperidone does not readily cross the blood–brain barrier (BBB), so it is much less likely to cause extrapyramidal side effects than is metoclopramide. In addition to prokinetic actions in the stomach, domperidone exhibits antiemetic properties via action on the area postrema, a brainstem region with a porous BBB. Side effects include galactorrhea and amenorrhea, a prolonged QT interval, and cardiac arrhythmias [14].

The FDA has developed a program for physicians who would like to prescribe domperidone for patients with severe upper GI motility disorders that are refractory to standard therapy even though it is not approved in the United States. Use of this investigational new drug (IND) mechanism for use of domperidone requires Institutional Review Board (IRB) approval, and the patient must pay for the medication. The dose is 10 mg three times a day, increasing if needed to 20 mg four times a day.

Antiemetic Agents

Antiemetic agents are given acutely for symptomatic nausea and vomiting (Table 21.2). The principal classes of drugs that have been used for symptomatic treatment of nausea and vomiting are phenothiazines, antihistamines, anticholinergics, dopamine receptor antagonists, and, more recently, serotonin receptor antagonists. The antiemetic action of phenothiazine compounds appears to be mediated primarily through a central antidopaminergic mechanism in the area postrema of the brain. Commonly used agents include prochlorperazine, trimethobenzamide, and promethazine.

Serotonin (5-HT-3) receptor antagonists, such as ondansetron and granisetron, have been shown to be helpful in treating or preventing chemotherapy-induced nausea and vomiting. The primary site of action of these compounds is probably the chemoreceptor trigger zone, since there is a high density of 5-HT-3 receptors in the area postrema. Ondansetron is now frequently used for nausea and vomiting of a variety of other etiologies.

Psychotropic Medications as Symptom Modulators

Tricyclic antidepressants have an uncertain benefit in suppressing symptoms in some patients with nausea and vomiting [15]. Doses are lower than those used to treat depression. A reasonable starting dose for a tricyclic drug is 10–25 mg at bedtime. If benefit is not observed in several weeks, this can be increased by 10 to 25 mg increments up to 50–100 mg. Side effects are common with use of tricyclic antidepressants and can interfere with management and lead to a change in medication in 25% of patients. The secondary amines, nortriptyline and desipramine, may have fewer side effects. A randomized trial of nortriptyline demonstrated no benefit over placebo in improving overall symptoms in patients with gastroparesis [16].

Pyloric Botulinum Toxin Injection

Gastric emptying is a highly regulated process, reflecting the integration of the propulsive forces of proximal fundic tone and distal antral contractions with the functional resistance provided by the pylorus. Manometric studies of patients with diabetic gastroparesis show prolonged periods of increased pyloric tone and phasic contractions, a phenomenon termed "pylorospasm." Botulinum toxin is a potent inhibitor of neuromuscular transmission and has been used to treat spastic somatic muscle disorders and achalasia. Several open-label studies have tested the effects of pyloric injection of botulinum toxin in small numbers of patients with diabetic and idiopathic gastroparesis and have observed mild improvements in gastric emptying and modest reductions in symptoms for several months. Two double-blind, placebo-controlled studies have shown an improvement in gastric emptying but no improvement in symptoms compared to placebo [17, 18]. Thus, botulinum toxin injection into the pylorus is not a long-term treatment option for gastroparesis.

Gastric Electric Stimulation

Gastric electric stimulation is an emerging treatment for refractory gastroparesis. Currently, it involves an implantable neurostimulator that delivers a high-frequency (12 cpm), low-energy signal with short pulses. With this device, stimulating wires are sutured into the gastric muscle along the greater curvature during laparoscopy or laparotomy. These leads are attached to the electric stimulator, which is positioned in a subcutaneous abdominal pouch. Based on initial studies that have shown symptom benefit, especially in patients with diabetic gastroparesis [19], the gastric electric neurostimulator has been granted humanitarian approval by the FDA for the treatment of chronic, refractory nausea and vomiting secondary to idiopathic or diabetic gastroparesis.

The main complication of the implantable neurostimulator is infection, which has necessitated device removal in approximately 5–10% of cases. More recently, a small minority of patients has, at times, experienced a shocking sensation.

Symptoms of nausea and vomiting can improve with gastric electric stimulation; however, abdominal pain often does not. In general, diabetic patients with primary symptoms of nausea and/or vomiting who are not taking narcotic pain medications and do not have an adequate response to antiemetic and prokinetic medications appear to have a favorable response to gastric electric stimulation [20]. Further investigation is needed to confirm the effectiveness of gastric stimulation in a long-term blinded fashion, the optimal electrode position, the optimal stimulation parameters, and which patients are likely to respond, none of which have been rigorously evaluated to date. Future improvements may include devices that can be implanted endoscopically and devices that sequentially stimulate the stomach in a peristaltic sequence to promote gastric emptying.

Take Home Points

- Diagnosis of a patient with gastroparesis consists of appropriate symptoms, negative endoscopy, and delayed gastric emptying.
- Dietary management and prokinetic and antiemetic agents are beneficial in treating patients with gastroparesis. The side effects of medications need to be discussed with the patient prior to their use.
- Treatment of refractory gastroparesis involves several options, including domperidone, symptom modulators, jejunostomy feeding tubes, and gastric electric stimulation.
- Botulinum toxin injection into the pylorus is not a long-term treatment option for gastroparesis. Though anecdotally it may provide short-term improvement in some patients, placebo-controlled studies have not demonstrated a significant clinical improvement of symptoms.
- Gastric electric stimulation is used for refractory gastroparesis. Generally, diabetic patients with refractory symptoms of nausea and vomiting respond best to this treatment.

References

1 Jung HK, Choung RS, Locke GR 3rd, *et al.* The incidence, prevalence, and outcomes of patients with gastroparesis in Olmsted County, Minnesota, from 1996 to 2006. *Gastroenterology* 2009; **136**(4): 1225–33.

2 Parkman HP. Idiopathic gastroparesis. *Gastroenterol Clin N Am* 2015; **44**(1): 59–68.

3 Parkman HP, Hasler WL, Fisher RS, American Gastroenterological Association. American Gastroenterological Association technical review on the diagnosis and treatment of gastroparesis. *Gastroenterology* 2004; **127**(5): 1592–622.

4 Soykan I, Sivri B, Sarosiek I, *et al.* Demography, clinical characteristics, psychological and abuse profiles, treatment, and long-term follow-up of patients with gastroparesis. *Dig Dis Sci* 1998; **43**(11): 2398–404.

5 Camilleri M, Shin A. Novel and validated approaches for gastric emptying scintigraphy in patients with suspected gastroparesis. *Dig Dis Sci* 2013; **58**(7): 1813–15.

6 Abell TL, Camilleri M, Donohoe K, *et al.* Consensus recommendations for gastric emptying scintigraphy: a joint report of the American Neurogastroenterology and Motility Society and the Society of Nuclear Medicine. *Am J Gastroenterol* 2008; **103**(3): 753–63.

7 Tougas G, Eaker EY, Abell TL, *et al.* Assessment of gastric emptying using a low fat meal: establishment of international control values. *Am J Gastroenterol* 2000; **95**(6): 1456–62.

8 Kuo B, McCallum RW, Koch KL, *et al.* Comparison of gastric emptying of a nondigestible capsule to a radio-labelled meal in healthy and gastroparetic subjects. *Aliment Pharmacol Ther* 2008; **27**(2): 186–96.

9 Bromer MQ, Kantor SB, Wagner DA, *et al.* Simultaneous measurement of gastric emptying with a simple muffin meal using [13C]octanoate breath test and scintigraphy in normal subjects and patients with dyspeptic symptoms. *Dig Dis Sci* 2002; **47**(7): 1657–63.

10 Abell TL, Bernstein RK, Cutts T, *et al.* Treatment of gastroparesis: a multidisciplinary clinical review. *Neurogastroenterol Motil* 2006; **18**(4): 263–83.

11 Quigley EM, Hasler WL, Parkman HP. AGA technical review on nausea and vomiting. *Gastroenterology.* 2001; **120**(1): 263–86.

12 Parkman HP, Yates KP, Hasler WL, *et al.* Dietary intake and nutritional deficiencies in patients with diabetic or idiopathic gastroparesis. *Gastroenterology* 2011; **141**(2): 486–98.e1–7.

13 Camilleri M. Clinical practice. Diabetic gastroparesis. *N Engl J Med* 2007; **356**(8): 820–9.

14 Sugumar A, Singh A, Pasricha PJ. A systematic review of the efficacy of domperidone for the treatment of diabetic gastroparesis. *Clin Gastroenterol Hepatol* 2008; **6**(7): 726–33.

15 Prakash C, Lustman PJ, Freedland KE, Clouse RE. Tricyclic antidepressants for functional nausea and vomiting: clinical outcome in 37 patients. *Dig Dis Sci* 1998; **43**(9): 1951–6.

16 Parkman HP, Van Natta ML, Abell TL, *et al.* Effect of nortriptyline on symptoms of idiopathic gastroparesis: the NORIG randomized clinical trial. *JAMA* 2013; **310**(24): 2640–9.

17 Arts J, Holvoet L, Caenepeel P, *et al.* Clinical trial: a randomized-controlled crossover study of intrapyloric injection of botulinum toxin in gastroparesis. *Aliment Pharmacol Ther* 2007; **26**(9): 1251–8.

18 Friedenberg FK, Palit A, Parkman HP, *et al.* Botulinum toxin A for the treatment of delayed gastric emptying. *Am J Gastroenterol* 2008; **103**(2): 416–23.

19 Abell T, McCallum R, Hocking M, *et al.* Gastric electrical stimulation for medically refractory gastroparesis. *Gastroenterology* 2003; **125**(2): 421–8.

20 Abell TL, Chen J, Emmanuel A, *et al.* Neurostimulation of the gastrointestinal tract: review of recent developments. *Neuromodulation* 2015; **18**(3): 221–7, disc. 227.

CHAPTER 22

Non-variceal Upper Gastrointestinal Bleeding

Thomas J. Savides

Division of Gastroenterology, University of California, San Diego, CA, USA

Summary

Upper gastrointestinal (GI) bleeding is a common problem in the United States, with an estimated annual hospitalization rate of 160 admissions per 100 000 population, with peptic ulcers being the most common lesion [1]. Despite advances in medical therapy, intensive care unit (ICU) care, and endoscopy, the mortality rate remains unchanged over the past 30 years at 5–10%, most likely due to the increasing number of elderly patients who die from comorbidities related to bleeding. This chapter focuses on severe acute bleeding from the esophagus, stomach, and duodenum that requires hospitalization.

Case

A 70-year-old man presents with melena and syncope. His past medical history is notable for coronary artery disease (CAD) and atrial fibrillation. He takes a baby aspirin and warfarin on a daily basis, and 3 weeks ago started ibuprofen for neck pain. On exam, he has orthostatic hypotension. His stool is black and guaiac-positive. Blood tests reveal hematocrit 25%, mean cell volume (MCV) 82 L, and International Normalized Ratio (INR) 3.1. He is admitted and transfused red blood cells (RBCs) and fresh frozen plasma (FFP). He is started on intravenous proton pump inhibitor (PPI) medication. Esophagogastroduodenoscopy (EGD) reveals a 15 mm duodenal ulcer with a visible vessel, which is endoscopically treated with epinephrine injection and a hemoclip. Gastric biopsies reveal no *Helicobacter pylori* infection. The patient is observed for the next 72 hours while being switched to an oral PPI and advancing diet. He is discharged home and advised to take long-term PPI medication.

Etiology

The most common cause of severe upper GI bleeding is peptic ulcer disease (gastric and duodenal ulcer), followed by a variety of other etiologies, including varices, esophagitis, Mallory–Weiss tear, Cameron erosions, and tumors. A careful history will narrow the differential diagnosis. Medical resuscitation with fluids and transfusions is the most important first step. Urgent endoscopy will diagnose the lesion and allow endoscopic treatment of lesions at highest risk for rebleeding. Pharmacologic therapy is playing an increasingly important role in the management of peptic ulcer and variceal bleeding. Interventional radiology and surgery are reserved only for rare cases not controlled medically and endoscopically.

Improvement in patient outcomes will occur with increased knowledge of risk factors for upper GI bleeding and with successful management of acute upper GI bleeding with medical and endoscopic therapy.

Initial Assessment and Management

There are several definitions of GI bleeding that are important in the initial assessment of a patient with upper GI bleeding (Figure 22.1). Hematemesis includes vomiting large amounts of red blood (which suggests active bleeding) or dark material ("coffee-ground emesis," which suggests older non-active bleeding) (see Chapter 13). Melena is defined as black tarry stool, which suggests passage of old blood, usually from an upper GI source, but possibly from the small bowel or proximal colon. Hematochezia is bright red blood per rectum, and will represent an upper GI source only if the patient is also hypotensive due to massive ongoing bleeding.

Initial patient assessment should focus on the history, paying particular attention to gastroesophageal reflux disease (GERD), peptic ulcers, abdominal pain, weight loss, aspirin/non-steroidal anti-inflammatory drugs (NSAIDs), alcohol abuse, cirrhosis, and abdominal aortic aneurysm. Physical examination focuses on the presence of orthostatic hypotension, which suggests significant volume depletion, as well as signs of chronic liver disease such as spider angiomas, palmar erythema, gynecomastia, ascites, and splenomegaly. Blood tests should include standard hematology, chemistry, liver, coagulation studies, and crossmatch for blood transfusion.

Nasogastric (NG) tube placement to aspirate and characterize gastric contents can be useful to determine whether large amounts of red blood, coffee grounds, or non-bloody fluid are present. Patients who have witnessed emesis do not need an NG tube for diagnostic purposes, but may need one to clear gastric contents before endoscopy and to minimize aspiration risk.

Initial medical resuscitation is usually performed in the emergency room. Intravenous saline is given to try to keep the systolic blood pressure >100 mHg and the pulse <100 bpm. Patients are transfused with packed RBCs, platelets, and FFP as necessary to keep the hematocrit ideally >21%, platelet count >50 000/mm³, and prothrombin time <15 seconds [2]. Patients with ongoing active bleeding (i.e., red blood in NG tube or hypotension) warrant ICU admission and urgent endoscopy, whereas patients with moderate bleeding (melena and resolved hypotension) are admitted to a

Practical Gastroenterology and Hepatology Board Review Toolkit, Second Edition. Edited by Nicholas J. Talley, Kenneth R. DeVault, Michael B. Wallace, Bashar A. Aqel and Keith D. Lindor.

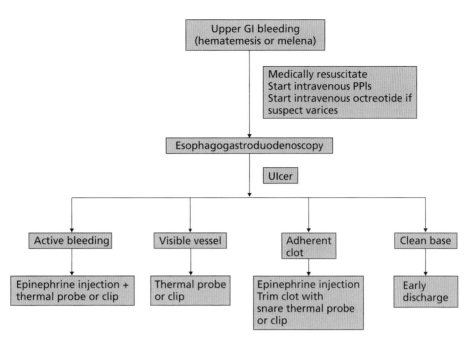

Figure 22.1 Algorithm for an approach to upper GI bleeding.

medical ward or intermediate care unit and undergo semi-urgent endoscopy.

Endotracheal intubation should be considered in patients with active, ongoing hematemesis and/or altered mental status in order to prevent aspiration pneumonia. Patients older than 60 years, with chest pain, or with a history of cardiac problems should also be evaluated for myocardial infarction with electrocardiograms (ECGs) and serial troponin measurements.

Patients with severe upper GI bleeding are usually started on intravenous PPI medications before endoscopy. Several studies and meta-analyses have shown that this accelerates the resolution of endoscopic stigmata of bleeding ulcers and reduces the need for endoscopic therapy, but does not result in improved clinical outcomes such as decreased transfusions, rebleeding, surgery, or death rates [3]. Patients with a strong suspicion for variceal bleeding should also be started on empirical intravenous octreotide, because this can reduce rebleeding to rates similar to those after endoscopic sclerotherapy [4].

Clinical scoring systems have been developed to try to determine which upper GI bleed patients are at highest risk for rebleeding and death. The most commonly used is the Rockall scoring system, which includes both clinical and endoscopic data [5]. Though important for research studies, the utility of scoring systems is limited in routine clinical practice.

Endoscopy

A large-channel therapeutic upper endoscope should be used to allow for rapid removal of bleed from the stomach and to utilize larger endoscopic hemostasis accessories. Well-trained assistants who are familiar with endoscopic hemostasis devices are critical to successful endoscopic hemostasis. At times, it may be worth delaying a procedure in order to utilize assistants who are competent at using accessories in emergency situations. A number of different endoscopic hemostasis devices have been developed over the past 20 years.

Thermal Contact Probes

These are the mainstay of endoscopic hemostasis. The most commonly used probes are bipolar probes, which create heat through a current flowing between two intertwined electrodes on the probe tip. These probes can be pressed against the bleeding lesion to physically tamponade the bleeding site, then the tip can be applied to thermally seal the underlying vessel (coaptive coagulation). Thermal contact probes can seal arteries up to 2 mm. The risks of thermal probes include perforation and induction of more bleeding.

Injection Therapy

This is performed using an endoscopic sclerotherapy needle to inject diluted epinephrine (1 : 10 000 or 1 : 20 000) into the submucosa around the bleeding site. The advantages are that it is widely available and relatively inexpensive, and it can be used in the setting of coagulopathy. In addition, it has less risk of perforation or subsequent thermal burn damage than with thermal contact probes. Injection can also be performed with a sclerosant, such as ethanolamine.

Endoscopic Clips

These are similar to surgical clips in that they apply mechanical pressure to a bleeding site. However, they differ in that they currently do not have as much compressive force and they do not have complete apposition of the prongs. Clips have the advantage of not causing thermal injury, but the disadvantage that they can be challenging to deploy, depending on scope position and lesion location.

Band Ligation

This involves aspiration of mucosa/submucosa into the tip of a plastic cap attached to the end of the scope, followed by pulling on a tripwire, which rolls a rubber band off the cylinder and over the mucosa/submucosa inside it. The rubber band ligates the lesion, and eventually the banded lesion sloughs off.

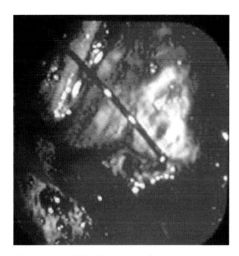

Figure 22.2 Active arterial bleeding peptic ulcer.

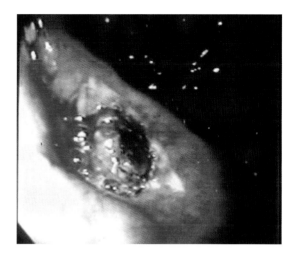

Figure 22.4 Adherent clot in peptic ulcer.

Peptic Ulcer Bleeding

Peptic ulcers are the most common source of upper GI bleeding. Most ulcers are caused by decreased mucosal defenses due to aspirin/NSAIDs and/or *H. pylori* infection. Resected bleeding ulcers reveal underlying exposed arteries (mean diameter 0.7 mm) or a small clot overlying the bleeding site in the vessel [6].

Poor prognostic factors for bleeding peptic ulcers include age >60 years, comorbid medical illness, orthostatic hypotension, coagulopathy, bleeding onset in the hospital, multiple blood transfusions, red blood in the NG tube, posterior duodenal bulb ulcer, and, most importantly, endoscopic findings of arterial bleeding or visible vessels.

Endoscopic stigmata of bleeding peptic ulcers provide excellent predictability of the likelihood of rebleeding (Figures 22.2, 22.3, 22.4, and 22.5). Table 22.1 shows that the ulcers at highest risk for rebleeding have active arterial bleeding, a non-bleeding visible vessel, and an adherent clot [7]. The risk of rebleeding is greatest in the first 72 hours after presentation.

Active Bleeding and Non-bleeding Visible Vessels

Many well-conducted randomized controlled trials (RCTs), meta-analyses, and consensus conferences have confirmed that endoscopic hemostasis with either epinephrine injection or coaptive probe therapy significantly decreases the rate of ulcer rebleeding, the need for urgent surgery, and mortality in patients with high-risk stigmata such as active bleeding and non-bleeding visible vessels (see Figures 22.2 and 22.3) [8,9]. The rebleeding rates of peptic ulcers with various endoscopic stigmata are shown in Table 22.2. Most of these studies were performed before the widespread use of PPIs, and predominantly used injection therapy, bipolar-probe coagulation therapy, or a combination of injection and probe therapy. In general, for the highest-risk lesions of active bleeding or non-bleeding visible vessels, endoscopic hemostasis alone will decrease the rebleed rate to approximately 20–25%. The adjunctive use of PPIs decreases this rate even further, as discussed later.

The most commonly used treatment in the world is injection therapy, because it is widely available, easy to perform, safe, and

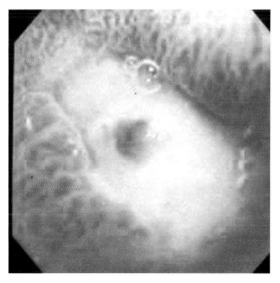

Figure 22.3 Non-bleeding visible vessel in peptic ulcer.

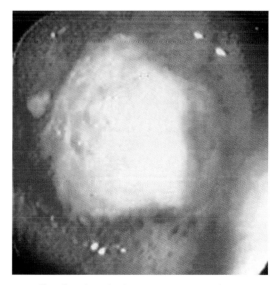

Figure 22.5 Clean-based peptic ulcer.

Table 22.1 Suspected sources of upper GI bleeding based on patient history.

Patient history and symptoms	Suspected source
Recurrent nose bleeds	Nasopharynx
Prior head and neck malignancy	
Hemoptysis	Lungs
Heavy alcohol use	Esophagitis
GERD	
Heartburn	
Dysphagia	Esophageal cancer
Weight loss	
Vomiting	Mallory–Weiss tear
Heavy alcohol use	
Liver disease	Esophageal or gastric varices/portal
Heavy alcohol use	hypertensive gastropathy
History of peptic ulcer disease	Peptic ulcer
Frequent aspirin or NSAID use	
Epigastric discomfort	
Recurrent severe acute unexplained bleeds	Dieulafoy lesion
	Aortoenteric fistula – primary
Early satiety	Gastric cancer
Weight loss	
Vomiting	Duodenal cancer
Weight loss	Gastric outlet obstruction
Prior abdominal aortic aneurysm surgical	Aortoenteric fistula – secondary
repair with synthetic graft	
Recent ERCP with sphincterotomy	Ampulla of Vater
Recent liver biopsy or cholangiogram	Bile duct system
Pancreatitis, pseudocyst, pancreatogram	Pancreatic duct system

GERD, gastroesophageal reflux disease; NSAID, non-steroidal anti-inflammatory drug; ERCP, endoscopic retrograde cholangiopancreatography.

inexpensive. Therapy with epinephrine alone seems more effective in high (13–20 mL) compared with low (5–10 mL) doses [10]. Injection of epinephrine will result in an increase in circulating plasma epinephrine, but rarely causes any clinically significant cardiovascular events. Though epinephrine injection alone is effective compared with placebo, numerous studies and meta-analyses have shown that the addition of a thermal or mechanical modality will further significantly decrease rebleeding, surgery, and mortality rates [11]. Several studies suggest that the only benefit of adding epinephrine injection to thermal probe therapy occurs in patients with active bleeding, and that there is no benefit in non-bleeding visible vessels [12].

Mechanical endoscopic clips have not been studied alongside injection and thermal probe techniques, but they seem to be more effective than epinephrine injection alone, and probably as effective as thermal probe therapy alone. Clips have the advantage of being usable in patients with severe coagulopathy with the risk of inducing bleeding. However, the disadvantage of clips is that they can be difficult to deploy, depending on the scope position required to reach an ulcer.

Adherent Clots

Adherent clots (see Figure 22.4) are blood clots that are resistant to several minutes of vigorous water irrigation. The rebleeding rate

Table 22.2 Peptic ulcer rebleeding rates.

	Rebleed rate (%)		
Endoscopic appearance	Without endoscopic treatment	After endoscopic treatment alone	After endoscopic treatment + intravenous PPI
Active arterial bleeding	90	25	<10
Visible vessel	50	25	<10
Adherent clot	25	<5	<5
Clean-based ulcer	<5	<5	<5

with medical therapy using H_2-receptor antagonists alone is approximately 30% [13]. RCTs have shown that endoscopic treatment of adherent clots can decrease the rebleeding rate to <5% [13,14].

Clean-based Ulcers

Patients with clean-based ulcers at endoscopy (see Figure 22.5) have a rebleed rate of <5%. Laine showed that there was no difference between immediate refeeding of these patients versus waiting several days to start eating [15]. Longstreth has shown that selected low-risk compliant patients with mild upper GI bleeds and clean-based ulcers can be discharged home safely with significant cost savings [16].

PPIs and Peptic Ulcer Bleeding

Gastric pH >6.8 is needed for optimal coagulation and clot formation. Intravenous H_2-receptor antagonists can raise the intragastric pH acutely, but tolerance rapidly develops. PPIs can consistently keep gastric pH >4–6 over a prolonged period. Several studies have found that PPIs initiated after endoscopic diagnosis of peptic ulcer bleeding significantly reduce rebleeding and surgery rates compared with placebo or H_2-receptor blockers [17]. The initiation of PPIs before endoscopy significantly decreases the proportion of patients with stigmata of a recent bleed (i.e., visible vessels) and the need for endoscopic hemostasis, but does not reduce mortality, rebleeding, or surgery risks compared with H_2-receptor blockers or placebo [2,3]. The effects of PPIs are more pronounced in Asian compared with non-Asian populations.

H. pylori Testing

Falsely negative histology for *H pylori*, as well as falsely negative rapid urease, urea breath test, and stool antigen testing, may occur in the setting of acute ulcer bleeding. If infection is not detected, it is important to repeat the evaluation at a later date to confirm the initial result.

Rebleeding after Peptic Ulcer Hemostasis

After successful endoscopic hemostasis and with the use of PPIs, the risk of rebleeding is <10% [18]. In the event of rebleeding, a second endoscopy should be performed rather than surgery, because the outcomes are generally similar with fewer complications. Patients who fail a second attempt at endoscopic hemostasis should undergo either angiography with embolization or surgery.

Variceal Bleeding

Esophageal variceal bleeding is the second most common cause of severe upper GI bleeding after peptic ulcers. Variceal bleeding is a manifestation of cirrhosis due to end-stage liver disease, with an estimated 1-year survival rate of 50%, and with most deaths occurring within the first 2 weeks of the bleed [19]. Patients can bleed from esophageal or gastric varices. Medical management of patients with variceal bleeding includes intravenous octreotide, which causes selective splanchnic vasoconstriction. A meta-analysis suggested that octreotide is as good as endoscopic sclerotherapy for controlling variceal bleeding and has fewer adverse events [20]. Patients with variceal bleeding should receive antibiotics, because up to 20% have bacterial infections at admission and antibiotics decrease bacterial infections and mortality [21].

Endoscopic hemostasis was initially performed most commonly with injection of sclerosants (i.e., ethanolamine), but this has mostly been replaced by rubber band ligation of varices, which has a similar acute hemostasis rate of 85% and a rebleed rate of 30% but fewer local complications such as esophageal strictures [22]. Gastric varices are much more difficult to treat, and the most successful endoscopic therapy is injection of cyanoacrylate glue, but this is not available in the United States as a result of the risk of embolization and scope damage.

Portosystemic shunts, in which portal pressure is reduced by bypassing the cirrhotic liver with a shunt between the portal and the hepatic veins, are very effective in stopping bleeding and reducing rebleeding. Initially, this was done surgically, but this has mostly been replaced by interventional radiologically placed transjugular intrahepatic portosystemic shunts (TIPSs), in which a percutaneously placed, self-expanding metal stent (SEMS) is placed between the hepatic and portal veins. A TIPS is more effective than endoscopic therapy for preventing variceal bleeding, but it has a slightly higher rate of hepatic encephalopathy and requires periodic checks or revisions to maintain stent patency.

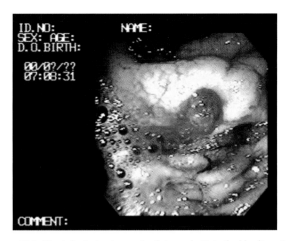

Figure 22.6 Dieulafoy lesion in proximal stomach. Note the bleeding site without adjacent ulceration or mass.

Esophagitis

Patients with severe erosive esophagitis can present with upper GI bleeding. Risk factors include alcohol abuse, cirrhosis, and anticoagulant use. This is treated with PPIs. Endoscopy is needed for diagnosis, but rarely for therapy. However, all patients with severe erosive esophagitis should undergo repeat EGD after 12 weeks of daily PPI therapy in order to make sure that there has been complete healing and there is no underlying Barrett's esophagus or malignancy.

Stress Ulcers

Stress ulcers occur in the upper GI tract of severely ill patients, most likely due to a combination of decreased mucosal protection and mucosal ischemia. They usually occur in the stomach or duodenum. Bleeding due to ICU stress ulcers occurs in 1.5% of ICU patients. Patients with the risk factors of coagulopathy or on mechanical intubation for >48 hours have a risk of clinically significant bleeding of 3.7%, compared with 0.1% without these risk factors [23]. Intravenous H_2-receptor blockers have been shown to decrease the risk of bleeding in these high-risk ICU patients compared with placebo. PPIs are as good as or better than intravenous H_2-receptor blockers at preventing stress ulcers in ICU patients. A potential risk of prophylactic acid suppression in ICU patients is that decreased gastric pH may allow bacteria to grow in the stomach, which can then be aspirated and cause ventilator-associated pneumonia.

Generally, patients with bleeding stress ulcers should be supported medically, and these ulcers will heal as the patient's overall medical status improves. These lesions tend to have high rebleeding rates and do not seem to respond as well to endoscopic therapy as peptic ulcers that start to bleed before hospitalization; they are better treated with clips than with thermal probes, which can cause perforation of the non-fibrotic ulcer base [24].

Dieulafoy Lesion

A Dieulafoy lesion (Figure 22.6) is a large (1–3 mm), aberrant, submucosal artery that protrudes through the mucosa but is not associated with ulceration. It can occur anywhere in the GI tract, though usually within the proximal stomach. The etiology is unknown, but may be congenital. Dieulafoy lesions can be difficult to identify due to intermittent bleeding. They are usually found when actively

bleeding, or in the setting of blood in the stomach and a protruding vessel. They can be successfully treated endoscopically with injection, thermal probes, clips, or band ligation. Though endoscopic hemostasis is usually successful and has low reported rebleeding risks, it is prudent to mark the area around a Dieulafoy lesion with a permanent endoscopic tattoo in case rebleeding that requires endoscopy or surgery occurs in the future.

Mallory–Weiss Tear

Mallory–Weiss tears (Figure 22.7) are mucosal lacerations that occur at the gastroesophageal junction (GEJ) and generally extend distally into a hiatus hernia. Patients generally present with hematemesis or coffee-ground emesis. Typically, there is a history of antecedent non-bloody vomiting or heavy alcohol use. Endoscopy can be used to treat the actively bleeding tears with epinephrine injection, thermal probe, or clips. Most tears are mild and will heal without treatment within 48 hours. Patients do not need long-term PPI treatment. Those patients who present with Mallory–Weiss tear

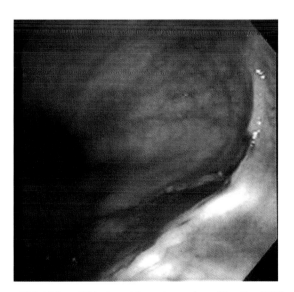

Figure 22.7 Mallory–Weiss tear at the gastroesophageal junction (GEJ).

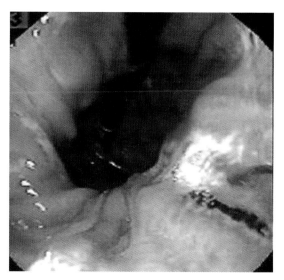

Figure 22.8 Cameron erosions caused by mucosal trauma from a hiatus hernia pinch.

and are also found to have esophageal varices should have therapy directed toward the varices with band ligation or sclerotherapy.

Cameron Erosions

Cameron erosions (Figure 22.8) are scattered linear erosions or ulcers located circumferentially in the proximal stomach at a hiatus hernia pinch. They are caused by mechanical mucosal trauma from the hiatus hernia compression. Though they can present as acute overt bleeding, they are more commonly a source of obscure bleeding with iron-deficiency anemia. Treatment is usually satisfactory with daily oral PPIs, but surgical correction of the hernia may be required.

Upper GI Malignancy

Malignancy accounts for 1% of severe upper GI bleeds, resulting from an esophageal, gastric, or duodenal cancer. Endoscopic hemostasis can be used to temporarily control bleeding, but long-term management requires medical or surgical oncologic treatment of the tumor. Angiography should be considered for patients with acute ongoing upper GI tumor bleeding that cannot be controlled endoscopically.

Gastric Antral Vascular Ectasia

Gastric antral vascular ectasia (GAVE; also known of "watermelon stomach") is characterized by rows of ectatic mucosal blood vessels that radiate from the pylorus proximally into the antrum. The etiology is unknown, but may represent mucosal trauma associated with antral contraction waves. It has been associated with older age, cirrhosis, chronic renal insufficiency, and systemic sclerosis. Endoscopic thermal therapy can generally control the bleeding, though several sessions may be required. Rarely, surgical antrectomy may be warranted to control bleeding.

Portal Hypertensive Gastropathy

Portal hypertensive gastropathy is characterized by a mosaic or snake-skin appearance of the proximal gastric body mucosa, resulting from high-pressure gastropathy caused by portal hypertension. Patients usually present with chronic blood loss but can have acute bleeding. Treatment is toward reducing portal pressure, either medically with β-blockers or with TIPS. Generally, there is no endoscopic role for treatment.

Hemobilia

Bleeding from the bile duct that exits the ampulla into the duodenum is usually iatrogenic, such as after a percutaneous liver biopsy or recent biliary endoscopic retrograde cholangiopancreatography (ERCP), but can also occur from hepatocellular carcinoma, cholangiocarcinoma, or biliary parasites. Patients often present with a combination of GI bleeding and increasing liver tests. Bleeding is usually self-limited, but if ongoing will generally be managed with angiographic embolization.

Hemosuccus Pancreaticus

Hemosuccus pancreaticus is bleeding from the pancreatic duct out of the ampulla and into the duodenum. This is best visualized with a side-viewing duodenoscope. It can occur in the setting of acute pancreatitis, chronic pancreatitis, pancreatic pseudocyst, pancreatic cancer, recent ERCP with pancreatic duct manipulation, or splenic artery aneurysm rupture in the pancreatic duct. Computed tomography (CT) can demonstrate pancreatic pathology if previously unsuspected. Management of ongoing bleeding is done with angiographic embolization or surgery.

Post-ERCP Sphincterotomy Bleeding

Post-ERCP sphincterotomy bleeding occurs in approximately 2% of patients [25]. Risk factors include coagulopathy, anticoagulation, portal hypertension, renal failure, intraprocedure bleeding, and particular types and lengths of sphincterotomy. Successful hemostasis of postsphincterotomy bleeding is usually achieved with endoscopic methods, such as injection of epinephrine, hemoclips, or bipolar probe coagulation. Rarely, angiographic embolization is needed.

Aortoenteric Fistula

Aortoenteric fistulas can be primary (new) or secondary (related to implanted graft). A primary aortoenteric fistula is a communication between the native abdominal aorta (usually an atherosclerotic abdominal aortic aneurysm) and the third portion of the duodenum [26]. Often, there will be a self-limited "herald bleed" hours to months before a more exsanguinating bleed. Occasionally, the diagnosis can be suspected by palpating a pulsatile abdominal mass. The endoscopic diagnosis can be difficult if not actively bleeding and not suspected. An abdominal CT scan showing an aneurysm suggests the diagnosis [27].

Secondary aortoenteric fistulas usually occur between the small intestine and an infected abdominal aortic aneurysm graft or stent. The fistula usually occurs between the third part of the duodenum and the proximal aspect of the graft, but may occur elsewhere in the GI tract as well. Fistulas usually form between 3 and 5 years after graft placement, though they have been reported earlier and later. Patients also often develop a subsequent "herald bleed," which is usually mild and self-limited, but can be intermittent [28]. A secondary fistula can occur between the third part of the duodenum and an endovascular stent, as a result of pressure from the graft on the duodenum, infection of the stent, or possibly expansion of the native aneurysm [29].

Patients with an acute upper GI bleed and a history of an aortic aneurysm repair should have an urgent CT scan and EGD to evaluate the third part of the duodenum for any compression or blood, as well as to rule out any other bleeding sources, and a vascular surgery consultation. CT may show inflammation around the graft. Surgical treatment is required, during which the infected graft is removed. There is no role for therapeutic endoscopy in the management of bleeding from aortoenteric fistulas.

Angiomas

Angiomas are occasional causes of upper GI bleeding, but usually occur as part of GAVE syndrome, or else are found in either the mid-distal small intestine or the right colon. If found in the upper GI tract, they can generally be treated with multipolar-probe endoscopic hemostasis.

Take Home Points

- The etiology of upper GI bleeding can be suspected by taking a good history.
- Peptic ulcers are the most common cause of severe upper GI bleeding.
- The endoscopic appearance of bleeding ulcers helps to predict the rebleeding rate.
- Endoscopic hemostasis can reduce the rebleeding rate from peptic ulcers.
- PPIs reduce rebleeding rates after endoscopic hemostasis.

References

1 Lewis JD, Bilker WB, Brensinger C, *et al.* Hospitalization and mortality rates from peptic ulcer disease and GI bleeding in the 1990s: relationship to sales of nonsteroidal anti-inflammatory drugs and acid suppression medications. *Am J Gastroenterol* 2002; **97**: 2540–9.

2 Villanueva C, Colomo A, Bosch A, *et al.* Transfusion strategies for acute upper gastrointestinal bleeding. *N Engl J Med* 2013; **368**: 11–21.

3 Lau JY, Leung WK, Wu JC, *et al.* Omeprazole before endoscopy in patients with gastrointestinal bleeding. *N Engl J Med* 2007; **356**: 1631–40.

4 Yan BM, Lee SS. Emergency management of bleeding esophageal varices: drugs, bands or sleep? *Can J Gastroenterol* 2006; **20**: 165–70.

5 Rockall TA, Logan RF, Devlin HB, Northfield TC. Risk assessment after acute upper gastrointestinal haemorrhage. *Gut* 1996; **38**: 316–21.

6 Swain CP, Storey DW, Bown SG, *et al.* Nature of the bleeding vessel in recurrently bleeding gastric ulcers. *Gastroenterology* 1986; **90**: 595–608.

7 Gralnek IM, Barkun AN, Bardou M. Management of acute bleeding from a peptic ulcer. *N Engl J Med* 2008; **359**: 928–37.

8 Laine L, Jensen DM. Management of patients with ulcer bleeding. *Am J Gastroenterol* 2012; **107**: 345–60.

9 Hwang JH, Fisher DA, Ben-Menachem T, *et al.* ASGE guideline: The role of endoscopy in the management of acute non-variceal upper GI bleeding. *Gastrointest Endosc* 2012; **75**(6): 1132–8.

10 Lin HJ, Hsieh YH, Tseng GY, *et al.* A prospective, randomized trial of large- versus small-volume endoscopic injection of epinephrine for peptic ulcer bleeding. *Gastrointest Endosc* 2002; **55**: 615–19.

11 Vergara M, Calvet X, Gisbert JP. Epinephrine injection versus epinephrine injection and a second endoscopic method in high risk bleeding ulcers. *Cochrane Database Syst Rev* 2007(**2**):CD005584.

12 Chung SS, Lau JY, Sung JJ, *et al.* Randomised comparison between adrenaline injection alone and adrenaline injection plus heat probe treatment for actively bleeding ulcers. *BMJ* 1997; **314**: 1307–11.

13 Jensen DM, Kovacs TO, Jutabha R, *et al.* Randomized trial of medical or endoscopic therapy to prevent recurrent ulcer hemorrhage in patients with adherent clots. *Gastroenterology* 2002; **123**: 407–13.

14 Bleau BL, Gostout CJ, Sherman KE, *et al.* Recurrent bleeding from peptic ulcer associated with adherent clot: a randomized study comparing endoscopic treatment with medical therapy. *Gastrointest Endosc* 2002; **56**: 1–6.

15 Laine L, Cohen H, Brodhead J, *et al.* Prospective evaluation of immediate versus delayed refeeding and prognostic value of endoscopy in patients with upper gastrointestinal hemorrhage. *Gastroenterology* 1992; **102**: 314–16.

16 Longstreth GF, Feitelberg SP. Successful outpatient management of acute upper gastrointestinal hemorrhage: use of practice guidelines in a large patient series. *Gastrointest Endosc* 1998; **47**: 219–22.

17 Leontiadis GI, Sharma VK, Howden CW. Proton pump inhibitor treatment for acute peptic ulcer bleeding. *Cochrane Database Syst Rev* 2006(**1**):CD002094.

18 Lau JY, Sung JJ, Lee KK, *et al.* Effect of intravenous omeprazole on recurrent bleeding after endoscopic treatment of bleeding peptic ulcers. *N Engl J Med* 2000; **343**: 310–16.

19 Graham DY, Smith JL. The course of patients after variceal hemorrhage. *Gastroenterology* 1981; **80**: 800–9.

20 D'Amico G, Pietrosi G, Tarantino I, Pagliaro L. Emergency sclerotherapy versus vasoactive drugs for variceal bleeding in cirrhosis: a Cochrane meta-analysis. *Gastroenterology* 2003; **124**: 1277–91.

21 Soares-Weiser K, Brezis M, Tur-Kaspa R, *et al.* Antibiotic prophylaxis of bacterial infections in cirrhotic inpatients: a meta-analysis of randomized controlled trials. *Scand J Gastroenterol* 2003; **38**: 193–200.

22 Laine L, el Newihi HM, Migikovsky B, *et al.* Endoscopic ligation compared with sclerotherapy for the treatment of bleeding esophageal varices. *Ann Intern Med* 1993; **119**: 1–7.

23 Cook DJ, Fuller HD, Guyatt GH, *et al.* Risk factors for gastrointestinal bleeding in critically ill patients. *Canadian Critical Care Trials Group. N Engl J Med* 1994; **330**: 377–81.

24 Jensen DM, Machicado GA, Kovacs TOG, *et al.* Current treatment and outcome of patients with bleeding "stress ulcers" (abstract). *Gastroenterology* 1988; **94**: A208.

25 Freeman ML, Nelson DB, Sherman S, *et al.* Complications of endoscopic biliary sphincterotomy. *N Engl J Med* 1996; **335**: 909–18.

26 Ihama Y, Miyazaki T, Fuke C, *et al.* An autopsy case of a primary aortoenteric fistula: a pitfall of the endoscopic diagnosis. *World J Gastroenterol* 2008; **14**: 4701–4.

27 Hagspiel KD, Turba UC, Bozlar U, *et al.* Diagnosis of aortoenteric fistulas with CT angiography. *J Vasc Interv Radiol* 2007; **18**: 497–504.

28 Odemis B, Basar O, Ertugrul I, *et al.* Detection of an aortoenteric fistula in a patient with intermittent bleeding. *Nat Clin Pract Gastroenterol Hepatol* 2008; **5**: 226–30.

29 Bergqvist D, Bjorck M, Nyman R. Secondary aortoenteric fistula after endovascular aortic interventions: a systematic literature review. *J Vasc Interv Radiol* 2008; **19**(2 Pt 1): 163–5.

CHAPTER 23

Other Gastric Tumors (Benign and Malignant)

Sun-Chuan Dai and Michael L. Kochman

Division of Gastroenterology, University of Pennsylvania Health System, Philadelphia, PA, USA

Summary

Gastric tumors, other than adenocarcinoma, are frequently encountered during clinical gastrointestinal (GI) practice. A variety of epithelial and subepithelial lesions may arise within the stomach. These are usually found incidentally during endoscopy or a radiographic study. They include both benign and malignant etiologies. Endoscopy alone is often insufficient in defining the full extent of the process, and endoscopic ultrasound (EUS) has become a mainstay in the evaluation of some of these pathologies. For the purposes of this chapter, these lesions have been classified as either mucosal or submucosal lesions.

Case

A 54-year-old male who has symptoms of reflux undergoes an endoscopy due to concern over Barrett's esophagus. His medications include a proton pump inhibitor (PPI) and two additional antibiotics, because the blood work shows that he "tested positive for *H. pylori*." He has a hiatal hernia but no evidence of esophagitis or Barrett's esophagus. An "incidental" 2 cm polypoid lesion is seen in the body of the stomach. Biopsies of the lesion demonstrate "normal mucosa," while biopsies from both the body and antrum reveal atrophic gastritis with *H. pylori*. The patient has a family history of stomach cancer and the question of a mucosa-associated lymphoid tissue (MALT) lymphoma is raised because of the *H. pylori*. Therefore, an EUS is scheduled. The lesion is determined to be submucosal, and endoscopic mucosal resection is performed. The pathology reveals that the lesion is a macrocarcinoid, which is thought to be related to high gastrin levels due to the atrophic gastritis. It is determined on pathologic exam that the entire lesion should be removed by endoscopic mucosal resection (EMR). Testing for multiple endocrine neoplasia type 1 (MEN1) syndrome is negative.

Mucosal Tumors

Some common etiologies that present as gastric tumors and thickened gastric folds are listed in Table 23.1.

Gastric Polyps

Gastric polyps are abnormal epithelial growths of the normally uniform and smooth lining of the gastric mucosa. On histology, they may be classified as hyperplastic, adenomatous, hamartomatous, fundic gland, or inflammatory fibroid polyps (Table 23.2). They may be sessile or pedunculated and single or multiple. Endoscopic and clinical features may be predictive in distinguishing the type of polyp, but tissue sampling or resection is often required for accurate diagnosis. Gastric polyps may be associated with syndromes including familial adenomatous polyposis (FAP), Peutz–Jeghers syndrome (PJS), and familial juvenile polyposis.

Fundic gland polyps (FGP) (Figure 23.1) are the most common type of gastric polyps observed in Western countries; their incidence has been reported to be 0.8–1.9% of all upper endoscopies [1]. Their histology comprises cystically dilated glands lined by gastric mucosa. FGP can be further classified as sporadic or associated with FAP. Sporadic FGP may be associated with PPI use or *H. pylori* infection, and dysplasia is rare, with an almost negligible malignant potential. In FAP, on the other hand, dysplasia can occur in 25–41% of FGP. The polyps are often multiple and may "carpet" the body and fundus of the stomach. Given their potential to harbor malignancy, surveillance esophagogastroduodenoscopy (EGD) is necessary, and resection is recommended if dysplasia is high-grade. Multiple FGP with dysplasia in the absence of PPI use should raise suspicion of FAP.

Hyperplastic polyps are the second most common polypoid lesions in the Western world (Figure 23.2). They are inflammatory proliferations of mucin-producing epithelial cells lining the gastric surface and consist of hyperplastic gastric glands with edematous stroma without change in the microcellular configuration. They are often referred to as "inflammatory polyps," though such nomenclature is discouraged as it may confuse these lesions with inflammatory fibroid polyps. There is a classic association of hyperplastic polyps with mucosal atrophy, often in the form of chronic atrophic gastritis, pernicious anemia, and *H. pylori* gastritis. The risk of malignant transformation is considered low (0.5–4.0%). In the setting of *H. pylori* gastritis, 80% of hyperplastic polyps will regress with complete eradication of infection [2]. In addition to resection of polyps and eradication of *H. pylori*, biopsies of the surrounding mucosa and any other abnormal areas should be performed to examine for chronic gastritis and intestinal metaplasia.

Adenomatous polyps are true neoplastic lesions with dysplastic epithelium and nuclear atypia. Histopathologically, they closely resemble colon adenomas, and are they classified as tubular, villous, and tubulovillous. In Western countries, gastric adenomas account for 6–10% of all gastric polyps, but they are more frequently identified in Asian countries, where rates of gastric cancer are higher. The malignant potential increases significantly in polyps >2 cm in diameter (up to 75% in some series), although adenomatous polyps

Practical Gastroenterology and Hepatology Board Review Toolkit, Second Edition. Edited by Nicholas J. Talley, Kenneth R. DeVault, Michael B. Wallace, Bashar A. Aqel and Keith D. Lindor.
© 2016 John Wiley & Sons, Ltd. Published 2016 by John Wiley & Sons, Ltd. Companion website: www.practicalgastrohep.com

CHAPTER 23

Table 23.1 Common etiologies that present as gastric tumors and thickened gastric folds.

Mucosal tumors	Submucosal tumors
Gastric polyps	Leiomyomas and leiomyosarcomas
Lymphoma	Lipoma and liposarcoma
MALT lymphoma	GIST
Ménétrier's disease	Gastric carcinoid
Zollinger–Ellison syndrome	Granular cell tumor
Kaposi's sarcoma	Pancreatic rest
Gastritis cystica profunda	Duplication cyst

MALT, mucosa-associated lymphoid tissue; GIST, gastrointestinal stromal tumor.

Table 23.2 Malignant potential and recommendations for resection of gastric polyps.

Polyp histology	Malignant potential	Resection?
Fundic gland polyp (sporadic)	Very low	Resect if >1 cm
FAP-associated fundic gland polyp	Low	Resect if >1 cm or high-grade dysplasia
Hyperplastic	Low	Resect if >2 cm, test for *H. pylori* and treat if positive
Adenomatous	Significant	Resect if histology confirmed
Hamartomatous	None	Resect if >1 cm and associated with PJS
Inflammatory fibroid	Very low	Resection only if symptomatic

Resection recommended for any dysplasia with symptoms or >2 cm, regardless of histology.
FAP, familial adenomatous polyposis; PJS, Peutz–Jeghers syndrome.

with carcinoma <2 cm have been reported. Like hyperplastic polyps, adenomatous polyps often occur in the background of mucosal atrophy and *H. pylori* infection, and therefore it is recommended that surrounding areas be biopsied after resection of the polyp. This is especially important as adenomatous polyps can also be associated with synchronous and metachronous gastric adenocarcinoma.

Hamartomatous polyps are uncommon. They may include sporadic juvenile polyps and may arise as manifestations of a congenital syndrome such as PJS, Cowden's syndrome, or juvenile polyposis

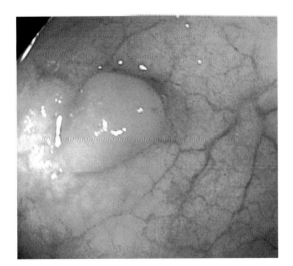

Figure 23.1 Endoscopic image demonstrating a fundic gland polyp (GFP). Notice the smooth borders and uniform "pits" on the surface.

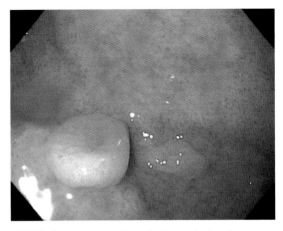

Figure 23.2 Endoscopic image of a typical hyperplastic polyp.

syndrome. Hamartomatous polyps consist of branching smooth-muscle bands surrounded by glandular epithelium. They have no malignant potential themselves [3, 4]. Endoscopic appearance and biopsy samples are sometimes insufficient to reliably diagnose polyp histology. For complete diagnosis, excision should be considered. Smaller polyps (<5 mm) may be removed with multiple biopsy forceps, while larger ones (>5 mm) may be resected with snare polypectomy. If multiple polyps are present, the larger lesions (>1 cm) should be resected to confirm histology and absence of dysplasia before treatment or surveillance strategies are chosen. EUS is a helpful adjunctive tool to use in delineating the layer of origin before resection. Surgical resection should be considered in those polyps thought to be too large to excise endoscopically.

Inflammatory fibroid polyps are extremely rare, accounting for less than 0.1% of all gastric polyps [5]. These lesions arise from the gastric submucosa but can resemble a mucosal lesion and may appear ulcerated. Histopathological features are distinct; they include spindle cell proliferation, small vessels, and a predominantly eosinophilic infiltrate. A common misnomer arising from the latter feature is "eosinophilic granuloma." Inflammatory fibroid polyps can be associated with chronic atrophic gastritis, and the malignant potential is extremely low. Therefore, resection is only recommended if they are symptomatic.

EUS is helpful when trying to determine whether a gastric lesion originates from the mucosal or submucosal layer. However, if a lesion is known to be a mucosal-based gastric polyp, EUS is not necessary as it has not been shown to prevent post-polypectomy bleeding during polyp resection and otherwise does not improve safety. If prior biopsies have confirmed a histological diagnosis of a mucosal based polyp, this further eliminates the need for EUS.

Generally, polyp resection is recommended in the presence of dysplasia, symptoms including gastric outlet obstruction or bleeding, or size >2 cm. Techniques include endoscopic mucosal resection, often with the assistance of a cap, band ligation system, or injection of normal saline mixed with methylene blue. The incidence of bleeding has been reported to be 6.0–7.2% [1], necessitating a histological diagnosis to determine management of polyps <2 cm in the absence of dysplasia or symptoms. To minimize the risk of sampling error from forceps biopsies, all adenomatous polyps and fundic gland and hamartomatous polyps >1 cm should be removed. If hamartomatous polyps are found in the context of juvenile polyposis or Cowden's disease, resection is not necessary. The cutoff size for resection of hyperplastic polyps remains to be determined, but size >2 cm or a pedunculated stalk is considered to hold great malignant risk [6].

Gastric Lymphoma and MALT lymphoma

Lymphomas of the stomach account for up to 5% of gastric malignancies and may be divided into primary gastric lymphomas and those with disseminated nodal disease and secondary gastric involvement [7]. More than 95% of gastric lymphomas are of the non-Hodgkin's type. Clinical presentation is similar to adenocarcinoma and the disease can be indolent in the early stage. Abdominal pain, weight loss, nausea, anorexia, and GI hemorrhage are the most common symptoms and signs. On endoscopy, they can appear as discrete polypoid lesions, ulcerated mass, or thickened gastric folds due to submucosal infiltration. Endoscopic forceps biopsies are not always diagnostic and snare biopsies or needle aspirates may be required. EUS is helpful in identifying submucosal involvement and perigastric lymph nodes. If the diagnosis remains elusive, surgical full-thickness biopsies may be considered [8, 9].

MALT lymphoma is classified as an extranodal marginal-zone lymphoma. Numerous lymphoid follicles, plasma cell infiltrates, and dense B-cell lymphocytic infiltrates are seen on histology. Clinical presentation may include bleeding from an ulcerated mass (Figure 23.3) or thickened gastric folds seen on endoscopy or cross-sectional imaging. Diagnosis is usually made on endoscopy with "jumbo" forceps biopsies. The majority of MALT lymphomas are low-grade, have an indolent course, and are associated with *H. pylori* infection. Gastric biopsies should also be performed to examine for atrophic gastritis, chronic active gastritis, and intestinal metaplasia. EUS is extremely useful in assessing the depth of invasion. Low-grade MALT lymphomas may demonstrate focal thickening of the mucosal and submucosal layers, while transmural thickening and perigastric lymphadenopathy indicate high-grade disease (Figure 23.4). Treatment options include *H. pylori* eradication, radiation, and chemotherapy. For low-grade disease limited to the submucosa, eradication of *H. pylori* may regress the tumor in 60–75% of patients. EUS is helpful in objective assessment of response to therapy post-treatment.

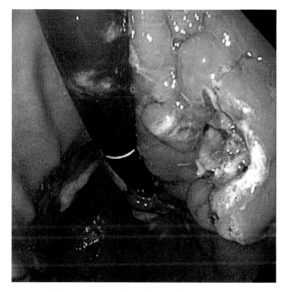

Figure 23.3 Endoscopic image of an ulcerated mass along the lesser curvature of the stomach. This patient presented with melena. Biopsies confirmed a diagnosis of a MALT lymphoma.

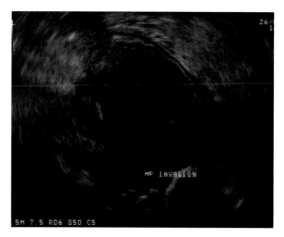

Figure 23.4 EUS image of the lesion in Figure 23.3. Note the extension of the mass through the muscularis propria.

Ménétrier's Disease

Ménétrier's disease is a condition characterized by marked foveolar hyperplasia with cystic dilation, resulting in giant gastric rugal folds with antral sparing. The submucosa may be penetrated, though this is rare. The pathogenesis is unclear and may involve transforming growth factor (TGF)-α. The symptoms may include abdominal pain, weight loss, GI hemorrhage, and protein leakage leading to hypoalbuminemia. EUS may demonstrate thickening of the deep mucosal layer and "jumbo" forceps biopsies or snare resection may be needed to confirm the diagnosis. The pathogenesis of Ménétrier's disease is poorly understood, though cytomegalovirus (CMV; particularly in the pediatric population) or *H. pylori* involvement has been postulated. Thus, testing for CMV and *H. pylori* and treating if either is positive is generally recommended. Other therapeutic options include antacids, H$_2$-receptor blockers, PPIs, steroids, prostaglandins, octreotide, and cetuximab, though trials have been small and/or have not shown any consistent benefit. Subtotal gastrectomy may be considered in refractory cases. The natural history is unclear, though some reports have demonstrated the evolution from Ménétrier's disease to gastric atrophy over a 4–8-year timespan, with return of the serum albumin concentration to normal. The risk of gastric cancer is also not well characterized, but is estimated at 2–15% [10].

In pediatric patients, the disease presents more acutely with abrupt-onset vomiting, abdominal pain, anorexia, and hypoproteinemia. Ascites and pedal edema may then occur, with laboratory values demonstrating hypoalbuminemia, a normocytic anemia, and peripheral eosinophilia. An additional histologic feature is intranuclear inclusion bodies consistent with CMV. Pediatric patients generally respond well to supportive treatment, with complete clinical resolution.

Zollinger–Ellison Syndrome

Zollinger–Ellison syndrome is a condition characterized by hyperplastic gastropathy of the body and fundus of the stomach, leading to hypersecretion of gastric acid due to a gastrinoma. Thickened proximal gastric folds are formed through parietal cell hyperplasia. The management of this entity is beyond the scope of this chapter. Most patients develop duodenal or jejunal ulcers, and diarrhea may be present; esophagitis and esophageal strictures may also be found at presentation [11]. Up to one-third of patients have metastatic disease at presentation (liver, axial skeleton), and the condition may be part of a MEN1 syndrome. Localization of the tumor is essential for curative resection and is generally achieved through a combination of somatostatin-receptor scintigraphic scanning, EUS examination of the pancreas, and intraoperative exploration. In patients with metastatic or MEN1 disease, medical therapy with PPIs is instituted.

Submucosal Tumors

Submucosal tumors are also listed in Table 23.1.

Leiomyoma

Leiomyoma is a gastric submucosal tumor, but is most often seen in the esophagus. EUS is highly accurate in defining the wall layer of origin and in differentiating from extraluminal compression or isolated gastric vascular structures such as varices. Leiomyomas are seen as hypoechoic lesions arising from the muscularis propria and may grow with either an intraluminal or an extraluminal pattern. They can range in size from <0.5 up to 30 cm and are most often associated with the esophagus. Microscopically, leiomyomas are formed of fascicles of benign-appearing spindle cells without nuclear atypia. Lesions <3 cm in size have a low risk for malignancy and can be observed with serial endosonography.

Gastrointestinal Stromal Tumor

Gastrointestinal stromal tumors (GISTs) are mesenchymal tumors thought to arise from the interstitial cells of Cajal (GI pacemaker cells). In the past, they were thought to be of smooth-muscle origin, but better understanding of the tumor biology has led to reclassification of many formerly diagnosed leiomyomas, leiomyosarcomas, schwannomas, and leiomyoblastomas as GISTs. Most (70%) GI-tract GISTs occur in the stomach in older patients (age 50–60), with a wide variety of sizes from a few millimeters to 30 cm. Gastric GISTs are believed to be less aggressive than those arising in the small bowel and rectum [12].

The endoscopic appearance is of a smooth submucosal mass (Figure 23.5). EUS findings include a hypoechoic, typically homogenous lesion with well-defined borders arising from the muscularis propria or muscularis mucosa (Figures 23.6 and 23.7).

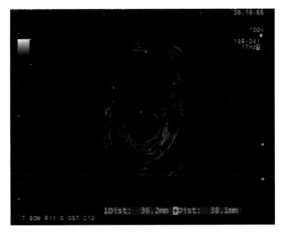

Figure 23.6 EUS image of the lesion in Figure 23.5. A hypoechoic mass measuring 36 × 38 mm arising from the muscularis propria is seen.

Larger lesions may show features of liquefactive necrosis, cystic, and hyaline degeneration. The malignant potential is difficult to predict without histologic evaluation; smaller lesions are typically benign in biologic behavior. EUS features (heterogeneous lesions >4 cm with irregular extraluminal borders and cystic spaces) may be suggestive of malignancy [13]. Typically, tumor size, location, and number of mitoses are factors in the risk stratification of GISTs.

GISTs are distinguishable by their molecular features. C-kit (a stem-cell receptor called CD117) or PDGFRA (platelet-derived growth factor-α receptor) expression is characteristic. Other markers found in GISTs include CD34, smooth-muscle actin, and s100 protein. Surgery is clearly indicated for lesions >3 cm or other malignant features. Unresectable lesions should be treated with a tyrosine kinase inhibitor, commonly imatinib mesylate (STI571; Gleevec, Novartis, USA). For small, asymptomatic, localized lesions, the management of GISTs is an area of controversy. While some advocate for resection due to malignant potential, others argue for observation because the malignant potential is low and the benefits of resection do not outweigh the risks. Multiple algorithms have been compiled for management, but none is universally accepted, and a lack of evidence has prevented gastroenterological societies from making definitive recommendations.

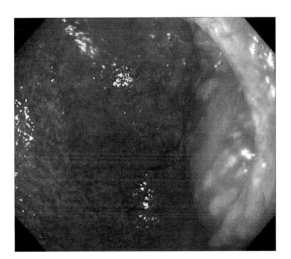

Figure 23.5 Endoscopic image demonstrating a submucosal mass in the antrum, with smooth, superficial mucosa.

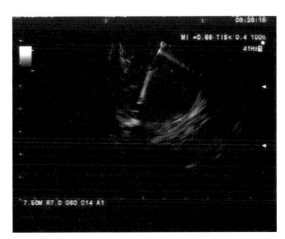

Figure 23.7 EUS guided fine-needle aspiration (FNA) of the lesion described in Figure 23.6.

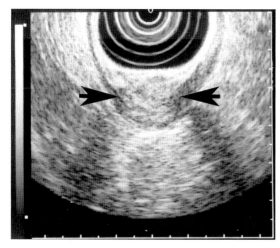

Figure 23.8 EUS image of gastric lipoma, demonstrating that it is relatively hyperechoic and found within the submucosa.

Lipoma

Lipomas are benign tumors composed of matures lipocytes. They are typically found incidentally on endoscopy and colonoscopy. Rarely, they may be symptomatic, presenting with bleeding, abdominal pain, or obstruction. Endoscopy will typically demonstrate an isolated solitary bulge with normal overlying mucosa, a yellowish hue, and a smooth, regular appearance. A "pillow" sign may be elicited when an indentation in created with palpation by an endoscopic device. EUS will demonstrate a hyperechoic lesion arising from the submucosa. Diagnosis is reliably made based on the typical endoscopic and EUS appearances (Figure 23.8). Expectant management is adequate, without any need for endoscopic surveillance. Excision should be performed if symptomatic (ulcerated or intussuscepting) or if unable to distinguish from a liposarcoma.

Gastric Carcinoids

Gastric carcinoids represent 2–3% of all GI carcinoids but only 0.3% of all gastric tumors. They are usually located in the body or fundus of the stomach, are generally submucosal, and may appear polypoid (Figure 23.9). They arise from GI neuroendocrine cells, and some are thought to develop as a result of high circulating gastrin, which is stimulating to the enterochromaffin cells of the proximal stomach. Therefore, pernicious anemia and chronic atrophic gastritis are risk factors for the typically benign macro- and microcarcinoids, but no such lesions have been reported in humans as a result of hypergastrinemia from PPI use. While circulating vasoactive peptides may be identified, they are frequently incidental, as true carcinoid syndrome does not develop without liver involvement. Endoscopy often demonstrates a submucosal mass with a central umbilication, and EUS is useful in defining wall-layer involvement. Carcinoids resulting from pernicious anemia and atrophic gastritis or MEN1 tend to have a benign course; for lesions <2 cm and without involvement of the muscularis propria, endoscopic resection may be the optimal therapy (Figure 23.10). Larger lesions may require surgical excision. Antrectomy to reduce G-cell burden may be effective in reducing smaller carcinoid tumors in this setting. Sporadic carcinoids, which are autonomous and present in the setting of gastric acid secretion and normal serum gastrin, should be treated as malignant and surgically excised, as they have a higher rate of regional lymph node involvement [14].

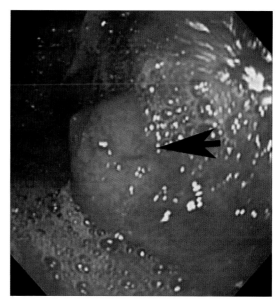

Figure 23.9 Endoscopic image of a gastric carcinoid with mucosal extension.

Granular Cell Tumor

Granular cell tumors (GCTs) are rare submucosal tumors of Schwann cell origin. Immunostaining is positive for s100 protein. They are generally benign, but malignant transformation for tumors >4 cm in size has been described. It may be possible to resect or ablate smaller lesions endoscopically, but larger lesions may need surgical resection.

Pancreatic Rest

Pancreatic rest is often referred to as "aberrant pancreas" or "ectopic pancreas." It is a rare submucosal lesion consisting of cystically dilated exocrine pancreatic glandular tissue. It is most commonly observed in the distal stomach or duodenum, and endoscopy shows a submucosal nodule with a central depression (Figure 23.11). EUS findings are an echovariable, hypoechoic, heterogeneous lesion with indistinct borders arising from the submucosa or muscularis propria. Diagnosis is made by forceps biopsy or snare excision. Management is expectant unless symptomatic or there is suspicion of malignancy.

Biopsy of Submucosal Tumors

While EUS can determine the originating layer of submucosal lesions and suggest a diagnosis, it is not definitive and may not preclude the need for future surveillance. Obtaining a definitive histologic diagnosis can often be challenging, and cold-forceps biopsies may not provide an adequate tissue sample. EUS-guided fine-needle aspiration (EUS-FNA) allows visualization of the needle biopsying the core of the lesion and is considered the gold standard, but is technically challenging in small, mobile nodules and the diagnostic yield has been reported to be as low as 38% [15]. Stacked "bite-on-bite" forceps biopsy has been routinely performed, but its diagnostic yield is low [16]. Innovative techniques for biopsy have been developed, including the use of multiple-forceps biopsies followed by FNA needle to "harpoon" the lesion, EUS-guided incision of the nodule with a needle knife followed by forceps biopsy (SINK), and drawing of the lesion into a cap for endoloop ligation followed by unroofing with a

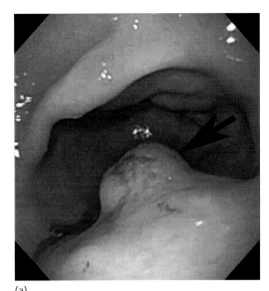

(a)

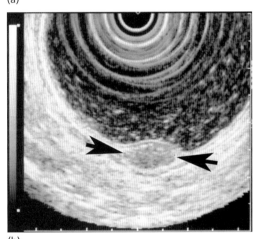

(b)

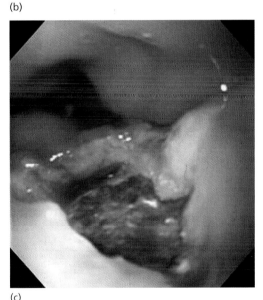

(c)

Figure 23.10 (a) Endoscopic image of a submucosal gastric carcinoid. (b) EUS image of the same gastric carcinoid, demonstrated to be in the submucosal layer. (c) Endoscopic image demonstrating clean endoscopic resection.

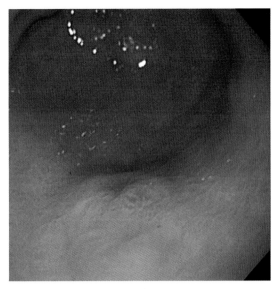

Figure 23.11 Endoscopic image showing a submucosal nodule with central dimpling. Biopsies confirmed the diagnosis of a pancreatic rest.

needle knife and forceps biopsy (SLUB) [16, 17]. These novel methods have only been described in single-center studies with a limited number of patients and are not yet routinely employed in practice as their safety and efficacy are not clear.

Take Home Points
- Most gastric mucosal and submucosal tumors are asymptomatic and found incidentally. Endoscopy alone is often insufficient for diagnosis. EUS is useful but may be of limited yield in certain situations and is not universally recommended.
- There are many types of gastric polyp, with varied malignant potential. In general, resection is recommended to establish diagnosis and for therapy.
- Most gastric lymphomas are of the non-Hodgkin's type and should be treated as such.
- For low-grade mucosa-associated lymphoid tissue (MALT) lymphomas, eradication of associated *H. pylori* infection may be sufficient, but chemotherapy or radiation is required for high-grade tumors.
- Apparent submucosal tumors may be intramural or may result from extramural causes.
- Leiomyomas and lipomas represent the most frequently encountered intramural submucosal tumors. They are generally benign when small.
- In general, undiagnosed submucosal tumors <3 cm can be managed expectantly, while larger ones should be evaluated for resection.

Videos of interest to readers of this chapter can be found by visiting the companion website at:

http://www.practicalgastrohep.com/

23.1 Endoscopic ultrasound (mechanical radial) of distal esophageal adenocarcinoma stage T3N1.

23.2 Endoscopic ultrasound-guided fine needle aspiration of mediastinal rounded hypoechoic lymph node.

23.3 Endoscopic mucosal resection of early adenocarcinoma in short-segment Barrett esophagus.

23.4 Endoscopic staging of gastric cancer.

23.5 Endoscopic treatment of gastric cancer (endoscopic submucosal dissection technique).

23.6 Endoscopic view of a submucosal lesion in the antrum causing mild distortion but not obstruction of the antrum and pylorus.

23.7 Endoscopic ultrasound examination of a submucosal lesion in the antrum.

References

1 Enestvedt BK, Chandrasekhara V, Ginsberg GG. Endoscopic ultrasonographic assessment of gastric polyps and endoscopic mucosal resection. *Curr Gastroenterol Rep* 2012; **14** 497–503.

2 Ohkusa T, Miwa H, Hojo M, *et al.* Endoscopic, histological and serologic findings of gastric hyperplastic polyps after eradication of *Helicobacter pylori*: comparison between responder and non-responder cases. *Digestion* 2003; **68**(2–3): 57–62.

3 Cristallini E, Ascani S, Bolis G. Association between histologic type of polyp and carcinoma of the stomach. *Gastrointest Endosc* 1992; **38**: 481–4.

4 Hirota WK, Zuckerman MJ, Adler DG, *et al.* ASGE guideline: the role of endoscopy in the surveillance of premalignant conditions of the upper GI tract. *Gastrointest Endosc* 2006; **63**: 570–80.

5 Hasgawa T, Yang P, Kagawa N, *et al.* Cd34 expression by inflammatory fibroid polyps of the stomach. *Mod Pathol* 1997; **10** 451–6.

6 Antonioli DA. Precursors of gastric carcinoma: a critical review with a brief description of early (curable) gastric cancer. *Hum Pathol* 1994; **25**(10): 994–1005.

7 Wotherspoon A. Gastric lymphoma of mucosa-associated lymphoid tissue and *Helicobacter pylori. Annu Rev Med* 1998; **49**: 289–99.

8 Kolve M, Fischbach W, Wilhelm M. Primary gastric non-Hodgkin's lymphoma: requirements for diagnosis and staging. *Recent Results Cancer Res* 2000; **156**: 63–8.

9 Amer MH, el-Akkad S. Gastrointestinal lymphoma in adults: clinical features and management of three hundred cases. *Gastroenterology* 1994; **106**: 846–58.

10 Scharschmidt B. The natural history of hypertrophic gastropathy (Ménétrier's diseases). *Am J Med* 1997; **63**: 644–52.

11 Roy PK, Venzon DJ, Shojamanesh H, *et al.* Zollinger–Ellison syndrome. Clinical presentation in 261 patients. *Medicine (Baltimore)* 2000; **79**: 379–411.

12 Chandrasekhara V, Ginsberg GG. Endoscopic management of gastrointestinal stromal tumors. *Curr Gastroenterol Rep* 2011; **13**: 532–9.

13 Chak A, Canto MI, Rosch T, *et al.* Endosonographic differentiation of benign and malignant stromal cells. *Gastrointest Endosc* 1997; **45**: 468–73.

14 Gilligan C, Lawton G, Tang L, *et al.* Gastric carcinoid tumors: the biology and therapy of an enigmatic and controversial lesion. *Am J Gastroenterol* 1995; **90**: 338–52.

15 Binmoeller KF, Shah JN, Bhat YM, *et al.* Suck-ligate-unroof-biopsy by using a detachable 20-mm loop for the diagnosis and therapy of small subepithelial tumors. *Gastrointest Endosc* 2014; **79**(5): 750–5.

16 Cantor MJ, Davila RE, Faigel DO. Yield of tissue sampling for subepithelial lesions evaluated by EUS: a comparison between forceps biopsies and endoscopic submucosal resection. *Gastroinest Endosc* 2006; **64**: 29–34.

17 de la Serna-Higuera C, Pereiz-Miranda M, Diez-Redondo P, *et al.* EUS-guided single–incision needle-knife biopsy: description and results of a new method for tissue sampling of subepithelial GI tumors. *Gastrointest Endosc* 2011; **74**: 672–6.

CHAPTER 23

Eosinophilic Gastroenteritis

Magnus Halland[1] and Nicholas J. Talley[2]

[1] Division of Gastroenterology and Hepatology, Mayo Clinic, Rochester, MN, USA
[2] Faculty of Health, University of Newcastle, Newcastle, NSW, Australia

Summary

Eosinophilic gastroenteritis (EG) is a rare and heterogeneous disorder characterized by gastrointestinal (GI) symptoms and eosinophilic infiltration of the GI tract. Symptoms are dependent upon the site of the GI tract involved and the depth of involvement. The diagnostic criteria include: (i) the presence of GI symptoms, (ii) histopathology demonstrating predominant eosinophilic infiltration, (iii) the absence of other conditions that cause eosinophilia, and (iv) no eosinophilic involvement of organs outside the GI tract.

Diagnosis requires a clinical history, physical exam, and documentation of any history of atopic disorders, allergies, and drug allergies. Laboratory evaluation includes a complete blood count (CBC) with differential to evaluate for peripheral eosinophilia. Endoscopic evaluation with random biopsies remains the cornerstone for diagnosis. Histopathologic diagnosis typically requires an infiltration level of 20 or more eosinophils per high-power field. Management strategies are based upon severity of symptoms and include antidiarrheals, dietary adjustments, and steroid therapy.

Case

A 41-year-old male presents with a 3-month history of recurring abdominal pain with nausea and vomiting. CBC is notable for peripheral eosinophilia at 5% of total leukocytes. He has traveled to South East Asia, but serologic and stool studies are negative for parasitic infection. Contrast-enhanced computed tomographic (CT) views of the abdomen demonstrates thickening of the antrum and the second part of the duodenum. The patient undergoes esophagogastroduodenoscopy (EGD), which reveals stenosis from the antrum through the pylorus and extending to the second portion of the duodenum. Antral and duodenal biopsies are obtained with histopathology, demonstrating marked eosinophilic infiltration of the lamina propria. The patient is started on steroid therapy with prednisone and has rapid clinical improvement with resolution of his previous symptoms.

Definition and Epidemiology

Unlike eosiniphiliic esophagitis (EoE), EG usually affects multiple portions of the GI tract and systemic eosinophilic is present in the majority of patients. The condition was originally described by Kaijser in 1937 [1], and EG has a myriad of clinical manifestations; symptoms are dependent upon both the site of the GI tract involved and the depth of involvement of the gut wall.

EG has been found to affect all age groups from infants to adults, though it usually presents in the third to fourth decade of life. It has been reported to have a slight male predominance [2,3,6].

Patients may present with a wide spectrum of symptoms, ranging from abdominal pain to ascites [2]. Concurrent extraintestinal manifestations have also been reported, including eosinophilic splenitis, hepatitis, and cystitis [7,8].

Pathophysiology

Currently, the pathophysiology of EG is suboptimally defined. Accumulation of eosinophils in the GI tract is a common finding in many GI disorders, such as parasitic infection, inflammatory bowel disease (IBD), and gastroesophageal reflux [9–13]. However, EG is a primary eosinophilic GI disorder, with histopathology demonstrating abundant accumulation of eosinophils. The pathogensis remains unclear, but an allergic component appears to play a role in at least half of patients. Food allergen-specific T-cells that express interleukin (IL)-5 are found in many patients [14]. Furthermore, though the exact etiopathogenesis for this disorder is unclear, it is believed that the eosinophilic infiltration of the GI tract secondary to food allergy, drugs, or toxins, or possibly unrecognized infection, results in an adverse immunologic response. Th-2 cytokines and the eotaxin subfamily of chemokines are implicated as eosinophil-specific mediators in regulating this accumulation [15–17]. Furthermore, there is also growing evidence of a specific interaction between eotaxin and expression of the CCR3 receptor, a 7-transmembrane-spanning G protein-coupled receptor expressed on eosinophils, in modulating eosinophil infiltration [15]. This has resulted in the consideration of eotaxin- or CC3-specific blocking agents as possible therapeutic interventions.

Following eosinophil localization in the GI tract, it is thought that cellular degranulation with release of cytotoxic proteins results in tissue destruction. Major basic protein (MBP) and eosinophil cationic protein are believed to play key roles and have been found at immunohistochemically elevated levels in the small-bowel tissue of patients with EG [15].

There appears to be evidence of an association between eosinophilic GI disorders and allergy, as many patients have coexisting atopic disorders, such as asthma, seasonal rhinitis, eczema,

Practical Gastroenterology and Hepatology Board Review Toolkit, Second Edition. Edited by Nicholas J. Talley, Kenneth R. DeVault, Michael B. Wallace, Bashar A. Aqel and Keith D. Lindor.

and food allergies [6, 15]. Allergy testing, such as patch, skin, or radioallergosorbent test (RAST), has not been reliably demonstrated to be able to identify culprit foods or environmental factors.

Clinical Features

The Klein classification system for EG, based upon depth of tissue infiltration, is the most widely accepted [18]. Patients are divided into those with disease of the mucosa, muscle layer, and serosa. Each group appears to have differing clinical symptoms. Predominant disease of the mucosa seems to be the most commonly reported subclass, but most data come from retrospective case series and should be interpreted with caution [3].

Mucosal involvement usually presents with non-specific symptoms of abdominal pain, nausea, vomiting, diarrhea, or anemia, or even malabsorption or protein-loss enteropathy with small-bowel involvement. Given these non-specific symptoms, patients may be inadvertently diagnosed with functional bowel disorder or IBD [3].

Eosinophilic infiltration of the muscular layer accounts often presents with symptoms of gastric outlet or small-intestinal obstruction [2, 3].

Finally, involvement of the serosal layer is most uncommon and typically presents as ascites [2, 3]. When compared to other types, serosal disease may have significantly higher levels of circulating eosinophils and may have a better treatment response to steroids [3].

Children with EG may present with growth failure, delayed puberty, or amenorrhea. More often, they have a history of allergy [19, 20].

Diagnosis

A careful clinical history and physical exam is paramount in the initial evaluation of a patient (Table 24.1). Inquire about a history of

Table 24.1 Generally accepted diagnostic criteria for eosinophilic gastroenteritis (EG).

1	Presence of GI symptoms
2	Biopsies with histopathology demonstrating predominant eosinophilic infiltration
3	Absence of parasitic or extraintestinal diseases that might cause eosinophilia
4	Absence of eosinophilic involvement of the heart or other organs outside the GI tract [2, 3]
5	Peripheral eosinophilia may be commonly found, but it is not required for diagnosis as it is not a universal finding [2, 4, 5]

atopic disorders or allergies. Any pets should be documented. Ask about travel history and exposures, in order to determine the likelihood of GI parasitosis. Consider drug allergies (e.g., recent use of azathioprine, co-trimoxazole).

Laboratory evaluations may include a CBC, and peripheral eosinophilia may alert the clinician but is absent in at least 20% of cases. In cases of elevated circulating eosinophils, other GI disorders associated with eosinophilia need to be excluded, including parasitic infections, malignancies, vasculitis such as Churg–Strauss syndrome, and IBD. Hypereosinophilic syndrome can be fatal if missed, and should be considered if the absolute eosinophil count is over 1500 cells/µL; a cardiac echo and other investigations are then needed to exclude suspected systemic disease.

Stool studies should be obtained to exclude parasites. In difficult cases, a duodenal aspirate for parasites can be helpful. Dog hookworm infestation classically causes ileocolonic disease; stool studies are usually negative but patients will typically respond to empiric mebendazole (100 mg twice daily for 3 days).

No pathognomonic features are found in radiographic studies. Findings of irregular and thickened intestinal walls have been reported [21]. Plain abdominal radiographs or CT scanning may demonstrate findings of bowel obstruction, as seen in EG with disease of the muscular layer (Figure 24.1). Abdominal ultrasound may also demonstrate ascites in serosal disease. Novel radiographic

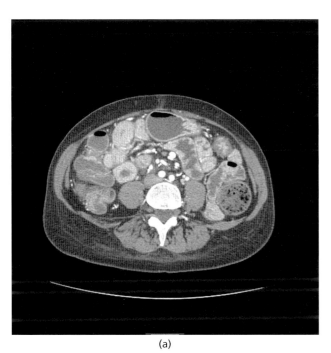
(a)

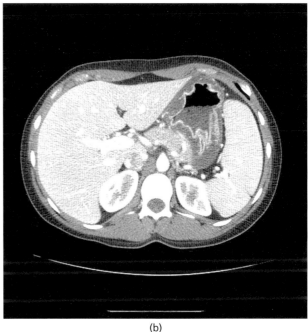
(b)

Figure 24.1 (a) CT enterography demonstrating thickened jejunal folds from eosinophilic gastroenteritis. (b) CT abdomen illustrating gastric-wall edema and hyperenhancement of the gastric mucosa from eosinophilic gastritis.

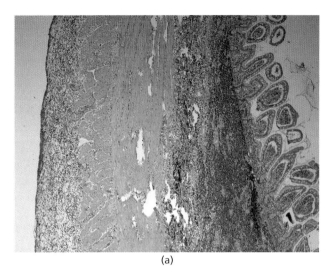 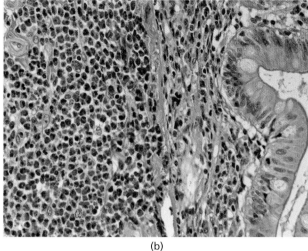

(a)   (b)

Figure 24.2 (a) Small-bowel biopsy from the jejunum, demonstrating dense eosinophilic infiltration involving the submucosa and the serosa. Note the dense "sheet-like" configuration of the eosinophils within the submucosa. (b) Higher-magnification view of the subserosa, demonstrating the significant submucosal accumulation of eosinophils. Source: Courtesy of Dr Thomas C. Smyrk, Mayo Clinic College of Medicine.

techniques previously used for IBD have been applied to EG, including bowel scintigraphy using radiolabeled granulocytes containing technetium-99 with hexamethyl-propylenamine oxime (Tc-99 HMPAO), which can be used to assess the extent of disease and the response to therapy [22].

Endoscopic evaluation with biopsies remains the cornerstone for diagnosis. Macroscopic abnormalities are only present in 50% of cases, however [23]. Thickened gastric or small-intestinal folds with or without nodules may be present; the differential diagnosis of enlarged small-bowel folds includes Whipple disease, amyloid, lymphoma, paraproteinemia, and intestinal lymphangiectasia. Random biopsies should be taken from both normal- and abnormal-appearing mucosa in the stomach and small intestine, as eosinophilic infiltration may exist despite a bland endoscopic appearance [24, 25] (Figure 24.2).

If endoscopic biopsies are negative but there remains a high level of clinical suspicion, then full-thickness laparoscopic biopsies can be considered. Biopsies should be sent for histopathology to evaluate for the degree of eosinophilic infiltration. Though no generally accepted histopathologic criteria for EG exist, many studies have taken 20 or more eosinophils per high-power field to meet diagnostic requirement [2, 25, 26]. At least two segments of the GI tract are involved in 70% of patients [23]. Ascites with suspected serosal EG should be evaluated with abdominal paracentesis and ascitic fluid should be evaluated for a high eosinophil count.

Therapeutics

Therapeutic strategies for EG are largely based upon anecdotal experience. There have not been any prospective, randomized controlled trials (RCTs) for potential therapies.

Common management strategies for EG revolve around the severity of symptoms and diseases. For patients with mild symptoms, symptomatic management can be attempted first (e.g., as-needed loperamide for diarrhea), followed by dietary adjustments and close observation, as some cases of EG spontaneously resolve without therapy [25]. Elimination diets may be an option, but there is insufficient evidence in adults.

The mainstay of therapy for patients with significant symptoms, such as obstruction or malabsorption, continues to be steroids. Though differing regimens have been reported, many recommend a prednisone taper therapy, with initial 8-week course of therapy with 1–2 mg/kg, to be followed with a 6–8-week taper; over 90% respond [3]. The largest natural history study to date followed 43 cases for a median of 13 years and found that approximately 40% had a single flare, while 40% relapsed and 20% had a more chronic course [23]. Repeated courses may be required, as recurrence has been reported either during the taper (15%) or following it (33–50%). For refractory cases where the patient cannot be tapered off oral prednisone, transition to budesonide has been reported as a possible alternative [27]. Other successful approaches include sodium cromoglycate or montelukast [28–31].

Take Home Points

Diagnosis:
- Clinical manifestations of eosinophilic gastroenteritis (EG) are dependent upon the site of disease involvement and on the depth of tissue involvement in the gut wall.
- Peripheral eosinophilia raises suspicion for EG but is not required for diagnosis.
- Gastric and/or duodenal biopsies with more than 20 eosinophils per high-power field are commonly accepted as confirming the diagnosis of EG, in the absence of parasitic infection.

Therapy:
- Mild disease may be monitored or symptomatically managed with dietary exclusions, as some cases resolve spontaneously.
- Steroids remain the cornerstone of therapy, with often dramatic clinical response.
- Relapse after steroid-induced remission occurs in up to 50% of cases. This usually responds to repeat treatment.

This chapter is modified from the original version by Joseph Y Chang and NJ Talley.

References

1 Kaijser R. Zur Kenntnis der allegischen Affektioner desima Verdauungskanal von Standpunkt desima Chirurgen aus. *Arch Klin Chir* 1937; **188**: 36–64.

2 Talley NJ, Shorter RG, Phillips SF, Zinsmeister AR. Eosinophilic gastroenteritis: a clinicopatholical study of patients with disease of the mucosa, muscle layer, and subserosal tissues. *Gut* 1990; **31**: 54–8.

3 Chang JY, Choung RS, Lee RM, *et al.* A shift in the clinical spectrum of eosinophilic gastroenteritis toward the mucosal disease type. *Clin Gastroenterol Hepatol* 2010; **8**: 669–75.

4 Zhang L, Duan L, Ding S, *et al.* Eosinophilic gastroenteritis: clinical manifestations and morphologic characteristics, a retrospective study of 42 patients. *Scand J Gastroenterol* 2011; **46**: 1074–80.

5 Johnstone J, Morson B. Eosinophilic gastroenteritis. *Histopathology* 1978; **2**: 335–48.

6 Kelly KJ. Eosinophilic gastroenteritis. *J Pediatr Gastroenterol Nutr* 2000; **30**: S28–S35.

7 Robert F, Mura E, Durant JR. Mucosal eosinophilic gastroenteritis with systemic involvement. *Am J Med* 1977; **62**: 39–43.

8 Gregg JA, Utz DC. Eosinophilic cystitis associated with eosinophilic gastroenteritis. *Mayo Clin Proc* 1974; **49**: 185–7.

9 Walsh RE, Gaginella TS. The eosinophil in inflammatory bowel disease. *Scand J Gastroenterol* 1991; **26**: 1217–24.

10 Sarin SK, Malhotra V, Sen Gupta S, *et al.* Significance of eosinophil and mast cell counts in rectal mucosa in ulcerative colitis: a prospective controlled study. *Dig Dis Sci* 1978; **32**: 363–7.

11 Winter HS, Madara JL, Stafford JL, *et al.* Intraepithelial eosinophils: a new diagnostic criterion for reflux esophagitis. *Gastroenterology* 1982; **83**: 818–23.

12 Brown LF, Goldman H, Antonioli DA. Intraepithelial eosinophils in endoscopic biopsies of adults with reflux esophagitis. *Am J Surg Pathol* 1984; **8**: 899–905.

13 Rothenberg ME, Mishra A, Brandt EB, *et al.* Gastrointestinal eosinophils. *Immunol Rev* 2001; **179**: 139–55.

14 Prussin C, Lee J, Foster B. Eosinophilic gastrointestinal disease and peanut allergy are alternatively associated with IL-5+ and IL-5(−) T(H)2 responses. *J Allergy Clin Immunol* 2009; **124**: 1326.

15 Rothenberg ME. Eosinophilic gastrointestinal disorders (EGID). *J Allergy Clin Immunol* 2004; **113**: 11–28.

16 Jose PJ, Griffiths-Johnson DA, Collins PD, *et al.* Eotaxin: a potent eosinophil chemoattractant cytokine detected in a guinea pig model of allergic airways inflammation. *J Exp Mode* 1994; **179**: 881–7.

17 Matthews AN, Fried DS, Zimmerman N, *et al.* Eotaxin is required for the baseline level of tissue eosinophils. *Proc Natl Acad Sci USA* 1998; **95**: 6273–8.

18 Klein NC, Hargrove RL, Sleisenger MH, *et al.* Eosinophilic gastroenteritis. *Medicine (Baltimore)* 1970; **49**: 299–319.

19 Goldman H, Proujansky R. Allergic proctitis and gastroenteritis in children: clinical and mucosal biopsy features in 53 cases. *Am J Surg Pathol* 1986; **10**: 75–86.

20 Moon A, Kleinman RE. Allergic gastroenteropathy in children. *Ann Allergy* 1995; **74**: 5–12.

21 Teele, RL, Katz AJ, Goldman H, *et al.* Radiographic features of eosinophilic gastroenteritis (allergic gastroenteropathy) of childhood. *Am J Roentgenol* 1979; **132**: 575–80.

22 Lee KJ, Hahm KB, Kim YS, *et al.* The usefulness of Tc-99m HMPAO labeled WBC SPECT in eosinophilic gastroenteritis. *Clin Nucl Med* 1997; **22**: 536–41.

23 Pineton de Chambrun G, Gonzalez F, Canva JY, *et al.* Natural history of eosinophilic gastroenteritis. *Clin Gastroenterol Hepatol* 2011; **9**(11): 950–6.

24 Straumann A, Spichtin HP, Bucher KA, *et al.* Eosinophilic esophagitis: red on microscopy, white on endoscopy. *Digestion* 2004; **70**: 109–16.

25 Lee M, Hodges WG, Huggins TL, *et al.* Eosinophilic gastroenteritis. *South Med J* 1996; **89**: 189–94.

26 Lee CM, Changchien CS, Chen PC, *et al.* Eosinophilic gastroenteritis: 10 years experience. *Am J Gastroenterol* 1993; **88**: 70–4.

27 Tan AC, Kruimel JW, Naber TH. Eosinophilic gastroenteritis treated with nonenteric coated budesonide tablets. *Eur J Gastroenterol Hepatol* 2001; **13**: 425–7.

28 Van Dellen RG, Lewis JC. Oral administration of cromolyn in a patient with protein-losing enteropathy, food allergy, and eosinophilic gastroenteritis. *Mayo Clin Proc* 1994; **69**: 441–4.

29 Perez-Millan A, Martin-Lorente JL, Lopez-Morante A, *et al.* Subserosal eosinophilic gastroenteritis treated efficaciously with sodium cromoglycate. *Dig Dis Sci* 1997; **42**: 342–4.

30 Neustrom MR, Friesen C. Treatment of eosinophilic gastroenteritis with montelukast. *J Allergy Clin Immunol* 1999; **104**: 506.

31 Schwartz DA, Pardi DS, Murray JA. Use of montelukast as steroid sparing agent for recurrent eosinophilic gastroenteritis. *Dig Dis Sci* 2001; **46**(8): 1787–90.

CHAPTER 24

Esophageal and Gastric Involvement in Systemic and Cutaneous Diseases

John M. Wo

GI Motility and Neurogastroenterology Unit, Division of Gastroenterology & Hepatology, Indiana University School of Medicine, Indiana University Hospital, Indianapolis, IN, USA

CHAPTER 25

Case

A 47-year-old female with scleroderma presents with complaints of dry mouth, dysphagia, heartburn, bloating, and effortless regurgitation at night. Her salivation is decreased and the test for Sjogren's is positive. At upper endoscopy, there is erosive esophagitis in the distal esophagus and undigested foods in the stomach. A standardized 4-hour gastric scintigraphy is performed [1]. Gastric retention after 2 hours is 48%, which is normal, but after 4 hours it is 32%, which is delayed. She later develops bloating and abdominal distension. Upper enteroscopy is performed, and quantitative aerobic and anaerobic culture of jejunal aspirate yields >10^5 CFU/mL of coliform Gram-negative bacilli. A diagnosis of small intestinal bacterial overgrowth is made, with impairment of small-bowel motility.

Connective-Tissue Diseases

The main features of connective-tissue diseases affecting the esophagus and stomach are listed in Table 25.1.

Systemic Sclerosis

Systemic sclerosis (SSc), also known as scleroderma, is a generalized disorder of the small arteries with proliferation of fibrosis affecting the skin and multiple organs. The gastrointestinal (GI) tract is the third most common organ affected after skin thickening and Raynaud's phenomenon. In the early stages of SSc, there are thickened capillary basement membrane, swollen endothelial cells, and arteriole sclerosis. In the later stages, there are extensive collagen infiltration in the lamina propria toward the muscularis mucosa in the esophagus and stomach. Esophageal involvement of SSc does not affect overall mortality [2]. However, esophageal manifestations of SSc are associated with an impairment of quality of life and with depressive symptoms [3,4].

Esophageal symptoms are common (Table 25.1), occurring in 50–80% of patients. The severity of gastroesophageal reflux disease (GERD) is correlated with diminished lower esophageal sphincter (LES) pressures and impairment of distal esophageal peristalsis (Figure 25.1b). Severe acid reflux, erosive esophagitis, and esophageal aperistalsis have been associated with interstitial lung disease in patients with SSc [5]. Patients with dysphagia are more likely to have decreased forced vital capacity by pulmonary function testing [6]. The extent of the GI dysmotility can be severe, involving the stomach and small bowel, and causing gastroparesis and chronic intestinal pseudo-obstruction (CIP). The presence of delayed gastric emptying in patients with SSc is indicative of significant impairment of the esophagus and stomach, based on esophageal and antroduodenal manometry [7].

Inflammatory Myopathies

Inflammatory myopathies consist of a heterogeneous group of acquired disorders, including polymyositis, dermatomyositis, and inclusion-body myositis. Polymyositis and dermatomyositis are characterized by proximal muscle weakness, with difficulty lifting the arms, climbing steps, and arising from chairs. Inclusion-body myositis involves mainly the distal muscles. The diagnosis of inflammatory myopathy is based on elevated muscle enzymes, electromyography, and muscle biopsy. Dermatomyositis affects both children and adults, and it is recognized by the characteristic heliotrope rash, periorbital edema, and papular scaly lesions over the knuckles (Gottren's signs) (Figure 25.2). There is a threefold increase in risk of cancer with the diagnosis of dermatomyositis in adults, especially for stomach, lung, ovarian, pancreatic, and colorectal cancers and non-Hodgkin's lymphoma [8,9]. Polymyositis affects patients in their second and third decade. Patients with inclusion body myositis are usually over 50 years old.

Reflux symptoms are less common in inflammatory myopathy than in SSc. However, gastroparesis and CIP may occur. Weak pharyngeal striated muscles, uncoordinated swallowing, and impaired upper esophageal sphincter (UES) relation can cause oropharyngeal dysfunction, which may be the presenting complaint rather than the proximal skeletal muscle weakness [10]. Dysphagia is progressive in patients with inclusion body myositis and may lead to aspiration pneumonia [11]. Prompt diagnosis of inflammatory myopathy is important, because it is a treatable condition [12,13].

Mixed Connective-Tissue Disease

Mixed connective-tissue disease (MCTD) is a syndrome characterized by overlapping features of SSc, systemic lupus erythematosus (SLE), inflammatory myopathy, and rheumatoid arthritis (RA). The systemic features of MCTD are Raynaud's phenomenon, polyarthritis, swelling of the hands, myalgia, and esophageal dysfunction. The

Practical Gastroenterology and Hepatology Board Review Toolkit, Second Edition. Edited by Nicholas J. Talley, Kenneth R. DeVault, Michael B. Wallace, Bashar A. Aqel and Keith D. Lindor.
© 2016 John Wiley & Sons, Ltd. Published 2016 by John Wiley & Sons, Ltd. Companion website: www.practicalgastrohep.com

Table 25.1 Connective-tissue diseases affecting the esophagus and stomach.

Clinical features	Diagnostic testing	Therapeutics
Systemic sclerosis (scleroderma) • Symptoms: heartburn, regurgitation, dysphagia, nausea, vomiting, early satiety, abdominal distension, weight loss, diarrhea, GI bleeding • Manifestations: GERD, gastroparesis, SIBO, CIP, gastric telangiectasia, iron-deficiency anemia	• EGD: esophagitis, reflux stricture, Barrett's esophagus uncommon, "watermelon" stomach • High-resolution esophageal manometry: diminished LES pressure, low DCI, absent peristalsis (see Figure 25.1) • pH-impedance monitoring: acid and non-acid reflux, especially at night • Others: increased esophageal wall stiffness, delayed gastric emptying • Serum: ACA, Scl-70 (anti-DNA topoisomerase I) antibodies	• Avoid eating late • PPI for GERD • Prokinetics for gastroparesis, avoid indigestible solids • Antibiotics for SIBO • Avoid antireflux surgery • Endoscopic therapy for "watermelon" stomach
Inflammatory myopathies (polymyositis, dermatomyositis, inclusion body myositis) • Symptoms: oropharyngeal dysphagia, aspiration, heartburn, regurgitation, nausea, vomiting, early satiety • Manifestations: oropharyngeal dysfunction, GERD, gastroparesis, SIBO, CIP	• EGD: esophagitis • Videofluoroscopy: poor UES relaxation, impaired muscle contraction, reduced hypolaryngeal excursion • Esophageal manometry: poor UES relaxation, diminished proximal and distal pressures • Scintigraphy: delayed gastric emptying • Serum: elevated CK and aldolase	• PPI for GERD • Prokinetics for gastroparesis • Swallowing therapy • Treatment for inflammatory myopathy • Look for paraneoplastic disease in dermatomyositis
Mixed connective-tissue disease • Symptoms and manifestations: similar to scleroderma and inflammatory myopathies	• Similar to scleroderma and inflammatory myopathies • Serum: ANA speckled pattern, anti-U1 RNP antibodies	• Similar to scleroderma and inflammatory myopathies
Sjögren's syndrome • Symptoms: dysphagia, heartburn, dyspepsia, nausea • Manifestations: chronic atrophic gastritis, MALT lymphoma	• Esophageal manometry: variable, simultaneous contractions, absent peristalsis rare • Serum: antibodies to Ro/SSA and La/SSB	• Correct lack of saliva: chew sugarless gum, mucous-containing lozenges, cholinergic agonists • Increase fluid intake
Systemic lupus erythematosus • Symptoms: heartburn, chest pain, nausea, vomiting, epigastric pain • Manifestations: GERD, gastroparesis, gastric ulcer, vasculitis	• Esophageal manometry: variable, low LES pressure, impaired distal esophageal peristalsis • Scintigraphy: delayed gastric emptying • Serum: ANA, antibodies to antiphospholipid, ds (double-strand) DNA and anti-Smith	• PPI for GERD • Prokinetics for gastroparesis

GI, gastrointestinal; GERD, gastroesophageal reflux disease; SIBO, small-intestinal bacterial overgrowth; CIP, chronic intestinal pseudo-obstruction; EGD, esophagogastroduodenoscopy; LES, lower esophageal sphincter; DCI, distal contractile integral; ACA, anticentromere antibody; PPI, proton pump inhibitor; UES, upper esophageal sphincter; CK, creatinine kinase; RNP, ribonucleoprotein; MALT, mucosa-associated lymphoid tissue; SSA, Sjögren's syndrome type A; SSB, Sjögren's syndrome type B; ANA, antinuclear antibodies.

upper GI manifestations of MCTD are also an overlap of the neural dysfunction and smooth-muscle atrophy of SSc and the striated proximal muscle weakness of polymyositis. Heartburn and regurgitation are common, occurring in up to half of patients with MCTD [14, 15]. As in SSc, the presence of impaired esophageal motility in patients with MCTD is associated with interstitial lung disease [16].

Sjögren's Syndrome

Sjögren's syndrome is a chronic autoimmune disorder associated with the destruction of salivary and lacrimal glands. It can present as a primary disorder or associated with other connective-tissue disorders. It is believed that the absence of saliva, acting as a lubricant, may lead to impaired solid bolus transit through the esophagus. Most patients localize the dysphagia sensation to the pharyngeal region [17]. Chronic atrophic gastritis and secondary hypergastrinemia may be present. Sjögren's syndrome has been associated with mucosa-associated lymphoid tissue (MALT) lymphoma, a form of non-Hodgkin's B-cell lymphoma of the salivary glands and other mucosal extranodal sites, including the stomach.

Systemic Lupus Erythematosus

Anorexia, nausea, vomiting, and abdominal pain are common complaints in patients with SLE. The precise cause of anorexia and abdominal pain is difficult to identify. Some patients with SLE have overlapping features of SSc, polymyositis, and MCTD, which can all

affect the esophagus. Salivary gland dysfunction may contribute to symptoms of dysphagia or impaired acid clearance. Esophageal and gastric manifestations of SLE are very variable. Esophageal aperistalsis, gastroparesis, and CIP are uncommon but have been reported in patients with SLE.

Endocrine and Metabolic Diseases

The main features of endocrine and metabolic diseases affecting the esophagus and stomach are listed in Table 25.2.

Diabetes Mellitus

Diabetes affects multiple levels in the neuromuscular motor and sensory control of the esophagus and stomach. The pathology of diabetic gastroparesis consists of demyelination of the vagus nerve, loss of parasympathetic and sympathetic fibers, and degeneration of the interstitial cells of Cajal in the enteric nervous system. Reflux symptoms in diabetics are unreliable predictors for the presence of GERD. Patients with type 2 diabetes mellitus and obesity are less likely to respond to proton pump inhibitors (PPIs) [18].

The clinical presentation of diabetic gastroparesis is heterogeneous (see Table 25.2). The presence of delayed gastric emptying does not always imply a diagnosis of gastroparesis. In studies of unselected diabetics, delayed gastric emptying can be found in 40–50% of patients, and many have no gastric symptoms. Gastroparesis is

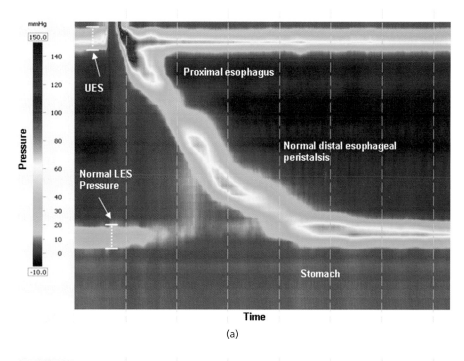

(a)

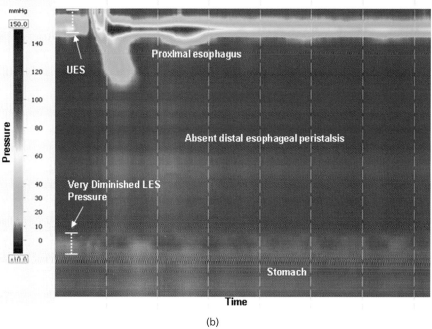

(b)

Figure 25.1 Pressure topography from high-resolution esophageal manometry in (a) an asymptomatic volunteer with normal esophageal peristalsis and (b) a patient with systemic scleroderma (SSc) who has very diminished lower esophageal sphincter (LES) pressure and absent esophageal peristalsis. Note that the pressures of the upper esophageal sphincter (UES) and proximal esophagus are preserved in SSc.

a clinical syndrome with chronic and recurrent symptoms. Establishing the cause and effect between delayed gastric emptying and symptom generation can be difficult because the pathophysiology of upper GI symptoms is multifactorial. These symptoms involve gastric motor and sensory function, the enteric nervous system, and the interaction between the central nervous system (CNS) and the stomach. This may explain why the severity of delayed gastric emptying, a measurement of motor dysfunction only, correlates poorly with symptom severity.

Hypothyroidism

Oropharyngeal dysphagia has been reported in patients with myxedema associated with edematous facies and periorbital edema. Dysphagia responds well to thyroid replacement therapy, and the manometric abnormalities are reversible. Hypothyroidism has been associated with impairment of esophageal and gastric transit by scintigraphy and general hypomotility of the GI tract, causing small-bowel ileus and constipation [19]. Cases of GI involvement are now rare, because hypothyroidism is easily detected and treated. The

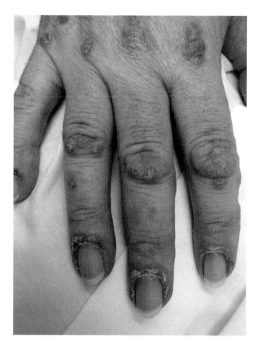

Figure 25.2 Papular scaly lesions over the knuckles (Gottren's signs) in a patient with dermatomyositis. Source: Courtesy of Dr. Jeff Callen, University of Louisville, Louisville, KY.

underlying histology in myxedema small-bowel ileus is the infiltration of the stroma, muscle fibers, and myenteric plexus by mucinous protein complexes. Patients with autoimmune thyroid disease, either Hashimoto's thyroiditis or Graves' disease, may develop histologic proven autoimmune gastritis during long-term follow-up [20]. However, the clinical implication of autoimmune gastritis in these patients is unclear.

Hyperthyroidism

Symptoms of overt hyperthyroidism are very variable, and include anxiety, emotional labiality, weakness, tremor, palpitations, heat intolerance, palpation, and weight loss. Hyperthyroidism can cause

a variety of neurologic manifestations, including thyrotoxic myopathy and periodic paralysis. The precise cause of oropharyngeal dysphagia may be difficult to determine, because myasthenia gravis, hypercalcemia, and hypokalemia can coexist in thyrotoxicosis. Patients with dysphagia have marked weight loss and muscle wasting associated with severe hyperthyroidism. Abnormal vagal autonomic function and gastric myoelectrical activity have been described [21]. However, the effects on gastric emptying have been mixed. Vomiting has been reported in case reports of patients with hyperthyroidism.

Inflammatory Diseases

The main features of inflammatory diseases affecting the esophagus and stomach are listed in Table 25.3.

Crohn's Disease

Crohn's disease is a systemic inflammatory disorder affecting the entire GI tract. Esophageal and gastric involvement occurs in only 0.2–11.0% of adults and is always associated with ileocolonic involvement. In children, the prevalence of esophageal Crohn's is 6–42%. Many children with esophageal Crohn's by esophagogastroduodenoscopy (EGD) have minimal or no upper GI symptoms [22]. Coexisting gastric and duodenal involvement may be common if children have esophageal Crohn's.

The esophageal inflammation can be superficial, with chronic inflammatory infiltration in the lamina propria without basal cell hyperplasia or transmural causing extensive fibrosis and fistula formation to the bronchopulmonary tree, mediastinum, and pleura. Dysphagia can be severe, with weight loss in patients with long narrowed esophageal stricture. Barium esophagram is helpful to determine the length of esophageal stricture and the presence of fistula. Endoscopic findings are variable. They may consist of prominent esophageal scarring with or without active ulcerations (Figure 25.3). Adult patients with Crohn's disease have more dyspepsia than the general population, even when the inflammation is controlled. Delayed gastric emptying has been indicated in vomiting patients with inactive Crohn's, despite no evidence of intestinal obstruction [23].

Table 25.2 Endocrine and metabolic diseases affecting the esophagus and stomach.

Clinical features	Diagnostic testing	Therapeutics
Diabetes mellitus • Symptoms: heartburn, regurgitation, dysphagia, chest pain, nausea, vomiting, dyspepsia, early satiety, weight loss • Manifestations: GERD, "silent" reflux, aspiration, gastroparesis, impaired gastric accommodation	• Esophageal manometry: variable, low LES pressure, impaired peristalsis, spastic contractions • Scintigraphy and breath test: delayed gastric emptying • Others: abnormal slow-wave frequency and diminished postprandial power by EGG, abnormal gastric barostat	• Antiemetics for nausea and vomiting • Treat hyperglycemia • PPI for GERD • Prokinetics for gastroparesis • Gastric electrical stimulation
Hypothyroidism • Symptoms: oropharyngeal dysphagia • Manifestations: oropharyngeal dysfunction, esophageal aperistalsis, autoimmune atrophic gastritis	• Videofluoroscopy: oropharyngeal dysfunction, poor UES relaxation • Esophageal manometry: reduced LES pressure, low amplitude • Serum: high TSH on screening test, low free T4	• Thyroid hormone replacement • Identify and treat underlying cause
Hyperthyroidism • Symptoms: oropharyngeal dysphagia, dysphonia, nasal regurgitation, choking, weight loss, muscle wasting, vomiting • Manifestations: oropharyngeal dysfunction	• Videofluoroscopy: oropharyngeal dysfunction • Others: delayed gastric emptying, abnormal EGG • Serum: low TSH on screening test, high free T4, high T3	• Treat hyperthyroidism • Identify and treat underlying cause, such as Graves' disease

GERD, gastroesophageal reflux disease; LES, lower esophageal sphincter; EGG, electrogastrography; PPI, proton pump inhibitor; UES, upper esophageal sphincter; TSH, thyrotropin; T4, thyroxine; T3, triiodothyronine.

Table 25.3 Inflammatory diseases affecting the esophagus and stomach.

Clinical features	Diagnostic testing	Therapeutics
Crohn's disease • Symptoms: dysphagia, odynophagia, chest pain, epigastric pain, hematemesis, dyspepsia, vomiting, weight loss • Manifestations: esophageal ulcers, long esophageal stricture, fistula; esophageal and gastric Crohn's is rare in adults	• Barium esophagram: shallow ulcers, irregular mucosa, stricture, fistula • EGD: erythema, esophageal aphthous ulcers, superficial erosions, ulcers, cobblestone mucosa, prominent scarring, polypoid lesions (Figure 25.3) • Biopsy: chronic lymphohistocytic inflammation, non-caseating granuloma uncommon	• Treat underlying Crohn's • Esophageal dilation • Surgery may be needed if fistula refractory to treatment for Crohn's
Behçet's disease • Symptoms: oral pain, chest pain, dysphagia, odynophagia, epigastric pain, hematemesis • Manifestations: oral and esophageal ulcers, esophageal stricture, fistula, esophageal varices from superior vena cava thrombosis	• Similar to Crohn's disease • Biopsies: non-specific ulcerations with neutrophilic inflammatory infiltrate • Positive pathergy skin test (a pustule developing in 24–48 hrs after a needle prick)	• Corticosteroids may be helpful • Esophageal dilation
Sarcoidosis • Symptoms: dysphagia, early satiety, epigastric pain, nausea, vomiting, weight loss, hematemesis • Manifestations: extrinsic compression of esophagus, infiltration of esophagus and stomach, involvement of enteric nervous system, laryngeal involvement (Figure 25.4), subglottic stenosis	• Barium esophagram: narrowing at level of carina, mimic achalasia • EGD: esophageal stricture, extrinsic esophageal compression, gastric nodule or mucosal nodularity, gastric ulcers mimicking adenocarcinoma • Biopsy: non-caseating, giant-cell granuloma, granulomatous gastritis • Esophageal manometry: variable, impaired LES relaxation, reduced amplitude, aperistalsis • Others: chest X-ray, CT scan shows mediastinal and/or retroperitoneal lymphadenopathy, luminal wall thickening of esophagus or antrum	• Treat underlying sarcoidosis • Treat impaired LES relaxation with botulinum toxin injection • Relieve obstruction

EGD, esophagogastroduodenoscopy; LES, lower esophageal sphincter; CT, computed tomography.

Behçet's Disease

Behçet's disease is an idiopathic systemic vasculitis with chronic relapsing symptoms. Systemic vasculitis, hyperfunction of neutrophils, and autoimmune inflammatory response are the predominant features. Patients with Behçet's disease cluster along the ancient Silk Road from eastern Asia to the Mediterranean basin, especially in Turkey, Japan, Korea, China, Iran, and Saudi Arabia. The diagnostic criteria according to the International Study Group for Behçet's Disease are recurrent oral ulcers for at least three times per year, plus two or more of the following: recurrent genital ulcerations, eye lesions (uveitis or retinal vasculitis), skin lesions (erythema nodosum, pseudofolliculitis, papulopustular lesions, acneiform nodules), and a positive pathergy skin prick test.

The prevalence of GI involvement varies among countries, with the highest in Japan (50–60%). Behçet's disease may affect the GI tract as small-blood-vessel disease with mucosal inflammation causing ulceration or as large-blood-vessel disease resulting in intestinal ischemia and infarction. Many aspects are similar to Crohn's disease. Penetrating ulcers can develop into fistulas. Esophageal ulcers usually parallel oral ulcers in Behçet's disease. Unfortunately, there is no sign, laboratory test, or histology specific for Behçet's disease.

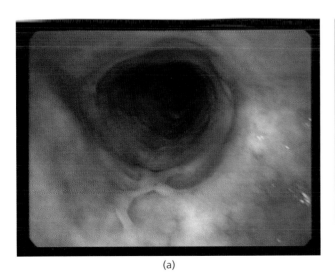
(a)

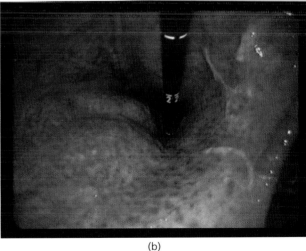
(b)

Figure 25.3 Endoscopic findings in a patient with Crohn's disease complaining of dysphagia. (a) Prominent scaring without active ulceration in the mid-esophagus. (b) Diffuse, non-specific granularity in the stomach. Source: Courtesy of Dr. Gerald Dryden, University of Louisville, Louisville, KY.

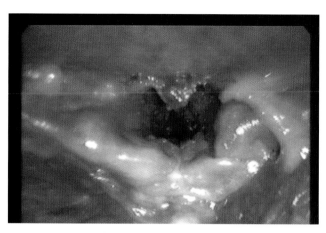

Figure 25.4 Sarcoid inflammatory infiltration of the larynx, identified during upper endoscopy.

Sarcoidosis

Sarcoidosis is a systemic disorder of unknown etiology characterized by accumulation of T-lymphocytes, macrophages, and non-caseating epithelial granuloma. It can occur in nearly all ages, ethnicities, and geographical regions. It affects the lungs in 90% of patients, and less frequently the lymph nodes, skin, eyes, nasopharynx (Figure 25.4), and liver. Direct granulomatous infiltration of the esophagus can result in a markedly thickened esophagus with extensive demyelinization and axonal loss of the myenteric plexus. The stomach, especially the antrum, is the most common site of GI involvement, and sarcoidosis may present as a subclinical, ulcerative, or infiltrative process mimicking gastric carcinoma. Endoscopic biopsy may reveal the typical non-caseating, granulomatous inflammation, but special stains are needed to exclude tuberculosis and histoplasmosis. If bronchoscopy is non-diagnostic, endoscopic ultrasound-guided biopsy can obtain adequate tissue from

adenopathy to diagnose sarcoidosis [24]. In rare cases of secondary achalasia, botulinum toxin injection and Heller myotomy may improve dysphagia, but symptoms usually persist.

Neuromuscular Diseases

Neuromuscular diseases represent a category of acquired and primary disorders affecting the motor neurons, peripheral nerves, neuromuscular junctions, and muscles (Table 25.4). Any abnormality involving the parasympathetic, sympathetic, and enteric nervous systems can potentially affect the esophagus and stomach.

American Trypanosomiasis (Chagas' Disease)

A Brazilian, Carlos Chagas, first described the tropical protozoan parasitic infection caused by *Trypanosoma cruzi*, which is an endemic disease in rural Central and South America. Transmission to humans occurs when the feces of reduviid insects containing *T. cruzi* contaminate a bite, mucosal surface, or the conjunctiva. Infection can also be transmitted from the mother to her fetus, through blood transfusion or organ donation, and by accidental exposure in laboratory workers. The parasite then spreads hematogeneously to internal organs. Acute Chagas' disease consists of 4–6 weeks of fever, malaise, and generalized lymphadenopathy. During the indeterminate phase, infected individuals are asymptomatic with low-grade parasitemia and detectable *T. cruzi* antibodies. Most individuals remain in the indeterminate phase, but 10–30% progress to chronic Chagas' disease. The cause of chronic Chagas' disease is likely infection-induced, immune-mediated tissue damage. Denervation of inhibitory and excitatory myenteric neurons has been described, followed by the replacement of neural structures by fibrosis.

The esophagus is affected in 7–10% of chronic *T. cruzi*-infected individuals in the endemic areas. Dysphagia is mostly intermittent and mild in early disease, when the esophagus is not dilated. In the late stages, megaesophagus develops, and dysphagia becomes

Table 25.4 Neuromuscular diseases affecting the esophagus and stomach.

Clinical features	Diagnostic testing	Therapeutics
American trypanosomiasis (Chagas' disease) • Symptoms: dysphagia, odynophagia, chest pain, regurgitation, aspiration, weight loss • Manifestations: esophageal aperistalsis, megaesophagus	• Barium esophagram: dysrhythmic contractions, dilated esophagus, mimic achalasia • Esophageal manometry: diminished LES pressure, impaired LES relaxation, low peristaltic amplitude, aperistalsis, HRM shows type I and II achalasia by Chicago classification • Others: abnormal EGG, impaired gastric accommodation • Serum: IgG antibodies to *T. cruzi*	• Benznidazole, nifurtimox for *T. cruzi*, but not effective in chronic disease • Pneumatic esophageal dilation, botulinum toxin injection to LES, laparoscopic myotomy, esophageal resection for megaesophagus
Amyloidosis • Symptoms: hoarseness, dysarthria, heartburn, dysphagia, nausea, vomiting, weight loss, hematemesis • Manifestations: oropharyngeal dysfunction, infiltration of oropharynx and thyroid, mimic achalasia, gastric lymphoma, gastric outlet obstruction	• Barium esophagram: mimic achalasia • Esophageal manometry: diminished peristalsis, aperistalsis, impaired LES relaxation • EGD: esophageal and gastric mucosal granularity, erosions, ulcers, gastric polyps, large gastric folds • Biopsy from rectum, abdominal fat pad, bone marrow or sural nerve: amorphous protein deposit staining pink by H&E (Figure 25.6) or apple-green appearance by Congo red under polarized light • Others: delayed gastric emptying, impaired autonomic testing	• Identify and treat underlying cause • Look for multiple myeloma • Prokinetics for gastroparesis
Paraneoplastic syndromes • Symptoms: dysphagia, regurgitation, weight loss, early satiety, nausea, vomiting • Manifestations: esophageal aperistalsis, gastroparesis	• Esophageal manometry: impaired LES relaxation, simultaneous contractions, aperistalsis • EGD: usually normal • Serum: paraneoplastic autoantibodies • Others: imaging to look for underlying cancer	• Identify and treat underlying cancer are essential • Prokinetics for gastroparesis

LES, lower esophageal sphincter; HRM, high-resolution manometry; EGG, electrogastrography; IgG, immunoglobulin G; EGD, esophagogastroduodenoscopy.

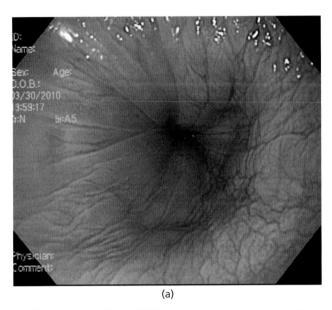
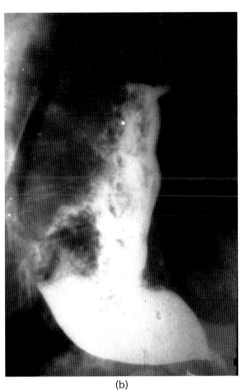

(a)   (b)

Figure 25.5 (a) Endoscopic finding and (b) barium esophagram in a patient with megaesophagus from chronic *Trypanosoma cruzi* infection (Chagas' disease). Source: Courtesy of Dr. Paulo Sakai, University of Sao Paulo Medical School, Sao Paulo, Brazil.

persistent, with regurgitation, aspiration, and weight loss (Figure 25.5). T-lymphocytic infiltration, myositis, enteric ganglionitis, and reduction of interstitial cells of Cajal have been described [25, 26]. Aperistalsis is a universal finding in patients with a megaesophagus. High-resolution esophageal manometric findings are similar to those in idiopathic achalasia, but the baseline LES pressure and swallowing-induced LES residual pressure are lower in Chagas' esophagus [27]. LES relaxation with swallowing can be normal in some patients with Chagas' disease.

Chronic infection can be detected by serum antibodies, but false-positive reaction may occur in connective-tissue diseases, leishmaniasis, malaria, and syphilis. Humoral response may not develop in some patients with chronic infection of *T. cruzi*, despite detection of the parasite's DNA by polymerase chain reaction (PCR) [28]. Medical treatment with benznidazole and nifurtimox eradicates *T. cruzi* in only <50% of patients, and the chronic clinical course is not affected. Laparoscopic myotomy has been successful in patients with Chagas' esophagus. In end-stage megaesophagus, surgical resection may be required, but perioperative mortality is significant [29]. Laparoscopic transhiatal subtotal esophagectomy through a left cervicotomy is a feasible approach, but surgical expertise is required [30].

Amyloidosis

Amyloidosis is a heterogeneous group of disorders caused by the deposition of insoluble fibril proteins that are resistant to proteolysis. There are six subtypes of amyloid: primary, secondary, hemodialysis-related, hereditary, senile, and localized. The most common is primary amyloidosis associated with amyloid light chain (AL) from primary idiopathic amyloidosis or multiple myeloma. Secondary amyloidosis (AA) is associated with various chronic inflammatory, infectious, and neoplastic diseases. The amyloid protein has been found in the esophagus and stomach within the mucosa, submucosa, and smooth muscle. The myenteric neural elements usually remain intact, but loss of interstitial cells of Cajal has been described in hereditary transthyretin (TTR) amyloidosis [31].

The most common site of GI involvement is the rectum, followed by the colon, small intestine, esophagus, and stomach. Only 8% of patients with primary amyloidosis have GI involvement, and only 1% have symptomatic gastric amyloidosis [32]. Upper GI symptoms of amyloidosis are non-specific (Table 25.4). Delayed gastric emptying has been described, but many patients do not have symptoms of gastroparesis [33]. Congo red staining of the endoscopic biopsies is often diagnostic, showing the characteristic apple-green birefringence under polarized light. Rectal biopsy and abdominal fat pad aspiration can be obtained if needed (Figure 25.6). Treatment of amyloidosis should be directed toward the primary cause, though effective treatment is not available.

Paraneoplastic Syndromes

Paraneoplastic syndromes encompass the remote effects of malignancy on various organ systems. Cancer cells express antigens mimicking neuronal tissues, thus producing an autoimmune response. Small-cell lung cancer accounts for approximately 80% of the paraneoplastic syndromes, followed by breast, ovarian, and Hodgkin's lymphoma. The myenteric plexus is infiltrated with lymphocytes and plasma cells associated with neuronal degeneration. The GI manifestations are very variable and often present before the cancer can be detected. Many patients may be misdiagnosed with primary achalasia or idiopathic gastroparesis. Paraneoplastic syndrome should be considered in patients with new onset of severe GI dysmotility of unclear etiology, especially in older individuals with

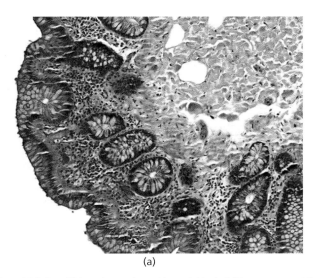
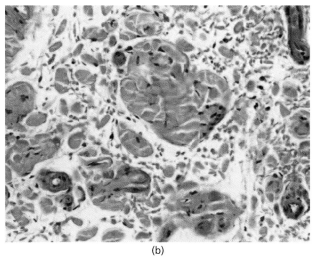

(a)   (b)

Figure 25.6 Rectal biopsy in a patient with amyloidosis. (a) Low-power and (b) high-power fields of light microscopy shows the pink, homogeneous protein deposit in the submucosa using routine hematoxylin and eosin staining. Source: Courtesy of Dr. Walter Jones, Floyd Memorial Hospital, New Albany, IN.

weight loss and in patients at risk for lung and breast cancers. Serum antineuronal antibodies may be present in some but not all patients with paraneoplastic involvement of the esophagus [34].

Cutaneous Syndromes

Many acquired and inherited cutaneous diseases may affect the oropharynx and the esophagus, since they share a similar stratified squamous epithelium (Table 25.5). The aim of this section is not to diagnose each of these dermatologic diseases, but to recognize the GI manifestations and to provide appropriate management and referral. Underlying causes should be identified in the acquired syndromes. The risk of oropharyngeal and GI cancers should be recognized.

Pemphigus

Pemphigus is a group of autoimmune intraepithelial blistering diseases involving the skin and mucous membrane. It may also affect the squamous mucosa of the oropharynx, larynx, esophagus, cervix, and anal canal. It is the result of the interaction between genetically predisposed individuals and an exogenous factor. Ethnic groups from the Mediterranean and South Asia are at increased risk. The autoantibodies of pemphigus disrupt the cell-to-cell adhesion to the epithelium, causing characteristic skin blisters, which may be several centimeters in size. Pemphigus vulgaris is the most common form, with painful oropharyngeal erosions (Figure 25.7), which may precede the skin blisters by weeks or months. Paraneoplastic pemphigus has been described in lymphoproliferative disorders, melanoma, carcinoid, and gastric, lung, and ovarian cancers.

Esophageal involvement may be present in patients with pemphigus vulgaris, despite a lack of esophageal symptoms [35]. Esophageal biopsy, using a "rocking" forcep to maximize the mucosal contact and the depth of the biopsy specimen, can identify the suprabasilar acanthosis by histology and intraepithelial immune complexes by immunofluorescence to diagnose pemphigus [36]. Indirect immunohistochemical staining can be performed from a paraffin block of past specimens.

Pemphigoid

Pemphigoid is a group of autoimmune subepithelial blistering diseases with autoantibodies disrupting the adhesion of the epithelium to the basement membrane, resulting in dermal–epidermal separation and skin blisters. Bullous pemphigoid affects older patients and is the most common autoimmune blistering disorder, but mucosal involvement is rare. Mucous-membrane pemphigoid (cicatricial pemphigoid) has a 2 : 1 predilection for women. Paraneoplastic pemphigoid has also been reported with lymphoma and with gastric and renal cancers. Esophageal manifestations of pemphigoid have been reported in case reports; they are similar to pemphigus. Desquamative gingivitis and conjunctivitis are common in mucous membrane pemphigoid. Cutaneous and mucosal scaring is more prominent. Esophageal biopsies can identify the subepithelial immune complexes of pemphigoid by immunohistology, in contrast to the intraepithelial deposits in patients with pemphigus.

Acquired and Inherited Epidermolysis Bullosa

Epidermolysis bullosa acquisita is an acquired mucocutaneous syndrome characterized by skin fragility and spontaneous and trauma-induced mucocutaneous blisters. It is associated with autoimmunity to type VII collagen, the anchoring protein for attachment of the epidermis to the dermis layer. Tense blisters tend to occur on trauma-prone areas, such as the palms, soles, elbows, and knees. Esophageal mucosa may be damaged by the endoscope itself.

Inherited epidermolysis bullosa is a group of rare inherited syndromes affecting children, with variable extracutaenous manifestations. Some children may have severe dysphagia with long and tight esophageal strictures, requiring multiple dilations and gastrostomy placement to provide enteral nutrition [37, 38]. The clinical and immunohistological findings of epidermolysis bullosa mimic mucous membrane pemphigoid, because they both cause subepithelial blisters.

Lichen Planus

Lichen planus is a chronic, presumed autoimmune, inflammatory disorder of the skin, nails, and mucous membrane. It causes mucocutaneous ulceration without blistering by a T-lymphocytic

Table 25.5 Cutaneous autoimmune diseases affecting the oropharynx and esophagus.

Clinical features	Diagnostic testing	Therapeutics
Pemphigus (pemphigus vulgaris, paraneoplastic, drug-induced)		
• Symptoms: oral and buccal burning, dysphagia, odynophagia, hematemesis, weight loss • Manifestations: blistering skin lesions, buccal mucositis (Figure 25.7), esophagitis dissecans superficialis, esophageal strictures, subglottic stenosis	• EGD: proximal esophageal bullae, raised white blisters, erosions, ulcers, webs, proximal stricture, linear furrows, white pseudomembrane, exfoliated mucosa sloughing • Histology: suprabasilar acantholysis (separation at the suprabasal level of epithelium), clumps of acantholytic cells within blister (Tzank cells), intraepithelial mononuclear inflammation, intraepithelial deposits of IgG and C3 in intercellular space by immunofluorescence • Serum: ELISA for anti-Dsg3 and anti-Dsg1 antibodies	• Identify and treat underlying cause, such as paraneoplastic, drugs (penicillamine, ACE-inhibitors, rifampin, fludarabine) • Treatment for pemphigus (steroid, immunomodulating agents) • Endoscopic dilation • Maintain nutrition
Pemphigoid (bullous pemphigoid, mucous membrane pemphigoid, paraneoplastic, drug-induced)		
• Symptoms: similar to pemphigus • Manifestations: similar to pemphigus, except more prominent oral ulcers, desquamative gingivitis, conjunctivitis, eruptions may be generalized	• EGD: similar to pemphigus • Biopsy: subepithelial mononuclear inflammation, subepithelial deposits of IgG, IgA, and C3 along basement membrane zone by immunofluorescence • Serum: ELISA for bullous pemphigoid antigen-2 antibodies	• Identify and treat underlying cause, such as paraneoplastic, drugs (penicillamine, ACE-inhibitors, rifampin, fludarabine) • Treatment for pemphigoid (steroid, dapsone, others)
Epidermolysis bullosa (acquired, inherited)		
• Symptoms: similar to pemphigus; children with inherited epidermolysis bullosa may have severe dysphagia and malnutrition • Manifestations: similar to pemphigus, mechanical or trauma-induced skin and mucosal blisters with scarring	• EGD: similar to pemphigus; endoscope may cause further mucosa damage • Biopsy: similar to pemphigus • Serum: antibodies for basement membrane zone antibody	• Identify and treat underlying cause, such as amyloidosis, multiple myeloma, IBD • Dilation may induce mucosal bullae
Lichen planus		
• Symptoms: oral pain, dysphagia, odynophagia, weight loss • Manifestations: non-blistering skin lesions, nail changes, similar to pemphigus but always associated with oral lichen planus	• EGD: can involve proximal and distal esophagus, esophageal lacy white (patches) papules, pinpoint erosions, desquamation, pseudomembrane, stricture of proximal esophagus • Biopsy: prominent band-like lymphohistocytic infiltration of the epithelium and lamina propria, cytotoxic T-cells (CD 8 staining), Civatte bodies (apoptosis of keratinocytes)	• Exclude secondary lichenoid esophagitis from hepatitis C, HIV, medications (chloroquine, methyldopa, penicillamine), syphilis • Topical: corticosteroids, calcineurin inhibitors • Phototherapy • Systemic treatment: steroids, cyclosporine, thalidomide, mycophenolate mofetil, TNF-α inhibitors (etanercept, adalimumab)

EGD, esophagogastroduodenoscopy; IgG, immunoglobulin G; ELISA, enzyme-linked immunosorbent assay; ACE, angiotensin-converting enzyme; IgA, immunoglobulin A; IBD, inflammatory bowel disease; HIV, human immunodeficiency virus; TNF, tumor necrosis factor.

cell-mediated response against the basal epithelium. The mean age of onset is 40–50 years old. The skin findings consist of the five Ps of lichen planus: **p**ruritic, **p**lanar (flat), **p**olygonal, and **p**urple **p**apules. There are various forms of lichen planus, from a few localized lesions to a more generalized eruption.

Esophageal lichen planus causes proximal esophageal ulceration and strictures, and distal esophageal involvement has been reported [39]. It is mostly found in women and is often misdiagnosed as reflux esophagitis. Using magnification chromoendoscopy, esophageal lichen planus may be more common than previously recognized [40]. Histology of esophageal lichen planus is characterized by striking epithelium apoptosis and a band-like lymphohistocytic inflammation at the interface of the squamous epithelium and lamina propria. Esophageal lichen planus should be differentiated from lichenoid esophagitis of various infections (Table 25.5) [41]. Malignant transformation to oral and esophageal squamous carcinomas has been reported in patients with mucosal lichen planus.

Cutaneous Hyperkeratosis Syndromes

Cutaneous hyperkeratosis syndromes are rare inherited or acquired disorders with a thickening of the skin and squamous mucosa with or without hyperpigmentation (Table 25.6). Mucosa hyperkeratosis may be present with an acellular keratin layer on the stratified squamous epithelium of the oropharynx and esophagus. These hyperkeratosis syndromes should be differentiated from isolated esophageal hyperkeratosis associated with squamous papilloma, papilloma from human papilloma virus, vitamin A deficiency, and GERD [42].

Endoscopy may be the first sign of the syndrome, finding esophageal and gastric benign or malignant lesions. It is important to recognize these syndromes, because patients are at risk for developing GI and other systemic cancers. Management depends on making the right diagnosis, identifying the underlying cause, providing proper surveillance, and providing genetic counseling for the family.

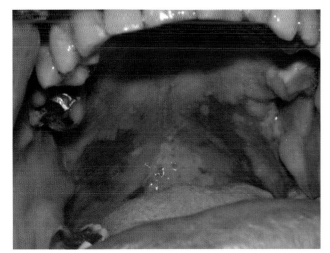

Figure 25.7 Oral ulceration and buccal mucositis in a patient with pemphigus vulgaris. Source: Courtesy of Dr. Jeff Callen, University of Louisville, Louisville, KY.

Table 25.6 Cutaneous hyperkeratosis syndromes involving the esophagus and stomach.

Summary	Clinical features	Diagnostic testing	Therapeutics
Hyperkeratosis plantaris and palmaris (tylosis) • Rare, autosomal-dominant inherited mucocutaneous syndrome • Tylosis-esophageal cancer gene on chromosome 17q25 locus • Lifetime risk for esophageal squamous carcinoma is very high in affected family members	• Symptoms: may be asymptomatic, dysphagia, weight loss • Manifestations: symmetric focal or diffuse hyperkeratosis of palms and soles, pruritic and painful dermal fissures, esophageal and oral cancers	• EGD: esophageal patchy or confluent smooth areas with raised edges, fissures, esophageal cancer; NBI with magnification with distorted intrapapillary capillary loop changes showing dysplasia [43] • Biopsy: acellular keratin on squamous epithelium	• Surveillance for esophageal cancer for at-risk family members • Genetic counseling
Acanthosis nigricans • Rare acquired syndrome with or without hyperpigmentation • Paraneoplastic is common (gastric, uterine, liver, renal, breast, and lung cancer) • Cancer secretes tumor growth factors to mimic epidermal growth factor • May progress to oral and esophageal squamous cancers	• Symptoms: may be asymptomatic, dysphagia, weight loss • Manifestations: small, hyperpigmented raised plaques of flexor surfaces (palm, neck, arms, axilla), esophageal papillomas, esophageal squamous cancer	• EGD: similar to tylosis, esophageal papillomatosis, esophageal cancer • Biopsy: papilloma, no significant inflammation	• Identify and treat underlying cause (scleroderma, dermatomyositis, lupus, paraneoplastic from gastric cancer)
Multiple hamartoma syndrome (Cowden's syndrome) • Autosomal-dominant inheritance, mutation of PTEN tumor-suppressor gene on chromosome 10q23 • Increased cancer risk for breast, thyroid, uterus, colon • Mixed upper and lower GI polyps (hyperplastic and hemartomas) [44]	• Symptoms: dysphagia, abdominal pain, GI bleeding • Manifestations: hyperkeratosis of soles, palms, oropharyngeal papillomas, hamartomas (GI tract, breast, thyroid, skin, uterus)	• EGD: esophageal and gastric polyps • Biopsy: epithelial hyperplasia, hemartomas, esophageal glycogen acanthosis	• Identify and screen for cancers • Genetic testing available • Genetic counseling for patient and family
Dyskeratosis congenita • Congenital syndromes with variable inheritance • Telomerase deficiency, resulting in accelerated cell loss (skin, mucosal lining) • Increased risk for bone-marrow failure and cancer	• Symptoms: dysphagia, fatigue • Manifestations: skin pigmentation, nail dystrophy, oral leucoplakia, esophageal strictures	• EGD: proximal esophageal webs	• Endoscopic dilation • Genetic counseling for patient and family
Acrokeratosis paraneoplastica (Bazex syndrome) • Rare, acquired paraneoplastic cutaneous syndrome • Skin lesion may precede aerodigestive tract cancer (oral cavity, larynx, pharynx, lung, esophagus) • Affects mostly men	• Symptoms: asymptomatic, dysphagia • Manifestations: scaly, psoriasis-like skin lesions of the ears, nose, hands, feet, nails; hyperkeratosis of plaques of palms, soles	• EGD: primary esophageal cancer	• Identify and treat underlying cancer • Skin lesions improve with cancer treatment

EGD, esophagogastroduodenoscopy; NBI, narrow-band imaging; GI, gastrointestinal; PTEN, phosphatase and tensin homolog gene.

CHAPTER 25

Take Home Points

- Gastroesophageal reflux disease (GERD), esophageal aperistalsis, gastroparesis, and chronic intestinal pseudo-obstruction (CIP) are gastrointestinal (GI) manifestations of systemic sclerosis (SSc).
- There is a threefold increase in the risk of cancer in patients with dermatomyositis, especially for ovarian, lung, pancreatic, stomach, and colorectal cancers and non-Hodgkin's lymphoma.
- Crohn's disease, Behçet's disease, and sarcoidosis are systemic inflammatory diseases that affect the esophagus and stomach.
- The esophagus is affected in 7–10% of chronic *T. cruzi*-infected individuals in areas endemic with Chagas' disease.
- Neuromuscular diseases represent a category of acquired and primary disorders affecting the motor neurons, peripheral nerves, neuromuscular junctions, and muscles. Any abnormality involving the parasympathetic, sympathetic, and enteric nervous systems can affect the esophagus and stomach.
- Paraneoplastic syndrome should be considered in patients with new onset of severe GI dysmotility of unclear cause, especially in older individuals with weight loss and in patients at risk for lung and breast cancer.

References

1 Abell TL, Camilleri M, Donohoe K, *et al.* Consensus recommendations for gastric emptying scintigraphy: a joint report of the American Neurogastroenterology and Motility Society and the Society of Nuclear Medicine. *Am J Gastroenterol* 2007; **102**: 1–11.

2 Ioannidis JP, Vlachoyiannopoulos PG, Haidich AB, *et al.* Mortality in systemic sclerosis: an international meta-analysis of individual patient data. *Am J Med* 2005; **118**: 2–10.

3 Omair MA, Lee P. Effect of gastrointestinal manifestations on quality of life in 87 consecutive patients with systemic sclerosis. *J Rheumatol* 2012; **39**: 992–6.

4 Bodukam V, Hays RD, Maranian P, *et al.* Association of gastrointestinal involvement and depressive symptoms in patients with systemic sclerosis. *Rheumatology (Oxford)* 2011; **50**: 330–4.

5 Marie I, Ducrotte P, Denis P, *et al.* Oesophageal mucosal involvement in patients with systemic sclerosis receiving proton pump inhibitor therapy. *Aliment Pharmacol Ther* 2006; **24**: 1593–601.

6 Zhang XJ, Bonner A, Hudson M, *et al.* Association of gastroesophageal factors and worsening of forced vital capacity in systemic sclerosis. *J Rheumatol* 2013; **40**: 850–8.

7 Marie I, Gourcerol G, Leroi AM, *et al.* Delayed gastric emptying determined using the 13C-octanoic acid breath test in patients with systemic sclerosis. *Arthritis Rheum* 2012; **64**: 2346–55.

8 Azuma K, Yamada H, Ohkubo M, *et al.* Incidence and predictive factors for malignancies in 136 Japanese patients with dermatomyositis, polymyositis and clinically amyopathic dermatomyositis. *Mod Rheumatol* 2011; **21**: 178–83.

9 So MW, Koo BS, Kim YG, *et al.* Idiopathic inflammatory myopathy associated with malignancy: a retrospective cohort of 151 Korean patients with dermatomyositis and polymyositis. *J Rheumatol* 2011; **38**: 2432–5.

10 Oh TH, Brumfield KA, Hoskin TL, *et al.* Dysphagia in inflammatory myopathy: clinical characteristics, treatment strategies, and outcome in 62 patients. *Mayo Clin Proc* 2007; **82**: 441–7.

11 Oh TH, Brumfield KA, Hoskin TL, *et al.* Dysphagia in inclusion body myositis: clinical features, management, and clinical outcome. *Am J Phys Med Rehabil* 2008; **87**: 883–9.

12 Dobloug C, Walle-Hansen R, Gran JT, *et al.* Long-term follow-up of sporadic inclusion body myositis treated with intravenous immunoglobulin: a retrospective study of 16 patients. *Clin Exp Rheumatol* 2012; **30**: 838–42.

13 Marie I, Menard JF, Hatron PY, *et al.* Intravenous immunoglobulins for steroid-refractory esophageal involvement related to polymyositis and dermatomyositis: a series of 73 patients. *Arthritis Care Res (Hoboken)* 2010; **62**: 1748–55.

14 Marshall JB, Kretschmar JM, Gerhardt DC, *et al.* Gastrointestinal manifestations of mixed connective tissue disease. *Gastroenterol* 1990; **98**: 1232–8.

15 Maldonado ME, Perez M, Pignac-Kobinger J, *et al.* Clinical and immunologic manifestations of mixed connective tissue disease in a Miami population compared to a Midwestern US Caucasian population. *J Rheumatol* 2008; **35**: 429–37.

16 Fagundes MN, Caleiro MT, Navarro-Rodriguez T, *et al.* Esophageal involvement and interstitial lung disease in mixed connective tissue disease. *Respir Med* 2009; **103**: 854–60.

17 Mandl T, Ekberg O, Wollmer P, *et al.* Dysphagia and dysmotility of the pharynx and oesophagus in patients with primary Sjogren's syndrome. *Scand J Rheumatol* 2007; **36**: 394–401.

18 Hershcovici T, Jha LK, Gadam R, *et al.* The relationship between type 2 diabetes mellitus and failure to proton pump inhibitor treatment in gastroesophageal reflux disease. *J Clin Gastroenterol* 2012; **46**: 662–8.

19 Yaylali O, Kirac S, Yilmaz M, *et al.* Does hypothyroidism affect gastrointestinal motility? *Gastroenterol Res Pract* 2009; **Article ID** 529802.

20 Tozzoli R, Kodermaz G, Perosa AR, *et al.* Autoantibodies to parietal cells as predictors of atrophic body gastritis: a five-year prospective study in patients with autoimmune thyroid diseases. *Autoimmun Rev* 2010; **10**: 80–3.

21 Barczynski M, Thor P. Reversible autonomic dysfunction in hyperthyroid patients affects gastric myoelectrical activity and emptying. *Clin Auton Res* 2001; **11**: 243–9.

22 Ammoury RF, Pfefferkorn MD. Significance of esophageal Crohn disease in children. *J Pediatr Gastroenterol Nutr* 2011; **52**: 291–4.

23 Nobrega AC, Ferreira BR, Oliveira GJ, *et al.* Dyspeptic symptoms and delayed gastric emptying of solids in patients with inactive Crohn's disease. *BMC Gastroenterol* 2012; **12**: 175.

24 Annema JT, Veselic M, Rabe KF. Endoscopic ultrasound-guided fine-needle aspiration for the diagnosis of sarcoidosis. *Eur Respir J* 2005; **25**: 405–9.

25 Cobo EC, Silveira TP, Micheletti AM, *et al.* Research on *Trypanosoma cruzi* and analysis of inflammatory infiltrate in esophagus and colon from chronic chagasic patients with and without mega. *J Trop Med* 2012; **2012**: 232646.

26 Carlucci W, Ceneviva R, Ferreira SH, *et al.* Histological, biochemical and pharmacological characterization of the gastric muscular layer in Chagas disease. *Acta Cir Bras* 2011; **26**(Suppl. 2): 74–8.

27 Vicentine FP, Herbella FA, Allaix ME, *et al.* Comparison of idiopathic achalasia and Chagas' disease esophagopathy at the light of high-resolution manometry. *Dis Esophagus* 2014; **27**(2): 128–33.

28 Batista AM, Aguiar C, Almeida EA, *et al.* Evidence of Chagas disease in seronegative Brazilian patients with megaesophagus. *Int J Infect Dis* 2010; **14**: e974–7.

29 Pinotti HW, Felix VN, Zilberstein B, *et al.* Surgical complications of Chagas' disease: megaesophagus, achalasia of the pylorus, and cholelithiasis. *World J Surg* 1991; **15**: 198–204.

30 Crema E, Ribeiro LB, Terra JA Jr., *et al.* Laparoscopic transhiatal subtotal esophagectomy for the treatment of advanced megaesophagus. *Ann Thorac Surg* 2005; **80**: 1196–201.

31 Wixner J, Obayashi K, Ando Y, *et al.* Loss of gastric interstitial cells of Cajal in patients with hereditary transthyretin amyloidosis. *Amyloid* 2013; **20**: 99–106.

32 Menke DM, Kyle RA, Fleming CR, *et al.* Symptomatic gastric amyloidosis in patients with primary systemic amyloidosis. *Mayo Clin Proc* 1993; **68**: 763–7.

33 Wixner J, Karling P, Rydh A, *et al.* Gastric emptying in hereditary transthyretin amyloidosis: the impact of autonomic neuropathy. *Neurogastroenterol Motil* 2012; **24**: 1111–e568.

34 Katzka DA, Farrugia G, Arora AS. Achalasia secondary to neoplasia: a disease with a changing differential diagnosis. *Dis Esophagus* 2012; **25**: 331–6.

35 Su O, Onsun N, Meric TA, *et al.* Upper airway tract and upper gastrointestinal tract involvement in patients with pemphigus vulgaris. *Eur J Dermatol* 2010; **20**: 792–6.

36 Galloro G, Diamantis G, Magno L, *et al.* Technical aspects in endoscopic biopsy of lesions in esophageal pemphigus vulgaris. *Dig Liver Dis* 2007; **39**: 363–7.

37 Fantauzzi RS, Maia MO, Cunha FC, *et al.* Otorhinolaryngological and esophageal manifestations of epidermolysis bullosa. *Braz J Otorhinolaryngol* 2008; **74**: 657–61.

38 Haynes L, Mellerio JE, Martinez AE. Gastrostomy tube feeding in children with epidermolysis bullosa: consideration of key issues. *Pediatr Dermatol* 2012; **29**: 277–84.

39 Katzka DA, Smyrk TC, Bruce AJ, *et al.* Variations in presentations of esophageal involvement in lichen planus. *Clin Gastroenterol Hepatol* 2010; **8**: 777–82.

40 Quispel R, van Boxel OS, Schipper ME, *et al.* High prevalence of esophageal involvement in lichen planus: a study using magnification chromoendoscopy. *Endosc* 2009; **41**: 187–93.

41 Salaria SN, Abu Alfa AK, Cruise MW, *et al.* Lichenoid esophagitis: clinicopathologic overlap with established esophageal lichen planus. *Am J Surg Pathol* 2013; **37**: 1889–94.

42 Taggart MW, Rashid A, Ross WA, *et al.* Oesophageal hyperkeratosis: clinicopathological associations. *Histopathology* 2013; **63**(4): 463–73.

43 Smart H, Kia R, Subramanian S, *et al.* Defining the endoscopic appearances of tylosis using conventional and narrow-band imaging: a case series. *Endosc* 2011; **43**: 727–30.

44 Heald B, Mester J, Rybicki L, *et al.* Frequent gastrointestinal polyps and colorectal adenocarcinomas in a prospective series of PTEN mutation carriers. *Gastroenterol* 2010; **139**: 1927–33.

PART 6

Functional Disease of the Esophagus and Stomach

26 Functional Esophageal Disorders, 169
  Ellionore Jarbrink-Sehgal, Kenneth R. DeVault, and Nicholas J. Talley

Functional Esophageal Disorders

Ellionore Jarbrink-Sehgal,[1] Kenneth R. DeVault,[2] and Nicholas J. Talley[3]

[1] Baylor College of Medicine, Houston, TX, USA
[2] Division of Gastroenterology and Hepatology, Mayo Clinic, Jacksonville, FL, USA
[3] Faculty of Health, University of Newcastle, Newcastle, NSW, Australia

Summary

Functional esophageal disorders (FEDs) affect a large proportion of the population and represent a major clinical challenge. The FEDs are defined by chronic symptoms suggestive of esophageal disease without identifiable structural or mucosal abnormalities. They comprises four major disorders: functional heartburn (FH), functional chest pain of presumed esophageal origin (FCP), functional dysphagia, and globus.

Prior to diagnosing any FED, gastroesophageal reflux disease (GERD) and primary esophageal motility abnormalities should be excluded. The etiology and pathogenesis of these disorders is poorly understood and likely multifactorial. Visceral hypersensitivity to acid or other stimuli is one of the main theories in pathogenesis. Current management strategies are based on limited evidence.

Case

A 49-year-old female pharmacist presents for evaluation of frequent and persistent retrosternal heartburn and regurgitation for more than 9 months. She was initially treated with omeprazole 20 mg daily (40 minutes prior to breakfast) for 8 weeks. Since she did not respond, her physician increased omeprazole to 20 mg twice daily (40 minutes before breakfast and dinner). After an additional 8 weeks of therapy, she seeks consultation for unabated symptoms. An esophagogastroduodenoscopy (EGD) is performed and shows normal results. Esophageal biopsies are negative for eosinophilic esophagitis. A pH impedance test reveals excellent acid inhibition on double-dose proton pump inhibitor (PPI) therapy, no evidence of non-acid reflux, and multiple symptomatic episodes, none correlating with acid or non-acid reflux. An esophageal motility test and a gastric emptying study at 4 hours are normal. A diagnosis of functional heartburn is made.

Definitions

FEDs represent chronic symptoms suggestive of esophageal disease without identifiable structural or mucosal abnormalities. There are four categories [1, 2]:

1 **Functional heartburn (FH):** Heartburn and regurgitation, but with normal endoscopy, normal acid contact time on pH testing, and negative symptom index correlation.
2 **Functional chest pain of presumed esophageal origin (FCP):** Midline chest pain that is not of burning quality, absence of evidence that GERD is the cause of symptoms, and absence of histopathology-based esophageal motility disorders.
3 **Functional dysphagia:** An abnormal sensation of bolus transit through the esophagus body in the absence of GERD, structural lesions, and motility disorders.
4 **Globus:** A persistent or intermittent, non-painful sensation of a lump or foreign body in the throat. It is episodic, frequently improved with food intake, with absent dysphagia or odynophagia (and there is no evidence for gastroesophageal reflux as the cause of symptoms and absence of histopathology based esophageal motility disorders).

All functional gastrointestinal (GI) disorders have in common that they are chronic; that is, symptoms last for at least 3 months, with symptom onset at least 6 months prior to diagnosis.

Epidemiology

Limited epidemiological data exists on FEDs. Further, differentiation of FH from non-erosive reflux disease (NERD) is poor and the actual prevalence of FH remains undetermined. However, a US household national survey (n = 5430) showed that up to 69% of the population reported suffering from at least one of 20 possible functional digestive symptoms, with 42% specifically complaining of possible functional esophageal symptoms (heartburn in 32.6% and dysphagia in 7.5%) [3]. Globus is a common symptom and has been reported by up to 46% of apparently healthy individuals, with a peak incidence in middle age and with three of four subjects seeking health care being women [4].

Pathophysiology

The etiology of FH and FCP is unknown. One of the main theories for both disorders is visceral hypersensitivity, with defective sensory perception at the esophageal or central nervous system (CNS) level. Other proposed causes include: increased susceptibility of the esophageal mucosa to reflux from acid, disrupting the intercellular connections of the squamous esophageal mucosa and exposing nociceptive nerve fibers; and non-acid triggering factors such as stress and longitudinal muscle contraction of the esophagus. Longitudinal muscle contraction of the esophagus, detected by intraluminal ultrasound, has been found to produce the sensation of heartburn [5].

Practical Gastroenterology and Hepatology Board Review Toolkit, Second Edition. Edited by Nicholas J. Talley, Kenneth R. DeVault, Michael B. Wallace, Bashar A. Aqel and Keith D. Lindor.

Among patients with esophageal symptoms refractory to PPI therapy, pH impedance on medication suggests refractory acid reflux explains symptoms in 11% of cases. By contrast, non-acid reflux events potentially explains symptoms in 31% [6]. The preponderance of "non-acid events" is understandable as this study reports pH testing on PPIs, which should drastically decrease acid-associated events. These observations underscore the role of mechanisms other than acid or non-acid reflux in causing symptoms and help explain the heterogeneous response of patients with NERD to acid-suppressive therapy.

The mechanism underlying functional dysphagia is poorly understood. Intraesophageal balloon-distension studies have shown an increased threshold perception consistent with a defect in visceral sensitivity [7]. Other studies using balloon-distension techniques have shown both reproduction of dysphagia and generation of abnormal motility patterns, suggesting a defect in the neural circuit of the esophagus [8]. A number of investigators have reproduced patients' dysphagia and identified an abnormal esophageal motor response during food-provoked but not water-provoked swallows [9]. In addition, patients with non-obstructive dysphagia show a defect in the triggering of secondary peristalsis and functional clearance by impedance manometry [10,11]. Increased stress can also induce abnormal esophageal motility responses [12], but no direct link to functional dysphagia exists.

Clinical Features and Diagnosis

Functional Heartburn

Heartburn is defined as burning retrosternal discomfort that may radiate toward the neck and is typically worst postprandially, during exercise, or in a supine position [1]. Heartburn is a typical symptom of GERD, and hence a PPI trial is recommended as the first step. If symptoms persist without alarm symptoms (dysphagia, odynophagia, anorexia, weight loss, or upper GI bleeding) despite a compliant patient, then doubling the dose of PPI or switching to a different PPI is often recommended, though well-designed trials proving the efficacy of this approach are lacking. If symptoms persist, ambulatory esophageal pH testing is helpful in excluding GERD and differentiating between NERD and FH. It is the general consensus of most experts that taking patients off reflux medications prior to such testing provides the greatest diagnostic yield [13].

Functional Chest Pain

Patients typically present after extensive cardiac workup for further evaluation. Treatment for esophageal spasm was often suggested in the past, but current data indicate that GERD is a more common etiology. Hence, an accepted initial management includes an empiric trial of high-dose (twice-daily) PPI. If symptoms persist, endoscopy, pH, or impedance-pH testing with symptom-association analyses and manometry can be used to exclude GERD and motility disorders.

Functional Dysphagia

Dysphagia is an alarm symptom. Hence, initial workup should include EGD or a radio-opaque bolus-challenge barium swallow to exclude intrinsic structural-related lesions (strictures, web, tumor, etc.) and GERD. Biopsies at endoscopy are recommended to exclude eosinophilic esophagitis. A carefully obtained barium swallow with a solid bolus may help confirm FD, especially if the patient reports dysphagia despite normal bolus transit (including solids). If these studies are non-diagnostic, esophageal manometry should be considered to exclude motility disorders (achalasia, distal esophageal spasm (DES), nutcracker or jackhammer esophagus). If the patient has reflux symptoms despite negative workup, a PPI trial or ambulatory pH testing is a reasonable diagnostic/therapeutic alternative [4].

Globus

Globus is a relatively benign condition. The main differential diagnoses include coexisting dysphagia, extrinsic causes, and GERD. Hence, a workup with a comprehensive history and a physical, directed workup including ear, nose, and throat (ENT) evaluation, EGD, and a PPI trial are sufficient [4].

Differential Diagnosis

Table 26.1 illustrates the differential diagnosis for FEDs.

Therapeutics

Functional Heartburn

Treatment of FH (where PPIs have failed) remains poorly studied [4]. As severe sustained stress exposure has been linked to

Table 26.1 Differential diagnosis and diagnostic tools.

		Differential diagnosis	Diagnostic tools
Functional esophageal disorder	Functional heartburn (FH)	GERD (high acid exposure and positive symptom associations)	PPI trial
		NERD (normal acid exposure but positive symptom association)	EGD
		Esophageal motor disorder (achalasia, DES)	Ambulatory or impedance pH test
			Esophageal manometry
	Functional chest pain of presumed esophageal origin (FCP)	Cardiac etiology	Cardiac diagnostics
		GERD	PPI trial, high-dose
		Esophageal motor disorder (nutcracker, DES)	EGD
			Ambulatory pH test
			Esophageal manometry
	Functional dysphagia	Intrinsic structural lesions (strictures, web, tumor)	EGD with biopsies
		Eosinophilic esophagitis	Barium swallow
		Esophageal motor disorder (achalasia, DES, aperistalsis)	Esophageal manometry
		Cricopharyngeal bar, Zenkers diverticulum	Video swallow
	Globus	Coexisting dysphagia	Extensive H&P
		GERD	EGD
			ENT evaluation

GERD, gastroesophageal reflux disease; NERD, non-erosive reflux disease; DES, diffuse esophageal spasm; PPI, proton pump inhibitor; EGD, esophgaoduodenoscopy; ENT, ear, nose, and throat.

increased heartburn, relaxation training has been recommended. However, its efficacy is in patients with GERD but not FH. Pharmacological options include esophageal pain modulators (tricyclic antidepressants (TCAs) and selective serotonin reuptake inhibitors (SSRIs)), which have shown efficacy in hypersensitivity esophagus [14].

Functional Chest Pain

Current treatment options are similar to those for FH. In patients with reflux excluded as an etiology, management options include: (i) pharmacotherapy, (ii) cognitive behavioral therapy (CBT), and (iii) hypnotherapy. Pharmacotherapy includes esophageal pain modulators such as theophylline a TCA (imipramine) or sertraline; and venlafaxine (serotonin-norepinephrine reuptake inhibitors (SNRIs)) have both shown significant symptom improvement on randomized controlled trials (RCTs) but have limited use due to side effects [15]. CBT may be superior to placebo in pain relief and autonomic symptoms [16]. Hypnotherapy may reduce pain intensity and provide improvement in overall well-being [17].

Functional Dysphagia

No RCTs for the management of patients with FD exists. Anecdotal therapies include reassurance, careful food mastication, and avoidance of any precipitating factors. Pain modulators such as low-dose trazodone, TCAs, and SSRIs may have an effect in hypersensitive esophagus. Another therapeutic option is empiric dilation, which has been shown to be helpful in some, but not all studies [18,19].

Globus

Explanation, reassurance, empiric trials of antidepressants, and speech therapy may be of help. However, 45% remain symptomatic at 7–8 years' follow-up. Reassurance of the benign nature of the symptom may be of benefit.

Take Home Points

- Functional esophageal disorders (FEDs) include functional heartburn (FH), functional chest pain (FCP), functional dysphagia, and globus sensation and are diagnoses by exclusion.
- Overlap and coexistence with other functional gastrointestinal (GI) disorders may occur.
- Pathogenesis is still unknown, but visceral hypersensitivity likely plays a role.
- Cognitive behavioral therapy (CBT), pain modulators (tricyclic antidepressants, selective serotonin reuptake inhibitors (SSRIs), and serotonin-norepinephrine reuptake inhibitors (SNRIs)) can reduce pain levels in a hypersensitive esophagus (e.g., FH or FCP).
- Globus (which is benign) should not be confused with dysphagia.
- Empiric dilatation is not of proven value in functional dysphagia.

References

1 Vakil N, van Zanten SV, Kahrilas P, *et al.* The Montreal definition and classification of gastroesophageal reflux disease: a global evidence-based consensus. *Am J Gastroenterol* 2006; **101**(8): 1900–20.

2 Galmiche JP CLouse RE, Balint A, *et al.* Functional esophageal disorders. *Gastroenterology* 2006; **130**: 1459–65.

3 Drossman DA, Li Z, Andruzzi E, *et al.* US householder survey of functional gastrointestinal disorders. Prevalence, sociodemography, and health impact. *Dig Dis Sci* 1993; **38**: 1569–80.

4 Kumar AR, Katz PO. Functional esophageal disorders: a review of diagnosis and management. *Expert Rev Gastroenterol Hepatol* 2013; **7**(5): 453–61.

5 Mittal RK. Longitudinal muscle of the esophagus: its role in esophageal health and disease.*Curr Opin Gastroenterol* 2013; **29**: 421–30.

6 Mainie I, Tutuian R, Shay S, *et al.* Acid and non-acid reflux in patients with persistent symptoms despite acid suppressive therapy: a multicentre study using combined ambulatory impedance-pH monitoring. *Gut* 2006; **55**: 1398–402.

7 Bohn B, Bonaz B, Gueddah N, *et al.* Oesophageal motor and sensitivity abnormalities in non-obstructive dysphagia. *Eur J Gastroenterol Hepatol* 2002; **14**: 271–7.

8 Deschner WK, Maher KA, Cattau EL Jr, *et al.* Manometric responses to balloon distention in patients with nonobstructive dysphagia. *Gastroenterology* 1989; **97**: 1181–5.

9 Cordier L, Bohn B, Bonaz B, *et al.* Evaluation of esophageal motility disorders triggered by ingestion of solids in the case of non-obstructive dysphagia. *Gastroenterologie Clinique Biologique* 1999; **23**: 200–6.

10 Schoeman MN, Holloway RH. Secondary oesophageal peristalsis in patients with non-obstructive dysphagia. *Gut* 1994; **35**: 1523–8.

11 Chen CL, Szczesniak MM, Cook IJ. Identification of impaired oesophageal bolus transit and clearance by secondary peristalsis in patients with non-obstructive dysphagia. *Neurogastroenterol Motil* 2008; **20**: 980–8.

12 Valori RM. Nutcracker, neurosis, or sampling bias? *Gut* 1990; **31**: 736–7.

13 Richter JE, Pandolfino JE, Vela MF, *et al.* Utilization of wireless pH monitoring technologies: a summary of the proceedings from the Esophageal Diagnostic Working Group. *Dis Esophagus* 2013; **8**: 755–65.

14 Weijenborgn PW, de Schepper HS, Smout AMPM, Bredenoord AJ. Effects of antidepressants in patients with functional esophageal disorders or gastroesophageal reflux disease: a systematic review. *Clin Gastroenterol Hepatol* 2015; **13**: 260–2.

15 Coss-Adame E, Erdogan A, Rao SSC. Treatment of esophageal (noncardiac) chest pain: an expert review. *Clin Gastroenterol Hepatol* 2014; **12**: 1224–45.

16 Chambers JB, Marks EM, Russel V, Hunter MS. A multidisciplinary, biopsychosocial treatment for non-cardiac chest pain. *Int J Clin Pract* 2015; **69**(9): 922–7.

17 Adachi R, Fujino H, Hakae A, *et al.* A meta-analysis of hypnosis for chronic pain problems: a comparison between hypnosis, standard care and other psychological interventions. *Int J Clin Exp Hypn* 2014; **62**: 1–18.

18 Colon VJ, Young MA, Ramirez FC. The short- and long-term effiacy of empirical esophageal dilation in patients with nonobstructive dysphagia: a prospective, randomized study. *Am J Gastroenterol* 2000; **95**: 910–13.

19 Scolapio JS, Goustout CJ, Schroeder KW, *et al.* Dysphagia without endoscopically evident disease: to dilate or not. *Am J Gastroenterol* 2001; **96**: 327–30.

SECTION III

Intestine and Pancreas

Editor Michael Wallace

Part 1 Pathobiology of the Intestine and Pancreas, 175

Part 2 Problem-Based Approach to Diagnosis and Differential Diagnosis, 201

Part 3 Diseases of the Small Intestine, 271

Part 4 Diseases of the Colon and Rectum, 321

Part 5 Diseases of the Pancreas, 369

Part 6 Functional Diseases of the Small and Large Intestine, 389

Part 7 Transplantation, 415

PART 1

Pathobiology of the Intestine and Pancreas

27 Clinical Anatomy, Embryology, and Congenital Anomalies, 177
Advitya Malhotra and Joseph H. Sellin

28 Small-Intestinal Hormones and Neurotransmitters, 181
James Reynolds

29 Mucosal Immunology of the Intestine, 187
Maneesh Dave and William A. Faubion

30 Motor and Sensory Function, 191
Vineet S. Gudsoorkar and Eamonn M.M. Quigley

31 Neoplasia, 198
John M. Carethers

CHAPTER 27

Clinical Anatomy, Embryology, and Congenital Anomalies

Advitya Malhotra[1] and Joseph H. Sellin[2]

[1]Coastal Gastroenterology Associates PA, Webster, TX, USA
[2]Division of Gastroenterology, Baylor College of Medicine, Houston, TX, USA

Summary

As clinicians and educators we update ourselves routinely with various aspects of our practicing field. Mainly, the focus is centered on the pathogenesis, diagnosis, and management aspects of the clinical problem. Rarely, we delve in to the anatomy of the organ system responsible for the presentation. However, some embryological anomalies can present in later decades of life and present unexpected and difficult challenges in both diagnosis and management. Hence, a practical working knowledge on this subject is critical for the clinical gastroenterologist.

We have compiled a chapter that deals succinctly with the clinical anatomy, embryology, and congenital anomalies of the gastrointestinal (GI) tract. The main body of the chapter is in line with the evolving division of the GI tract of the embryo into foregut, midgut, and the hindgut. We briefly cover the anatomy, embryogenesis, and the congenital anomalies of each derivative of the germ layer starting from the foregut, and ending with the Hirschsprung disease (HSCR), a congenital anomaly of the ganglion cells of the hindgut. Some of the more commonly seen anomalies, such as pancreas divisum (PD), are dealt in detail wherever required.

Small and Large Intestine

Anatomy and Embryogenesis

At 4 weeks of gestation, the alimentary tract is divided into three parts: foregut, midgut, and hindgut. The duodenum originates from the terminal portion of the foregut and cephalic part of the midgut. With rotation of the stomach, the duodenum becomes C-shaped and rotates to the right. The midgut gives rise to the duodenum distal to the ampulla, to the entire small bowel, and to the cecum, appendix, ascending colon, and the proximal two-thirds of the transverse colon. The distal third of the transverse colon, the descending colon and sigmoid, the rectum, and the upper part of the anal canal originate from the hindgut. The anal canal's proximal portion is formed from the hindgut endoderm whereas the distal portion arises from the ectoderm of the cloacal membrane.

The colon has a rich blood supply, with a specific vascular arcade formed by union of branches of superior mesenteric, inferior mesenteric, and internal iliac arteries. Despite its presence, the colon vasculature has two weak points: the splenic flexure and the rectosigmoid junction which are supplied by the narrow terminal branches of superior mesenteric artery (SMA) and inferior mesenteric artery (IMA), respectively. These two watershed areas are most vulnerable to ischemia during systemic hypotension.

Aberrations in midgut development may result in a variety of anatomic anomalies (Table 27.1), and these are broadly classified as:
- Rotation and fixation
- Duplications
- Atresias and stenoses: these occur most frequently and are either due to failure of recanalization or a vascular accident. Atresias have a reported incidence rate of 1 in 300 to 1 in 1500 live births, and are more common than stenoses. Atresias are more common in black infants, low birth-weight infants, and twins. Clinically, the presentation is that of a proximal intestinal obstruction with bilious vomiting on the first day of life. Treatment is surgical correction.

The other major congenital anomalies of the intestine and abdominal cavity are related to abnormalities with development of abdominal wall, the vitelline duct, and innervation of the GI tract.

Abdominal Wall Congenital Anomalies

The congenital anomalies of the abdominal wall are:
- Gastrochisis: caused by an intact umbilical cord with evisceration of the bowel, but no covering membranes, through a defect in the abdominal wall [1]. Gastrochisis is commonly associated with intestinal atresia and cryptorchism.
- Omphalocele: characterized by herniation of the bowel, liver, and other organs into the intact umbilical cord; unlike gastrochisis, these tissues are covered by a membrane formed from fusion of the amnion and peritoneum.

Diagnosis

An abdominal wall defect may be diagnosed during routine prenatal ultrasonography. Both gastroschisis and omphalocele are associated with elevation of maternal serum α-fetoprotein.

Table 27.1 Congenital anomalies of upper GI tract.

Anomaly	Incidence	Symptoms and Signs	Treatment
Esophageal stenosis	1 : 25 000 to 50 000	Emesis dysphagia	Dilation, myotomy, or resection with anastomosis
Esophageal duplication	1 : 8000	Respiratory symptoms, vomiting, neck mass	Resection
Gastric, antral, or pyloric atresia	3 : 100 000, when combined with webs	Non-bilious emesis	Gastroduodenostomy, gastrojejunostomy
Pyloric or antral membrane	As above	Failure to thrive, emesis	Incision or excision, pyloroplasty
Microgastria	Rare	Emesis, malnutrition	Continuous-drip feedings or jejunal reservoir pouch
Pyloric stenosis	US, 3 : 1000 (range, 1–8 : 1000 in various regions); male/ female, 4 : 1	Non-bilious emesis	Pyloromyotomy
Gastric duplication	Rare male/female, 1 : 2	Abdominal mass, emesis, hematemesis	Excision or partial gastrectomy
Gastric volvulus	Rare	Emesis, feeding refusal	Reduction of volvulus, anterior gastropexy
Duodenal atresia or stenosis	1 : 20 000	Bilious emesis, upper abdominal distension	Duodenojejunostomy or gastrojejunostomy
Annular pancreas	1 : 10 000	Bilious emesis, failure to thrive	Duodenojejunostomy
Duodenal duplication	Rare	Pain, GI bleeding	Excision
Malrotation and midgut volvulus	Rare	Abdominal distension, bilious emesis	Reduction, division of bands, possibly resection

Management

Recommended management for both these conditions is operative reduction of the contents back in to the abdominal cavity. The size of the omphalocele determines whether a primary repair or delayed primary closure is selected as the surgical approach.

Vitelline Duct Congenital Anomalies

Persistence of the duct communication between the intestine and the yolk sac beyond the embryonic stage may result in several anomalies of the omphalomesenteric or vitelline duct.

The most common congenital abnormality of the GI tract is omphalomesenteric duct, or Meckel diverticulum, which results from the failure of the vitelline duct to obliterate during the fifth week of fetal development [2].

Clinical presentation

Meckel diverticulum may remain completely asymptomatic or it may mimic such disorders as Crohn disease, appendicitis, and peptic ulcer disease. Bleeding is the most common complication of Meckel diverticulum, related to acid-induced ulceration of adjacent small intestine from the presence of ectopic gastric mucosa. Obstruction, intussusception, diverticulitis, and perforation may also occur, especially in adults, due to the active ectopic pancreatic tissue or gastric mucosa.

Diagnosis

The most useful method of detection of a Meckel diverticulum is technetium-99m pertechnetate scanning. Technetium uptake depends on the presence of heterotopic gastric tissue. The test has 85% sensitivity and 95% specificity. The sensitivity of the scan can be increased minimally with use of cimetidine [3]. Other tests useful in diagnosis are superior mesenteric artery angiography, laparoscopy, and double balloon enteroscopy.

Management

Meckel diverticulectomy either by laparoscopy or open laparotomy approach is the procedure of choice for symptomatic diverticulum.

Less Common Vitelline Duct Abnormalities

Other, less common congenital abnormalities of vitelline duct include:

- Omphalomes-enteric or vitelline cyst: central cystic dilatation in which the duct is closed at both ends but patent in its center

- Umbilical-intestinal fistula: a patent duct throughout its length
- Omphalomesenteric band: complete obliteration of the duct, resulting in a fibrous cord or ligament extending from the ileum to the umbilicus.

Enteric Nervous System Anomalies

The most common enteric nervous system congenital anomaly is Hirschsprung (HSCR) disease; other associated anomalies include intestinal neuronal dysplasia (IND) and chronic intestinal pseudo-obstruction.

HSCR is characterized by the absence of ganglion cells in the submucosal (Meissner) and myenteric (Auerbach) plexuses along a variable length of the hindgut. It is classified as short-segment HSCR (80% of cases), when the aganglionic segment does not extend beyond the upper sigmoid, and long-segment HSCR when aganglionosis extends proximal to the sigmoid. Twelve percent of children with Hirschsprung disease have chromosomal abnormalities, 2 to 8% of which are trisomy 21 (Down syndrome) [4].

Clinical Presentation

In most cases, HSCR presents at birth as non-passage of meconium, abdominal distension, feeding difficulties, and/or bilious emesis. Some patients are diagnosed later in infancy or in adulthood with severe constipation, chronic abdominal distension, vomiting, and failure to thrive.

Diagnosis

The diagnosis in a symptomatic individual may be made by one or a combination of the following tests: barium enema, rectal biopsy, and anal manometry.

Management

Definitive treatment of Hirschsprung disease is surgical, and the specific method of surgery is operator dependent.

Pancreas

Anatomy and Embryogenesis

The pancreas first appears during the fourth week of gestation as ventral and dorsal outpouchings from the endodermal lining of

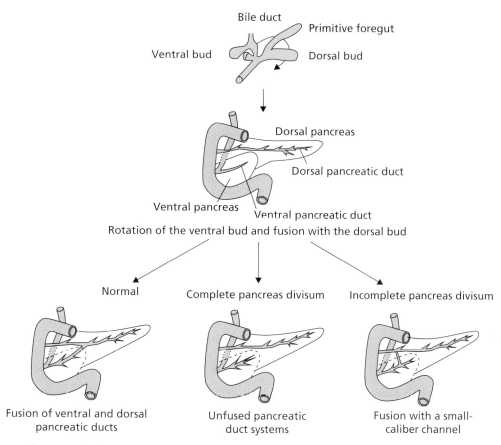

Figure 27.1 Schematic illustration of embryology of normal pancreas and pancreas divisum. Source: Kamisawa 2004 [6]. Reproduced with permission of Springer Science+Business Media.

the duodenum. The normal adult pancreas results from the fusion of these dorsal and ventral pancreatic buds during the second month of fetal development. The tail, body, and part of the head of the pancreas are formed by the dorsal component; the remainder of the head and the uncinate process derive from the ventral pancreas.

The dorsal duct arises directly from the duodenal wall, and the ventral duct arises from the common bile duct. On fusion of the ventral and dorsal components of the pancreas, the ventral duct anastomoses with the dorsal one, forming the main pancreatic duct of Wirsung (Figure 27.1). The proximal end of the dorsal duct becomes the accessory duct of Santorini in the adult [5]. The pancreatic acini appear in the third month of gestation as derivatives of the side ducts and termini of these primitive ducts.

Pancreas Divisum (PD)

PD occurs when the dorsal and ventral ducts fail to fuse; the dorsal duct drains the majority of the pancreas via the minor papilla, while the short ventral duct drains the inferior portion of the head via the major papilla (Figure 27.1). Pancreas divisum has been observed in 5 to 10% of autopsy series and in about 2 to 7% of patients undergoing endoscopic retrograde cholangiopancreatography (ERCP) [7]. Most patients with pancreas divisum are asymptomatic, and the diagnosis is made incidentally. However, some patients develop abdominal pain, recurrent acute pancreatitis, or chronic pancreatitis. The causal relationship between divisum and pancreatitis is still

a matter of debate. PD is usually diagnosed by ERCP although endoscopic ultrasonography and magnetic resonance cholangiopancreatography (MRCP) may be useful for diagnosis [8]. Therapeutic intervention (either endoscopic sphincterotomy with placement of stents through the accessory papilla or surgical sphincteroplasty of the accessory papilla) may benefit some patients with PD and recurrent, acute pancreatitis associated with accessory papilla stenosis [9].

Ectopic Pancreas

Ectopic pancreas is pancreatic tissue found outside the usual anatomic confines of the pancreas. Although it may occur throughout the GI tract it is most commonly found in the stomach and small intestine. Usually an incidental finding, it may rarely become clinically evident when complicated by inflammation, bleeding, obstruction, or malignant transformation [10].

Pancreatic Agenesis

Agenesis of the pancreas is very rare and may be associated with other congenital disease states. In addition, isolated agenesis of the dorsal or, less commonly, the ventral pancreas can occur as silent anomalies [11].

Congenital Cysts

Congenital cysts of the pancreas are rare and are distinguished from pseudocysts by the presence of an epithelial lining. True congenital cysts occur as a result of developmental anomalies related to the sequestration of primitive pancreatic ducts. They are generally asymptomatic, although abdominal distension, vomiting, jaundice, or pancreatitis can be observed requiring surgical removal.

Anomalous Pancreaticobiliary Ductal Union (APBDU)

APBDU is a congenital malformation of the confluence of the pancreatic and bile ducts. A classification has been developed for APBDU: if the pancreatic duct appears to join the common bile duct, this is classified as a P–B type. If the common bile duct joins the main pancreatic duct, this is a B–P type. A long common channel is denoted Y type. The frequency of APBDU varies from 1.5 to 3 2%. APBDU is associated with pancreatitis (with long >21 mm and wide >5 mm common channel), choledochal cysts, and neoplastic abnormalities like cholangiocarcinoma and pancreatic cancer in adults [12].

Videos of interest to readers of this chapter can be found by visiting the companion website at:

http://www.practicalgastrohep.com/

27.1 Identification and intubation of the ileocecal valve with visualization of the terminal ileum.

27.2 Inspection of the colonic mucosa with identification of a colonic lesion.

27.3 Use of an irrigation pump to allow visualization of the colonic mucosa.

27.4 Visualization of colon lesions with white-light and narrow-band imaging.

Take Home Points

Small and large intestine:
- The colon vasculature has two weak points; the splenic flexure and the rectosigmoid junction which are supplied by the narrow terminal branches of SMA and IMA, respectively. These two watershed areas are most vulnerable to ischemia during systemic hypotension.
- The two common congenital anomalies of the abdominal wall presenting at birth are gastrochisis and omphalocele.
- The most common congenital abnormality of the gastrointestinal (GI) tract is omphalomesenteric duct, or Meckel diverticulum, which results from the failure of the vitelline duct to obliterate during fetal development.
- The most common enteric nervous system congenital anomaly is Hirschsprung (HSCR) disease, which is characterized by the absence of ganglion cells in the submucosal (Meissner) and myenteric (Auerbach) plexuses along a variable length of the hindgut.

Pancreas:
- Pancreas divisum occurs when the dorsal and ventral ducts fail to fuse; the dorsal duct drains the majority of the pancreas via the minor papilla, while the short ventral duct drains the inferior portion of the head via the major papilla.

References

1 Weber T, Au-Fliegner M, Downard C, Fishman S. Abdominal wall defects. *Curr Opin Pediatr* 2002; **14**: 491–7.

2 Turgeon D, Barnett J. Meckel's diverticulum. *Am J Gastroenterol* 1990; **85**: 777–81.

3 Petrokubi R, Baum S, Rohrer G. Cimetidine administration resulting in improved pertechnetate imaging of Meckel's diverticulum. *Clin Nucl Med* 1978; **3**: 385–8.

4 Skinner M. Hirschsprung's disease. *Curr Probl Surg* 1996; **33**: 389–460.

5 Kleitsch W. Anatomy of the pancreas; a study with special reference to the duct system. *AMA Arch Surg* 1955; **71**: 795–802.

6 Kamisawa T. Clinical significance of the minor duodenal papilla and accessory pancreatic duct. *J Gastroenterol* 2004; **39**: 606.

7 Delhaye M, Engelholm L, Cremer M. Pancrease divisum: congenital anatomic variant or anomaly? Contribution of endoscopic retrograde dorsal pancreatography. *Gastroenterology* 1985; **89**: 951–8.

8 Bret P, Reinhold C, Taourel P, *et al.* Pancreas divisum: evaluation with MR cholangiopancreatography. *Radiology* 1996; **199**: 99–103.

9 Lans J, Geenen J, Johanson J, Hogan W. Endoscopic therapy in patients with pancreas divisum and acute pancreatitis: a prospective, randomized, controlled clinical trial. *Gastrointest Endosc* 1992; **38**: 430–4.

10 Eisenberger C, Gocht A, Knoefel W, *et al.* Heterotopic pancreas—clinical presentation and pathology with review of the literature. *Hepatogastroenterology* 2004; **51**: 854–8.

11 Fukuoka K, Ajiki T, Yamamoto M, *et al.* Complete agenesis of the dorsal pancreas. *J Hepatobiliary Pancreat Surg* 1999; **6**: 94–7.

12 Wang H, Wu M, Lin C, *et al.* Pancreaticobiliary diseases associated with anomalous pancreaticobiliary ductal union. *Gastrointest Endosc* 1998; **48**: 184–9.

Small-Intestinal Hormones and Neurotransmitters

James Reynolds

Department of Medicine, Drexel University College of Medicine, Philadelphia, PA, USA

Summary

The gastrointestinal (GI) tract is the largest endocrine organ, producing more than 100 bioactive peptides, which regulate motility, secretion, absorption and growth of the gut. These peptides are secreted from specialized endocrine cells that are interspersed throughout the luminal digestive tract and the pancreas. Several peptide hormones are used in a variety of diagnostic and therapeutic applications. Regulation of GI hormone secretion is tightly controlled and involves complex interaction between nutrient stimuli, the enteric nervous system (ENS) and the central nervous system (CNS). Alteration in either hormone secretion or action results in rare but classic syndromes, which can be clinically symptomatic or silent. In this chapter, we describe the key peptide hormones, their physiologic and pathophysiologic role, and their clinical applications.

Introduction

The epithelium of the GI tract comprises multiple cell types, including specialized cells termed "entero-endocrine cells," which number less than 1% of cell population and yet form the largest endocrine system of the body. They are mainly located in the stomach, small intestine, and pancreas, but can be found scattered throughout the GI tract [1].

Entero-endocrine cells produce chemical transmitters that are involved in GI motility, secretion, absorption, and regulation of appetite. These transmitters are predominantly small polypeptides, which are also found in the ENS and the CNS. Though GI peptides are typically thought of as hormones and are referred to as such in this chapter, not all peptides act through the traditional endocrine pathway, by which they are secreted into the bloodstream and act at a distant site; several function in an autocrine, paracrine, or neurocrine manner [2].

Peptide hormone synthesis begins with transcription of genomic DNA into messenger RNA (mRNA), which is then translated into a precursor protein called prohormone. Post-translational processing occurs in the Golgi apparatus, which is critical in the biologic activity of the peptide. After various enzymatic cleavages, the hormones are packaged into secretory granules before exocytosis at the apical surface, allowing luminal contents to influence their secretion [3].

Regulation of GI hormone secretion is complex. It involves intrinsic mechanisms such as the ENS and paracrine mediators secreted by neighboring epithelial cells, as well as extrinsic regulators, most notably the autonomic nervous system (ANS) and endocrine glands that reside outside of the GI tract.

The field of GI endocrinology began after the discovery of secretin by Starling and Bayliss in 1902 [4]. In 1905, Edkins discovered a substance that stimulates gastric secretion and called it gastrin, and later, in 1928, Ivy discovered cholecystokinin (CCK). Despite an early start, gut endocrinology was neglected until the 1960s, when purification and sequencing of these peptides catalyzed an exponential development and enhanced understanding of the complex physiology [2]. To date, more than 30 gut peptide hormone genes, which express more than 100 bioactive peptides, have been discovered. They are grouped into "families" according to their primary structure (Table 28.1) and function (Table 28.2). A detailed description of all such peptides is beyond the scope of this chapter, but the most clinically important will be reviewed in the next section. The role of leptin and other hormones involved in regulation of appetite is discussed elsewhere.

Specific Peptides

Gastrin

Gastrin is the product of a single gene located on chromosome 17. Several bioactive forms exist, whcih vary by the length of the peptide, but all share the same amidated tetrapeptide at the carboxyl terminus. The two major biologically active forms have chains of 17 and 34 amino acids. The longer chain has a halftime that is five times longer than the short chain [5].

Gastrin is produced mainly in the G cells of the gastric antrum in response to a meal, with levels tripling within 30–60 minutes after ingestion. Stimuli include high gastric pH, calcium, and amino acids, particularly aromatic amino acids such as tryptophan and phenylalanine [6]. G cells are tightly regulated by two counterbalancing hormones: gastrin-releasing peptide, which is stimulatory, and somatostatin, which is a potent inhibitor. Additionally, vagal inputs from the parasympathetic nervous system have complex influences on gastrin secretion. Receptors for gastrin and CCK are related and constitute the "CCK/gastrin" receptor family. CCK1 has increased affinity for CCK, whereas gastrin preferentially binds to CCK2/gastrin receptor.

Gastrin is a major mediator of gastric acid secretion. It binds to CCK2/gastrin receptors located on histamine-containing

Practical Gastroenterology and Hepatology Board Review Toolkit, Second Edition. Edited by Nicholas J. Talley, Kenneth R. DeVault, Michael B. Wallace, Bashar A. Aqel and Keith D. Lindor.

Table 28.1 GI peptide families and endocrine cell locations.

Hormone family	Members	Cell type and location
CCK/gastrin	Gastrin	G cells in gastric antrum
	CCK	I cells in proximal small bowel
Secretin/glucagon	Secretin	S cells in proximal small bowel
	GLP-1&2	L cells in small intestine and B cells of pancreatic islets
	VIP	
	Glucagon	A cells in pancreatic islets
	GHRH	
	PACAP	
	PP	Pancreatic islet cells
Pancreatic polypeptide	PYY	L cells in ileum
	NPY	Sympathetic neurons
	Substance P	
Tachykinin	Neurokinins	
	Somatostatin	D cells in intestines and pancreas
Somatostatin	Ghrelin	X/A-like endocrine cells in stomach
Ghrelin	Motilin	M cells in proximal small intestine
	Epidermal growth factor	
Growth factors	Transforming growth factor	
Insulin	Insulin	B cells in pancreatic islets
	Insulin-like growth factor	

CCK, cholecystokinin; GLP, glucagon-like peptide; VIP, vasoactive intestinal polypeptide; GHRH, growth hormone-releasing hormone; PACAP, pituitary adenylate cyclase-activating peptide; PP, pancreatic polypeptide; PYY, peptide YY; NPY, neuropeptide Y.

enterochromaffin cells and induces both the secretion and the synthesis of histamine in enterochromaffin-like (ECL) cells. Histamine, in turn, stimulates HCl secretion in a paracrine manner by binding to the H_2 receptor on nearby parietal cells, which possess receptors for histamine, acetylcholine, and gastrin. Though activation of all three receptors can stimulate acid secretion, the most important step for acid release is the stimulation of the ECL cell to secrete histamine. Gastrin also increases parietal cell secretion of intrinsic factor through a mechanism that is not linked to proton pump activity and is involved in promoting cell growth.

Pathophysiology

The most common cause of elevated gastrin level is the use of acid-suppressive medications – specifically proton pump inhibitors (PPIs). Hypergastrinemia occurs as a result of the alkaline environment produced by the potent acid inhibition, which also decreases somatostatin release from the antral D-cells. Short-term PPI treatment may induce a two- to fourfold increase, whereas long-term therapy may lead to marked hypergastrinemia (often exceeding 400 pmol/L) [7]. Another important cause of hypergastrinemia is atrophic gastritis, often associated with *H. pylori* infection or

pernicious anemia. Zollinger–Ellison syndrome (ZES), a rare disorder, is caused by a gastrin-producing tumor. Such tumors are commonly located in the gastrinoma triangle, bound by the neck of the pancreas, the duodenum, and the cystic and common bile ducts. The serum gastrin in patients with a gastrinoma can be higher than 1000 pmol/L. ZES typically presents with peptic ulcers, diarrhea, and abdominal pain. Other rare causes of hypergastrinemia include retained antral tissue in patients with partial gastrectomy, short gut syndrome, antral G-cell hyperplasia, gastric outlet obstruction, hypercalcemia, and chronic renal failure.

Gastrin and Carcinogenesis

Aside from regulating acid secretion, gastrin has growth-promoting properties, through stimulation of cell proliferation and inhibition of apoptosis. Gastrin-knockout mice display poorly differentiated gastric mucosa, with a reduced number of ECL and parietal cells. In contrast, patients suffering from ZES exhibit hypertrophy and hyperplasia of the gastric mucosa, as well as enlarged submucosal rugal folds. There is growing evidence to suggest that elevated gastrin levels may favor the development of certain neoplasms in the GI tract and even outside the GI tract. A CCK2 receptor

Table 28.2 Clinically important peptide hormones and associated disease states.

Peptide	Disease state	Clinical application
Gastrin	(↑) Zollinger–Ellison syndrome (ZES) – severe peptic ulcer disease, diarrhea	Pentagastrin (analogue), used to assess acid secretory capacity and provoke bioactive neuropeptide secretion in VIPoma and medullary carcinoma of the thyroid
CCK	(↓) Seen in bulimia, celiac disease, delayed gastric emptying	Evaluation of gallbladder contractility in HIDA scan and sphincter of Oddi manometry
VIP	(↑) Verner–Morrison syndrome – voluminous diarrhea, hypokalemia, flushing	VIP-based radionuclide imaging used to locate and guide resection of VIP-secreting tumors, pancreatic adenocarcinomas, and carcinoid tumors that express VIP receptors
	(↓) Hirschsprung disease, achalasia	
Secretin	Not described	Used to assess exocrine pancreatic function; secretin-stimulation test used to diagnose gastrinomas; aids in cannulation of pancreatic duct during ERCP
Somatostatin	(↑-) Somatostatinoma – diabetes, diarrhea	Octreotide (analog):
	Gallstone disease	Diagnostics – Diagnosis and localization of NETs
		Therapeutics – Secretory diarrheas, variceal bleeding, certain NETs
Motilin	Not described	Macrolide antibiotics (Erythromycin) stimulate motilin receptors and are used in diabetic gastroparesis. Also used to clear gastric contents and increase visibility in emergent endoscopy for upper GI bleed

HIDA scan, hepatobiliary scan; VIP, vasoactive intestinal polypeptide; ERCP, endoscopic retrograde cholangiopancreatography; NET, neuroendocrine tumor; GI, gastrointestinal.

variant referred to as the "CCK2R receptor" has been found in colorectal tumors, pancreatic cancers, and Barrett's metaplasia of the esophagus, but not in normal adjacent tissues [8]. Alternatively, some tumors produce their own gastrin, which can promote tumor growth in an autocrine manner [9]. Though both *in vitro* and *in vivo* animal model studies support an association between a rise in gastrin levels and a higher risk of cancer development, it is still unclear in human beings and remains a key target for further investigation.

Clinical Uses

The gastrin analogue pentagastrin has clinical uses in various diagnostic tests. It is used to assess acid-secretory capacity after surgical vagotomy and to provoke bioactive neuropeptide secretion in patients with vasoactive intestinal polypeptide-secreting tumors. It is also used to provoke calcitonin secretion in order to diagnose medullary carcinoma of the thyroid.

Gastrin receptor antagonists are being investigated for their acid-suppressive activity, which avoids hypergastrinemic states. These agents may have application in the treatment of GI malignancies that express gastrin receptors. Netazepide, an oral potent and highly selective CCK2/gastrin receptor antagonist, has shown promise in recent early phase studies [10].

Cholecystokinin

CCK is a peptide produced by the I cells of the duodenum and jejunum. Five distinct CCK peptides are present as a result of post-translational processing. The principal form is composed of 58 amino acids, with a five-amino-acid carboxyl terminus identical to that of gastrin. CCK-containing cells are concentrated in the proximal small intestine and decrease in number toward the distal jejunum and ileum. CCK is also found in the CNS and peripheral nerves, innervating the intestine and mesenteric vessels predominantly as CCK8. It functions as a neurotransmitter in these areas. This makes it a member of the family of "brain–gut" peptides, in which the same transmitter is found in the intestine and CNS and likely has a role in regulation of food intake. Two types of G protein-linked CCK receptor have been identified based upon receptor binding characteristics: CCK1 receptors (formerly known as CCK-A) and CCK2 receptors (formerly known as CCK-B/gastrin receptor). The CCK1 receptor is abundant in the pancreas and gallbladder and has a 1000-fold higher affinity for CCK.

CCK, along with secretin, regulates pancreatic and gallbladder function during the intestinal digestive period. The primary stimulus for CCK secretion is the presence of long-chain fatty acids, monoglycerides, or proteins in the small intestine, which increases the plasma CCK concentration by 5–10-fold. The mechanism for secretion is not well understood, but appears to be related to CCK-releasing peptides (CCK-RPs), which are released luminally from enterocytes and stimulate CCK release through binding to CCK-RP receptors on the apical membranes of I cells. Degradation of these releasing peptides by pancreatic enzymes halts this process and controls the release via a negative-feedback regulation. CCK is a potent stimulator of gallbladder contraction, but also stimulates rhythmic contraction of the common bile duct and relaxation of the sphincter of Oddi, which facilitates flow of bile into the intestine. Secretion of pancreatic enzymes, and to a lesser extent fluid and bicarbonate secretion, is stimulated directly by circulating CCK and by CCK-mediated release of acetylcholine by the vagus nerve. CCK is a potent inhibitor of acid secretion, through activation of somatostatin release via CCK 1 receptors. Over the past few decades,

understanding of CCK's role in the regulation of meal ingestion satiety has increased. Following postprandial secretion, it delays gastric emptying. CCK also acts on vagal afferent nerve fibers and sends signals to the dorsal hindbrain to reduce meal size and increase the intermeal interval [11].

Pathophysiology

There is no known clinical entity caused by the oversecretion of CCK, but low levels have been reported in patients with bulimia nervosa and celiac disease. Genetic polymorphisms or reduced expression of the CCK1 receptors have been associated with increased gallstone formation and have been observed in some obese individuals.

Clinical Uses

CCK is primarily used clinically for diagnostic purposes. It is commonly used in CCK-stimulated cholescintigraphy to estimate the gallbladder ejection fraction. CCK alone or combined with secretin can be used to assess the secretory capacity of the pancreas. It also aids in the diagnosis of sphincter of Oddi dyskinesia, where a paradoxical rise in the sphincter of Oddi pressure is demonstrated following administration of CCK-octapeptide. Therapeutic applications, however, are limited. Earlier studies had suggested use of CCK injections to reduce gallbladder sludge and gallstone formation in patients on long-term parenteral nutrition [12]. Current studies are focused on development of peptides that are able to regulate appetite

Secretin

Secretin is a peptide secreted by the S cells in the duodenum and jejunum. Similar to other GI peptides, secretin is amidated at the C-terminus. The secretin receptor is a member of the family of G protein-coupled receptors (GPCRs) that activate adenylate cyclase. These receptors are abundant on pancreatic acinar cells and ducts. Secretin receptors are also present in brain cells, the vagus nerve, and other cells of the GI tract.

Secretin release is controlled by a peptidase-sensitive negative-feedback regulatory mechanism, similar to CCK. The primary stimulus for secretin release is a decrease in duodenal pH to less than 4.5. Circulating secretin levels increase rapidly after acidified chyme passes through the pyloric sphincter into the duodenum. The exact mechanism by which H^+ induces secretin release from S cells is unclear. There is evidence for a direct action of H^+ on S cells, as well as evidence for indirect actions through enteric neurons and through a phospholipase A_2-like secretin-releasing peptide (SRP). The primary physiologic action of secretin is stimulation of pancreatic fluid and bicarbonate secretion, leading to neutralization of acidic chyme in the intestine. Secretin also stimulates fluid and bicarbonate release from biliary ducts, duodenal mucosa, and Brunner's glands, while inhibiting gastric acid release and intestinal motility. The bicarbonate that is released into the duodenum neutralizes gastric acid and raises the duodenal pH, thereby "turning off" secretin release via a negative-feedback mechanism.

Pathophysiology

Hypersecretinemia can be seen in patients with advanced renal failure due to impaired clearance and in untreated ZES. Hyposecretinemia is seen in untreated celiac disease resulting from loss of S cells, related to proximal small-bowel mucosal atrophy. This contributes to the maldigestion but is reversed upon institution of gluten-free diet. Lack of postprandial rise in secretin is also seen in patients with achlorhydria.

Verner–Morrison-like syndrome, with watery diarrhea, hypokalemia, and hypochlorhydria, has been described in a patient with a neuroendocrine tumor (NET) that secreted high levels of secretin and only modest levels of vasoactive intestinal polypeptide (VIP).

Administered in pharmacologic doses, secretin appears to lower esophageal sphincter pressure, delay gastric emptying, increase intestinal motility, and promote growth of the pancreas. Furthermore, it may have anorectic properties [13].

Clinical Use

Secretin has been used in the diagnosis of pancreatic disease since the 1930s. With the availability of human synthetic secretin, the intraductal secretin test and endoscopic secretin test have replaced the conventional double-lumen-tube secretin test for exocrine pancreatic secretion. Furthermore, secretin is used in magnetic resonance imaging (MRI) of the pancreas during functional testing to evaluate pancreatic secretion and ductal obstruction. It is particularly useful in detecting congenital, inflammatory, and neoplastic conditions of the pancreas. Secretin also aids in ductal cannulation during endoscopic retrograde cholangiopancreatography, by temporarily dilating pancreatic ducts.

Another important application of secretin is in the diagnosis of ZES. Secretin normally inhibits gastrin release and gastric acid secretion, but in patients with ZES it causes a significant paradoxical increase in both gastric acid secretion and serum gastrin concentration. This novel finding has been recognized as the most sensitive and specific diagnostic method for ZES.

The efficacy of intravenous synthetic human secretin for the treatment of autism spectrum disorders (ASDs) had been investigated extensively in multiple randomized controlled trials (RCTs) since 1998, but no significant improvements have been observed and secretin is not currently recommended for the treatment of ASDs [14]. Secretin in pharmacological doses is being investigated for a possible relief of chronic pancreatitis-associated severe pain, but larger studies are still needed before it can see clinical use [13].

Peptide YY

Peptide YY (PYY) belongs to the pancreatic polypeptide (PP) family of peptides, which includes PP and neuropeptide Y (NPY). Despite sharing structural similarities and the same 36-amino acid length, they vary in their biological functions and locations.

PYY is secreted from L cells in the ileum and H cells in the colon in response to an oral nutrient load. PYY levels start to rise within 15 minutes of any caloric ingestion – long before the nutrients themselves reach the distal gut – implying other neural or hormonal mechanisms are involved in its release. The actions of PYY include potent inhibition of gastric acid secretion, reduction in gastric emptying, inhibition of pancreatic exocrine secretion, and a delay of intestinal transit: the so-called "ileal brake."

PP is secreted by specialized pancreatic islet cells and inhibits gallbladder contraction and pancreatic exocrine secretion.

NPY is a neurotransmitter that is predominantly found in sympathetic neurons and is the most potent known stimulant of food intake.

PYY, along with NPY and PP, binds to a family of G protein-linked receptors (called Y receptors). At present, five receptor subtypes have been identified.

Pathophysiology

Plasma PYY levels are increased in patients with celiac disease who have diarrhea associated with malabsorption of fat and in patients with postgastrectomy dumping syndrome. This is probably due to an increased load of unabsorbed nutrients in the distal intestine, which stimulates PYY secretion. Conversely, both basal plasma PYY and postprandial PYY levels are reduced in morbidly obese patients, despite increased food intake.

Clinical Use

Despite having a clear role in feeding behavior and theoretical antiobesity effects, no member of the PP family of peptides has been able to be used clinically as a therapeutic agent. Investigation is underway, however, to develop methods of delivering these peptides at stable levels for extended periods of time in a safe and acceptable manner [15].

Somatostatin

Somatostatin is distributed throughout the entire body, but is particularly concentrated in nervous tissue of the cortex, hypothalamus, brainstem, and spinal cord. It has also been localized in nerves of the heart, thyroid, skin, eye, and thymus. Somatostatin is abundant in the GI tract and pancreas, where it is produced by paracrine D cells. In the nervous system, it functions as a neurotransmitter. Somatostatin exists in two active forms, 14 and 28 amino acids in length, generated by post-translational processing from a single precursor. The somatostatin receptor is a typical GPCR. At present, there are five known subtypes of the somatostatin receptor. In the GI tract, somatostatin secretion is stimulated by meal ingestion and gastric acid secretion. Additionally, GI somatostatin production is regulated by the ANS, with catecholamines inhibiting and cholinergic mediators stimulating the release. Somatostatin is a key inhibitory peptide. It decreases endocrine and exocrine secretion, reduces GI motility and blood flow, and inhibits gallbladder contraction and secretion of most GI hormones.

Pathophysiology

Only one clinical entity, somatostatinoma, causes excess somatostatin. It is a rare disorder that presents with a triad of diabetes mellitus, diarrhea secondary to malabsorption, and gallstone disease. Somatostatin deficiency may be seen in chronic *H. pylori* gastritis.

Clinical Use

The clinical utility of somatostatin is limited by its very short half-life of less than 3 minutes. The synthetic analogue octreotide acetate is much more potent and stable, however, remaining active for over 90 minutes in the circulation. Newer analogues such as somatostatin LAR and lanreotide-PR are slow-release formulations that require only monthly injections, supplying high-dose, stable serum levels of octreotide. Octreotide is used in the treatment of secretory diarrhea (VIPoma, carcinoid, human immunodeficiency virus (HIV), graft-versus-host disease (GVHD)) and variceal GI bleeding. Somatostatin analogues and somatostatin receptor agonists have been investigated in a number of disorders of the pancreas, including prevention of post-endoscopic retrograde cholangiopancreatography (ERCP) pancreatitis and treatment of acute pancreatitis, but the studies do not indicate clear benefit [16]. In contrast, Pasireotide, a somatostatin analogue, has been shown to decrease the rate of clinically significant postoperative pancreatic fistula [17].

Overexpression of somatostatin-receptor subtypes on the membrane of the neuroendocrine cells provides the rationale for the use of radiolabeled octreotide to image these tumors. Somatostatin-receptor scintigraphy provides a more sensitive tool for detecting tumors that are too small to be visualized by conventional imaging techniques such as computed tomography (CT), ultrasound, or MRI.

Somatostatin analogues inhibit the growth of some NETs by reducing hormonal overproduction and thereby achieving symptomatic relief in most cases. Several studies have shown that long-acting somatostatin analogues can significantly lengthen progression-free survival in patients with functionally active and inactive metastatic midgut NET [18]. Furthermore, radiolabeled somatostatin analogues can be used to deliver isotopes to tumors that contain somatostatin receptors through somatostatin receptors on tumor cells.

Vasoactive Intestinal Polypeptide

VIP is a neuropeptide widely expressed in the peripheral nervous system, ENS, and CNS. Peptide histidine isoleucine (PHI) is an alternative peptide derived from the VIP gene. There are two known receptor types (VPAC1 and VPAC2), found in various tissues, including the GI tract, where it serves multiple functions. It stimulates GI epithelial secretion and promotes fluid and bicarbonate secretion from bile duct epithelium. It is a potent smooth-muscle relaxant, particularly in the LES and colon. It is a powerful vasodilator and may have a role in stimulating the growth of certain adenocarcinomas. Its immunomodulatory properties have recently ignited research into the pathogenesis of inflammatory bowel disease (IBD).

Pathophysiology

Excessive, unregulated secretion of VIP occurs in VIPoma, a rare NET that usually arises in the pancreas. The majority of patients present with voluminous diarrhea and the VIPoma syndrome, also called the "pancreatic cholera syndrome," "Verner–Morrison syndrome," and the "watery diarrhea, hypokalemia, and hypochlorhydria or achlorhydria (WDHA) syndrome." Therefore, serum VIP quantitation aids in the evaluation of chronic secretory or high-volume diarrhea. On the other hand, deficiency of VIP-secreting neurons has been implicated in Hirschsprung's disease and achalasia. Radionuclide imaging has been used to locate and guide resection of VIP-secreting tumors, pancreatic adenocarcinomas, and carcinoid tumors that express VIP receptors. Moreover, a variety of VIP antagonists have been developed and are being evaluated for VIP receptor-targeted therapy [19].

Motilin

Motilin is a peptide produced from prepromotilin secreted by the M cells of the proximal small intestine. It is released in the interdigestive state triggered by luminal alkalinization and bile. However, the presence of nutrients or acid in the small intestine strongly suppresses the endogenous release of motilin in a digestive state. The motilin receptor is a GPCR that activates the phospholipase C-signaling pathway expressed in nerves and smooth muscles. Circulating motilin levels peak every 1–2 hours in fasting individuals. Motilin is thought to facilitate phase III migrating motor complex, often known as the "intestinal housekeeper," a strong contraction that begins at the LES and progresses down the GI tract, sweeping non-digestible solid residue toward the colon and preventing colonic bacteria from migrating into the small bowel [20].

Clinical Use

The motilin receptor also binds and is activated by the macrolide antibiotic erythromycin, which is used in the off-label treatment of delayed gastric emptying seen in diabetes mellitus and in patients with duodenectomy. However, its broad range of activities limits long-term use. Alternative motilin agonists have been developed but haven't reached clinical use at this time.

Gastropancreatic Neuroendocrine Tumors

NETs of the digestive system include genetically diverse solid tumors arising from secretory cells of the neuroendocrine cells in the tubular GI tract and the pancreas. They produce peptides causing characteristic hormonal syndromes, which can be clinically symptomatic (i.e., "functioning") or silent (i.e. "non-functioning").

Classification

Based on embryological origin, NETs used to be classified as foregut (thymus, esophagus, lung, stomach, duodenum, pancreas), midgut (appendix, ileum, cecum, ascending colon), or hindgut (distal large bowel, rectum). However, current best practice is to describe NETs according to their location of primary origin (e.g., pancreas, duodenum, small intestine, etc.) and include reference to the resultant hormone secretion or symptoms (e.g., gastrinoma, insulinoma, carcinoid syndrome). In 2010, the World Health Organization (WHO) adopted a staging scheme similar to that used for other types of epithelial neoplasm, accompanied by a histologic grading system that separates well-differentiated tumors into low-grade and intermediate-grade categories and classifies all poorly differentiated NETs as high-grade.

Incidence

Gastropancreatic NETs are relatively rare, representing only 2% of all GI tumors. However, recent survey data from the Surveillance, Epidemiology, and End Results (SEER) Program indicate that the incidence is increasing [21]. This may partly be due to increased physician awareness and improved diagnostic techniques.

Functioning Gastropancreatic NETs

Carcinoids are the most common NET. The majority (55%) arise from the GI tract, commonly in the distal small bowel. "Carcinoid syndrome" refers to the set of symptoms characterized by flushing, diarrhea, abdominal pain, telangiectasia, and bronchoconstriction. It is mainly associated with small-bowel carcinoid, and patients almost always have hepatic metastasis.

Pancreatic NETs are the most common functioning NETs and cause various well-established syndromes. Insulinomas cause hypoglycemia through excess insulin, while glucagonomas produce cause hyperglycemia through excess glucagon, which is also associated with diabetes mellitus, thrombosis, anemia, and a typical skin rash. Other important examples include VIPomas and gastrinomas, which have already been described.

Non-functioning Gastropancreatic NETs

Non-functioning GI NETs are not associated with a distinct hormonal syndrome and thus are more difficult to detect than functioning GI NETs. As a result, patients generally present late with weight loss, abdominal pain, and bleeding caused by large primary tumors and advanced disease. These tumors primarily arise in the pancreas, duodenum, colon, and rectum.

Biomarker Tests

The various peptides and biogenic amines secreted from the neuroendocrine cells are tumor-specific and may serve as markers for the diagnosis and follow-up of treatment. Some are general markers, such as chromogranin and PP, while others are specific, such as 5-hydroxyindole acetic acid (5 HIAA), gastrin, and VIP.

Tumor Localization

Common imaging techniques include CT and MRI scans. Positron emission tomography (PET) scans are often used to complement information gathered from physical examination, CT, and MRI. Somatostatin receptor scintigraphy (SRS) allows NETs to be localized through the high-affinity binding of somatostatin to its receptors on the NET surfaces. SRS is indicated as the first staging procedure and is one of the most sensitive single-screening methods for extra hepatic disease. Whole-body imaging enables the identification of distant metastases.

Treatment

Surgery is the first-line therapy for a possible curative approach; however, most patients with NETs are diagnosed once metastases have occurred. Even then, there is evidence for a survival advantage, with a low procedure-related mortality, in patients with metastatic NETs and liver metastases who have undergone resection of their primary tumor [22]. Somatostatin analogues can improve the symptoms of carcinoid syndrome and stabilize tumor growth in many patients [18].

An antiproliferative effect can also be achieved with the m-TOR inhibitor everolimus, alone or in combination with octreotide LAR [23]. The vascular endothelial growth factor-inhibitor sunitinib has demonstrated antitumor effects in pancreatic NETs.

- General biochemical markers such as chromogranin A and 5-hydroxyindole acetic acid (5 HIAA) and specific markers such as gastrin and VIP assist in the diagnosis of several NETs and offer prognostic information.

> **Take Home Points**
>
> - The gastrointestinal (GI) tract represents the largest endocrine organ, producing more than 100 bioactive peptides.
> - Gastrin is the major mediator of gastric acid. Proton pump inhibitors (PPIs) are potent acid suppressors and are the most common cause of hypergastrinemia.
> - Cholecystokinin (CCK) is the primary hormone responsible for gallbladder contraction and delays gastric emptying. It is widely used as an aid to radiographic examination of the gallbladder and in diagnostic tests for pancreatic exocrine function and sphincter of Oddi dyskinesia.
> - Secretin plays a key role in the postprandial stimulation of pancreatic fluid and bicarbonate secretion. The most common clinical application of secretin is in the diagnosis of Zollinger–Ellison syndrome (ZES) using the secretin stimulation test.
> - Somatostatin and its analogues are the most widely used gut peptides, with a broad range of activities that include diagnosis and localization of neuroendocrine tumors (NETs) and treatment of diarrheal states, variceal hemorrhage, and certain endocrine tumors.
> - Gastropancreatic NETs arise from secretory endocrine cells throughout the GI tract and pancreas, producing peptides that cause characteristic hormonal syndromes such as carcinoid syndrome, ZES, and the Verner–Morrison syndrome.

References

1 Fujita T, Kobayashi S. Structure and function of gut endocrine cells. *Int Rev Cytol Suppl* 1977; **6**: 187–233.

2 Rehfeld JF. The new biology of gastrointestinal hormones. *Phys Rev* 1998; **78**(4): 1087–108.

3 Park JJ, Koshimizu H, Loh YP. Biogenesis and transport of secretory granules to release site in neuroendocrine cells. *J Mol Neurosci* 2009; **37**(2): 151–9.

4 Bayliss WM, Starling EH. The mechanism of pancreatic secretion. *J Physiol* 1902; **28**(5): 325–53.

5 Walsh JH, Isenberg JI, Ansfield J, Maxwell V. Clearance and acid-stimulating action of human big and little gastrins in duodenal ulcer subjects. *J Clin Invest* 1976; **57**(5): 1125–31.

6 McArthur KE, Isenberg JI, Hogan DL, Dreier SJ. Intravenous infusion of L-isomers of phenylalanine and tryptophan stimulate gastric acid secretion at physiologic plasma concentrations in normal subjects and after parietal cell vagotomy. *J Clin Invest* 1983; **71**(5): 1254–62.

7 Singh P, Indaram A, Greenberg R, *et al.* Long term omeprazole therapy for reflux esophagitis:follow-up in serum gastrin levels, EC cell hyperplasia and neoplasia. *World J Gastroenterol* 2000; **6**(6): 789–92.

8 Chueca E, Lanas A, Piazuelo E. Role of gastrin-peptides in Barrett's and colorectal carcinogenesis. *World J Gastroenterol* 2012; **18**(45): 6560–70.

9 Kovac S, Xiao L, Shulkes A, *et al.* Gastrin increases its own synthesis in gastrointestinal cancer cells via the CCK2 receptor. *FEBS Lett* 2010; **584**(21): 4413–18.

10 Moore AR, Boyce M, Steele IA, *et al.* Netazepide, a gastrin receptor antagonist, normalises tumour biomarkers and causes regression of type 1 gastric neuroendocrine tumours in a nonrandomised trial of patients with chronic atrophic gastritis. *PloS One* 2013; **8**(10): e76462.

11 Rehfeld JF. Clinical endocrinology and metabolism. Cholecystokinin. *Best Pract Res Clin Endocrinol Metab* 2004; **18**(4): 569–86.

12 Sitzmann JV, Pitt HA, Steinborn PA, *et al.* Cholecystokinin prevents parenteral nutrition induced biliary sludge in humans. *Surg Gynecol Obstet* 1990; **170**(1): 25–31.

13 Chey WY, Chang TM. Secretin: historical perspective and current status. *Pancreas* 2014; **43**(2): 162–82.

14 Williams K, Wray JA, Wheeler DM. Intravenous secretin for autism spectrum disorders (ASD). *Cochrane Database Syst Rev* 2012(4):CD003495.

15 Troke RC, Tan TM, Bloom SR. The future role of gut hormones in the treatment of obesity. *Ther Adv Chronic Dis* 2014; **5**(1): 4–14.

16 Concepcion-Martin M, Gomez-Oliva C, Juanes A, *et al.* Somatostatin for prevention of post-ERCP pancreatitis: a randomized, double-blind trial. *Endoscopy* 2014; **46**(10): 851–6.

17 Allen PJ, Gonen M, Brennan MF, *et al.* Pasireotide for postoperative pancreatic fistula. *N Engl J Med* 2014; **370**(21): 2014–22.

18 Caplin ME, Pavel M, Cwikla JB, *et al.* Lanreotide in metastatic enteropancreatic neuroendocrine tumors. *N Engl J Med* 2014; **371**(3): 224–33.

19 Tang B, Yong X, Xie R, *et al.* Vasoactive intestinal peptide receptor-based imaging and treatment of tumors (review). *Int J Oncol* 2014; **44**(4): 1023–31.

20 Poitras P, Peeters TL. Motilin. *Curr Opin Endocrinol Diabetes Obes* 2008; **15**(1): 54–7.

21 Tsikitis VL, Wertheim BC, Guerrero MA. Trends of incidence and survival of gastrointestinal neuroendocrine tumors in the United States: a seer analysis. *J Cancer* 2012; **3**: 292–302.

22 Ahmed A, Turner G, King B, *et al.* Midgut neuroendocrine tumours with liver metastases: results of the UKINETS study. *Endocr Relat Cancer* 2009; **16**(3): 885–94.

23 Pavel ME, Hainsworth JD, Baudin E, *et al.* Everolimus plus octreotide long-acting repeatable for the treatment of advanced neuroendocrine tumours associated with carcinoid syndrome (RADIANT-2): a randomised, placebo-controlled, phase 3 study. *Lancet* 2011; **378**(9808): 2005–12.

CHAPTER 29
Mucosal Immunology of the Intestine

Maneesh Dave and William A. Faubion

Division of Gastroenterology and Hepatology, Mayo Clinic, Rochester, MN, USA

Summary

In the intestine, the mucosal immune system is separated from a significant bacterial and dietary antigen load by an epithelial cell layer. The immunologic tone is one of tolerance toward non-pathogenic bacteria and food antigens. However, the system maintains the capacity to exclude and eliminate pathogenic microbes. This tolerance exists as a result of multiple innate and adaptive responses, but the presence of adequate regulatory cells, which are common in mucosal sites, is probably the most important factor. Defects in mucosal tolerance underlie the development of inflammatory intestinal diseases such as inflammatory bowel disease (IBD), celiac disease, and food allergy.

Mucosal and Epithelial Barrier

Barriers to entry for pathogenic bacteria or toxins include pancreatic and gastric proteases, bile acids, and extremes of pH in the intestine, such as the harsh acidic environment of the stomach and the alkaline pH in the upper small bowel.

Another key barrier is the goblet cell-produced mucus layer, which lines the surface epithelium from the nasal cavity to the rectum. MUC2 is the main mucin glycoprotein secreted by goblet cells, while MUC3A and B are two predominant, membrane-bound isoforms [1]. Bacteria, particles, and viruses are trapped in this layer of mucus and are expelled by the peristaltic contractions of the gut.

Another family of secreted goblet cell proteins, called trefoil factors, promotes restoration of the barrier in response to injury. Trefoil factors bind mucin to form the hydrophobic mucus barrier [2]. In the absence of these factors, the host is susceptible to uncontrolled inflammation.

The main component of the barrier is the epithelial cell. Tight junctions between epithelial cells prevent passage of macromolecules that might elicit antigenic responses. Defects in the tight-junction barrier may be involved in the aberrant immune responses seen in IBD, food allergy, and celiac disease [3, 4]. Agents that affect the epithelial barrier, such as non-steroidal anti-inflammatory drugs (NSAIDs), antibiotics, and microbial infections, are common triggers of IBD. Certain pathogenic bacteria mediate their damage through tight-junction and barrier disruption. For example, enteropathogenic E. coli dephosphorylates and dissociates occludin from the epithelial tight junctions [5]. In addition, intestinal epithelial cells are immunologically active. They process and present antigen and secrete cytokines and chemokines, which initiate protective immune responses [6, 7].

Innate Immune System

The innate immune response is the body's first line of defense against invading microbes. Its objective is to localize and eradicate threats quickly.

Paneth cells are unique intestinal epithelial cells that participate in innate immunity and inhibit excessive microbial growth by secreting α-defensins, which are cationic antimicrobial peptides. The importance of paneth cells has been emphasized by reports that defensins confer protection from Salmonella typhi infection [8]. A recent study has implicated paneth cell dysfunction as responsible for ileal Crohn's disease [9], with abnormal paneth cell phenotype (histologic) linked to shorter time to Crohn's disease recurrence after surgery [10].

The cells of the innate immune system have a rapid and reasonably non-specific response to invading microorganisms or toxic macromolecules that is mediated by pathogen recognition receptors (PRRs), which are either membrane-bound (i.e., toll-like receptors (TLRs), C-type lectin receptors (CLRs)) or cytoplasmic (i.e., nucleotide-binding oligomerization-domain family members (NODs)). As an example, TLR4 and TLR5 recognize lipopolysaccharides and flagellin, respectively, while the intracellular sensor CARD15/NOD2 recognizes peptidoglycan and muramyl dipeptide. These receptors are expressed on epithelial cells and other innate immune cells, and their trigger leads to a proinflammatory response. NOD2/CARD15 mutations were the first genetic susceptibility locus to be identified in Crohn's disease [7]. The NOD2 mutation may affect the innate system's ability to localize and eradicate bacteria that gain entry to the host. The resulting persistence of a microbial stimulus may lead to an adaptive immune response toward something that is otherwise harmless. Interestingly, patients with genetic defects in innate immunity, such as chronic granulomatous disease or Herman–Pudlak syndrome, can have an IBD-like disease [11].

Antigen Uptake and Induction of a Mucosal Immune Response

Peyer patches and mesenteric lymph nodes are the main inductive sites of the mucosal immune system. Peyer patches are aggregates of lymphoid tissue composed of a large B-cell follicle, an interfollicular T-cell zone, and interspersed dendritic cells and macrophages.

Antigen uptake in the gut occurs through a number of different mechanisms. Dendritic cells underneath the epithelium of the

Practical Gastroenterology and Hepatology Board Review Toolkit, Second Edition. Edited by Nicholas J. Talley, Kenneth R. DeVault, Michael B. Wallace, Bashar A. Aqel and Keith D. Lindor.
© 2016 John Wiley & Sons, Ltd. Published 2016 by John Wiley & Sons, Ltd. Companion website: www.practicalgastrohep.com

distal small bowel insert dendrites between intestinal epithelial cells to sample luminal content [9]. Specialized epithelial cells known as microfold (M) cells overlie Peyer patches and mediate the uptake of luminal antigen (particulate) and microorganisms, as well as their transfer to subepithelial dendritic cells and B cells for further processing [12]. Finally, intestinal epithelial cells ingest soluble antigen by fluid-phase endocytosis. This is a slow and stable process, the kinetics of which is dependent on solubility, not size.

Naïve lymphocytes home to Peyer patches, and are exposed to antigen. They then traffic to mesenteric lymph nodes, where there is further antigen exposure, expansion, and maturation. These newly activated T cells leave the mesenteric lymph nodes and enter into the circulation through the thoracic duct, where they subsequently home back to all mucosal effector sites (lamina propria) under the guidance of tissue-specific integrins on the high endothelial venules (HEVs). This last step is mediated by the interaction between the $\alpha_4\beta_7$ integrin, expressed on mucosally derived lymphocytes, and mucosal addressin cell adhesion molecule MadCAM-1, expressed on HEVs in the lamina propria [13]. Activation of mucosal lymphocytes at any site along the intestine can generate protective responses at all mucosal sites.

Adaptive Immune System

The adaptive immune system is characterized by specificity and memory, which is largely mediated by T and B cells. T cells produce cytokines, thereby orchestrating an organized and directed immune response that eradicates infections and gives rise to memory cells (Figure 29.1).

Exposed to a vast array of microbial and food antigens, the mucosal immune system mounts a constant "controlled" immune response, as evidenced by the presence of activated CD4+ helper T cells [14]. This suppression is characterized by hyporesponsive lymphocytes and antigen-presenting cells (APCs) [15] and is mediated by a variety of regulatory cells that produce immunosuppressive cytokines such as transforming growth factor (TGF)-β and interleukin (IL)-10.

CD4+ T helper 1 (Th1) cells are characterized by the production of interferon (IFN)-γ, tumor necrosis factor (TNF)-α, and IL-2. APC-derived IL-12 drives their differentiation. The cytokines stimulate enhanced intracellular killing (IFN-γ, TNF-α), inflammatory cell recruitment (TNF-α), and tissue destruction. The Th1 response leads to the formation of granulomas, whose chief role is to wall off infectious agents. Tissues from patients with graft-versus-host disease (GVHD), transplant rejection, and celiac disease also display Th1 cytokine profiles.

Crohn's disease was initially thought to be the result of aberrant Th1 responses, due to increased mucosal levels of IFN-γ, IL-2, and IL-12 and the presence of mucosal granulomas in patients. However, evidence has steadily accumulated to support a prominent role for a second T-helper subset, Th17. IL-17 and IL-22 are increased in inflamed Crohn's mucosa [16]. A genome-wide association study showed that mutation in the IL-23 receptor protects hosts from developing Crohn's disease [17].

Th2 cells produce cytokines IL-4, IL-5, and IL-13 and are involved in hypersensitivity reactions, food allergy, helminthic infections, and ulcerative colitis (UC). UC was previously thought to be a Th2-mediated disease, due to increased mucosal levels of IL-5 and IL-13

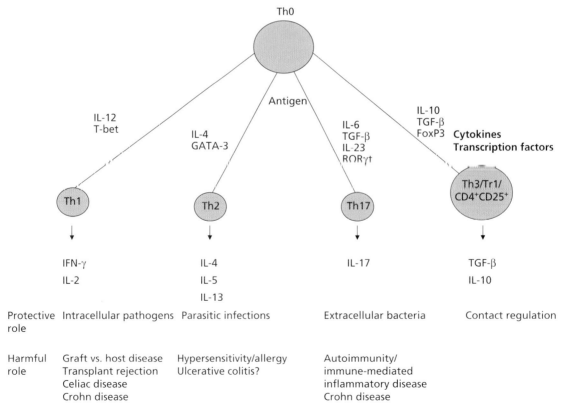

Figure 29.1 CD4+ helper T cells differentiate along different pathways and assume various protective or harmful roles. IFN, interferon; IL, interleukin; TGF, transforming growth factor.

[18]. However, patients with UC exhibit decreased production of mucosal IL-4 (Th2 cytokine), and biopsies from UC patients cultured *ex vivo* release IFN-γ (Th1 cytokine) in similar amounts to those from celiac patients [19]. Natural killer T cells may be responsible for the aberrant production of IL-13, which targets epithelial cells of the mucosal barrier to become dysfunctional. This may explain why UC is a superficial epithelial injury disorder [13].

Humoral Response and Secretory IgA

The mucosal immune system is characterized by secretory IgA, which is produced more than any other antibody in the body and is transported by intestinal epithelial cells. It is protected from luminal proteases by an epithelial-derived glycoprotein known as secretory component that envelops the Fc portion of sIgA and protects potential proteolytic cleavage sites. Secretory IgA functions mainly to inhibit the adhesion of viruses and bacteria to the epithelium by agglutinating the bacteria and other antigens, trapping them in the mucus layer and facilitating their removal from the host [20].

Secretory IgA derived from breast milk provides newborns with passive immunity against pathogens. It may also aid tolerance by preventing exposure of the immune system to commensal bacteria and food antigen, a process known as immune exclusion. In IgA deficiency, there is a greater incidence of serum antibody to food antigen. However, it is unknown whether this plays a role in food allergy, since the majority of patients with food allergy are not IgA-deficient.

IgE is not a dominant antibody of the gastrointestinal (GI) tract. In food allergy, however, IgE is present in the GI tract and facilitates antigen uptake and transepithelial transfer to mucosal mast cells [21].

Tolerance and Regulatory T Cells

Tolerance to non-pathogenic bacteria and food antigens is mediated by regulatory cells, and is perhaps the most critical immune pathway in the intestine.

Oral tolerance is defined as a lack of systemic immune response to orally introduced antigen. Tolerance is dependent on a number of factors, including the dose of the antigen. High-dose antigen leads to anergy or deletion of responsive T cells [22], while low-dose antigen activates regulatory T cells, which secrete IL-10 and TGF-β [23].

The regulatory T cells in the gut include Tr1, Th3, and CD4+CD25+ T cells. CD4+ Tr1 T cells secrete IL-10, which suppresses the response to flora [24]. Interestingly, IL-10-deficient mice develop a Crohn's-like inflammatory disorder [25]. CD4+ Th3 cells produce TGF-β, which promotes IgA production and inhibits T- and B-cell activation. CD4+CD25+ Treg cells are located systemically and are dependent on the transcription factor forkhead box P3 (FoxP3). FoxP3 deficiency leads to a life-threatening systemic polyautoimmune disease in humans known as immune dysregulation, polyendocrinopathy, enteropathy, X-linked (IPEX) syndrome [26]. Populations of CD8+ regulatory T cells have also been described in the gut, and have been shown to be deficient in IBD patients [27].

Tolerance to food and/or bacteria is broken in disease states such as IBD and celiac disease. Antibodies against microbial products such as anti-Saccharomyces cerevisiae (ASCA) [28] and the anti-flagellin antibody Cbir1 [29] have been found in the serum of IBD patients. Furthermore, defective oral tolerance has been demonstrated in both IBD patients and healthy relatives [29].

Celiac disease is characterized by an immune response to gluten that involves aberrant IL-15 production by intestinal epithelial cells and aberrant IFN-γ production by T cells. This results in flattening of the villi of the upper small intestine, crypt hyperplasia, and intraepithelial lymphocytosis [30].

Commensal Flora

The human intestinal tract is colonized by a complex community of microorganisms collectively called "microbiota" that outnumbers human cells by a factor of 10. The intestinal flora plays a major role in both immune system development and defense. In addition, it performs a variety of beneficial functions, including maintenance of intestinal epithelial integrity, provision of an energy source, vitamin biosynthesis, bile salt transformation, provision of a barrier to colonization by microbial pathogens, and xenobiotic metabolism [31]. As an example, the commensal flora occupies all available ecological niches of the intestine, preventing outgrowth of pathogenic bacteria such as *Clostridium difficile* [32]; when the flora is altered (e.g., antibiotics), outgrowth of pathogenic bacteria may occur, leading to leading to *C. difficile* colitis.

Studies show that germ-free animals are relatively immunodeficient, and colonization of these animals with normal flora establishes both the mucosal and the systemic immune system [33]. It is believed that an interaction between host genetics and environmental factors (microbiota) mediated through the human immune system has led to an increase in the incidence of complex immunologically mediated diseases such as IBD, type I diabetes, and asthma over the last few decades [34]. The study of microbiota is an area of intense ongoing investigation [35].

> ### Take Home Points
>
> - In the intestine, the mucosal immune system is separated from a vast bacterial and dietary antigen load by an epithelial cell layer.
> - The immunologic tone in the intestine is one of suppression, with tolerance and controlled physiologic inflammation being examples of this suppressed state.
> - Tolerance exists as a result of multiple innate and adaptive responses, but the presence of adequate regulatory cells is probably the most important factor.
> - Defects in mucosal tolerance, as well as underlying deficits in the innate and adaptive immune response, lead to the unchecked inflammation that results in intestinal diseases such as IBD, celiac disease, and food allergy.

References

1 Kyo K, Muto T, Nagawa H, *et al.* Associations of distinct variants of the intestinal mucin gene MUC3A with ulcerative colitis and Crohn's disease. *J Hum Genet* 2001; **46**(1): 5–20.

2 Sands B, Podolsky D. The trefoil peptide family. *Ann Rev Physiol* 1996; **58**(1): 253–73.

3 de Boissieu D, Matarazzo P, Rocchiccioli F, Dupont C. Multiple food allergy: a possible diagnosis in breastfed infants. *Acta Paediatr* 1997; **86**(10): 1042–6.

4 Fasano A, Shea-Donohue T. Mechanisms of disease: the role of intestinal barrier function in the pathogenesis of gastrointestinal autoimmune diseases. *Nat Clin Pract Gastroenterol Hepatol* 2005; **2**(9): 416–22.

5 Simonovic I, Rosenberg J, Koutsouris A, Hecht G. Enteropathogenic *Escherichia coli* dephosphorylates and dissociates occludin from intestinal epithelial tight junctions. *Cell Microbiol* 2000; **2**(4): 305–15.

6 Kagnoff MF, Eckmann L. Epithelial cells as sensors for microbial infection. *J Clin Invest* 1997; **100**(1): 6.

7 Gunther C, Martini E, Wittkopf N, *et al.* Caspase-8 regulates TNF-alpha-induced epithelial necroptosis and terminal ileitis. *Nature* 2011; **477**(7364): 335–9.

8 Salzman NH, Ghosh D, Huttner KM, *et al.* Protection against enteric salmonellosis in transgenic mice expressing a human intestinal defensin. *Nature* 2003; **422**(6931): 522–6.

9 Adolph TE, Tomczak MF, Niederreiter L, *et al.* Paneth cells as a site of origin for intestinal inflammation. *Nature* 2013; **503**(7475): 272–6.

10 VanDussen KL, Liu TC, Li D, *et al.* Genetic variants synthesize to produce paneth cell phenotypes that define subtypes of Crohn's disease. *Gastroenterology* 2014; **146**(1): 200–9.

11 Korzenik J. Is Crohn's disease due to defective immunity? *Gut* 2007; **56**(1): 2–5.

12 Miller H, Zhang J, KuoLee R, *et al.* Intestinal M cells: the fallible sentinels? *World J Gastroenterol* 2007; **13**(10): 1477.

13 Newberry RD, Lorenz RG. Organizing a mucosal defense. *Immunol Rev* 2005; **206**: 6–21.

14 Macdonald TT, Monteleone G. Immunity, inflammation, and allergy in the gut. *Science* 2005; **307**(5717): 1920–5.

15 Smythies LE, Sellers M, Clements RH, *et al.* Human intestinal macrophages display profound inflammatory anergy despite avid phagocytic and bactericidal activity. *J Clin Invest* 2005; **115**(1): 66–75.

16 Fujino S, Andoh A, Bamba S, *et al.* Increased expression of interleukin 17 in inflammatory bowel disease. *Gut* 2003; **52**(1): 65–70.

17 Duerr RH, Taylor KD, Brant SR, *et al.* A genome-wide association study identifies IL23R as an inflammatory bowel disease gene. *Science* 2006; **314**(5804): 1461–3.

18 Heller F, Florian P, Bojarski C, *et al.* Interleukin-13 is the key effector Th2 cytokine in ulcerative colitis that affects epithelial tight junctions, apoptosis, and cell restitution. *Gastroenterology* 2005; **129**(2): 550–64.

19 Rovedatti L, Kudo T, Biancheri P, *et al.* Differential regulation of interleukin 17 and interferon gamma production in inflammatory bowel disease. *Gut* 2009; **58**(12): 1629–36.

20 Cunningham-Rundles C. Physiology of IgA and IgA deficiency. *J Clin Immunol* 2001; **21**(5): 303–9.

21 Berin MC, Kiliaan AJ, Yang PC, *et al.* Rapid transepithelial antigen transport in rat jejunum: impact of sensitization and the hypersensitivity reaction. *Gastroenterology* 1997; **113**(3): 856–64.

22 Benson JM, Campbell KA, Guan Z, *et al.* T-cell activation and receptor downmodulation precede deletion induced by mucosally administered antigen. *J Clin Invest* 2000; **106**(8): 1031–8.

23 Neurath MF, Fuss I, Kelsall BL, *et al.* Experimental granulomatous colitis in mice is abrogated by induction of TGF-beta-mediated oral tolerance. *J Exp Med* 1996; **183**(6): 2605–16.

24 Groux H, O'Garra A, Bigler M, *et al.* A CD4+ T-cell subset inhibits antigen-specific T-cell responses and prevents colitis. *Nature* 1997; **389**(6652): 737–42.

25 Kuhn R, Lohler J, Rennick D, *et al.* Interleukin-10-deficient mice develop chronic enterocolitis. *Cell* 1993; **75**(2): 263–74.

26 Bennett CL, Christie J, Ramsdell F, *et al.* The immune dysregulation, polyendocrinopathy, enteropathy, X-linked syndrome (IPEX) is caused by mutations of FOXP3. *Nat Genet* 2001; **27**(1): 20–1.

27 Allez M, Brimnes J, Dotan I, Mayer L. Expansion of CD8+ T cells with regulatory function after interaction with intestinal epithelial cells. *Gastroenterology* 2002; **123**(5): 1516–26.

28 Landers CJ, Cohavy O, Misra R, *et al.* Selected loss of tolerance evidenced by Crohn's disease-associated immune responses to auto- and microbial antigens. *Gastroenterology* 2002; **123**(3): 689–99.

29 Lodes MJ, Cong Y, Elson CO, *et al.* Bacterial flagellin is a dominant antigen in Crohn disease. *J Clin Invest* 2004; **113**(9): 1296–306.

30 Kagnoff MF. Celiac disease: pathogenesis of a model immunogenetic disease. *J Clin Invest* 2007; **117**(1): 41–9.

31 Dave M, Higgins PD, Middha S, Rioux KP. The human gut microbiome: current knowledge, challenges, and future directions. *Transl Res* 2012; **160**(4): 246–57.

32 Reeves AE, Theriot CM, Bergin IL, *et al.* The interplay between microbiome dynamics and pathogen dynamics in a murine model of *Clostridium difficile* infection. *Gut Microbes* 2011; **2**(3): 145–58.

33 Sartor RB. Microbial influences in inflammatory bowel diseases. *Gastroenterology* 2008; **134**(2): 577–94.

34 Bach JF. The effect of infections on susceptibility to autoimmune and allergic diseases. *N Engl J Med* 2002; **347**(12): 911–20.

35 Human Microbiome Project Consortium. Structure, function and diversity of the healthy human microbiome. *Nature* 2012; **486**(7402): 207–14.

Motor and Sensory Function

Vineet S. Gudsoorkar and Eamonn M.M. Quigley

Division of Gastroenterology, Department of Medicine, Houston Methodist Hospital and Weill Cornell College of Medicine, Houston, TX, USA

Summary

Motor activity of the small intestine and colon has evolved to subserve the basic physiological functions of these parts of the gastrointestinal (GI) tract. In the small intestine, motility propels food, chime, and stool along the gut, promotes mixing of chyme with intestinal enzymes to facilitate digestion, and increases contact time between luminal contents and the mucosa, thereby promoting absorption [1]. In the colon, in contrast, tone is an important feature, permitting changes in volume to accommodate stool; the colon is also capable of periodically generating high-amplitude phasic contractions that traverse the organ and propel stool into the rectum. Coordinated activity in the rectum, anal sphincters, pelvic floor, and abdominal musculature and diaphragm affects defecation and maintains continence [2].

Neuromuscular Apparatus

Anatomy and Morphology

Throughout the small intestine, gut muscle is arranged in two circumferential layers: an outer longitudinal and an inner circular layer. In the cecum and colon, the longitudinal layer is condensed into three bands, the tenia coli, which are arrayed equidistant from one another along the length of the large intestine as far as the rectum, where they are replaced by a complete longitudinal layer. In the anorectum, smooth-muscle fibers of the internal anal sphincter function in concert with striated muscle of the external anal sphincter and pelvic floor musculature to maintain continence and participate in the act of defecation.

Gut smooth-muscle cells (SMCs) in the small intestine generate an omnipresent slow wave: a persistent resting membrane potential that does not reach the critical level for firing of the action potential. While slow waves do not generate contractions, they do determine the frequency of contractions, given that the action potentials that do cause contractions occur on the summits of slow waves. In this manner, the frequency of phasic contractions, in a given part of the gut, is "phase-locked" to its slow-wave frequency. Slow waves originate in the proximal 1 cm of the duodenum and propagate distally, with their frequency falling from approximately 12 Hz in the duodenum and proximal jejunum to 9 Hz in the distal ileum.

Colonic smooth-muscle electrophysiology is more complex, including differences in electrical activity between the longitudinal and circular muscle layers. Unlike in the small intestine, slow-wave activity in colonic circular muscle is more variable in frequency and amplitude, averaging between two and four cycles per minute, is not omnipresent, is sensitive to stretch and is markedly altered by excitatory and inhibitory substances: *in vitro* properties that mirror the sensitivity of the colon to such factors as stress and meal ingestion in life [3]. Again, in contrast to the small intestine, tone, a state of more sustained contraction, is an important function in the colon and is critical to the function of its sphincters.

Smooth-Muscle Cells

Gut SMCs respond to pacemaker currents from interstitial Cajal cells (ICCs). Areas of close contact (nexi) between SMCs facilitate the transmission of electrical events between SMCs, allowing smooth muscle to function as a syncytium. Action potentials may result from neurogenic or neurochemical stimuli; the response of the SMC to an incoming stimulus may also be influenced by modulatory events at the neuromuscular junction. Like other contractile cells, gut SMCs possess motor units comprising actin and myosin chains that cross-bridge upon generation of an action potential, resulting in a coordinated phasic contraction and relaxation. This excitation–contraction coupling appears to be more complex in gut SMCs than was previously thought. Briefly, the action potential is generated when an influx of positive charges (mainly, calcium and sodium) occurs across the cell membrane, creating a potential gradient. The majority of calcium influx takes place through voltage-dependent L-type calcium (Ca^{2+}) channels, though a role for another, less well-defined T-type Ca^{2+} channel has been postulated. An efflux of positive charge results in repolarization and hyperpolarization, a role performed mainly by voltage-dependent potassium (K^+) channels. Voltage-gated sodium (Na^+) and chloride (Cl^-) channels, non-selective ion channels, transient receptor potentials (TRPs), the Na^+-K^+ pump and Na^+-Ca^{2+} exchanger, and organelles such as the sarcoplasmic reticulum and various excitatory and inhibitory neurotransmitters, play key roles in pacemaker current generation and excitation–contraction coupling [4].

Interstitial Cajal Cells

ICCs are found at various locations in the gut wall, including the myenteric plexus (ICC-MY) and submucosa (ICC-SM), as well as intramuscularly (ICC-IM). They are directly innervated by nerve varicosities from the enteric nervous system (ENS) and have gap junctions with SMCs. ICCs are pacemakers and actively propagate electrical slow waves. In the small bowel, electrical slow waves

Practical Gastroenterology and Hepatology Board Review Toolkit, Second Edition. Edited by Nicholas J. Talley, Kenneth R. DeVault, Michael B. Wallace, Bashar A. Aqel and Keith D. Lindor.

are generated by ICC-MYs; slow waves in the colon, in contrast, originate in ICC-SMs and actively propagate along the submucosal surface into the circular muscle [5].

The release of Ca^{2+} from inositol triphosphate receptor-operated stores is responsible for the pacemaker currents that generate slow waves. Ca^{2+}-activated Cl^- channels play an important role in this process. One such channel, anoctamin 1 (ANO1), has emerged as being highly expressed in ICCs [6]. Encoded by the transmembrane protein 16A (Tmem16a) gene, ANO1 appears to be an important component of the pacemaker machinery of ICCs. While current data support the concept of ICCs as neuromodulators integrating excitatory and inhibitory neurotransmission, their exact role in the modulation of neurotransmission remains to be defined [7].

Platelet-Derived Growth Factor Alpha Cells

These "fibroblast-like" cells also lie near the terminals of motor neurons and form gap junctions with SMCs [8]. They express platelet-derived growth factor alpha (PDGFRα+) and small-conductance Ca^{2+}-activated K^+ channels. They respond to purinergic inhibitory stimuli, presumably by forming large-amplitude K^+ currents, resulting in hyperpolarization.

Enteric Nervous System

The ENS is an elaborate network of neurons and glial cells that lies within the wall of the intestine and controls multiple aspects of intestinal physiology [9]. The total number of neurons in the ENS is approximately 500 million, which outnumbers the sympathetic and parasympathetic nervous systems combined. Inhibitory neurotransmission is mediated by nitric oxide, purines, and peptides, such as vasoactive intestinal polypeptide (VIP) or pituitary adenylate cyclase-activating polypeptide, whereas acetylcholine and neurokinins, such as substance P or neurokinin A, are excitatory neurotransmitters. The heuristics of the ENS are similar to that of the central nervous system (CNS), wherein sensory neurons, interneurons, and motor neurons are synaptically connected, creating directional flow of information from sensory neurons to effector organs via interneurons, leading to the concept of the "brain in the gut." Indeed, the ENS is capable of regulating basic intestinal functions even when completely separated from the CNS and has a complete reflex circuitry (including a sensory limb and a motor limb) to coordinate the behavior of the effector system, comprising smooth muscle, glands, and blood vessels.

The ENS is derived from the neural crest. Its constituent cells migrate radially along the gut, forming two layers of ganglionic plexi: the myenteric (Auerbach's) plexus and the submucosal (Meissner's) plexus. The myenteric plexus lies between the inner circular and the outer longitudinal muscle layers, while the submucosal plexus, as the name suggests, lies beneath the mucosal surface. The plexi are continuous along the length and around the circumference of the gut wall, though there are regional differences in the ultrastructure, such as the absence of a ganglionated submucosal plexus in the esophagus and stomach. The two plexi are connected by interplexus neurons running between them, creating synaptic cross-talk. Through variations in morphology and in the interconnections between neurons and plexi, as well as through the presence of a wide variety of neurotransmitters and neuromodulators, the ENS is capable of exhibiting striking plasticity in generating responses to stimuli, be their origin in the lumen, in the gut wall, or external to the gut. This plasticity is illustrated by the regulation and modulation of transmission of an electrical signal within the ENS.

Such transmission may be influenced at either the presynaptic or postsynaptic level. For example, inhibitory or excitatory postsynaptic potentials may either "downregulate" or "upregulate" the postsynaptic neuron and, thereby, either diminish or accentuate, respectively, the likelihood of an action potential's traveling down the presynaptic neuron and generating a response in the postsynaptic neuron.

In the small intestine, the ENS, in conjunction with ICCs, is the principal driver of various motility patterns, such as peristalsis, segmentation, the migrating motor complex (MMC), and retropulsion in response to noxious stimuli. Ganglia are partially enclosed by interstitial cells and connective tissue elements found between the muscle layers or in the submucosa. The lack of a continuous connective tissue sheath means that neuronal cell bodies, dendrites, and glial cells, covered only by a basal lamina, are exposed to the extracellular milieu. Therefore, neurohumoral agents in the interstitial fluid have ready access to cells of the ganglia. Small blood vessels, in close proximity to ganglia of the myenteric plexus, create periganglionic networks in some species.

The organization of the plexus differs in the distal colon, where bundles, referred to as "shunt fascicles," convey myelinated (parasympathetic and sympathetic efferents) and unmyelinated (arising from the intrinsic nerves of the plexus) fibers from the hypogastric plexi that lie on the ganglia of the myenteric plexus. Again, the ENS plays a key role in colonic motility. Indeed, the absence of an ENS in the colon results in Hirschsprung's disease, whereas its degeneration results in Chagas' disease and other enteric neuropathies.

Glial Cells

Enteric glia comprises stellate-shaped cells that are present beneath the mucosa, in the intramuscular layer, and inside the enteric ganglia, in close association with ENS neurons [10]. Enteric glia are densely innervated by nerve processes. They appear to respond in a context-specific manner to strong purinergic and nicotinergic stimuli. The exact purpose of this neuromodulation is not clear at present, but it may be hypothesized that glia act as a relay center for enteric and sympathetic neural signals, modulating the final response. Additionally, considering their structural homology with astrocytes in the CNS, their role in intestinal epithelial injury and repair, neuronal survival, and regeneration is being explored with great interest.

Autonomic Nervous System

The "extrinsic" or autonomic nervous system (ANS) is divided into sympathetic and parasympathetic parts. The sympathetic supply of the GI tract is derived from abdominal prevertebral ganglia: the celiac, superior mesenteric, and inferior mesenteric ganglia. Neurons of the prevertebral ganglia receive synaptic inputs from the preganglionic sympathetic fibers arising from cell bodies in the inferomediolateral columns of the thoracolumbar spinal cord. They also receive inputs from afferent neurons located in the wall of the gut. Postganglionic sympathetic fibers from these ganglia make up the adrenergic nerve supply of the gut. The parasympathetic supply is carried by vagal efferent fibers arising from cell bodies in the dorsal motor nucleus of the vagus and the nucleus ambiguous. Those originating in the dorsal motor nucleus are preganglionic parasympathetic fibers that project to the smooth-muscle esophagus, the stomach, the small intestine, and the proximal half of the colon. The pelvic plexus is a ganglionated plexus that is located on either side of the rectum. Nerves from this plexus project to the aboral part of the GI tract and to the urogenital organs. The ganglia serve as integrating centers between the CNS and ENS for regulation of intestinal motility, blood flow, and secretion. Tracer studies have indicated that both sympathetic and parasympathetic fibers synapse with enteric neurons, and in this way influence intestinal motility, regional blood flow, epithelial transport, and both endocrine and immune functions indirectly through the enteric neurons rather than directly on the relevant effector cell(s) [11].

The CNS and the ENS, facilitated by the proximity of their neurons to intestinal immune cells, can modulate immune responses. Thus, both noradrenergic and cholinergic neurons can influence the cytokine profiles, migration, proliferation, and antibody production of lymphocytes and the phagocytic activity of macrophages. The ENS also receives input from both autonomic branches and through various non-cholinergic, non-adrenergic neuromodulators such as VIP, nitric oxide, substance P, neuropeptide Y (NPY), peptide YY (PYY), and serotonin; inputs that can significantly affect the immune system [12].

Gut Sensation: Neurobiology

Sensory output from the GI tract is a complex process mediated or modulated by neural, hormonal, immunological, and psychological inputs/factors. In addition to food, nutrients, pathogens, and foreign antigens, factors that evoke sensory responses in the gut include temperature, osmolarity, acidity, mechanical distortion, stretch, and tension [13]. Nutrient receptors are mostly located on, but not limited to, the enteroendocrine cells that, in turn, secrete various (>20) hormones which can both locally modulate intestinal functions and also act at distal sites such as the pancreas, to modulate insulin secretion, and the CNS, to influence appetite and satiety.

Both extrinsic and intrinsic neuronal pathways carry sensation from the GI tract [11]. The first-order neurons carrying this information are referred to as "primary afferent neurons." These are large multipolar neurons that are contained entirely within the gut wall, without any projections to the CNS [13]. They are present in myenteric and submucosal ganglia and respond to luminal chemical stimuli, mechanical deformation of the mucosa, and muscle stretch and tension. They also respond to noxious stimuli to initiate tissue-protective propulsive and secretory reflexes and so rid the gut of pathogens. Afferent input is then conveyed to the CNS by rapidly conducting myelinated A-delta fibers and slower, non-myelinated C fibers. These nerve fibers reach the CNS via the vagus nerve and spinal afferents. Spinal afferents have their cell bodies in the dorsal root ganglia. The second-order neuron is the dorsal-horn neuron in the spinal cord, which sends information along the lateral spinothalamic or spinoreticular tracts. In addition, there is a midline dorsal-column nociceptive pathway conveying pain sensation from abdominal and pelvic viscera to brainstem centers. Third-order neurons project from the latter to cortical or subcortical centers, which convey the specific sensation and associated symptoms such as affective responses, appetite changes, or autonomic features. Each region of the gut receives a dual sensory innervation: from the vagus and thoracolumbar afferents in the proximal part of the GI tract (esophagus, stomach, small intestine, and proximal colon) and from thoracolumbar and lumbosacral afferents in the remaining colon and rectum. Often, the afferent and efferent pathways are shared by the same nerve trunk, imparting significant connectivity between the two.

Gut Motility

Small Intestine

The first detailed observations of small-intestinal motor patterns were those performed by Walter Cannon in the non-anesthetized cat almost a century ago [14]. Currently, recordings of small-intestinal motor activity in humans are performed using either low-compliance perfusion or solid-state systems. While initially limited to a maximum of eight sensors, recent progress in the development of solid-state systems for esophageal manometry has seen the incorporation of 36 solid-state sensors in a single assembly. The data from all sensors is interpolated and computed in a graphical representation, which is referred to as "high-resolution manometry" [15].

Multichannel impedance records resistance to alternating currents measured between multiple electrode pairs. A change in impedance occurs whenever the electrodes come in contact with materials with different electrical conductances. Thus, after recording the baseline impedance of the gut tissue itself, any changes in impedance can be inferred as bolus transit. This technology has been used to record pharyngoesophageal and duodenal motility [16].

Impedance planimetry measures the area of a plane as registered by changes in electrical impedance during distension of a fluid-filled bag placed inside the viscus. Data on the cross-sectional area of the bag (and hence indirectly the organ under study) are extrapolated from the electrical potential difference between the electrodes inside the bag. These data then can be combined with pressure measurements to compute the wall tension, as well as contractility, in response to a standard force or stretch [17].

Magnetic resonance imaging (MRI) and ultrasound rely on their ability to image the intestinal wall and or wall/lumen interface and to dynamically assess changes in wall diameter over time; both modalities benefit from being non-invasive, reproducible, and not associated with radiation exposure. While MRI can provide high-resolution images and MRI studies have provided valuable information on gut volume and transit [18, 19], dynamic acquisition rates are slow and hence not cost-effective for the assessment of motility. While ultrasound imaging is quicker, cheaper, and more readily available, a high degree of interobserver variability and the occurrence of image artifacts are limiting factors [20].

Recently, images obtained from capsule endoscopy have been analyzed to provide an assessment of intestinal motion [21] and a wireless motility capsule with pH, temperature, and pressure sensors has been developed for the measurement of whole-gut and regional transit times [22]. The latter capsule transmits data to an external receiver, which can then be downloaded and analyzed.

Regardless of the system used, the basic motor patterns recorded are similar, being organized, in the fasted state, into recurring cycles of the MMC and featuring a fed response to meal administration. Each MMC cycle comprises three phases, which occur in sequence and continue to recur as long as the individual remains fasted (Figure 30.1). Each cycle begins with a period of quiescence (phase 1), followed by a period of apparently irregular contractions, which increase in frequency and amplitude (phase 2), and culminates in a burst of uninterrupted phasic activity (phase 3), which slowly migrates along the intestine from the proximal duodenum [23]. Simultaneous with the onset of phase 3 activity in the duodenum, related activity occurs in the stomach, gallbladder, and biliary tree. Following the administration of a meal of adequate caloric composition, two things happen; first, the MMC is interrupted, and, second, it is replaced by the fed pattern: a period of irregular

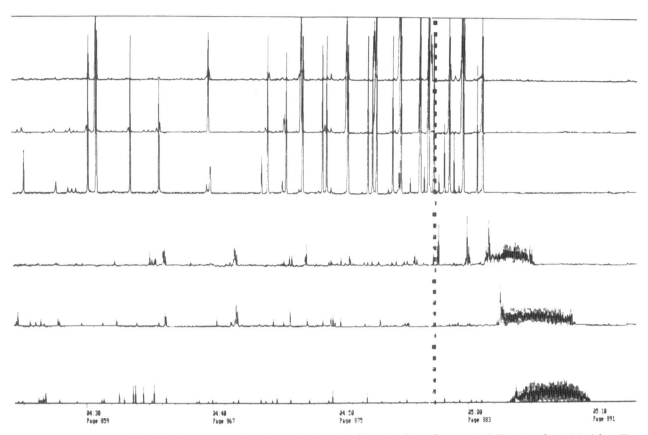

Figure 30.1 Fasting motor activity in the human antrum (top three tracings) and small intestine (lower three tracings). Note irregular activity (phase 2) recorded at all sites, culminating in a burst of rhythmic activity (phase 3), which slowly traverses the segment and is followed by quiescence (phase 1) of the next cycle.

but intense contractions that last from 2 to 6 hours, depending on meal size and content (Figure 30.2).

The extreme variability in the frequency of the MMC has been revealed by 24-hour recordings of normal individuals going about their usual activities in a fully ambulatory state; the number recorded in a single day, in a given individual, varying from as few as one to as many as eight [24].

These 24-hour studies also emphasize the significance of diurnal variations in normal small-bowel motility. Other factors also contribute to variability. For example, recordings performed along the length of the small intestine have revealed the extent of regional variations. In humans, the ileocolonic junctional region demonstrates quite different patterns; here, the MMCs peter out and are replaced by irregular activity, grouped or clustered contractions, and occasional high-amplitude, prolonged, propagated contractions [25]. Clustered activity is also prominent in the proximal duodenum, where motor activity is closely synchronized with that of the distal antrum. Gender may also be relevant; variations in such motor parameters as gastric emptying have been demonstrated in relation to the phase of the menstrual cycle, as well as during pregnancy. Finally, both acute and chronic stressors have been shown to be capable of causing significant disruption to motor patterns in the stomach and small intestine. Certain stresses can, indeed, completely interrupt the postprandial response and lead to its replacement by phase 3-type activity. Given the invasive nature of small-intestinal manometry, one cannot discount the possible – and variable – effects of stress on recorded motor activity.

Large Intestine

Colonic motility in humans presents alternating periods of activity and quiescence. Some recognizable patterns have been described in the active periods: individual phasic contractions, propagating contractions, propagating bursts or clusters of contractions, and, most recognizable of all, high-amplitude propagating contractions (HAPCs) (Figure 30.3a). HAPCs are the manometric equivalents of mass movements and originate primarily in the proximal colon; they occur infrequently (mean frequency 9.9/24 hours), last for a brief time (20–30 seconds), have an average propagation velocity of 1.0–1.5 cm/s, and have an average amplitude of 100 mmHg. HAPCs are suppressed during sleep and increase upon awakening, likely contributing to the urge to defecate commonly experienced on rising. HAPCs can be elicited by cholinergic agonists such as neostigmine, by eating, and by the instillation of short-chain fatty acids and laxatives such as bisacodyl. There is a general increase in colonic motor activity on eating a meal: the gastrocolonic response (Figure 30.3b). Other motor patterns identified include, in the colon: isolated pressure waves, propagating pressure waves, periodic colonic motor activity, discrete random bursts of phasic and tonic pressure waves, and retrograde pressure waves; and in the rectum: periodic rectal motor activity and discrete rectosigmoid bursts of phasic and tonic pressure waves.

With the advent of high-resolution colonic manometry, we now know that the most prevalent motor pattern in the colon comprises retrograde propagation of pressure waves; a phenomenon that serves to regulate transit through the colon [15]. In the colon, tone

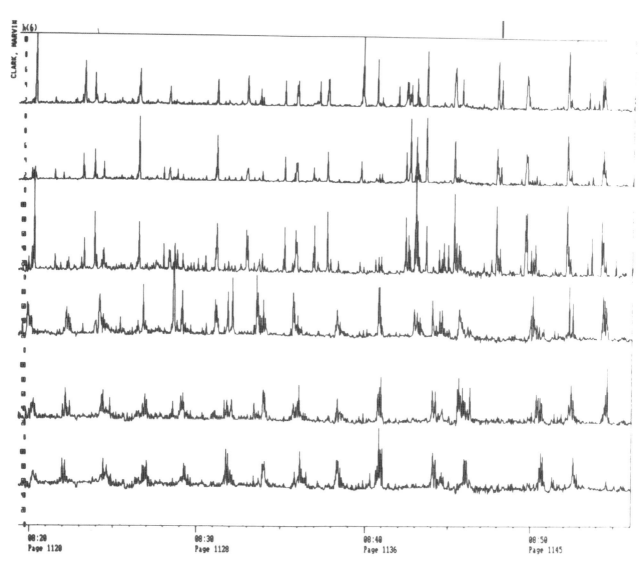

Figure 30.2 Fed motor pattern, from the same recording sites as Figure 30.1. The migrating motor complex (MMC) has been abolished and is replaced by intense, irregular activity at all sites.

is low during sleep, rises on waking, and increases further following meal ingestion or the instillation of short-chain fatty acids.

Motor Activity of the Anorectum

When colonic contents reach the rectum, a sensation of rectal fullness is generated by rectal afferents, probably arising from activation of stretch receptors in the mesentery or pelvic floor muscles. In response to this, a "sampling" reflex, also known as the rectoanal inhibitory or rectosphincteric reflex, is generated, which leads to internal anal sphincter relaxation and external sphincter contraction. At this stage, the individual can decide to postpone or – if it is considered socially acceptable – proceed with defecation. To facilitate the process, the puborectalis muscle and external anal sphincter relax, thereby straightening the rectoanal angle and opening the anal canal. The propulsive force for defecation is then generated by contractions of the diaphragm and the muscles of the abdominal wall, which now propel the rectal contents through the open sphincter. The internal anal sphincter is a continuation of the smooth

muscle of the rectum and is under sympathetic control. It provides approximately 80% of normal resting anal tone. The external anal sphincter and pelvic floor muscles are striated muscles, innervated, respectively, by sacral roots 3 and 4 and the pudendal nerve. The anorectum represents, therefore, the other site of convergence of the somatic nervous system and ANS, and is susceptible to disorders of both striated and smooth muscle, as well as to diseases of the CNS, peripheral nervous system, and ANS. Recently, based on high-resolution anorectal manometric findings, three distinct phenotypes of disordered defecation, based upon anorectal pressure changes at rest and during evacuation, have been proposed [26].

Intestinal Microbiota in Motility and Sensation

The human gut harbors approximately 100 trillion microorganisms, comprising more than 1000 bacterial species and encoding a collective genome 150 times larger than the human genome [27]. It is now evident that the microbiota can influence motility and sensation. It

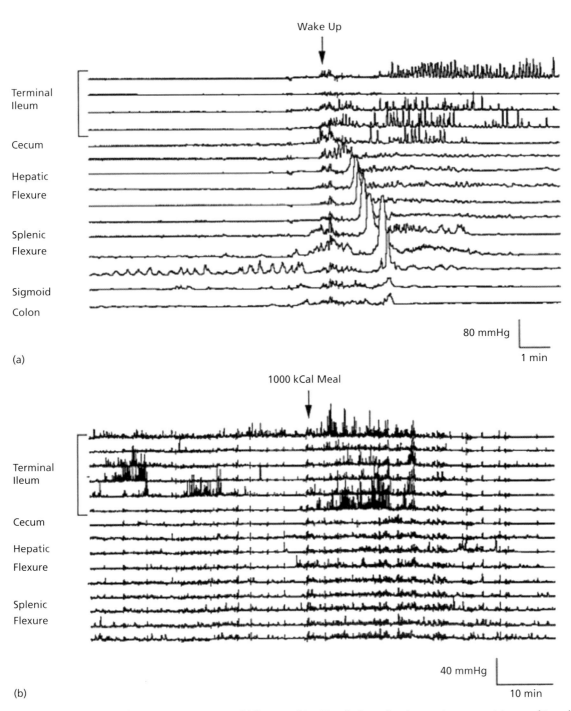

Figure 30.3 Colonic motor activity. (a) Motor activity prior to and following waking. Note the immediate increase in motor activity on waking, which includes a high-amplitude propagating contraction (HAPC) in the more distal sites. (b) Fed motor response. Note the immediate increase in motor activity. Source: Bampton 2001. Reproduced with permission of Nature Publishing Group.

can influence colonic sensation and motility directly through the elaboration of neuromodulatory molecules or indirectly through its intraluminal modulation of short-chain fatty acid or bile salt metabolism, or else via the generation of various gases [28]. Indeed, the microbiota is essential for the development of afferent neuron excitability [29]. The very novel concept of the microbiota–gut–brain axis is based on observations of the ability of modifications of the microbiota to influence behavior and effect changes in brain function, morphology, and biochemistry [30].

Take Home Points

- Gut smooth muscle, interstitial Cajal cells (ICCs), and the enteric nervous system (ENS) work in unison to generate, propagate, and modulate most motor events in the small intestine and colon.
- Extrinsic neural influences exert a greater impact on the colon than the small intestine.
- Sensation is an important but poorly understood phenomenon in the normal colon and small intestine.

- During fasting, motor activity in the small intestine is organized into recurring cycles of the migrating motor complex (MMC); on meal ingestion, these are abolished and replaced by the fed motor response.
- Motor activity in the colon is more complex and less readily characterized but features diurnal variation, a meal response, and powerful contractions that can traverse much of the colon and induce an urge to defecate.
- Less invasive methods have been introduced that may provide more insights into motility in health and disease.
- Interactions between the ENS and the musculature of the gut, on the one hand, and luminal contents and the microbiota (in particular), on the other, are emerging as important factors in the regulation of small-intestinal and colonic motor activity.

References

1 Quigley EMM. Gastric and small intestinal motility in health and disease. *Gastro Clin North Am* 1996; **25**: 113–46.

2 Quigley EMM. Colonic motility and colonic motor function. In: Pemberton JH, Swash M, Henry MM, eds. *The Pelvic Floor, Its Function and Disorders.* Philadelphia, PA: WB Saunders, 2002: 84–93.

3 Gudsoorkar VS, Quigley EM. Colorectal sensation and motility. *Curr Opin Gastroenterol* 2014; **30**: 75–83

4 Sanders KM, Koh SD, Ro S, Ward SM. Regulation of gastrointestinal motility – insights from smooth muscle biology. *Nat Rev Gastroenterol Hepatol* 2012; **9**: 633–45

5 Quigley EM. What we have learned about colonic motility: normal and disturbed. *Curr Opin Gastroenterol* 2010; **26**: 53–60.

6 Sanders KM, Zhu MH, Britton F, *et al.* Anoctamins and gastrointestinal smooth muscle excitability. *Exp Physiol* 2012; **97**: 200–6.

7 Klein S, Seidler B, Kettenberger A, *et al.* Interstitial cells of Cajal integrate excitatory and inhibitory neurotransmission with intestinal slow-wave activity. *Nat Commun* 2013; **4**: 1630.

8 Kurahashi M, Zheng H, Dwyer L, *et al.* A functional role for the "fibroblast-like cells" in gastrointestinal smooth muscles. *J Physiol* 2011; **589**: 697–710.

9 Furness JB. The enteric nervous system and neurogastroenterology. *Nat Rev Gastroenterol Hepatol* 2012; **9**: 286–94.

10 Gulbransen BD, Sharkey KA. Novel functional roles for enteric glia in the gastrointestinal tract. *Nat Rev Gastroenterol Hepatol* 2012; **9**: 625–32

11 Brookes SJ, Spencer NJ, Costa M, Zagorodnyuk VP. Extrinsic primary afferent signalling in the gut. *Nat Rev Gastroenterol Hepatol* 2013; **10**: 286–96.

12 de Jonge WJ. The gut's little brain in control of intestinal immunity. *ISRN Gastroenterol* 2013; **2013**: 630159.

13 Furness JB, Rivera LR, Cho HJ, *et al.* The gut as a sensory organ. *Nat Rev Gastroenterol Hepatol* 2013; **10**: 729–40.

14 Quigley EMM. Intestinal manometry in man: an historical and clinical perspective. *Dig Dis* 1994; **12**: 199–209.

15 Dinning PG, Arkwright JW, Gregersen H, *et al.* Technical advances in monitoring human motility patterns. *Neurogastroenterol Motil* 2010; **22**: 366–80.

16 Chaikomin R, Wu KL, Doran S, *et al.* Concurrent duodenal manometric and impedance recording to evaluate the effects of hyoscine on motility and flow events, glucose absorption, and incretin release. *Am J Physiol Gastrointest Liver Physiol* 2007; **292**: G1099–104.

17 Gregersen H, Liao D, Pedersen J, Drewes AM. A new method for evaluation of intestinal muscle contraction properties: studies in normal subjects and in patients with systemic sclerosis. *Neurogastroenterol Motil* 2007; **19**: 11–19.

18 Pritchard SE, Marciani L, Garsed KC, *et al.* Fasting and postprandial volumes of the undisturbed colon: normal values and changes in diarrhea-predominant irritable bowel syndrome measured using serial MRI. *Neurogastroenterol Motil* 2014; **26**: 124–30.

19 Chaddock G, Lam C, Hoad CL, *et al.* Novel MRI tests of orocecal transit time and whole gut transit time: studies in normal subjects. *Neurogastroenterol Motil* 2014; **26**: 205–14.

20 Richburg DA, Kim JH. Real-time bowel ultrasound to characterize intestinal motility in the preterm neonate. *J Perinatol* 2013; **33**: 605–8.

21 Malagelada C, De Iorio F, Azpiroz F, *et al.* New insight into intestinal motor function via noninvasive endoluminal image analysis. *Gastroenterology* 2008; **135**: 1155–62.

22 Kloetzer L, Chey WD, McCallum RW, *et al.* Motility of the antroduodenum in healthy and gastroparetics characterized by wireless motility capsule. *Neurogastroenterol Motil* 2010; **22**: 527–33.

23 Husebye E. The patterns of small bowel motility: physiology and implications in organic disease and functional disorders. *Neurogastroenterol Motil* 1999; **11**: 141–61.

24 Wilson P, Perdikis G, Hinder RA, *et al.* Prolonged ambulatory antroduodenal manometry in humans. *Am J Gastroenterol* 1994; **89**: 1489–95.

25 Quigley EMM, Borody TJ, Phillips SF, *et al.* Motility of the terminal ileum and ileocaecal sphincter in healthy man. *Gastroenterology* 1984; **87**: 857–66.

26 Ratuapli SK, Bharucha AE, Noelting J, *et al.* Phenotypic identification and classification of functional defecatory disorders using high-resolution anorectal manometry. *Gastroenterology* 2013; **144**: 314–22.e2.

27 Aziz Q, Doré J, Emmanuel A, *et al.* Gut microbiota and gastrointestinal health: current concepts and future directions. *Neurogastroenterol Motil* 2013; **25**: 4–15.

28 Quigley EM. Microflora modulation of motility. *J Neurogastroenterol Motil* 2011; **17**: 140–7.

29 McVey Neufeld KA, Mao YK, Bienenstock J, *et al.* The microbiome is essential for normal gut intrinsic primary afferent neuron excitability in the mouse. *Neurogastroenterol Motil* 2013; **25**: e183–8

30 Cryan JF, Dinan TG. Mind-altering microorganisms: the impact of the gut microbiota on brain and behaviour. *Nat Rev Neurosci* 2012; **13**: 701–12.

CHAPTER 31

Neoplasia

John M. Carethers

Division of Gastroenterology, Department of Internal Medicine, University of Michigan, Ann Arbor, MI, USA

Summary

Neoplasia, the abnormal proliferation of cells, causes a macroscopic tumor that is often benign initially but can progress to malignancy through successive waves of clonality caused by genomic instability. The genetic damage that causes the genomic instability comes from environmental and other local stresses, which damage a stem cell's DNA and allow it to evade the mechanisms that normally regulate its growth and proliferation. Neoplasms can occur anywhere in the gastrointestinal (GI) tract, and each affected organ has different gender distributions and different prognoses. Benign neoplasms are often found incidentally or at screening, while malignant neoplasms typically present symptomatically. Multiple neoplasms in a single person and family history can identify individuals at high risk who should be targeted for surveillance. GI neoplasms can be removed surgically or at endoscopy, but malignant ones may need additional chemotherapy and/or radiation treatment. Precision medicine takes into account genetic information on both the patient and the tumor to provide an optimized outcome.

Definition and Epidemiology

"Neoplasia" refers to an abnormal proliferation of cells. At the macroscopic level, neoplasia results in a neoplasm, or tumor. Neoplasms within the GI tract generally start out as benign lesions, which, if discovered and treated, have no untoward effect on patient survival. Often, however, neoplasms grow indolently and transform into malignant tumors, which can threaten survival [1].

The GI tract, including the hollow organs of the gut, pancreas, liver, and biliary tree, is the site of more cancers and the source of more cancer mortality than any other organ system in the body. As shown in Table 31.1, the incidence of GI tract cancer in the United States was over 289 000 cases in 2014 [2]. However, this number greatly underestimates the incidence for all GI neoplasms, because those that are benign or remain indolent are not included; if they were included, they would probably increase the incidence at least fivefold. Table 31.1 also shows that there are differences in incidence between men and women and between relatively benign and deadly cancers (the latter including esophageal, pancreas, and liver cancers). These differences may be related to a multitude of factors, including: (i) gender and hormone differences, (ii) differing levels of exposure to environmental carcinogens, (iii) the late clinical presentation and discovery of certain neoplasms, (iv) genetic factors, and (v) the response to therapy of specific cancers [1].

Malignant neoplasms such as hepatocellular carcinoma are on the rise, due to the prevalence of hepatitis C infection, while colorectal neoplasms are on the decline, in part due to systematic screening efforts [2].

Clinical Features

Benign neoplasms are often asymptomatic and are typically discovered incidentally or during screening or surveillance. The best recognized benign lesion in the GI tract is the colonic adenoma, due to screening of all persons over the age of 50 years, with only a few per cent progressing to cancer. The size and histology of adenomas can predict future risk for colon cancer, and these features are used in algorithms for surveillance [1, 3]. Other GI organs may begin as benign neoplasms prior to malignancy; these include pancreatic intraepithelial neoplasia, adenomas of the stomach, small intestine, and colon, and benign neuroendocrine tumors. Inflammation can be a common precursor to many neoplasms of the GI tract, including Barrett's metaplasia before esophageal adenocarcinoma, *H. pylori*-induced inflammation before gastric cancer, hepatitis B or C infection and inflammation prior to liver cancer, recurrent pancreatitis before pancreatic adenocarcinoma, and chronic inflammation of inflammatory bowel disease (IBD) before intestinal cancer.

Malignant neoplasms can be discovered incidentally, but are more often brought to medical attention due to patient symptoms. Esophageal cancers often present with solid-food dysphagia. Pancreatic, liver, and gastric cancers may present with abdominal pain and weight loss. Colon and small-intestinal cancers may present with weight loss, bowel obstruction, and iron-deficiency anemia. Anal cancers may present with rectal pain and bleeding.

In some cases, which it is important to recognize, there may be a familial component to GI-tract and other cancers [4]. Clues such as young age of presentation, a strong family history for cancers, multiple neoplasms in a single individual, and some clinical features help determine whether a patient should be evaluated for genetic counseling and genetic testing. Identifying these high-risk individuals helps target them for regular surveillance strategies, which will extend their life span [5].

Pathophysiology

The abnormal cellular growth that defines neoplasia is born out of alterations to normal cellular proteins, which change normal

Practical Gastroenterology and Hepatology Board Review Toolkit, Second Edition. Edited by Nicholas J. Talley, Kenneth R. DeVault, Michael B. Wallace, Bashar A. Aqel and Keith D. Lindor.

Table 31.1 Incidence and mortality of GI cancers in the United States (2014). Source: Adapted from Siegel 2014 [2]. Reproduced with permission of Wiley.

Cancer	Incidence	Male incidence	Female incidence	Deaths	Annual deaths/incidence
Esophagus	18 170	14 660	3510	15 450	85%
Stomach	22 220	13 730	8490	10 990	49%
Small intestine	9160	4880	4280	1210	13%
Pancreas	46 420	23 530	22 890	39 590	85%
Liver and intrahepatic duct	33 190	24 600	8590	23 000	69%
Gallbladder and biliary ducts	10 650	4960	5690	3630	34%
Colon and rectum	136 830	71 830	65 000	50 310	37%
Anus and anorectum	7210	2660	4550	950	13%
Other digestive organs	5760	1880	3880	2130	37%
Total	**289 610**	**162 730**	**126 880**	**147 260**	**51%**

cellular responses and checkpoints in cells. The alterations may occur via environmental factors (e.g., toxin exposure, such as tobacco or alcohol, for pancreatic, liver, and esophageal squamous cell cancer; acidic bile exposure for esophageal adenocarcinoma; ingested fats and microbiome changes for colorectal cancer; certain viral etiologies for liver and anal cancers; and *Helicobacter pylori* for gastric cancer), as well as through inherited genetic factors that affect key growth-regulatory genes in affected patients, predisposing them to neoplastic growth [5–8].

The paradigm of environmental or inherited genetic damage to a stem cell (termed "genomic instability") [1, 7, 9, 10], followed by clonal expansion with continued genetic alteration during accelerated cellular proliferation, transforming normal cells to an initially benign but rapidly malignant tumor capable of metastasizing to distant organs, holds for most GI neoplasms [1]. Stem-cell proteins can ultimately be altered by a number of DNA damage mechanisms, including mutation, loss of heterozygosity or chromosome breakage, rearrangement, amplification, methylation,

acetylation and deacetylation, inactivation of DNA repair mechanisms, and telomerase damage, as well as non-DNA mechanisms such as microRNA expression [1, 7, 9–11]. Damaged cells have deregulated growth pathways, subvert normal cell-cycle checkpoints, and avoid programmed cell death mechanisms. The best studied of these is the adenoma-to-carcinoma sequence in the colon, due to the accessibility of the colon with colonoscopy. Specific genetic changes have been detected and can be predicted during each wave of clonal expansion, matching the histology of the growing adenoma and its transformation into cancer [1, 3, 7, 9, 10]. As depicted in Figure 31.1, sporadic colon adenomas may take 3–5 decades of life to form and another 1–2 decades to become malignant, and may be a consequence of environmental exposure in the colon plus some genetic factors. In familial adenomatous polyposis (FAP), the development of adenomas is greatly accelerated by an inherited germline mutation in the *APC* gene, but the malignant transformation rate is the same as that in the sporadic condition. With Lynch syndrome, adenomas form at the same rate

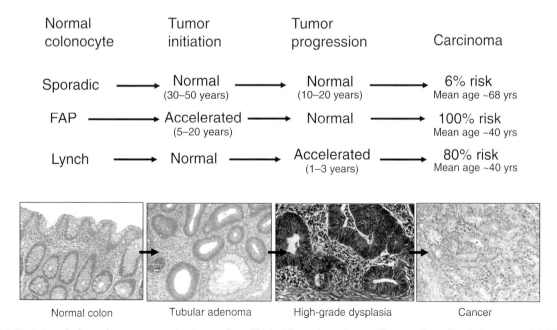

Figure 31.1 Depiction of colorectal tumor progression in sporadic and high-risk genetic syndromes. The general paradigm is that a tumor is initiated from a normal colonocyte stem cell that has sustained genetic damage over time from the local environment and any germline genetic mutation that may have been inherited. The damaged DNA provides a growth advantage that drives tumor progression as successive clonal outgrowths are generated, ultimately forming carcinoma. In familial adenomatous polyposis (FAP), tumor initiation is accelerated by the inheritance of a germline *APC* mutation, and in Lynch syndrome, tumor progression is accelerated by the hypermutable phenotype that occurs with loss of DNA mismatch repair. Photomicrographs depict, in order, normal colon, tubular adenoma, high-grade dysplasia, and cancer.

Table 31.2 Potential biomarker material for neoplasia detection and prognosis.

Luminal sources	Non-luminal sources (blood/plasma/serum/saliva/urine/sweat)
Fecal DNA	Circulating tumor cells (CTCs)
Brushings (exfoliated cells)	DNA
Biopsies (cells and histology)	RNAs (messenger RNA, microRNA, etc.)
	Oncofetal proteins and other proteins (cancer proteome)
	Metabolites (metabolomics)

as sporadic ones, but malignant transformation is accelerated by loss of function of the DNA mismatch repair system [1, 7].

Diagnosis

Because of the internal nature of the organs that make of the GI tract, diagnosis of neoplasms involves the use of radiologic imaging studies (e.g., computed tomography (CT), magnetic resonance imaging (MRI), ultrasound, contrast X-ray), direct endoscopic viewing (e.g., esophagogastroduodenoscopy, colonoscopy wireless capsule video endoscopy, double-balloon enteroscopy), or combined radiologic and endoscopic modalities (e.g., endoscopic ultrasound, endoscopic retrograde cholangiopancreatography (ERCP)). Many of these modalities allow tissue sampling for pathological diagnosis.

Many GI neoplasms exfoliate and extravasate cells, usually in their malignant stage (Table 31.2). These cells and their associated nucleic acids and proteins can act as biomarkers that are useful in confirming a diagnosis or a cancer, or can be used in surveillance for recurrence [12]. Information from these cells may be utilized for precision medicine [13].

Treatment

Most GI neoplasms are removed at surgery or at endoscopy. Patients are cured of their neoplasm if a benign lesion is completely removed. Malignant neoplasms will often require surgery for attempted cure, and depending on the staging of the patient's tumor, may require pre- and or postsurgical chemoradiation [13–15]. Chemoprevention may be effective in some patients who belong to high-risk groups, such as FAP [16]. Advances in the understanding of the molecular pathogenesis of some tumors have led to the development of targeted drugs that can dramatically shrink a tumor, such as imatinib for GI stromal tumors [12, 17]. Using information derived from the patient and the malignant tumor allows a personalized approach to therapy: precision medicine [13].

Acknowledgements

Supported by the United States Public Health Service (DK067287 and CA162147).

Take Home Points

- Abnormal cell growth, or neoplasia, can occur anywhere in the gastrointestinal (GI) tract, from the mouth to the anus.
- Neoplasia can commence as a benign but altered growth process or can form as a mass, and can progress to a malignant process, eventually affecting patient survival.
- Neoplasms reflect altered cellular processes that change the balance of cell proliferation and cell death in favor of proliferation, and potential local or distant spread when malignant.
- Genetic predisposition and environmental factors affect an individual's neoplastic risk, and surveillance programs for high-risk individuals may improve detection and survival.
- Malignant neoplasms release cells that contain proteins and nucleic acids, which may be helpful diagnostically and may prognosticate patient outcome.
- Precision medicine approaches for patients with malignant neoplasia take into account the individual's and the tumor's genetic information to optimize care and outcome.

References

1 Grady WM, Carethers JM. Genomic and epigenetic instability in colorectal cancer pathogenesis. *Gastroenterology* 2008; **135**: 1079–99.

2 Segal R, Ma J, Zou Z, Jemal A. Cancer statistics, 2014. *CA Cancer J Clin* 2014; **64**: 9–29.

3 Carethers JM. One colon lumen but two organs. *Gastroenterol* 2011; **141**: 411–12.

4 Carethers JM. Differentiating Lynch-like from Lynch syndrome. *Gastroenterol* 2014; **146**: 602–4.

5 Boland CR, Koi M, Chang DK, Carethers JM. The biochemical basis of microsatellite instability and abnormal immunohistochemistry and clinical behavior in Lynch syndrome: from bench to bedside. *Fam Cancer* 2008; **7**: 41–52.

6 Anderson AR, Weaver AM, Cummings PT, Quaranta V. Tumor morphology and phenotypic evolution driven by selective pressure from the microenvironment. *Cell* 2006; **127**: 905–15.

7 Fearon ER. Molecular genetics of colorectal cancer. *Annu Rev Pathol* 2011; **6**: 479–507.

8 Cancer Genome Atlas Network. Comprehensive molecular characterization of human colon and rectal cancer. *Nature* 2012; **487**: 330–7.

9 Vogelstein B, Fearon ER, Hamilton SR, *et al.* Genetic alterations during colorectal-tumor development. *N Engl J Med* 1988; **319**: 525–32.

10 Issa JP. CpG island methylator phenotype in cancer. *Nat Rev Cancer* 2004; **4**: 988–93.

11 Kim DH, Rossi JJ. Strategies for silencing human disease using RNA interference. *Nat Rev Genet* 2007; **8**: 173–84.

12 Carethers JM. DNA testing and molecular screening for colon cancer. *Clin Gastroenterol Hepatol* 2014; **12**: 377–81.

13 Carethers JM. Proteomics, genomics, and molecular biology in the personalized treatment of colorectal cancer. *J Gastrointest Surg* 2012; **16**(9): 1648–50.

14 Carethers JM. Systemic treatment of advanced colorectal cancer – tailoring therapy to the tumor. *Ther Adv Gastroenterol* 2008; **1**: 33–42.

15 Potti A, Dressman HK, Bild A, *et al.* Genomic signatures to guide the use of chemotherapeutics. *Nat Med* 2006; **12**: 1294–300.

16 Steinbach G, Lynch PM, Phillips RK, *et al.* The effect of celecoxib, a cyclooxygenase-2 inhibitor, in familial adenomatous polyposis. *N Engl J Med* 2000; **342**: 1946–52.

17 Heinrich MC, Blanke CD, Druker BJ, Corless CL. Inhibition of KIT tyrosine kinase activity: a novel molecular approach to the treatment of KIT positive malignancies. *J Clin Oncol* 2002; **20**: 1692–703.

PART 2

Problem-Based Approach to Diagnosis and Differential Diagnosis

32 General Approach to Relevant History-Taking and Physical Examination, 203
Christopher L. Steele and Suzanne Rose

33 Acute Diarrhea, 213
John R. Cangemi

34 Chronic Diarrhea, 218
Lawrence R. Schiller

35 Loss of Appetite and Loss of Weight, 223
Angela Vizzini and Jaime Aranda-Michel

36 Gastrointestinal Food Allergy and Intolerance, 227
Mark T. DeMeo

37 Obesity: Presentations and Management Options, 231
Andres Acosta, Todd A. Kellogg, and Barham K. Abu Dayyeh

38 Hematochezia, 237
Lisa L. Strate

39 Obscure Gastrointestinal Bleeding, 241
R. Sameer Islam and Shabana F. Pasha

40 Constipation, 246
Arnold Wald

41 Perianal Disease, 251
Leyla J. Ghazi and David A. Schwartz

42 Fecal Incontinence, 256
David Prichard and Adil E. Bharucha

43 Colorectal Cancer Screening, 261
Katherine S. Garman and Dawn Provenzale

44 Endoscopic Palliation of Malignant Obstruction, 266
Todd H. Baron

CHAPTER 32

General Approach to Relevant History-Taking and Physical Examination

Christopher L. Steele[1] and Suzanne Rose[2]

[1]Resident, Osler Medical Training Program, The Johns Hopkins University School of Medicine, Baltimore, MD

[2]Office of Academic Affairs and the Department of Medicine, Division of Gastroenterology, University of Connecticut School of Medicine, Farmington, CT, USA

Summary

Taking a comprehensive history and performing a thorough physical examination are essential to the evaluation and management of patients presenting with a gastrointestinal (GI) complaint. The line of questioning should focus on the concern, but should be comprehensive enough to rule out both non-GI and GI causes, as well as systemic problems. Superb communication skills will support a trusting patient–physician relationship, resulting in better care. This chapter offers strategies for approaching specific complaints, reviews the pertinent features of the physical examination, discusses advancements in medical simulation, and reviews current preventative guidelines applicable to the field of gastroenterology.

Introduction to History Taking

The ability to solicit a good history comes from a combination of clinical knowledge and the development of a strong doctor–patient relationship. It is important for the health care provider to introduce him or herself, maintain eye contact, identify his/her role, ensure a private setting, and be aware of both verbal and non-verbal cues during the interaction [1]. Initially, questions should be open-ended, allowing the patient to freely express him or herself. Later, a perceptive historian will refine the line of questioning, using more directed questions to narrow the differential diagnosis. Simply asking the patient if he/she has had or has been seen for this illness before can help tremendously. It is important to conduct an appropriate review of the possible organ systems that may be involved and then to consider the physiologic processes (e.g., inflammatory, infectious, neoplastic, congenital, etc.) in order to narrow the differential and discover any other underlying ailments. One good strategy is to review the patient's story and ask if there is anything additional that should have been discussed. Often enough, the patient will provide valuable information. For more detail, see Table 32.1 for general questioning strategies and an initial approach to diagnosing any patient complaint.

In addition to great communication, a practitioner must recognize the most common conditions seen in their field. Tables 32.2 and 32.3 are summaries of the top 10 most common gastroenterology chief complaints and medical diagnoses encountered in an outpatient clinic setting [2]. The following section expands upon the most common reasons for patients to present with a GI complaint and discusses the appropriate history, physical examination techniques, and maneuvers for each concern.

Patient Concerns

Abdominal Pain

Abdominal pain is the most common gastroenterology chief complaint, making up nearly 15.9 million visits annually [2]. The causes for a patient's abdominal pain can be extensive, making it a true challenge to formulate the correct diagnosis. The source may actually not be in the GI system, but could be a manifestation of cardiopulmonary disease, dermatologic problems, or musculoskeletal issues. A strategy for an initial approach to the patient with abdominal pain may be to determine the source and, if the problem is of GI origin, to evaluate whether the patient's symptom can be identified as either visceral or parietal in nature. Visceral pain is the result of distension and spasm of an organ's lumen or covering. The pain is usually poorly localized and is described as aching, dull, or a cramping midline sensation. On the other hand, parietal pain results from peritoneal inflammation and is commonly described as severe, sharp, and a well-localized sensation. Referred pain is the product of crosstalk between visceral sensory nerves and somatic sensory nerves of the same vertebral level and is described as aching, burning, or a gnawing feeling. The classic example of this is the pain felt below the right scapula as a result of biliary colic. The quality and severity of abdominal pain may vary between individuals, based on clinical environment, culture, personality, mental status, medications, and past experiences with pain [3]. Take note of the patient's body position, as this may provide information about the severity of the pain. Table 32.4 provides questions to be asked in order to define abdominal pain [3,4].

Another way of establishing a differential diagnosis is to determine the region where the abdominal pain is experienced. Figure 32.1 shows the four-quadrants approach, while Figure 32.2 demonstrates the nine-regions approach to describing the location of abdomen pain. Table 32.5 indicates abdominal anatomic regions with possible etiologies of pain in those regions.

Practical Gastroenterology and Hepatology Board Review Toolkit, Second Edition. Edited by Nicholas J. Talley, Kenneth R. DeVault, Michael B. Wallace, Bashar A. Aqel and Keith D. Lindor.
© 2016 John Wiley & Sons, Ltd. Published 2016 by John Wiley & Sons, Ltd. Companion website: www.practicalgastrohep.com

Table 32.1 General history-taking.

Onset: When did the symptoms begin? How frequent are they?
Precipitating/palliation: Does anything make it worse? Anything make it better?
Quality: How would you describe the symptoms?
Region: Where is the pain located?
Severity: On a scale from 1 (not at all) to 10 (severely), how do these symptoms interfere with your daily life?
Timing: How long does this last? Does it vary over the day?
Have you ever had these symptoms before? If so, what happened?
Is there any association with eating, bowel movements, flatulence, or belching?
Do you have close contacts with similar symptoms?

Table 32.2 Top 10 most common GI chief complaints [2].

Rank	Chief complaint
1	Abdominal pain
2	Diarrhea
3	Constipation
4	Vomiting
5	Nausea
6	Indigestion
7	Rectal bleeding
8	Other GI symptoms (unspecified)
9	Dysphagia
10	GI bleeding

Table 32.3 Top 10 most common GI medical diagnoses [2].

Rank	Medical diagnosis
1	Gastroesophageal reflux disease (GERD)
2	Abdominal pain
3	Gastroenteritis/dyspepsia
4	Constipation
5	Abdominal wall hernia
6	Diverticular disease
7	Diarrhea
8	Inflammatory bowel disease (IBD)
9	Colorectal neoplasm
10	Nausea/vomiting

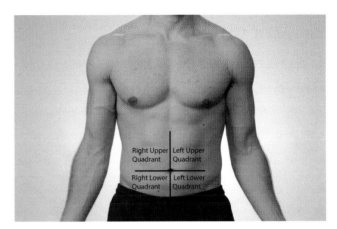

Figure 32.1 Four quadrants of the abdomen.

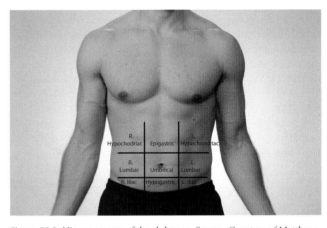

Figure 32.2 Nine segments of the abdomen. Source: Courtesy of Matthew Sara, MD.

Bowel Complaints

Diarrhea and constipation can result from alterations in the balance of intestinal secretion, absorption, surface area, bacterial flora, transit time, and neurological and muscular function. Patients may describe bowel complaints in terms of stool consistency, frequency, or volume, or in terms of sensation of stool passage [5–7]. A thorough history will elicit the time course and detailed characteristics of the stool changes. Table 32.6 shows the Bristol Stool Form Scale, which is a tool to help patients further describe stool consistency to their provider [8, 9]. It has been shown that this scale correlates

Table 32.4 Questions targeted to define abdominal pain.

Question	Indication
Where do you feel the pain?	See Table 32.5, Figures 32.1 and 32.2
Has the pain radiated or moved since onset?	Appendicitis begins at umbilicus and later causes right lower-quadrant pain
	Aortic dissection begins as chest pain and later causes abdominal or back pain
	Biliary colic radiates to the right scapula
	Pancreatitis radiates to the back
How severe is the pain from 0 to 10?	Very severe pain is seen with intestinal perforation, peritonitis, or volvulus
How does the pain feel?	Differentiate between visceral, parietal, and referred pain
	Colicky pain often has a crescendo–decrescendo pattern
Is the pain associated with meals?	Worsens after fatty meals with biliary disease
	Worsens after meals with gastric peptic ulcers and mesenteric ischemia [4]
	Improves after meals with duodenal peptic ulcers [3, 4]
Is the pain associated with nausea and vomiting?	Biliary disease, acute pancreatitis, appendicitis, peritonitis, intestinal obstruction, and ectopic pregnancy
Does the pain disrupt your sleep?	Duodenal peptic ulcers and GERD
Is the pain out of proportion to physical exam?	Mesenteric ischemia
Does anything make it worse or better?	Biliary colic is made worse with fatty meals
	Gastric ulcers are worse with eating, while duodenal are relieved with food
	Consumption history: alcoholic gastritis, aspirin-induced ulcers

GERD, gastroesophageal reflux disease.

Table 32.5 Differential diagnosis of pain, based on etiology and location. NB: Neoplasms and musculoskeletal pathology can also cause pain in any of the locations.

Location of the pain	GI causes					Non-GI causes
	Inflammatory or infectious	Vascular	Mechanical	Congenital	Functional	
Left upper quadrant (LUQ)	Splenic infection Gastritis Gastric ulcer Pancreatitis	Splenic infarction	Volvulus		Gastroparesis	Myocardial infarction Pneumonia
Right upper quadrant (RUQ)	Hepatitis Cholecystitis Cholangitis Pancreatitis	Budd–Chiari Ischemic hepatopathy	Biliary colic Volvulus		IBS	Subdiaphragmatic abscess Pneumonia Empyema Fitz-Hugh–Curtis
Left lower quadrant (LLQ)	Diverticulitis IBD	Ischemia	Inguinal hernia		IBS	Pelvic inflammatory disease Ectopic pregnancy Mittelschmerz Endometriosis Ovarian cysts Nephrolithiasis Pyelonephritis
Right lower quadrant (RLQ)	Late appendicitis Colitis IBD Pseudoappendicitis (Yersinia)	Intestinal ischemia	Inguinal hernia Intestinal obstruction	Meckel's diverticulitis	IBS	Pelvic inflammatory disease Ectopic pregnancy Mittelschmerz Endometriosis Ovarian cysts Nephrolithiasis Pyelonephritis
Umbilical	Early appendicitis Gastroenteritis	Aortic aneurysm or dissection	Intestinal obstruction Umbilical hernia			
Epigastric	Peptic ulcer disease Gastritis Pancreatitis Esophagitis	Aortic aneurysm or dissection	Gastroparesis Abdominal hernia	Lactase deficiency	GERD Gastroparesis Non-ulcer dyspepsia Malabsorption	Myocardial infarction Pericarditis Costochondritis Anxiety Pneumonia
Hypogastric					IBS	Cystitis Endometriosis Urethral obstruction
Diffuse	Gastroenteritis Malaria Peritonitis	Mesenteric ischemia	Intestinal obstruction Volvulus	Acute intermittent porphyria	IBS	

IBS, irritable bowel syndrome; IBD, inflammatory bowel disease; GERD, gastroesophageal reflux disease.

with colonic transit time, such that type 1 stool suggests a slow transit, while type 7 stool suggests rapid transit [10]. Table 32.7 lists questions to use in clarifying the symptoms of bowel complaints [4,7,11].

Both diarrhea and constipation can be characterized as either acute or chronic in onset. Most causes of acute diarrhea are infectious in nature, requiring a detailed social history regarding recent travel, sick contacts, food consumption, and medication use. On the other hand, chronic diarrhea tends to be non-infectious in nature. It can be separated into categories of secretory and osmotic, or further characterized related to the etiology, such as

secondary to an inflammatory process, to malabsorption, or due to a motility disorder [12]. Common causes of constipation include poor fiber intake and lack of time set aside for a bowel movement; true dehydration may also lead to this symptom. Medications such as opioids and exogenous iron are known to cause constipation as well. The line of questioning should always include ruling out alarm signs suggestive of colon cancer or other malignancies. These alarm symptoms have been delineated, particularly for constipation, and include weight loss of more than 4.5 kg (10 pounds), blood in the stool, anemia, a family history of colon cancer, fever, bowel symptoms, lack of response to treatment, and new-onset symptoms in an elderly patient without evidence of a primary cause [6,7].

Embarrassing symptoms, such as fecal incontinence, may not be voluntarily disclosed by some patients. It is a good strategy to either ask directly or include these symptoms as part of a general survey of questions asked of every patient. For a patient with constipation, a question related to digitation or manual maneuvers should be asked explicitly. Dyschezia, or difficulty defecating, as distinguished from constipation, may suggest pelvic-floor dysfunction, such as dyssynergic defecation. The treatment for this etiology of constipation is specific to the cause, and therefore identifying this problem is crucial for proper therapy.

Table 32.6 Bristol Stool Form Scale [8, 9].

Type	Stool description
1	Separate hard lumps, like nuts or pellets, which are difficult to pass
2	Lumpy, but with a sausage-shape
3	Sausage-shaped with cracks on its surface
4	Smooth and soft, sausage-shaped
5	Soft pieces with clear-cut edges, which can be passed with ease
6	Ragged edges, fluffy pieces, "mushy"
7	Watery, entirely liquid stool with no solid pieces

CHAPTER 32

Table 32.7 Questions targeted to define bowel complaints.

Question	Indication
When was your most recent bowel movement?	Determine whether the complaint is acute or chronic in nature
Describe the stool consistency and size	Utilize the Bristol Stool Form Scale (see Table 32.6)
	Thin stools with colon malignancy or with spasm
	Watery stool with infection or ingestion of indigestible particles [7]
	Greasy or floating stool with pancreatitis
Do you experience bouts of both diarrhea and constipation?	IBS, diverticulitis, and colon malignancy [4]
Have you experienced fecal incontinence?	A positive reply requires a comprehensive dietary history, gynecologic history, and neurologic history
Are you passing more or less gas than usual?	Unable to pass gas with complete intestinal obstruction
	Excessive gas with malabsorption, maldigestion, or heavy ingestion of carbonated beverages (e.g. lactose intolerance or pancreatitis)
Is there blood and/or mucus in the stool?	Blood and mucus with ulcerative colitis, radiation colitis, pseudomembranous colitis, or villous adenomas
	Blood with hemorrhoids, anal pathology, diverticula, malignancy, or vascular lesions
	Blood with invasive infections, such as Shigella, E. coli, Salmonella, Yersinia, and amoeba [11]
What is the color of the stool?	Black or tarry stool with proximal GI bleed
	Light brown or gray stool with biliary obstruction
	Red stool may indicate distal GI bleed or may occur after eating large amounts of beets or food dye
Does the stool have an unusual foul odor?	Maldigestion of dietary fat with pancreatitis
Are the symptoms associated with eating certain types of food?	Wheat, barley, rye, and gluten-containing foods associated with celiac disease [11]
	Milk products associated with lactose intolerance
	Diarrhea after ingestion of caffeinated beverages, artificial sweeteners, or fruit products [7]
Do you experience rectal fullness or incomplete emptying?	Often a manifestation of visceral hypersensitivity and IBS
Do you feel the need to strain or digitate to pass stool?	May indicate pelvic-floor dysfunction

IBS, irritable bowel syndrome; GI, gastrointestinal.

Nausea and Vomiting

Vomiting is coordinated by both the vomiting center in the medulla and the chemoreceptor trigger zone near the fourth ventricle in response to signals from the GI tract, blood, cerebrospinal fluid, and inner ear [13]. Pain, visual, gustatory, and olfactory stimuli, as well as memories, contribute to the individual experience of nausea and vomiting. Nausea and vomiting are GI symptoms, but there are many non-GI causes that can either be easily explained or suggest systemic disease. Table 32.8 provides a list of non-GI causes for nausea and vomiting.

Table 32.8 Differential diagnosis for non-GI causes of nausea and vomiting. Source: Quigley 2001 [14]. Reproduced with permission of Elsevier.

Category	Examples
1 Medications	Dopamine agonists
	Nicotine
	Opiates
	Others: digoxin, NSAIDs, erythromycin
2 Cancer therapy	Chemotherapy (cisplatin)Radiation
3 Infectious	Otitis media
4 Substance abuse	Ethanol
5 Central nervous system	Migraines, increased cranial pressure (malignancy, meningitis, etc.), seizures, labyrinth disorders (Meniere's, labyrinthitis, etc.)
6 Endocrine	Uremia, diabetic ketoacidosis, hyperparathyroidism, hyperthyroidism, Addison's disease, acute intermittent porphyria
7 Postoperative vomiting	History of recent surgery and/or anesthesia for a procedure
8 Cyclic vomiting syndrome	Marijuana use
9 Psychiatric	Anxiety, pain, emotional stress, bulimia/anorexia
10 Pregnancy	Normal pregnancy
	Hyperemesis gravidarum
11 Other	Cardiac (CHF, MI)
	Starvation

NSAID, non-steroidal anti-inflammatory drug; CHF, congestive heart failure; MI, myocardial infarction.

The first step in the evaluation should be to obtain a detailed history, which will help distinguish nausea and vomiting from rumination, regurgitation, and retching, while ruling out any "do not miss" diagnoses. Red-flag symptoms, such as poor hydration resulting in moderate to severe hypotension, intense abdominal pain, chest pain, or the presence of acute nausea and vomiting in any elderly patient, should lead to possible hospital admission for treatment and further evaluation. Table 32.9 lists questions that may be asked to characterize a complaint of nausea or vomiting [14, 15].

GI Bleeding

Bleeding from the GI tract is classified as stemming from either the upper or the lower GI tract, depending upon whether the source is proximal or distal to the ligament of Treitz. The ligament of Treitz originates at the right crus of the diaphragm and inserts upon the third to fourth portion of the duodenum. A detailed history may help distinguish these forms of bleeding, though manifestations of a GI bleed depend on the rate, source, and location. For example, hematemesis is the vomiting of bright red blood and melena is black, tarry stool with a characteristic odor. The former definitively indicates an upper GI source, but the latter could indicate either. Hematochezia is the passage of bloody bowel movements from the rectum, and though a lower GI source is often found to be the etiology, hematochezia can be the manifestation of a rapid upper GI bleed secondary to varices or bleeding from an arterial source. Occult bleeding may occur from anywhere in the GI tract and is usually detected with the presentation of chronic anemia or by testing the stool for occult blood.

Common sources of upper GI bleeding include esophageal varices, peptic ulcers, Mallory–Weiss tears, gastric cancer, and erosive gastritis. It is important to ask about alcohol consumption and non-steroidal anti-inflammatory drug (NSAID) use, because the source of the bleed can be related to these substances. Lower GI bleeding may result from diverticulosis, polyps and colon cancer, inflammatory bowel disease (IBD), infectious causes, anal fissures,

Table 32.9 Questions targeted to define nausea and vomiting.

Question	Indication
How frequently are you vomiting?	Continuous vomiting with ingestion of toxic substances [4]
	Abrupt, forceful vomiting with increased intracranial pressure or other CNS lesions [15]
	Early-morning vomiting with metabolic disturbances or pregnancy
Have you taken recent steroids or pain medicines?	Nausea is an early sign of steroid, opioid, or sedative withdrawal
Do you have dizziness or difficulty with balance?	Vestibular or CNS lesion
Describe the color and consistency of the vomitus	Green or yellow vomitus with biliary disease
	Bloody vomitus with acute bleed of esophageal varices or peptic ulcer
	Coffee-ground vomitus with upper GI bleed
	Feculent vomitus with ileus or intestinal obstruction
	Large-volume vomitus with gastric outlet obstruction
	Undigested vomitus with achalasia and incompletely digested vomitus with gastroparesis
	Food particles on the pillow can be a sign of Zenker diverticulum
Has the color of your stool or urine changed?	Light stools and dark urine with biliary obstruction
Does anyone close to you have similar symptoms?	After meals with foodborne illness
	Gastroenteritis
Is the vomiting associated with abdominal pain?	Onset of pain occurs before onset of vomiting with appendicitis [4], can be a sign of early obstruction [14]
	Consider pancreatitis

CNS, central nervous system; GI, gastrointestinal.

or hemorrhoids. Vascular ectasias can be found throughout the GI tract [16]. Table 32.10 provides a list of questions to ask a patient presenting with a GI bleed, remembering that the ABCs of resuscitation and assessment of the status of the patient are the key first step [4,17].

Jaundice

Jaundice is the yellowing of the skin and sclera of the eyes due to excess bilirubin from disruption in the uptake, conjugation, or excretion of bilirubin by the liver. Therefore, jaundice may be the result of damage to hepatocytes, impaired liver cell function due to internal or external blockage of the bile ducts, or excessive breakdown of red blood cells (RBCs). Inherited defects of bilirubin metabolism (Dubin–Johnson, Crigler–Najjar, Gilbert's) may also present as jaundice. Like jaundice, increased carotene intake can also affect skin coloring, but it does not cause discoloration of the sclera. The symptoms associated with jaundice may be specific to the cause, and frequently labs and imaging such as ultrasonography are necessary to establish the diagnosis [18]. See Table 32.11 for

specific questions that should be asked related to the presentation of jaundice.

Other Symptoms

An allergy and medication list should be obtained for all patients. A pertinent family history should be documented, along with a social history that includes tobacco, alcohol and drug use, occupation, living environment, stressors, sick contacts, and sexual activity.

A history of abuse is more common in patients with functional GI complaints. There is a high prevalence of abuse that spans the ages, socioeconomic lines, and gender, though it is more common in women. The elicitation of a history of abuse or domestic violence should be considered for all patients. It is important to gain the trust of the patient; often, a more personal history is obtained on a second or subsequent visit. It is crucial that the interviewer be nonjudgmental and have resources available to help patients who have a positive response to this line of questioning (e.g., referral to a collaborative psychiatric support team) [19]. Table 32.12 presents general history questions that should be asked of all patients.

CHAPTER 32

Table 32.10 Questions targeted to define GI bleeding.

Question	Indication
Do you have a history of GI bleed?	At times, patients can provide a past diagnosis associated with bleeding, such as diverticulosis,
What is your past medical history?	malignancy, ulcers, hemorrhoids, or anal fissures
How did you first notice the blood?	Blood combined with stool in ulcerative colitis, diverticula, infection [4], and malignancy
	Blood droplets or streaks on toilet paper with external hemorrhoids
	Blood on undergarments or bedsheets with a brisk bleed from malignancy
How would you describe the blood?	Dark red, maroon, or black blood usually with more proximal GI bleed [17]
Do you have black, tarry stools or red blood in the stool?	Bright red blood with hemorrhoids, diverticula, malignancy, ulcerative colitis, or brisk upper GI bleed
What is your alcohol consumption?	Overuse can result in liver failure, leading to esophageal varices
Have you been vomiting recently?	Erosive gastritis and Mallory–Weiss tears
Have you vomited blood?	
Do you vomit material resembling coffee grounds?	
Do you or your close family members have a history of colon cancer?	One must assume bleeding from a lower GI source is malignancy until proven otherwise in adults over 40 years of age
When was your last colonoscopy?	
What were the results of your last exam?	
Are you taking any medications?	NSAIDs can result in erosive gastritis and ulcers
	Anticoagulants
	Bismuth, iron, and charcoal can cause stool to turn black
Are there any associated symptoms?	Painless bleeds are associated with diverticulosis
	Changes in bowel habits, weight loss, and fatigue can suggest malignancy

GI, gastrointestinal; NSAID, non-steroidal anti-inflammatory drug.

Table 32.11 Questions targeted to define jaundice.

Question	Indication
Does anyone in your family have a history of jaundice?	Inherited disorders of metabolism of bilirubin
	Inherited disorders of the liver: alpha-1-antitrypsin, hemochromatosis
Is your jaundice associated with abdominal pain?	RUQ pain with biliary obstruction or hepatitis
Do you have fever?	Biliary obstruction, hepatitis
	Fever, jaundice, and RUQ abdominal pain is the Charcot triad, indicating ascending cholangitis [18]
Is jaundice associated with nausea, vomiting, or itching?	Severe itching with biliary obstruction, primary biliary cirrhosis
Has the color of your stool or urine changed?	Light brown or gray stool with biliary obstruction and liver, biliary, or pancreatic malignancy
Have you been feeling tired?	Fatigue with hemolytic anemia, malignancy, or hepatitis
What is the risk of infectious hepatitis?	Intravenous or nasal drug use, unsafe sexual practices, tattoos, blood transfusions, recent travel [4]
What is the risk of exposure to hepatotoxic substances?	Exposure associated with occupation, recreation (solvents related to paints), accidents, or environment
	Use of alcohol or acetaminophen, any new medications or over the counter supplements or medications
Is there a history of IBD?	Primary sclerosing cholangitis
What is the patient's mental health status?	Acetaminophen overdose (and other substance ingestion) can be a cause of acute fulminant liver failure

RUQ, right upper quadrant; IBD, inflammatory bowel disease.

Physical Examination

This section will focus on the abdominal and rectal examination. In general, one should first visually inspect, then auscultate, and finally palpate the abdomen. Touching before listening can disturb the GI tract, with alteration of bowel sounds. It is important to rule out other non-GI diagnoses with other physical exam techniques. For example, a cardiac examination should be part of the evaluation of every patient presenting with acute epigastric pain.

Abdominal Examination

Inspection

- **Scars:** Prior procedures and increased risk for abdominal adhesions.
- **Striae:** Exogenous or endogenous steroids, weight loss or gain, or prior pregnancy.
- **Rashes and abnormal skin color or texture.**
- **Distended veins**: Portal hypertension and perihepatic disease.
- **Enlarged abdomen:** Intestinal obstruction, constipation, hepatosplenomegaly, masses, and peritoneal fluid.
- **Asymmetry and irregular shape:** Masses, hernias, or intestinal obstruction.

Auscultation

- **Types of bowel sounds:** Normoactive, hyperactive, absent, hypoactive, rushes, borborygmi, and tinkling.
- **Normoactive bowel sounds:** Heard every 5–10 seconds [4].

- **Absent or hypoactive bowel sounds:** Intestinal perforation, peritonitis, impaired motility, and prolonged intestinal obstruction.
- **Hyperactive bowel sounds:** Onset of intestinal obstruction, IBD, infectious gastroenteritis, and bleeding.

Percussion and Palpation

- **Tympani:** Free air or intestinal gas.
- **Dullness:** Fluid, stool, or solid mass.
- Assess for masses, hepatosplenomegaly, and texture of liver edge.
- Examine the patient's facial expression to assess discomfort or pain during light and deep palpation in all four quadrants.
- Always examine the painful or tender region of the abdomen last, in order to optimize the patient's comfort level [4].

Table 32.13 indicates additional special maneuvers and signs on physical examination. Table 32.14 is a list of GI disorders that present with extraintestinal findings, which may help a practitioner come to the right diagnosis [11,20].

Digital Rectal Examination

Before Digital Examination

- First inspect the external anal region to assess for masses, fissures, scars, skin tags, condyloma, hemorrhoids, skin infections, mucus, and blood. Rectal prolapse may also be evident.
- The "anal wink" reflex can be elicited by gently scratching the external area adjacent to the anal opening. This reflexive contraction of the external sphincter indicates an intact sacral reflex arc [21].

During Digital Examination

- Assess the entire circumference of the rectum for masses, tenderness, impacted stool, muscle tone, and contractility.
- Assess the internal anal sphincter to determining muscle strength at rest. The patient should then be asked to squeeze, so that the examiner may appreciate contraction strength.
- At resting state, ask the patient to bear down and try to expel the examining finger. Providing precise instructions is important as many patients interpret "bearing down" as squeezing instead of an attempt to mimic what the patient might do with these muscles during defecation.
  - A normal performance excludes dyssynergic defecation.
  - A sensation of increased pressure could indicate dyssynergia defecation, but other factors such as embarrassment may also play a role. A normal performance excludes dyssynergia.

Table 32.12 General history questions that should be asked of all patients.

Do you have any medical illnesses or chronic conditions?
Have you had any surgeries or procedures specific to the abdomen or pelvis?
Do you take any prescriptions, over-the-counter medications, or herbal supplements?
Are symptoms associated with changes in your menstrual cycle?
Are there medical illnesses that run in your family?
Do you use alcohol, tobacco, or illicit or recreational drugs?
Where have you traveled in the last year?
What is your usual diet?
Do you engage in any unsafe sexual practices?
Have you ever had or are you at risk of having any sexually transmitted infections?
Have you experienced recent life changes or stress?
Have you been feeling depressed or have you felt that activities do not seem as enjoyable lately? Do you feel your life is worth living?
Have you ever witnessed or experienced physical, emotional, or sexual abuse? (Note: Consider providing a safe and trusting environment and timing this discussion as noted in the text.)

Table 32.13 Special maneuvers and signs on physical examination.

Sign or special maneuver	Technique/indication	Positive finding
Carnett sign	Palpate abdomen at the site of discomfort while the patient engages the abdominal muscles and raises their upper body from a horizontal position	Abdominal wall pathology
Costovertebral tenderness	Tap the posterior thorax with a closed fist while stabilizing the patient	Kidney disease
Courvoisier sign	Palpation of RUQ of abdomen reveals an enlarged gall bladder	Gallbladder mass or cancer
Cullen sign	Blue or purple color around the umbilicus	Peritoneal blood, as with pancreatitis
Grey–Turner sign	Blue or purple color around the flanks	Pancreatitis
Guarding	Patient tenses abdominal muscles to protect the area	Peritonitis
McBurney point	Tenderness at location of appendix – one-third of the way from the anterior superior iliac crest to the umbilicus	Appendicitis
Murphy sign	Palpation of RUQ of abdomen during inspiration elicits pain and abrupt arrest of inspiration	Cholecystitis
Psoas sign	Patient flexes hip against resistance	Left – diverticulitis Right – appendicitis
Rebound tenderness	Apply deep, slow pressure to abdomen away from site of discomfort and then quickly remove the examining hand	Peritonitis
Rosving sign	Patient experiences RLQ pain as examiner applies pressure in LLQ	Appendicitis
Shifting dullness	Percuss the abdomen with patient supine and then partially rolled toward the lateral position	Peritoneal fluid, as with liver disease
Succussion splash	Auscultate upper abdomen while gently moving patient from side to side	Gastric outlet obstruction

RUQ, right upper quadrant; RLQ, right lower quadrant; LLQ, left lower quadrant.

- ◦ The degree of perineal descent may also be assessed (normal 1.0–3.5 cm) [6,21].
- For males, assess the prostate gland for enlargement or irregularities.
- After withdrawing the gloved finger, assess the color of stool and presence of blood or mucus.

Ultrasonography and the Physical Examination

Advancements in color Doppler, higher-resolution imaging, and handheld devices have allowed ultrasound to be a good complement to a thorough physical examination. Sonography allows the health care provider to view both solid and liquid structures instantaneously, allowing for symptoms to correlate to physical findings. It is regarded as a first-line option for imaging pathology for the liver and biliary tract. Unfortunately, ultrasound cannot penetrate gas or structures filled with air, such as bowel, making it nearly impossible to visualize deep organs such as the pancreas [22].

Ultrasonography has been shown as a great educational tool by which to improve learners' physical exam techniques. First-year medical students trained in ultrasonography scored higher in accuracy during the abdominal exam than their counterparts without training [23]. Furthermore, ultrasonography carried out by novice operators has been shown to be superior in measuring liver size when compared to a physical exam done by an experienced clinician [24]. Though not a regular part of the routine physical examination, the use of bedside ultrasound has been employed in acute care settings such as the emergency department (ED) and intensive care unit (ICU). The emergence of handheld ultrasonography opens the possibility for health care practitioners to incorporate this modality into the physical examination, allowing for enhanced accuracy and diagnostic capabilities.

Table 32.14 GI disorders and the extraintestinal complaints and findings that may be associated with them [11,20].

Disease process	Extraintestinal physical findings
Celiac disease	Dermatitis herpetiformis, polyarthralgia
Cowden's disease	Craniomegaly, skin manifestations, breast and other cancers
Crohn's disease	Erythema nodosum, pyoderma gangrenosum, axial arthritis
Cronkhite–Canada syndrome	Hyperpigmentation, nail and hair loss
Enteric infections	Keratoderma blenorrhagica, reactive arthritis
Familial adenomatous polyposis (FAP)	Thyroid and pancreatic cancer, hepatoblastomas, CNS tumors, various benign tumors, dental abnormalities
Gardner syndrome	Supernumerary teeth, osteomas, fibromas, epithelial cysts
Henoch–Schönlein purpura	Palpable purpura, arthralgias
Hepatitis B	Livedo reticularis, mononeuritis multiplex
Hepatitis C	Mixed cryoglobulinemia, palpable purpura
Neuroendocrine tumor or carcinoid	Flushing, wheezing, palpitations, right-sided heart murmur
Peutz–Jegher syndrome	Genital tract tumors and other tumors, pigmented cutaneous manifestations
Turcot syndrome	CNS tumors, café au lait spots, cutaneous port-wine stain, focal nodular hyperplasia
Ulcerative colitis	Erythema nodosum, pyoderma gangrenosum, axial arthritis, peripheral arthritis
Whipple disease	Polyarthralgia, lymphadenopathy

CNS, central nervous system.

Medical Simulation in Gastroenterology

The use of simulation is a growing part of medical education and fellowship training in gastroenterology. Medical simulation is broadly defined as the imitation of specific clinical encounters and procedures in a controlled, scripted environment aimed at providing education, self-improvement, and a focus on patient safety. Simulated clinical encounters are generally of two types: (i) utilizing standardized patients or actor patients, sometimes known as patient instructors, who follow structured scripts as either a teaching or an assessment tool; and (ii) utilizing avatars or mannequins, which are digitally programmed to respond to the learner's activity during the scenario. A combination of standardized patients and the technology-assisted devices is becoming more common.

The types of standardized patient encounter are endless, and can range from basic outpatient complaints to counseling, breaking of bad news, patient education, and high-stress emergency situations. Participants are evaluated not only on their accuracy of diagnosis, but also on their ability to take a history, how they carry out

Table 32.15 Selected USPSTF grades A and B guidelines for preventable services for the field of gastroenterology (Last Update: Feb 2016) [27].*
http://www.uspreventiveservicestaskforce.org/Page/Name/uspstf-a-and-b-recommendations/

Topic	Description	Grade[a]	Release Date of Current Recommendation
Abdominal aortic aneurysm screening: men	*The USPSTF recommends one-time screening for abdominal aortic aneurysm by ultrasonography in men ages 65 to 75 years who have ever smoked.	B	June 2014
Blood pressure screening in adults	*The USPSTF recommends screening for high blood pressure in adults aged 18 years or older. The USPSTF recommends obtaining measurements outside of the clinical setting for diagnostic confirmation before starting treatment.	A	October 2015
Cholesterol Screening	*Men >35 or older or Women >45 or older. Men and Women 20 and older should be screened if they are at higher risk for CAD.	Evidence A. for 35/45 age and B for 20 or older.	Jun-08
Colorectal cancer screening[b]	*The USPSTF recommends screening for colorectal cancer using fecal occult blood testing, sigmoidoscopy, or colonoscopy in adults beginning at age 50 years and continuing until age 75 years. The risks and benefits of these screening methods vary. *Fecal occult blood testing (FOBT)-Annually *Sigmoidoscopy-Every 5 years (with FOBT done every 3) *Colonoscopy-Every 10 years *Screening should be earlier or more frequent depending on risk factors, family history and past history of polyps or colon cancer.	A	Oct-08
Diabetes screening	*The USPSTF recommends screening for abnormal blood glucose as part of cardiovascular risk assessment in adults aged 40 to 70 years who are overweight or obese. Clinicians should offer or refer patients with abnormal blood glucose to intensive behavioral counseling interventions to promote a healthful diet and physical activity.	B	October 2015
Healthy diet counseling	*The USPSTF recommends offering or referring adults who are overweight or obese and have additional cardiovascular disease (CVD) risk factors to intensive behavioral counseling interventions to promote a healthful diet and physical activity for CVD prevention.	B	August 2014
Hepatitis B Screening: Pregnancy women	*The USPSTF strongly recommends screening for hepatitis B virus infection in pregnant women at their first prenatal visit.	A	June 2009
Hepatitis B screening	*The USPSTF recommends screening for hepatitis B virus infection in persons at high risk for infection.	B	May 2014
Hepatitis C virus infection screening: adults	*The USPSTF recommends screening for hepatitis C virus (HCV) infection in persons at high risk for infection. The USPSTF also recommends offering one-time screening for HCV infection to adults born between 1945 and 1965.	B	Jun-13
Obesity screening and counseling: adults	*The USPSTF recommends screening all adults for obesity. Clinicians should offer or refer patients with a body mass index of 30 kg/m^2 or higher to intensive, multicomponent behavioral interventions.	B	Jun-12
Obesity screening and counseling: children	*The USPSTF recommends that clinicians screen children age 6 years and older for obesity and offer them or refer them to comprehensive, intensive behavioral interventions to promote improvement in weight status.	B	Jan-10

[a]**Grade A**, The USPSTF recommends the service. There is high certainty that the net benefits are substantial; **Grade B**, The USPSTF recommends the service. There is high certainty that the net benefit is moderate or there is moderate certainty that the net benefit is moderate to substantial.
For all clinical recommendations, see full list of USPSTF guidelines.
[b]For more recommendations for high-risk patients see the ACS Guidelines for colon cancer:
http://www.cancer.org/cancer/colonandrectumcancer/moreinformation/colonandrectumcancerearlydetection/colorectal-cancer-early-detection-acs-recommendations

Table 32.16 Recommended vaccinations for the field of gastroenterology (last update: January 2014). Source: Bridges 2013 [28].

Vaccination	Indications	Dose	Contraindications
Influenza	All age groups annually	1 dose IM	Allergic to eggs Past history of GBS
HPV	**Females:** 13–26 years old **Males:** 13–21 years old Men who have sex with men (all ages)	3 doses IM	
Hepatitis A	**Strongly recommended in the following situations:** Men who have sex with men Chronic liver disease	2 doses IM	
Hepatitis B	**Strongly recommended in the following situations:** Men who have sex with men Patients with HIV Chronic liver disease Diabetes Health care personnel Kidney failure, hemodialysis recipient, or end-stage renal disease	3 doses IM	

IM, intramuscular injection; GBS, Guillain–Barré syndrome; HPV, human papilloma virus. For a complete list of recommended vaccines, refer to reference [28].

a physical exam, their communication skills, their professionalism, and their time-management skills. These simulations also provide a friendly environment for self-reflection, constructive criticism by faculty, and practice of communication skills around difficult subjects, such as death and medical mistakes. Research has shown that these encounters are an effective means of assessing communication skills and professionalism (e.g., Accreditation Council for Graduate Medical Education competencies in the field of gastroenterology) [25]. Many academic medical centers now have clinical skills centers available to their faculty and students.

The strong push for patient safety has led to the incorporation of simulated procedures into early training in gastroenterology. Techniques such as endoscopy, sigmoidoscopy, and colonoscopy can now be practiced using simulation manikins and virtual-reality simulators, further supplementing patient-based training. Early use of simulated procedures has been shown to build basic skillsets, decrease user time, improve identification of anatomy, develop confidence, and decrease errors among novice operators, when supplemented with patient-based training. These types of activities can also be used for team training, which is the direction of enhanced patient care in all health settings. Though promising, more research needs to be conducted to see the long-term effects on clinical training [26].

Current Preventive Guidelines in Gastroenterology

The Affordable Care Act has placed a strong emphasis on the use of preventative services in the general population. Early detection has been proven to be one of the best methods by which to prevent disease, and a working knowledge of the suggested guidelines is essential for quality care. It is a practitioner's job to determine whether their patients are up to date on all of the recommended vaccinations and screening exams. Table 32.15 provides a summary of the US Preventive Services Task Force (USPSTF) grade A and B recommendations for current preventative screening exams that apply to the field of gastroenterology [27]. Table 32.16 provides a summary of all pertinent recommended vaccines for adult patients seen by a gastroenterologist, with the caveat that the patient should have a comprehensive primary care assessment of all preventative needs [28].

Conclusion

The history and physical examination are the initial key factors in characterizing and determining the etiology of a patient's complaint. A careful and comprehensive history will help guide the focus of the physical examination. In addition to mastering the techniques of questioning and the skills of performing a physical examination, attention must be paid to other important factors, including communication skills, professionalism, and appropriate sensitivity to sex-based differences in health and disease, as well as gender-related problems and cultural differences [29]. Awareness of health care disparities and health literacy, combined with a conscious effort to address such challenges, will promote the ideal patient–physician relationship and result in enhanced health care.

Acknowledgments

The authors gratefully acknowledge the work of Dr. Sheryl A. Tulin-Silver (Serbowicz) in preparing the first-edition version of this chapter.

Take Home Points

- Taking a history is a key component in determining a patient's problem and requires that the health care provider:
  - Establishes a strong doctor–patient relationship.
  - Listens.
  - Asks open-ended questions.
  - Focuses questions to elucidate the patient's symptoms.
- Physical examination can further define the etiology of a symptom. There are four key components of an effective and complete abdominal examination:
  - Inspection.
  - Auscultation.
  - Percussion.
  - Palpation.
- Communication of findings procured from the history and physical examination is crucial in being able to participate in patient-centered, team-based care, especially for patients with complex problems or multiple complaints, and should include:
  - Oral presentation.
  - A written record.
  - Sensitivity to the patient's needs.
- It is important to recognize and implement the National Guidelines for vaccinations and screening.

References

1 Bickley L. Interviewing and the health history. In: Bickley LS, Szilagy PG, eds. *Bates' Guide to Physical Examination and History Taking*, 9th edn. Philadelphia, PA: Lippincott Wiliams & Wilkins, 2007.

2 Perry A, Shaheen N. Burden of gastrointestinal disease in the united states: 2012 update. *Gastroenterology* 2012; **143**: 1179–87.

3 Millham FH. Acute abdominal pain. In: Feldman M, Friedman LS, Brant LJ, eds. *Sleisenger and Fordtran's Gastrointestinal and Liver Disease: Pathophysiology/Diagnosis/Management*, 9th edn. Philadelphia, PA: WB Saunders Company, 2010.

4 Swartz M. The abdomen. In: Swartz MH, ed. *Textbook of Physical Diagnosis History and Physical Exam*, 4th edn. Philadelphia, PA: WB Saunders Company, 2002.

5 Schiller L. Diarrhea. *Med Clin N Am* 2000; **84**:1259–574.

6 Lembo A, Camilleri M. Chronic constipation. *N Engl J Med* 2003; **349**: 1360–8.

7 Longstreth G, Thompson W, Chey W. Functional bowel disorders. *Gastroenterology* 2006; **130**: 1480–91.

8 Heaton K, Ghosh S, Braddon F. How bad are the symptoms and bowel dysfunction of patients with the irritable bowel syndrome? A prospective, controlled study with emphasis on stool form. *Gut* 1991; **32**: 73–9.

9 Lewis S, Heaton K. Stool form scale as a useful guide to intestinal transit time. *Scand J Gastroenterol* 1997; **32**: 920–4.

10 Saad R, Rao SS, Koch KL, *et al.* Do stool form an frequency correlate with whole-gut and colonic transit? Results from a multicenter study in constipated individuals and health controls. *Am J Gastroenterol* 2010; **105**: 403–11.

11 Karnath B, Sunkureddi P, Nguyen-Oghalia T. Extraintestinal manifestations of hepatogastrointestinal diseases. *Hospital Physician* 2006; **42**: 61–6.

12 Binder H. Causes of chronic diarrhea. *N Engl J Med* 2009; **355**: 236–9.

13 Fraga X, Malagelada J. Nausea and vomiting. *Curr Treat Options Gastroenterol* 2002; **5**: 241–50.

14 Quigley E, Hasler W, Parkman H. AGA technical review on nausea and vomiting. *Gastroenterology* 2001; **120**: 263–86.

15 Malagelada J, Malagelada C. Nausea and vomiting. In: Feldman M, Friedman LS, Brant LJ, eds. *Sleisenger and Fordtran's Gastrointestinal and Liver Disease: Pathophysiology/Diagnosis/Management*, 8th edn. Philadelphia, PA: Saunders, 2006.

16 Marek T. Gastrointestinal bleeding. *Endoscopy* 2007; **39**: 998–1004.

17 Madoff R, Fleshman J. Clinical practice committee, american gastroenterological association. american gastroenterological association technical review on the diagnosis and treatment of hemorrhoids. *Gastroenterology* 2004; **126**: 1463–73.

18 Roach S, Kobos R. Jaundice in the adult patient. *Am Fam Physician* 2004; **69**: 299–304.

19 Drossman D, Talley N, Leserman J, *et al.* Sexual and physical abuse and gastrointestinal illness: review and recommendations. *Ann Intern Med* 1995; **123**: 782–94.

20 Rustgi A. Hereditary polyposis and nonpolyposis syndromes. *N Engl J Med* 1994; **331**: 1694–702.

21 Talley N. How to do and interpret a rectal examination in gastroenterology. *Am J Gastroenterol* 2008; **103**: 820–2.

22 Kim D, Pickhardt P. Diagnostic imaging procedures in gastroenterology. In: Goldman L, Ausiello D, eds. *Cecil Medicine*, 24th edn. Philadelphia, PA: Saunders Elsevier, 2011.

23 Butter J, Grant TH, Egan M, *et al.* Does ultrasound training boost year 1 medical student competence and confidence when learning abdominal examination? *Med Educ* 2007; **41**: 843–8.

24 Mouratev G, Howe D, Hoppmann R, *et al.* Teaching medical students ultrasound to measure liver size: Comparison with experienced clinicians using physical examination alone. *Teach Learn Med* 2013; **25**(1): 84–8.

25 Chander B, Kule R, Baiocco P, *et al.* Teaching the competencies: using objective structured clinical encounters for gastroenterology fellows. *Clin Gastroenterol Hepatol* 2009; **7**: 509–14.

26 Walsh C, Sherlock M, Ling S, Carnahan H. Virtual reality simulation training for health professions trainees in gastrointestinal endoscopy. *Cochrane Database Syst Rev* 2012(6):CD008237.

27 US Preventive Services Task Force. Recommendations for primary care practice. Available from: http://www.uspreventiveservicestaskforce.org/Page/Name/uspstf-a-and-b-recommendations/ (last accessed February 15, 2016).

28 Bridges C, Woods L, Coyne-Beasley T. Advisory committee on immunization practices (ACIP) recommended immunization schedule for adults aged 19 years and older – United States. *MMWR Surveill Summ* 2013; **62**(1): 9–19.

29 Talley N, O'Connor S. The general principles of history taking. In: O'Connor S, ed. *Clinical Examination: A Systematic Guide to Physical Diagnosis*, 6th edn. Philadelphia, PA: Elsevier, 2010.

CHAPTER 32

Acute Diarrhea

John R. Cangemi

Division of Gastroenterology and Hepatology, Department of Internal Medicine, Mayo Clinic, Jacksonville, FL, USA

Summary

Acute diarrhea is a common, primarily self-limited illness, which can be managed most often with supportive care. Stool cultures are rarely indicated early on unless the patient has the presence of fever, abdominal pain, or bloody diarrhea, suggestive of a bacterial etiology. The focus of treatment should be on replacement of fluid and electrolytes, especially in the young or elderly, who are at increased risk of excessive morbidity and mortality. Empiric antibiotic therapy, with few exceptions, should be given in the setting of severe dysentery or in patients with significant comorbidities. Specific antibiotic therapy is determined by the organism identified. Any decision to treat must carefully weigh the potential benefits and risks, particularly if the patient is at risk for Shiga toxin-producing *Escherichia coli*.

Case

A 42-year-old female presents to the emergency room with acute onset of diarrhea shortly after attending a summer church picnic. That evening she was awakened by significant lower abdominal crampy pain and multiple loose, non-bloody, liquid bowel movements. She had no complaints of fever or chills. She felt somewhat nauseated from the cramping but did not vomit. She is on no new medications and has not traveled recently.

On physical examination, she appears comfortable, with a heart rate of 86 and a blood pressure without orthostatic change. Abdominal examination is benign, rectal examination is normal. Her laboratory profile reveals a normal hemoglobin of 13.2, white count of 6.4, and creatinine of 0.9. Multiple stool studies are obtained and results are pending.

Definition and Epidemiology

Acute diarrhea is defined as an increase in stool frequency (more than three loose bowel movements per day) or volume (>200 g daily) for 14 days or fewer. The majority of cases are of infectious origin, primarily bacterial or viral, but it may also result from a drug reaction, food allergy, or an underlying systemic illness. In the United States, it is difficult to estimate the actual frequency, as most cases are not reported, so fewer than 3% are diagnosed. In one population-based telephone survey in the United States, the rate was estimated to be 0.72 episodes per person-year [1]. Approximately 179 million cases of acute gastroenteritis occur yearly, resulting in 500 000 hospitalizations and more than 5000 deaths [2]. Fortunately, the majority of cases are self-limited, with morbidity and mortality primarily seen in the immunocompromised patient or at extremes of age. Fecal–oral transmission accounts for most cases, due to contaminated water, food, or direct person-to-person contact. The cause of diarrhea in each case varies with the specific pathogen, whether toxin-mediated or through direct invasion.

Pathophysiology

There are essentially three mechanisms by which enteric pathogens can cause diarrhea. The first involves ingestion of a food contaminated with a preformed toxin produced within it prior to ingestion. The second is caused by production of the toxin by the pathogen after consumption. The third, and potentially most significant, is the diarrhea produced by an organism that either damages or invades the mucosal surface. The actual impact on the host varies per organism. Toxin-mediated diarrhea leads to activation of adenylate cyclase, with resultant increase in intracytoplasmic cyclic adenosine monophosphate (cAMP) concentration and subsequent increase in chloride secretion. Chloride secretion may also be induced by activation of guanylate cyclase C receptors (e.g., from the heat-stable enterotoxin of *E. coli*). Invasive organisms, in addition to toxin production, will cause direct damage to the mucosal surface, with altered permeability, increased calcium influx, or altered protein synthesis, resulting in an increase in fluid loss. Enhanced mucin secretion, activation of motor mechanisms, and inhibition of bile acid absorption may also contribute to the volume of diarrhea [3].

Clinical Features

The diagnosis is often gleaned from the history, based on the disease presentation, travel history, type of living conditions, medication use, and potential exposures. A food history may provide important clues as to the diagnosis, specifically relating the onset of symptoms to the timing of the meal (e.g. *Staphylococcus aureus* or *Bacillus cereus*). Is the diarrhea accompanied by nausea and vomiting? Is there a fever, suggesting infection with an invasive organism? The onset of bloody diarrhea serves to further narrow the differential (Table 33.1). It is important to determine the frequency and characteristics of the diarrhea: is it large-volume and watery, suggestive of a small-bowel source, or frequent, urgent, and involving small-volume bowel movements, consistent with colonic involvement? Special attention should be paid to the patient's

Practical Gastroenterology and Hepatology Board Review Toolkit, Second Edition. Edited by Nicholas J. Talley, Kenneth R. DeVault, Michael B. Wallace, Bashar A. Aqel and Keith D. Lindor.
© 2016 John Wiley & Sons, Ltd. Published 2016 by John Wiley & Sons, Ltd. Companion website: www.practicalgastrohep.com

Table 33.1 Common pathogens in acute diarrhea.

Pathogen	Source	Indicated therapy	Antibiotic (alternative)
Norovirus	Institutions, cruise ships, common outbreaks	Supportive	
Salmonella	Poultry, eggs, raw milk, beef, vegetables	Not indicated in healthy hosts with no risk of sepsis	Fluoroquinolones (trimethoprim-sulfamethoxazole)
Shigella	Person to person, vegetables	Indicated	Fluoroquinolones (trimethoprim-sulfamethoxazole)
Campylobacter	Poultry, raw milk	Only in severe cases	Erythromycin (fluoroquinolones?)
Vibrio parahemolyticus	Raw seafood, shellfish	Not indicated in healthy host	Tetracycline
Enterotoxigenic E. coli	Travelers	Not indicated in healthy host	Fluoroquinolones (trimethoprim-sulfamethoxazole)
Enteroinvasive E. coli	Milk, cheese	Indicated	Fluoroquinolones (trimethoprim-sulfamethoxazole)
Enterohemorrhagic E. coli	Beef, pork, lettuce, milk, cheese, raw seed sprouts	Avoid antibiotics – can induce Shiga toxin (HUS)	
Yersinia	Beef, pork, milk, cheese	Only in severe cases	Doxycycline (trimethoprim-sulfamethoxazole)
Giardia	Contaminated water	Indicated	Metronidazole (tinidazole, quinicrine HCl)
Cryptosporidium	Contaminated water	Not proven effective	Paromomycin plus azithromycin (nitazoxanide)
Cyclospora	Imported fruit	Indicated	Trimethoprim-sulfamethoxazole
Entamoeba histolytica	Travelers	Indicated	Metronidazole plus iodoquinol (paromomycin)

HUS, hemolytic uremic syndrome.

volume status. The abdomen should be assessed for the presence of tenderness, peritoneal signs, or progressive distention.

Diagnosis

As the majority of episodes of acute diarrhea are of viral origin and self-limited, there is no evidence to support stool cultures in all patients in the acute setting (Figure 33.1). The diagnostic yield overall ranges from 1.5 to 5.6% [4]. However, if a patient presents with fever, dehydration, blood or pus in the stool, or large-volume diarrhea of several days' duration, then stool cultures are warranted. The exception should be made for those who have significant comorbidities or those who are elderly or immunocompromised, where early diagnosis has important implications for therapy. Also, patients who are hospitalized or have recently used antibiotics should be tested early for C. difficile toxin. In the appropriate setting, a fecal lactoferrin may help to distinguish inflammatory from non-inflammatory diarrhea with a sensitivity and specificity ranging from 79 to 92% [5]. If the clinical history, physical examination, or fecal lactoferrin yields positive findings, as just outlined, then stool cultures are warranted. Routine cultures will identify most organisms, but special stains may be required for specific pathogens (Yersinia, cold enrichment; E. coli 0157:H7, sorbitol MacConkey agar). Up to 40% of acute infectious diarrhea cases will escape diagnosis even with appropriate cultures.

There are limited circumstances in which ova and parasites should be part of the diagnostic algorithm of acute diarrhea. Travelers with exposure to untreated water (Giardia, Cryptosporidium, or Cyclospora), patients with persistent diarrhea, and immunocompromised patients should all be tested. Enzyme-linked immunosorbent assay is the preferred method of testing, with a sensitivity of >95%.

Endoscopic procedures are rarely indicated in the evaluation of acute diarrhea. Sigmoidoscopy or colonoscopy could be considered in the patient with bloody diarrhea who does not respond appropriately to therapy.

Differential Diagnosis

Watery Diarrhea

If vomiting is a predominant symptom associated with non-bloody loose stools, then either viral or toxin-induced food poisoning should be suspected. Viral illnesses are the most common cause of acute diarrhea in the United States, and the majority of infections are from norovirus: 60–90% of outbreaks that are not bacterial in origin are caused by norovirus [6, 7]. These outbreaks tend to occur more commonly during the winter months and are seen in institutions, cruise ships, social events, and vacation settings. The illness is generally self-limited, lasting 24–48 hours after an incubation period of 1–3 days. Transmission typically occurs via water, fresh food (e.g., shellfish), prepared food, food handlers, personal contact, or contaminated environmental services. Symptoms early on include vomiting followed by several days of watery diarrhea.

Foodborne bacterial toxins have a shorter incubation phase (B. cereus and S. aureus: 2–7 hours; Clostridium perfringens: 8–14 hours) and are less severe. B. cereus has been commonly associated with contaminated fried rice and vegetables sprouts. Neither S. aureus nor its enterotoxin is destroyed by cooking, and both proliferate at room temperatures. Infections may be associated with prepackaged meat of high salt content, particularly ham, but any number of food products (e.g., dairy, produce, eggs, salad) may be contaminated. C. perfringens is one the most common pathogens worldwide. It is a diverse species, with at least five different strains, depending on the type of toxin produced. Infection occurs when food (e.g., meat or poultry) infected with C. perfringens spores is allowed to cool slowly after cooking. The ingested organism sporulates within the small intestine, producing the enterotoxin. Diarrhea and cramping typically begin within 8–12 hours and resolve in 24 hours, rarely producing significant morbidity. Parasites are less common pathogens in acute gastroenteritis, but foodborne transmission may occur. Parasites include Cryptosporidium parvum (water, unpasteurized milk, fresh produce) and Cyclospora cayetanensis (imported fruits and vegetables). C. cayetanensis may produce a prolonged diarrhea, lasting more than 3 weeks, which responds effectively to trimethoprim-sulfamethoxazole.

Enterotoxigenic E. coli is the most common cause of traveler's diarrhea and is a growing cause of concern for foodborne transmission in the United States [8]. The bacterium adheres to the surface of the small-bowel mucosa, where it produces two separate plasmid-encoded enterotoxins: heat-stable and heat-labile. This produces a secretory diarrhea that is non-bloody and may be associated with headache, fever, nausea, and vomiting. It has a short intubation period of 1–2 days and typically resolves within 3–4 days. Enteropathogenic E. coli also produces a secretory diarrhea, which may be more severe, with symptoms including diarrhea, anorexia, rapid wasting, and even death. It too is a self-limited disease, responding primarily to rehydration.

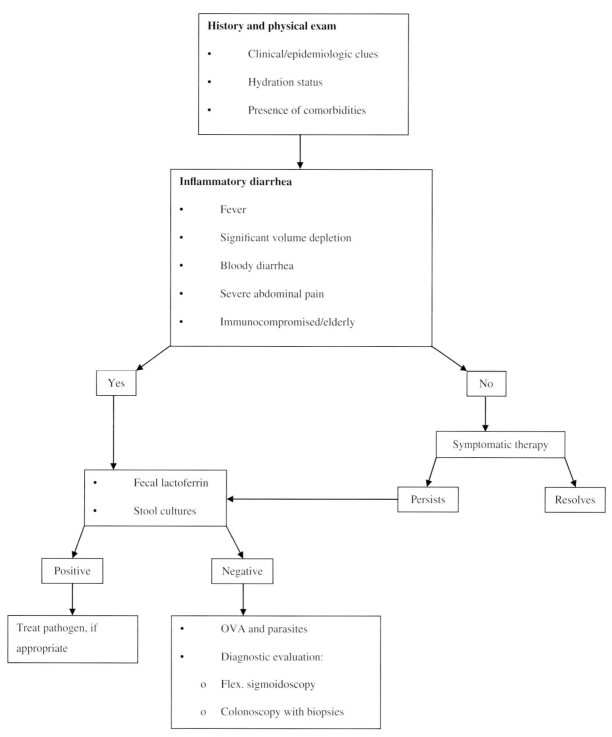

Figure 33.1 Approach to the treatment of acute diarrhea.

Inflammatory Diarrhea

Inflammatory diarrhea, or dysentery, is often characterized by the passage of bloody stools, seen in association with significant abdominal pain with or without the presence of a fever. Among patients presenting to the emergency department with bloody diarrhea in the United States, Shigella *species* is the most common pathogen identified (15.3%), followed by Salmonella (5.8%), Campylobacter (6.2%), and Shiga toxin-producing *E. coli* (2.6%) [9]. *Vibrio parahemolyticus* is rarely seen except in coastal areas. More than 5.2 million cases of bacterial diarrhea occur

each year in the United States, accounting for up to 1500 deaths annually [10].

Shigella

There are four separate species of Shigella (*S. dysenteriae, S. boydii, S. sonnei,* and *S. flexneri*) that are capable of causing diarrhea in humans. As few as 10 organisms can initiate diarrhea, so there is a high risk of either person-to-person spread or infection through ingestion of contaminated food, including poultry, dairy products, salads, and fresh vegetables. The organism initially multiplies in the small intestine and eventually passes into the colon, where it invades the colonic mucosa. It spreads from cell to cell, allowing it to avoid the normal luminal defenses. Shigella produces species-specific enterotoxins, which inhibit protein synthesis and stimulate intestinal secretion. The diarrhea typically resolves within 7 days with supportive treatment only.

Non-typhoid Salmonella

Transmission is caused by ingestion of contaminated food, mainly of animal origin, including poultry, meat, eggs, and dairy products. It is the leading cause of foodborne disease in the United States. After invading the mucosal surface, it survives within macrophages, where it can replicate and control cell function. The most common serotypes are *S. enteritidis* and *S. typhimurium*. Most infections are mild to moderate in severity, but they may be severe, with up to 15 000 hospitalizations annually and 400 deaths. Multidrug resistance is an increasing problem, with the resistant strains more often associated with morbidity and mortality.

Campylobacter

Campylobacter is transmitted via the fecal–oral route, with the majority of cases related to either *C. jejuni* or *C. coli*; 80% of cases relate to foodborne transmission, with improperly cooked chicken the primary source. The organism invades the mucosal surface through the M cells of the Peyer's patch and may infect the small or, more commonly, the large intestine. It produces cytolethal distending toxin, which arrests the cell cycle, resulting in DNA damage. Most cases are self-limited and do not require antibiotic therapy.

Shiga Toxin-Producing *E. coli*

Infection may cause a wide range of clinical symptoms, ranging from mild gastroenteritis to hemolytic uremic syndrome (HUS). The clinical spectrum can arise from either *E. coli* 0157:H7 or non-0157 strains. Infections in the United States are split equally between serotypes. Infection is usually associated with ground beef, but may be found in unpasteurized juice, fresh fruits, and vegetables. Diarrhea is quite common with this organism and is typically bloody within 5 days of onset; it results from the production of two separate cytotoxins and direct invasion of the small intestinal mucosa via a plasmid-encoded pilus. Commercially available immunoassays of Shiga toxins 1 and 2 may be the preferred initial test over culture on sorbitol MacConkey plates.

Yersinia

Yersinia enterocolitica is the most common form of Yersinia induced gastroenteritis. It has an incubation period of 4–6 days and may produce a prolonged diarrhea, lasting up to 22 days. It is most commonly attributed to the consumption of undercooked or raw pork products. In addition to diarrhea, acute clinical symptoms may include pharyngitis or right lower quadrant pain masquerading as acute appendicitis.

Drug-Induced Diarrhea

Drug-induced diarrhea is an important aspect of the differential diagnosis of acute diarrhea. [11]. Over 700 drugs have been listed as a potential cause for diarrhea, and it is essential that a careful history focus on both prescribed drugs and non-prescription drugs and supplements.

Treatment

Early management of the patient with acute diarrhea should focus on appropriate replacement of fluid and electrolytes. Oral rehydration is adequate in most settings, unless the patient is incapable of retaining fluids (severe nausea and vomiting) or is severely dehydrated or comatose. This should consist of a glucose-based solution, as glucose facilitates absorption of sodium and water even in the face of a secretory process. The World Health Organization (WHO) recommends oral rehydration solution with 3.5 g sodium chloride, 2.5 g sodium bicarbonate, 1.5 g potassium chloride, and either 20 g glucose or 40 g sucrose per liter of fluid. This should be given at 1.5 times the volume of stool lost over 24 hours. A number of effective commercial products are available. When intravenous hydration is required, Ringer's lactate should be used, and at least half the calculated deficit should be administered in the first 4 hours. If tolerated, the diet should be continued, as adequate nutrition is important. Early feeding may also be beneficial, by decreasing the intestinal permeability induced by the infection and decreasing the duration of the illness [12]. In acute infection, secondary lactose intolerance may occur, due to the loss of brush-border enzymes; this can last up to several weeks, requiring lactose restriction.

The use of anti-diarrheal medication in patients with acute diarrhea is controversial. In a systematic review of adjunctive loperamide with antibiotics in traveler's diarrhea, antibiotic therapy plus loperamide was more effective than antibiotics alone in terms of decreasing duration of illness and achieving an earlier cure [13]. However, these agents should not be used in the setting of fever, bloody diarrhea, or significant abdominal pain [14]. In these settings, antimotility agents may enhance the severity of the illness by delaying excretion of the organism. Their use may result in prolonged fever plus increased risk of toxic megacolon or HUS in patients infected with *E. coli* 0157:H7 and should be avoided. Bismuth subsalicylate is an alternative choice, but it has a slower onset and is less effective in comparative trials [15].

Most cases of acute diarrhea resolve spontaneously, and antibiotics are not required. Yet, if treatment is considered, often the decision is made prior to isolation of the specific pathogen. In this case, it is important to weigh the risks (e.g., prolonged carriage of Salmonella, induction of Shiga toxin) versus the benefit of an earlier response in a susceptible organism. Empiric therapy is generally recommended in the treatment of severe dysentery characterized by fever with or without bloody stools, except in cases of suspected Shiga toxin-producing *E. coli*. Those patients with large-volume diarrhea resulting in volume depletion, prolonged symptoms, or immunocompromise should be treated in most circumstances. Fluoroquinolones for 3–5 days is the treatment of choice for empiric therapy, though increased resistance has been identified in infections with Campylobacter in travelers to South East Asia and India [16].

Antibiotic therapy is most effective when given at the onset of symptoms. However, treatment of non-typhoidal Salmonella may actually prolong shedding of the organism and is rarely required unless the host is immunocompromised or bacteremia is suspected. Treatment of Shiga toxin-producing *E. coli* may induce the production of Shiga toxin and result in HUS. Shigella, on the other hand, responds well to therapy with a fluoroquinolone, and treatment will shorten the period of diarrhea by 2.4 days and is therefore recommended in the presence of progressive dysentery. Campylobacter will typically clear without therapy and should not be treated unless associated with a prolonged, severe illness, or in an immunocompromised patient. Figure 33.1 presents an algorithm by which to outline the approach to therapy of acute diarrhea.

Special consideration needs to be given to the elderly patient with acute diarrhea [17]. Older patients are at increased risk secondary to achlorhydria, altered gut motility, frequent antibiotic exposure, and serious comorbidities. Morbidity and mortality are significantly increased, which requires aggressive supportive care and early institution of therapeutic measures.

Case Continued

The patient is dismissed from the emergency room feeling much improved after being given intravenous (IV) fluids as her only form of therapy. Stool cultures are reported later to be all negative. The patient recalls eating a pasta salad that had been sitting out in the sun. The assumed diagnosis is food poisoning associated with *S. aureus*. She recovers uneventfully within 24 hours.

Take Home Points

- Most cases of acute diarrhea are self-limited and require no therapy.
- Most common pathogens in acute diarrhea are viral (norovirus), and early stool cultures yield <6% and are not cost-effective.
- The most important aspect of management early on is repletion of fluids and electrolytes. In the majority of cases, this can be done with oral rehydration solution.
- Fecal lactoferrin is both sensitive and specific for identifying inflammatory diarrhea.
- Elderly patients are at increased risk of morbidity and mortality from acute diarrhea and require special consideration.
- Even with a suspected bacterial pathogen, empiric antibiotic therapy should be withheld in most settings unless the patient exhibits fever, severe abdominal pain, or bloody diarrhea.
- Antibiotic therapy should be withheld in cases of suspected Shiga toxin-producing *E. coli* or non-typhoid Salmonella unless bacteremia suspected.

References

1 Cohen ML. The epidemiology of diarrheal diseases in the United States. *Infect Dis Clin North Am* 1988; **2**: 557.

2 Bresee JS, Marcus R, Venezia RA, *et al.* The etiology of severe acute gastroenteritis among adults visiting emergency departments in the United States. *J Inf Dis* 2012; **205**: 1374–81.

3 Camilleri M, Nullens S, Nelsen T. Enteroendocrine and neuronal mechanisms in pathophysiology of acute infectious diarrhea. *Dig Dis Sci* 2012; **57**: 19–27.

4 Guerrant RL, Vangilder T, Steiner TS, *et al.* Practice guidelines for the management of infectious diarrhea. *Clin Inf Dis* 2001; **32**: 331–51.

5 Kane SV, Sandborn WJ, Ruffo PA, *et al.* Fecal lactoferrin is a sensitive and specific marker in identifying intestinal inflammation. *Am J Gastro* 2003; **98**: 1309.

6 Marcos LA, DuPont HL. Advances in defining etiology and new therapeutic approaches in acute diarrhea. *J Infect* 2007; **55**: 385–93.

7 Goodgame R. Norovirus gastroenteritis. *Curr Gastroenterol Rep* 2006; **8**: 401–8.

8 Arenas-Hernandez M, Martinez-Laguna Y, Torres AG. Clinical implications of enteroadherent *Escherichia coli*. *Curr Gastroenterol Rep* 2012; **14**: 386–94.

9 Talan DA, Moran GJ, Newdow M, *et al.* Etiology of bloody diarrhea among patients presenting to United States emergency departments: prevalence of *Escherichia coli* 0157: H7 and other enteropathogens. *Clin Infect Dis* 2001; **32**: 573–80.

10 DuPont HL. Bacterial diarrhea. *N Engl J Med* 2009; **361**: 1560–9.

11 Abraham B, Sellin JH. Drug-induced diarrhea. *Curr Gastroenterol Rep* 2007; **9**: 365–72.

12 Gadewar S, Fasano A. Current concepts in the evolution, diagnosis and management of acute infectious diarrhea. *Curr Opin Pharmacol* 2005; **5**: 559–65.

13 Riddle M, Arnold, Trible S. Effects of adjuvant loperamide in combination with antibiotics on treatment outcomes in traveler's diarrhea: a systematic review and meta-analysis. *Clin Infect Dis* 2008; **47**: 1007–14.

14 Ross AG, Olds GR, Cripps AW *et al.* Enteropathogens and chronic illness in returning travelers. *N Engl J Med* 2013; **368**: 1817–25.

15 De Bruyn G. Diarrhea in adults (acute). *Am Fam Physician* 2008; **78**: 263–6.

16 Kollaritsch H, Paulke-Korinek M, Wiedermann U. Traveler's diarrhea. *Infect Dis Clin N Am* 2012; **26**: 691–706.

17 Trinh C, Prabhakar K. Diarrheal diseases in the elderly. *Clin Geriat Med* 2007; **23**: 833–56.

CHAPTER 34

Chronic Diarrhea

Lawrence R. Schiller

Division of Gastroenterology, Baylor University Medical Center, Dallas, TX, USA

Summary

Chronic diarrhea is a common clinical problem, most inclusively defined as frequent passage of fluid stools lasting more than 1 month. A comprehensive history is the best start to the evaluation. Probably the most important features to define are the onset (acute or gradual), pattern (continuous or intermittent), severity (causing dehydration or not), and type of stool produced (watery, fatty, or inflammatory). Coexisting symptoms, such as weight loss or abdominal pain, may be important clues to etiology. Patients with irritable bowel syndrome (IBS) should be identified by the presence of characteristic abdominal pain associated with variable stool form or frequency, and should be distinguished from others with chronic diarrhea. The differential diagnosis of continuing chronic diarrhea is broad, but targeted evaluation is often rewarded with a diagnosis that can be treated.

Case

A 78-year-old woman presents with a 3-year history of diarrhea. The problem began gradually and is now complicated by episodes of fecal incontinence. She has watery stools every day, moves her bowels up to five times a day, and has lost about 2 kg (5 pounds). She has no abdominal pain, never sees blood in her stools, and has never been hospitalized for dehydration. Occasional loperamide reduces stool frequency and urgency of defecation, but does not eliminate loose stools. She has taken non-steroidal anti-inflammatory drugs (NSAIDs) for arthritis, but uses no other scheduled medications. Physical examination is unremarkable, except for reduced anal sphincter tone and squeeze.

Definition and Epidemiology

Chronic diarrhea is best described as frequent passage of loose stools for more than 1 month [1]. Some patients confuse fecal incontinence with diarrhea and a few consider frequent passage of formed stool to be diarrhea, but otherwise patient reports of diarrhea are usually valid. For clinical purposes, it is best to distinguish chronic diarrhea from IBS with diarrhea, in which abdominal pain is prominent [1, 2]. IBS tends to have more variable stool frequency and form, typically runs a benign course without medical complications, and does not need an extensive diagnostic evaluation. In contrast, patients with chronic diarrhea typically always have loose stools, may have medical complications, and often have treatable causes for chronic diarrhea that can be discovered [3–5]. Therefore, efforts to make a diagnosis will be rewarded. Surveys suggest that 3–5% of the population has chronic diarrhea in any given year. It is unclear how many of these people have IBS as opposed to other causes of chronic diarrhea.

Pathophysiology

At a fundamental level, diarrhea is caused by excess water in stools resulting from decreased absorption of fluid from the lumen or increased secretion of fluid into the lumen [5]. This may occur because of toxins, hormones, neurotransmitters, bile acids, or cytokines that affect mucosal absorption directly; because rapid motility hurries fluid past the absorptive surface; because the absorptive surface area is reduced or bypassed; or because poorly absorbed substances are ingested and hold water within the lumen osmotically.

Clinical Features

Diarrhea is a symptom that most people experience transiently from time to time, and so there is a universal appreciation of acute diarrhea. Chronic diarrhea is less common, and patients are often bewildered when it does not go away spontaneously. Other symptoms may be present, such as weight loss, evidence of malnutrition, cramps, bleeding, fecal incontinence, and abdominal pain, which can produce substantial disability.

While most patients know diarrhea when they have it, few have a good idea about its severity. Many view the number of stools per day, coexisting urgency or incontinence, or the intensity of cramps as key measures. Researchers often consider stool weight (>200 g/24 hours) to be critical – and in some ways it is – because stool weights >1000 g may be associated with dehydration and electrolyte depletion. However, patients have no idea what their stool weights are and clinicians typically do not measure stool weight, depending instead upon weight loss, dehydration, and the intensity of patient complaints in deciding how severe diarrhea is.

Clinical signs associated with chronic diarrhea are often sparse, though when present they may be helpful [1,5] (Figure 34.1).

Practical Gastroenterology and Hepatology Board Review Toolkit, Second Edition. Edited by Nicholas J. Talley, Kenneth R. DeVault, Michael B. Wallace, Bashar A. Aqel and Keith D. Lindor.
© 2016 John Wiley & Sons, Ltd. Published 2016 by John Wiley & Sons, Ltd. Companion website: www.practicalgastrohep.com

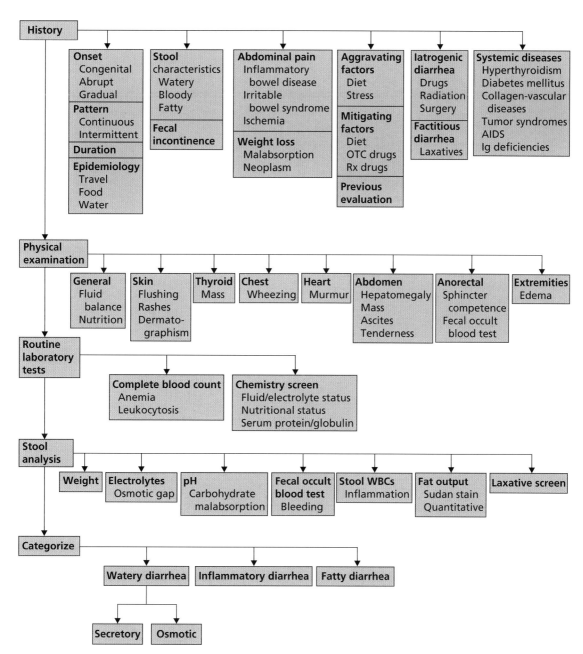

Figure 34.1 Initial diagnostic approach to chronic diarrhea. OTC, over-the-counter; Rx, prescription; AIDS, acquired immunodeficiency syndrome; Ig, immunoglobulin; WBC, white blood cell. Source: Fine 1999. Reproduced with permission of the American Gastroenterological Association.

Diagnosis and Differential Diagnosis

Chronic diarrhea can be a symptom of many different conditions that have multiple diagnostic pathways [5]. Given this complexity, even experienced clinicians worry about getting the diagnosis right. Three general approaches can be recommended, depending upon circumstances [6]:

- **Presumptive diagnosis:** When the temporal association of events and onset, course of illness, and clinical features are characteristic, making a specific diagnosis likely, *and* definitive diagnostic tests are not readily available or are imprecise, *and* therapy is not risky, a presumptive diagnosis can be made and a therapeutic trial should be instituted.

- **Directed evaluation:** When the clinician has a good idea of the diagnosis or a limited differential diagnosis *and* a definitive

diagnostic test is available, that diagnostic test should be done to confirm the diagnosis and to direct further management.

- **Categorization and algorithmic evaluation:** When no particular diagnosis is especially likely, categorizing diarrhea as watery (with subtypes of secretory and osmotic), inflammatory, or fatty by simple tests can lead to a series of diagnostic tests that may yield a diagnosis. A retrospective review from a tertiary referral center highlights the potential of stool analysis in categorizing the potential causes of diarrhea [7].

Presumptive diagnosis might be used, for example, in a patient who developed chronic diarrhea shortly after a cholecystectomy. If the diarrhea had the expected characteristics of watery stools that were more numerous in the morning, a therapeutic trial of bile acid-binding resin would be warranted, since no definitive diagnostic test is available and the therapeutic trial would not be risky or expensive. If the patient improved, the diagnosis of postcholecystectomy diarrhea would be likely.

Directed evaluation might be employed in a patient who was likely to have celiac disease based on a characteristic history of weight loss, bloating, and fatty stools. Serological testing and small-bowel biopsy have a very high true-positive rate and would confirm the diagnosis if positive [8]. The thoughtful clinician would obtain those tests early in the evaluation and proceed on to long-term treatment with confidence.

Categorization and algorithmic evaluation make sense when there is no dominant diagnosis [4]. In this scenario, the extensive differential diagnosis of chronic diarrhea is limited by categorizing the type of stool produced as watery, inflammatory, or fatty and then looking for the specific problems causing that type of diarrhea. This categorization is done by gross inspection of stools and by analyzing stools for blood, white blood cells (WBCs) (or a surrogate marker, such as fecal lactoferrin or calprotectin), and fat (Figure 34.1). Watery stools are easily pourable and have no blood or pus. Inflammatory stools have blood or pus. Fatty stools have excess fat or oil.

Watery stools can be subdivided into secretory diarrhea or osmotic diarrhea based on stool electrolyte analysis [9]. Secretory diarrhea is caused by incomplete absorption of electrolytes, making the stools are electrolyte-rich. Osmotic diarrhea is caused by ingestion of a poorly absorbed substance that obligates water retention within the lumen to maintain osmotic equilibration with serum (the intestine is too permeable to water to allow an osmotic gradient to develop between the lumen and serum). Electrolyte absorption is unaffected, so stools have very low electrolyte concentrations. This distinction can be quantitated by calculating the fecal osmotic gap (FOG), which estimates the contribution of non-electrolytes to stool osmolality:

$$FOG = 290 - 2([Na^+] + [K^+]),$$

where 290 is the assumed luminal osmolality and $2([Na^+] + [K^+])$ represents an estimate of the total cations and anions present in stool water. A FOG >100 mosm/kg suggests osmotic diarrhea, while a FOG below 25 mosm/kg suggests secretory diarrhea.

Once the diarrhea has been categorized, the differential diagnosis becomes more manageable (Table 34.1) and algorithmic approaches to each subtype are feasible (Figure 34.2).

Case Continued

Because there is no dominant diagnosis, this patient is most appropriately evaluated by categorizing the diarrhea and using an algorithmic approach. Routine laboratory tests, including complete blood count (CBC), metabolic profile, and C-reactive protein, are unremarkable. A 48-hour stool collection yields 550 g/24 hours of watery diarrhea. Fecal occult blood test is negative, fecal lactoferrin is negative, and stool fat excretion is 2 g/24 hours. Fecal [Na⁺] is 40 mmol/L and fecal [K⁺] is 100 mmol/L, making the FOG = 10 mosm/kg, consistent with a secretory diarrhea. Flexible sigmoidoscopy reveals normal appearances, but biopsies are interpreted as showing collagenous colitis.

Therapeutics

The treatment of chronic diarrhea ultimately depends on the underlying condition. For some conditions, therapy can be *curative* (e.g., a

Table 34.1 Differential diagnosis of chronic diarrhea. Source: Fine 1999. Reproduced with permission of the American Gastroenterological Association.

Osmotic diarrhea	Osmotic laxative abuse: Mg^{++}, SO_4^{-2}, PO_4^{-3}, lactulose, mannitol, sorbitol, PEG
	Carbohydrate malabsorption: lactose, fructose, others
Secretory diarrhea	Congenital chloridorrhea
	Chronic infections
	IBD: ulcerative colitis, Crohn's disease (ileum), microscopic colitis (lymphocytic colitis, collagenous colitis), diverticulitis
	Drugs and poisons: stimulant laxative abuse
	Disordered regulation: postvagotomy, postsympathectomy, diabetic neuropathy, IBS
	Ileal bile acid malabsorption
	Endocrine diarrhea: hyperthyroidism, Addison's disease
	Neuroendocrine tumors: gastrinoma, VIPoma, somatostatinoma, mastocytosis, carcinoid syndrome, medullary carcinoma of the thyroid
	Other neoplasia: colon carcinoma, lymphoma, villous adenoma
	Idiopathic secretory diarrhea: epidemic (Brainerd)
	Sporadic
Fatty diarrhea	Malabsorption syndromes: mucosal diseases, SBS, postresection diarrhea, small-bowel bacterial overgrowth, mesenteric ischemia
	Maldigestion: pancreatic insufficiency
	Reduced luminal bile acid
Inflammatory diarrhea	IBD: ulcerative colitis, Crohn's disease, diverticulitis, ulcerative jejunoileitis
	Infections: invasive bacterial infection (*Clostridium*, *E. coli*, tuberculosis, others), ulcerating viral infection (CMV, herpes simplex), invasive parasites (amebiasis, strongyloides)
	Ischemic colitis
	Radiation enterocolitis
	Neoplasia: carcinoma of colon
	Lymphoma

PEG, percutaneous endoscopic gastrostomy; IBD, inflammatory bowel disease; IBS, irritable bowel syndrome; VIP, vasoactive intestinal polypeptide; SBS, short-bowel syndrome; CMV, cytomegalovirus.

gluten-free diet for celiac disease) [8]. For relapsing conditions, such as collagenous colitis, appropriate therapy can *induce remission* [10]. For all others, *symptomatic therapy* can diminish the impact of diarrhea on quality of life, both while evaluation is ongoing and chronically [11] (Table 34.2).

The most important issue to address is rehydration. Intravenous fluid is used in hospitalized patients. Oral rehydration can correct even serious fluid depletion [12]. Intraluminal agents can modify stool texture, but may not reduce stool output.

The most effective and most widely applicable symptomatic therapy is antidiarrheal opiates [13]. Low-potency opiates include loperamide and diphenoxylate plus low-dose atropine (to reduce abuse potential). The key difference in using these agents to treat chronic rather than acute diarrhea is giving the antidiarrheal on a scheduled basis (e.g., before each meal) instead of on an "as-needed" basis. Antidiarrheal drugs work best if given before meals, when they can blunt the physiological stimulus for defecation.

When low-potency opiate antidiarrheal drugs fail to control diarrhea, higher-potency ones, such as codeine, morphine, or deodorized tincture of opium, should be used [11]. These agents should be started at a low dose and titrated up slowly to allow tolerance to sedative effects to develop in the brain. Tolerance does not develop to the constipating effects of these agents, so an effective dose that will control diarrhea but not produce sedation can usually be achieved.

Clonidine and octreotide have non-specific antidiarrheal activity, but should be reserved for special cases, such as those that fail opiate therapy [11].

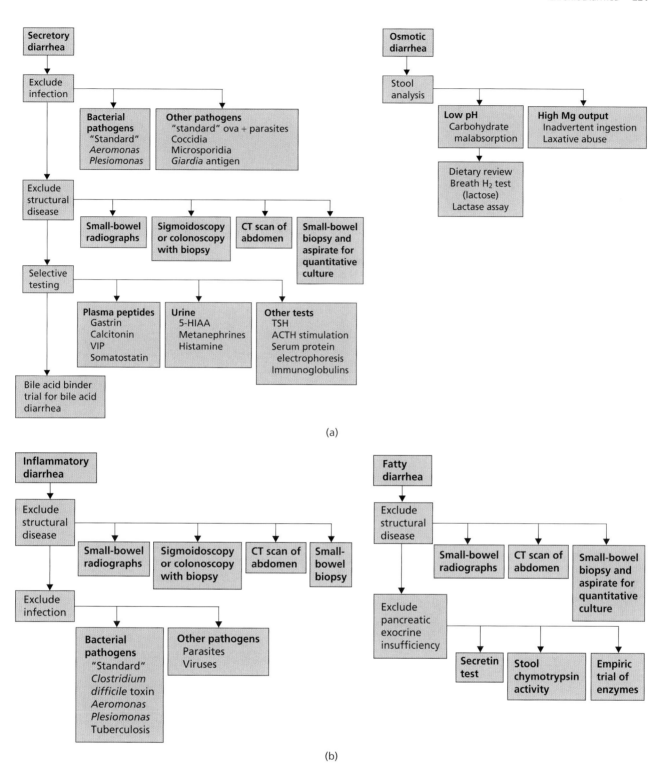

Figure 34.2 Algorithmic evaluation of subtypes of chronic diarrhea. CT, computed tomography; TSH, thyroid-stimulating hormone; ACTH, adrenocorticotropic hormone. Source: Fine 1999. reproduced with permission of the American Gastroenterological Association.

CHAPTER 34

Table 34.2 Non-specific treatment of diarrhea.

Category	Treatment	Typical adult dose
Rehydration	Intravenous fluid	1–5 L/24 hours
	Oral rehydration solution	1–5 L/24 hours
Intraluminal agents	Adsorbents (kaolin–pectin)	15–60 mL QID
	Bismuth subsalicylate	30 mL QID
	Texture modifiers (psyllium)	15–30 g/24 hours
Drugs that inhibit transit		
Potent opiates	Deodorized tincture of opium (10 mg morphine/mL)	5–20 drops QID
	Morphine sulfate (20 mg/mL)	2–10 drops QID
	Codeine phosphate or sulfate	15–60 mg QID
Less potent opiates	Diphenoxylate with atropine	1–2 tablets QID
	Difenoxin with atropine	1–2 tablets QID
	Loperamide (2 mg)	1–2 tablets QID
Others	Clonidine	0.1–0.3 mg TID
	Octreotide injection	50–200 µg TID

QID, four times per day; TID, three times per day.

Case Continued

The patient is started on loperamide 4 mg three times per day as symptomatic therapy after the stool collection is completed. Stool frequency decreases from five to two bowel movements daily, but stools remains fluid. When the biopsy is reported as showing collagenous colitis, the patient is started on oral budesonide 9 mg daily, a drug shown to work well for this condition by meta-analysis [10]. Her diarrhea resolves and budesonide is tapered.

Prognosis

Diarrhea resolves or is controlled in most patients with chronic diarrhea. The prognosis depends on the underlying diagnosis and the availability of treatment for the condition.

Take Home Points

- Chronic diarrhea is a common condition that is defined as having loose stools for more than 4 weeks.
- A detailed history provides valuable clues to the diagnosis.

- Irritable bowel syndrome (IBS) should be distinguished from chronic diarrhea by its characteristic historical criteria.
- Approaches to management include presumptive diagnosis and empiric treatment, directed evaluation, and categorization of diarrhea as watery, inflammatory, or fatty using algorithmic evaluation.
- Watery diarrhea can be subdivided into osmotic and secretory types by measuring fecal electrolytes and calculating the fecal osmotic gap (FOG).
- Therapy depends upon the specific diagnosis. Non-specific therapy with antidiarrheal drugs can provide symptomatic relief.

References

1 Schiller LR, Pardi DS, Spiller R, *et al.* Gastro 2013 APDW/WCOG Shanghai Working Party Report: Chronic diarrhea: definition, classification, diagnosis. *J Gastroenterol Hepatol* 2014; **29**: 6–25.

2 Longstreth GF, Thompson WG, Chey WD, *et al.* Functional bowel disorders. *Gastroenterology* 2006; **130**: 1480–91.

3 Tack J. Functional diarrhea. *Gastroenterol Clin North Am* 2012; **41**: 629–37.

4 Schiller LR. Definitions, pathophysiology, and evaluation of chronic diarrhea. *Best Pract Res Clin Gastroenterol* 2012; **26**: 551–62.

5 Schiller LR, Sellin JH. Diarrhea. In: Feldman M, Friedman L, Brandt LJ, eds. *Sleisenger & Fordtran's Gastrointestinal and Liver Disease: Pathophysiology/Diagnosis/Management*, 9th edn. Philadelphia, PA: Saunders Elsevier, 2010: 211–32.

6 Schiller LR. Management of diarrhea in clinical practice: strategies for primary care physicians. *Rev Gastroenterol Disord* 2007; **7**(Suppl. 3): S27–38.

7 Steffer KJ, Santa Ana CA, Cole JA, Fordtran JS. The practical value of comprehensive stool analysis in detecting the cause of idiopathic chronic diarrhea. *Gastroenterol Clin North Am* 2012; **41**(3): 539–60.

8 Freeman HJ. Pearls and pitfalls in the diagnosis of adult celiac disease. *Can J Gastroenterol* 2008; **22**: 273–80.

9 Eherer AJ, Fordtran JS. Fecal osmotic gap and pH in experimental diarrhea of various causes. *Gastroenterology* 1992; **103**: 545–51.

10 Chande N, McDonald JW, MacDonald JK. Interventions for treating collagenous colitis. *Cochrane Database Syst Rev* 2008(2):CD003575.

11 Schiller LR. Chronic diarrhea. *Curr Treat Options Gastroenterol* 2005; **8**: 259–66.

12 Hartling L, Bellemare S, Wiebe N, *et al.* Oral versus intravenous rehydration for treating dehydration due to gastroenteritis in children. *Cochrane Database Syst Rev* 2006(3): CD004390.

13 Hanauer SB. The role of loperamide in gastrointestinal disorders. *Rev Gastroenterol Disord* 2008; **8**: 15–20.

CHAPTER 35

Loss of Appetite and Loss of Weight

Angela Vizzini[1] and Jaime Aranda-Michel[2]

[1] Department of Dietetics, Mayo Clinic, Jacksonville, FL, USA
[2] Gastroenterology, Hepatology and Liver Transplant, Swedish Health Systems, Seattle, WA, USA

Summary

The evaluation of unintentional weight loss can be intriguing and challenging; therefore, a systematic approach is required to avoid lengthy workups (which can lead to overutilization of health resources) and to uncover the correct diagnosis. There are essentially *four* primary reasons for weight loss: (i) reduced caloric intake; (ii) decreased caloric "utilization" (i.e., maldigestion/malabsorption); (iii) increased energy expenditure (organic illness); and (iv) increased losses (enteric fistulas). Evaluation should include: (i) detailed medical and dietetic history and physical examination; (ii) laboratory and radiographic testing; and (iii) gastrointestinal (GI) testing. In many cases, weight loss can be treated by increasing nutrition orally to meet demand. Use of liquid nutritional supplements to supplement dietary intake is an effective way of increasing calories and reversing weight loss. In patients with anorexia, the use of appetite stimulants may need to be considered. Finally, in some cases, for patients with functional deficits, the use of enteral or parenteral nutrition may be necessary.

Case

A 50-year-old female patient presents with a 10 kg weight loss over a period of 6 months. Her usual weight is 61 kg. A detailed history notes that the patient has a normal appetite and is eating an estimated 1800 calories per day. Her body mass index (BMI) is 27. On further review of systems, she notes five to ten liquid bowel movements a day. She has had no previous GI surgeries and denies abdominal bloating or postprandial abdominal pain. Her physical examination is unremarkable. Routine laboratory blood testing is unremarkable, including normal thyroid function studies. Given her history, a 72-fecal fat study is performed to exclude intestinal malabsorption. Her fecal fat level is found to be elevated at 17 g. Upper endoscopy with a small-bowel aspirate is done to exclude bacterial overgrowth and a small-intestine biopsy is taken to exclude celiac disease. Aspirate is normal; however, the small-intestine biopsy reveals total villous atrophy consistent with celiac disease. The patient is referred to a registered dietician for instruction on a gluten-free diet; 2 weeks later, the patient's diarrhea resolves, and over a period of 12 weeks she returns to her usual weight.

Introduction

Unintentional weight loss is a powerful indicator of nutrition risk and nutrition-associated complications and is an independent predictor of increased morbidity and mortality [1]. The prevalence of the different etiologies of weight loss varies among studies. In several studies, the most common causes of weight loss are organic illness *without* cancer (13–36%), cancer alone (6–38%), psychiatric illness (9–42%), and non-malignant GI-tract disorders (9–19%) [2]. In 5–38% of patients with unintentional weight loss, no cause can be identified despite extensive testing [2]. It is very important to carefully evaluate a patient with unintentional weight loss, as significant weight loss carries a very high mortality. This chapter will present an overview of the evaluation and causes of unintentional weight loss.

History and Physical Exam

The first step when evaluating a patient with unintentional weight loss is to take a thorough medical history, with focus on the patient's weight history. It is very important to ask the patient if they have been trying to lose weight (intentional) or if the weight loss has occurred without their trying (unintentional). Most studies suggest a weight loss of 4.5 kg (10 lb) is significant and a weight loss of >10% body weight is prognostic of clinical outcomes [3]. Weight loss greater than 10% is associated with protein–energy malnutrition, while weight loss of more than 20% from baseline usually indicates severe protein–energy malnutrition. Most physiological body functions will show some degree of impairment at this level of weight loss [4]. In addition to a history of weight loss, it is important to consider physical findings such as loss of subcutaneous fat and muscle mass. Rapidly dividing cells are more prone to show nutrition, vitamin, and mineral deficiencies. Clinicians should exam the oral mucosa, hair, and nails for signs of deficiency. Physical assessment of lean muscle mass with triceps skinfold thickness using a caliper or body-fat analysis using bioelectrical impedance is useful in determining overall nutrition stores. Peripheral edema may mask weight loss and confound weight measurements [3]. Baseline determination of non-fat muscle mass with a body composition allows future determinations of nutrition interventions and goals. A decline is muscle mass is frequently accompanied by a decrease in functional status.

The associated risk of weight loss depends greatly on the patient's overall stores and on timeline: the faster the weight loss, the more pronounced metabolic derangements are likely to occur (e.g., non-alcoholic fatty liver disease (NAFLD), non-alcoholic steatohepatitis

Practical Gastroenterology and Hepatology Board Review Toolkit, Second Edition. Edited by Nicholas J. Talley, Kenneth R. DeVault, Michael B. Wallace, Bashar A. Aqel and Keith D. Lindor.

Table 35.1 Body mass index (BMI).

BMI <18.5	Low body weight
BMI 18.6–24.9	Normal body weight
BMI 25.0–29.9	Overweight
BMI 30.0–34.9	Obese class I
BMI 35.0–39.9	Obese class II
BMI >40	Obese class III

(NASH)). Patients with a low BMI (<18.5) are at greater risk [5]. BMI can be calculated as follows:

$$weight~(kg)/height~(m)^2$$

or as:

$$weight~(lbs)/height~(in)^2 \times 703$$

See Table 35.1 for interpretation.

Causes of Unintentional Weight Loss

In obtaining the patient history, the clinician needs to look for clues as to the cause of the weight loss. There are essentially four primary reasons for weight loss: (i) reduced caloric intake; (ii) decreased caloric "utilization" (i.e., maldigestion/malabsorption); (iii) increased energy expenditure (organic illness); and (iv) increased losses (enteric fistulas). Patients usually have a good sense of what category they belong to, if asked appropriately. Once a category is determined, the etiology and evaluation are greatly simplified. It is important to mention that patients with chronic diseases may think that they are eating enough but be found not to be meeting their caloric and, especially, protein requirements upon measurement.

Reduced Caloric Intake

An obvious but often overlooked component of weight loss is a decrease in the amount of food, and particularly the caloric and protein value of the food, that a patient is consuming. Changes in caloric intake can take place gradually, and patients may not be weighing themselves frequently enough to notice the impact immediately. It has been estimated that caloric intake may decrease by as much as 30% between the ages of 20 and 80 years, with weight loss of as much as 4% per year after age 65 [6]. A dietetic consult by a registered dietitian can be extremely helpful in determining deficits in a patient's intake compared to their estimated energy needs. A prospective rather than retrospective caloric count is the best way of accurately measuring per os intake. A 250 calorie reduction per day can create significant changes in weight in as little as 6 months [7]. Over time, these seemingly small changes in intake can create more dramatic weight loss and overall health risk, especially in the elderly population.

Along with age come a number of functional disabilities that may impact a patient's ability to consume adequate calories. A decline in general oral health, including loss of teeth, ill-fitting dentures, and pain while eating, has been identified as a strong predictor of weight loss [8]. Difficulty chewing and swallowing may limit the patient's choice of foods, making eating less pleasurable, especially if modified diets such as puréed or thickened liquids are used. Motor skill disabilities, visual impairment, dementia, and inability to prepare food may also be a factor. The elderly population may experience social isolation, leading to depression and decreased oral intake.

Dysgeusia and anosmia may also result in a significant decrease in caloric intake through a decline in the patient's enjoyment of eating and through increased food aversions. Dysguesia is a common side effect in cancer patients. For non-cancer patients, taste changes can occur with aging, with medication use in various chronic illnesses (e.g., cirrhosis, chronic obstructive pulmonary disease (COPD)) [10], and with infections such as oral thrush.

Loss of appetite with early satiety is frequently described by patients as the primary cause of a decrease in caloric intake. Chronic illnesses such as human immunodeficiency virus (HIV), chronic kidney disease, cancer, cirrhosis, and COPD are all associated with anorexia. However, loss of appetite alone is not usually enough to cause significant weight loss, and there are often other mechanisms associated with these chronic illnesses, such as altered metabolism, disruption in GI digestion/absorption, and side effects of treatment, that also have an effect on weight [9].

Clinical depression and medication side effects are very important and often overlooked causes of lack of taste and, consequently, weight loss. An estimated 10% of unintentional weight loss cases can be attributed to psychological causes [1]. National Health and Nutrition Examination Survey (NHANES) data published by the Centers for Disease Control and Prevention (CDC) report more than 1 out of 20 Americans aged 12 years and older have suffered from depression [11]. Depression can result in apathy toward life, as well as food, and lead to a patient's gradual disinterest in their own well-being. Many adults will never visit a mental health professional for their depression, leaving the diagnosis to the primary-care provider. Understanding the symptoms of depression and how they may be affecting eating habits and weight loss is essential for diagnosis. Depression may also lead to substance abuse, where use of the substance can act as an anorexic agent or replace the enjoyment of eating. Social isolation in patients with mental disorders may worsen depression and further decrease oral intake.

Decreased Caloric Utilization

Various GI illnesses can result in intestinal malabsorption. It is crucial in the medical history to ask the patient if they are having diarrhea and/or changes in stool consistency. If the patient admits to frequent stooling and has stool characteristics of steatorrhea, intestinal malabsorption is the most likely culprit of their weight loss.

Chronic pancreatitis can result in weight loss through exocrine function and subsequent malabsorption of all macronutrients and fat soluble vitamins. The clinical manifestations include postprandial abdominal pain (which may limit oral intake of food), steatorrhea, and anorexia. The diagnosis may be late in the illness, as >90% of the pancreatic exocrine function is usually lost before signs and symptoms are clinically observed. Chronic alcoholism usually compounds the malnutrition in this group of patients through concomitant liver disease and a decrease in oral intake.

Bacterial overgrowth of the small bowel can cause malabsorption of intraluminal nutrients and decreased oral intake of food due to bloating symptoms. Common causes of bacterial overgrowth may include small-intestinal diverticulosis, surgically created blind loops, small-bowel strictures, and small-bowel motility disorders. The symptoms are non-specific, and the diagnosis is established with breath tests and/or small-bowel aspirate.

Short-bowel syndrome (SBS), GI surgery, and disorders affecting the motor function of the stomach and small bowel can result in unintentional weight loss as well. A thorough history and review of surgical reports is needed to make an appropriate diagnosis. Disorders that can result in weight loss include gastric surgery (pyloroplasty, gastrojejunostomy, subtotal gastric resection, and total gastrectomy) and small-bowel resections (short bowel syndrome). SBS usually becomes clinically significant when more than two-thirds of the small bowel has been removed. Review of operative reports is critical to determination of a patient's prognosis and management. Rarely, short-bowel syndrome can be caused by a dysfunction of large segments of the small intestine, leading to intestinal failure (bowel obstruction and dysmotility syndromes).

Gastroparesis and chronic intestinal pseudo-obstruction may also result in significant weight loss. A history of diabetes and early satiety, persistent nausea, and vomiting should provide the pointed clues necessary to make a diagnosis of gastroparesis. Many of these patients will require dietary counseling (i.e., small, frequent meals and, occasionally, the use of an enteral feeding tube beyond the pylorus for nutritional delivery). Patients with scleroderma and amyloidosis frequently have involvement of the intestinal system and signs and symptoms of pseudo-obstruction. Often, dietary counseling on an oral diet is not enough, and these patients may require enteral feeding and occasionally parenteral nutrition.

Many diseases discussed in other chapters of this book may cause gastric and intestinal mucosal disruption and subsequent weight loss by immunological (Crohn's disease, celiac disease, autoimmune enteritis, eosinophillic gastroenteritis), infectious (tropical sprue, acquired immunodeficiency syndrome (AIDS) enteropathy), ischemic (chronic mesenteric ischemia), and radiation-induced (radiation enteritis) injury. These diagnoses usually require a thorough medical history, physical examination, and laboratory, radiological, and endoscopic evaluation. Radiation enteritis and chronic mesenteric ischemia are two diagnoses that are frequently overlooked.

Radiation enteritis may not present with weight loss until 20 years following treatment. Frequently, this piece of information is not gathered during the history of a patient. Such patients may present with diarrhea or obstructive symptoms. They are usually women who have been treated with radiation for ovarian cancer or men who have been treated with radiation for testicular cancer years prior. Chronic mesenteric ischemia should be suspected in patients with postprandial pain (more than 30 minutes following a meal) in the *absence* of bloating. These patients are usually smokers and may have a history of peripheral vascular disease. An abdominal bruit may or may not be heard on physical examination.

Increased Energy Expenditure

When energy demand exceeds energy intake, weight loss will occur over time in direct relation to the degree of deficit. Generally, a deficit of about 500 kilocalories per day equates to approximately 0.45 kg (1 lb) of weight loss per week. Patients who develop hypermetabolism usually experience weight loss in the absence of reduced oral intake. In other words, they have a good appetite. Common causes of unintentional weight loss in this category may include cancer, chronic infection, hyperthyroidism, liver disease, COPD, and cystic fibrosis. The degree of hypermetabolism is hard to ascertain unless measurements such as indirect calorimetry are performed. Use of illicit drugs, alternative non-prescribed medications, and weight loss stimulants should be questioned in select patients.

Increased Losses

Patients with a previous history of pancreatic surgery (Whipple's procedure), Crohn's disease, ischemic bowel injury, previous small-bowel surgery, or complicated bariatric surgery and trauma can develop GI fistulas. Fistulas are the abnormal communication between the GI tract and other areas. Fistulas can be internal – between two hollow organs (entero-entero fistula) – or external – typically to the skin (enterocutaneous fistula). Enterocutaneous fistulas that are considered high-output (>500 mL/day) may lead to electrolyte abnormalities, dehydration, and malnutrition by bypassing intestinal absorption. Patients with pancreato-cutaneous fistulas and, in particular, pancreatic leaks can develop malnutrition through impaired digestion and consequent malabsoprtion of fat.

Patients with refractory ascites (due to liver disease) requiring frequent large-volume paracentesis are also at risk for malnutrition. Frequent abdominal paracentesis can lead to removal of albumin and proteins present in the ascitic fluid.

Evaluation of Unintentional Weight Loss

The evaluation of unintentional weight loss can be challenging; however, a systematic approach avoids lengthy workups, which can lead to overutilization of health resources. For the purpose of this review, we have divided the approach into three steps.

Step 1: Detailed History and Physical Examination

A detailed history and physical examination can identify the etiology of unintentional weight loss in a majority of patients. As already described, the focus of history-taking and physical examination should not be solely on the exploration of medical causes, but should also include psychosocial and nutritional causes. The patient's history should begin with documentation of accurate weights over time, particularly in patients with fluid retention, and should include a prospective caloric count, a diet diary, or recall over the past month. It is helpful to place a patient in one of the three categories previously discussed.

In select patients, the flowing steps should be undertaken.

Step 2: Laboratory and Radiographic Testing

Laboratory testing may include complete blood count (CBC) with differential, comprehensive erythrocyte profile, International Normalized Ratio (INR) for vitamin K deficiency, thyroid-stimulating hormone (TSH) plus T4 measurement, iron studies, fecal occult blood testing (FOBT), and urinalysis. Additional testing can be obtained based on the clinical history; this may include 48-or 72-hour stool collection for fat, tissue transglutaminase (tTG) antibodies for celiac disease, protein electrophoresis for age-related occult cancer and amyloidosis, and HIV antibodies in high-risk patients. Other tests can be directed for diagnosis of suspected malignancies (colorectal cancer, prostate cancer, lung cancer, breast cancer) based on the clinical situation.

A chest X-ray is usually included in the initial evaluation. Additional testing should be based on the clinical situation; for example, a mammogram can be obtained in women with risk of breast cancer (abnormal breast examination, personal or family history of breast cancer, age >40 years), while computed tomography (CT) or magnetic resonance imaging (MRI) of the neck, chest, or abdomen can be conducted for occult cancers.

Step 3: GI Testing

If the diagnosis is not obvious after the first two steps, further testing, including endoscopic procedures, may be required. Usually, an esophagogastroduodenoscopy (EGD) with small-bowel biopsies and colonoscopy is the initial step. If routine endoscopies are negative, additional testing, including capsule endoscopy and GI motility studies, may be required in select patients.

Patients with a negative evaluation are unlikely to have a serious organic explanation for weight loss. In one out of four patients, a cause is not identified. These patients should be followed up in 3–6 months.

Nutrition Management of Unintentional Weight Loss

Management of unintentional weight loss is largely dependent on the findings of evaluation. Though specific therapy will be needed to address the cause of weight loss, appropriate nutrition support is essential to halting and improving any nutrition deficiencies. Attention should be given to the principles of reduced caloric intake, decreased caloric utilization, increased energy expenditure, and increased losses. Following these principles allows the physician to target better nutrition support.

If there are deficits in caloric intake but no functional impairments, use of an oral calorie–protein supplement is the first line of intervention. Most over-the-counter (OTC) oral supplements (e.g., Boost (Abbott Nutrition, Abbott Park, IL) or Ensure (NestleHealthScience, Florham Park, NJ)) provide 1 kcal/mL and 10 g of protein per 8 fl oz. The standard supplement should be taken in addition to meals and should not be used as a meal replacement. For patients with severe early satiety or anorexia, there are supplements that provide as much as 2 kcal/mL and 20 g of protein per unit. Evidence from two separate reviews demonstrates that use of supplements in addition to dietary counseling is more beneficial than dietary counseling alone, and that nutritional supplements can be used effectively to promote small but consistent weight gain [12, 13]. In addition, patients found to have inadequate intakes should take a daily multivitamin.

In patients with inadequate intake, the clinician may also consider an appetite stimulant. Megestrol acetate, dronabinol, and oxandrolone are options. While these have been investigated in patients with cancer cachexia and HIV, studies are lacking for their use in treating non-organic weight loss. Each has significant side effects, so their use should be determined on a case-by-case basis.

Patients with functional deficits without evidence of small-bowel pathology affecting absorption will most likely require nutrition support such as tube feeds or parenteral nutrition; the latter is reserved for a very select group of patients, as enteral feeding is the preferred route. The length of time for which a patient is expected to require nutrition support with feeding should dictate whether a nasoenteric feeding tube or a percutaneous placed tube is used: if the feeding device is expected to be needed only on a short-term basis (generally <4 weeks) then a nasoenteric feeding tube is recommended; if therapy is expected to last >4 weeks then an endoscopically or fluoroscopically placed gastrostomy or jejunostomy tube may be necessary [14]. When oral or enteral tube feeding cannot be achieved, total parenteral nutrition (TPN) has been shown to be an adequate and important source of nutrition. Patients with short-bowel syndrome, intestinal disease, and obstruction and severely malnourished patients may require long-term TPN. Given the risk of catheter sepsis, TPN should only be used when oral nutrition and tube feeds have failed or cannot be used. Patients with problems in digestion and absorption, such as pancreatic insufficiency, may need pancreatic supplementation. The dosage of pancreatic enzymes should be routinely monitored and adjusted according to the patient's meal pattern, fat intake, and GI symptoms.

Follow-up with a Registered Dietitian is essential not only in assessing patients with decreased appetite, but also in determining whether caloric and protein goals have been met. Continued evaluation will determine whether patients require enteral feeding as a supplement to oral intake.

Take Home Points

- The evaluation of unintentional weight loss can be intriguing and challenging; therefore, a systematic approach is required to avoid lengthy workups, which can lead to overutilization of health resources.
- There are essentially four primary reasons for weight loss: (i) reduced caloric intake; (ii) decreased caloric "utilization" (i.e., maldigestion/malabsorption); (iii) increased energy expenditure (organic illness); and (iv) increased loses (enteric fistulas).
- Non-organic causes of weight loss account for up to 46% of cases. Consult psychiatry or a psychologist with interest in eating disorders
- Evaluation should include: (i) a detailed history and physical examination; (ii) laboratory and radiographic testing; and (iii) gastrointestinal (GI) testing.

Videos of interest to readers of this chapter can be found by visiting the companion website at:

http://www.practicalgastrohep.com/

35.1 Conversion of a percutaneous endoscopic gastrostomy to a percutaneous endoscopic gastrojejunostomy.

References

1 Reife CM. Involuntary weight loss. *Med Clin N Am* 1995; **79**: 299–313.
2 Vanderschueren S, Greens E, Knockaert D, Bobbaers H. The diagnostic spectrum of unintentional weight loss. *Eur J Intern Med* 2005; **16**: 160–4.
3 Jensen GL, Hsiao PY, Wheeler D. Nutrition screening and assessment. In: Gottschlich MM, ed. *The ASPEN Adult Nutrition Core Curriculum*, 2nd edn. ASPEN, 2012: 155–69.
4 Jeejeebhoy KN, Detsky AS, Baker JP. Assessment of nutritional status. *J Parenter Enteral Nutr* 1990; **15**(5 Suppl.): 193S–6S.
5 Nightingale JMD, Walsh N, Bullock ME, Wicks AC. Three simple methods of detecting malnutrition on medical wards. *J Royal Soc Med* 1996; **89**: 144–8.
6 Chapman IM. Nutritional disorders in the elderly. *Med Clin N Am* 2006; **90**: 887–907.
7 Gans KM, Wylie-Rosett J, Eaton CB. Treating and preventing obesity through diet: practical approaches for family physicians. *Clin Fam Pract* 2002; **4**: 391.
8 Sullivan DH, Martin W, Flaxman N, *et al.* Oral health problems and involuntary weight loss in a population of frail elderly. *J Am Geriatr Soc* 1993; **41**: 725–31.
9 Delano MJ, Moldawer LL. The origins of cachexia and chronic inflammatory diseases. *Nutr Clin Pract* 2006; **21**: 68–81.
10 Dahlin C, Lynch M, Szmuilowicz E, Jackson V. Management of symptoms other than pain. *Anesthesiol Clin N Am* 2006; **24**: 39–60.
11 Pratt LA, Brody DJ. Depression in the United States household population, 2005–2006. *NCHS Data Brief* 2008(7): 1–8.
12 Milne AC, Potter J, Vivanti A, Avenall A. Protein and energy supplementation in elderly people at risk from malnutrition. *Cochrane Database Syst Rev* 2009(2):CD003288.
13 Baldwin C, Weekes CE. Dietary advice for illness-related malnutrition in adults. *Cochrane Database Syst Rev* 2008(1):CD002008.
14 Bankhead RR, Fang JC. Enteral access devices. In: Gottschlich MM, ed. *The ASPEN Adult Nutrition Core Curriculum*. ASPEN, 2007.

CHAPTER 35

Gastrointestinal Food Allergy and Intolerance

Mark T. DeMeo

Division of Gastroenterology, Hepatology and Nutrition, Department of Medicine, Rush University Medical Center, Chicago, IL, USA

Summary

Adverse reactions to food are a large and growing problem in developed countries. Symptoms can be immune-mediated or not, and differentiating between these two broad categories can be difficult at the time of presentation. The gastrointestinal (GI) system is reported to be involved in approximately 50% of cases. GI symptoms are dependent on the site of involvement and can include dysphagia, nausea, vomiting, abdominal cramping, and diarrhea. These reactions can be mild and self-limited or can result in anaphylaxis and death. A careful history and physical exam, complemented by a careful food/GI event diary, can help identify the culpable food antigen. This association can be further defined through more objective measures, such as blood/skin testing or food challenges. The cornerstone of therapy is avoiding the offending food or foods. However, medications that suppress the inflammatory response or control the mediators can dampen or abolish clinical symptoms.

Case

A 28-year-old Caucasian female with a history of asthma and irritable bowel syndrome (IBS) presents with complaints of diarrhea. She states that during the winter she did not seem to have as much problem, but now she can move her bowels three or four times per day. The stool consistency is "mudlike" and though there is no associated blood, there is mucous in her stool. She denies weight loss or nocturnal diarrhea. She feels that her symptoms are worse with ingestion of dairy products. She is concerned that she may have lactose intolerance or celiac disease.

Overview of Food Allergies and Food Intolerances

Adverse reactions to food are common complaints in the general population, and GI symptoms are predominant in up to 50% of those affected [1, 2]. The difference between these entities is based on the ability to associate symptoms with a definable immune response. Specifically, food allergies have been defined as "an adverse health effect" arising from a specific immune response that occurs reproducibly on exposure to a given food. Conversely, food intolerances, though also characterized by a reproducible adverse reaction to a particular food or food component, do not have a likely or established immunologic mechanism [1].

Adverse reactions to food are a significant health problem in the United States. A recent study, in a pediatric population, demonstrated that the prevalence of food allergy has increased 18% between 1997 and 2007 [3]. Similar increases in prevalence are also believed to have occurred in adults [1]. In spite of issues with reporting, a reasonable estimate suggests a prevalence of food allergy of between 2 and 10% of the population [4, 5].

Are There Predisposing Factors in Food Allergies?

The GI tract is constantly exposed to bacterial and dietary antigens. However, it must also respond with tolerance or hyporesponsiveness to commensal bacteria, nutrients, and innocuous antigens. The "default mechanism" of the maturing GI tract is biased toward immune suppression or tolerance.

Unfortunately, it has been difficult to precisely define what interventions will protect against or render the individual more susceptible to food allergies. Breast-feeding confers passive immunity through the immunoglobulin A (IgA) present in breast milk and can deliver early antigen exposure from maternally digested proteins. Though this intervention should improve tolerance, it has been associated with a decreased, neutral, and increased risk of subsequent food allergies. Some studies have suggested that delayed introduction of a food antigen is protective, while others have suggested that it is associated with an increased risk of allergy or intolerance.

The role of the host's microflora has also been a subject of interest regarding food allergies. The hygiene hypothesis proposes that changes in the intestinal colonization pattern during infancy are an important reason for the increased prevalence of food allergies. These changes in the gut microbiota can be caused by caesarian section (increases the risk of food allergy), the presence of siblings (older siblings may delay but not necessarily prevent food allergy), antibiotic use (increased risk of food allergy), child care, and pet/farm animal exposure (tends to decrease the incidence of food allergy, at least if the exposure occurs at an early age). Collectively, the risk of food allergies appears to decrease as the diversity of the microbial flora in the individual increases [6]. Other interesting associations include obesity (proinflammatory state) and alcohol consumption (possible increased intestinal permeation). These discrepant findings and interesting observations highlight the complexity of the factors associated with food allergies and suggest

Practical Gastroenterology and Hepatology Board Review Toolkit, Second Edition. Edited by Nicholas J. Talley, Kenneth R. DeVault, Michael B. Wallace, Bashar A. Aqel and Keith D. Lindor.
© 2016 John Wiley & Sons, Ltd. Published 2016 by John Wiley & Sons, Ltd. Companion website: www.practicalgastrohep.com

that further modifying influences such as age, gender, family history of allergy, existence of other allergic diseases, and genetic background will also influence the risk of food allergy [6].

Immune-Mediated GI Adverse Reactions to Food

IgE-Mediated

IgE-mediated food allergy is the result of host "re-exposure" to a particular food antigen. Re-exposure of an antigen to primed effector cells results in release of vasoactive mediators. The major stored mediator of the mast cell, histamine, causes symptoms within minutes to 2 hours after ingestion of the offending agent. Symptoms include vasodilatation, mucus production, and smooth-muscle spasm. The amount of antigen exposure determines the severity of the systemic response, which may affect many organ systems, including the GI, integumentary, pulmonary, and cardiovascular systems. A more sustained or "late-phase" response occurs 2–24 hours after exposure to the antigen. This reaction develops as the result of mast cell production of leukotrienes and consequent recruitment of eosinophils and other inflammatory cells to the site [7]. The most common food allergens in the United States that mediate this type of immune reaction include egg, milk, soy, peanut, tree nut, wheat, fish, and shellfish. Milk, egg, and peanut account for the vast majority of IgE-mediated allergic reactions in children, while peanuts, tree nuts, and seafood account for the majority of these reactions in teens and adults [1]. Allergies to egg, milk, and soy usually appear during infancy, and 80% resolve by adulthood. However, allergies to tree nuts, peanuts, and shellfish are less likely to resolve. A severe allergic response can result in anaphylaxis.

Oral allergy syndrome (OAS) may represent the most common food allergy in adults. Early studies described oral-pharyngeal symptoms provoked by exposure to specific food allergens. These symptoms typically included tingling and itching of the mouth, lips, and throat, but could also involve swelling of the lips and tongue. While the oral–pharyngeal symptoms do not progress in some patients, in others these clinical symptoms represent the initial presentation, which subsequently progresses to include GI manifestations such as nausea, diarrhea, and abdominal pain, urticaria or angioedema, and rarely anaphylaxis [8]. OAS is caused by an IgE crossreactivity between a previously sensitized aeroallergen and a homologous food allergen, typically a plant protein. The lability of many of these proteins in the face of denaturation or proteolysis may help explain why these allergic reactions are limited to the oral–pharyngeal area. Though OSA is most frequently used to describe the relationship between ingestion of plant antigens and oral–pharyngeal symptoms following cross-sensitization by pollen antigens, other non-plant allergens can produce similar oral–pharyngeal manifestations. Therefore, a more specific term, "pollen-food allergy syndrome," has been introduced to describe the particular association between pollen sensitivity and allergy to raw fruits, vegetables, and species caused by crossreactive allergens [9].

Mixed IgE- and Non-IgE-Mediated

Abnormally high infiltration of eosinophils in the stomach or small intestine characterizes eosinophilic GI disease [10]. Presenting symptoms are dependent on the site and depth of infiltration of the GI tract. Specifically, mucosal infiltration can present as N/V, diarrhea, and malabsorption, whereas motility disorders can be present if the muscularis is involved. Serosal involvement can result in eosinophilic ascites, gastric involvement can present with nausea and vomiting, small-bowel involvement can result in malabsorption and diarrhea, colonic involvement can present with diarrhea and blood in the stool, and rectal involvement can display blood in the stool and incontinence. The diagnosis is established through biopsy (>20 eosinophils per high-power field (HPF)). Involvement may be patchy, so multiple biopsies should be obtained. Blood eosinophilia can be seen in approximately 60% of patients with eosinophilic gastroenteritis. Generally, steroids provide a quick and effective response, but symptoms often recur with withdrawal of the agent. Other medications that have been used include cromolyn sulfate (a mast-cell stabilizer) and mepolizumab (a monoclonal antibody against interleukin (IL)-5, a major cytokine in the TH2 reaction) [10].

Non-IgE-Mediated

Non-IgE-mediated food allergy (NFA) has been attributed to aberrant cell-mediated immunity against food proteins in the absence of food allergen-specific IgE antibodies [11]. NFA most commonly affects only the GI tract. The clinical presentation can be highly variable, ranging from mild enterocolitis or proctitis with rapid resolution of symptoms with food avoidance to severe intolerance of multiple foods for a prolonged period of time. In rare cases, NFA can manifest as an acutely severe response, resembling anaphylaxis. A severe form of NFA is food protein-induced enterocolitis syndrome (FPIES) [12]. FPIES occurs in infants, usually in response to milk and soy proteins, but also with other protein antigens. The clinical manifestations can include vomiting, diarrhea, failure to thrive, and even hematochezia and melena. Treatment is based on eliminating the offending food antigen. Most children will become tolerant to the offending food antigen by the age of 3 [12].

Another entity has recently been described, in which patients feel that ingestion of gluten is associated with both GI and extraintestinal symptoms. Additionally, a gluten-free diet leads to improvement in symptoms. These patients, by definition, have negative serologies for celiac disease and are without villous damage on small-bowel biopsies. The entity has been termed "non-celiac gluten sensitivity" (NCGS) or, more recently, "non-celiac wheat sensitivity" (NCWS) [13]. Multiple mechanistic explanations have been offered, ranging from gluten-associated stimulation of an immune response to the effects of gluten on the microbial flora. A related theory suggests that symptoms do not arise from gluten but from the associated dietary fermentable oligo-di-monosaccharides and polyols (FODMAPs; see later) [14–16].

Non-Immune-Mediated GI Adverse Reactions to Food

Food Poisoning

Food poisoning occurs when food contaminated with bacteria, bacterial toxins, viruses, parasites, or chemicals is consumed. The timing of the clinical symptoms will vary between hours and days, depending on whether a toxin or a pathogen is ingested. Additionally, resolution of symptoms can take place within a few hours but can also last for days to weeks.

Lactose Intolerance

Lactose intolerance is a common adverse reaction to food. The majority of the world's population will experience decreases in lactase enzyme shortly after weaning. In this setting, lactose is not broken down to its component monosaccharides (glucose and galactose) by this enzyme, and hence absorption is compromised. Bacterial metabolism of the unabsorbed sugars results in the production of hydrogen, methane, and short-chain fatty acids, which are responsible for the symptoms, including bloating, diarrhea, and abdominal pain. Symptoms can be worsened by an additional acquired deficiency of lactase enzyme. As lactase is in the brush border of the small bowel, inflammatory conditions of the small bowel, such as celiac disease and viral gastroenteritis, can further exacerbate the deficiency of this enzyme [17].

FODMAPs

Diets that contain a high amount of short-chain carbohydrates and sugar alcohols have been associated with symptoms in susceptible individuals. Representative carbohydrates in this group include fructose, lactose, sorbitol, and manitol. The characteristics of these substances that contribute to GI symptoms include their poor absorption in the small intestine, their osmotic activity, and their rapid fermentation by intestinal bacteria. GI symptoms associated with ingestion of these carbohydrates include bloating, pain, and nausea, as well as disturbed bowel habits (constipation and/or diarrhea). These symptoms can occur in many people, but are especially troublesome in patients with visceral hypersensitivity. FODMAPs are widely distributed in the North American diet [18]. A recent controlled crossover study of patients with IBS demonstrated that a diet low in FODMAPs significantly reduced functional symptoms in this population [19].

Toxic Reactions to Foods

Food substances that have been prepared by a fermentative process or have been exposed to microbial contamination during aging or storage are likely to contain biogenic amines. Histamine and tyramine are two biogenic amines that have been linked to symptoms in humans.

Histamine toxicity or scombroid fish poisoning is associated with consumption of spoiled fish with toxic histamine levels (>500 mg/kg). Scromboid fish, such as tuna and mackerel, naturally have high quantities of free histadine in their tissue as a precursor of histamine. This process is exacerbated with spoilage. Histamine is heat–resistant, and cooking does not eliminate previously formed toxin. The reaction to the ingested fish simulates an allergic reaction, as it is associated with histamine. Symptoms usually occur within 10–30 minutes of ingestion and consist of skin flushing, headache, oral burning, abdominal cramps, nausea, diarrhea, and palpations; they are usually self-limited. However, in severe reactions, there can be life-threatening cardiovascular collapse. Some patients have reduced diamine oxidase activity or are on inhibitors; in these patients, even low dietary exposure can induce symptoms of histamine intolerance or even histamine poisoning [20].

Tyramine reactions have also been reported; these consist of acute blood pressure elevation, headache, flushing, and allergic-like reactions. Tyramine intolerance can be caused by genetic predisposition or diminished catabolism (drugs that inhibit monoamine oxidase). In this setting, tyramine-rich foods such as smoked or pickled fish, cheese, sausage, and soy sauce should be avoided [20].

Food Aversion

When intake of a certain food produces an unpleasant taste or texture, or is associated with unpleasant GI symptoms, the individual learns to avoid eating that or similar foods.

Diagnosis

A medical history is very useful in defining the allergen responsible for a patient's adverse food reaction. Food allergy should be suspected by the clinician when there are specific cutaneous, ocular, respiratory, cardiovascular, or GI symptoms following ingestion of a specific food on more than one occasion [1]. The patient will occasionally, but not invariably, have an idea of the culpable food, which may or may not be accurate. Therefore, a food diary coupled with a listing of adverse GI symptoms is an invaluable tool not only in helping to define the causative food but also in determining the time interval between ingestion and associated symptoms. Immediate food-induced allergic reactions occur within minutes to a few hours following ingestion of a particular food or food additive. These reactions are typically IgE-mediated. Delayed food reactions can occur several hours to a few days following ingestion and are typically felt to involve cellular mechanisms. This information provides a foundation for subsequent testing aimed at better defining the allergic reaction.

As immediate food allergies are IgE-mediated, IgE levels to various antigens have been measured in the blood or as a skin reaction to intradermally placed antigens. Measurement of total IgE is of little clinical utility, as studies suggest that high levels have a low positive predictive value (PPV) for food allergies, and even low serum IgE values have a low negative predictive value (NPV) for elevation of specific elevated IgE levels [21]. Measurement of blood levels of IgE to specific allergens and skin prick testing are much more accurate tests. However, false positives can be a problem with both testing methods; these are more common than false negatives. Specifically, patients can show evidence of sensitization to an allergen in both of these tests without having a clinical allergic reaction to that allergen. These tests thus cannot be used to confirm an allergic association but can support the clinical history. However, high titer-specific IgE measurements and strongly positive wheal diameters (greater than 8 mm) on skin prick testing are highly predictive of clinical allergy, at least to certain allergens. Tests that are not recommended in this setting include IgG anti-food antibodies (poor specificity), IgG4 antibodies, basophil activation, and leukotriene-release assays. Additionally, other "alternative" diagnostic procedures, such as applied kinesiology, the leukocytotoxic test, electrodemal testing, and hair analysis, do not, as yet, have enough scientific merit to advocate their use [22].

The atopy patch test is an epicutaneous application that was initially used to evaluate the cutaneous reaction to aero-allergens placed on the skin of patients with atopic dermatitis. This test differs from IgE-based testing in that it is designed to evaluate the delayed, cellular response to allergens. It has recently been expanded to evaluate the delayed reaction to certain food antigens and provide complementary yet different information to supplement IgE testing [20]. However, a recent publication of an expert panel did not recommend its use either alone or in combination with IgE testing [1].

The most specific test in determining and confirming the responsible antigen in food allergies is a double-blind, placebo-controlled food challenge. However, due to the expense and inconvenience of this test, single-blinded and open-food challenges can be used in the clinical setting instead [1]. Alternately, if a particular food or several foods have been implicated by the patient or through their history/food diary, an elimination diet of the identified foods can be undertaken [1].

In addition to these tests designed to diagnose specific food allergens, other basic testing should also be performed. A complete blood count (CBC) should be obtained in order to determine peripheral eosinophilia. If GI eosinophilia is suspected then, depending on the presumed site of involvement, an esophagogastroduodenoscopy (EGD) with esophageal biopsies plus gastric and small-bowel biopsies should be obtained. Small-bowel biopsies can also be used in the evaluation of celiac disease. If diarrhea is the predominant symptom, a colonoscopic evaluation is also indicated and biopsies should be obtained. Lactose intolerance can be evaluated with a lactose breath test, but a trial of a lactose-free diet seems a reasonable initial step, with the breath test to be scheduled if clinical confusion remains.

Management of Adverse Reactions to Foods

The mainstay of food allergy management is the identification and avoidance of specific food allergens that incite symptoms. Unfortunately, food allergen avoidance can be difficult, because food allergens are often hidden or undeclared in commercial foods. If an allergen is accidentally ingested, epinephrine, antihistamines, and steroids can be used to treat the allergic reaction [8]. In addition to acute interventions, the author uses antihistamines and cromolyn sulfate to decrease GI symptoms from accidental exposures that do not reach anaphylactic levels.

It is also possible to use immune desensitization to dampen the immune response. This involves oral or sublingual delivery of small, increasing amounts of food allergen on a regular basis in order to desensitize and potentially "tolerize" the patient to the implicated food [23]. However, there are questions about the long-term safety and efficacy of this approach. A possible alternative or adjunctive therapy to oral immunotherapy in patients with milk or egg allergy is excessive heating of the milk and egg protein. The heating process alters protein conformation and so decreases IgE binding. Additionally, omalizumab, a recombinant humanized anti-IgE antibody, has been used as another intervention that can increase the reaction threshold to peanut oral food challenges. Though these interventions all seem promising, additional studies are needed before any can be recommended [23].

In addition to these interventions, advocacy, from grassroots efforts to organizational lobbying at the national level, has been a vital part of the growing awareness of and research into food allergy. A leader in increasing awareness of food allergies is Food Allergy Research and Education (FARE; www.foodallergy.org), which is an important resource for patients with food allergies and their families [24].

- Fermentable oligo-di-monosaccharides and polyols (FODMAPs) cause symptoms in susceptible individuals, due to their poor absorption, high osmolality, and rapid fermentation.
- Blood IgE levels to certain food allergens and skin-prick allergen testing generally do not establish the culpability of a particular food, but rather support the clinical suspicion.
- The cornerstone of treatment is avoidance of the culpable food/food component, but medications can be used to dampen the immune response or the consequences of accidental exposure.

References

1 Boyce JA, Assa'ad A, Burkes AW, *et al.* Guidelines for the diagnosis and management of food allergy in the United States: report of the NIAID-Sponsored Expert Panel. *J Allergy Clin Immunol* 2010; **126**(Suppl.): S1–58.

2 Eswaran S, Tack J, Chey WD. Food: the forgotten factor in the irritable bowel syndrome. *Gastroenterol Clin N Am* 2011; **40**: 141–62.

3 Branum AM, Lukacs SL. Food allergy among children in the United States. *Pediatrics* 2009; **124**: 1549–55.

4 Rona RJ, Keil T, Summers C, *et al.* The prevalence of food allergies: a meta-analysis. *J Allergy Clin Immunol* 2007; **120**: 638–46.

5 Schneider Chafen JJ, Newberry SJ, Riedl DM, *et al.* Diagnosing and managing food allergies: a systemic review. *JAMA* 2010; **303**: 1848–56.

6 Hong X, Wang X. Early life precursors, epigenetics, and the development of food allergy. *Semin Immunopathol* 2012; **34**: 655–69.

7 Palomares O. The role of regulatory T cells in IgE mediated food allergy. *J Investig Allergol Clin Immunol* 2013; **23**: 371–82.

8 Webber CM, England RW. Oral allergy syndrome: a clinical, diagnostic, and therapeutic challenge. *Ann Allergy Asthma Immunol* 2010; **104**: 101–8.

9 Katelaris CH. Food allergy and oral allergy or pollen-food syndrome. *Curr Opin Allergy Clin Immunol* 2010; **10**: 246–51.

10 Bischoff SC. Food allergy and eosinophilic gastroenteritis and colitis. *Curr Opin Allergy Clin Immunol* 2010; **10**: 238–45.

11 Jyonouchi H. Non-IgE mediated food allergy – update of recent progress in mucosal immunity. *Inflamm Allergy Drug Targets* 2012; **11**: 382–96.

12 Guandalini S, Newland C. Differentiating food allergies from food intolerances. *Curr Gastroenterol Rep* 2011; **13**: 426–34.

13 Carroccio A, Mansueto P, D'Alcamo A, Iacono G. Non-celiac wheat sensitivity as an allergic condition: personal experience and narrative review. *Am J Gastroenterol* 2013; **108**: 1845–52.

14 Verdu EF, Armstrong D, Murray JA. Between celiac disease and irritable bowel syndrome: the "no man's land" of gluten sensitivity. *Am J Gastroenterol* 2009; **104**: 1587–94.

15 Boettcher E, Crowe SE. Dietary proteins and functional gastrointestinal proteins. *Am J Gastroenterol* 2013; **108**: 728–36.

16 Biesiekierski JR, Peters SL, Newnham ED, *et al.* No effects of gluten in patients with self-reported non-celiac gluten sensitivity after dietary reduction of fermentable poorly absorbed short chain carbohydrates. *Gastroenterology* 2013; **145**: 320–8.

17 Levitt M, Wilt T, Shaukat A. Clinical implications of lactose malabsorption versus lactose intolerance. *J Clin Gastroenterol* 2013; **47**: 471–80.

18 Gibson PR, Shepherd SJ. Evidence-based dietary management of functional gastrointestinal symptoms: the FODMAP approach. *J Gastroenterol Hepatol* 2010; **25**: 252–8.

19 Halmos EP, Power VA, Shepherd SJ, *et al.* A diet low in FODMAPs reduces symptoms of irritable bowel syndrome. *Gastroenterology* 2014; **146**: 67–75.

20 Prester L. Biogenic amines in fish, fish products and shellfish: a review. *Food Addit Contam* 2011; **28**: 1547–60.

21 Lock RJ, Unsworth DJ. Food allergy: which tests are worth doing and which are not? *Ann Clin Biochem* 2011; **48**: 300–9.

22 Wollenberg A, Vogel S. Patch testing for noncontact dermatitis: the atopy patch test for food and inhalants. *Curr Allergy Asthma Rep* 2013; **13**: 539–44.

23 Kim EH, Burks AW. Managing food allergy in childhood. *Curr Opin Pediatr* 2012; **24**: 615–20.

24 Jones SM, Burks AW. The changing CARE for patients with food allergy. *J Allergy Clin Immunol* 2013; **131**: 3–11.

Take Home Points

- Food allergy is common, affecting between 2 and 10% of the general population.
- Adverse reactions to food can either be mediated by the immune system or cause symptoms through metabolic, toxic, physiologic, pharmacologic, or psychological mechanisms.
- Milk, eggs, and peanuts account for the vast majority of immunoglobulin E (IgE)-mediated allergic reactions in children, while peanuts, tree nuts, and seafood account for the majority of these reactions in teens and adults.
- Oral allergy syndrome (OAS) is caused by an IgE crossreactivity between a previously sensitized aeroallergen and a homologous food allergen, typically a plant protein.

Obesity: Presentations and Management Options

Andres Acosta,[1] Todd A. Kellogg,[2] and Barham K. Abu Dayyeh[3]

[1] Department of Gastroenterology and Hepatology, Mayo Clinic, Rochester, MN, USA
[2] Department of Subspeciality General Surgery, Mayo Clinic, Rochester, MN, USA
[3] Mayo Clinic Hospital, Saint Mary's Campus, Rochester, MN, USA

Summary

Obesity has reached pandemic proportions. Mirroring this rise in obesity prevalence is a rise in its associated comorbid conditions, including type 2 diabetes mellitus (T2DM) and cardiovascular disease (CVD). Gastrointestinal (GI) disorders associated with obesity are more frequent and present earlier than T2DM and CVD. Diseases such as gastroesophageal reflux disease (GERD), cholelithiasis, and non-alcoholic steatohepatitis (NASH) are directly related to body weight and abdominal adiposity. There are still no low-cost, safe, effective treatments for obesity and its complications. Currently, bariatric surgical approaches targeting the GI tract are more effective than non-surgical approaches in inducing weight reduction and resolving obesity-related comorbidities. The purpose of this chapter is to review the subject of obesity, including current treatments, with a focus on bariatric (metabolic) surgery.

Case

A 48-year-old female presents with morbid obesity with a body mass index (BMI) of 45 kg/m² (height 5 foot 1 inch, weight 238 lb). She has been obese since adolescence and has failed multiple attempts at weight loss with supervised diets and exercise. She also has diabetes mellitus, hypertension on two medications, hyperlipidemia, GERD, and sleep apnea.

She is evaluated at a bariatric center-of-excellence program and undergoes laparoscopic Roux-en-Y gastric bypass (RYGB). She develops progressive dysphagia 5 weeks after surgery and is diagnosed with a stricture at her gastrojejunostomy, which is successfully treated with single endoscopic balloon dilation. No other complications occur. After 1 year, she has lost a total of 36 kg (80 lb; corresponding to 60% excess weight loss (EWL), BMI 30), is euglycemic off medication with a glycosylated hemoglobin of 5.9, no longer requires a continuous positive airway pressure (CPAP) machine, has no heartburn, and is only on a single agent for hypertension.

Definitions and Epidemiology

Obesity is defined as the amount of excess adipose tissue at which your health risks increase [1]. Normal weight, overweight, and obesity can be measured by BMI (weight in kilograms divided by the square of the height in meters). The BMI for an adult healthy weight is from 18.5 to 24.9 kg/m², overweight is from 25.0 to 29.9 kg/m², and obese is 30 kg/m² or above. Obesity is considered morbid or severe when BMI is higher than 40 kg/m² [2]. In children, obesity is measured as BMI higher than the 95th percentile related to their age and sex [3]. Obesity can also be measured by waist circumference, defined as larger than 102 cm in men and 88 cm in women.

Obesity has reached epidemic proportions in developed countries, and its prevalence is increasing in developing countries. In the United States, the adult's overweight prevalence is 64%, while obese prevalence is 32.2% among adult men and 35.5% among adult women [4]. In children and adolescents, the obesity prevalence has increased to 17.1% [5]. According to the World Health Organization (WHO) 2010 Global Burden of Disease Study, obesity and its associated conditions are now among the highest contributors to the global burden of disease [6]. The American Medical Association (AMA) recognizes obesity as a disease requiring a range of interventions.

Obesity affects almost every organ system in the body and increases the risk of numerous diseases, including T2DM, hypertension, dyslipidemia, CVD, and cancer (Table 37.1). Increased severity of obesity correlates with a higher prevalence of the associated comorbidities. Likewise, obesity increases the risk of premature mortality [7]. It is estimated that a man in his 20s with a BMI over 45 will have a 22% reduction (13 years) in life expectancy [8].

GI Comorbidities

GI disorders associated with obesity are more frequent and present earlier in the course of disease than in normal weight. Diseases such as GERD, cholelithiasis, and NASH are directly related to body weight and abdominal adiposity [9] (Table 37.2). In fact, non-alcoholic fatty liver disease (NAFLD) has become the most common cause of chronic liver disease, and obesity – through the associated development of NAFLD and NASH – has replaced alcohol as the most common cause of hepatic cirrhosis in the United States; it is projected that NAFLD will be the most common indication for liver transplantation by 2020 [10]. Furthermore, obesity is a state of low-grade chronic inflammation that affects the whole body, including GI organs. Compared to individuals of lean body weight, overweight and obese individuals have increased tissue inflammatory cytokines, activated immune responses, and altered cell

Practical Gastroenterology and Hepatology Board Review Toolkit, Second Edition. Edited by Nicholas J. Talley, Kenneth R. DeVault, Michael B. Wallace, Bashar A. Aqel and Keith D. Lindor.

Table 37.1 Comorbidities associated with obesity.

Cardiovascular	Genitourinary
Hypertension, hyperlipidemia, coronary artery disease, left ventricular hypertrophy, heart failure, venous stasis, thrombophlebitis	Stress urinary incontinence, urinary tract infections
Pulmonary	**Obstetric/gynecologic**
Obstructive sleep apnea, asthma, obesity hypoventilation syndrome	Infertility, miscarriage, fetal abnormalities
Endocrine	**Musculoskeletal**
Insulin resistance, type 2 diabetes, polycystic ovarian syndrome	Degenerative joint disease, gout, plantar fasciitis, carpal tunnel syndrome
Hematopoietic	**Neurologic**
Deep venous thrombosis, pulmonary embolism	Stroke, pseudotumor cerebri, migraine headaches
Psychiatric	**Increased cancer risk**
Depression, anxiety, binge-eating disorder	Endometrial, ovarian, breast, prostate, kidney, liver, esophagus, colon, pancreas

signaling of their metabolic pathways, which has been associated with cancer development. The increased prevalence of GI morbidity in the general population may be related to the increased prevalence of obesity in Western countries. Thus, it is important to recognize the role of higher BMI and, particularly, increased abdominal adiposity in the development of GI morbidity [9].

Management Options

Lifestyle Modification

Lifestyle modification is the cornerstone of any treatment approach to obesity. All other approaches, including surgery, have adopted

Table 37.2 Quantified risk ratios of GI disorders in obesity. Source: Acosta 2014 [9]. Reproduced with permission of Wiley.

GI disease	Obesity as risk factor Risk (OR or RR)	Confidence interval
Esophagus		
GERD	OR = 1.94	95% CI, 1.46–2.57
Erosive esophagitis	OR = 1.87	95% CI, 1.51–2.31
Barrett's esophagus	OR = 4.0	95% CI, 1.4–11.1
Esophageal adenocarcinoma	Men: OR = 2.4	95% CI: 1.9–3.2
	Women: OR = 2.1	95% CI: 1.4–3.2
Stomach		
Erosive gastritis	OR = 2.23	95% CI: 1.59–3.11
Gastric cancer	OR = 1.55	95% CI: 1.31–1.84
Small intestine		
Diarrhea	OR = 2.7	95% CI: 1.10–6.8
Colon and rectum		
Diverticular disease	RR = 1.78	95% CI: 1.08–2.94
Polyps	OR = 1.44	95% CI: 1.23–1.70
Colorectal cancer	Men: RR = 1.95	95% CI: 1.59–2.39
	Women: RR=1.15	95% CI: 1.06–1.24
Liver		
NAFLD	RR = 4.6	95% CI: 2.5–110
Cirrhosis	RR = 4.1	95% CI: 1.4–11.4
Hepatocellular carcinoma	RR = 1.89	95% CI: 1.51–2.36
Gallbladder		
Gallstones disease	Men: RR = 2.51	95% CI: 2.16–2.91
	Women: RR = 2.32	95% CI: 1.17–4.57
Pancreas		
Acute pancreatitis	RR = 2.20	95% CI: 1.82–2.66
Pancreatic cancer	Men: RR = 1.10	95% CI: 1.04–1.22
	Women: RR = 1.13	95% CI: 1.05–1.18

OR, odds ratio; RR, relative risk; GERD, gastroesophageal reflux disease; CI, confidence interval; NAFLD, non-alcoholic fatty liver disease.

lifestyle changes (Table 37.3). Guidelines published by the American Heart Association (AHA), American College of Cardiology (ACC), and the Obesity Society in 2013 suggest "that a 10 percent reduction in body weight reduces disease risk factors. Weight should be lost at a rate of 1 to 2 pounds per week based on a calorie deficit of 500–1000 kcal/day" [2]. The guidelines also recommend increasing physical activity up to 150 minutes per week during the weight-loss phase and up to 250 minutes per week during the maintenance phase. This approach has been efficacious in multiple large-scale clinical trials: the Diabetes Prevention Program showed that intense lifestyle modification reduced the incidence of diabetes by 58% when compared to placebo controls; similarly, the Look Ahead Trial showed that intense lifestyle intervention resulted in 7% weight loss and improved diabetes control [2].

Pharmacotherapy

Current recommendations for the pharmacologic treatment of obesity limit its use to patients with BMI >30 kg/m² or to those with BMI >27 kg/m² plus significant obesity comorbidities who have previously failed behavioral and lifestyle approaches alone [2]. The standard Food and Drug Administration (FDA) benchmark for the clinical efficacy of antiobesity drugs is a loss of initial body weight of 5% more than that produced by placebo treatment in the same study. However, in clinical practice the most common criterion is a 1.8 kg (4 lb) weight loss per month for at least 3 months. Maintaining this weight loss after the first 3 months is used as an indication for continued treatment.

Pharmacological approaches have shown encouraging early results followed by alarming side effects, triggering withdrawal of a number of agents from the market, including sibutramine, rimonabant, and fenfluramine/phentermine (Fen-Phen). Those pharmacological options that are currently available in the US market can be classified as being approved for short-term (less than 12 weeks) versus long-term use.

Short-Term Weight-Loss Medications

Phentermine (Adipex-P, Fastin) and diethylpropion (Tenuate) are amphetamine analogues that activate the sympathetic nervous system through increased norepinephrine and dopamine release, resulting in decreased appetite and increased basal energy expenditure.

Long-Term Weight-Loss Medications

Orlistat (Alli, Xenical) is an inhibitor of pancreatic and intestinal lipases that causes decreased hydrolysis of ingested triglycerides to absorbable fatty acids and monoacylglycerol, thus inducing malabsorption of calorie dense fats [11].

Lorcaserin (Belviq) is a serotonin 2c (5-HT2C) receptor agonist that activates pro-opiomelanocortin (POMC) neurons of the hypothalamic arcuate nucleus, thus decreasing appetite [12] and resulting in an average 5.8% weight loss when compared to placebo. Lorcaserin's side effects are mainly headaches and nausea [13].

Phentermine plus extended-release topiramate (Qsymia) capitalizes on the apparent synergy between these two medications, using smaller doses of each than are used alone and so reducing the risk of side effects. In clinical trial, this slow-release formulation produced 8–10% weight loss when compared to placebo [14]. The most common adverse events are dry mouth, paresthesia, constipation, insomnia, dizziness, and dysgeusia.

Table 37.3 Treatment recommendation for obesity. Source: Data from Jensen 2013 [2].

Treatment	BMI category (kg/m²)				
	25.0–26.9	27.0–29.9	30.0–34.9	35.0–39.9	>40.0
Diet, physical activity, and behavior therapy	With comorbidities	With comorbidities	+	+	+
Pharmacotherapy		With comorbidities	+	+	+
Surgery				With comorbidities	+

Bariatric (Metabolic) Surgery

Lifestyle modification and current pharmacological approaches for the treatment of obesity are generally associated with modest (average 5 kg) weight loss that is poorly sustained in a majority of patients. The reasons for this are multifactorial, and include the redundancy of pathways regulating energy intake and expenditure and the counterproductive response to weight loss that often leads to increased hunger and decreased energy expenditure, resulting in regain of the lost weight [15, 16].

Bariatric surgery remains the most effective treatment option for obese patients with a BMI >35 kg/m². Available procedures include RYGB, vertical-sleeve gastrectomy, adjustable gastric band, and biliopancreatic diversion with duodenal switch (Figure 37.1). Currently, 90% of weight loss operations are performed laparoscopically. The RYGB is currently the most commonly performed bariatric surgical procedure and is considered the "gold standard." In a meta-analysis of 164 studies including 161 756 patients, RYGB resulted in an average excess body weight loss of 67.5% at 1 year, with remission of diabetes in 94%, of hypertension in 80%, of obstructive sleep apnea in 95%, and of dyslipidemia in 72% of cases [17]. Unlike medications and lifestyle modifications, the effects of bariatric surgery seem to be sustained in the long term. The recently updated Swedish Obese Subjects Study demonstrated mean changes in body weight after bariatric surgery (13% RYGB, 19% gastric banding, 68% vertical-banded gastroplasty (VBG)) at 2, 10, 15, and 20 years of −23, −17, −16, and −18%, respectively [18].

The new obesity management guidelines suggest that bariatric surgery is appropriate for carefully selected patients with clinically severe obesity (BMI >40, or >35 with comorbid conditions) when medical and behavioral methods of weight loss have failed and the patient is at high risk for obesity-associated morbidity or mortality [2].

Roux-en-Y Gastric Bypass

RYGB accounts for approximately 80% of all bariatric surgeries in the United States. It is almost exclusively done laparoscopically (LRYGB). RYGB surgery is a complex procedure with at least four distinct components, all of which may have biological relevance in the induction of weight loss or amelioration of hyperglycemia: (i) isolation of the gastric cardia by creation of a small gastric pouch (15–30 mL); (ii) exclusion of the distal stomach from contact with food; (iii) exclusion of the proximal small intestine from contact with food by bypassing the duodenum and the proximal jejunum with a Roux limb (typically 75–150 cm long); and (iv) exposure of the jejunum to partially digested nutrients. Each of these components has the potential to alter appetite, energy absorption and expenditure, and glucose homeostasis.

The %EWL observed after RYGB is about 70% [19]. In general, 80% of the weight loss occurs in the first 12 months and the final 20% by 18–24 months postoperatively. In severely obese patients with type 2 diabetes, RYGB results in better glucose control and diabetes improvement than medical therapy [20]. Similarly, type 2 diabetic patients with mild to moderate obesity also benefit substantially after RYGB [21]. The mortality rate associated with LRYGB is about 0.28%. Postoperative complications following LRYGB can be categorized as early or late. Early postoperative complications

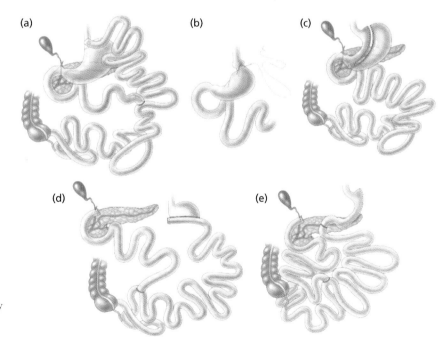

Figure 37.1 Standard bariatric surgery procedures: (a) Roux-en-Y gastric bypass (RYGB), (b) laparoscopic adjustable gastric banding, (c) sleeve gastrectomy, (d) biliopancreatic diversion, (e) biliopancreatic diversion with duodenal switch. Source: Bardley 2012 [37]. Reproduced with permission of Elsevier.

include anastomotic leak, hemorrhage, thromboembolic events, and wound infection. Late postoperative complications include anastomotic stricture, marginal ulcer, bowel obstruction, abdominal hernia, micronutrient and vitamin deficiency, and weight regain. Anastomotic leaks generally occur less than 1% of the time after LRYGB. Most large series report leak rates of 0.5–2.0%. The most common site is at the gastrojejunostomy. Persistent tachycardia, tachypnea, or hypoxia should alert the clinician to look for a leak even when other symptoms or laboratory abnormalities are absent. Pulmonary embolism after LRYGB occurs 0.5–1.0% of the time but is highly lethal when it does, as these patients have little pulmonary reserve. This complication accounts for 30–50% of all deaths after gastric bypass. Bleeding complications occur in about 0.5% of patients. Postoperative bleeding can be from mesenteric or omental vessels within the peritoneal cavity or from an anastomosis or staple line. Marginal ulceration occurs at the gastrojejunostomy less than 5% of the time after laparoscopic gastric bypass and is associated with ischemia at the anastomosis, smoking, excessive acid exposure (gastrogastric fistula), non-steroidal anti-inflammatory drug (NSAID) use, foreign material at the anastomosis (such as non-absorbable suture), *H. pylori* infection, and type 2 diabetes. This complication typically occurs within 2 months after surgery, but can occur years later. Treatment includes removing the inciting factor, sucralfate, and acid suppression. Other late complications of RYGB include bowel obstruction and anastomotic stricture. Bowel obstruction after LRYGB is most commonly secondary to an internal hernia. Patients who develop internal hernias may not present with the typical symptoms of abdominal bloating and vomiting seen with an adhesive obstruction and may only report vague, intermittent, crampy abdominal pain. The incidence of gastrojejunal stricture is 5–10% and varies with the technique used to create the anastomosis [22]. The use of a circular stapler, particularly the 21 mm size, is associated with higher stricture rates than other techniques. This complication is easily managed with endoscopic dilation. Weight loss following gastric bypass is accompanied by increased incidence of cholelithiasis: 38–52% of patients develop stones within 1 year of surgery. Between 15 and 28% of all patients require urgent cholecystectomy within 3 years. This incidence can be reduced by using ursodiol for 6 months postoperatively during the period of most rapid weight loss. Finally, the incidence of macro- and micronutrient deficiency after RYGB is up to 15%.

Laparoscopic-Sleeve Gastroplasty

Laparoscopic-sleeve gastroplasty (LSG) has gained popularity recently as a minimally invasive and successful standalone weight loss procedure with excellent safety profile. LSG reduces the gastric volume by 75–80% by removing the majority of the gastric fundus and body along the great curvature and creating a narrow tube from the gastroesophageal junction (GEJ) to the antrum. In a systemic review of randomized trials, LSG %EWL ranged from 49 to 81%, with a follow-up ranging from 6 months to 3 years [23]. Long-term (≥5 years) weight loss results showed a 53–69% EWL. T2DM remission rate ranging from 26.5 to 75.0%.

The associated mortality rate is about 0.2%. Complications after LSG include leakage (2%), bleeding (2%), and stricture (0.63%).

Laparoscopic Adjustable Gastric Banding

Approved for use in the United States in 2001, the laparoscopic adjustable gastric band (LAGB) is a silastic ring with an inflatable inner balloon. The size of the inner diameter is adjusted by adding or removing fluid through a subcutaneous port to produce

about 0.5-1kg weight loss per week. The adjustable nature of the LAGB is a major advantage over previous non-adjustable bands and the degree of gastric restriction can be titrated to minimize side effects and maximize weight loss. Percent EWL reported with LAGB ranges from 40-70% [24]. Early, major postoperative complications following LAGB are rare and include bleeding (0.1%), iatrogenic bowel perforation (0.5%), deep venous thrombosis (0.1%), and pulmonary embolism (0.1%). Band-related complications can occur in the early or late postoperative period. Among 8504 patients studied by Chapman et al. [25] tube or port malfunction requiring reoperation occurred in 1.7% of cases, band erosion into the gastric lumen occurred in 0.6% of patients, and pouch dilation or band slippage occurred in 5.6%. In the short term, the LAGB has the best safety profile of the bariatric procedures offered today. However, over the long-term, complications requiring an operation can occur in up to 50% of patients [26].

Vertical-Banded Gastroplasty

VBG was developed in 1980 but is no longer performed. Long-term weight loss was generally poor and many patients developed complications such as staple-line failure or band stenosis that required reoperation [27].

Biliopancreatic Diversion with Duodenal Switch

Biliopancreatic diversion with duodenal switch (BPD-DS) is a powerful malabsorptive operation. This procedure is technically demanding to perform and has a higher incidence of perioperative complications and nutritional deficiencies compared to other procedures. As such, the BPD-DS only accounts for about 5% of all bariatric procedures performed in the United States.

Endoscopic Treatments

Despite proven efficacy, it is estimated that less than 1% of obese subjects who qualify for bariatric surgery will undergo such intervention [28]. This mismatch is fueled by high surgical costs and by morbidity and mortality associated with surgical interventions. Our understanding of the mechanisms by which bariatric surgery works has evolved from mechanical restriction and malabsorption to anatomical surgical manipulations resulting in physiological alterations in gut neuroendocrine signaling, GI motility, autonomic nervous system (ANS) signaling, bile acid production and absorption, and gut microbiota, leading to weight loss and diabetes resolution. Emerging endoscopic technologies have opened the door to using endoscopic approaches and devices to reproduce many of the anatomical alterations of bariatric surgery endoscopically and thereby contribute to the effective treatment of obesity and its associated conditions [29]. Early results are encouraging and suggest that endoscopy-based intraluminal therapies may provide the next major treatment advance in this area by providing cost-effective and minimally invasive treatment options to a wider segment of the obese and overweight population, to vulnerable populations such as children and adolescents, and to at-risk super-obese individuals.

Intragastric Balloons

Endoscopically placed intragastric balloons (IGBs) may serve as a primary weight-loss procedure or as a "bridge therapy" prior to bariatric surgery, used to decrease the perioperative surgical risk. Currently available IGBs are generally designed to remain within the stomach for up to 6 months prior to removal. Several small prospective randomized trials with mid-term follow-up reported the safety and efficacy of IGB for weight reduction, improvement of metabolic syndrome [30], and NASH. When compared to sham, pharmacotherapy, and one- or two-balloon insertion in sequence, about 10% of body weight loss appears to be maintained at 6–12 months after balloon removal [31]. Nausea, abdominal pain, acid reflux, and vomiting are common complaints after IGB placement, but the majority of these symptoms seem to improve with time and medical therapy, without necessitating early balloon removal.

Endoscopic Gastroplasty Techniques

Primary Obesity Surgery Endolumenal Procedure
Primary obesity surgery endolumenal (POSE) procedures use a peroral Incisionless Operating Platform (IOP) (USGI Medical, San Clemente, CA) to place transmural tissue anchor plications that reduce gastric fundus accommodation and parts of the distal gastric body. Results of a single-center, open-label, prospective trial enrolling 45 obese patients mostly with mild to moderate obesity demonstrated the feasibility and safety of the technique. A mean of 8.2 suture anchors were placed in the fundus and 3 in the distal body. Mean operative time was about 69 minutes and all patients were admitted for observation. Patients lost about 13 kg at 6 months, representing 49% EWL. The procedure was well tolerated [32].

Endoscopic-Sleeve Gastroplasty
Using an FDA-approved and commercially available endoscopic suturing device (Overstitch; Apollo Endosurgery, Austin, TX), Abu Dayyeh and colleagues demonstrated the feasibility of transoral endoscopic gastric volume reduction in a fashion similar – but not identical – to sleeve gastrectomy, accomplished by a series of endoluminally placed, free-hand, full-thickness, closely spaced sutures through the gastric wall from the prepyloric antrum to the GEJ [33]. A multicenter trial of this technique is ongoing, and early results are encouraging.

Aspiration Therapy

Aspiration therapy is a novel treatment approach for obesity that allows obese patients to dispose of a portion of their ingested meal by placing a specially designed gastrostomy tube, known as the A-Tube, in the stomach. The aspiration procedure is performed about 20 minutes after the entire meal is consumed and takes about 5–10 minutes to complete. The apparatus that enables patients to aspirate is known as the Aspire Assist (Aspire Bariatrics, King of Prussia, PA). This approach provides an effective mean of portion control and has been efficacious in a pilot prospective trial: 18 subjects were randomized in a 2 : 1 ratio to 1 year of aspiration therapy (AT) plus lifestyle intervention (BMI = 42.0 ± 4.7 kg/m^2) or lifestyle intervention alone (LIA) (BMI = 43.4 ± 5.3 kg/m^2). The AT group was permitted to continue therapy for an additional 1 year (2 years total); 7 of 11 patients randomized to AT opted to continue for 2 years. The initial 1 year was completed by 10 of 11 AT and 4 of 7 LIA subjects. Among completers, AT and LIA subjects lost $18.3 \pm 7.6\%$ ($49.0 \pm 24.4\%$ EWL) and $5.9 \pm 10.0\%$ ($14.9 \pm 24.6\%$ EWL) body weight, respectively. The seven subjects who completed 2 years of AT maintained a $20.1 \pm 9.3\%$ body weight loss ($54.6 \pm 31.7\%$ EWL) at 2 years [34]. A pivotal multicenter, randomized, controlled, open-label, 52-week trial to support FDA approval of this device is currently underway in the United States.

EndoBarrier GI Liner

Endoscopic implantation of a duodenal-jejunal bypass sleeve made from a Teflon liner (EndoBarrier; GI Dynamics, Lexington, MA) shows promise and efficacy in the management of obesity and associated diabetes [35]. When deployed in the duodenal bulb under endoscopic and fluoroscopic guidance, this impermeable fluoropolymer sleeve, extending 60 cm into the small bowel, creates a mechanical barrier that allows food to bypass the duodenum and proximal jejunum, thus potentially manipulating the enteroinsulin system. Several prior studies have documented the technique's feasibility and efficacy in weight loss and in improving obesity comorbidity (especially diabetes and NASH) [36]. This device has a favorable safety profile. A pivotal US multicenter FDA registry trial is currently underway.

Conclusion

The prevalence of obesity and diabetes is increasing dramatically in the United States and worldwide. Recommendations for treatment are: intense lifestyle modification for BMI >27 kg/m^2, pharmacological approach plus intense lifestyle modification for BMI >30 kg/m^2, and bariatric (metabolic) surgery plus lifestyle modification for BMI >40 kg/m^2. In patients with obesity-associated comorbidities, recommendations are intense lifestyle modification for BMI >25 kg/m^2, pharmacological approach plus intense lifestyle modification for BMI BMI >27 kg/m^2, and metabolic surgery plus lifestyle modification for BMI BMI >35 kg/m^2. Bariatric surgery is currently the only effective and durable therapy for obesity; it results in improvements in all major obesity-related comorbidities. The majority of bariatric procedures are performed laparoscopically, and the two most common – LRYGB and LSG – can be performed with low complication rates. Emerging endoscopic technologies have opened the door to using endoscopic approaches and devices to reproduce many of the anatomical alterations of bariatric surgery endoscopically and thereby contribute to the effective treatment of obesity and its associated conditions. Early results are encouraging, and suggest that endoscopy-based intraluminal therapies may provide a major treatment advance in this area.

Take Home Points

- The prevalence of obesity has markedly increased in the United States and worldwide; one-third of adult Americans are obese.
- Bariatric surgery remains the only therapy that affords significant and durable weight loss.
- Weight loss following bariatric surgery is associated with improvement and resolution of multiple comorbidities and reduction in long-term mortality.
- When performed in experienced centers, bariatric surgery is associated with low complication rates.
- Emerging endoscopic techniques and technologies may provide a minimally invasive and effective treatment approach to obesity.

References

1 Yach D, Stuckler D, Brownell KD. Epidemiologic and economic consequences of the global epidemics of obesity and diabetes. *Nat Med* 2006; **12**(1): 62–6.

2 Jensen MD, Ryan DH, Apovian CM, *et al.* 2013 AHA/ACC/TOS guideline for the management of overweight and obesity in adults: a report of the American College of Cardiology/American Heart Association Task Force on Practice Guidelines and The Obesity Society. *Circulation* 2014; **129**(25 Suppl. 2): S102–38.

3 Daniels SR, Jacobson MS, McCrindle BW, *et al.* American Heart Association Childhood Obesity Research Summit: executive summary. *Circulation* 2009; **119**(15): 2114–23.

4 Flegal KM, Carroll MD, Kit BK, Ogden CL. Prevalence of obesity and trends in the distribution of body mass index among US adults, 1999–2010. *JAMA* 2012; **307**(5): 491–7.

5 Ogden CL, Carroll MD, Kit BK, Flegal KM. Prevalence of obesity and trends in body mass index among US children and adolescents, 1999–2010. *JAMA* 2012; **307**(5): 483–90.

6 Lim SS, Vos T, Flaxman AD, *et al.* A comparative risk assessment of burden of disease and injury attributable to 67 risk factors and risk factor clusters in 21 regions, 1990–2010: a systematic analysis for the Global Burden of Disease Study 2010. *Lancet* 2012; **380**(9859): 2224–60.

7 Hensrud DD, Klein S. Extreme obesity: a new medical crisis in the United States. *Mayo Clin Proc* 2006; **81**(10 Suppl.): S5–10.

8 Fontaine KR, Redden DT, Wang C, *et al.* Years of life lost due to obesity. *JAMA* 2003; **289**(2): 187–93.

9 Acosta A, Camilleri M. Gastrointestinal morbidity in obesity. *Ann N Y Acad Sci* 2014; **1311**: 42–56.

10 Wree A, Broderick L, Canbay A, *et al.* From NAFLD to NASH to cirrhosis-new insights into disease mechanisms. *Nat Rev Gastroenterol Hepatol* 2013; **10**(11): 627–36.

11 Padwal RS, Majumdar SR. Drug treatments for obesity: orlistat, sibutramine, and rimonabant. *Lancet* 2007; **369**(9555): 71–7.

12 Sohn JW, Xu Y, Jones JE, *et al.* Serotonin 2C receptor activates a distinct population of arcuate pro-opiomelanocortin neurons via TRPC channels. *Neuron* 2011; **71**(3): 488–97.

13 Smith SR, Weissman NJ, Anderson CM, *et al.* Multicenter, placebo-controlled trial of lorcaserin for weight management. *N Engl J Med* 2010; **363**(3): 245–56.

14 Allison D, Gadde K, Garvey W, *et al.* Controlled-release phentermine/topiramate in severely obese adults: a randomized controlled trial (EQUIP). *Obesity (Silver Spring)* 2012; **20**(2): 330–42.

15 Sumithran P, Prendergast LA, Delbridge E, *et al.* Long-term persistence of hormonal adaptations to weight loss. *N Engl J Med* 2011; **365**(17): 1597–604.

16 Acosta A, Abu Dayyeh BK, *et al.* Recent advances in clinical practice challenges and opportunities in the management of obesity. *Gut* 2014; **63**(4): 687–95.

17 Chang SH, Stoll CR, Song J, *et al.* The effectiveness and risks of bariatric surgery: an updated systematic review and meta-analysis, 2003–2012. *JAMA Surg* 2014; **149**(3): 275–87.

18 Sjöström L. Review of the key results from the Swedish Obese Subjects (SOS) trial – a prospective controlled intervention study of bariatric surgery. *J Int Med* 2013; **273**(3): 219–34.

19 Schneider BE, Villegas L, Blackburn GL, *et al.* Laparoscopic gastric bypass surgery: outcomes. *J Laparoendosc Adv Surg Tech A* 2003; **13**(4): 247–55.

20 Ikramuddin S, Korner J, Lee WJ, *et al.* Roux-en-Y gastric bypass vs intensive medical management for the control of type 2 diabetes, hypertension, and hyperlipidemia: the Diabetes Surgery Study randomized clinical trial. *JAMA* 2013; **309**(21): 2240–9.

21 Schauer PR, Bhatt DL, Kirwan JP, *et al.* Bariatric surgery versus intensive medical therapy for diabetes – 3-year outcomes. *N Engl J Med* 2014; **370**(21): 2002–13.

22 Podnos YD, Jimenez JC, Wilson SE, *et al.* Complications after laparoscopic gastric bypass: a review of 3464 cases. *Arch Surg* 2003; **138**(9): 957–61.

23 Trastulli S, Desiderio J, Guarino S, *et al.* Laparoscopic sleeve gastrectomy compared with other bariatric surgical procedures: a systematic review of randomized trials. *Surg Obes Relat Dis* 2013; **9**(5): 816–29.

24 Nguyen N, DeMaria EJ, Ikramuddin S, Hutter MM, eds. *The SAGES Manual: A Practical Guide to Bariatric Surgery.* New York, NY: Springer, 2008.

25 Chapman AE, Kiroff G, Game P, *et al.* Laparoscopic adjustable gastric banding in the treatment of obesity: a systematic literature review. *Surgery* 2004; **135**(3): 326–51.

26 Kellogg TA. Revisional bariatric surgery. *Surg Clin North Am* 2011; **91**(6): 1353–71, x.

27 Ramsey-Stewart G. Vertical banded gastroplasty for morbid obesity: weight loss at short and long-term follow up. *Aust N Z J Surg* 1995; **65**(1): 4–7.

28 Buchwald H, Oien D. Metabolic/bariatric surgery worldwide 2011. *Obes Surg* 2013; **23**(4): 427–36.

29 Abu Dayyeh BK, Thompson CC. Obesity and bariatrics for the endoscopist: new techniques. *Therap Adv Gastroenterol* 2011; **4**(6): 433–42.

30 Fuller NR, Pearson S, Lau NS, *et al.* An intragastric balloon in the treatment of obese individuals with metabolic syndrome: a randomized controlled study. *Obesity* 2013; **21**(8): 1561–70.

31 Mathus-Vliegen EM. Obesity: intragastric balloons – a bubble to combat the obesity bubble? *Nat Rev Gastroenterol Hepatol* 2010; **7**(1): 7–8.

32 Espinos JC, Turro R, Mata A, *et al.* Early experience with the Incisionless Operating Platform (IOP) for the treatment of obesity: the Primary Obesity Surgery Endolumenal (POSE) procedure. *Obes Surg* 2013; **23**(9): 1375–83.

33 Abu Dayyeh BK, Rajan E, Gostout CJ. Endoscopic sleeve gastroplasty: a potential endoscopic alternative to surgical sleeve gastrectomy for treatment of obesity. *Gastrointest Endosc* 2013; **78**(3): 530–5.

34 Sullivan S, Stein R, Jonnalagadda S, *et al.* Aspiration therapy leads to weight loss in obese subjects: a pilot study. *Gastroenterology* 2013; **145**(6): 1245–52, e1–5.

35 Gersin KS, Rothstein RI, Rosenthal RJ, *et al.* Open-label, sham-controlled trial of an endoscopic duodenojejunal bypass liner for preoperative weight loss in bariatric surgery candidates. *Gastrointest Endosc* 2010; **71**(6): 976–82.

36 Patel SR, Hakim D, Mason J, Hakim N. The duodenal-jejunal bypass sleeve (EndoBarrier Gastrointestinal Liner) for weight loss and treatment of type 2 diabetes. *Surg Obes Relat Dis* 2013; **9**(3): 482–4.

37 Bradley D, Magkos F, Klein S. Effects of bariatric surgery on glucose homeostasis and type 2 diabetes. *Gastroenterology* 2012; **143**(4): 897–912.

Hematochezia

Lisa L. Strate

University of Washington School of Medicine, Harborview Medical Center, Seattle, WA, USA

Summary

Hematochezia is a very common gastrointestinal (GI) problem, especially among the elderly. Most patients with hemotachezia have colonic sources of bleeding, such as diverticular bleeding, ischemic colitis, or hemorrhoids. However, it is important to exclude an upper GI source in patients with significant blood loss. Colonoscopy is the best strategy for most patients with acute hematochezia, because of its diagnostic and therapeutic possibilities and relative safety. Colonoscopy should generally be performed within 24 hours of presentation or close to the onset of bleeding, and after a thorough bowel preparation. Radiographic interventions, including angiography, radionuclide scintigraphy, and multidetector computed tomography (CT) scanning, are useful for patients who cannot be stabilized or who have failed endoscopic diagnosis or treatment. Aggressive resuscitation and management of other comorbid illnesses are important.

Case

An 80-year-old female is admitted to the hospital with 2 days of hematochezia and lightheadedness. She has a history of arthritis and hypertension and reports a normal colonoscopy 5 years previously. She takes a daily aspirin (81 mg), an angiotensin-converting enzyme (ACE) inhibitor, and acetaminophen as needed for pain. She lives independently. On physical examination, she is an elderly woman in no distress. Her blood pressure is 118/80 mmHg and her heart rate is 105 bpm. She has no abdominal tenderness. There is maroon stool on rectal exam. The remainder of the exam is unremarkable. Her admission hematocrit is 25% (a drop of 14% from her recent baseline). Her platelets and prothrombin time are normal. Her creatinine is 1.8 mg/dL (an increase from 1.1 mg/dL) and her blood urea nitrogen (BUN) is 7 mg/dL. She passes another bloody stool in the emergency department.

Definition and Epidemiology

Hematochezia is defined as the passage of red or maroon blood per rectum. It is most often associated with lower intestinal bleeding (bleeding beyond the ligament of Treitz) but can represent bleeding from any source, depending on the amount of bleeding and transit time. An upper GI source of bleeding is found in 5–15% of individuals with hematochezia, and 5–10% have small-bowel sources [1]. It can be difficult to determine whether hematochezia is from the upper GI tract, the mid-bowel, or the colon based on the initial presentation. This review will focus on hematochezia from a colonic source or lower intestinal bleeding.

Historically, lower intestinal bleeding was felt to be much less common than upper GI bleeding. However, recent studies in the United States and Europe indicate that the incidence of these disorders is similar, due to an increase in the incidence of lower intestinal bleeding and a decrease in upper GI bleeding [2, 3]. The majority of patients with lower intestinal bleeding have at least one comorbid condition, which adds to the complexity of this disorder.

Clinical Features

There are a number of clinical features that can guide the diagnosis and management of hematochezia. The character, volume, frequency, and duration of the bleeding can help determine its source and severity. Typically, small amounts of bright red blood indicate an anal or rectal source, whereas larger amounts of maroon stool signify a brisk bleed from a more proximal source. Rectal symptoms such as pain with the passage of stool, presence of hemorrhoids, and tenesmus are also clues to a rectal source. However, symptoms and clinical features alone cannot be used to exclude lesions in the proximal colon [4]. The presence of abdominal pain and tenderness usually reflects mucosal injury, such as inflammatory bowel disease (IBD) or ischemic colitis. A prior or family history of intestinal disorders (IBD, cancer), radiation treatment (radiation colitis), or abdominal surgeries (aortoenteric fistula, anastomotic bleeding) may also allude to specific sources.

A number of risk models or scores have been developed for prediction of poor outcome in lower intestinal bleeding [5–8]. Predictors common to each of these studies include indicators of hemodynamic instability (hypotension, tachycardia, syncope, and orthostasis), ongoing rectal bleeding, and the presence of comorbid illness. Older age, the use of aspirin or anticoagulants, a non-tender abdominal exam, and a past history of bleeding from diverticulosis or angiodysplasia were also predictive in one or more of the studies. In one study, the number of risk factors correlated with the risk of poor outcome [7]. These risk factors can assist in decision-making – particularly at the point of first medical contact – regarding which patients will benefit from intensive care and urgent interventions.

Practical Gastroenterology and Hepatology Board Review Toolkit, Second Edition. Edited by Nicholas J. Talley, Kenneth R. DeVault, Michael B. Wallace, Bashar A. Aqel and Keith D. Lindor.
© 2016 John Wiley & Sons, Ltd. Published 2016 by John Wiley & Sons, Ltd. Companion website: www.practicalgastrohep.com

References

1 Jensen DM, Machicado GA. Diagnosis and treatment of severe hematochezia. *The role of urgent colonoscopy after purge. Gastroenterology* 1988; **95**(6): 1569–74.

2 Laine L, Yang H, Chang SC, Datto C. Trends for incidence of hospitalization and death due to GI complications in the United States from 2001 to 2009. *Am J Gastroenterol* 2012; **107**(8): 1190–5, quiz 6.

3 Lanas A, Garcia-Rodriguez LA, Polo-Tomas M, *et al.* Time trends and impact of upper and lower gastrointestinal bleeding and perforation in clinical practice. *Am J Gastroenterol* 2009; **104**(7): 1633–41.

4 Fine KD, Nelson AC, Ellington RT, Mossburg A. Comparison of the color of fecal blood with the anatomical location of gastrointestinal bleeding lesions: potential misdiagnosis using only flexible sigmoidoscopy for bright red blood per rectum. *Am J Gastroenterol* 1999; **94**(11): 3202–10.

5 Das A, Ben-Menachem T, Cooper GS, *et al.* Prediction of outcome in acute lower-gastrointestinal haemorrhage based on an artificial neural network: internal and external validation of a predictive model. *Lancet* 2003; **362**(9392): 1261–6.

6 Kollef MH, O'Brien JD, Zuckerman GR, Shannon W. BLEED: a classification tool to predict outcomes in patients with acute upper and lower gastrointestinal hemorrhage. *Crit Care Med* 1997; **25**(7): 1125–32.

7 Strate LL, Saltzman JR, Ookubo R, *et al.* Validation of a clinical prediction rule for severe acute lower intestinal bleeding. *Am J Gastroenterol* 2005; **100**(8): 1821–7.

8 Velayos FS, Williamson A, Sousa KH, *et al.* Early predictors of severe lower gastrointestinal bleeding and adverse outcomes: a prospective study. *Clin Gastroenterol Hepatol* 2004; **2**(6): 485–90.

9 Green BT, Rockey DC, Portwood G, *et al.* Urgent colonoscopy for evaluation and management of acute lower gastrointestinal hemorrhage: a randomized controlled trial. *Am J Gastroenterol* 2005; **100**(11): 2395–402.

10 Jensen DM, Machicado GA, Jutabha R, Kovacs TO. Urgent colonoscopy for the diagnosis and treatment of severe diverticular hemorrhage. *N Engl J Med* 2000; **342**(2): 78–82.

11 Schmulewitz N, Fisher DA, Rockey DC. Early colonoscopy for acute lower GI bleeding predicts shorter hospital stay: a retrospective study of experience in a single center. *Gastrointest Endosc* 2003; **58**(6): 841–6.

12 Strate LL, Syngal S. Timing of colonoscopy: impact on length of hospital stay in patients with acute lower intestinal bleeding. *Am J Gastroenterol* 2003; **98**(2): 317–22.

13 Hunter JM, Pezim ME. Limited value of technetium 99m-labeled red cell scintigraphy in localization of lower gastrointestinal bleeding. *Am J Surg* 1990; **159**(5): 504–6.

14 Laine L, Shah A. Randomized trial of urgent vs. elective colonoscopy in patients hospitalized with lower GI bleeding. *Am J Gastroenterol* 2010; **105**(12): 2636–41, quiz 42.

15 Jensen DM, Machicado GA. Colonoscopy for diagnosis and treatment of severe lower gastrointestinal bleeding. Routine outcomes and cost analysis. *Gastrointest Endosc Clin N Am* 1997; **7**(3): 477–98.

16 Zuckerman GR, Prakash C. Acute lower intestinal bleeding: part I: clinical presentation and diagnosis. *Gastrointest Endosc* 1998; **48**(6): 606–17.

17 Kuo WT, Lee DE, Saad WE, *et al.* Superselective microcoil embolization for the treatment of lower gastrointestinal hemorrhage. *J Vasc Interv Radiol* 2003; **14**(12): 1503–9.

18 Strate LL, Ayanian JZ, Kotler G, Syngal S. Risk factors for mortality in lower intestinal bleeding. *Clin Gastroenterol Hepatol* 2008; **6**(9): 1004–10, quiz 955.

19 Longstreth GF. Epidemiology and outcome of patients hospitalized with acute lower gastrointestinal hemorrhage: a population-based study. *Am J Gastroenterol* 1997; **92**(3): 419–24.

CHAPTER 39

Obscure Gastrointestinal Bleeding

R. Sameer Islam and Shabana F. Pasha

Division of Gastroenterology, Mayo Clinic, Scottsdale, AZ, USA

Summary

Obscure gastrointestinal bleeding (OGIB) constitutes 5% of all gastrointestinal (GI) bleeding. The majority of lesions are located in the small bowel. Angioectasias are the most common lesion in older patients, and small-bowel tumors in younger patients. The newer endoscopic and radiologic small-bowel modalities have transformed our approach to the management of this disorder. Capsule endoscopy (CE) is the diagnostic test of choice after a negative esophagogastroduodenoscopy (EGD) and colonoscopy. Computed tomographic enterography (CTE) is complementary to CE in the diagnostic evaluation of OGIB. Device-assisted enteroscopy (DAE) is useful for therapeutic interventions and in the evaluation of patients with a high suspicion of a small-bowel lesion despite negative diagnostic evaluation. The role of intraoperative enteroscopy is reserved for the management of refractory bleeding and small-bowel lesions not accessible to endoscopy. Supportive management may be appropriate for patients with multiple lesions or significant comorbidities.

Case

A 67-year-old male presents with melena and iron-deficiency anemia. He reports intermittent melena and fatigue for the past 12 months. His medical history includes gastroesophageal reflux disease (GERD), asthma, hypertension, and hypothyroidism. His medications include a beta-blocker, synthroid, proton pump inhibitor (PPI), and oral iron supplements. He avoids all non-steroidal anti-inflammatory drugs (NSAIDs) and has recently stopped the prophylactic use of aspirin. Physical examination is unremarkable, except for melenic stools on digital rectal exam. His hematocrit is 35%, iron 45 mcg/dL, transferrin saturation 7%, and ferritin 15 mcg/L. He had an EGD and ileocolonoscopy a year ago, which were within normal limits. A repeat bidirectional endoscopy performed at his current presentation is also unrevealing for an etiology of GI bleeding.

Definition and Epidemiology

Approximately 10–20% of patients who present with GI bleeding have no identifiable etiology on initial evaluation. Recurrent or persistent bleeding occurs in half of these patients (5%) and poses a challenge to diagnosis and treatment [1]. OGIB is defined as bleeding from the GI tract that persists or recurs after a negative initial evaluation with bidirectional endoscopy and small-bowel follow-through (SBFT) or enteroclysis [2]. OGIB is classified according to clinical presentation as overt (clinically perceptible bleeding) or occult (unexplained iron-deficiency anemia, suspected to be caused by chronic blood loss) [2, 3]. With respect to location, GI bleeding is classified as upper (proximal to ampulla of Vater), mid (ampulla of Vater to ileocecal valve), or lower (colon) [2, 4]. The majority of lesions in patients with OGIB are located in the small intestine, with the remainder constituting missed lesions within reach of standard endoscopy.

Clinical Features

Hematemesis generally indicates a bleeding source proximal to the ligament of Treitz. Hematochezia and melena may represent an upper, small-bowel, or colon source. Other clinical symptoms include abdominal pain, weight loss, and unexplained iron-deficiency anemia. Patients with aortic stenosis, renal failure, or von Willebrand's disease may be predisposed to bleeding from angioectasias. A history of NSAID use raises the possibility of small-bowel ulcerations. A physical examination may be useful in the diagnosis of systemic syndromes (e.g., hereditary hemorrhagic telangiectasias, amyloidosis, and blue-rubber bleb nevus syndrome).

Case Continued

A CE is performed. The first duodenal image is at 0 hours, 12 minutes, 5 seconds and the first cecal image at 5 hours, 10 minutes, 12 seconds. Multiple angioectasias are seen in the proximal and mid small bowel from 0 hours, 50 minutes, 10 seconds to 2 hours, 50 minutes, 15 seconds.

Diagnosis

A second-look EGD and colonoscopy should be considered to evaluate for missed lesions. There is a high yield of 35–75% on repeat EGD and 6% on repeat colonoscopy [5–8].

CE is the preferred test of choice for evaluation of the small bowel after negative bidirectional endoscopy. The diagnostic yield of CE is 38–83% [9], with a high positive predictive value (PPV; 94–97%) and a high negative predictive value (NPV; 83–100%) in OGIB [10, 11]. There is a higher likelihood of positive CE findings in patients with a hemoglobin level <10 g/dL, longer duration of

Practical Gastroenterology and Hepatology Board Review Toolkit, Second Edition. Edited by Nicholas J. Talley, Kenneth R. DeVault, Michael B. Wallace, Bashar A. Aqel and Keith D. Lindor.

bleeding (>6 months), more than one episode of bleeding, overt bleeding, and the use of CE within 2 weeks of the bleeding episode [12–14]. Additional evaluation can usually be deferred due to low rebleeding rates (6–11%) after a negative CE [15, 16]. In patients with recurrent bleeding after a negative or non-diagnostic CE, the yield of repeat CE is 49–75% [17,18], particularly in patients whose presentation changed from occult to overt bleed and in those with a drop in hemoglobin of more than 4 g/dL [19].

The limitations of CE include a lack of therapeutic capabilities, a high rate of false-positive findings and the potential for missed lesions, including 19% of small-bowel tumors. CE may be complicated by retention, and is therefore contraindicated in patients with suspected small-bowel obstruction or stricture [20–24].

Push enteroscopy (PE) allows only a limited evaluation of the proximal small bowel (50–100 cm distal to ligament of Treitz). A meta-analysis of 14 studies showed a higher yield for clinically significant lesions with CE (56%) compared to PE (26%) [25]. CE has largely replaced PE in the diagnostic evaluation of OGIB. PE may be useful for endoscopic treatment in patients with proximal small-bowel lesions detected on non-invasive testing.

In a study comparing CE to CTE and mesenteric angiography, CE detected more bleeding lesions – predominantly angioectasias [26]. CTE has a yield of 25–45% in OGIB, with a significantly higher yield in patients with overt versus occult bleed. CTE usually detects small-bowel tumors missed on CE [27–29] and is thus considered complementary to CE in the diagnostic evaluation of OGIB. This may be the preferred test in patients with a suspected small-bowel tumor or obstruction [30] (see Figure 39.1).

DAE is useful for the performance of therapy in patients with a positive CE or CTE, and for evaluation of patients with a negative CE and CTE but high clinical suspicion for a small-bowel lesion.

Though double-balloon enteroscopy (DBE) may have a higher rate of total enteroscopy, the diagnostic and therapeutic yield is comparable to that of single-balloon enteroscopy (SBE) [31–33]. A recent multicenter trial showed no difference in depth of intubation, total enteroscopy rate, and diagnostic yield between these tests [34]. Studies have also found no difference in the yield of SE when compared to DBE and SBE [35, 36]. The device-assisted enteroscope of choice depends upon local experience and availability, but DBE may be preferred when total enteroscopy is the desired goal.

Two meta-analyses compared CE and DBE in patients with suspected small-bowel disorders and found no difference in their yield [37, 38]. CE did have a significantly higher yield when compared to DBE by a single approach, but there was no difference between the tests when DBE was performed using a combined antegrade and retrograde approach. Another meta-analysis that compared the tests in patients with OGIB also showed no difference in their diagnostic yield (62% with CE and 56% with DBE). The yield of DBE was significantly higher after a positive (75%) versus a negative (27.5%) CE [39].

Cost-minimization analyses indicate that the optimal strategy may be initial DBE, particularly if therapeutics or a definitive diagnosis is necessary [40]. However, CE remains the initial test of choice for most patients because it is non-invasive, widely available, and more reliable in visualizing the entire small bowel. CE is also useful as a screening tool for determining the route of DAE, based upon capsule transit times. There is a higher yield with antegrade DAE when a lesion is suspected to lie within the proximal 75% of the small bowel, whereas the retrograde route is used for more distal lesions [41]. Radionuclide scintigraphy and angiography require active bleeding, and are usually reserved for patients with massive bleeding who may be too hemodynamically unstable

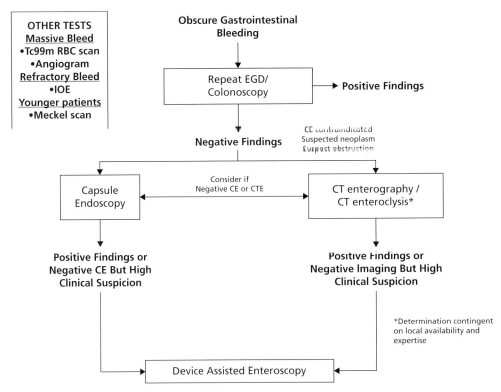

Figure 39.1   Treatment algorithm for OGIB.

Table 39.1 Etiologies of OGIB.

Vascular lesions	Angioectasias
	Dieulafoy lesions
	Portal hypertensive gastropathy
	Varices: esophageal, gastric, small bowel, colon
	Hemorrhoids
	Meckel's diverticulum
	Radiation enteritis
Inflammatory lesions	Esophagitis
	Peptic ulcer disease
	Celiac disease
	Cameron erosions
	IBD
	Meckel's diverticulum
	NSAID-related enteropathy
Neoplastic	Carcinoid
	GIST
	Adenocarcinoma
	Lymphoma
	Ampullary adenoma/carcinoma
	Metastatic lesions
Extraluminal lesions	Hemobilia
	Hemosuccus pancreaticus
	Aortoenteric fistulas
Rare etiologies	Hereditary hemorrhagic telangiectasia
	Von Willebrand's disease
	Pseudoxanthoma elasticum
	Amyloidosis
	Blue-rubber bleb nevus syndrome

IBD, inflammatory bowel disease; NSAID, non-steroidal anti-inflammatory drug; GIST, gastrointestinal stromal tumor.

to undergo endoscopic evaluation [30, 42, 43]. The role of intraoperative enteroscopy is limited to management of severe recurrent bleeding with transfusion dependency and of those with a small-bowel lesion not accessible with DAE [44].

Differential Diagnosis

Small-bowel lesions account for the majority of the etiologies of OGIB (~75%), and predominantly include vascular lesions in Western populations and ulcerations in Asian populations [4]. Angioectasias and NSAID-related ulcerations are more common in the elderly, while Crohn's disease and tumors occur more commonly in younger patients (<40 years) presenting with OGIB; therefore, careful evaluation and follow-up is necessary. Cameron erosions, Dieulafoy lesions, and angioectasias are commonly missed on upper endoscopy. Extraluminal sources such as hemobilia and hemosuccus pancreaticus are other etiologies, while Meckel's diverticulum should be considered in young patients [2]. The common etiologies of OGIB are outlined in Table 39.1.

Case Continued

An antegrade balloon-assisted enteroscopy is performed. Multiple angioectasias are noted in the jejunum and are treated with argon plasma coagulation (APC). The melena resolves and the hemoglobin returns to normal in 3 months. The hemoglobin remains stable without iron supplementation at 1-year follow-up.

Management

In patients with OGIB, management should be individualized according to the clinical situation. Patients with acute bleeding require resuscitation. In the setting of brisk or massive bleeding or hemodynamic instability, one can pursue a radioisotope bleeding scan and/or angiography to localize and treat the bleeding source. If the patient is hemodynamically stable, endoscopic evaluation may

Table 39.2 Advantages and disadvantages of various methods of evaluation of OGIB.

Method	Advantages	Disadvantages
Push enteroscopy (PE)	• Commonly available • No additional training necessary	• Not able to reach or detect lesions beyond proximal jejunum
Intraoperative enteroscopy	• High diagnostic yield for OGIB	• Invasive, with adverse events (less invasive modalities available)
Video capsule endoscopy (CE)	• Safe, non-invasive evaluation of entire small bowel	• Capsule retention in subset of patients (Crohn's) • Can miss lesions • Quality of exam determined by adequacy of small-bowel preparation • False-positive findings
Computed tomographic enterography (CTE)	• Detection of hypervascular small-bowel masses • Allows extraluminal visualization	• Incomplete bowel distension can limit the study • Ionizing radiation exposure
Computed tomographic enteroclysis	• Same as CTE • Allows distension of small bowel due to nasojejunal tube	• Ionizing radiation exposure • Patient discomfort due to placement of nasojejunal tube
Double-balloon enteroscopy (DBE)	• Both diagnostic and therapeutic • Higher rate of total enteroscopy than other DAE modalities	• Invasive and time-consuming • Not available at all centers • Adverse events, including perforation • Additional training may be necessary • Cannot be performed in patients with latex allergy (currently)
Single-balloon enteroscopy (SBE)	• Both diagnostic and therapeutic • Can be performed in patients with latex allergy	• Invasive and time-consuming • Not available at all centers • Adverse events, including perforation • Additional training may be necessary • Total enteroscopy rate not as high as in DBE
Spiral enteroscopy	• Both diagnostic and therapeutic • Can be performed in patients with latex allergy • Early studies suggest fewer adverse events	• Invasive and time-consuming • Not available at all centers • Adverse events, including perforation • Additional training may be necessary • Total enteroscopy rate not as high as in DBE

DAE, device-assisted enteroscopy.

CHAPTER 39

be pursued with CE. Therapeutics can then be performed using PE or DAE. Intraoperative enteroscopy should be reserved for management of patients with small-bowel tumors, refractory bleeding, and transfusion dependency and those with a small-bowel lesion not accessible with DAE. Supportive management with iron supplementation and packed red blood cell (PRBC) transfusions may be appropriate for patients with multiple vascular lesions or significant comorbidities. There are few data to suggest a benefit of medical therapy with hormonal agents, somatostatin, or thalidomide (Table 39.2).

Prognosis

Patients with small-bowel bleeding tend to require more diagnostic examinations, blood transfusions, and hospitalizations than patients with lower GI bleeding [45]. Outcomes can vary with the etiology of the bleed. Recurrent bleeding is a common problem despite endoscopic management in patients with angioectasias [46].

Take Home Points

- Repeat bidirectional endoscopy should be performed, due to the high rate of missed lesions with standard endoscopy.
- Capsule endoscopy (CE) is the initial test of choice for small-bowel evaluation after negative bidirectional endoscopy.
- CE can guide the route and modality of therapy for obscure gastrointestinal bleeding (OGIB), as it allows non-invasive evaluation of the entire small bowel.
- Computed tomographic enterography (CTE) is complementary to CE. It is the initial test of choice when a small-bowel tumor or obstruction is suspected.
- Device-assisted enteroscopy (DAE) allows endoscopic treatment of lesions detected on non-invasive testing.
- DAE is also useful for evaluation following negative CE and CTE in patients with recurrent bleeding or high suspicion for a small-bowel lesion.
- Radionuclide scintigraphy and angiography are reserved for patients with massive bleeding or hemodynamic instability.
- Intraoperative enteroscopy is reserved for the management of small-bowel tumors, refractory bleeding, and small-bowel lesions not accessible with DAE.
- Supportive management may be appropriate for patients with multiple vascular lesions or significant comorbidities.

References

1 Lin S, Rockey DC. Obscure gastrointestinal bleeding. *Gastroenterol Clin North Am* 2005; **34**(4): 679–98.

2 Raju GS, Gerson L, Das A, Lewis B. American Gastroenterological Association (AGA) Institute technical review on obscure gastrointestinal bleeding. *Gastroenterology* 2007; **133**(5): 1697–717.

3 Fisher L, Lee Krinsky M, Anderson MA, et al. The role of endoscopy in the management of obscure GI bleeding. *Gastrointest Endosc* 2010; **72**(3): 471–9.

4 Ell C, May A. Mid-gastrointestinal bleeding: capsule endoscopy and push-and-pull enteroscopy give rise to a new medical term. *Endoscopy* 2006; **38**(1): 73–5.

5 Zaman A, Katon RM. Push enteroscopy for obscure gastrointestinal bleeding yields a high incidence of proximal lesions within reach of a standard endoscope. *Gastrointest Endosc* 1998; **47**(5): 372–6.

6 Descamps C, Schmit A, Van Gossum A. "Missed" upper gastrointestinal tract lesions may explain "occult" bleeding. *Endoscopy* 1999; **31**(6): 452–5.

7 Leaper M, Johnston MJ, Barclay M, et al. Reasons for failure to diagnose colorectal carcinoma at colonoscopy. *Endoscopy* 2004; **36**(6): 499–503.

8 Spiller RC, Parkins RA. Recurrent gastrointestinal bleeding of obscure origin: report of 17 cases and a guide to logical management. *Br J Surg* 1983; **70**(8): 489–93.

9 Rondonotti E, Villa F, Mulder CJ, et al. Small bowel capsule endoscopy in 2007: indications, risks and limitations. *World J Gastroenterol* 2007; **13**(46): 6140–9.

10 Pennazio M, Santucci R, Rondonotti E, et al. Outcome of patients with obscure gastrointestinal bleeding after capsule endoscopy: report of 100 consecutive cases. *Gastroenterology* 2004; **126**(3): 643–53.

11 Delvaux M, Fassler I, Gay G. Clinical usefulness of the endoscopic video capsule as the initial intestinal investigation in patients with obscure digestive bleeding: validation of a diagnostic strategy based on the patient outcome after 12 months. *Endoscopy* 2004; **36**(12): 1067–73.

12 Bresci G, Parisi G, Bertoni M, et al. The role of video capsule endoscopy for evaluating obscure gastrointestinal bleeding: usefulness of early use. *J Gastroenterol* 2005; **40**(3): 256–9.

13 Carey EJ, Leighton JA, Heigh RI, et al. A single-center experience of 260 consecutive patients undergoing capsule endoscopy for obscure gastrointestinal bleeding. *Am J Gastroenterol* 2007; **102**(1): 89–95.

14 May A, Wardak A, Nachbar L, et al. Influence of patient selection on the outcome of capsule endoscopy in patients with chronic gastrointestinal bleeding. *J Clin Gastroenterol* 2005; **39**(8): 684–8.

15 Macdonald J, Porter V, McNamara D. Negative capsule endoscopy in patients with obscure GI bleeding predicts low rebleeding rates. *Gastrointest Endosc* 2008; **68**(6): 1122–7.

16 Lai LH, Wong GL, Chow DK, et al. Long-term follow-up of patients with obscure gastrointestinal bleeding after negative capsule endoscopy. *Am J Gastroenterol* 2006; **101**(6): 1224–8.

17 Jones BH, Fleischer DE, Sharma VK, et al. Yield of repeat wireless video capsule endoscopy in patients with obscure gastrointestinal bleeding. *Am J Gastroenterol* 2005; **100**(5): 1058–64.

18 Bar-Meir S, Eliakim R, Nadler M, et al. Second capsule endoscopy for patients with severe iron deficiency anemia. *Gastrointest Endosc* 2004; **60**(5): 711–13.

19 Viazis N, Papaxoinis K, Vlachogiannakos J, et al. Is there a role for second-look capsule endoscopy in patients with obscure GI bleeding after a nondiagnostic first test? *Gastrointest Endosc* 2009; **69**(4): 850–6.

20 Goldstein JL, Eisen GM, Lewis B, et al. Video capsule endoscopy to prospectively assess small bowel injury with celecoxib, naproxen plus omeprazole, and placebo. *Clin Gastroenterol Hepatol* 2005; **3**(2): 133–41.

21 Lewis BS, Eisen GM, Friedman S. A pooled analysis to evaluate results of capsule endoscopy trials. *Endoscopy* 2005; **37**(10): 960–5.

22 Fry LC, De Petris G, Swain JM, Fleischer DE. Impaction and fracture of a video capsule in the small bowel requiring laparotomy for removal of the capsule fragments. *Endoscopy* 2005; **37**(7): 674–6.

23 Cheifetz AS, Kornbluth AA, Legnani P, et al. The risk of retention of the capsule endoscope in patients with known or suspected Crohn's disease. *Am J Gastroenterol* 2006; **101**(10): 2218–22.

24 Um S, Poblete H, Zavotsky J. Small bowel perforation caused by an impacted endocapsule. *Endoscopy* 2008; **40**(Suppl. 2): E122–3.

25 Triester SL, Leighton JA, Leontiadis GI, et al. A meta-analysis of the yield of capsule endoscopy compared to other diagnostic modalities in patients with obscure gastrointestinal bleeding. *Am J Gastroenterol* 2005; **100**(11): 2407–18.

26 Saperas E, Dot J, Videla S, et al. Capsule endoscopy versus computed tomographic or standard angiography for the diagnosis of obscure gastrointestinal bleeding. *Am J Gastroenterol* 2007; **102**(4): 731–7.

27 Huprich JE, Fletcher JG, Alexander JA, et al. Obscure gastrointestinal bleeding: evaluation with 64-section multiphase CT enterography initial experience. *Radiology* 2008; **246**(2): 562–71.

28 Agrawal JR, Travis AC, Mortele KJ, et al. Diagnostic yield of dual-phase computed tomography enterography in patients with obscure gastrointestinal bleeding and a non-diagnostic capsule endoscopy. *J Gastroenterol Hepatol* 2012; **27**(4): 751–9.

29 Lee SS Oh TS, Kim HJ, et al. Obscure gastrointestinal bleeding: diagnostic performance of multidetector CT enterography. *Radiology* 2011; **259**(3): 739–48.

30 Graca BM, Freire PA, Brito JB, et al. Gastroenterologic and radiologic approach to obscure gastrointestinal bleeding: how, why, and when? *Radiographics* 2010; **30**(1): 235–52.

31 May A, Farber M, Aschmoneit I, et al. Prospective multicenter trial comparing push-and-pull enteroscopy with the single- and double-balloon techniques in patients with small-bowel disorders. *Am J Gastroenterol* 2010; **105**(3): 575–81.

32 Landaeta JL, Dias C, Rodriguez MJ. Double balloon enteroscopy vs single balloon enteroscopy in obscure gastrointestinal bleeding. *Gastrointest Endosc* 2009; **69**: AB187.

33 Takano N, Yamada A, Watabe H, et al. Single-balloon versus double-balloon endoscopy for achieving total enteroscopy: a randomized, controlled trial. *Gastrointest Endosc* 2011; **73**(4): 734–9.

34 Domagk D, Mensink P, Aktas H, et al. Single- vs. double-balloon enteroscopy in small-bowel diagnostics: a randomized multicenter trial. *Endoscopy* 2011; **43**(6): 472–6.

35 Frieling T, Heise J, Sassenrath W, *et al.* Prospective comparison between double-balloon enteroscopy and spiral enteroscopy. *Endoscopy* 2010; **42**(11): 885–8.

36 Khashab MA, Lennon AM, Dunbar KB, *et al.* A comparative evaluation of single-balloon enteroscopy and spiral enteroscopy for patients with mid-gut disorders. *Gastrointest Endosc* 2010; **72**(4): 766–72.

37 Pasha SF, Leighton JA, Das A, *et al.* Double-balloon enteroscopy and capsule endoscopy have comparable diagnostic yield in small-bowel disease: a meta-analysis. *Clin Gastroenterol Hepatol* 2008; **6**(6): 671–6.

38 Chen X, Ran ZH, Tong JL. A meta-analysis of the yield of capsule endoscopy compared to double-balloon enteroscopy in patients with small bowel diseases. *World J Gastroenterol* 2007; **13**(32): 4372–8.

39 Teshima CW, Kuipers EJ, van Zanten SV, Mensink PB. Double balloon enteroscopy and capsule endoscopy for obscure gastrointestinal bleeding: an updated meta-analysis. *J Gastroenterol Hepatol* 2011; **26**(5): 796–801.

40 Somsouk M, Gralnek IM, Inadomi JM. Management of obscure occult gastrointestinal bleeding: a cost-minimization analysis. *Clin Gastroenterol Hepatol* 2008; **6**(6): 661–70.

41 Gay G, Delvaux M, Fassler I. Outcome of capsule endoscopy in determining indication and route for push-and-pull enteroscopy. *Endoscopy* 2006; **38**(1): 49–58.

42 Wang CS, Tzen KY, Huang MJ, *et al.* Localization of obscure gastrointestinal bleeding by technetium 99m-labeled red blood cell scintigraphy. *J Formos Med Assoc* 1992; **91**(1): 63–8.

43 Lau WY, Ngan H, Chu KW, Yuen WK. Repeat selective visceral angiography in patients with gastrointestinal bleeding of obscure origin. *Br J Surg* 1989; **76**(3): 226–9.

44 Cave DR, Cooley JS. Intraoperative enteroscopy. Indications and techniques. *Gastrointest Endosc Clin N Am* 1996; **6**(4): 793–802.

45 Prakash C, Zuckerman GR. Acute small bowel bleeding: a distinct entity with significantly different economic implications compared with GI bleeding from other locations. *Gastrointest Endosc* 2003; **58**(3): 330–5.

46 Samaha E, Rahmi G, Landi B, *et al.* Long-term outcome of patients treated with double balloon enteroscopy for small bowel vascular lesions. *Am J Gastroenterol* 2012; **107**(2): 240–6.

CHAPTER 39

Constipation

Arnold Wald

Division of Gastroenterology and Hepatology, University of Wisconsin School of Medicine and Public Health, Madison, WI, USA

Summary

Constipation is a common complaint that can be either primary (idiopathic or functional) or associated with a number of disorders or medications. Symptomatic treatment (e.g., fiber supplements, laxatives) is often effective. Functional constipation that fails to respond to symptomatic treatment should be investigated initially with anorectal manometry and balloon expulsion to assess for a defecation disorder. If this is normal, a colon-transit study using radiopaque markers should be obtained. Slow-transit constipation ("colonic inertia") is defined by an abnormal transit study and normal manometry and balloon expulsion; it is often difficult to treat and sometimes requires surgery. Subtotal colectomy with ileorectal anastomosis should be reserved for those few patients with intractable slow-transit constipation without disordered defecation or generalized gastrointestinal (GI) dysmotility and in whom abdominal pain is not a prominent complaint. Defecation disorders may be caused by poor relaxation or inappropriate contraction of the pelvic floor muscles, with or without inadequate propulsion. They are best treated with biofeedback therapy, which teaches the patient to better control the muscles used in defecation.

Case

A 36-year-old woman consults with a gastroenterologist for chronic constipation. She has had one to two bowel movements weekly for the past 6 years, often with straining and a sense of incomplete evacuation. She denies abdominal pain, blood per rectum, nausea, weight change, diarrhea, fecal or urinary incontinence, dry skin, cold intolerance, or neuromuscular symptoms. Except for mild hypertension, for which she takes a beta-blocker, she is otherwise healthy and takes no other medications. She has had no abdominal surgeries. On the advice of her primary-care physician, she has increased fiber intake and exercise, to no avail. She has also tried over-the-counter (OTC) laxatives such as bisacodyl, senna, magnesium citrate, and polyethylene glycol, which have all been ineffective.

Definition and Epidemiology

Though most individuals have a bowel movement at least three times per week, infrequent defecation alone is very uncommon among constipated persons. Most constipated patients have other symptoms, such as straining or stools that are perceived as too hard or too small. Consensus guidelines [1] define functional constipation as a combination of symptoms (Table 40.1). Prevalence in many studies ranges from 5 to as high as 28%. Constipation is more common in women and the elderly, and accounts for 2.5 million physician visits each year in the United States, mainly to primary-care physicians and gastroenterologists [2].

Pathophysiology

Constipation may be associated with a systemic disorder, such as hypothyroidism, neurologic diseases, or collagen vascular diseases, and is associated with many drugs (Table 40.2). It may be precipitated or exacerbated by physical or behavioral disorders that interfere with toileting. Low income, low education, physical inactivity, depression, and low calorie intake are known risk factors for constipation. Two subgroups of constipation require special attention.

Slow-Transit Constipation ("Colonic Inertia")

Patients with slow-transit constipation often have unremitting constipation characterized by infrequent defecation in the absence of a defecation disorder. These individuals often lack the increase in colonic motility ordinarily promoted by stimulants, such as eating, cholinergic agents, and stimulant laxatives. Patients with colonic inertia have delayed passage of radiopaque markers in the proximal colon. Histologic studies in severe cases have shown a decrease in enteric "pacemaker" neurons (interstitial Cajal cells, ICCs) and the presence of support cells that form myelin sheaths and modulate neurotransmitter concentrations (enteric glial cells). This may account for the often poor response to laxatives and dietary measures [3].

Defecation Disorders

Normal defecation involves coordinated actions, including: (i) increase in intra-abdominal pressure; (ii) relaxation of the anal sphincters to reduce resistance to elimination; and (iii) relaxation of the puborectalis muscle to widen the anorectal angle. Constipation may result when this process is disordered. Disordered defecation can be divided into: (i) dyssynergic defecation, which results from poor relaxation or inappropriate contraction of the pelvic floor muscles; and (ii) inadequate propulsive forces. Both lead to ineffective evacuation of the rectum and distal colon [4]. Patients with defecation disorders may exhibit slow colonic transit, which can normalize after successful treatment. This is why testing for a defecation disorder is the first evaluation in a patient with constipation refractory to conservative therapy.

Practical Gastroenterology and Hepatology Board Review Toolkit, Second Edition. Edited by Nicholas J. Talley, Kenneth R. DeVault, Michael B. Wallace, Bashar A. Aqel and Keith D. Lindor.

© 2016 John Wiley & Sons, Ltd. Published 2016 by John Wiley & Sons, Ltd. Companion website: www.practicalgastrohep.com

Table 40.1 Rome III diagnostic criteria for functional constipation (criteria fulfilled for the last 3 months with symptom onset at least 6 months prior to diagnosis) [1].

Must include two or more of the following:
- Straining during at least 25% of defecations.
- Lumpy or hard stools in at least 25% of defecations.
- Sensation of incomplete evacuation for at least 25% of defecations.
- Sensation of anorectal obstruction/blockage for at least 25% of defecations.
- Manual maneuvers to facilitate at least 25% of defecations (e.g., digital evacuation, support of the pelvic floor).
- Fewer than three defecations per week.

- Lack of loose stools without the use of laxatives.
- Insufficient criteria for IBS.

Table 40.2 Common medications associated with constipation.

Opiates
Antipsychotics
Anticholinergics
Tricyclic antidepressants
Calcium channel blockers
Iron
5-HT$_3$ antagonists (i.e., ondansetron)
Anticonvulsants
Diuretics
Antineoplastic agents

Clinical Features

Most patients with constipation respond to OTC medications. When a patient consults with a physician for problematic symptoms, a detailed history and focused examination are important. This includes characterizing the frequency and nature of the patient's bowel movements, including what the patient means by "constipation" and what is the major concern. A 2-week prospective diary detailing food and beverage intake and the frequency and characteristics of bowel movements may be useful in refractory cases. The initial assessment should explore for possible underlying disorders by inquiring about abdominal pain, weight gain or loss, eating disorders, and clues to disorders associated with constipation. Review of symptoms should also inquire about "alarm symptoms": anorexia, blood in stools, recent changes in bowel habits, nausea, and vomiting. Other important aspects of the history include previous abdominal surgeries, medications, and a family history of colon cancer.

Physical exam should include an abdominal exam to assess for distension, hernias, abdominal muscle strength and integrity, and masses; and an anorectal exam to assess for fissures, mass, sphincter tone, rectocele, prolapse, and occult blood. The rectal exam should also assess for puborectalis muscle and anal sphincter responses

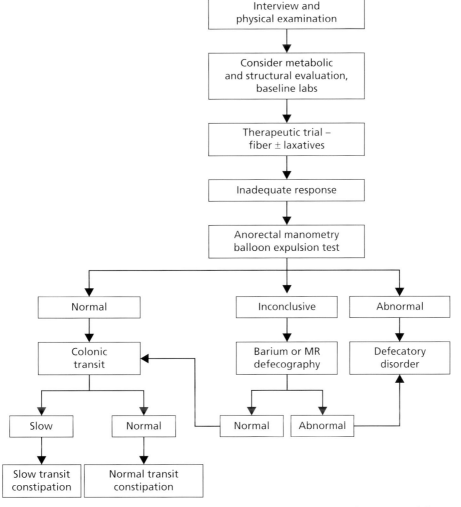

Figure 40.1   Management algorithm for chronic constipation. Source: Bharucha 2013 [5]. Reproduced with permission of Elsevier.

when bearing down as if to defecate. In appropriate cases, a neurologic assessment may uncover an underlying disorder associated with constipation.

Diagnosis

Patients with chronic constipation and without alarm symptoms may be treated empirically and generally do not require further diagnostic tests. In those who do not respond to conservative therapy, history alone often does not distinguish the etiology of constipation. Abdominal X-rays may confirm the presence of excessive stool in the colon, while colonoscopy or barium radiograph may identify an anatomic cause of constipation. These tests are not recommended routinely unless alarm features are present or a patient is eligible for routine colon cancer screening [5]. This is because colon polyps and cancers are no more common in constipated patients than the normal population. Useful diagnostic tests by which to assess anorectal and colonic function include a colon-transit study, balloon expulsion, anorectal manometry, and, in selected cases, defecography, which allows differentiation into colonic versus anorectal dysfunction (Figure 40.1). These tests are indicated only when patients do not respond to conservative measures. Characterizing these disorders is important, as management differs [5].

Diagnosis of Colonic Inertia

In a colon-transit study, patients ingest radiopaque markers and abdominal X-rays are obtained at various time points according to different protocols. The "Hinton technique" involves ingestion of 24 markers on day 0 and an abdominal X-ray (110 keV) on day 5 [6]. Slow transit is defined as the presence of >20% [5] markers on day 5. Colon-transit studies are normal in many patients with constipation. An abnormal colon-transit study cannot reliably differentiate between colonic inertia and a defecation disorder; however, patients with disordered defecation may exhibit a predominance of markers in the left or rectosigmoid colons. It is important to emphasize that anorectal manometry and balloon expulsion should be obtained before considering a diagnosis of colonic inertia [5]. If correction of the defecation disorder fails to normalize constipation, a colon-transit study should be obtained [5].

Diagnosis of Disordered Defecation

Disordered defecation has also been called "outlet obstruction" or "pelvic floor dyssynergia" [7]. It is suspected when a patient contracts or fails to relax the external anal sphincter and puborectalis muscle on digital rectal exam when asked to bear down. A colon-transit study may be normal or slow. Anorectal manometry may demonstrate weak expulsion effort and/or inappropriate anal sphincter contraction, or no sphincter relaxation during simulated defecation. However, many patients with abnormal manometry have normal defecation due to the artificial setting of the manometry study. Abnormal expulsion of a 50 mL water filled balloon from the rectum (>60 seconds) supports the diagnosis of disordered defecation [8]. If the results of manometry and balloon expulsion differ, defecography should be performed. Defecography may confirm or refute manometry or balloon expulsion, or may show structural abnormalities such as an enterocele that are not diagnosable by functional testing.

Differential Diagnosis

Irritable Bowel Syndrome

Constipation occurs in some patients with irritable bowel syndrome (IBS). IBS is differentiated from functional constipation by the predominance of abdominal pain, though recent studies indicate that there is some overlap of the two disorders

Megarectum and Megacolon

Some patients with constipation have chronic megacolon or megarectum [9]. These disorders are often seen in patients with psychosis, dementia, and diseases such as Parkinsonism, as well as in the institutionalized elderly. Megacolon and megarectum are associated with myogenic dysfunction, increased colonic or rectal compliance, and blunted rectal sensation. The diagnosis is usually made by radiographic studies, but may be suggested by a rectal exam in an unprepared patient.

Hirschsprung Disease (Aganglionic Megacolon)

This is a rare congenital disease that often presents with severe constipation, most often in male infants. Manometry shows no relaxation of the internal anal sphincter in response to rectal distension, the result of a congenital absence of enteric neurons in the distal bowel. Deep rectal biopsies are needed to confirm the diagnosis. Of clinical importance, the presence of internal anal sphincter relaxation in response to rectal distension can be used to exclude Hirschsprung disease, thus obviating the need for rectal biopsies in most patients. An equally important point is that biopsies obtained during colonoscopy or flexible sigmoidoscopy are insufficient, because they are too superficial to evaluate the myenteric and submucosal plexuses.

Case Continued

On physical exam, blood pressure and pulse are normal, as are cardiac, pulmonary, thyroid, skin, and neurologic exams. Abdominal exam reveals normal bowel sounds, with no tenderness, guarding, masses, or hepatosplenomegaly. Rectal exam reveals no perianal disease, prolapse, or rectocele. Stool is brown and hemoccult negative. On rectal exam, there is an increase in both the external anal sphincter and puborectalis pressures when the patient bears down as if to simulate defecation.

Dyssynergic defecation is suspected and appropriate studies are ordered at a laboratory center that is experienced in performing them. Anorectal manometry shows inappropriate anal sphincter contraction during straining. The patient is unable to expel a 50 mL water balloon within 60 seconds on two attempts. She is diagnosed with dyssynergic defecation and referred for biofeedback therapy.

Therapy

Initial therapy includes alteration of lifestyle, such as regular exercise and increased dietary fiber [3]. Patients who do not improve should be started on a laxative (Table 40.3). A good first choice is the osmotic laxative, polyethylene glycol (PEG), as its side effects are minimal compared to lactulose and sorbitol, which often result in undesirable gas and bloating. Stimulant laxatives such are senna and bisacodyl are also inexpensive options. The chronic use of senna and other anthraquinones is associated with melanosis coli, a benign dark pigmentation of the colonic mucosa. Magnesium salts may be used episodically but should be avoided in the presence of

Table 40.3 OTC medications for constipation.

Medication	Grade[a] [14]	Dose (daily)	Cost ($)[b]	Notes and side effects
Bulking agents				
Psyllium	B	20–30 g	7.80–15.60	Avoid in patients with IBS, megacolon, colonic inertia
Methylcellulose	C	19 g	9.33–21.00	
Stool softener				
Docusate	C	200 mg	6.00	Abdominal cramps
Stimulant laxatives				
Senna	C	17.2 mg	3.72	Melanosis coli
Bisacodyl	A	10 mg	15.00	
Osmotic laxatives				
Polyethylene glycol (PEG)	A	17 g	14.00–52.00	Nausea, abdominal cramps
Magnesium citrate	C	150 mg	3.75	Avoid in renal failure
Lactulose	B	10 g (15 mL)	18.90	Bloating, gas

[a]Based on strength of evidence and grading of recommendations as utilized by the US Preventive Services Task Force. Grade A: Good evidence in support of the use of a modality in the treatment of constipation. Grade B: Moderate evidence in support of the use of a modality in the treatment of constipation. Grade C: Poor evidence to support a recommendation for or against the use of a modality.
[b]Dollar amount obtained from www.northwestpharmacy.com in February 2014 and based on a 30-day supply.
IBS, irritable bowel syndrome.

renal insufficiency. Many of these relatively inexpensive and easily obtained medications work well and should be used as first-line agents, either alone or together [10, 11]. Lubiprostone, which stimulates intestinal chloride-2 channels to increase intraluminal fluid, is a more expensive agent for chronic constipation (as well as IBS-C) and has been approved for constipation associated with opiate use. The major side effects are nausea and headaches. Tegaserod, a partial 5-HT$_4$ agonist used for chronic constipation, was withdrawn from the market in 2007 after reports of increased cardiovascular events; it is now approved as an investigational drug for constipated women aged less than 55 years who have no cardiovascular risk factors and have failed all other agents. Linaclotide is a guanylate cyclase-C receptor agonist that increases intestinal intracellular cyclic guanosine monophosphate to increase general secretion of chloride and secretion of water into the GI lumen (Table 40.4). It was released in 2013 after receiving approval from the Food and Drug Administration (FDA) for both constipation and IBS-C [12, 13]. No trials have compared linaclotide or lubiprostone with established non-prescription agents such as bisacodyl or PEG.

Slow-Transit Constipation

Misoprostol can be very effective in slow-transit constipation, often combined with small doses of PEG, with titration of doses as tolerated. It should be used with caution in women of childbearing age as it is an abortifacient. It is given as a single morning dose of 400–1200 μg and has proved effective in approximately 40% of cases (personal experience). In severe, refractory cases of colonic inertia, subtotal colectomy with ileorectostomy should be considered. Ideal candidates for this surgery should have normal anorectal function and absence of GI dysmotility, as established with esophageal, gastric, and small-bowel motility studies. Pain should not be a major complaint, as there is a high incidence of pain after surgery. If a patient has a coexistent defecation disorder that is not responsive to treatment or exhibits evidence of diffuse GI dysmotility, a diverting ileostomy may be considered.

Disordered Defecation

At least four studies have convincingly shown that biofeedback of pelvic floor dyscoordination by muscle retraining is effective in many patients. Patients undergo 30–60 minute sessions up to several times a week to enhance rectal perception of rectal distension and relax the pelvic floor using instrumental feedback provided by manometry or electromyographic recordings [14, 15]. The overall response rate in published studies is approximately 70–80% and is durable. In patients who relapse, repeat biofeedback is often effective.

Case Continued

The patient undergoes weekly biofeedback training with supplemental education regarding diet, exercise, pelvic floor exercises, and toileting habits. After four training sessions by a therapist who employs techniques consistent with those reported in the literature, her bowel movements increase to three to four times weekly. On a follow-up visit 6 months later, she continues to be satisfied with her bowel habit and uses laxatives only once or twice monthly.

Prognosis

Constipation is often controlled with change in diet and lifestyle and using medications such as bulking agents, stimulant laxatives, and osmotic laxatives. Newer agents may sometimes be helpful, either alone or in combination with established OTC laxatives. Biofeedback is often effective in selected patients with dyssynergic defecation, and many patients with slow colonic transit may be treated successfully with misoprostol and small amounts of PEG. In carefully selected patients who respond to no pharmacologic interventions, surgical intervention is often effective.

Table 40.4 Prescription drugs for constipation.

Medication	Evidence	Grade[a]	Dose	Cost ($)[b]	Side effects
Tegaserod	5 RCTs (n = 3341) Duration = 4–12 weeks	A	4–6 mg twice daily	N/A	Headache, nausea
Lubiprostone	2 RCTs (n = 371) Duration = 3–4 weeks	A	24 μg twice daily	290.00	Headache, nausea
Linaclotide	2 RCTs (n=1276) Duration =12 weeks	A	145–290 μg daily	270.00	Diarrhea

[a]Based on strength of evidence and grading of recommendations as utilized by the US Preventive Services Task Force. Grade A: Good evidence in support of the use of a modality in the treatment of constipation. Grade B: Moderate evidence in support of the use of a modality in the treatment of constipation. Grade C: Poor evidence to support a recommendation for or against the use of a modality.
[b]Dollar amount obtained from www.drugstore.com in February 2014 and based on a 30-day supply.
RCT, randomized, placebo-controlled, double-blinded trial; N/A, not applicable.

CHAPTER 40

Take Home Points

- Constipation is a common disorder and may be functional or associated with systemic disorders or medications.
- Constipation is usually treated symptomatically with non-prescription stimulant or osmotic laxatives and with newer secretory agents.
- Patients with chronic constipation unresponsive to laxatives should undergo diagnostic testing with anorectal manometry and a balloon expulsion study. If these are normal or if they are abnormal and correctable, colon-transit studies can determine whether transit is normal or slow.
- Colonoscopy is not part of the routine workup for chronic constipation unless a patient has alarm symptoms or needs colon cancer screening.
- Slow-transit constipation is diagnosed by colon-transit study and the exclusion of a defecation disorder.
- Defecation disorders are characterized by balloon expulsion study and anorectal manometry.
- Biofeedback therapy is often effective for patients with disordered defecation and is considered the treatment of choice.

References

1 Longstreth GF, Thompson WG, Chey WD, et al. Functional bowel disorders. *Gastroenterology* 2006; **130**: 1480–91.

2 Higgins PD, Johanson JF. Epidemiology of constipation in North America: a systematic review. *Am J Gastroenterol* 2004; **99**: 750–9.

3 Wald A. Pathophysiology, diagnosis and current management of chronic constipation. *Nat Clin Pract Gastroenterol Hepatol* 2006; **3**: 90–100.

4 Bharucha AE, Wald A, Enck P, Rao S. Functional anorectal disorders. *Gastroenterology* 2006; **130**: 1510–18.

5 Bharucha AE, Dorn SD, Lembo A, et al. AGA medical position statement on constipation. *Gastroenterology* 2013; **144**: 211–17.

6 Hinton JM, Lennard-Jones JE, Young AC. A new method for studying gut transit times using radioopaque markers. *Gut* 1969; **10**: 842–7.

7 Bharucha AE, Rao SS. An update on anorectal disorders for gastroenterologists. *Gastroenterology* 2014; **146**: 37–45.

8 Minguez M, Herreros B, Sanchiz V, et al. Predictive value of the balloon expulsion test for excluding the diagnosis of pelvic floor dyssynergia in constipation. *Gastroenterology* 2004; **126**: 57–62.

9 Hanauer S, Wald A. Acute and chronic megacolon. *Curr Treat Options Gastroenterol* 2007; **10**: 237–47.

10 Muller-Lissner SA, Kamm MA, Scarpignato C, Wald A. Myths and misconceptions about chronic constipation. *Am J Gastroenterol* 2005; **100**: 232–42.

11 Ford AC, Suares NC. Effect of laxatives and pharmacologic therapies in chronic idiopathic constipation. *Gut* 2011; **60**: 209–18.

12 Lembo AJ, Schneier HA, Shiff SJ, et al. Two randomized trials of linaclotide for chronic constipation. *N Engl J Med* 2011; **365**: 27–36.

13 Johnston JM, Shiff SJ, Quigley EM. A review of the efficacy of linaclotide in irritable bowel syndrome with constipation. *Curr Med Res Opin* 2013; **29**: 149–60.

14 Heymen S, Scarlett Y, Jones K, et al. Randomized, controlled trial shows biofeedback to be superior to alternative treatments for patients with pelvic floor dyssynergia-type constipation. *Dis Colon Rectum* 2007; **50**: 428–41.

15 Rao SS, Seaton K, Miller M, et al. Randomized controlled trial of biofeedback, sham feedback, and standard therapy for dyssynergic defecation. *Clin Gastroenterol Hepatol* 2007; **5**: 331–8.

Perianal Disease

Leyla J. Ghazi[1] and David A. Schwartz[2]

[1] Division of Gastroenterology, Vanderbilt University, Nashville, TN, USA
[2] Division of Gastroenterology and Hepatology, University of Maryland School of Medicine, Baltimore, MD, USA

Summary

Perianal disease is a common manifestation of Crohn's disease. Fistulas may be associated with active or quiescent intestinal inflammation. The diagnosis of fistula is made clinically and confirmed by exam under anesthesia and/or other imaging modality (either endoscopic ultrasound (EUS) or magnetic resonance imaging (MRI)). Treatment depends on severity of disease and complexity of the fistula. Combined medical and surgical treatment is typically the preferred approach. Anti-tumor necrosis factor (TNF) drugs are the most efficacious medical therapy available.

Case

A 38-year-old woman presents with history of colonic Crohn's disease of 5 years' duration. Her main symptoms include diarrhea and occasional blood in her stool. She is currently on 5-aminosalicylic acid therapy alone. She presents to the office with stool "incontinence." She describes staining of her undergarments every day with small amounts of yellowish discharge, without the sensation of defecation. She has some discomfort when she defecates, and has no fevers or chills.

Definition and Epidemiology

Crohn's disease can lead to a variety of perianal complications, including skin tags, hemorrhoids, anal fissure, anal ulcer, anorectal stricture, and perirectal ulcers. In this section, we will focus on perianal fistulas. Fistulas are abnormal connections between two epithelium-lined organs that normally do not connect: in this case the colon/rectum and the perianal skin.

Fistulas can be grouped into two categories: simple or complex. A simple fistula is superficial, intersphincteric, or low trans-sphincteric, has only one external opening, and is not associated with an abscess or connected to an adjacent structure. A complex fistula involves more of the anal sphincters (i.e., high trans-sphincteric, extrasphincteric, or suprasphincteric), may have multiple openings, "horseshoes" (crosses the midline either anteriorly or posteriorly), is associated with a perianal abscess, and/or connects to an adjacent structure such as the vagina or bladder [1] (Figure 41.1).

The frequency of perianal fistulas in Crohn's disease has been estimated to be 20% [2]. Distal disease is more likely to result in perianal fistula; for example, colonic disease with rectal involvement (92% have fistulas) versus isolated disease of ileum (12% have fistulas) [3].

Pathophysiology

There are two proposed mechanisms for fistula development (Figures 41.2 and 41.3): fistulas may develop as ulcers that extend over time as stool is forced into the ulcer with the pressure of defecation or as anal gland abscesses that originate from the intersphincteric space.

Clinical Features

Perianal Crohn's disease often presents as anorectal abscess, fistulas, or fissures. Symptoms usually include rectal pain, fever, fluctuance, and/or drainage of stool or purulent material. A majority of patients experience acute relapses of their symptoms, some despite medical therapy. It is common for fistulas to be more actively draining during periods of increased disease activity, such as when patients have diarrhea. Occasionally, perianal fistula may be the initial or only manifestation of a patient's Crohn's disease (occurs in ~5%).

Typically, surgical incision and drainage of perianal abscesses relieves the severity of pain, but a sequela of perianal drainage/leakage, odor, and scarring can persist. Surgical intervention is necessary for a majority of patients with fistulizing Crohn's disease. Over 70% of patients with perianal fistulas require an operation; major operations such as proctectomy and diverting ileostomy are needed in 32% of patients [2].

Diagnosis

The type of fistula (simple vs. complex) and the degree of luminal inflammation will determine the initial choice of therapy (Figure 41.4). Initial diagnostic testing should include a thorough physical examination of the perianal region and documentation of the location, activity, and severity (i.e., presence of fluctuance, ulcer, or anal stenosis and number of fistula openings) of the disease. The Fistula Drainage Assessment Measure (FDAM) classifies fistulas as improved (i.e., decrease from baseline in number of open draining

Practical Gastroenterology and Hepatology Board Review Toolkit, Second Edition. Edited by Nicholas J. Talley, Kenneth R. DeVault, Michael B. Wallace, Bashar A. Aqel and Keith D. Lindor.
© 2016 John Wiley & Sons, Ltd. Published 2016 by John Wiley & Sons, Ltd. Companion website: www.practicalgastrohep.com

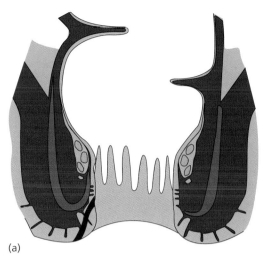
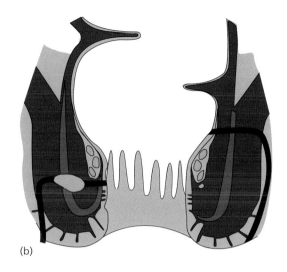

(a)   (b)

Figure 41.1 (a) Complex fistula. (b) Simple fistula.

fistulas by ≥ 50%) or in remission (i.e., closure of all fistulas). It is important to remember that the term "closed" is only clinically relevant. Imaging studies with EUS or MRI have demonstrated persistent fistula activity for months after a fistula stops draining [4]. Alternatively, the Perianal Disease Activity Index (PDAI) measures fistulas according to five categories: discharge, pain, restriction of sexual activity, type of perianal disease, and degree of induration. A high score indicates greater activity of disease [5].

Endoscopic evaluation can assess for concomitant luminal disease activity. Because of the presence of scarring and induration, digital rectal examination or exam under anesthesia is not always an accurate way of assessing fistulas. Therefore, imaging should be performed in nearly all situations. Fistulography and computed tomography (CT) of the pelvis have fallen out of favor as a result of significant limitations in the accurate detection of perianal abscesses and classification of fistula anatomy.

MRI and EUS have been studied extensively and have been shown to be very accurate for evaluating Crohn's-disease fistulas [6, 7]. When EUS or MRI is combined with exam under anesthesia, the accuracy in diagnosing fistulas is 100% [8]. The type of imaging chosen can also be used to follow fistula disease activity over time after institution of medical and surgical therapy.

Case Continued

On exam, the patient has an obvious draining perirectal fistula. Colonoscopy is performed, revealing pancolitis of moderate intensity. Rectal EUS is then performed and reveals a complex fistula (high trans-sphincteric fistula without associated abscess).

Therapeutics

The management of perianal fistulizing disease can oftentimes be daunting. A number of medical options exist for the treatment of Crohn's-disease perianal fistula (Table 41.1). Commonly used therapies include antibiotics, immunomodulators, cyclosporine, tacrolimus, and anti-TNF-α antibodies.

Antibiotics such as metronidazole 750–1000 g/day or ciprofloxacin 1000–1500 g/day are most commonly used with short-term benefit. Several open-label studies support the observation that metronidazole may lead to cessation of fistula drainage in 34–50% of patients [9, 10]. Typically, patients will have clinical improvement after 6–8 weeks of therapy, but reoccurrence is frequently noted after cessation of therapy. Ciprofloxacin has been

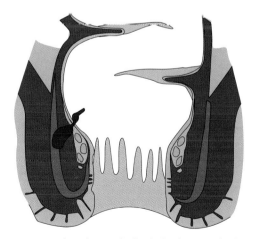

Figure 41.2 Proposed mechanism for fistula development: fistula beginning as an abscess.

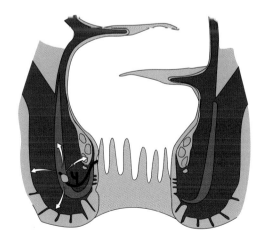

Figure 41.3 Proposed mechanism for fistula development: fistula beginning as an ulcer.

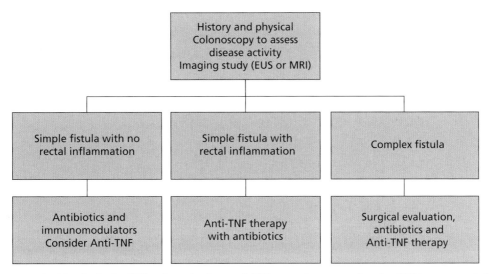

Figure 41.4 Management algorithm for fistulas. EUS, endoscopic ultrasound; MRI, magnetic resonance imaging; TNF, tumor necrosis factor.

used as an alternative to metronidazole for perianal disease, though no controlled trials have been performed to support its use in this setting. Alternative oral antibiotics, including amoxicillin-clavulanic acid, trimethoprim-sulfamethoxazole, and rifaximin, have also been used; these have not been studied for this indication in the literature.

Immunomodulators – specifically 6-mercaptopurine (6-MP) and azathioprine (AZA) – have been studied for the treatment of perianal disease. A meta-analysis of patients with luminal Crohn's disease with fistula response as a secondary end point demonstrated a 54% response rate in the AZA group compared to only 21% in the placebo group. The pooled odds ratio was 4.44 in favor of fistula healing [11]. Antibiotic use (ciprofloxacin or metronidazole) combined with 6-MP or AZA has also been associated with better response rates, especially in patients with simple fistulas [12]. The efficacy persisted when patients were maintained on AZA after antibiotics were stopped. A lack of controlled trials and the small volume of existing data do not support the use of methotrexate as monotherapy for perianal disease. Methotrexate can be considered in patients intolerant or refractory to 6-MP/AZA when used in combination with anti-TNF therapy.

Tacrolimus has been studied for fistulizing Crohn's disease in a randomized, double-blinded, placebo-controlled trial [13]. In this trial, 43% of patients treated with 0.20 g/kg/day of tacrolimus improved, compared with 8% of placebo-treated patients. However, only 10% of tacrolimus-treated patients had complete fistula closure, versus 8% of placebo-treated patients. At the present time, tacrolimus is reserved for non-responders to anti-TNF therapy.

The anti-TNF-α drugs have changed the management of perianal fistulizing disease. Biologic therapies (a.k.a., anti-TNF agents) currently available for the treatment of Crohn's disease include infliximab (a chimeric monoclonal antibody to TNF-α), adalimumab (a fully human immunoglobulin IgG1 anti-TNF-α monoclonal antibody), and certolizumab pegol (a humanized anti-TNF Fab' monoclonal antibody fragment linked to polyethylene glycol).

The initial short-term infliximab fistula trial showed a 68% response rate for those who received the induction sequence of infliximab of 5 g/kg at weeks 0, 2, and 6, compared to 26% response in the placebo cohort [14]. The ACCENT II trial investigated whether cessation of fistula drainage could be preserved with infliximab maintenance therapy given every 8 weeks. Patients who had active fistulas and responded to the induction sequence of infliximab of 5 g/kg at weeks 0, 2, and 6 were randomized to receive infliximab or placebo every 8 weeks. After 54 weeks, 36% of patients in the infliximab group maintained complete fistula closure, compared with 19% in the placebo arm (p = 0.009) [15].

The adalimumab maintenance trial (CHARM) looked at fistula healing as a secondary end point [13]. Complete fistula closure at 56 weeks was 33%, as compared to 13% in the placebo arm (p = 0.016). Additional data revealed that early closure of draining

Table 41.1 Options for the treatment of Crohn's-disease perianal fistulas.

Reference	Year	Therapy	No. of patients	Response (%)	Comment
Present *et al.* [15]	1980	Mercaptopurine	36	Therapy: 31 Placebo: 6	Daily 6-mercaptopurine or placebo for 1 year, before crossing over to the other arm of the study for an additional year
Sandborn *et al.* [10]	2003	Tacrolimus	48	Therapy: 43 Placebo: 8	Fistula remission similar between groups (10 vs. 8%)
Present *et al.* [11]	1999	Infliximab	94	Therapy: 68 Placebo: 26	Closure of all fistulas in 55% of therapy group, as compared to 13% with placebo
ACCENT II [12]	2004	Infliximab	195	Therapy: 36 Placebo: 19	Maintenance of fistula closure at 54 weeks
CHARM [13]	2007	Adalimumab	117	Therapy: 33 Placebo: 13	Durable response: all with response at week 26 had continued response at week 56
PRECISE [18]	2011	Certolizumab	58	Therapy: 36 Placebo: 17	Closure of draining fistulas at 26 weeks predictive of a durable response of 60% at 2 years

fistulas at 26 weeks was predictive of a durable response of 60% at 2 years [16,17]. Similarly, fistula healing has been examined as a secondary end point in certolizumab maintenance trials (PRECISE), but these were underpowered to show the efficacy of certolizumab in fistula closure. Subgroup analysis of patients with draining fistulas revealed that 36% had complete fistula closure versus 17% of the placebo group at week 26 [18]. There has not been and probably will not be a head-to-head trial looking at the efficacy of the three anti-TNF therapies in fistula healing.

Though a thorough discussion of surgical options is beyond the scope of this chapter, conservative surgical procedures such as the placement of draining or non-cutting seton, fistulotomy, or incision and drainage of abscess are necessary components of fistula management and allow for control of infection and fistula/abscess healing during medical treatment. Adjunctive surgical procedures help medications work more effectively and optimize outcomes. A retrospective study of patients with Crohn's-disease perianal fistulas treated with infliximab demonstrated that patients who underwent exam under anesthesia with seton placement prior to receiving infliximab had nearly half the recurrence rate of those treated with infliximab alone (44 vs. 79%). Alternatively, surgical options for those who are surgically refractory include advancement flaps, fibrin glue, and fistula plugs, while options for those who are medically refractory include diverting ileostomy and proctectomy.

Case Continued

The patient is sent for exam under anesthesia with seton placement and is started on infliximab. Drainage stops in 4 weeks, and after 8 weeks no material can be expressed from fistula on exam. EUS reveals fistula inactivity 12 weeks later and the seton is removed.

Management

An examination of the perianal anatomy is paramount, using physical examination, endoscopy, and imaging such as MRI of the pelvis or EUS. A simple fistula without luminal disease should be treated with antibiotics and immunosuppressive therapy (6-MP/AZA). Early anti-TNF therapy should be considered if patients are intolerant to 6-MP/AZA, if there is no response within approximately 3 months, or if proctitis or other luminal disease is present. If a complex fistula is associated with an abscess, then a surgical consult for EUA should be obtained, with the goal of abscess drainage and seton placement prior to the initiation of medical therapy [20]. In this setting, antibiotics should be initiated for a duration dependent upon response. Complex fistulas should be treated with anti-TNF therapy, preferably in combination with immunomodulator (6-MP 1.0–1.5 mg/kg; AZA 2.0–2.5 mg/kg), if tolerated. Setons should be maintained if there is persistent purulent drainage or if imaging shows ongoing fistula activity. A discussion regarding alternative surgical approaches, such as fibrin plug, advancement flap, or fecal diversion, should take place if patients have refractory perianal disease.

Take Home Points

- Perianal fistulas are a frequent manifestation in Crohn's disease.
- Fistulas result in significant morbidity and often lead to a need for surgical intervention.

- Exam and imaging with endoscopic ultrasonography (EUS) or magnetic resonance imaging (MRI) are recommended modalities for the evaluation of fistulas.
- Patients should be stratified into one of three groups: simple fistula and no proctitis; simple fistula and concomitant proctitis; and complex fistula.
- Simple fistulas and no proctitis can be treated with antibiotics and immunomodulators.
- Simple fistulas in the setting of proctitis can be treated with biologic agents.
- Complex fistulas commonly require surgical intervention.
- A combined medical and surgical approach is the preferred management strategy.

Videos of interest to readers of this chapter can be found by visiting the companion website at:

http://www.practicalgastrohep.com/

41.1 Endoscopic ultrasound for fistula.

References

1 American Gastroenterological Association. American Gastroenterological Association medical position statement: perianal Crohn's disease. *Gastroenterology* 2003; **125**: 1503–7.

2 Schwartz DA, Loftus EV Jr., Tremaine WJ, *et al.* The natural history of fistulizing Crohn's disease in Olmsted County, Minnesota. *Gastroenterology* 2002; **122**: 875–80.

3 Hellers G, Bergstrand O, Ewerth S, *et al.* Occurrence and outcome after primary treatment of anal fistulae in Crohn's disease. *Gut* 1980; **21**: 525–7.

4 Schwartz DA, White CM, Wise PE, *et al.* Use of endoscopic ultrasound to guide combination medical and surgical therapy for patients with perianal fistulas. *Inflamm Bowel Dis* 2005; **11**: 727–32.

5 Irvine EJ. Usual therapy improves perianal Crohn's disease as measured by a new disease activity index. McMaster IBD Study Group. *J Clin Gastroenterol* 1995; **20**(1): 27–32.

6 Haggett PJ, Moore NR, Shearman JD, *et al.* Pelvic and perineal complications of Crohn's disease: assessment using magnetic resonance imaging. *Gut* 1995; **36**: 407–10.

7 Tio TL, Mulder CJ, Wijers OB, *et al.* Endosonography of peri-anal and pericolorectal fistula and/or abscess in Crohn's disease. *Gastrointest Endosc* 1990; **36**: 331–6.

8 Schwartz DA, Wiersema MJ, Dudiak KM, *et al.* A comparison of endoscopic ultrasound, magnetic resonance imaging, and exam under anesthesia for evaluation of Crohn's perianal fistulas. *Gastroenterology* 2001; **121**: 1064–72.

9 Jakobovits J, Schuster MM. Metronidazole therapy for Crohn's disease and associated fistulae. *Am J Gastroenterol* 1984; **79**: 533–40.

10 Brandt LJ, Bernstein LH, Boley SJ, *et al.* Metronidazole therapy for perineal Crohn's disease: a follow-up study. *Gastroenterology* 1982; **83**: 383–7.

11 Pearson DC, May GR, Fick GH, *et al.* Azathioprine and 6-mercaptopurine in Crohn disease. A meta-analysis. *Ann Intern Med* 1995; **123**: 132–42.

12 Dejaco C, Harrer M, Waldhoer T, *et al.* Antibiotics and azathioprine for the treatment of perianal fistulas in Crohn's disease. *Aliment Pharmacol Ther* 2003; **18**(11–12): 1113–20.

13 Sandborn WJ, Present DH, Isaacs KL, *et al.* Tacrolimus for the treatment of fistulas in patients with Crohn's disease: a randomized, placebo-controlled trial. *Gastroenterology* 2003; **125**: 380–8.

14 Present DH, Rutgeerts P, Targan S, *et al*. Infliximab for the treatment of fistulas in patients with Crohn's disease. *N Engl J Med* 1999; **340**: 1398–405.

15 Sands BE, Anderson FH, Bernstein CN, *et al*. Infliximab maintenance therapy for fistulizing Crohn's disease. *N Engl J Med* 2004; **350**: 876–85.

16 Colombel JF, Sandborn WJ, Rutgeerts P, *et al*. Adalimumab for maintenance of clinical response and remission in patients with Crohn's disease: the CHARM trial. *Gastroenterology* 2007; **132**: 52–65.

17 Panacionne R, Colombel JF, Sandborn WJ, *et al*. Adalimumb sustains clinical remission and overall clinical benefit after 2 years of therapy for Crohn's disease. *Aliment Pharmacol Ther* 2010; **31**(12): 1296–309.

18 Schreiber S, Lawrance IC, Thomsen OØ, *et al*. Randomised clinical trial: certolizumab pegol for fistulas in Crohn's disease – subgroup results from a placebo-controlled study. *Aliment Pharmacol Ther* 2011; **33**(2): 185–93.

19 Regueiro M, Mardini H. Treatment of perianal fistulizing Crohn's disease with infliximab alone or as an adjunct to exam under anesthesia with seton placement. *Inflamm Bowel Dis* 2003; **9**: 98–103.

20 Siemanowski B, Regueiro M. Management of perianal fistula in Crohn's disease. *Inflamm Bowel Dis* 2008; **14**: S266–8.

21 Present DH, Korelitz BI, Wisch N, *et al*. Treatment of Crohn's disease with 6-mercaptopurine. A long-term, randomized, double-blind study. *N Engl J Med* 1980; **302**: 981–7.

CHAPTER 41

Fecal Incontinence

David Prichard and Adil E. Bharucha

Division of Gastroenterology and Hepatology, Mayo Clinic, Rochester, MN, USA

Summary

Fecal incontinence (FI) is commonly defined as the involuntary loss of feces. It has significant psychosocial consequences. Several factors – in particular anal sphincter trauma secondary to obstetric injury – have been implicated as causes of FI. Clinical evaluation is very useful for assessing symptom severity and guiding management. Testing is guided by clinical features and the response to therapy. It generally begins with anorectal manometry. Additional tests (e.g., endoanal ultrasound, defecography, pelvic magnetic resonance imaging (MRI), and anal electromyography (EMG)) are useful in selected cases. In approximately 25% patients, education and management of disordered bowel habits are very useful in improving fecal continence. Pelvic floor retraining may be useful for patients who do not respond to these measures. Though anal sphincteroplasty improves fecal continence in the short term, the beneficial effects wane over time. Perianal injectable bulking agents and sacral nerve stimulation are options for selected patients with refractory FI.

Case

A 67-year-old female presents with incontinence for small amounts of formed stool on an average of 3 days a week for 6 months. This leakage is not associated with urgency and often occurs shortly after defecation. She uses a protective panty liner, which she changes once daily. The rectal examination is notable for reduced anal resting tone, an impaired puborectalis lift during voluntary contraction of pelvic floor muscles, and reduced perineal descent during simulated evacuation. The anal wink reflex is absent despite normal perianal sensation.

Anal manometry demonstrates reduced anal resting and squeeze pressures, with normal thresholds for sensation, desire to defecate, and urgency. The rectoanal inhibitory reflex is present. A rectal balloon expulsion test is abnormal. Anal surface EMG discloses increased resting activity, appropriate activation of pelvic floor and accessory muscles, and a tendency to paradoxically co-contract abdominal and pelvic floor muscles during simulated evacuation.

Nine sessions of pelvic floor retraining by biofeedback therapy are provided over 1 week. After 3 months, she is passing an average of two large formed bowel movements daily and has an average of fewer than two episodes of FI per month.

Definition and Epidemiology

FI is defined by the unintentional loss of solid or liquid stool. It occurs in a variety of disorders associated with pelvic floor weakness and/or altered bowel habits. It can significantly impair a patient's social habits and quality of life.

The prevalence in the community is variable, ranging from 2.2 to 15.0%. In nursing homes, the prevalence may be up to 50% [1]. Prevalence is related to age, with 7% of women in the 3rd decade and 22% in the 6th decade reporting symptoms. Above this age, the prevalence plateaus. A majority of people with FI in the community have symptoms which are of mild (43%) or moderate (49%) severity. Though most attention has focused on women, the prevalence of FI is similar in men [2,3].

Etiology

FI is attributable to anorectal sensorimotor dysfunctions and/or altered bowel habits, which may be caused by a variety of conditions [4] (Table 42.1). While women with severe obstetric trauma (e.g., third- or fourth-degree lacerations) may develop FI shortly after vaginal delivery, most present 2–3 decades after delivery; the median age of FI onset is the 6th decade [3]. Obstetric injury is not a significant risk factor for delayed-onset FI in women [6,7] (Table 42.2).

Age, female gender, poor general health, physical limitations, obesity, loose stools, urgency, perianal injury, and anorectal surgery are all risk factors for FI. Diarrhea, irritable bowel syndrome (IBS), prior cholecystectomy, and rectal urgency are the factors most strongly associated with FI [6,7]. In people aged 65 years and older, self-reported diabetes mellitus, self-reported stroke, and certain medications (antiparkinsonian, hypnotic, and antipsychotic medications) are also risk factors [8].

Mechanisms of Normal Fecal Continence

Fecal continence is maintained by anatomical factors, rectoanal sensation, and rectal compliance [9]. The internal anal sphincter, which is made of circular smooth muscle, maintains approximately 70% of anal resting tone. The external anal sphincter, made of striated muscle, accounts for the remaining component of resting tone. The puborectalis is a U-shaped component of the levator ani complex that maintains a relatively acute rectoanal angle at rest. The external sphincter, puborectalis, and levator ani contract further when necessary to preserve continence.

Rectal distension by stool induces rectal contraction, the sensation of urgency, reflex relaxation of the internal anal sphincter, and

Practical Gastroenterology and Hepatology Board Review Toolkit, Second Edition. Edited by Nicholas J. Talley, Kenneth R. DeVault, Michael B. Wallace, Bashar A. Aqel and Keith D. Lindor.

Table 42.1 Etiology of FI. Source: Bharucha 2003 [5]. Reproduced with permission of Elsevier.

Anal sphincter weakness
Injury: obstetric trauma, related to surgical procedures (e.g., hemorrhoidectomy internal sphincterotomy, fistulotomy, anorectal infections)
Non-traumatic: scleroderma, internal sphincter thinning of unknown etiology
Neuropathy: stretch injury, obstetric trauma, diabetes mellitus
Anatomical disturbances of pelvic floor: fistula, rectal prolapse, descending perineum syndrome
Inflammatory conditions: Crohn's disease, ulcerative colitis, radiation proctitis
Central nervous system (CNS) disease: dementia, stroke, brain tumors, spinal cord lesions, multiple system atrophy (Shy–Drager syndrome), multiple sclerosis
Diarrhea: irritable bowel syndrome (IBS), postcholecystectomy diarrhea

Table 42.2 Relationship between obstetric history, anorectal injury, and incontinence.

Ultrasound reveals anal sphincter defects – which are often clinically occult – in 25–50% of women after a vaginal delivery
External sphincter defects are more likely to cause anal weakness than injury to the longitudinal muscle and transverse perinei
Incident postpartum FI is uncommon (10% or less of all vaginal deliveries); it is more likely (15–59%) in women who sustain a third- or fourth-degree anal sphincter tear during vaginal delivery
A higher body mass index (BMI), white race, antenatal urinary incontinence, and older age at delivery are risk factors for FI in women with anal sphincter tears
Obstetric risk factors for anal sphincter tears vary among studies
The use of forceps is a consistent risk factor
There is no difference between restrictive episiotomy practices versus midline versus mediolateral episiotomies
The risk of FI is not lower after cesarean section than after vaginal delivery

semivoluntary relaxation of pelvic floor muscles, prompting defecation if socially convenient. If not, defecation can be deferred by voluntary contraction of the external anal sphincter and puborectalis muscles; rectal contraction and the sensation of urgency generally subside as the rectum accommodates to continued distension.

Pathophysiology

Anal Sphincter Weakness

A majority of women with FI have reduced anal resting and/or squeeze pressures, reflecting weakness of the internal and/or external anal sphincters, respectively [10,11]. In addition to anal sphincter injury, FI is also associated with atrophy, denervation, and impaired function of the puborectalis muscle. Generalized pelvic floor weakness is often associated with pelvic organ prolapse affecting the anterior and/or middle compartments. Additionally, excessive straining may cause increased perineal descent, which can

stretch and thereby damage the pudendal nerve and make the anorectal angle more obtuse.

Rectal Sensorimotor Dysfunctions

Patients with FI may have normal, reduced, or increased rectal sensation [10]. When rectal sensation is reduced, the external anal sphincter may not contract promptly when the rectum is distended by stool. Conversely, rectal hypersensitivity in FI may be partly secondary to an exaggerated contractile response to distension and/or increased rectal tone with reduced capacity.

Impaired Rectal Evacuation

FI may be associated with features of disordered evacuation [10]. Such patients may benefit from biofeedback retraining, not only to improve rectal sensation and rectal coordination, but also to improve abdominopelvic coordination during defecation.

Clinical Features

In patients presenting with bowel dysfunction, it is imperative to inquire about symptoms of FI. A majority of patients do not volunteer FI symptoms to physicians. Patients with this condition may prefer the descriptive term "accidental bowel leakage." A detailed history is required to determine the etiology and severity of FI and to guide diagnostic testing and treatment. Stool form and consistency should preferably be characterized by pictorial stool scales (e.g., Bristol Stool Scale). "Staining," "soiling," "seepage," and "leakage" are terms used to indicate the severity of incontinence [12]. "Soiling" indicates more leakage than staining of underwear; it can be specified further as soiling of the underwear, of outer clothing, or of furnishing/bedding. "Seepage" refers to leakage of small amounts of stool. Leakage of solid stool probably reflects more severe anal weakness than isolated leakage of liquid stool.

Patients can present with urge incontinence, passive incontinence, or a combination [10]. Those who report that they "leak liquid or solid stool without any warning" either often (>25% of time) or usually (>75% of time) are considered to have passive incontinence. Patients often or usually experiencing "an urgent need to empty their bowels" are considered to have rectal urgency. The objective severity of FI can be scored by standardized scoring systems [3,13,14] (Table 42.3). The impact of FI on a patient's quality of life should be ascertained [15].

After anal inspection, a digital rectal examination should be performed to gauge anal sphincter and puborectalis function. The resistance to anal digital insertion provides a measure of anal resting pressure. Voluntary contraction should lift the examining finger anteriosuperiorly (i.e., toward the umbilicus). Conversely, simulated

Table 42.3 Symptom Severity Scale in FI. The score was derived using a physician-assigned value (i.e., the symptom severity score) for each of the four self-reported symptoms of FI. Maximum total score = 13. Scores of 4–6, 7–10, and 11–13 are categorized as mild, moderate, and severe FI, respectively. Source: Bharucha 2006 [14]. Reproduced with permission of Elsevier.

| Symptom | Symptom severity score | | | |
	1	2	3	4
Frequency	<1/month	<1/month to several times per week	Daily	
Composition	Mucus/liquid stool	Solid stool	Liquid and solid stool	
Amount	Small (i.e., staining only)	Moderate (i.e., requiring change of underwear)	Large (i.e., requiring change of all clothes)	
Urge or passive incontinence	Neither	Passive	Urge	Combined (i.e., passive and urge)

defecation should be accompanied by 2–4 cm of perineal descent and puborectalis relaxation [16]. Further examination in the seated position on a commode may reveal rectal prolapse or excessive perineal descent that is not evident when supine.

Diagnostic Testing

The extent of diagnostic testing is tailored to the patient's age, probable etiological factors, symptom severity, impact on quality of life, response to conservative medical management, and availability of tests.

Anal Manometry

Assessment of anal pressures by manometry is a starting point for diagnostic testing in FI. Manometry should be interpreted with reference to normal values in age- and gender-matched subjects. Anal resting and squeeze pressures are frequently reduced in FI, reflecting underlying neuromuscular pathology. Anorectal testing (i.e., anal manometry, rectal balloon expulsion test) can also identify a rectal evacuation disorder, which may coexist with FI.

Rectal Sensation and Compliance

Rectal sensation is assessed by distending a balloon manually, or with a barostat. Volume thresholds for first perception, desire to defecate, and severe urgency are measured during distension. Thresholds for rectal sensation may be normal, reduced, or increased in FI, as already discussed.

Rectal compliance is optimally measured by assessing rectal pressure–volume relationships with a barostat [10]. Reduced compliance may cause symptoms of rectal urgency and frequent defecation.

Endoscopy

Endoscopic assessment of the rectosigmoid mucosa should be considered in some patients, particularly those with new-onset constipation and/or diarrhea, in order to exclude neoplastic or inflammatory processes.

Endoanal Ultrasound

Endoanal ultrasound identifies anal sphincter thinning and defects, which are often clinically unrecognized and may be amenable to surgical repair. Whereas endoanal ultrasound reliably identifies anatomic defects or thinning of the internal sphincter, interpretation of external sphincter images is more subjective, operator-dependent, and confounded by normal anatomical variations in the external sphincter.

Dynamic Proctography (Defecography)

Dynamic proctography is useful when clinical features suggest excessive perineal descent, internal rectal intussusception, rectoceles, sigmoidoceles, or enteroceles. Puborectalis dysfunction during squeeze and evacuation can also be characterized. Contrast retention and evacuation, the anorectal angle, and the position of the anorectal junction are tracked at rest and while patients squeeze and subsequently strain to expel barium paste from the rectum.

Pelvic MRI

Pelvic MRI is the only imaging modality that can visualize both anal sphincter anatomy and global pelvic floor motion in real time, without radiation exposure. MRI performs the same or better than ultrasound in assessing the external sphincter [10]. Endoanal MRI may also reveal puborectalis defects (atrophy/injury) in FI [10]. Dynamic MRI provides a unique appreciation of pelvic anatomy and function, because the urological and gynecological structures within the pelvis are also readily visualized.

Needle EMG of the External Sphincter

Needle EMG provides a sensitive measure of denervation and can usually identify myopathic damage, neurogenic damage, or mixed injury affecting the external anal sphincter. Anal EMG should be considered in patients with clinically suspected neurogenic sphincter weakness.

Management

Dietary and Pharmacological Approaches

Modifying irregular bowel habits is the cornerstone of effective management of FI (Figure 42.1). A detailed dietary history is useful for identifying excessive ingestion of foods that might cause or aggravate diarrhea, such as those that contain fructose and sorbitol. Loperamide increases stool consistency and slightly increases internal anal sphincter tone, thereby reducing FI [4]. Adequate doses are essential (i.e., 2–4 mg 30 minutes before meals; up to 16 mg daily). Taking loperamide before social occasions may reduce the risk of having an accident outside the home. Diphenoxylate and amitriptyline are alternative options for diarrhea; amitriptyline may also reduce rectal urgency. Though its use is restricted, the 5-HT$_3$ antagonist alosetron may be useful for managing refractory functional diarrhea. Patients with constipation, fecal impaction, and overflow incontinence might benefit from an evacuation program that includes one or more of the following measures: using timed evacuation by bisacodyl or glycerol suppositories, fiber supplementation, and judicious use of oral laxatives.

Pelvic Floor Exercises and Biofeedback Therapy

Pelvic floor exercises entail contraction of the external anal sphincter and pelvic floor muscles but not the abdominal wall. Biofeedback therapy is generally performed by providing patients with feedback, usually visual, from anal manometric or surface EMG sensors. Patients learn to coordinate sphincter contraction during rectal distension. If rectal sensation is reduced, patients are taught to recognize rectal distension with progressively smaller volumes, generally beginning with 50 mL and declining to 10 mL or lower. In general, biofeedback is more effective than pelvic floor exercises alone for patients with FI who do not respond to routine medications and educational and behavioral strategies [18, 19].

Incontinence Products

Perineal protective devices include disposable and reusable body-worn products (diaper-type garments or pads) and disposable and reusable underpads (also called bed pads). Many patients wear panty liners, often lined with toilet paper. Anal plugs are available in Europe but not in the United States.

Surgical Approaches

Anal Sphincteroplasty

Consideration should be given to repairing external sphincter defects in women with postpartum FI. Outside of this circumstance, the benefit of repairing defects with overlapping anterior

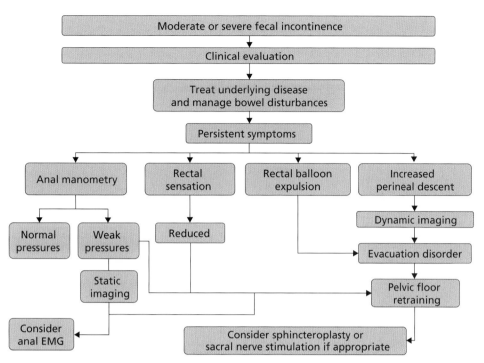

Figure 42.1 Simplified algorithm for managing FI. The choice of investigations is guided by the clinical features, as detailed in the text, and by the response to conservative measures, particularly management of bowel disturbances. Thereafter, further measures (e.g., pelvic floor retraining) may be necessary. EMG, electromyography. Source: Stoker 2008 [17]. Fig 6.2.8. Reproduced with permission of Springer Science + Business Media.

sphincteroplasty is not clear, because the initial improvement in fecal continence is not often sustained. A 50% failure rate after 40–60 months has been reported [20].

Other Surgical Approaches

Dynamic graciloplasty involves continuous electrical stimulation of the gracilis muscle, which is surgically transposed around the anal canal [4]. Though fecal continence may improve, both graciloplasty and artificial sphincter implantation are associated with significant morbidity. Therefore, these procedures are not widely used in the United States. A colostomy is the last resort for patients with severe FI.

Perianal Injectable Bulking Agents

Few trials have assessed the use of perianal injectable bulking agents for the treatment of FI [21]. In the largest randomized placebo-controlled trial, 80% of patients received two injections. A greater proportion of patients who received dextranomer in stabilized hyaluronic acid (52 vs. 31%) reported a ≥50% reduction in incontinence episodes at 12 months [22]; 6% of patients became completely continent. However, quality of life did not improve significantly with active treatment versus placebo. Moreover, limited data regarding the baseline severity of the cohorts were reported, making interpretation of this data challenging [23, 24].

Sacral Nerve Stimulation

A North American multicenter study of 120 patients with FI demonstrated that 83% of subjects achieved therapeutic success (95% CI: 74–90%), defined as a 50% or greater reduction in the number of weekly incontinent episodes at 12 months. The response appears durable up to 5 years from implantation. However, complications, which are mostly not severe (device revision, implant site pain,

paresthesia, infection), may occur in up to one-quarter of patients [25, 26]. The mechanisms of action of sacral nerve stimulation are not understood, as effects on anal pressures and rectal sensation are inconsistent across studies.

Conclusion

FI is a common and often devastating symptom. Because people with FI are often reluctant to acknowledge the symptom, physicians must inquire of patients with risk factors (e.g., diarrhea, urinary incontinence) whether they have FI. The clinical assessment is extremely useful for understanding the circumstances and severity surrounding FI. It also provides considerable information about the pathophysiology of FI. Diagnostic testing should be guided by the clinical features and the response to previous therapy. Management should initially focus on regulation of bowel disturbances. Pelvic floor retraining, surgery, and sacral nerve stimulation may also be helpful in selected patients.

Take Home Points

Diagnosis:
- It is imperative to ask patients if they have fecal incontinence (FI) and to obtain a detailed history.
- A careful digital rectal examination is useful for assessing anal sphincter functions and rectal evacuation.
- Assessment of anal resting and squeeze pressures by manometry is a starting point for diagnostic testing in FI.
- Depending on the clinical features, anorectal imaging (ultrasound, defecography, and pelvic magnetic resonance imaging (MRI)) and electromyography (EMG) may also be useful.

Therapy:

* Modifying irregular bowel habits is the cornerstone of effective management of FI in most patients.
* Biofeedback therapy should be considered in patients who do not respond to conservative management.
* Surgery, perianal injectable bulking agents, and sacral nerve stimulation may be considered in patients refractory to medical therapy and physical therapy.

References

1 Nelson RL. Epidemiology of fecal incontinence. *Gastroenterology* 2004; **126** (1 Suppl. 1): S3–7.

2 Whitehead WE, Borrud L, Goode PS, *et al.* Fecal incontinence in US adults: epidemiology and risk factors. *Gastroenterology* 2009; **137**(2): 512–17.

3 Bharucha AE, Zinsmeister AR, Locke GR, *et al.* Prevalence and burden of fecal incontinence: a population based study in women. *Gastroenterology* 2005; **129**: 42–9.

4 Andrews CN, Bharucha AE. The etiology, assessment, and treatment of fecal incontinence. *Nat Clin Pract Gastroenterol Hepatol* 2005; **2**(11): 516–25.

5 Bharucha AE. Fecal incontinence. *Gastroenterology* 2003; **124**(6): 1672–85.

6 Bharucha AE, Zinsmeister AR, Schleck CD, Melton LJ 3rd. Bowel disturbances are the most important risk factors for late onset fecal incontinence: a population-based case-control study in women. *Gastroenterology* 2010; **139**(5): 1559–66.

7 Bharucha AE, Fletcher JG, Melton LJ 3rd, Zinsmeister AR. Obstetric trauma, pelvic floor injury and fecal incontinence: a population-based case-control study. *Am J Gastroenterol* 2012; **107**(6): 902–11.

8 Quander CR, Morris MC, Melson J, *et al.* Prevalence of and factors associated with fecal incontinence in a large community study of older individuals. *Am J Gastroenterol* 2005; **100**(4): 905–9.

9 Bharucha AE. Pelvic floor: anatomy and function. *Neurogastroenterol Motil* 2006; **18**(7): 507–19.

10 Bharucha AE, Fletcher JG, Harper CM, *et al.* Relationship between symptoms and disordered continence mechanisms in women with idiopathic fecal incontinence. *Gut* 2005; **54**: 546–55.

11 Bharucha AE, Rao SSC. An update on anorectal disorders for gastroenterologists. *Gastroenterology* 2014; **146**(1): 37–45.e2.

12 Perry S, Shaw C, McGrother C, *et al.* Prevalence of faecal incontinence in adults aged 40 years or more living in the community. *Gut* 2002; **50**(4): 480–4.

13 Rockwood TH. Incontinence severity and QOL scales for fecal incontinence. *Gastroenterology* 2004; **126**: S106–13.

14 Bharucha AE, Zinsmeister AR, Locke GR, *et al.* Symptoms and quality of life in community women with fecal incontinence. *Clin Gastroenterol Hepatol* 2006; **4**(8): 1004–9.

15 Norton NJ. The perspective of the patient. *Gastroenterology* 2004; **126**(1 Suppl. 1): S175–9.

16 Wald A, Bharucha AE, Cosman BC, Whitehead WE. ACG clinical guideline: management of benign anorectal disorders. *Am J Gastroenterol* 2014; **109**(8): 1141–57.

17 Bharucha AE, Fletcher JG. Investigation of FI. In: Stoker J, Taylor SA, DeLancey JOL, eds. *Medical Radiology: Diagnostic Imaging and Radiation Oncology; Imaging and Pelvic Floor Disorders*, 2nd revised edn. Philadelphia, PA: Springer, 2008: 229–43.

18 Norton C, Cody JD, Hosker G. Biofeedback and/or sphincter exercises for the treatment of faecal incontinence in adults. *Cochrane Database Syst Rev* 2006(3):CD002111.

19 Norton C, Hosker G, Brazzelli M. Biofeedback and/or sphincter exercises for the treatment of faecal incontinence in adults. *Cochrane Database Syst Rev* 2000(2):CD002111.

20 Brown SR, Wadhawan H, Nelson RL. Surgery for faecal incontinence in adults. *Cochrane Database Syst Rev* 2010(9):CD001757.

21 Maeda Y, Laurberg S, Norton C. Perianal injectable bulking agents as treatment for faecal incontinence in adults. *Cochrane Database Syst Rev* 2013(2):CD007959.

22 Graf W, Mellgren A, Matzel KE, *et al.* Efficacy of dextranomer in stabilised hyaluronic acid for treatment of faecal incontinence: a randomised, sham-controlled trial. *Lancet* 2011; **377**(9770): 997–1003.

23 Norton C. Treating faecal incontinence with bulking-agent injections. *Lancet* 2011; **377**(9770): 971–2.

24 Wald A. New treatments for fecal incontinence: update for the gastroenterologist. *Clin Gastroenterol Hepatol* 2014; **12**(11): 1783–8.

25 Mowatt G, Glazener C, Jarrett M. Sacral nerve stimulation for fecal incontinence and constipation in adults: a short version Cochrane review. *Neurourol Urodyn* 2008; **27**(3): 155–61.

26 Mellgren A, Wexner SD, Coller JA, *et al.* Long-term efficacy and safety of sacral nerve stimulation for fecal incontinence. *Dis Colon Rectum* 2011; **54**(9): 1065–75.

Colorectal Cancer Screening

Katherine S. Garman[1] and Dawn Provenzale[2,3]

[1] Division of Gastroenterology and Institute for Genome Sciences and Policy, Veterans Affairs Medical Center, Duke University Medical Center, Durham, NC, USA
[2] VA Cooperative Studies Epidemiology Center
[3] Veterans Affairs Medical Center, Division of Gastroenterology, Duke University Medical Center, Durham, NC, USA

Summary

Colorectal cancer screening is an important mission for a practicing gastroenterologist. Several different screening modalities are available: fecal occult blood testing (FOBT), flexible sigmoidoscopy, colonoscopy, barium enema, and, more recently, computed tomography (CT)-colonography and stool DNA tests. The physician is charged with weighing the pros and cons of the different screening methods and selecting the most appropriate for each patient.

Case

A 35-year-old man with positive family history of colorectal cancer, diagnosed in his father at age 53, presents for information about colorectal cancer screening. He is in good health, with hypertension controlled on hydrochlorothiazide. What recommendations should be provided in terms of screening? What other information should be gathered from the patient?

Introduction

Screening applies to healthy, asymptomatic individuals and should improve life expectancy. Surveillance applies to the follow-up of patients at increased risk for colorectal cancer, including those with a personal or family history of colorectal cancer or polyps or with a history of inflammatory bowel disease (IBD).

Formal recommendations for colorectal screening began in 1980, with the first guidelines for screening issued by the American Cancer Society, initiating a series of guidelines aimed at reducing colorectal cancer mortality [1]. Since then, guidelines have become numerous and increasingly complex, culminating in a Joint Guideline by the US Multi-Society Task Force on Colorectal Cancer and the American College of Radiology [2], released in 2008, and the updated National Comprehensive Cancer Network Guidelines [3], released in 2010.

Review of Screening Methods

Stool-Based Tests

The studies that primarily detect cancer are stool-based. The two tests designed to detect blood in the stool are the guaiac-based fecal occult blood test (gFOBT) and the fecal immunochemical test (FIT). DNA-based stool tests are designed to test for the presence of DNA carrying some of the genetic mutations common in colorectal cancer.

The gFOBT was the first screening test shown to decrease mortality from colorectal cancer [4–6]. The test is inexpensive and easy to perform, making it ideal for population-based screening programs. It is important to note that there is no role for office-based gFOBT in colorectal cancer screening; it should be sent home with the patient and completed using two samples from each of three consecutive bowel movements. Sensitivity for cancer in the gFOBT ranges from 37.1 to 79.4% [7], and it is recommended that the gFOBT be repeated annually. Specificity for detection of cancer ranges from 86.7 to 97.7% [7].

The FIT represents a variation on the FOBT. It has not been studied in randomized controlled trials (RCTs), but has been evaluated in a population based screening program in Taiwan. A prospective cohort study of the follow up of a screened group who underwent biennial FIT was compared to an unscreened group. The mortality reduction in the screened group, compared to the unscreened group, was 0.38 (95% CI; 0.35–0.42) consistent with the mortaltly reduction seen in clinical trials of gFOBT [8]. The Joint Guideline [2] indicates that two samples may be better than one, but the ideal regimen has not been established. As with gFOBT, immunochemical stool tests should be repeated annually, and a positive test should always be followed with a colonoscopy. The stool DNA test considers that most colorectal cancers acquire a series of mutations that can be detected by the presence of abnormal DNA in stool [9]. One commercially available stool DNA test examines mutations in *APC*, K-*ras*, *TP53*, and *BAT26*. A stool specimen is collected and mailed to a central lab. In a large prospective study using stool DNA to screen average-risk individuals [10], 51.6% of invasive cancers, 32.5% of adenomas with high-grade dysplasia, and 18.2% of all advanced adenomas were detected. Specificity was high at 94.4%. A recent randomized trial of multitarget stool DNA testing (KRAS mutations, aberrant NDRG4 and BMP3 methylation and B-actin, plus a hemoglobin assay) compared one-time stool DNA and FIT, with colonoscopy as the gold standard. The sensitivity for detecting colorectal cancer was 92.3% with DNA testing and 73.8% with FIT (p = 0.002). The sensitivity for detecting advanced precancerous lesions was 42.4% with DNA testing and 23.8% with FIT

Practical Gastroenterology and Hepatology Board Review Toolkit, Second Edition. Edited by Nicholas J. Talley, Kenneth R. DeVault, Michael B. Wallace, Bashar A. Aqel and Keith D. Lindor.

(p < 0.001). The rate of detection of polyps with high-grade dysplasia was 69.2% with DNA testing and 46.2% with FIT (p = 0.004). The rate of detection of serrated sessile polyps measuring ≥1 cm was 42.4% with DNA testing and 5.1% with FIT (p < 0.001). Specificities with DNA testing and FIT were 86.6 and 94.9%, respectively, among participants with non-advanced or negative findings (p < 0.001) and 89.8 and 96.4%, respectively, among those with negative results on colonoscopy (p < 0.001). This stool DNA test has been approved by the FDA (Cologard) and accepted by the Centers for Medicare and Medicaid Services (CMS) for coverage as a Medicare benefit, with a testing interval of 3 years. While this is a promising test, there are several unanswered questions about its effectiveness in practice. The interval for screening has not been tested. The sensitivity of a FIT increases with annual screening, but the performance of the stool DNA test in a screening program is unknown. The adherence rate for the stool DNA test has not been measured. Recommendations for follow-up for a positive stool DNA test with a subsequent negative colonoscopy have not been established. Finally, the test is expensive, and its use in a screening program has not been determined. The Joint Guideline [2] includes the stool DNA test as an acceptable screening test, but the US Preventive Services Task Force (USPSTF) Guidelines do not, citing lack of evidence [11].

Endoscopic Screening Tests

Flexible sigmoidoscopy has been associated with a significantly decreased risk of and mortality from colorectal cancer. Flexible sigmoidoscopy can be performed in an office setting by a broad set of providers. However, because screening is limited to the distal colon, the main impact is in reducing mortality associated with left-sided colorectal cancer. Guidelines recommend a 5-year follow-up after a normal flexible sigmoidoscopy. In one study, the combination of flexible sigmoidoscopy and one-time FOBT increased the sensitivity of advanced adenoma detection from 70.3% for screening flexible sigmoidoscopy alone to 75.8% for both tests combined [12].

Colonoscopy has become the gold standard to which other colorectal cancer screening tests are compared, yet direct evidence for colonoscopy as a screening tool is limited. Colonoscopy is the screening test of choice for most gastroenterologists because it provides a complete exam of the colon with the opportunity for polypectomy and diagnostic biopsy of any suspicious lesion. There have been no prospective RCTs demonstrating a reduced cancer incidence or mortality benefit from screening colonoscopy.

Several studies have evaluated colonoscopy miss rates. For large adenomas, the colonoscopy miss rate has been estimated at 6–12% [2,13], and for colorectal cancers, as high as 4% [14,15].

Recent data suggest that the colonoscopy miss rate may be higher for lesions in the proximal colon compared to the distal colon. In a cohort of Ontario residents, while the relative risk of colorectal cancer after colonoscopy was 0.21 (95% CI: 0.05–0.36), colorectal cancers diagnosed after a negative colonoscopy were more likely to be located in the proximal colon compared with the control group [16]. In this same cohort, colonoscopy performed by a non-gastroenterologist was more likely to be associated with finding colorectal cancer after negative colonoscopy [17]. In a cross-sectional German cohort, the prevalence of colorectal cancer in patients who had undergone colonoscopy in the past 10 years was decreased compared to that in those without previous colonoscopy, with an adjusted prevalence ratio 0.54 (95% CI: 0.39–0.75). However, the adjusted prevalence ratio for right-sided lesions was 1.05 (95% CI: 0.63–1.76), indicating no protective effect in the proximal colon after colonoscopy [18] There are many potential reasons for higher miss rates in the proximal colon, including the quality of right-sided bowel preparation, different tumor biologies in the proximal and distal colon, an increased likelihood of flat lesions in the proximal colon, and factors related to the endoscopist [19].

Compared to the other available screening tests, colonoscopy carries a higher burden of complications. Bleeding is a risk after polypectomy, and the risk of perforation is 1/1000 in the Medicare population [20]. Additional adverse events, including cardiac arrhythmias, may result from the use of sedation for colonoscopy.

Most guidelines recommend a 10-year interval for follow-up after a normal colonoscopy. This interval is based on reports that suggest a slow growth rate of adenomatous polyps, some of which will eventually develop into cancers, but there are few data to support it.

Recently, studies have compared FIT to colonoscopy. An RCT of asymptomatic adults compared a colonoscopy with FIT every 2 years [21]. Cancer detection rates were similar in both groups. Screening was more likely to be performed in patients randomized to FIT. Only 19% of those randomized to colonoscopy actually underwent a colonoscopy, but adenoma detection was higher in the colonoscopy arm. This report is an interim analysis of participation rates. The study is ongoing, with colorectal cancer mortality as its end point. A US study, the Colonoscopy versus Fecal Immunochemical Test in Reducing Mortality from Colorectal Cancer (CONFIRM) Trial (a large, multicenter, randomized trial), is actively recruiting within the Department of Veterans Affairs (DVA). Its goal is to compare annual FIT screening to screening colonoscopy in individuals at average risk for colorectal cancer, with a primary end point of 10-year colorectal cancer mortality. We expect results to be informative on the question of FIT versus colonoscopy.

Imaging Tests

Imaging tests have been recommended as a primary screening modality by some [2,22], but the recent USPSTF Guidelines concluded that there is insufficient evidence to recommend CT colonography for screening for colorectal cancer [23].

A double-contrast barium enema (DCBE) can be a primary screening modality or can be used to complete a failed colonoscopy. Data are limited on the use of this modality for cancer screening. With the advent of other imaging techniques, DCBE is being performed less frequently. While DCBE is still included as a potential screening modality in most guidelines, its use is likely to continue to decline, as reflected in the recent omission of DCBE from the USPSTF Guidelines [11]. It may be more appropriate to consider DCBE as a means of completely examining the colon when a complete colonoscopy is indicated but cannot be performed.

CT colonography is a new and minimally invasive method of examining the colon and the rectum. It has only recently been incorporated into the Joint Guideline [2] as an acceptable form of colorectal cancer screening. However, the USPSTF Guidelines do not include CT colonography as a recommended screening method, due to lack of evidence [11].

As with DCBE, the patient requires colon preparation. In addition, the patient must consume an oral contrast agent to tag the stool. The interpretation of CT colonography is time-consuming, which may limit its use in clinical settings. As with colonoscopy, there have been no RCTs demonstrating that CT colonography can reduce morbidity and mortality from colorectal cancer. A recent multisite American College of Radiology Imaging Network (ACRIN) study of asymptomatic people undergoing routine colorectal cancer screening via CT colonography demonstrated 65% sensitivity for detection of polyps of size 5 mm or larger, with 89%

specificity; for polyps of 9 mm or larger, sensitivity improved to 90%, with 86% specificity [24]. One cancer was missed by CT colonography in 2531 participants.

At this time, several factors limit CT colonography. The optimal interval between screening CT colonography exams has not yet been established, but the Joint Guideline suggests 5 years. This is particularly important, as small polyps <5 mm are not reported and sensitivity for 5 mm polyps is only 65%.

Finally, the radiation-related risks from repeat CT scans have not been established.

Discussion of the Guidelines

Several different organizations and professional societies have created guidelines for colorectal screening and surveillance. Table 43.1 reviews the different screening modalities recommended in the different guidelines. In general, the Joint Guideline [2] includes many different screening modalities, including newer options such as CT colonography and stool DNA, while the USPSTF [11,23,25,26] and National Comprehensive Cancer Network (NCCN) Colorectal Cancer Screening [3] Guidelines favor better-studied screening methods such as FOBT and colonoscopy.

The guidelines vary slightly as to when to initiate colorectal cancer screening, though for most asymptomatic individuals with a negative family history, screening should begin at age 50. The American College of Gastroenterology (ACG) recommends beginning screening at age 45 for African Americans [27]. The screening guidelines also differ in the management of patients who are at increased risk of colorectal cancer due to a personal history of IBD or a positive family history for colorectal cancer. It is important to recall that 35% of colorectal cancer is associated with some hereditary factor, even if it is not part of an established familial colorectal cancer syndrome [28]. A thorough family history, including age of diagnosis and type of cancer for each affected family member, should be considered an important part of cancer screening for every individual; those with significant family histories may warrant more aggressive screening. The NCCN Guidelines provide information on the collection and integration of a family history into colorectal cancer screening [3].

The 2008 USPSTF Guidelines recommend against routine screening in persons age 75–85 and against any screening for those older than 85 [11].

Once polyps or cancer has been diagnosed, the patient enters into a program of surveillance by colonoscopy. The guidelines for surveillance are included in Table 43.2 for comparison.

Case Continued

Cancer screening by colonoscopy should begin at age 40 or at 10 years younger than the youngest family member with colorectal cancer. If normal, it should be repeated in 5 years. Otherwise, follow-up is indicated by the findings at colonoscopy. It would be helpful to obtain a more detailed family history, asking about any family members with high polyp burden, other family members with colorectal cancer, or any of the hereditary non-polyposis colorectal cancer (HNPCC)-associated tumors (colorectal, endometrial, stomach, ovarian, pancreas, ureter, renal pelvis, biliary tract, brain, small intestine, sebaceous gland adenomas, and keratoacanthomas [3]). If suspicion is raised for a familial syndrome, then genetic counseling should be offered.

Conclusion

Colorectal cancer screening has assumed two goals: reduction of mortality due to colorectal cancer and prevention of colorectal cancer through the removal of polyps. FOBT and flexible sigmoidoscopy, both beginning at age 50, with follow-up colonoscopy for a positive test have been shown to reduce colorectal cancer mortality in RCTs. The effectiveness of FIT in reducing colorectal cancer mortality has been demonstrated in a prospective cohort study [8]. Colonoscopy has long been considered the gold standard for polyp detection and removal, though miss rates for even the detection of cancer have been reported to be as high as 4% [14, 15]. In addition, emerging evidence suggests that the effectiveness of colonoscopy as a colorectal cancer prevention tool is reduced, particularly in the right colon [16–19]. Newer, less-invasive tests, such as stool DNA and CT colonography, represent additional modes of screening, and we can expect more debate regarding the role of these new modalities in screening programs in the coming years. Average-risk individuals age 50 and older should be encouraged to participate in colorectal cancer screening. Patients at high risk due to family history of cancer or polyps or a personal history of longstanding IBD should be encouraged to adhere to a regular program of surveillance through colonoscopy.

There are a variety of recommended modalities for colorectal cancer screening. Some are more acceptable to patients and more feasible for health care systems [2]. Ideally, the choice of screening modality should be screened and provider-based. Future research should focus on interventions aimed at implementing appropriate screening and should identify ways to reduce the need for more invasive and expensive tests.

Table 43.1 Choice of colorectal screening modality by guideline.

Guideline	Year	FOBT	Stool DNA	DCBE	Flexible sigmoidoscopy	Combination FS and FOBT	Colonoscopy	CT colonography
Joint Guideline [2]	2008	Annually, using guaiac-based test or immunochemical test	Interval uncertain	Every 5 years	Every 5 years		Every 10 years	Every 5 years
USPSTF [11]	2008	Annually	Insufficient evidence	No longer recommended		FS every 5 years and high-sensitivity FOBT every 3 years	Every 10 years	
NCCN [3]	2015	Annually, using guaiac-based test or immunochemical test	Not considered screening test		Every 5 years	FS ± intervals of stool testing at 3 years	Every 10 years	No consensus on use as a primary screening modality

FOBT, fecal occult blood test; DCBE, double-contrast barium enema; FS, flexible sigmoidoscopy; CT, computed tomography; USPSTF, US Preventive Services Task Force; NCCN, National Comprehensive Cancer Network.

Table 43.2 Colonoscopy surveillance by guideline.

Guideline	Hyperplastic polyps	1–2 small adenomas	Advanced adenomas	>10 adenomas at a single exam	Sessile polyps removed piecemeal	Personal history of colorectal cancer
Joint Guideline [2, 29]	Small rectal hyperplastic polyps: follow average screening guidelines	1–2 small tubular adenomas: 5–10 years after initial polypectomy	3–10 adenomas or 1 adenoma >1 cm or any adenoma with villous features or high-grade dysplasia: 3 years after initial polypectomy; if polyps are removed and follow-up is normal or if there are 1–2 small polyps, repeat in 5 years	<3 years after initial polypectomy: consider familial syndrome	< 1 year	3–6 months after surgery or intraoperatively for perioperative clearing and then 1 year after surgical resection or the perioperative clearing exam
ACG [30]		1 or 2 adenomas <1 cm in size and no family history: repeat in 5 years	>2 adenomas, adenoma ≥1 cm, high-grade dysplasia, villous histology, or positive family history: repeat in 3 years and, if normal, again in 5 years		3–6 months	Malignant polyps: 3 months after endoscopic resection
NCCN [3]	Hyperplastic: 10 years	≤2 polyps <1 cm: repeat in 5 years and, if normal, again every 10 years	3–10 adenomas, adenoma ≥1 cm, high-grade dysplasia, or villous features: repeat within 3 years and, if normal, again in 5 years	>10 cumulative adenomas: individual management; consider polyposis syndrome	2–6 months	Colonoscopy within 1 year (or within 3–6 months if no complete preoperative colonoscopy)
SSAT [31]		2 small <1 cm polyps: repeat in 3 years				

ACG, American College of Gastroenterology; NCCN, National Comprehensive Cancer Network; SSAT, Society for Surgery of the Alimentary Tract.

Take Home Points

- Colorectal cancer screening has been shown to reduce mortality from colorectal cancer.
- There are multiple recommended screening modalities, including fecal occult blood testing (FOBT) fecal immunochemical testing (FIT), stool DNA tests, flexible sigmoidoscopy, computed tomography (CT) colonography, colonoscopy, and barium enema, with different levels of evidence to support the efficacy of each. These tests need to be repeated at their suggested intervals in order for screening to be effective.
- The choice of screening modality should be based on risk assessment by the provider. Risk assessment will determine whether the individual is eligible for screening (e.g., does not have life-limiting comorbidities that would diminish the effectiveness of screening). Furthermore, risk assessment is critical to determining whether the individual to be screened is at average or high risk for developing colorectal cancer based on personal or family history.
- Once an assessment of the individual's risk for colorectal cancer has been performed, the choice of screening modality should be based on a shared decision between the provider and the patient.
- Population-based colorectal cancer screening requires a substantial investment of patient, provider, and health system time and resources. Screening must be offered to the patient. The patient must accept screening and comply with appropriate instructions for the screening test. Positive tests must be followed up in a timely manner, in order to diagnose colorectal cancer in an early and treatable stage. Some colorectal cancer screening tests are more acceptable to patients and more feasible for health care systems. In systems or settings where resources are limited, any of the approved modalities is preferable to the alternative of no screening.

References

1 Eddy DM. *Screening for Cancer: Theory, Analysis, and Design.* Englewood Cliffs, NJ: Prentice-Hall, 1980: xii, 308.

2 Levin B, Lieberman DA, McFarland B, *et al.* Screening and surveillance for the early detection of colorectal cancer and adenomatous polyps, 2008: a joint guideline from the American Cancer Society, the US Multi-Society Task Force on Colorectal Cancer, and the American College of Radiology. *CA Cancer J Clin* 2008; **58**: 130–60.

3 National Comprehensive Cancer Network. *Colorectal Cancer Screening. NCCN Clinical Practice Guidelines in Oncology J Natl Compr Canc Netw* 2015; **13**: 959–68.

4 Scholefield JH, Moss S, Sufi F, *et al.* Effect of faecal occult blood screening on mortality from colorectal cancer: results from a randomised controlled trial. *Gut* 2002; **50**: 840–4.

5 Jorgensen OD, Kronborg O, Fenger C. A randomised study of screening for colorectal cancer using faecal occult blood testing: results after 13 years and seven biennial screening rounds. *Gut* 2002; **50**: 29–32.

6 Vernon SW, Meissner H, Klabunde C, *et al.* Measures for ascertaining use of colorectal cancer screening in behavioral, health services, and epidemiologic research. *Cancer Epidemiol Biomarkers Prev* 2004; **13**: 898–905.

7 Allison JE, Tekawa IS, Ransom LJ, *et al.* A comparison of fecal occult-blood tests for colorectal-cancer screening. *N Engl J Med* 1996; **334**: 155–9.

8 Chiu HM, Chen SL, Yen AM, *et al.* Effectiveness of fecal immunochemical testing in reducing colorectal cancer mortality from the One Million Taiwanese Screening Program. *Cancer* 2015; **121**(18): 3221–9.

9 Osborn NK, Ahlquist DA. Stool screening for colorectal cancer: molecular approaches. *Gastroenterology* 2005; **128**: 192–206.

10 Imperiale TF, Wagner DR, Lin CY, *et al.* Risk of advanced proximal neoplasms in asymptomatic adults according to the distal colorectal findings. *N Engl J Med* 2000; **343**: 169–74.

11 U.S. Preventive Services Task Force. Screening for Colorectal Cancer: US Preventive Services Task Force Recommendation. *Ann Intern Med* 2008; **149**: 627–37.

12 Rex DK, Lieberman DA. Feasibility of colonoscopy screening: discussion of issues and recommendations regarding implementation. *Gastrointest Endosc* 2001; **54**: 662–7.

13 Rex DK, Cutler CS, Lemmel GT, *et al.* Colonoscopic miss rates of adenomas determined by back to back colonoscopies. *Gastroenterology* 1997; **112**: 24–8.

14 Bressler B, Paszat LF, Vinden C, *et al.* Colonoscopic miss rates for right-sided colon cancer: a population-based analysis. *Gastroenterology* 2004; **127**: 452–6.

15 Rex DK, Rahmani EY, Haserman JH, *et al.* Relative sensitivity of colonoscopy and barium enema for detection of colorectal cancer in clinical practice. *Gastroenterology* 1997; **112**: 17–23.

16 Lakoff J, Paszat LF, Saskin R, Rabeneck L. Risk of developing proximal versus distal colorectal cancer after a negative colonoscopy: a population-based study. *Clin Gastroenterol Hepatol* 2008; **6**: 1117–21, quiz 1064.

17 Rabeneck L, Paszat LF, Saskin R. Endoscopist specialty is associated with incident colorectal cancer after a negative colonoscopy. *Clin Gastroenterol Hepatol* 2010; **8**: 275–9.

18 Brenner H, Hoffmeister M, Arndt V, *et al.* Protection from right- and left-sided colorectal neoplasms after colonoscopy: population-based study. *J Natl Cancer Inst* 2010; **102**: 89–95.

19 Hewett DG, Kahi CJ, Rex DK. Does colonoscopy work? *J Natl Compr Canc Netw* 2010; **8**: 67–76, quiz 77.

20 Gatto NM, Frucht H, Sundararajan V, *et al.* Risk of perforation after colonoscopy and sigmoidoscopy: a population-based study. *J Nat Cancer Instit* 2003; **95**: 230–6.

21 Quintero E, Castells A, Bujanda L, *et al.* Colonoscopy versus fecal immunochemical testing in colorectal cancer screening. *N Engl J Med* 2012; **366**(8): 697–706.

22 Heiken JP, Bree RL, Foley WD, *et al. Colorectal cancer screening.* Reston, VA: American College of Radiology (ACR), 2006. Available from: http://www.dcamedical.com/webdocuments/appropriateness-criteria-colonrectal-cancer-screening.pdf (last accessed February 12, 2016).

23 Whitlock EP, Lin JS, Liles E, *et al.* Screening for colorectal cancer: US Preventive Services Task Force recommendation statement. *Ann Intern Med* 2008; **149**: 639–58.

24 Johnson CD, Chen M, Toledo AY, *et al.* Accuracy of CT colonosgraphy for detection of large adenomas and cancers. *N Engl J Med* 2008; **359**: 1207–17.

25 US Preventive Services Task Force. Screening for colorectal cancer: recommendation and rationale. *Ann Intern Med* 2002; **137**: 129–45.

26 Pignone M, Rich M, Teutsch SM, *et al.* Screening for colorectal cancer in adults at average risk: a summary of the evidence for the US Preventive Services Task Force. *Ann Intern Med* 2002; **137**: 132–41.

27 Agrawal S, Bhupinderjit A, Bhutani MS, *et al.* Colorectal cancer in African Americans. *Am J Gastroenterol* 2005; **100**: 515–23, disc. 514.

28 Lichtenstein P, Holm NV, Verkasalo PK, *et al.* Environmental and heritable factors in the causation of cancer – analyses of cohorts of twins from Sweden, Denmark, and Finland. *N Engl J Med* 2000; **343**: 78–85.

29 Lieberman DA, Rex DK, Winawer SJ, *et al.* Guidelines for colonoscopy surveillance after screening and polypectomy: a consensus update by the US Multi-Society Task Force on Colorectal Cancer. *Gastroenterology* 2012; **143**(3): 844–57.

30 Bond JH. Polyp guideline: diagnosis, treatment, and surveillance for patients with colorectal polyps. Practice Parameters Committee of the American College of Gastroenterology. *Am J Gastroenterol* 2000; **95**(11): 3053–63.

31 Society for Surgery of the Alimentary T. SSAT patient care guidelines. Management of colonic polyps and adenomas. *J Gastrointest Surg* 2007; **11**(9):1197–9.

CHAPTER 45

Endoscopic Palliation of Malignant Obstruction

Todd H. Baron

Division of Gastroenterology and Hepatology, Mayo Clinic, Rochester, MN, USA

Summary

Endoscopy plays a major role in the palliation of malignant obstruction, both luminal and biliary. Endoscopic palliation of malignant biliary obstruction is discussed in Chapter 74. There are a variety of endoscopic methods for the endoscopic palliation of esophageal obstruction, including simple dilation, expandable stent placement, photodynamic therapy (PDT), argon plasma coagulation (APC), and brachytherapy. However, palliation of lumenal obstruction beyond the esophagus and in the colon is achieved through the use of self-expanding metal stents (SEMS). Finally, endoscopic placement of gastrostomy tubes for supplemental nutrition and/or decompression can be used for palliation of obstruction.

> ### Case
>
> A 75-year-old man presents with progressive dysphagia. He can only swallow liquids. An esophagogastroduodenoscopy (EGD) reveals a malignant-appearing mass at the gastroesophageal junction (GEJ). Biopsies reveal adenocarcinoma. Computed tomography (CT) scan of the abdomen reveals a large, locally invasive mass at the GEJ with liver metastases. A SEMS is placed for palliation of dysphagia, after which he can swallow semisolid food until death 12 weeks later.

Equipment and Review of Technology

Endoscopic palliation of luminal obstruction is primarily achieved using SEMS. There are a variety of types of SEMS, particularly for use within the esophagus [1]. SEMS are composed of alloys, most commonly Nitinol, a nickel–titanium alloy. The stents have a lattice configuration and are preloaded on to a delivery system in a constrained fashion. When the constraining system is released, the stent expands. Almost all esophageal SEMS have a covering to allow closure of fistula and prevention of tissue ingrowth through the lattice of the stent. A removable, expandable, fully covered plastic esophageal stent is available. SEMS used outside the esophagus do not have a covering, because of a high rate of migration. Newer esophageal and non-esophageal SEMS are also available in a predeployed diameter small enough to pass through the endoscope channel.

PDT requires the use of a photosensitizing agent and a laser fiber, which emits a wavelength of light that activates the drug. This results in release of cytotoxic oxygen radicals, which kill tumor cells in the areas where light exposure occurs.

APC palliation involves a specialized electrosurgical generator equipped with argon gas. A probe that passes through the endoscope channel allows necrosis and ablation of tissue at high power settings.

Endoscopic placement of brachytherapy catheters can deliever radiation therapy to the esophagus and provide palliation of malignant dysphagia [2].

How to Place SEMS

Most SEMS are placed under endoscopic and fluoroscopic guidance, though esophageal stents can be placed without fluoroscopy [1]. The endoscope is passed to the site of the lesion. A guidewire is used to traverse the malignant obstruction. When non-through-the-scope (TTS) esophageal stents are placed, the endoscope is removed and the stent passed over the wire, since most of these predeployed stents are not small enough to pass through the endoscope. The endoscope can be passed alongside the stent so that the stent is deployed under direct endoscopic visualization. Alternatively, the stent can be deployed under fluoroscopic guidance alone. The approach to malignant obstruction when TTS stents are used is similar, though the endoscope is not usually removed; the predeployed stent is passed through the channel of the endoscope and deployed under endoscopic view. Currently, one covered TTS esophageal stent and several uncovered TTS stents are available for duodenal and colonic use.

PDT is performed at 48–72 hours following infusion of a photosensitizing agent. The endoscope is passed into the esophagus to the level of the tumor. A laser-diffusion fiber is inserted through the endoscope and positioned across the stricture for a defined period of time.

Argon beam coagulation has replaced laser in most endoscopy units and is applied by passing the probe into the esophagus. At high power settings and in close proximity to the lesion, the tissue is coagulated to induce necrosis of the tumor [3].

Brachytherapy is performed by endoscopically placing a guidewire into the stomach and positioning the catheter fluoroscopically. The catheter remains in place for a defined period of time [2].

Malignant Dysphagia

In patients with advanced disease, palliation of dysphagia is performed to improve quality of life and nutritional status and to prevent aspiration pneumonia (Table 44.1). Simple dilation using

Practical Gastroenterology and Hepatology Board Review Toolkit, Second Edition. Edited by Nicholas J. Talley, Kenneth R. DeVault, Michael B. Wallace, Bashar A. Aqel and Keith D. Lindor.

Table 44.1 Methods of palliation of esophageal cancer.

Simple dilation (balloon or bougie)
Expandable stent placement (plastic or metal)
Photodynamic therapy (PDT)
Argon plasma coagulation (APC)
Gastrostomy tube placement

Table 44.2 Complications of expandable stents (early and delayed).

Esophageal stents	Airway obstruction
	Aspiration
	Tracheoesophageal fistula
	Chest pain
	Reflux with aspiration, esophagitis
	Food impaction
All stents	Obstruction: tumor ingrowth, overgrowth, tissue hyperplasia
	Bleeding
	Migration
	Perforation
Colonic stents	Tenesmus, incontinence (rectal stent placement)

balloon or bougie can allow brief relief of dysphagia. Endoscopically placed stents apply internal radial forces to the esophagus, mechanically widening the esophageal lumen (Figure 44.1). Stents are useful for palliating malignant dysphagia from both intrinsic tumors of the esophagus and malignant extrinsic compression. Unlike feeding tubes, stents can produce palliation of dysphagia, allowing peroral nutrition. Covered metal stents and an expandable plastic stent allow closure of tracheoesophageal fistulas. Dysphagia has been shown to be effectively and reliably relieved after insertion of SEMS [1]. Early complications after esophageal stent placement may include perforation, aspiration, chest pain, malpositioning of the stent, and acute airway obstruction (Table 44.2). Late stent complications may occur as a result of SEMS placement (Table 44.2), including gastroesophageal reflux and aspiration when a stent traverses the GEJ. Stent occlusion can result from an impacted food bolus or from tumor ingrowth or tissue hyperplasia (through the uncovered portions of metal stents). Additional stents can be placed to restore luminal patency through the previous stent (or after removal of fully covered SEMS or self-expanding plastic stents (SEPS)). Covered metal stents placed across the GEJ and plastic stents in any location are more prone to migration [4, 5]. Major bleeding can result from erosion of the stent through the esophagus and into the aorta. Tracheoesophageal fistulas can result from stent erosion into the respiratory tree.

Placement of SEMS after prior administration of radiation and/or chemotherapy may result in a higher complication rate [6, 7]. There is little information about the effect of concomitant radiation and stent placement [8].

PDT allows successful palliation in the majority of patients with intrinsic esophageal lesions [9], though chest pain and fever are common. Ambient-light photosensitivity occurs for up to 8 weeks. Mediastinitis is an uncommon complication.

Single-dose brachytherapy allows successful palliation of malignant dysphagia. Compared to stent placement, the effects are delayed, but more durable palliation can be achieved [2].

Malignant Gastric Outlet Obstruction

Malignant gastric outlet obstruction (GOO) produces postprandial abdominal pain, early satiety, vomiting, and intolerability of oral intake. In the United States, SEMS are placed for palliation of malignant GOO most often in the setting of pancreatic cancer. Other malignancies include gastric cancer, cholangiocarcinoma, gallbladder cancer, and metastatic disease. Technical success, defined as successful stent placement and deployment, can be achieved in up to 97% of cases [10]. Clinical success, defined as relief of symptoms and improved oral intake, occurs in about 90%. Stent occlusion occurs in about 20%, due to tumor ingrowth. Migration occurs in 5% of patients. Compared to surgical bypass (gastroenterostomy) for palliation of malignant GOO, SEMS placement results in a shorter time to oral intake and a shorter initial hospital stay [11]. However, patients who live longer experience a higher recurrence of obstruction and need for reintervention.

Many patients with GOO may also need biliary stent placement (Figure 44.2), which should be done prior to gastroduodenal stent

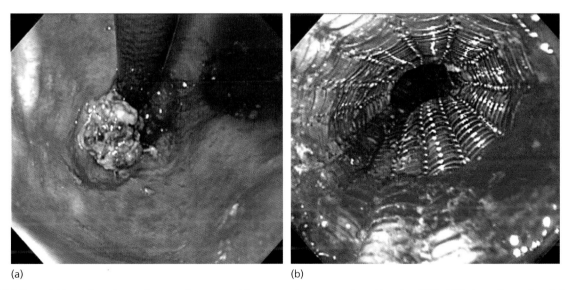

(a)   (b)

Figure 44.1 Expandable esophageal stent placement for unresectable tumor at the gastroesophageal junction (GEJ). (a) Endoscopic retroflexed view in the stomach, showing obstructing mass. (b) Endoscopic view from the esophagus immediately after placement of a covered self-expanding metal stent (SEMS).

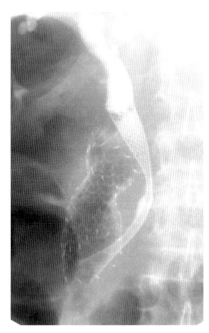

Figure 44.2 Endoscopic palliation of malignant gastric outlet obstruction (GOO) and malignant biliary obstruction. Radiographic image shows a duodenal stent and biliary stent. Contrast is still visible in the biliary tree.

placement, since the duodenal portion of the stent can cover the papilla and make it inaccessible.

Colonic Obstruction

Patients with malignant colonic obstruction may present with minimal symptoms or with subtotal or complete obstruction. Mortality associated with acute malignant colonic obstruction is high. Endoscopic stent placement can be used for palliation of widespread, obstructive colorectal malignancy and in patients who are poor candidates for surgery, and can allow avoidance of a colostomy (Figure 44.3). Extrinsic compression from pelvic malignancies and lymphadenopathy may also be palliated with stents. Use of a

covered stent in the rectum can allow closure of fistulas to the vagina and bladder [12].

Technical success rate for stent placement can be achieved in 93% and clinical success in 91% of cases [13]. Perforation during or after stent placement usually requires emergency surgery. Reobstruction due to tumor ingrowth occurs in about 8% of patients, at a median time of 24 weeks. Other causes of obstruction include fecal impaction, tumor overgrowth, and peritoneal metastasis in other areas of the gastrointestinal (GI) tract. Stent placement in the right colon is also effective [14].

The complications of expandable enteral stents are listed in Table 44.2.

Enteral Tubes

Enteral tubes can be used to palliate obstruction [15]. Percutaneous endoscopic gastrostomy (PEG) tubes can be used to supplement nutrition in patients with esophageal cancer. Simultaneous endoscopic placement of jejunal feeding tubes and gastric decompression tubes can be used to palliate malignant gastroduodenal obstruction. Finally, in patients with extensive peritoneal carcinomatosis, PEG tubes can be used as a final way of providing comfort care, as an alternative to nasogastric decompression.

> **Take Home Points**
>
> - Palliation of malignant esophageal obstruction can be achieved endoscopically using a variety of techniques.
> - Self-expanding esophageal stents are used as the primary modality for palliation of malignant esophagorespiratory fistulas.
> - Esophageal stents are effective in the palliation of malignant dysphagia, due to extrinsic compression of the esophagus.
> - Expandable metal stents allow effective palliation of malignant gastroduodenal obstruction, with an efficacy similar to that of surgical bypass.
> - Colonic stents are useful for palliation of malignant colonic obstruction and can allow avoidance of a permanent colostomy.
> - Endoscopically placed feeding and decompression tubes can be used as standalone or supplemental measures for palliation of malignancy.

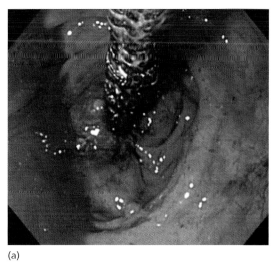

(a)

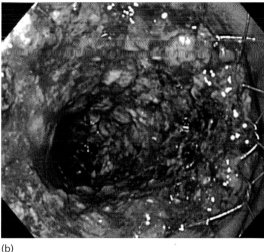

(b)

Figure 44.3 Palliation of malignant rectal stricture. (a) Endoscopic view of an obstructive mass, with predeployed stent visible. (b) Endoscopic view taken immediately after stent placement, With widely patent lumen inside the stent visible.

Videos of interest to readers of this chapter can be found by visiting the companion website at:

http://www.practicalgastrohep.com/

44.1 Endoscopic palliation of dysphagia.

References

1 Papachristou GI, Baron TH. Use of stents in benign and malignant esophageal disease. *Rev Gastroenterol Disord* 2007; **7**: 74–88.

2 Homs MY, Steyerberg EW, Eijkenboom WM, *et al.* Single-dose brachytherapy versus metal stent placement for the palliation of dysphagia from oesophageal cancer: multicentre randomised trial. *Lancet* 2004; **364**: 1497–504.

3 Eriksen JR. Palliation of non-resectable carcinoma of the cardia and oesophagus by argon beam coagulation. *Dan Med Bull* 2002; **49**: 346–9.

4 Vakil N, Morris AI, Marcon N, *et al.* A prospective, randomized, controlled trial of covered expandable metal stents in the palliation of malignant esophageal obstruction at the gastroesophageal junction. *Am J Gastroenterol* 2001; **96**: 1791–6.

5 Conio M, Repici A, Battaglia G, *et al.* A randomized prospective comparison of self-expandable plastic stents and partially covered self-expandable metal stents in the palliation of malignant esophageal dysphagia. *Am J Gastroenterol* 2007; **102**: 2667–77.

6 Kinsman KJ, DeGregorio BT, Katon RM, *et al.* Prior radiation and chemotherapy increase the risk of life-threatening complications after insertion of metallic stents for esophagogastric malignancy. *Gastrointest Endosc* 1996; **43**: 196–203.

7 Lecleire S, Di Fiore F, Ben-Soussan E, *et al.* Prior chemoradiotherapy is associated with a higher life-threatening complication rate after palliative insertion of metal stents in patients with oesophageal cancer. *Aliment Pharmacol Ther* 2006; **23**: 1693–702.

8 Ludwig D, Dehne A, Burmester E, *et al.* Treatment of unresectable carcinoma of the esophagus or the gastroesophageal junction by mesh stents with or without radiochemotherapy. *Int J Oncol* 1998; **13**: 583–8.

9 Litle VR, Luketich JD, Christie NA, *et al.* Photodynamic therapy as palliation for esophageal cancer: experience in 215 patients. *Ann Thorac Surg* 2003; **76**: 1687–92.

10 Dormann A, Meisner S, Verin N, Wenk Lang A. Self-expanding metal stents for gastroduodenal malignancies: systematic review of their clinical effectiveness. *Endoscopy* 2004; **36**: 543–50.

11 Jeurnink SM, Steyerberg EW, Hof G, *et al.* Gastrojejunostomy versus stent placement in patients with malignant gastric outlet obstruction: a comparison in 95 patients. *J Surg Oncol* 2007; **96**: 389–96.

12 Repici A, Reggio D, Saracco G, *et al.* Self-expanding covered esophageal ultraflex stent for palliation of malignant colorectal anastomotic obstruction complicated by multiple fistulas. *Gastrointest Endosc* 2000; **51**: 346–8.

13 Sebastian S, Johnston S, Geoghegan T, *et al.* Pooled analysis of the efficacy and safety of self-expanding metal stenting in malignant colorectal obstruction. *Am J Gastroenterol* 2004; **99**: 2051–7.

14 Repici A, Adler DG, Gibbs CM, *et al.* Stenting of the proximal colon in patients with malignant large bowel obstruction: techniques and outcomes. *Gastrointest Endosc* 2007; **66**: 940–4.

15 Holm AN, Baron TH. Palliative use of percutaneous endoscopic gastrostomy and percutaneous endoscopic cecostomy tubes. *Gastrointest Endosc Clin N Am* 2007; **17**: 795–803.

CHAPTER 44

PART 3

Diseases of the Small Intestine

45 Crohn's Disease, 273
Kara M. De Felice and Sunanda V. Kane

46 Small-Bowel Tumors, 279
Nadir Arber and Menachem Moshkowitz

47 Small-Intestinal Bacterial Overgrowth, 285
Johanna Iturrino and Madhusudan Grover

48 Celiac Disease and Tropical Sprue, 291
Alberto Rubio-Tapia and Joseph A. Murray

49 Whipple's Disease, 296
Seema A. Patil and George T. Fantry

50 Short-Bowel Syndrome, 299
Alan L. Buchman

51 Protein-Losing Gastroenteropathy, 304
Lauren K. Schwartz and Carol E. Semrad

52 Acute Mesenteric Ischemia and Chronic Mesenteric Insufficiency, 308
Timothy T. Nostrant

53 Intestinal Obstruction and Pseudo-obstruction, 313
Magnus Halland and Purna Kashyap

CHAPTER 45

Crohn's Disease

Kara M. De Felice and Sunanda V. Kane

Division of Gastroenterology and Hepatology, Mayo Clinic, Rochester, MN, USA

Summary

Crohn's disease is a chronic idiopathic inflammatory condition that can affect the mucosa from mouth to anus. The presenting signs and symptoms can mimic a variety of other conditions, and a thorough workup, including complete history and physical examination, blood tests, imaging, and endoscopy with biopsies, needs to be performed to make the diagnosis. Treatment is based on disease location, behavior (inflammatory, stricturing, fistulizing), and severity. The goal of therapy is mucosal healing, with the intent to prevent complications.

Case

A 30-year-old male presents with diarrhea for 6 weeks. He has 8–10 non-bloody bowel movements per day associated with right lower quadrant pain and a 2.5 kg unintentional weight loss. He has also noticed perianal pain, erythema, and swelling with no drainage. He denies nausea, vomiting, fevers, or chills. He takes no medications and has no medication allergies. He smokes a half pack of cigarettes per day, drinks alcohol occasionally, and denies illicit drug use. He has no family history of gastrointestinal (GI) diseases. His physical exam is remarkable for mild tenderness in the right lower quadrant without rebound or guarding. Rectal exam shows a tender, erythematous, and fluctuant lesion in the 3 o' clock perianal position.

Definition and Epidemiology

Crohn's disease is a disorder characterized by asymmetric, transmural, and sometimes granulomatous inflammation that can occur anywhere in the GI tract.

It occurs at any age, with the highest incidence among adolescents (15–25 years) and a smaller peak between the 5th and 7th decades. There is a slight female predominance.

The incidence and prevalence of Crohn's disease worldwide are rising, affecting both developed and underdeveloped countries. The incidence and prevalence of Crohn's disease in North America are estimated to be 3.1–14.6 cases per 100 000 person years and 26–199 cases per 100 000 persons, respectively [1].

Pathophysiology

The pathogenesis of Crohn's disease is unknown, but it is thought to manifest from abnormal interactions between the immune system, microbiota, and environmental factors in a genetically susceptible host. Environmental factors trigger the onset or reactivation of disease by transiently breaking the mucosal barrier and activating the immune response [2] (Figure 45.1).

About 15% of patients will have a relative with inflammatory bowel disease (IBD), mainly Crohn's disease. The NOD2/CARD15 gene is present in up to 17% of Crohn's disease patients; it has been associated with early-onset Crohn's disease, fibrostenotic disease, ileal Crohn's disease, and a family history of Crohn's disease. Other single-nucleotide polymorphisms in the SLC22A4 and IL-23 genes have also been associated with Crohn's disease.

Smoking, geographic location (colder climates), westernization of lifestyle, and industrialization of developing countries have been implicated as potential environmental risk factors.

Clinical Features

Symptoms vary according to disease location and behavior (inflammatory, stricturing, and penetrating/fistulizing disease). Locations includes ileal (30%), colonic (20%), ileocolonic (40%), and upper GI (<5%) disease.

Common symptoms include chronic diarrhea, abdominal pain, fever, and weight loss. Hematochezia points toward colonic disease. Perianal pain, drainage, and fevers are characteristic of perianal fistulas with or without abscesses. Esophageal Crohn's disease can present as dysphagia, odynophagia, chest pain, and gastroesophageal reflux disease (GERD). Gastric and duodenal Crohn's disease are marked by epigastric pain, nausea, vomiting, or gastric outlet obstruction. Obstructive symptoms can be seen in stricturing disease affecting the upper or lower GI tract.

Extraintestinal manifestations include peripheral arthritis, spondylarthritis (sacroiliitis and ankylosing spondyloarthropathy), ocular inflammation (uveitis, scleritis, and episcleritis), cutaneous manifestations (erythema nodosum and pyoderma gangrenosum), primary sclerosing cholangitis, and hypercoagulability. Adenocarcinoma of the GI tract is associated with longstanding Crohn's disease. Other associated disease manifestations such as anemia, osteoporosis, osteopenia, cholelithiasis, and nephrolithiasis can occur.

Disease Severity

Remission can be described as clinical, endoscopic, or surgical. The Crohn's Disease Activity Index (CDAI) is a validated tool for

Practical Gastroenterology and Hepatology Board Review Toolkit, Second Edition. Edited by Nicholas J. Talley, Kenneth R. DeVault, Michael B. Wallace, Bashar A. Aqel and Keith D. Lindor.

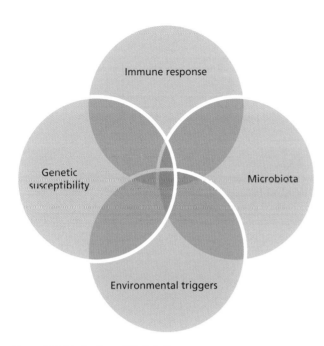

Figure 45.1 Mechanisms of Crohn's disease.

measuring clinical severity (Table 45.1). Clinical remission is defined as being asymptomatic due to medical or surgical therapy (corresponding to a CDAI < 150). Asymptomatic but steroid-dependent patients are not considered to be in clinical remission.
- **Mild to moderate disease (CDAI 150–220):** No systemic symptoms, abdominal pain, painful mass, obstructive symptoms, or >10% weight loss.
- **Moderate to severe disease (CDAI 220–450):** Failed therapy for mild to moderate disease and systemic symptoms, abdominal pain, obstructive symptoms, significant weight loss, or anemia.

Table 45.1 Crohn's Disease Activity Index (CDAI).

Variable	Descriptor	Score	Multiplier
Number of liquid stools	Sum of 7 days		×2
Abdominal pain	Sum of 7 days' ratings	0 = none 1 = mild 2 = moderate 3 = severe	×5
General well being	Sum of 7 days' ratings	0 = generally well 1 = slightly under par 2 = poor 3 = very poor 4 = terrible	×7
Extraintestinal complications	Number of listed complications	Arthritis/arthralgia, iritis/ uveitis, erythema nodosum, pyoderma gangrenosum, apthous stomatitis, anal fissure/ fistula/abscess, fever >37.8 °C	×20
Antidiarrheal drugs	Use in the previous 7 days	0 = no 1 = yes	×30
Abdominal mass		0 = no 2 = questionable 5 = definite	×10
Hematocrit	Expected– observed hematocrit	Males: 47 observed Females: 42 observed	×6
Body weight	Ideal/observed ratio	(1 – (ideal/observed)) × 100	1 (not < –10)

- **Fulminant disease (CDAI > 450)** no response to corticosteroids or biologic agents (infliximab, adalimumab, certolizumab, vedolizumab or natalizumab). Toxic-appearing with systemic symptoms, abdominal pain and guarding, evidence of an abscess, persistent obstructive symptoms, and evidence of intestinal obstruction [3].

Diagnosis

The diagnosis is based on a combination of clinical symptoms, endoscopy, imaging, and histology [4]. The sequence of testing is based on the clinical symptoms and physical exam findings. Genetic testing and serological studies (anti-*Saccharomyces cerevisiae* antibody (ASCA), antineutrophil cytoplasmic antibody (pANCA), etc.) should not be used as screening tools for the diagnosis of Crohn's disease.

Laboratory Findings

Erythrocyte sedimentation rate, C-reactive protein (CRP), and high fecal calprotectin levels can be good indicators of intestinal inflammation but are non-specific. Serologic markers including ASCA, perinuclear antineutrophil cytoplasmic antibody (pANCA), and antibodies directed against CBir1 and OmpC are supportive of Crohn's disease but are not diagnostic.

An elevated white blood cell (WBC) count can be seen in active luminal disease or an abscess. Anemias are frequently seen and can be secondary to blood loss, iron deficiency, vitamin B12 deficiency, or folate deficiency, or a result of chronic inflammatory disease. In severe cases, hypoalbuminemia, hypokalemia, and metabolic acidosis can be found.

Endoscopy

Colonoscopy with biopsies can determine the location, extent, and severity of disease (Figure 45.2). Terminal ileum intubation with biopsies is key to accurately defining distal small-bowel involvement. Upper GI endoscopy can confirm the presence of Crohn's disease in the esophagus, stomach, and duodenum. Video-capsule endoscopy can be used to help define GI involvement between the duodenum and distal ileum, where upper and lower endoscopy cannot reach. Video-capsule endoscopy is contraindicated in stricturing Crohn's disease.

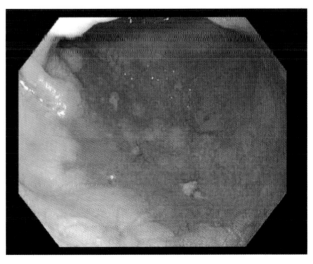

Figure 45.2 Colonoscopy showing discrete patchy erythema involving the ascending colon and distal ileum in a skip pattern.

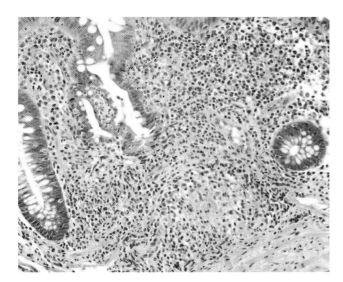

Figure 45.3 Biopsy showing chronic colitis with crypt distortion, cryptitis, and non-caseating granulomas.

Characteristic lesions at endoscopy are superficial ulcers, deep linear or serpiginous ulcers, pseudopolyps, and strictures.

Radiographic Findings

Computed tomographic (CT) enterography or magnetic resonance (MR) enterography can be used to assess the extent, location, and complications (fistula, abscess, strictures) of small-bowel Crohn's disease. Magnetic resonance imaging (MRI) can be used to evaluate perianal (fistulas and abscesses) Crohn's disease. A barium swallow with small-bowel follow-through can be used to assess esophageal, stomach, duodenal, and small-bowel disease.

Histology

In early Crohn's disease, the histopathology is characterized by an acute inflammatory infiltrate and crypt abscesses (Figure 45.3). Later on, there is distortion of mucosal crypt architecture, lymphocytic inflammatory infiltrate, crypt abscesses, and, in some subjects, non-caseating granulomas. Non-caseating granulomas are not unique to Crohn's disease but help distinguish Crohn's disease from ulcerative colitis.

> ### Case Continued
>
> Stool studies are negative for common bacterial pathogens and *Clostridium difficile*. Blood work is notable for a normocytic anemia with a hemoglobin of 10 g/dL and a CRP of 26.3 mg/L. Colonoscopy shows discrete patchy erythema involving the ascending colon and distal ileum in a skip pattern. Biopsies are obtained and reveal chronic colitis with crypt distortion, cryptitis, and non-caseating granulomas (Figure 45.3). An MRI of the pelvis shows a complex perianal fistula with abscess. The findings are suggestive of Crohn's disease. The patient is counseled on quitting smoking.

Differential Diagnosis

Crohn's disease should be differentiated from other infectious and non-infectious inflammatory disorders that can affect the small bowel and colon (Table 45.2).

Table 45.2 Infectious and non-infectious inflammatory disorders affecting the small bowel and colon.

Infections	Bacterial
	Enterohemorrhagic *E.coli*
	Campylobacter jejuni
	Yersinia
	Clostridium difficile
	Mycobacterium tuberculosis
	Salmonella
	Shigella
	Viral
	Cytomegalovirus (CMV)
	Herpes simplex virus (HSV)
	Fungal
	Histoplasma capsulatum
	Parasites
	Entamoeba histolytica
Non-infectious disorders	*Vascular*
	Wegner's granulomatosis
	Behçet's disease
	Churg–Strauss syndrome
	Henoch–Schönlein purpura
	Systemic lupus erythematosus (SLE)
	Polyarteritis nodosa
	Ischemia
	Neoplasia
	Carcinoid
	Carcinoma
	Lymphoma
	Medications/toxins
	Non-steroidal anti-inflammatory drugs (NSAIDs)
	Radiation
	Inflammatory
	Appendicitis
	Diverticular disease
	Celiac disease
	Microscopic colitis
	Miscellaneous
	Solitary rectal ulcer syndrome

Therapeutics

A combination of medical and surgical treatment is often needed to induce and maintain remission in Crohn's disease. Modifiable risk factors such as smoking should be discussed as part of the treatment algorithm (Figure 45.4).

Medical Therapy

The aim of medical therapy is to induce and maintain clinical remission, with the ultimate goal of achieving mucosal healing. The choice of medical therapy depends on the location and severity of disease and on disease-associated complications (Table 45.3).

Aminosalicylates

Sulfasalazine, oral mesalamine (Pentasa, Asacol, Lialda, Apriso), rectal mesalamine (Canasa, Rowasa), olsalazine (Dipentum), and balsalazide (Colazal) are drugs that deliver 5-aminosalicylate. Data suggest that oral mesalamine is minimally effective versus placebo and less effective than budesonide or corticosteroids. Sulfasalazine has only modest efficacy for inducing remission in mild to moderate ileocolonic and colonic Crohn's disease when compared to placebo [5].

Mesalamine, olsalazine, and balsalazide are better tolerated than sulfasalazine (headache, nausea, vomiting, rash). Rash, alopecia, and hypersensitivity reaction resulting in worsening diarrhea can occur. Severe adverse events such as interstitial nephritis, pancreatitis, and pneumonitis can rarely occur. Yearly urinalysis and creatinine should be checked for patients on mesalamine products.

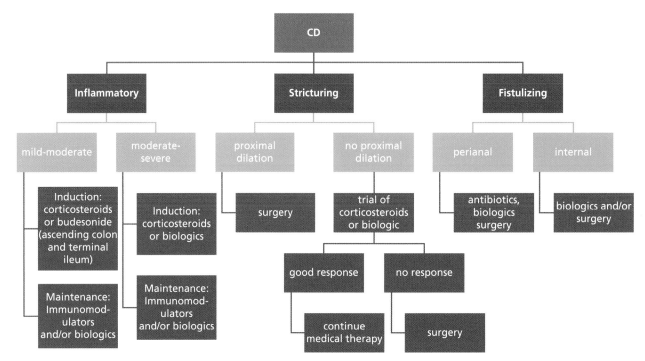

Figure 45.4 Algorithm for the management of Crohn's disease.

Antibiotics

Antibiotic therapy for luminal disease is widely debated. Antibiotics such as metronidazole and ciprofloxacin are used for perianal Crohn's disease. Metronidazole helps prevent 1 year-postoperative recurrence of Crohn's disease when given after surgery [6].

Corticosteroids

Oral prednisone at a dose of 40–60 mg daily is effective for inducing remission in mild to moderate Crohn's disease. However, prednisone is not effective for maintenance of remission. Long-term prednisone use is associated with increased risk of infection,

Table 45.3 Medications used in Crohn's disease.

Drug	Dose	Release site
5-aminosalicylates		
Sulfasalazine (Azulfidine)	2–6 g/day	Colon
Mesalamine (Asacol, Lialda)	2.4–4.8 g/day	Distal ileum, colon
Mesalamine (Pentasa)	2–4 g/day	Duodenum, jejunum, ileum, colon
Olsalazine (Dipentum)	1–3 g/day	Colon
Balsalazide (Colazal)	6.25 g/day	Colon
Mesalamine (Rowasa) enema	4g/day	Rectum, sigmoid
Mesalamine (Canasa) suppository	1 g/day	Rectum
Corticosteroids		
Budesonide (Entocort)	Induction: 9 mg/day orally	Small intestine, right colon
	Maintenance: 3–6 mg/day orally	
Prednisone	40–60 mg/kg/day orally	Systemic
Methylprednisolone	40–60 mg/day IV	Systemic
Immunomodulators		
6-mercaptopurine	1–1.5 mg/kg daily	Systemic
Azathioprine	2–2.5 mg/kg daily	Systemic
Methotrexate	Induction: 25 mg SC/IM every week for 4 months	Systemic
	Maintenance: 15 mg SC/IM every week	
Biologics		
Infliximab	Induction: 5 mg/kg IV at weeks 0, 2, and 6	Systemic
	Maintenance: 5 mg/kg IV every 8 weeks	
Adalimumab	Induction: 160 mg SC at week 0, 80 mg at week 2	Systemic
	Maintenance: 40 mg SC every other week	
Certolizumab pegol	Induction: 400 mg SC at weeks 0, 2, and 4	Systemic
	Maintenance: 400 mg SC every 4 weeks	
Natalizumab	Induction: 300 mg IV at weeks 0, 4, and 8	Systemic
	Maintenance: 300 mg IV every 4 weeks	
Vedolizumab	Induction: 300 mg IV at weeks 0, 2, and 6	Systemic
	Maintenance: 300 mg IV every 8 weeks	

IV, intravenous; SC, subcutaneous; IM, intramuscular; FDA, Food and Drug Administration.

diabetes mellitus, osteoporosis, osteonecrosis, cataracts, glaucoma, and myopathy. Corticosteroids are associated with serious infections and increase risk of mortality – long-term corticosteroid use should be minimized [7].

Controlled-release oral budesonide at 9 mg daily has been demonstrated to be more effective than placebo and mesalamine and as equally effective as oral corticosteroids for induction of remission of mild to moderate Crohn's disease involving the distal ileum and/or right colon. Long-term budesonide use is not recommended for maintenance therapy [8]. Budesonide MMX is an extended-release formulation of budesonide that is released in the colon; it is Food and Drug Administration (FDA)-approved for ulcerative colitis. Budesonide has a high first-pass metabolism and therefore a more desirable side-effect profile when compared to oral corticosteroids.

Thiopurines

Azathioprine and 6-mercaptopurine are not more effective than placebo in inducing remission of Crohn's disease. Thiopurines (2.0–2.5 mg/kg for azathioprine and 1.0–1.5 mg/kg 6-mercaptopurine daily) are effective in maintaining a steroid-induced remission of Crohn's disease [9]. The primary enzyme that metabolizes azathioprine/6-mercaptopurine is thiopurine methyltransferase (TPMT). The FDA recommends measuring TPMT prior to starting therapy with azathioprine/6-mercaptopurine in order to help determine whether patients are rapid or slow metabolizers.

Side effects associated with thiopurine use include allergic reactions, pancreatitis, myelosuppression, nausea, infections, hepatotoxicity, and malignancy – particularly lymphoma. Routine labs such as complete blood cell (CBC) count and liver enzymes need to be done to monitor for myelosuppression and drug-induced hepatitis.

Methotrexate

Methotrexate is not more effective than placebo in inducing remission of Crohn's disease [9]. Methotrexate at doses of 15–25 mg subcutaneously or intramuscularly weekly has been shown to be effective at maintaining steroid-induced remission in moderate to severe Crohn's disease [10]. Adverse events include rash, nausea, diarrhea, myelosuppression, hepatic fibrosis, and rarely hypersensitivity pneumonitis. A baseline chest X-ray is recommended prior to initiation of therapy. Risk factors for methotrexate hepatotoxicity include diabetes, obesity, baseline high liver enzymes, excessive or long-term alcohol use, daily methotrexate use, and a cumulative dose of methotrexate exceeding 1.5 g total drug. Baseline liver biopsy is indicated for those with chronic liver disease, elevated liver enzymes, or one or more risk factors for hepatotoxicity. Routine monitoring for leukopenia and drug-induced hepatitis is recommended.

Anti-TNF agents

Infliximab, adalimumab, and certolizumab have been approved for the induction and maintenance of moderate to severe Crohn's disease [11]. These drugs are also effective in treating fistulizing and perianal disease.

Infliximab is an infusion given at 5 mg/kg at weeks 0, 2, and 6 for induction, then every 8 weeks for maintenance. Combination therapy of thiopurines and infliximab is superior to either therapy alone [12]. Adalimumab is administered subcutaneously at a dose of 160 mg at week 0 and 80 mg at week 2 for induction, followed by 40 mg every other week for maintenance [13]. Certolizumab is administered subcutaneously at a dose of 400 mg at weeks 0, 2, and 4 for induction, then 400 mg every 4 weeks for maintenance [14].

Adverse events include infections (tuberculosis, fungal infections, etc.), autoantibody formation, psoriasis, drug-induced lupus, infusion reactions (infliximab), injection-site reaction (adalimumab and certolizumab), delayed hypersensitivity reaction (infliximab), and lymphoma (higher in combination therapy). Tuberculosis testing and screening for hepatitis B should be done prior to initiation of anti-tumor necrosis factor (TNF) agents.

Natalizumab

Natalizumab is a humanized monoclonal antibody against alpha-4 integrin and is effective in the induction and maintenance of remission in moderate to severe Crohn's disease. Natalizumab is administered intravenously at doses of 300 mg at weeks 0, 4, and 8 for induction, followed by 300 mg monthly for maintenance [15]. Natalizumab is associated with the reactivation of human JC polyoma virus, which leads to fatal progressive multifocal leukoencephalopathy (PML). Therefore, natalizumab is only given once patients have failed other therapies (steroids, immunomodulators, anti-TNF agents). To minimize the risk of PML, natalizumab is given as monotherapy, and only to those who are JC virus antibody-negative at baseline [16]. Other side effects include infusion reaction, hepatotoxicity, infections, and autoantibody formation.

Vedolizumab

Vedolizumab is a humanized antibody to α4β7 integrin. It modulates lymphocyte trafficking in the gut and not the brain, making it theoretically less likely to cause PML. Studies show that vedolizumab is effective in the induction and maintenance of remission in moderate to severe Crohn's disease. Vedolizumab is an infusion given at 300 mg at week 0, 2, and 6 weeks for induction and 300 mg every 8 weeks thereafter for maintenance [17]. The most common side effects are nasopharyngitis and transient elevations in liver enzymes. No cases of PML has been reported to date.

Surgery

About two-thirds of Crohn's disease patients will require surgery for their Crohn's disease in their lifetime. Surgical resection, stricturoplasty, or drainage of abscesses is indicated to treat medically refractory disease or complications. Fistulizing and perianal Crohn's disease is often treated with a combination of surgery and medical therapy.

Patients should be evaluated 6–12 months after surgical resection for recurrence of disease. They should be risk-stratified based on their disease behavior (penetrating disease), duration of disease (short), smoking status, and number of prior surgeries. Moderate-to high-risk patients should be treated with immunomodulators and/or biologics to prevent recurrence of disease [18].

Case Continued

Exam under anesthesia with drainage of the abscess and seton placement is performed. The patient is started on a course of antibiotics with ciprofloxacin. Combination therapy with azathioprine 2 mg/kg and infliximab 5 mg/kg is initiated. He has a good clinical response, with cessation of diarrhea and weight gain at 6 weeks. Repeat colonoscopy at 6 months shows mucosal healing. MRI shows successful healing of his perianal fistula, and his seton is removed. He successfully quits smoking by participating in a smoking cessation program.

Prognosis

Crohn's disease is a multisystem disorder with potential for systemic and extraintestinal complications. Patients with Crohn's disease have a slightly higher morbidity and mortality risk compared to the general population. Treatment of Crohn's disease with corticosteroids or narcotics is associated with an increase in mortality risk. Treatment with infliximab and immunomodulators in a 5-year follow-up study did not show an increase in mortality [19].

Aggressive medical and/or surgical treatment is required to induce and maintain remission, minimize complications, and improve quality of life.

Take Home Points

- Crohn's disease is a disorder of the immune system that leads to asymmetric, transmural, and sometimes granulomatous inflammation, which can occur anywhere in the gastrointestinal (GI) tract.
- Symptoms of Crohn's disease vary with disease location, behavior (inflammatory, stricturing, penetrating/fistulizing disease), and complications.
- The diagnosis of Crohn's disease is based on a combination of clinical symptoms, endoscopy, imaging, and histology.
- Crohn's disease should be differentiated from other infectious and non-infectious inflammatory disorders that can affect the small bowel and colon.
- A combination of medical and surgical treatment is often needed to induce and maintain remission in Crohn's disease.
- Modifiable risk factors such as smoking and the use of non-steroidal anti-inflammatory drugs (NSAIDs) should be eliminated as part of the treatment algorithm for Crohn's disease.
- Long-term corticosteroid use and narcotics should be minimized, as they increase mortality risk in Crohn's disease patients.

References

1 Loftus E. Clinical epidemiology of inflammatory bowel disease: Incidence, prevalence, and environmental influences. *Gastroenterology* 2004; **126**: 1504–17.

2 Sartor R. Mechanisms of disease: pathogenesis of Crohn's disease and ulcerative colitis. *Nat Clin Pract Gastroenterol Hepatol* 2006; **3**: 390–407.

3 Lichtenstein G, Hanauer S, Sandborn W; Practice Parameters Committee of American College of Gastroenterology. Management of Crohn's disease in adults. *Am J Gastroenterol* 2009; **104**: 465.

4 Stange E, Travis SPL, Vermeire S, *et al.* European evidence based consensus on the diagnosis and management of Crohn's disease: definitions and diagnosis. *Gut* 2006; **55**(Suppl. 1): 15.

5 Ford AC, Kane SV, Khan KJ, *et al.* Efficacy of 5-aminosalicylates in Crohn's disease: systematic review and meta-analysis. *Am J Gastroenterol* 2011; **106**: 617–29.

6 Rutgeerts P, Van Assche G, Vermeire S, *et al.* Ornidazole for prophylaxis of postoperative Crohn's disease recurrence: a randomized, double-blind, placebo-controlled trial. *Gastroenterology* 2005; **128**: 856–61.

7 Irving P, Gearry R, Sparrow M, Gibson P. Review article: appropriate use of corticosteroids in Crohn's disease. *Aliment Pharmacol Ther* 2007; **26**: 313–29.

8 Kane SV, Schoenfeld P, Sandborn WJ, *et al.* The effectiveness of budesonide therapy for Crohn's disease. *Aliment Pharmacol Ther* 2002; **16**: 1509–17.

9 Dassopoulos T, Sultan S, Falck-Ytter YT, *et al.* American Gastroenterological Association Institute technical review on the use of thiopurines, methotrexate, and anti-TNF-alpha biologic drugs for the induction and maintenance of remission in inflammatory Crohn's disease. *Gastroenterology* 2013; **145**: 1464–78, e1461–5.

10 Feagan BG, Fedorak RN, Irvine EJ, *et al.* A comparison of methotrexate with placebo for the maintenance of remission in Crohn's disease. North American Crohn's Study Group Investigators. *N Engl J Med* 2000; **342**: 1627–32.

11 Peyrin-Biroulet L, Deltenre P, de Suray N, *et al.* Efficacy and safety of tumor necrosis factor antagonists in Crohn's disease: meta-analysis of placebo-controlled trials. *Clin Gastroenterol Hepatol* 2008; **6**: 644–53.

12 Colombel JF, Sandborn WJ, Reinisch W, *et al.* Infliximab, azathioprine, or combination therapy for Crohn's disease. *N Engl J Med* 2010; **362**: 1383–95.

13 Colombel JF, Sandborn WJ, Rutgeerts P, *et al.* Adalimumab for maintenance of clinical response and remission in patients with Crohn's disease: the CHARM trial. *Gastroenterology* 2007; **132**: 52–65.

14 Sandborn WJ, Feagan BG, Stoinov S, *et al.* Certolizumab pegol for the treatment of Crohn's disease. *N Engl J Med* 2007; **357**: 228–38.

15 Targan SR, Feagan BG, Fedorak RN, *et al.* Natalizumab for the treatment of active Crohn's disease: results of the ENCORE Trial. *Gastroenterology* 2007; **132**: 1672–83.

16 Van Assche G, Van Ranst M, Sciot R, *et al.* Progressive multifocal leukoencephalopathy after natalizumab therapy for Crohn's disease. *N Engl J Med* 2005; **353**: 362–8.

17 Sandborn W, Feagan BG, Rutgeerts P, *et al.* Vedolizumab as induction and maintenance therapy for Crohn's disease. *N Engl J Med* 2013; **369**: 711–21.

18 Regueiro M. Management and prevention of postoperative Crohn's disease. *Gastroenterol Hepatol* 2011; **7**: 170–2.

19 Lichtenstein GR, Feagan BG, Cohen RD, *et al.* Serious infection and mortality in patients with Crohn's disease: more than 5 years of follow-up in the TREAT registry. *Am J Gastroenterol* 2012; **107**: 1409–22.

Small-Bowel Tumors

Nadir Arber and Menachem Moshkowitz

Tel-Aviv Sourasky Medical Center, Sackler Faculty of Medicine, Tel-Aviv University, Tel Aviv, Israel

Summary

Tumors of the small bowel, both benign and malignant, are relatively uncommon but may cause significant morbidity and mortality if undetected. These tumors present a diagnostic challenge as their symptoms are often vague. Small bowel tumors have a poor prognosis because most patients present with advanced disease. Surgical resection remains the cornerstone of therapy for these malignancies. New endoscopic modalities such as capsule endoscopy and double balloon enteroscopy allow full examination of the small bowel with improved diagnosis. Advanced endoscopic interventions are likely to broaden the endoscopic management of small bowel tumors.

Case

A 51-year-old woman presented with general malaise, loss of weight, and vomiting. At 18 years of age she had first presented with abdominal pain, diarrhea, and general malaise. Barium follow-through examination showed Crohn disease of the terminal ileum. She was treated with sulfasalazine and corticosteroids. In the following years, the patient experienced repeated episodes of abdominal pain without diarrhea.

Two years ago, the severity of the abdominal pain increased and she underwent ileocolonoscopy, which yielded no suspicious macroscopic or histopathologic findings. Blood tests showed mild iron deficiency and hypoalbuminemia. C-reactive protein (CRP) and erythrocyte sedimentation rate (ESR) were within normal limits. The recommended enteroclysis of the small bowel was not performed. In order to taper her steroids, azathioprine was initiated (3 mg/kg/ day). Recently, she presented again with abdominal pain, vomiting, and distended abdomen. Enteroclysis revealed a dilated intestinal loop of the ileum and a pseudotumor in the right abdomen with two stenotic areas. Prednisone was increased to 50 mg/day, in addition to metronidazole and ciprofloxacine. Three weeks later due to signs of intestinal obstruction, the patient underwent exploratory laparotomy.

The resected small intestinal specimen showed multiple strictures and sacculation with superficial ulceration and fissures, mucosal edema, and fibrosis. There was an ulcerated lesion (3 x 2 cm) 3 cm from the distal end of the resected specimen. Histologic examination showed adenocarcinoma of the small intestine complicating Crohn disease.

Introduction

Small bowel tumors are extremely rare and account for only 1–2% of all gastrointestinal (GI) malignancies [1, 2]. It was estimated that there will be 5640 new cases and 1090 deaths in the United States in 2007, making it one of the most uncommon types of cancer. This low incidence is intriguing, considering the fact that the small bowel comprises 75% of the length and 90% of the mucosal surface area of the alimentary tract. Various theories have been proposed to explain this resistance to carcinogenesis, among them the short contact time with potential carcinogens, reduced intestinal concentrations of inherent potential carcinogens, high concentrations of biliary and pancreatic secretions, low concentration of bacteria, and well-developed local immunoglobulin A antibody (IgA)-mediated immune and lymphatic systems [3].

Practical Gastroenterology and Hepatology: Small and Large Intestine and Pancreas, 1st edition. Edited by Nicholas J. Talley, Sunanda V. Kane and Michael B. Wallace. © 2010 Blackwell Publishing Ltd.

The non-specific symptoms and the lack of typical laboratory and physical signs serve to explain the long latency period before establishing the diagnosis. This delay in identifying the pathology contributes to the poor prognosis and presence of metastases in 50% of the subjects at the time of diagnosis. Approximately two-thirds of all small bowel tumors are malignant, although benign tumors are detected in up to 0.3% of all primary tumors of the small intestine [4].

Benign Tumors of the Small Intestine

Benign tumors of the small intestine include adenomas, leiomyomas, lipomas, hamartomas, desmoid tumors, hemangiomas, lymphangiomas, neurofibromas, and ganglioneuromas, depending on their cell of origin [5].

Adenomas usually appear in the duodenum, mostly on the medial wall, around the ampulla of Vater. A more distal location is rather unusual. Similar to colonic polyps, they are classified as tubular, villous, or tubulovillous. They follow the adenoma–carcinoma sequence, as is seen in colorectal cancer (CRC) [6]. Tubular adenomas bear a relatively low malignant potential, while villous adenomas carry a significant risk of malignant transformation. A focus of carcinoma *in situ* can be detected in 40% of these villous adenomas [7], and synchronous colonic polyps are frequently detected as well. A colonoscopy is a must in these patients. Duodenal adenomas often develop in familial adenomatous polyposis (FAP) syndrome, in which there is a greater risk for malignant transformation than in sporadic cases.

Leiomyomas are true smooth muscle cell tumors arising from the muscularis propria. They are usually small and well-circumscribed. The peak incidence is seen in the sixth decade. Malignant transformation is unusual when they are less than 4 cm in diameter. They need to be differentiated from gastrointestinal stromal tumors (GISTs).

Brunner gland hyperplasia is defined as benign hyperplasia of the exocrine glandular structures in the postpyloric part of the duodenum. It carries no malignant risk. Systemic neurofibromatosis (von Recklinghausen disease) involves the small bowel in up to 25% of the patients. The submucosal neurofibromas tend mostly to be asymptomatic, but ulceration of the overlying mucosa may be a cause of GI bleeding.

Hamartomas are found in Peutz–Jeghers syndrome (PJS), a rare autosomal dominant disorder characterized by multiple hamartomatous (non-neoplastic) GI polyps that are spread throughout the entire GI tract and which have characteristic mucocutaneous melanin pigmentation. These hamartomatous polyps arise in the stromal tissue of the muscularis mucosae and vary in size from a few millimeters up to 5 cm. They have normal overlying mucosa, and develop as early as the first decade of life. They become symptomatic by the age of 10–30 years, and are characterized by signs of intussusception, intestinal obstruction, or ulceration with bleeding. A germline mutation in the *LKB1/STK11* gene can be found in 50% of the families. Hamartomas *per se* do not harbor any cancer risk, but adenomatous tissue can be formed in 5% of them. Up to 90% of patients with PJS carry a lifetime risk for cancer, including colon, small bowel, pancreatic, cervical, uterine, ovarian, breast, testicular, and lung cancers [8].

Malignant Small Bowel Tumors

Small bowel cancer has four major histologic subtypes: adenocarcinoma is the most common malignancy (accounting for 40–50% of all primary small bowel neoplasm) [3], followed by neuroendocrine tumors (20–40%, mostly carcinoids that are located in the ileum), lymphomas (14%) and GISTs (11–13%).

The mean age at diagnosis is 57 years (median 67 years), males are slightly more affected, and African Americans have almost twice the incidence compared to caucasians [2].

Adenocarcinoma of the Small Bowel

This malignancy occurs most frequently within the duodenum (49%), particularly around the ampulla of Vater, and with decreasing frequency in the jejunum (21%) and ileum (15%) [9]. It is more common in men than in women and twice as common in African Americans. In Crohn-associated cases, 70% of adenocarcinomas are found in the ileum [10]. Risk factors for this type of tumor include: Crohn disease [11], FAP [12], and hereditary non-polyposis colorectal cancer syndrome. Smoking, alcohol use, high intake of sugar, red meat, salt cured/ smoked foods or low intake of fish, fruit, and vegetables, and environmental factors, such as radiation therapy, have all been associated with increased risk for small bowel tumors [13,14].

Neuroendocrine Tumors

The term "neuroendocrine tumor (NET)" (also called carcinoid and APUDoma) is used for all endocrine tumors of the digestive system that derive from the intestinal neuroendocrine system [15]. The mucosa of the GI tract contains at least 15 different endocrine cell types that produce hormonal peptides and/or biogenic amines

[16]. NETs are more common in the ileum (mostly located within 60 cm of the ileocecal valve). The clinical picture is characterized by sluggish biologic behavior. The vast majority of the tumors are carcinoids with some gastrinomas located in the duodenum. Other types of NETs are quite rare in the small bowel. Most of the cases are sporadic, but some are associated with inherited syndromes, with multiple endocrine neoplasia type 1 being the most significant among them. Diagnostic strategies include ultrasonography (US), computerized tomography (CT), magnetic resonance imaging (MRI), bone scanning, angiography, and, in rare cases, selective venous sampling for hormonal gradients. Somatostatin receptor scintigraphy has begun to play a central role as well [17].

Gastrointestinal Stromal Tumors

Mesenchymal tumors of the small bowel comprise a widely diverse group of neoplasms (leiomyoma, schwannoma, neurofibroma, sarcoma, and others). GISTs are the most common subtype of mesenchymal neoplasm, and they are derived from the interstitial cells of Cajal. They occur anywhere within the GI tract, but are most common in the stomach (60–70%) and small bowel (20–25%) [18]. GISTs may be benign or malignant, depending on their size and mitotic index. They are submucosal, highly vascular tumors ranging in size from 1 to 40 cm. Ulceration of these lesions is common, and intestinal bleeding is a frequent symptom. GISTs also may invade adjacent organs directly or spread via peritoneal seeding. Compared with gastric GISTs, small bowel GISTs tend to be more aggressive and have a worse prognosis. Metastases develop in nearly 50% of patients, primarily via the hematogenous route, commonly involving the liver and peritoneum. GISTs smaller than 2 cm with a low mitotic index are generally considered benign with a very low risk of recurrence. About 5% of GIST cases are multiple, and an increased incidence is seen in patients with neurofibromatosis type 1. Gain-of-function mutations in exon 11 of the *c-kit* proto-oncogene are associated with most cases of GISTs [19].

Primary Lymphomas

Up to 40% of lymphomas develop in sites other than the lymph nodes, with the gut being the most common extralymphatic site [20]. Several patterns of small bowel lymphoma have been identified, including an infiltrating pattern which appears as wall thickening, an exophytic mass that sometimes simulates an adenocarcinoma or GIST, multifocal submucosal nodules within the small bowel, and single mass lesions which can lead to intussusceptions.

Four different histologic types of lymphomas may be found in the small bowel:

Celiac-Associated T-cell High-Grade Lymphoma

Enteropathy-associated T-cell lymphoma is a rare form of high-grade T-cell non-Hodgkin lymphoma (NHL) of the upper small intestine that is associated with celiac disease [21]. An abnormal clonal intraepithelial lymphocyte cell population is diffusely present throughout the GI tract in approximately 80% of refractory celiac disease cases. These cells are characterized by a low ratio of $CD_8{}^+/CD_3{}^+$ and T cell receptor (TCR)-γ gene rearrangement [22]

Burkitt-Type Lymphoma of the Small Intestine

Burkitt lymphoma is an aggressive type of B-cell lymphoma that has two major forms: endemic (African) and non-endemic (sporadic). The sporadic form usually involves abdominal organs, with the most common being the distal ileum, cecum, or mesentery. Burkitt lymphoma is a childhood tumor that can also be observed in adult patients. It is characterized by a high rate of malignant cell proliferation (indicated by ki-67 expression) and by morphologic features that are distinct from diffuse large B-cell lymphoma. Burkitt lymphoma can be seen in the setting of acquired immune deficiency syndrome (AIDS) or chronic immunosuppression [23].

Mucosa-Associated Lymphoid Tissue Lymphoma – Maltoma

Maltoma was first defined as a primary low-grade gastric B-cell lymphoma and immunoproliferative small intestinal disease. This definition was later extended to include several other extranodal low-grade B-cell NHLs. The gastric form is the most common and best characterized maltoma. These tumors tend to stay localized in the mucosal wall without involvement of regional lymph nodes. This type of malignancy has recently been linked with the response to bacterial infections [24].

Immunoproliferative Small Intestinal Disease (Mediterranean Lymphoma)

This is an unusual intestinal B-cell lymphoma that occurs mostly in children and young adults of Mediterranean ancestry, and is associated with a single protein abnormality. The mucosal IgA α-heavy chain has a deletion in its variable region [25]. Treatment with antibiotics can lead to remission, suggesting that the proliferative burst is due to an aberrant immunogenic response to bacterial infection. *Campylobacter jejuni* was shown to play a role in this disease, similar to the role of *Helicobacter pylori* in gastric MALT lymphoma [26].

Clinical Features

Small bowel tumors are usually asymptomatic in the early stages. The rarity of these tumors and the subtle and non-specific presenting symptoms may delay the diagnosis. The most frequent are abdominal pain, nausea, vomiting, and intestinal obstruction (50% of the patients undergo emergency surgery for intestinal obstruction) [27]. The nature of the symptoms depends mainly on the size and location of the tumor, with lesions distal to the ligament of Treitz tending to present with either obstruction or bleeding, while GISTs more commonly present with acute GI bleeding. The most common laboratory abnormality is hypochromic microcytic anemia, and many of these patients have a positive test for fecal occult blood. Direct hyperbilirubinemia and increased alkaline phosphatase are usually found in cases of duodenal tumors as a consequence of extrahepatic biliary obstruction. Clinical features of small-bowel tumors are listed in Table 46.1.

Diagnosis

Early detection of a small bowel neoplasm is certainly desirable but a challenging prospect. The detection of small intestinal tumors by traditional imaging modalities is often compromised by overlapping bowel loops and suboptimal bowel distension. Newer techniques are expected to improve diagnostic capabilities.

Imaging Modalities

Small Bowel Follow-Through

This is the oldest barium study traditionally used for evaluation of the small bowel. The true value of this non-invasive test is open to question due to the reported wide range of sensitivity for tumor detection (30–90%) [29].

Table 46.1 Staging of small bowel carcinoma. Source: Greene 2002 [28]. Reproduced by permission of Springer.

Primary tumor stage (T)	
TX	Primary tumor cannot be assessed
T0	No evidence of primary tumor is present
Tis	Carcinoma *in situ* is present
T1	Tumor invades the lamina propria or submucosa
T2	Tumor invades the muscularis propria
T3	Tumor invades through the muscularis propria into subserosa or into nonperitonealized perimuscular tissue (mesentery or retroperitoneum), with extension of < 2 cm
T4	Tumor penetrates the visceral peritoneum or directly invades other organs or structures

Regional lymph nodes (N)	
NX	Regional lymph nodes cannot be assessed
N0	No regional lymph node metastasis is present
N1	Regional lymph node metastasis has occurred

Distant metastases (M)	
MX	Presence of distant metastasis cannot be assessed
M0	No distant metastasis is present
M1	Distant metastasis has occurred

Stage grouping	T	N	M
Stage 0	Tis	N0	M0
Stage I	T1-2	N0	M0
Stage II	T3-4	N0	M0
Stage III	Any T	N1	M0
Stage IV	Any T	Any N	M1

Enteroclysis

This is considered superior to small bowel followthrough due to the minute mucosal detail that can be demonstrated, its specificity and sensitivity. It is, however, a more difficult procedure for both the radiologist and the patient, requiring nasojejunal intubation and oral administration of large volumes of contrast material. The sensitivity of enteroclysis is as high as 95%, with 90% correct estimation of the actual size of the tumor.

Multidetector Computed Tomography Scans

Multidetector CT scans (MDCTs) produce high-resolution crosssectional imaging of the abdomen and small bowel. The lumen of the small bowel must be distended with orally administered contrast material to demonstrate the wall thickening that characterizes small bowel tumors on CT. An MDCT allows multiplanar visualization of small bowel tumors, and demonstrates signs of small bowel obstruction as well as the mural and extramural extent of small bowel malignancies.

Multidetector Computed Tomography Enteroclysis

Multidetector CT enteroclysis (MDCT-E) shares the advantages of both conventional enteroclysis and crosssectional imaging. This technique is more sensitive than conventional barium studies and less invasive than enteroscopy, and lesions as small as 5 mm can be identified. MDCT-E studies have shown 100% sensitivity and 85–95% concordance with enteroscopy [30]. The recent introduction of cellulose as the contrast material has significantly increased the sensitivity and specificity of CT enterography.

Magnetic Resonance Imaging and Magnetic Resonance Enteroclysis

The advantages of MRI over CT include excellent soft tissue contrast, absence of exposure to radiation and iodine contrast, and multiple contrast sources. MR enteroclysis includes small bowel intubation and the administration of a biphasic contrast agent. This protocol can provide anatomic demonstration of the normal intestinal wall, identification of wall thickening or timorous lesions, lesion characterization or evaluation of disease activity, and assessment of exoenteric/mesenteric disease extension [31].

FDG-Positron Emission Tomography

The role of positron emission tomography (PET) in the initial diagnosis of small bowel malignant tumors has not yet been established. It can serve to monitor response to treatment and is highly sensitive and specific for the evaluation of nodal and extranodal patients with malignant lymphomas [32].

Push Enteroscopy

Push enteroscopy permits evaluation of the proximal one-third of the small intestine to a distance that is approximately 50–100 cm beyond the ligament of Treitz. The diagnostic yield of this technique is reported to increase with a greater depth of scope insertion. Data on the diagnostic yield of small bowel tumors and polyps are limited to studies that have investigated push enteroscopy in the context of obscure GI bleeding, with a reported yield in the range of 1–5% [33, 34].

Video Capsule Endoscopy

Video capsule endoscopy (VCE) is safe, easy, minimally invasive, and patient-friendly, and has become a first-line tool in imaging and managing small bowel pathologies [35]. The utility of VCE has more than doubled the rate of detection of small bowel tumors from the precapsule endoscopy era of approximately 3% to today's 6–9% prevalence rate, when the procedure is done for obscure GI bleeding. The detected small bowel tumors are malignant in more than 50% of cases [36]. VCE examinations reach the cecum about 80% of the time and luminal debris and bubbles interfere with viewing in some patients. Capsule retention is the major and, for all practical purposes, the only complication of VCE. The reported incidence of capsule retention ranges from 0% in healthy volunteers to 2% in obscure GI hemorrhage, reaching up to 21% in individuals with suspected small bowel obstruction. The retention rate in patients with small bowel tumors may be around 10%.

Double Balloon Enteroscopy

Double balloon enteroscopy (DBE) is a novel endoscopic insertion technique that uses a high-resolution, dedicated video endoscope with a working length of 200 cm and two soft latex balloons, one attached to the tip of the endoscope and the other to the distal end of a soft, flexible overtube. The balloons can be inflated and deflated using an air pump that is controlled by the endoscopist while monitoring air pressure. DBE has been shown to be of both diagnostic and therapeutic value. DBE was found to be accurate in demonstrating the bleeding sites in 115 (75.7%) patients with obscure bleeding, of which 45 (39.1%) were due to small bowel tumors [37]. There are limitations associated with DBE, including concerns about the learning curve, the need for endoscopy on two separate days (transoral and then transanal approaches), limitations in visualization of the entire small bowel, miss rates for subepithelial lesions due to inadequate insufflation, its being a time-consuming procedure that requires a high level of ancillary staffing, the high level of sedation requirements, and patient tolerance and preferences. In addition, although uncommon, the reported incidence of severe complications associated with DBE ranges from 0% to 2.5% and these include pancreatitis, perforations, bleeding, abdominal pain, and fever.

Intraoperative Enteroscopy

This has been utilized since the 1980s and is an important diagnostic and potentially therapeutic endoscopic modality in suspected small bowel polyps and tumors [38]. It is considered to be the ultimate endoscopic evaluation of the small bowel. The reported complications include mucosal lacerations, perforations, prolonged ileus, abdominal abscess, and bowel ischemia.

Therapy

Benign Tumors

A simple endoscopic snare polypectomy is the treatment of choice for adenomatous polyps located within the reach of esophagogastroduodenoscopy. If this is not technically feasible, a local surgical excision is indicated, and close endoscopic follow-up is warranted. All patients with duodenal adenomas should undergo colonoscopy to rule out polyposis syndromes, especially FAP.

Lipomas should not be resected unless they are symptomatic.

Benign leiomyomas should be resected only if they are symptomatic, if they cannot be differentiated from GISTs, or if there is doubt about their being benign or malignant.

Neurofibromatas in patients with von Recklinghausen disease are considered to be benign and should not be resected unless they are symptomatic.

Hamartomatous polyps in PJS generally are not premalignant and they should only be resected if they become symptomatic (bleeding, intussusceptions, obstruction), if their size exceeds 15 mm, or if they reveal macroscopic or microscopic features that are suspicious for malignant degeneration. Since polyps in PJS patients are abundant, and considering the high lifetime risk for having multiple interventions, appropriate surgical management consists of surgical enterectomy and polypectomy. If bowel resection is required, an absolute minimum length of bowel should be sacrificed in order to limit the risk for development of short bowel syndrome. Appropriate surveillance of the proband and his/ her first-degree relatives is warranted.

Adenocarcinoma

Wide surgical resection of early lesions is the sole potentially curative treatment, but it is possible only in a minority of patients. The rarity of these tumors has resulted in a paucity of information on the benefits of adjuvant chemotherapy. There are reports of better overall survival for patients who receive combination treatment consisting of 5-fluorouracil (5-FU) alone or in combination with a variety of other agents [38]. In metastatic disease, a palliative surgical resection of the primary tumor and palliative chemotherapeutic treatment are frequently needed in order to prevent or treat complications, such as bowel obstruction or bleeding. Since there are no randomized clinical trials in the setting of small bowel tumors [39], the approach is similar to that of CRC.

Neuroendocrine Tumors

Surgery is the most effective treatment for the control of both local tumor effect and of endocrinopathy-related symptoms in the setting of unresectable or metastatic disease [40]. A thorough presurgical examination is essential to rule out synchronous or metachronous tumors (most likely adenocarcinomas), not only along the GI tract, but also in the lung, prostate, cervix, and ovary. If liver metastases are present at diagnosis, the primary tumor should still be resected in order to avoid later complications, which may include obstruction, bleeding, and perforation.

In patients with moderate-to-severe symptoms, treatment with the somatostatin analogs, octreotide, and lanreotide is considered to be gold standard. The addition of interferon-α has shown to be effective in controlling carcinoid-related symptoms in patients resistant to somatostatin analogs [41]. Hepatic artery embolization or chemoembolization should be reserved for patients who have unresectable liver metastases without extrahepatic spread or for progressive disease and/or severe symptoms not responding to somatostatin analogs or interferon.

Lymphoma

The majority of primary intestinal low-grade lymphomas can be cured by surgery alone (resection of the affected segment of small bowel together with its adjacent mesentery). Aggressive chemotherapy is the mainstay of treatment in more advanced stages, while complete surgical resection is usually performed in order to alleviate symptoms of mass effect and to avoid complications during chemotherapy, even in advanced stages.

Remission can be induced by antibiotic treatment alone in Mediterranean lymphoma or in immunoproliferative small intestinal disease restricted to the mucosa and/or submucosa.

Gastrointestinal Stromal Tumors

The mainstay of resectable GIST treatment has been and continues to be surgery. The resectability of the tumor and the ability of the patient to tolerate a major resection must be carefully assessed. It is important to stress that although GISTs may present as a huge lesion, the "pushing" nature of tumor growth may allow adequate *en bloc* resection, leaving the pseudocapsule intact, thus avoiding intra-abdominal tumor spillage. Unlike adenocarcinoma or carcinoid tumor that spread thorough lymphatics, GISTs metastasize hematogenously, obviating the need for removal of lymphatic drainage in the mesentery. Dense adhesions often hamper resection. In the presence of metastatic disease, a local resection of the primary tumor may be considered for control of bleeding or relief of obstruction. Imatinib mesylate (Gleevec®), a selective tyrosine kinase inhibitor, has been shown to be effective in metastatic disease. It may also be used as a neoadjuvant drug in an attempt to downstage a borderline case to the point of making it resectable.

Take Home Points

- Small bowel tumors are extremely rare and account for only 1–2% of all gastrointestinal (GI) malignancies. Two-thirds of these tumors are malignant.
- Adenocarcinoma is the most common malignancy (40%), followed by neuroendocrine tumors (carcinoid) (20–40%), lymphomas (14%), and gastrointestinal stromal tumors (GISTs) (11–13%).
- Small bowel tumors are usually asymptomatic in the early stages. The most frequent presenting symptoms are abdominal pain, nausea, vomiting, and intestinal obstruction.
- The diagnostic strategies include conventional non-invasive imaging (small bowel barium series, enteroclysis, computerized tomography, and magnetic resonance imaging), as well as the push, double balloon and video-capsule endoscopic modalities. The newer techniques have improved diagnostic accuracy.
- Since there are no data from clinical trials, therapy of small bowel adenocarcinoma is similar to that of colorectal cancer.

References

1 Jemal A, Siegel R, Ward E, Murray T, Xu J, Thun MJ. Cancer statistics, 2007. *CA Cancer J Clin* 2007; **57**: 43–66.

2 Hatzaras I, Palesty JA, Abir F, *et al*. Small-bowel tumors: epidemiologic and clinical characteristics of 1260 cases from the Connecticut tumor registy. *Arch Surg* 2007; **142**:229–35.

3 Neugut AI, Jacobson JS, Suh S, Mukherjee R, Arber N. The epidemiology of cancer of the small bowel. *Cancer Epidemiol Biomarkers Prev* 1998; **7**: 243–51.

4 Ciresi DL, Scholten DJ. The continuing clinical dilemma of primary tumors of the small intestine. *Am Surg* 1995; **61**: 698–702; discussion 702–3.

5 Minardi AJ Jr, Zibari GB, Aultman DF, McMillan RW, McDonald JC. Small-bowel tumors. *J Am Coll Surg* 1998; **186**: 664–8.

6 Seifert E, Schulte F, Stolte M. Adenoma and carcinoma of the duodenum and papilla of Vater: a clinicopathologic study. *Am J Gastroenterol* 1992; **87**: 37–42.

7 Whiteman BJ, Janssens AR, Griffioen G, Lamers CB.Villous tumors of the duodenum. An analysis of the literature with emphasis on malignant transformation. *Neth J Med* 1993; **42**: 5–11.

8 Wirtzfeld DA, Petrelli NJ, Rodriguez-Bigas MA. Hamartomatous polyposis syndromes: molecular genetics, neoplastic risk, and surveillance recommendations. *Ann Surg Oncol* 2001; **8**: 319–27.

9 Dabaja BS, Suki D, Pro B, Bonnen M, Ajani J. Adenocarcinoma of the small bowel: presentation, prognostic factors, and outcome of 217 patients. *Cancer* 2004; **101**: 518–26.

10 Michelassi F, Testa G, Pomidor WJ, Lashner BJ, Block GE. Adenocarcinoma complicating Crohn's disease. *Dis Colon Rectum* 1993; **36**: 654–61.

11 Kaerlev L, Teglbjaerg PS, Sabroe S, *et al*. Medical risk factors for small-bowel adenocarcinoma with focus on Crohn disease: a European population-based case-control study. *Scand J Gastroenterol* 2001; **36**: 641–6.

12 Offerhaus GJ, Giardiello FM, Krush AJ, *et al*. The risk of upper gastrointestinal cancer in familial adenomatous polyposis. *Gastroenterology* 1992; **102**: 1980–2.

13 Wu AH, Yu MC, Mack TM. Smoking, alcohol use, dietary factors and risk of small intestinal adenocarcinoma. *Int J Cancer* 1997 **70**: 512–7.

14 Negri E, Bosetti C, La Vecchia C, Fioretti F, Conti E, Franceschi S. Risk factors for adenocarcinoma of the small intestine. *Int J Cancer* 1999; **82**: 171–4.

15 Polak JM. *Diagnostic Histopathology of Neuroendocrine Tumours*. Edinburgh: Churchill-Livingstone, 1993.

16 Rindi G, Capella C, Solcia E. Pathobiology and classification of digestive endocrine tumors. In: Mignon M, Colombel JF (eds). *Recent Advances in the Pathophysiology of Inflammatory Bowel Disease and Digestive Endocrine Tumors*. Montrouge: John Libbey Eurotext, 1999: 177–91.

17 Lebtahi R, Cadiot G, Sarda L, *et al*. Clinical impact of somatostatin receptor scintigraphy in the management of patients with neuroendocrine gastroenteropancreatic tumors. *J Nucl Med* 1997; **38**: 853–8.

18 Pidhorecky I, Cheney RT, Kraybill WG, Gibbs JF. Gastrointestinal stromal tumors: current diagnosis, biologic behavior, and management. *Ann Surg Oncol* 2000; **7**: 705–12.

19 Hirota S, Isozaki K, Moriyama Y, *et al*. Gain-of-function mutations of c-kit in human gastrointestinal stromal tumors. *Science* 1998; **279**: 577–80.

20 Crump M, Gospodarowicz M, Shepherd FA. Lymphoma of the gastrointestinal tract. *Semin Oncol* 1999; **26**: 324–37.

21 Catassi C, Bearzi I, Holmes GK. Association of celiac disease and intestinal lymphomas and other cancers. *Gastroenterology* 2005; **128** (4 Suppl 1): S79–86.

22 Verkarre V, Romana SP, Cellier C, *et al*. Recurrent partial trisomy 1q22-q44 in clonal intraepithelial lymphocytes in refractory celiac sprue. *Gastroenterology* 2003; **125**: 40–6.

23 Bishop PC, Rao VK, Wilson WH. Burkitt's lymphoma: molecular pathogenesis and treatment. *Cancer Invest* 2000; **18**: 574–583.

24 Isaacson P, Wright DH. Malignant lymphoma of mucosaassociated lymphoid tissue. A distinctive type of B-cell lymphoma. *Cancer* 1983; **52**: 1410–6.

25 Salem PA, Estephan FF. Immunoproliferative small intestinal disease: current concepts. *Cancer J* 2005; **11**: 374–82.

26 Lecuit M, Abachin E, Martin A, *et al*. Immunoproliferative small intestinal disease associated with *Campylobacter jejuni*. *N Engl J Med* 2004; **350**: 239–48.

27 Dabaja BS, Suki D, Pro B, Bonnen M, Ajani J. Adenocarcinoma of the small bowel: presentation, prognostic factors, and outcome of 217 patients. *Cancer* 2004; **101**: 518–26.

28 Greene FL, Page DL, Fleming ID, *et al. AJCC Cancer Staging Manual*, 6th edn. New York, NY: Springer, 2006.

29 Korman MU. Radiologic evaluation and staging of small intestine neoplasms. *Eur J Radiol* 2002; **42**: 193–205.

30 Horton, KM; Fishman, EK Multidetector-row computed tomography and 3-dimensional computed tomography imaging of small bowel neoplasms: Current concept in diagnosis. *J Comput Assist Tomogr* 2004; **28**: 106–16.

31 Semelka RC, John G, Kelekis NL, Burdeny DA, Ascher SM. Small bowel neoplastic disease: demonstration by MRI. *J Magn Reson Imaging* 1996; **6**: 855–60.

32 Kumar R, Xiu Y, Potenta S, *et al*. 18F-FDG PET for evaluation of the treatment response in patients with gastrointestinal tract lymphomas. *J Nucl Med* 2004; **45**: 1796–803.

33 Bessette, JR, Maglinte DD, Kelvin FM, Chernish SM. Primary malignant tumors in the small bowel: a comparison of the small-bowel enema and conventional follow-through examination. *AJR Am J Roentgenol* 1989; **153**: 741–4.

34 Chak A, Koehler MK, Sundaram SN, *et al*. Diagnostic and therapeutic impact of push enteroscopy: analysis of factors associated with positive findings. *Gastrointest Endosc* 1998; **47**: 18–22.

35 Triester SL, Leighton JA, Grigoris LI, *et al*. A meta-analysis of the yield of capsule endoscopy compared to other diagnostic modalities in patients with obscure gastrointestinal bleeding. *Am J Gastroenterol* 2005; **100**: 2407–18.

36 Pennazio M, Rondonotti E, de Franchis R. Capsule endoscopy in neoplastic diseases. *World J Gastroenterol* 2008; **14**: 5245–53.

37 Sun B, Rajan E, Cheng S, *et al*. Diagnostic yield and therapeutic impact of double-balloon enteroscopy in a large cohort of patients with obscure gastrointestinal bleeding. *Am J Gastroenterol* 2006; **101**: 2011–5.

38 Matsumoto T, Esaki M, Yanaru-Fujisawa R, *et al*. Smallintestinal involvement in familial adenomatous polyposis: evaluation by double-balloon endoscopy and intraoperative enteroscopy. *Gastrointestinal Endosc* 2008; **68**: 911–9.

39 Singhal N, Singhal D. Adjuvant chemotherapy for small intestine adenocarcinoma. *Cochrane Database Syst Rev* 2007: CD005202.

40 Kulke MH, Mayer RJ. Carcinoid tumors. *N Engl J Med* 1999; **340**: 858–68.

41 Modlin IM, Lye KD, Kidd M. A 5-decade analysis of 13,715 carcinoid tumors. *Cancer* 2003; **97**: 934–59.

CHAPTER 46

Small-Intestinal Bacterial Overgrowth

Johanna Iturrino and Madhusudan Grover

Division of Gastroenterology and Hepatology, Mayo Clinic, Rochester, MN, USA

Summary

Small-intestinal bacterial overgrowth (SIBO) can cause a wide range of clinical and nutritional manifestations. Clinical suspicion must be high in patients with disorders that disrupt normal defenses of the small intestine. Though an association between SIBO and irritable bowel syndrome (IBS) has been suggested, the available evidence is not conclusive. There is no currently available test that can be considered an adequate gold standard for the diagnosis of SIBO. Small-bowel culture is highly specific but lacks sensitivity, particularly for distal SIBO. Carbohydrate breath tests are non-invasive and simple to perform but lack standardization and have not been adequately validated as a reliable surrogate means of identifying SIBO. Therapy consists of antibiotics to decontaminate the small intestine, nutritional support to address the consequences of longstanding SIBO, and, when possible, correction of the underlying cause.

Case

A 45-year-old woman is referred with complaints of bloating and chronic diarrhea. She reports passing three to four loose bowel movements per day. She states that her stools occasionally float in the toilet bowl. She reports abdominal distension, which can be severe enough to require loosening of the beltline of her pants. She also describes early satiety and malodorous flatus. Her symptoms worsen after eating a meal. She reports the onset of difficulty driving at night and numbness and tingling of her lower extremities over the past few weeks. She has self-medicated with over-the-counter (OTC) remedies, including simethicone, loperamide, and antacids, without benefit to her symptoms. She has a history of systemic sclerosis. Her current medications include methotrexate 25 mg/week, folate 1 mg/day, aspirin 81 mg/day, and verapamil 180 mg once daily.

She has no history of abdominal surgery or family history of gastrointestinal (GI) cancer.

Physical examination reveals a thin Caucasian female in no distress. Positive findings include smooth, shiny skin with sclerodactyly (consistent with her diagnosis of systemic sclerosis), and there is an area of calcinosis cutis on her back. Her abdomen is moderately distended with decreased bowel sounds, but no succussion splash is appreciated. Abdominal palpation reveals no masses or tenderness. Digital rectal examination reveals normal anal sphincter tone and hemoccult-negative stool. Neurological examination reveals decreased sensation to pinprick in her lower extremities, but is otherwise non-focal.

Definition and Epidemiology

SIBO has traditionally been defined by quantitative culture of aspirated juice from the proximal jejunum. The most widely accepted definition of SIBO is $>10^5$ colony-forming units of bacteria per milliliter of aspirate (CFU/mL). Some have argued that a lower threshold may be appropriate ($>10^3$ CFU/mL) if the bacteria species identified are absent from the saliva and gastric juice or are similar to those found in the colon [1, 2]. SIBO is typically a byproduct of structural abnormalities involving the GI tract or alterations in gut motor, secretory, or immunological function.

The frequency of SIBO in healthy individuals is not well known, but it has been estimated to be up to 20% [3]. Estimates of the frequency of SIBO in at-risk populations vary widely depending on the disease entity, test, and diagnostic threshold used. For example, in patients with inflammatory bowel disease (IBD), those with Crohn's disease were more likely to show evidence of SIBO (45%) than those with ulcerative colitis (18%) [4]; in patients with IBS, a lactulose breath test (LBT) was positive for SIBO in 34% of cases, while only 6% tested positive on glucose breath test (GBT) [5].

Because symptoms of IBS and SIBO often overlap, a relationship has been proposed between the two [6]. Data suggest that anywhere from 4 to 64% of patients with IBS test positive for SIBO [7,8] – particularly those with diarrhea-predominant IBS [9]. However, because of the lack of symptomatic, psychological, and physiologic differences between IBS patients with and without SIBO, it is felt that SIBO is unlikely to contribute significantly to the pathogenesis of IBS [10]. Perhaps the commonplace use of proton pump inhibitors (PPIs) confounds the IBS/SIBO dilemma. Though some investigators have not found PPI use to be associated with SIBO [11, 12], findings of a recent meta-analysis would suggest that potent gastric acid suppression through PPI use is linked to a greater likelihood of SIBO [13]. However, it remains to be elucidated whether these changes can cause clinically meaningful phenotypic differences.

Pathophysiology

The quantity and species of bacterial flora vary from the proximal to distal small intestine. Normal colony counts are 10^2 CFU/mL in the proximal small intestine, increasing to as high as 10^9 CFU/mL in the terminal ileum. In the proximal small intestine, Gram-positive, aerobic bacterial species are most common, while Gram-negative,

Practical Gastroenterology and Hepatology Board Review Toolkit, Second Edition. Edited by Nicholas J. Talley, Kenneth R. DeVault, Michael B. Wallace, Bashar A. Aqel and Keith D. Lindor.

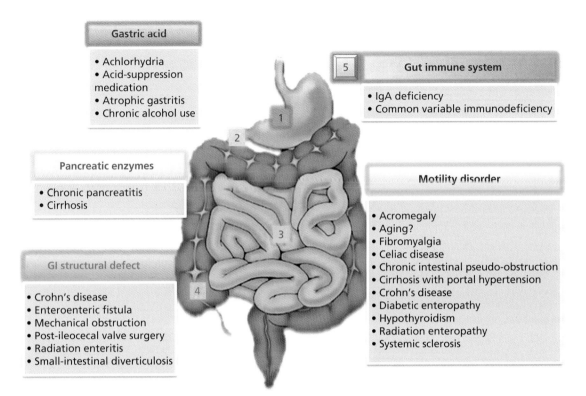

Gastric acid

• Achlorhydria
• Acid-suppression medication
• Atrophic gastritis
• Chronic alcohol use

Pancreatic enzymes

• Chronic pancreatitis
• Cirrhosis

GI structural defect

• Crohn's disease
• Enteroenteric fistula
• Mechanical obstruction
• Post-ileocecal valve surgery
• Radiation enteritis
• Small-intestinal diverticulosis

Gut immune system

• IgA deficiency
• Common variable immunodeficiency

Motility disorder

• Acromegaly
• Aging?
• Fibromyalgia
• Celiac disease
• Chronic intestinal pseudo-obstruction
• Cirrhosis with portal hypertension
• Crohn's disease
• Diabetic enteropathy
• Hypothyroidism
• Radiation enteropathy
• Systemic sclerosis

Figure 47.1 Mechanisms that maintain normal gut microflora.

anaerobic bacteria are more common distally. In healthy individuals, the normal gut microflora is maintained by five major mechanisms: gastric acid secretion, pancreatic enzyme secretion, small-intestinal motility, structural integrity of the GI tract, and an intact gut immune system [1, 14, 15]. The primary role of gastric acid is to reduce the bacterial content of food and suppress bacterial growth within the proximal small intestine. Pancreatic enzymes also exert an antimicrobial effect within the proximal small intestine. Normal fasting small-intestinal motility is critical to the prevention of bacterial overgrowth. Phase III of the migrating motor complex comprises frequent peristaltic contractions, which propel retained luminal debris and bacteria through the small intestine. Mechanical obstruction predisposes to intestinal stasis. Further, the ileocecal valve provides a physical barrier to reflux of colonic contents into the terminal ileum [16]. Disruption of any of these protective mechanisms can result in the development of SIBO (Figure 47.1).

Clinical Manifestations

SIBO can lead to both direct and indirect effects on the gut mucosa and luminal microenvironment. Bacterial adherence to the intestinal mucosa can result in direct injury, dysfunction, and alterations in gut immunology. Significant mucosal injury can lead to reduced brush-border disaccharidase activity. Bacterial metabolism and fermentation can compete with the host for nutritionally valuable substrates and lead to the production of byproducts that possess biologic activity or alter gut function (Figure 47.2). Though it has been speculated that SIBO might alter small-bowel permeability, data in IBS patients suggest that it does not [17].

The clinical consequences of SIBO span a spectrum ranging from asymptomatic to florid malabsorption. Most often, affected patients report non-specific symptoms, including bloating,

distension, abdominal cramping, and diarrhea. Diarrhea is usually multifactorial, with contributions from malabsorption, maldigestion, bile acid deconjugation, protein-losing enteropathy, and comorbid disease processes. Numerous nutritional deficiencies have been reported, the most notable of which include vitamin B_{12} and fat-soluble vitamins. Specific clinical features can raise suspicion for such nutritional deficiencies: macrocytic anemia and peripheral neuropathy can be an indicator of B_{12} deficiency, while night blindness and follicular hyperkeratosis can suggest vitamin A deficiency. Interestingly, levels of folate and vitamin K are usually normal or elevated in the setting of SIBO, as a consequence of either increased bacterial synthesis or increased dietary absorption [18].

SIBO has been linked to neurological diseases such as Parkinson's disease [19,20] and restless leg syndrome (RLS) [21,22]. While some have shown that treatment of SIBO improves neurological symptoms of Parkinson's disease [19] and RLS [21], others have shown the opposite [23].

Obesity has been related to SIBO, which in turn has been suggested as a putative pathophysiological mechanism for hepatic steatosis in this population, either from decreased intestinal motility or from changes in the inflammatory profile [24–26]. Likewise, in patients with cirrhosis, SIBO appears prevalent and has been implicated as a potential key driver of hepatic encephalopathy [27] and bacterial translocation [28]. Though some argue that SIBO does not appear to be related to the presence of ascites or to the etiology or severity of liver dysfunction [29], others have found it to be more common in the presence of ascites and advanced liver disease [30].

Diagnosis

Aspiration of jejunal fluid for quantitative culture has been considered the gold standard for the diagnosis of SIBO. Though this

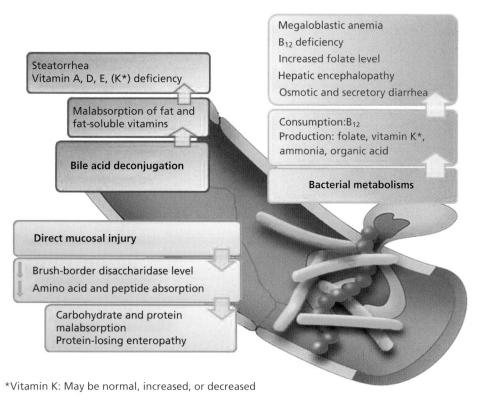

*Vitamin K: May be normal, increased, or decreased

Figure 47.2 Effects of bacteria on gut mucosa and clinical consequences of SIBO.

technique is highly specific, small-bowel aspiration for quantitative culture is far from perfect. Drawbacks include the invasive nature of sample collection, the contamination of aspirated material by oral flora, the lack of sensitivity for detecting distal SIBO, the expense, and the need for infrastructure and trained personnel in order to perform quantitative culture. Nowadays, despite being less extensively validated, endoscopic duodenal sampling has mostly replaced jejunal aspirates due to its sampling convenience. During endoscopy, the appearance of the small bowel is often normal and non-specific; villous blunting appears to be the only histopathological feature seen more frequently in SIBO patients when compared to controls [31].

Many investigators and clinicians have utilized carbohydrate breath tests as a surrogate means of identifying SIBO. Breath tests rely upon the ability of intestinal bacteria to metabolize various carbohydrate substrates to hydrogen and/or methane gas, which is rapidly absorbed across the intestinal epithelium and eventually excreted in the breath. After a carbohydrate load, a rapid rise in breath hydrogen or methane excretion may indicate the presence of SIBO [32] (Figure 47.3). The most commonly used substrates for commercially available breath tests include lactulose and glucose. Each substrate offers unique advantages and disadvantages.

In the absence of SIBO, lactulose is not fermented or absorbed within the small intestine. When exposed to bacteria within the small intestine, lactulose is fermented to short-chain fatty acids and a number of gases, including hydrogen and methane. Unfortunately, colonic bacteria will also ferment lactulose, making it difficult to interpret whether a positive breath test result truly represents SIBO or simply rapid orocecal transit [33]. The optimal way in which to define a positive LBT remains controversial [32, 34]. The effects of

GI transit on LBT [33] and the lack of well-defined criteria for interpretation are likely causes of the high rates of SIBO reported in IBS by some [35].

The other substrate commonly used to test for SIBO is glucose. Glucose is avidly absorbed in the proximal small intestine. Because glucose typically does not reach the distal small bowel, GBT may be less sensitive than LBT. On the other hand, GBT is likely more specific than LBT [32,34]. It is important to note that concurrent testing of breath methane levels should be performed, as approximately 15–20% of patients (particularly those with constipation-predominant IBS) [10,36] can have methanogenic bacteria that convert hydrogen into methane, yielding a false negative if only hydrogen breath levels are measured. The characteristics and performance of the tests commonly used for SIBO can be found in Table 47.1.

Other breath tests, using d-xylose, ^{13}C-xylose, and cholyglycine, have been described in the literature but have yielded conflicting results and are not widely available [32, 37]. With advances in our ability to understand and characterize the microbiota of the gut, we can anticipate that newer diagnostic modalities which employ metabolomic techniques will emerge and hopefully improve the diagnostic accuracy of SIBO [38]. The treatment of SIBO can be separated into several phases: acute antibiotic therapy, to decontaminate the small intestine; repletion of vitamin deficiencies and correction of malnutrition; and management of any underlying disease process that might have been responsible for the development of SIBO.

Treatment

Antibiotics are most commonly used to acutely decontaminate the small intestine (Figure 47.4). As a group, antibiotic therapy

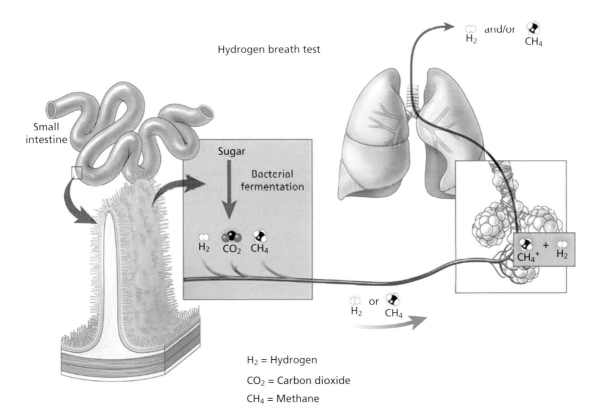

Hydrogen breath test

H_2 = Hydrogen

CO_2 = Carbon dioxide

CH_4 = Methane

Figure 47.3 Schematic for hydrogen breath testing. Source: Saad 2007 [32]. Reproduced with permission of Elsevier.

has been shown to normalize breath tests in about 51% of patients when compared to placebo, which yields about 10% normalization rates. Symptom improvement does not always follow breath-test normalization, but overall it tends to correlate with it [39]. An ideal antibiotic for SIBO should possess activity against both aerobic and anaerobic enteric bacteria. A variety of antibiotics have been used to treat SIBO, including amoxicillin–clavulanic acid, cefoxitin, ciprofloxacin, norfloxacin, metronidazole, neomycin, and doxycyclin. Most reports in the literature have recommended courses of 7–14 days. If a correctable underlying etiology for SIBO can be identified, a single course of antibiotics may result in a durable clinical response. In many cases, the underlying cause of SIBO cannot be identified or cannot be corrected. In these circumstances, repeated courses of antibiotics are often necessary. When SIBO is infrequent or only leads to mild clinical or nutritional consequences, it may be sufficient to wait for symptoms to recur before reinstituting a course of antibiotics. When patients have frequent or very severe bouts of SIBO, using

rotating courses of antibiotics every 4–6 weeks can be very effective. Concerns over such a strategy include the development of *Clostridium difficile* colitis and multidrug-resistant bacterial flora.

Special attention has been given to rifaximin, a semisynthetic, broad-spectrum, non-absorbable oral antibiotic, in the management of SIBO, particularly in patients with IBS [40, 41]. Pooled breath-test normalization rates of rifaximin have been in the range of 60% when compared to placebo [39]. To date, little in the way of resistance to rifaximin has been reported.

There are scant data on the role of diet in the development, perpetuation, or recurrence of SIBO. Based on GBT results, one study found SIBO to be more prevalent in subjects who consumed significantly less fiber, folic acid, and vitamins B_2 and B_6 than found in a normal diet [42]. In another study, an elemental diet led to normalization of abnormal LBT results and improved symptoms in patients with IBS [43]. It is likely that diet does play a role in SIBO, but further work is needed in this area.

Table 47.1 Comparison of diagnostic tests for SIBO.

	Small-intestinal aspiration for quantitative culture	Glucose breath test (GBT)	Lactulose breath test (LBT)
Advantages	Quantitative measurement Allows speciation of bacteria	Non-invasive, simple to perform, less costly than culture	
Disadvantages	Invasive High-cost Technically difficult	Need specialized equipment, space, and technical support Abnormal thresholds not well validated	
False-positive results	Contamination from bacteria in upper GI tract	Rapid small bowel transit time	
False-negative results	Inappropriate sample processing or culture techniques	Distal SIBO	Chronic lactose exposure
Sensitivity (%) [2, 34, 45]	56	20–93	16.7–68
Specificity (%) [2, 34, 45]	100	45–86	44–86

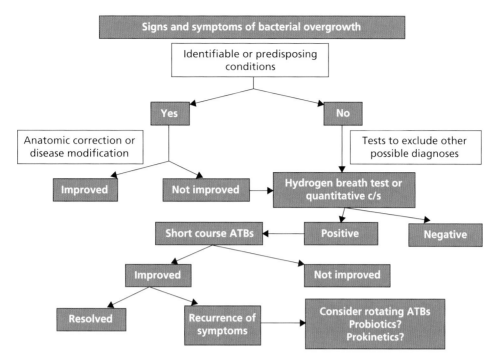

Figure 47.4 Algorithm for the treatment of SIBO. ATBs, antibiotics.

Though evidence of the effects of prebiotics and/or probiotics as treatment options for SIBO remains scant and is mostly limited to small pilot studies, the data obtained so far appear promising. The addition of a prebiotic (partially hydrolyzed guar gum) to rifaximin therapy led to an improved breath-test normalization rate of 85%, compared to 62% with rifaximin alone [44].

There are some data to suggest that prokinetic drugs, including motilin agonists and 5-HT$_4$ agonists, might offer a primary treatment option for SIBO in patients with abnormal motility. It has also been suggested that prokinetic therapy might offer a means by which to prolong the duration of therapeutic benefit following intestinal decontamination with antibiotics. The available literature consists of small, methodologically flawed studies [1]. Further practical issues regarding the development of tolerance with chronic dosing (motilides) and lack of availability (5-HT$_4$ agonists) limit the role of prokinetic therapy in clinical practice.

Case Continued

A comprehensive metabolic profile reveals a low albumin level of 3.2 g/dL (3.5–4.9 g/dL). B$_{12}$ level is decreased at 174 pg/mL (211–911 pg/mL). The patient undergoes serological testing for celiac disease, which is negative. Stool studies for leukocytes, ova and parasite examination, Giardia antigen, and *Clostridium difficile* antigen are all negative. A Sudan stain for qualitative fecal fat is positive. A glucose hydrogen breath test is positive, with a rise in breath hydrogen excretion of >20 ppm within 30 minutes of ingesting 50 g of glucose.

The patient is diagnosed with SIBO and started on a 10-day course of oral rifaximin 1.2 g/day, as well as selected vitamin and mineral supplements. Within a week, she experiences a dramatic improvement of her symptoms, including bloating, flatus, and diarrhea.

Take Home Points

- In healthy individuals, the normal gut microflora is maintained by five major mechanisms: gastric acid secretion, pancreatic enzyme secretion, small-intestinal motility, structural integrity of the GI tract, and an intact gut immune system. Abnormalities in any of these defensive mechanisms can lead to the development of SIBO.
- The clinical consequences of SIBO span a spectrum ranging from asymptomatic to florid malabsorption. Most commonly, patients present with non-specific symptoms such as bloating, cramping, and diarrhea.
- Aspiration of jejunal fluid for quantitative culture has been considered the gold standard for the diagnosis of SIBO. However, quantitative culture is invasive, complex to perform, expensive, and lacking in sensitivity, particularly for distal SIBO.
- Breath tests utilizing glucose and lactulose are non-invasive and easy to perform but difficult to interpret, due to a high false-positive rate.
- Therapy consists of antibiotics to decontaminate the small intestine, nutritional support to address the consequences of longstanding SIBO, and, when possible, correction of the underlying cause.
- All of the methods available for the diagnosis of SIBO have limitations, and a gold-standard diagnostic test for the condition may not exist. Accurate diagnosis of SIBO will require better tests, capable of identifying pathogenic bacterial colonization in the small intestine and of obtaining evidence of symptom response to treatment.

References

1 Quigley EMM, Quera R. Small intestinal bacterial overgrowth: roles of antibiotics, prebiotics, and probiotics. *Gastroenterology* 2006; **130**(2 Suppl. 1): S78–90.

2 Simrén M, Stotzer P-O. Use and abuse of hydrogen breath tests. *Gut* 2006; **55**: 297–303.

3 Grace E, Shaw C, Whelan K, Andreyev HJN. Review article: small intestinal bacterial overgrowth – prevalence, clinical features, current and developing diagnostic tests, and treatment. *Aliment Pharmacol Ther* 2013; **38**(7): 674–88.

4 Rana SV, Sharma S, Malik A, et al. Small intestinal bacterial overgrowth and orocecal transit time in patients of inflammatory bowel disease. *Dig Dis Sci* 2013; **58**(9): 2594–8.

5 Rana SV, Sharma S, Kaur J, et al. Comparison of lactulose and glucose breath test for diagnosis of small intestinal bacterial overgrowth in patients with irritable bowel syndrome. *Digestion* 2012; **85**(3): 243–7.

6 Chey WD, Spiegel B. Proton pump inhibitors, irritable bowel syndrome, and small intestinal bacterial overgrowth: coincidence or Newton's third law revisited? *Clin Gastroenterol Hepatol* 2010; **8**(6): 480–2.

7 Lupascu A, Gabrielli M, Lauritano EC, et al. Hydrogen glucose breath test to detect small intestinal bacterial overgrowth: a prevalence case-control study in irritable bowel syndrome. *Aliment Pharmacol Ther* 2005; **22**(11–12): 1157–60.

8 Quigley EMM. Small intestinal bacterial overgrowth: what it is and what it is not. *Curr Opin Gastroenterol* 2014; **30**(2): 141–6.

9 Pyleris E, Giamarellos-Bourboulis EJ, Tzivras D, et al. The prevalence of overgrowth by aerobic bacteria in the small intestine by small bowel culture: relationship with irritable bowel syndrome. *Dig Dis Sci* 2012; **57**(5): 1321–9.

10 Grover M, Kanazawa M, Palsson OS, et al. Small intestinal bacterial overgrowth in irritable bowel syndrome: association with colon motility, bowel symptoms, and psychological distress. *Neurogastroenterol Motil* 2008; **20**(9): 998–1008.

11 Choung RS, Ruff KC, Malhotra A, et al. Clinical predictors of small intestinal bacterial overgrowth by duodenal aspirate culture. *Aliment Pharmacol Ther* 2011; **33**(9): 1059–67.

12 Ratuapli SK, Ellington TG, O'Neill M-T, et al. Proton pump inhibitor therapy use does not predispose to small intestinal bacterial overgrowth. *Am J Gastroenterol* 2012; **107**(5): 730–5.

13 Lo W-K, Chan WW. Proton pump inhibitor use and the risk of small intestinal bacterial overgrowth: a meta-analysis. *Clin Gastroenterol Hepatol* 2013; **11**(5): 483–90.

14 Pignata C, Budillon G, Monaco G, et al. Jejunal bacterial overgrowth and intestinal permeability in children with immunodeficiency syndromes. *Gut* 1990; **31**(8): 879–82.

15 Riordan SM, McIver CJ, Wakefield D, et al. Serum immunoglobulin and soluble IL-2 receptor levels in small intestinal overgrowth with indigenous gut flora. *Dig Dis Sci* 1999; **44**: 939–44.

16 Miller LS, Vegesna AK, Sampath AM, et al. Ileocecal valve dysfunction in small intestinal bacterial overgrowth: a pilot study. *World J Gastroenterol* 2012; **18**(46): 6801–8.

17 Park JH, Park D Il, Kim HJ, et al. The relationship between small-intestinal bacterial overgrowth and intestinal permeability in patients with irritable bowel syndrome. *Gut Liver* 2009; **3**(3): 174–9.

18 Giuliano V, Bassotti G, Mourvaki E, et al. Small intestinal bacterial overgrowth and warfarin dose requirement variability. *Thromb Res* 2010; **126**(1): 12–17.

19 Fasano A, Bove F, Gabrielli M, et al. The role of small intestinal bacterial overgrowth in Parkinson's disease. *Mov Disord* 2013; **28**(9): 1241–9.

20 Gabrielli M, Bonazzi P, Scarpellini E, et al. Prevalence of small intestinal bacterial overgrowth in Parkinson's disease. *Mov Disord* 2011; **26**(5): 889–92.

21 Weinstock LB, Fern SE, Duntley SP. Restless legs syndrome in patients with irritable bowel syndrome: response to small intestinal bacterial overgrowth therapy. *Dig Dis Sci* 2008; **53**(5): 1252–6.

22 Weinstock LB, Walters AS. Restless legs syndrome is associated with irritable bowel syndrome and small intestinal bacterial overgrowth. *Sleep Med* 2011; **12**(6): 610–13.

23 Dobbs SM, Charlett A, Dobbs RJ, et al. Antimicrobial surveillance in idiopathic parkinsonism: indication-specific improvement in hypokinesia following *Helicobacter pylori* eradication and non-specific effect of antimicrobials for other indications in worsening rigidity. *Helicobacter* 2013; **18**(3): 187–96.

24 Sabaté J-M, Jouët P, Harnois F, et al. High prevalence of small intestinal bacterial overgrowth in patients with morbid obesity: a contributor to severe hepatic steatosis. *Obes Surg* 2008; **18**(4): 371–7.

25 Wu W-C, Zhao W, Li S. Small intestinal bacteria overgrowth decreases small intestinal motility in the NASH rats. *World J Gastroenterol* 2008; **14**(2): 313–17.

26 Shanab AA, Scully P, Crosbie O, et al. Small intestinal bacterial overgrowth in nonalcoholic steatohepatitis: association with toll-like receptor 4 expression and plasma levels of interleukin 8. *Dig Dis Sci* 2011; **56**(5): 1524–34.

27 Gupta A, Dhiman RK, Kumari S, et al. Role of small intestinal bacterial overgrowth and delayed gastrointestinal transit time in cirrhotic patients with minimal hepatic encephalopathy. *J Hepatol* 2010; **53**(5): 849–55.

28 Jun DW, Kim KT, Lee OY, et al. Association between small intestinal bacterial overgrowth and peripheral bacterial DNA in cirrhotic patients. *Dig Dis Sci* 2010; **55**(5): 1465–71.

29 Lakshmi CP, Ghoshal UC, Kumar S, et al. Frequency and factors associated with small intestinal bacterial overgrowth in patients with cirrhosis of the liver and extra hepatic portal venous obstruction. *Dig Dis Sci* 2010; **55**(4): 1142–8.

30 Pande C, Kumar A, Sarin SK. Small intestinal bacterial overgrowth in cirrhosis is related to the severity of liver disease. *Aliment Pharmacol Ther* 2009; **29**(12): 1273–81.

31 Lappinga PJ, Abraham SC, Murray JA, et al. Small intestinal bacterial overgrowth: histopathologic features and clinical correlates in an underrecognized entity. *Arch Pathol Lab Med* 2010; **134**(2): 264–70.

32 Saad RJ, Chey WD. Breath tests for gastrointestinal disease: the real deal or just a lot of hot air? *Gastroenterology* 2007; **133**(6): 1763–6.

33 Yu D, Cheeseman F, Vanner S. Combined oro-caecal scintigraphy and lactulose hydrogen breath testing demonstrate that breath testing detects oro-caecal transit, not small intestinal bacterial overgrowth in patients with IBS. *Gut* 2011; **60**(3): 334–40.

34 Corazza GR, Menozzi MG, Strocchi A, et al. The diagnosis of small bowel bacterial overgrowth. Reliability of jejunal culture and inadequacy of breath hydrogen testing. *Gastroenterology* 1990; **98**: 302–9.

35 Shah ED, Basseri RJ, Chong K, Pimentel M. Abnormal breath testing in IBS: a meta-analysis. *Dig Dis Sci* 2010; **55**: 2441–9.

36 Reddymasu SC, Sostarich S, McCallum RW. Small intestinal bacterial overgrowth in irritable bowel syndrome: are there any predictors? *BMC Gastroenterol* 2010; **10**: 23.

37 Romagnuolo J, Schiller D, Bailey RJ. Using breath tests wisely in a gastroenterology practice: an evidence-based review of indications and pitfalls in interpretation. *Am J Gastroenterol* 2002; **97**: 1113–26.

38 Leimena MM, Ramiro-Garcia J, Davids M, et al. A comprehensive metatranscriptome analysis pipeline and its validation using human small intestine microbiota datasets. *BMC Genomics* 2013; **14**: 530.

39 Shah SC, Day LW, Somsouk M, Sewell JL. Meta-analysis: antibiotic therapy for small intestinal bacterial overgrowth. *Aliment Pharmacol Ther* 2013; **38**(8): 925–34.

40 Yang J, Lee H-R, Low K, et al. Rifaximin versus other antibiotics in the primary treatment and retreatment of bacterial overgrowth in IBS. *Dig Dis Sci* 2008; **53**: 169–74.

41 Di Stefano M, Malservisi S, Veneto G, et al. Rifaximin versus chlortetracycline in the short-term treatment of small intestinal bacterial overgrowth. *Aliment Pharmacol Ther* 2000; **14**(5): 551–6.

42 Parlesak A, Klein B, Schecher K, et al. Prevalence of small bowel bacterial overgrowth and its association with nutrition intake in nonhospitalized older adults. *J Am Geriatr Soc* 2003; **51**: 768–73.

43 Pimentel M, Constantino T, Kong Y, et al. A 14-day elemental diet is highly effective in normalizing the lactulose breath test. *Dig Dis Sci* 2004; **49**: 73–7.

44 Furnari M, Parodi A, Gemignani L, et al. Clinical trial: the combination of rifaximin with partially hydrolysed guar gum is more effective than rifaximin alone in eradicating small intestinal bacterial overgrowth. *Aliment Pharmacol Ther* 2010; **32**(8): 1000–6.

45 Riordan SM, McIver CJ, Walker BM, et al. The lactulose breath hydrogen test and small intestinal bacterial overgrowth. *Am J Gastroenterol* 1996; **91**: 1795–803.

CHAPTER 47

Celiac Disease and Tropical Sprue

Alberto Rubio-Tapia and Joseph A. Murray

Division of Gastroenterology and Hepatology, Mayo Clinic, Rochester, MN, USA

Summary

Celiac disease and tropical sprue are the most frequent enteropathies that cause the malabsorption syndrome. While the pathophysiology of these disorders is quite different, some clinical manifestations – but especially the histologic findings – can be similar or even indistinguishable.

Case

A 50-year-old Caucasian man presents with involuntary loss of weight, diarrhea, and fatigue 3 months after a visit to southern Mexico, where his diarrhea began acutely. Macrocytic anemia and folic acid deficiency are detected. An esophagogastroduodenoscopy (EGD) with mucosal biopsies of the small intestine is performed, which reveals scalloping of the circular folds of the duodenum and partial villous atrophy in the microscopic evaluation, suggesting celiac disease or tropical sprue. Antibodies against endomysial and tissue transglutaminase are negative and the level of total immunoglobulin A is normal, making celiac disease unlikely. *Giardia* antigen and three stool samples are negative for the presence of cysts and trophozoites. The patient is successfully treated with folic acid and tetracycline.

Celiac Disease

Definition and Epidemiology

Celiac disease is an immune-mediated enteropathy induced by the ingestion of gluten (present in wheat, barley, and rye) in genetically susceptible individuals, which reverts to normal after the exclusion of gluten from the diet. It can affect any system or organ [1].

Epidemiological studies have shown that celiac disease is common (prevalence around 0.5–1.0%) in many developed and developing countries, but most cases remain unrecognized [2]. The high prevalence (>5%) of celiac disease among the African Saharawi population and recent evidence of a prevalence comparable to that in Western countries in the Middle East are especially interesting [3]. Celiac disease is more frequent in females (by about 2 : 1), with onset of symptoms occurring at all ages. The prevalence is higher in patients and family members of patients with type 1 diabetes mellitus (T1DM), thyroiditis, autoimmune liver disorders, infertility, and some chromosomal disorders than in the general population [1,4].

Clinical Features

Celiac disease has protean manifestations of variable severity that are summarized according to the "celiac iceberg" model as classical, atypical, silent, or latent [5]. "Classical celiac disease" refers to those patients with the florid malabsorption syndrome (this group is at the top of the iceberg). "Atypical celiac disease" refers to significant but generally monosymptomatic extraintestinal manifestations. "Silent celiac disease" refers to the presence of disease-specific autoimmunity with villous atrophy in the absence of any symptoms or apparent consequences. "Latent celiac disease" refers to genetically susceptible persons without symptoms or histological evidence of celiac disease who will ultimately go on to develop the disease. Further, "potential celiac disease" refers to patients who have positive celiac-specific serologies, particularly tissue transglutaminase immunoglobulin A (IgA) and endomysial IgA antibody, who lack symptoms and, when undergoing biopsies, do not have the histologic changes of celiac disease, or at the very most have increased intraepithelial lymphocytes with preserved architecture; a substantial portion – probably a third of these subjects – will proceed to develop full-blown celiac disease. In the iceberg model, some atypical cases, but most especially silent and latent celiac disease, are below the waterline [5]. Currently, non-classical symptoms are the clinical presentation in more than 50% of American patients with celiac disease [1].

Diagnosis

Serologic Tests

Celiac disease is characterized by the development of antibodies directed against the components of the environmental factor (gliadin) or connective tissue. The sensitivity and specificity may vary among the antibodies (Table 48.1). It is important that the patient not reduce or exclude gluten in the diet before testing, as all tests may become negative. Because of the inferior accuracy of the standard antigliadin assays, the use of this test is no longer recommended [6]. The use of deamidated gliadin antibodies increases accuracy compared to the antigliadin test for celiac disease [7]. The majority of the antibodies produced are of the IgA isotype, likely originating from the intestinal mucosa. Therefore, the first antibody test performed in celiac disease should be IgA-based. The utility of IgG-based testing for celiac disease, such as tissue transglutaminase IgG or deamidated gliadin IgG, is limited to those patients who have either low or deficient IgA. Approximately 3% of patients

Practical Gastroenterology and Hepatology Board Review Toolkit, Second Edition. Edited by Nicholas J. Talley, Kenneth R. DeVault, Michael B. Wallace, Bashar A. Aqel and Keith D. Lindor.

Table 48.1 Serologic tests and their diagnostic accuracy in celiac disease.

Test (all IgA isotype antibodies)[a]	Sensitivity (%)[b]	Specificity (%)[b]
Antigliadin [7]	<70	~90
Deamidated gliadin [7]	74	95
Endomysial [8]	91–98	99–100
Tissue transglutaminase [8]	95–98	94–98

[a]IgA (immunoglobulin A) isotype antibodies (tissue transglutaminase IgA and DGP IgG) are essentially useful only in patients with diminished or deficient IgA.
[b]Sensitivity and specificity vary between studies and according to the antigenic substrate used.

with celiac disease have selective IgA deficiency. Also, very young children (under the age of 1 year) often have quite low levels of IgA. Serologic testing should include a measure of IgA to detect IgA deficiency in patients where a pre-test prevalence of celiac disease is more substantial [8].

Tissue Transglutaminase Antibodies

The tissue transglutaminase antibody (tTGA) test by enzyme-linked immunosorbent assay is the screening test of choice for celiac disease, due to its technical simplicity and accuracy. The diagnostic performance is slightly better using human or human recombinant substrate (new-generation kits) than using guinea pig substrate. Overall, the tTGA sensitivity is in the range of 95–98% and the specificity >94% [9]. The positive predictive value (PPV) of tissue transglutaminase IgA testing in the general population is approximately 50%, assuming a pre-test prevalence of 1%. In circumstances where the pre-test prevalence or likelihood of celiac disease is much higher, even poorly performing serologic tests have a higher predictive value [10]. The higher the titer of tissue transglutaminase IgA antibodies, the greater the likelihood of celiac disease. The European Society of Paediatric Gastroenterology, Hepatology and Nutrition (ESPGHAN) has suggested that a tTGA 10 times the upper limit of normal followed by a positive endomysial antibody (EMA) and confirmatory or consistent human leukocyte antigen (HLA) genotype performed on a separate blood sample in patients who are symptomatic for celiac disease may obviate the need for intestinal biopsy in children. This view is not yet universally held.

Endomysial Antibodies

EMAs can be measured using an immunofluorescence technique. The overall sensitivity and specificity using monkey esophagus as substrate are 97 and 99%, respectively. The tests using human umbilical cord as substrate have a lower sensitivity (90%) [9]. While the very high specificity makes EMA a very powerful serologic test, there are some disadvantages: the test is time-consuming and resource-intensive, requires microscopy and monkey esophagus substrate, is semiquantitative at best, and is highly operator-dependent [9].

Genetic Testing

Celiac disease is strongly associated with two HLA haplotypes: DQ2 (encoded by DQA1*05 and DQB1*02) and DQ8 (encoded by DQA1*03 and DQB1*0302) [1]. Patients with celiac disease carry at least one of those two gene pairs (90–95% have DQ2). Typing of DNA from patients with celiac disease can be easily performed from whole blood using sequence-specific primers or allele-specific oligonucleotide probes. Though approximately 30–35% of the general Caucasian population carries either the HLA-DQ2 or the

HLA-DQ8 haplotype, only a small subset of these subjects have celiac disease [4]. Thus, HLA genotyping in a clinical setting is useful to practically exclude the diagnosis of celiac disease (high negative predictive value (NPV)) when the at-risk gene pairs are absent, especially when the diagnosis is uncertain [1,5]. Rare exceptions occur, however, and it should be recognized that HLA genotyping for risk of celiac disease has been applied largely in European populations, and unusual combinations of HLA type are possible. In the setting of an individual who has strongly positive celiac-specific serology and biopsies consistent with celiac disease (even if they lack the usual HLA types), celiac disease should be actively considered. A very tiny percentage of patients with celiac disease have half of one of the genes encoding DQ2 but not both genes. HLA genotyping may be beneficial in symptomatic patients already on gluten-free diet (GFD) who also have a history of tropical travel and perhaps did not have celiac serology before the diet. In this usually difficult clinical situation, the authors recommend carrying out both celiac serology and HLA typing, because: (i) if doubly negative, treatment for tropical sprue is indicated and a GFD is not necessary; but (ii) if celiac serology is negative but the patient is DQ2- or DQ8-positive, celiac disease cannot be concluded, but after treatment for tropical sprue a gluten challenge may be necessary to clarify whether the patient will require a lifelong GFD. HLA typing for celiac disease susceptibility may also be used in patients who have a diagnosis of celiac disease originally based on biopsies without confirmatory serology for whom an alternative explanation for the enteropathy could be forthcoming (e.g., drug-associated enteropathy, self-limited enteritis). The utility of HLA typing in family members of patients with celiac disease or in patients with type 1 diabetes is limited by a relatively high carriage rate of the at-risk genotypes in both of these populations. It is especially important that patients – and particularly parents – be counseled that the carriage of the gene pair associated with celiac disease risk alone does not equal disease and that the great majority of patients carrying these genetic susceptibility genotypes will never get celiac disease.

Histopathology

Small-bowel biopsy is the confirmatory test for celiac disease. Multiple biopsies (ideally four biopsies from the second part of the duodenum plus two additional biopsies from the duodenal bulb) are recommended, as the lesions may be patchy or short disease may occur [5,8]. Correct orientation – either in the endoscopy lab or, more often, during histopathology processing – is essential to accurate histological evaluation. Histologic findings include an increased number of intraepithelial lymphocytes (>25 for 100 epithelial cells), villous atrophy, and crypt hyperplasia. Biopsies may be classified according to one of several scales. The most common in use by clinicians is the modified Oberhuber–Marsh scale, which recognizes stage I where there is infiltration of the surface layer by intraepithelial lymphocytes, stage II where in addition to intraepithelial lymphocytes there is hyperplasia of the crypts, and stage III where there is villous atrophy in addition to the other changes. A subtyping of IIIA, IIIB, and IIIC represents mild villous blunting, partial villous atrophy, and total villous atrophy. Typically, histology is graded on the most advanced lesion seen. The original Marsh classification recognized a severe end-stage hypoplastic lesion (stage IV), which is very rare [11].

Gluten Challenge

It is no longer necessary to rechallenge most patients with a well-established diagnosis of celiac disease [1,6]. However, gluten

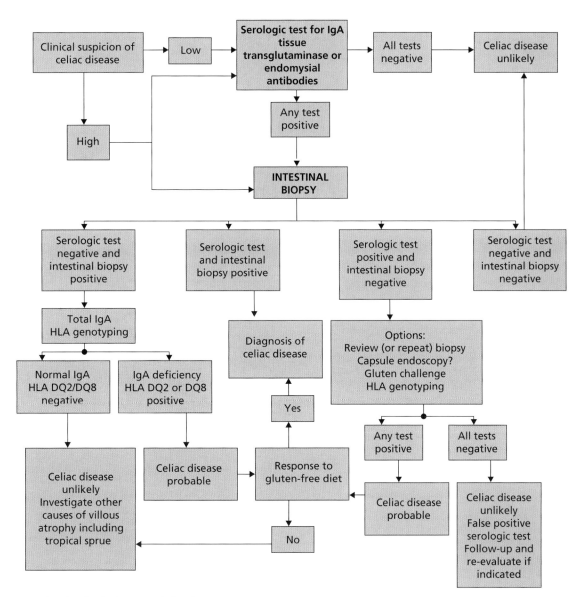

Figure 48.1   Algorithm for the detection of celiac disease.

challenge may be useful in patients started on a GFD without confirmatory histology (if the biopsy was taken elsewhere and is available for review, the challenge is unnecessary) or in those with an equivocal diagnosis. The standard challenge includes four slices (~12 g gluten) of whole-wheat bread per day, with serial clinical and serologic follow-up starting 4 weeks after reintroduction of gluten [5,8]. A lower-dose gluten challenge has also been proposed, wherein patients receive one or two slices of bread per day for a 2-week period and are followed with serology. If serology becomes positive, a biopsy can be scheduled; if not, the challenge is prolonged for 8 weeks and serology is repeated.

Suggested Diagnostic Approach
Celiac disease is most often detected with serologic tests [6]. However, serology alone is not sufficient for diagnosis. A presumptive and, indeed, definitive diagnosis of celiac disease can be made in patients who have a combination of positive celiac-specific serology, tissue transglutaminase IgA, and/or endomysial IgA followed by an

intestinal biopsy showing villous atrophy Marsh III. In patients who are seronegative but have consistent histology, celiac disease is still possible, but HLA typing and confirmation of a response to a GFD should be forthcoming. In patients with positive serology and minor degrees of change (such as Marsh I), HLA typing and response to a GFD will be required for diagnosis. Definitive diagnosis of celiac disease is established after demonstration of response to the GFD [5, 6]. Response to gluten withdrawal does not indicate celiac disease in the patient with self-diagnosis or poorly investigated gastrointestinal (GI) symptoms [5] (Figure 48.1).

Treatment
The management of celiac disease is a lifelong, medically supervised diet that is devoid of gluten [1]. Wheat (*Triticum* spp.), barley (*Hordeum vulgare*), and rye (*Secale cereale*) in all their forms are toxic to celiac patients [12]. Voluntary or accidental ingestion of gluten may occur as a result of a lack of readily available gluten-free foods, eating outside of the home, cross-contamination (trace

amounts of gluten in other non-gluten-containing foods), and hidden sources of gluten (e.g., some vitamins and prescription and over-the-counter (OTC) medications may contain gluten as an inactive ingredient) [12].

Other important components of the initial management include the aggressive correction of dehydration and nutritional deficiencies, when necessary [6]. All patients require assessment of the potential metabolic osteopathy by densitometry. Temporary restriction of lactose for a period of a few weeks may be beneficial in some cases [1].

Tropical Sprue

Definition and Epidemiology

Tropical sprue is an acquired disease of unknown etiology that affects residents and/or visitors of certain tropical areas (a zone centered on the equator and limited in latitude by the Tropic of Cancer in the northern hemisphere and the Tropic of Capricorn in the southern hemisphere). As infectious agents are the most frequent cause of chronic diarrhea in a tropical environment, the diagnosis of tropical sprue requires the exclusion of active infection, especially by protozoa [13, 14]. The prevalence of tropical sprue is unknown and may be different in different locations (e.g., high prevalence in South India and the Philippines and very low prevalence in Africa) [15]. The incidence of tropical sprue appears to have decreased during the past decade, possibly because of improved hygiene and, potentially, the widespread empiric use of antibiotics for the treatment of chronic diarrhea [14, 15].

Pathophysiology

The etiology of tropical sprue is not known [16]. The favored hypothesis is that tropical sprue is either initiated or sustained by complex interactions among as yet unidentified infectious agents, the enterocyte, and the immune system of the host [15, 16]. The host risk factors (e.g., immunologic status, genetics) remain obscure, as does the specific environmental trigger. Bacterial overgrowth, disturbed motility, and mucosal injury contribute to the manifestation of tropical sprue in a susceptible host [16]. The epidemiology of tropical sprue suggests an infectious etiology, but extensive investigations have not yet identified or isolated any consistent causal agent [13].

"Tropical enteropathy" describes non-specific changes in the intestine (usually mild inflammation and partial villous atrophy) of asymptomatic subjects residing in tropical areas and should not be confused with tropical sprue.

Clinical Features

The onset of tropical sprue is usually insidious and is characterized by diarrhea, steatorrhea, abdominal pain, weight loss, fatigue, glossitis, multiple nutritional deficiencies, and loss of appetite [16].

Diagnosis

Tropical sprue should be considered in the differential diagnosis of chronic diarrhea and especially steatorrhea in patients with a recent history of travel to or residence in tropical areas [17] (Table 48.2). The histologic findings are non-specific and may be indistinguishable from those seen in celiac disease [1]. The d-xylose test and folic acid levels are usually abnormally low. Macrocytic anemia is a common finding [13]. Other indirect markers of malabsorption may be present, such as hypoalbuminemia, prolonged prothrombin time, and a low level of β-carotene. Indirect pancreatic test (e.g.,

Table 48.2 Suggested diagnostic tests for subjects with chronic diarrhea following travel to tropical areas.

Test	Suggested diagnosis on positive test	Comment
tTGA IgA	Celiac disease	Requires intestinal biopsy as confirmatory test
Stool analysis for ova and trophozoites	Infectious diarrhea	The most common cause of persistent infectious diarrhea is protozoal infection
Giardia antigen in stool	Giardiasis	Stool analysis for cysts or trophozoites is not reliable
Endoscopy with intestinal biopsy and sampling of duodenal aspirate	Celiac disease Bacterial overgrowth Tropical sprue Giardiasis	An expensive and invasive test that requires case-by-case indication
Folic acid and β-carotene in serum	Malabsorption syndrome	Severe folic acid deficiency strongly suggests tropical sprue
–	All tests normal	Normal tests suggest postinfective IBS

tTGA, tissue transglutaminase antibody; IgA, immunoglobulin A; IBS, irritable bowel syndrome.

pancreolauryl test) may be abnormal in as many as 64% of cases due to reversible exocrine pancreatic insufficiency related to a low pancreatic hormonal stimulation caused by the loss of enterocytes [18]. While antigliadin antibodies can be positive (reflecting non-specific increased intestinal permeability), both tTGAs and EMAs are negative [5]. The HLA type for celiac disease may be absent in patients with tropical sprue, but it is certainly no more common than in the general population, so it can be quite effective for ruling out celiac disease (Table 48.3). It should be noted that in the context of extreme poverty, environmental enteropathy is a common condition that can cause inflammation and blunting in the intestine, and, while not associated with overt chronic diarrhea, it nevertheless can result in malnutrition and stunting of growth and intellectual development.

Treatment

Broad-spectrum antibiotics and folic acid are the treatment of choice [15]. The clinical response is usually rapid (within weeks) and complete. Recurrence is uncommon, especially if the patient is not a resident of or frequent traveler to tropical areas. Relapses are common in treated patients who return to, or remain in, tropical areas. Tetracycline is the antibiotic of choice and should be used

Table 48.3 Differences between features of celiac disease and tropical sprue.

Feature	Celiac disease	Tropical sprue
Etiology	Immune-mediated disease	Unknown (possibly infectious)
Family history	Yes	No
Residence in or travel to tropic areas	Not required	Yes
Gender difference	Yes (females)	No
Prevalence in the United States	1% of general population	Unknown
EMAs or tTGAs	Yes	No
Iron-deficiency anemia	Common	Infrequent
Severe folic acid deficiency	Rare	Common
HLA typing	All carry DQ2 or DQ8	Usual frequency of DQ2 and DQ8
Intestinal involvement	Proximal	Proximal and distal
Treatment	GFD	Oral tetracycline and folic acid

EMA, endomysial antibody; tTGA, tissue transglutaminase antibody; HLA, human leukocyte antigen; GFD, gluten-free diet.

for 3–6 months, usually in conjunction with folic acid [13,16]. Sulfonamide therapy may be an effective alternative in patients with allergy or other absolute contraindications for the use of tetracycline. Rifaximin, a non-absorbed antimicrobial drug with a broad spectrum of antimicrobial activity that is effective for treatment of pathogen-negative traveler's diarrhea, is an attractive alternative therapy for tropical sprue, but clinical trials are necessary to evaluate its safety and efficacy in tropical sprue. A GFD does not result in either clinical or histologic improvement in tropical sprue.

Take Home Points

Diagnosis:

- The diagnosis of celiac disease is based on specific serology and an intestinal biopsy as a confirmatory test.
- History of either residence in or recent travel to a tropical area may be a key to suspecting the diagnosis of tropical sprue.
- Marked folic acid deficiency is frequent in tropical sprue.
- Iron-deficiency anemia may be the only sign or a clinical component of celiac disease.
- Clinical, serologic, and histologic response to a gluten-free diet (GFD) is characteristic of celiac disease.
- In patients in whom tropical sprue is suspected who lack specific serology for celiac disease, therapy for tropical sprue should be initiated.

Therapy:

- Correction of dehydration and nutritional deficiencies is an important part of the management of both celiac disease and tropical sprue.
- A GFD is the treatment of choice for celiac disease.
- Broad-spectrum antibiotics and folic acid may lead to a prompt clinical and histologic response in tropical sprue.

References

1 Green PH, Cellier C. Celiac disease. *N Engl J Med* 2007; **357**: 1731–43.
2 Rubio-Tapia A, Ludvigsson JF, Brantner TL, *et al.* The prevalence of celiac disease in the United States. *Am J Gastroenterol* 2012; **107**: 1538–44
3 Catassi C. The world map of celiac disease. *Acta Gastroenterol Latinoam* 2005; **35**: 37–55.
4 Rubio-Tapia A, Van Dyke CT, Lahr BD, *et al.* Predictors of family risk for celiac disease: a population-based study. *Clin Gastroenterol Hepatol* 2008; **6**: 983–7.
5 Rostom A, Murray JA, Kagnoff MF. American Gastroenterological Association (AGA) Institute technical review on the diagnosis and management of celiac disease. *Gastroenterology* 2006; **131**: 1981–2002.
6 Schuppan D, Dennis MD, Kelly CP. Celiac disease: epidemiology, pathogenesis, diagnosis, and nutritional management. *Nutr Clin Care* 2005; **8**: 54–69.
7 Rashtak S, Ettore MW, Homburger HA, Murray JA. Comparative usefulness of deamidated gliadin antibodies in the diagnosis of celiac disease. *Clin Gastroenterol Hepatol* 2008; **6**: 426–32, quiz 370.
8 Rubio-Tapia A, Hill ID, Kelly CP, *et al.* American College of Gastroenterology Clinical Guidelines: diagnosis and management of celiac disease. *Am J Gastroenterol* 2013; **108**: 656–76
9 Lewis NR, Scott BB. Systematic review: the use of serology to exclude or diagnose coeliac disease (a comparison of the endomysial and tissue transglutaminase antibody tests). *Aliment Pharmacol Ther* 2006; **24**: 47–54.
10 Harewood GC, Murray JA. Diagnostic approach to a patient with suspected celiac disease: a cost analysis. *Dig Dis Sci* 2001; **46**: 2510–4.
11 Marsh MN. Gluten, major histocompatibility complex, and the small intestine. A molecular and immunobiologic approach to the spectrum of gluten sensitivity ("celiac sprue"). *Gastroenterology* 1992; **102**: 330–54.
12 See J, Murray JA. Gluten-free diet: the medical and nutrition management of celiac disease. *Nutr Clin Pract* 2006; **21**: 1–15.
13 Mathan VI. Diarrhoeal diseases. *Br Med Bull* 1998; **54**: 407–19.
14 Ramakrishna BS, Venkataraman S, Mukhopadhya A. Tropical malabsorption. *Postgrad Med J* 2006; **82**: 779–87.
15 Westergaard H. Tropical sprue. *Curr Treat Options Gastroenterol* 2004; **7**: 7–11.
16 Nath SK. Tropical sprue. *Curr Gastroenterol Rep* 2005; **7**: 343–9.

CHAPTER 48

Whipple's Disease

Seema A. Patil and George T. Fantry

Division of Gastroenterology, University of Maryland School of Medicine, Baltimore, MD, USA

Summary

Whipple's disease [1, 2] is a rare, chronic, systemic infection caused by *Tropheryma whipplei* [3–9]. The symptoms and clinical findings are caused by chronic infection of the small intestine and other extraintestinal sites. Immune evasion and host interaction are important in the pathogenesis of infection. Clinical features include gastrointestinal (GI) and extraintestinal symptoms, with diarrhea the most common presenting complaint, arthritis the most common extraintestinal symptom, and hyperpigmentation and peripheral lymphadenopathy the most common physical findings. Small-intestinal mucosal biopsy is the diagnostic test of choice. Infiltration of the lamina propria of the small intestine by large, foamy, periodic acid–Schiff (PAS)-positive macrophages containing Gram-positive, acid-fast-negative bacilli accompanied by lymphatic dilation is specific and diagnostic of Whipple's disease. Antibiotic therapy usually results in dramatic improvement. The prognosis for patients with Whipple's disease who receive effective antibiotic therapy is excellent.

Case

A 55-year-old Caucasian man presents with a longstanding history of seronegative arthritis, anemia, lethargy, and weight loss and recent intermittent fevers of uncertain etiology. He has visual disturbances and an unsteady gait. He has no GI symptoms. Physical exam reveals severe cachexia, axillary adenopathy, and ataxia. Abdominal exam is benign. Laboratory evaluation reveals severe anemia, hypoalbuminemia, and an elevated erythrocyte sedimentation rate. Abdominal computed tomography (CT) scan reveals thickening of jejunal folds and mesenteric adenopathy. Endoscopy reveals a normal duodenum. Duodenal biopsies reveal extensive infiltration of the lamina propria with PAS-positive, foamy macrophages. Electron microscopy reveals multiple bacilli with a characteristic cell wall and a pale central nucleoid. A diagnosis of Whipple's disease is made. Treatment is instituted with parenteral penicillin G and streptomycin for 14 days, followed by oral trimethoprim–sulfamethoxazole twice daily for 1 year. All symptoms rapidly improve over the course of a few weeks. Repeat endoscopy at 1 year reveals persistence of PAS-positive, foamy macrophages in the lamina propria; however, electron microscopy reveals no organisms consistent with treated Whipple's disease.

Definition and Epidemiology

Whipple's disease is most common between the 4th and 6th decades of life [10], with a male predominance. It occurs predominantly in Caucasians and is more common in farmers and individuals involved in farm-related trades.

Pathophysiology

Immune Response

The symptoms and clinical findings in Whipple's disease are caused by chronic infection of the small intestine and other extraintestinal sites with *T. whipplei*. *T. whipplei* DNA has been found in gastric fluid, saliva, and stool samples from asymptomatic patients, suggesting that *T. whipplei* may be a ubiquitous, commensal organism in the environment. Its mode of transmission and pathogenic role are uncertain, however. Immune evasion and host interaction are important in the pathogenesis of infection. There is evidence that abnormal host defense – specifically defects of monocyte/macrophage function – plays an important pathophysiologic role, leading to an inability of the host response to eliminate the bacteria [10].

Histopathology

The lamina propria of the small-bowel mucosa is infiltrated by large, foamy macrophages, which distort normal villous architecture, resulting in a blunted, club-like appearance. The cytoplasm of these macrophages is filled with large glycoprotein granules that stain with PAS. The lymphatic channels are dilated. Electron microscopy reveals rod-shaped bacillary bodies in the lamina propria. The bacilli have a characteristic cell wall and pale central nucleoid. The Whipple bacillus is acid-fast-negative. PAS-positive macrophages and the characteristic bacilli have been identified in many extraintestinal tissues, reflecting the systemic nature of the disease.

Clinical Features

GI Symptoms

Diarrhea or steatorrhea is the most common presenting complaint [11]; however, it is not invariably present. Other intestinal symptoms include abdominal bloating, cramps, and anorexia. Weight loss is the second most common presenting complaint and is present before the initial evaluation in the majority of patients [11] (Table 49.1).

Practical Gastroenterology and Hepatology Board Review Toolkit, Second Edition. Edited by Nicholas J. Talley, Kenneth R. DeVault, Michael B. Wallace, Bashar A. Aqel and Keith D. Lindor.
© 2016 John Wiley & Sons, Ltd. Published 2016 by John Wiley & Sons, Ltd. Companion website: www.practicalgastrohep.com

Table 49.1 Clinical manifestations of Whipple's disease.

GI symptoms	Extraintestinal symptoms
Diarrhea	Arthritis or arthralgias
Weight loss	Fever
Anorexia	Fatigue and lethargy
Abdominal cramps	Lymphadenopathy
Abdominal bloating	Hyperpigmentation
Hepatomegaly	Heart murmurs
Splenomegaly	Cognitive deficits
	Visual changes

Extraintestinal Symptoms

Arthritis is the most common extraintestinal symptom, affecting the majority of patients [11]. It often develops before the initial diagnosis of Whipple's disease and is typically an intermittent, migratory arthritis of both the large and small joints. Fever – usually low-grade and intermittent – is the second most common extraintestinal symptom [11]. Fatigue and generalized weakness are also common. Numerous other extraintestinal symptoms may develop, reflecting the systemic nature of the infection (Table 49.1). *T. whipplei* is a commonly found pathogen associated with culture-negative infective endocarditis [12].

Neurological Symptoms

Central nervous system (CNS) involvement is common; however, symptoms related to CNS Whipple's disease are present in a minority of patients. Neurological symptoms may occur with GI symptoms or as isolated symptoms. The most common CNS symptoms are dementia, paralysis of gaze, and myoclonus.

Physical Findings

Hyperpigmentation and peripheral lymphadenopathy are the most common physical findings [11]. Emaciation, muscle wasting, peripheral edema, and peripheral neuropathy are often present. Abdominal findings may include mild distension, tenderness, or mass. Ascites, hepatomegaly, and splenomegaly are uncommon.

Additional physical findings may include fever, peripheral arthritis, heart murmurs, pleural or pericardial friction rubs, ocular abnormalities, and neurologic findings suggestive of CNS or cranial nerve involvement.

Radiologic and Endoscopic Findings

A small-bowel series typically reveals marked thickening of the mucosal folds, most prominent in the proximal small bowel [11]. Abdominal CT often reveals small-bowel thickening and massive para-aortic and retroperitoneal adenopathy [11]. On endoscopy, a characteristic finding of pale, shaggy, yellow mucosa in the postbulbar duodenum may be seen [13].

Laboratory Findings

Laboratory abnormalities, including low serum carotene levels, hypoalbuminemia, and electrolyte disturbances, are common [11]. Anemia is usually present secondary to chronic disease or iron deficiency [10]. The erythrocyte sedimentation rate is often elevated and the prothrombin time is frequently prolonged.

Diagnosis

Small-intestinal mucosal biopsy is the diagnostic test of choice. Infiltration of the lamina propria of the small intestine by PAS-positive macrophages containing Gram-positive, acid-fast-negative bacilli accompanied by lymphatic dilation is specific and diagnostic of Whipple's disease. Electron microscopy should be performed to verify the presence of the characteristic bacillus. Rarely, the diagnosis of Whipple's disease is established in the absence of intestinal involvement by the identification of bacilli in involved tissues. Molecular diagnosis using polymerase chain reaction (PCR)-based diagnostic tests may be useful in confirming Whipple's disease and in monitoring the response to antibiotic treatment [14–17].

Differential Diagnosis

Malabsorptive and Infiltrative Diseases of the Small Bowel

Other malabsorptive and infiltrative diseases of the small bowel, such as celiac disease and lymphoma, may present in a similar manner to Whipple's disease. These diseases can be readily differentiated by small-intestinal mucosal biopsy.

Small-Bowel Infections

Mycobacterium avium complex (MAC) infection may mimic Whipple's disease by causing infiltration of the lamina propria with PAS-positive macrophages [18]; however, MAC bacilli are acid-fast. PAS-positive macrophages in the intestinal lamina propria can also be seen in systemic histoplasmosis, but large, PAS-positive, rounded, encapsulated *Histoplasma* organisms are easily seen in macrophages.

Therapeutics

Antibiotic therapy usually results in dramatic improvement. Given concern over CNS involvement, treatment with an antibiotic that readily crosses the blood–brain barrier (BBB) is appropriate [19, 20]. One double-strength tablet of trimethoprim–sulfamethoxazole (TMP–SMX) given twice daily for 1 year has been proposed to be the optimal long-term option [11,19]. Initial therapy with parenteral penicillin G and streptomycin, ceftriaxone, or meropenem for 10–14 days may be of additional benefit, resulting in a lower relapse rate [11, 19–21] (Table 49.2). In patients who are allergic to TMP–SMX, initial parenteral therapy followed by oral penicillin VK or ampicillin for 1 year is reasonable. Decreasing the duration of long-term therapy with TMP-SMX to 3 months following initial therapy, as opposed to 1 year, may be effective but is not routinely recommended [22].

Treatment of Whipple's disease can precipitate a syndrome of fever, rigors, and hypotension, known as the Jarisch–Herxheimer

Table 49.2 Treatment of Whipple's disease.

Medication	Dose/frequency	Duration
Procaine penicillin G +	1.2 million units/day	2 weeks
Streptomycin or	1 g daily	2 weeks
Ceftriaxone or	2 g daily	2 weeks
Meropenem plus	1 g three times daily	2 weeks
TMP–SMX	160 mg/800 mg twice daily	1 year

TMP–SMX, trimethoprim–sulfamethoxazole.

reaction. Patients may also develop an immune reconstitution inflammatory syndrome (IRIS), manifested by a high fever in the first few weeks following initiation of antibiotics. This is more common in patients with CNS involvement and in those who were on extended immunosuppressive therapy that was discontinued upon the start of antibiotics [23].

After 1 year of antibiotic therapy, a small-intestinal mucosal biopsy should be repeated to document the absence of residual bacilli. Though PAS-positive macrophages may be present in the lamina propria for many years in patients treated for Whipple's disease, the presence of bacilli on electron microscopy suggests inadequate treatment [24].

Prognosis

The prognosis for patients with Whipple's disease who receive effective antibiotic therapy is excellent, with rapid improvement in GI and extraintestinal symptoms. Relapses are common [11, 19]. Relapse of GI symptoms and arthritis may occur early or late and may respond favorably to further antibiotic treatment, whereas CNS relapses tend to occur late and respond poorly to additional antibiotic therapy. If relapse is suspected, small-intestinal biopsy should be repeated to assess for the presence of free bacilli. The treatment of a relapse of Whipple's disease is a repeat course of the initial antibiotic therapy.

Take Home Points

Diagnosis:
- Consider Whipple's disease in the setting of malabsorption, unexplained gastrointestinal (GI) symptoms, weight loss, seronegative arthritis, culture-negative endocarditis, and fever of unknown origin.
- Endoscopy with small-bowel biopsy is indicated to diagnose Whipple's disease.
- Characteristic, diagnostic, histopathologic, and electron microscopic features are present in the lamina propria of the duodenal mucosa.

Therapy:
- An initial 14 days of parenteral antibiotics followed by a 1-year course of oral antibiotics is highly effective in most patients.
- Relapse is common.

References

1 Whipple GH. A hitherto undescribed disease characterized anatomically by deposits of fat and fatty acids in the intestinal and mesenteric lymphatic tissues. *Bull Johns Hopkins Hosp* 1907; **18**: 382.

2 Dobbins WO III. Whipple's disease: a historical perspective. *QJM* 1985; **56**: 523–31.

3 Relman DA, Schmidt TM, MacDermott RP, Falkow S. Identification of the uncultured bacillus of Whipple's disease. *N Engl J Med* 1992; **327**: 293 301.

4 Wilson KH, Blitchington R, Frothingham R, Wilson JAP. Phylogeny of the Whipple's-disease-associated bacterium. *Lancet* 1991; **338**: 474–5.

5 Maiwald M, Ditton HJ, Von Herbay A, *et al.* Reassessment of the phylogenetic position of the bacterium associated with Whipple's disease and determination of the 16S-23S ribosomal intergenic spacer sequence. *Int J Syst Bacteriol* 1996; **46**: 1078–82.

6 Raoult D, Birg ML, La Scola B, *et al.* Cultivation of the bacillus of Whipple's disease. *N Engl J Med* 2000; **342**: 620–5.

7 Raoult D, La Scola B, Lecocq P, *et al.* Culture and immunological detection of *Tropheryma whippelii* from the duodenum of a patient with Whipple disease. *JAMA* 2001; **285**: 1039–43.

8 Fenollar F, Birg ML, Gauduchon V, Raoult D. Culture of *Tropheryma whipplei* from human samples: a 3-year experience (1999–2002). *J Clin Microbiol* 2003; **41**: 3816–22.

9 Bentley SD, Maiwald M, Murphy LD, *et al.* Sequencing and analysis of the genome of the Whipple's disease bacterium *Tropheryma whipplei. Lancet* 2003; **361**: 637–44.

10 Moos V, Schmidt C, Geelhaar A, *et al.* Impaired immune functions of monocytes and macrophages in Whipple's disease. *Gastroenterology* 2010; **138**: 210–20.

11 Fleming JL, Wiesner RH, Shorter RG. Whipple's disease: clinical, biochemical, and histopathologic features and assessment of treatment in 29 patients. *Mayo Clin Proc* 1988; **63**: 539–51.

12 Geissdorfer W, Moos V, Moter A, *et al.* High frequency of *Tropheryma whipplei* in culture-negative endocarditis. *J Clin Microbiol* 2012; **50**: 216–22.

13 Geboes K, Ectors N, Heidbuchel H, *et al.* Whipple's disease. Endoscopic aspects before and after therapy. *Gastrointest Endosc* 1990; **36**: 247–52.

14 Von Herbay A, Ditton HJ, Maiwald M. Diagnostic application of a polymerase chain reaction assay for the Whipple's disease bacterium to intestinal biopsies. *Gastroenterology* 1996; **110**: 1735–43.

15 Ramzan NN, Loftus E, Burgart LJ. Diagnosis and monitoring of Whipple's disease by polymerase chain reaction. *Ann Intern Med* 1997; **126**: 520–7.

16 Muller C, Petermann D, Stain C, *et al.* Whipple's disease: comparison of histology with diagnosis based on polymerase chain reaction in four consecutive cases. *Gut* 1997; **40**: 425–7.

17 Pron B, Poyart C, Abachin C, *et al.* Diagnosis and follow-up of Whipple's disease by amplification of the 16S rRNA gene of *Tropheryma whippelii. World J Clin Microbiol Infect Dis* 1999; **18**: 62–5.

18 Gillin JS, Urmacher C, West R, Shike M. Disseminated *Mycobacterium avium-intracellulare* infection in acquired immunodeficiency syndrome mimicking Whipple's disease. *Gastroenterology* 1983; **85**: 1187–91.

19 Keinath RD, Merrell DE, Vlietstra R, Dobbins WO III. Antibiotic treatment and relapse in Whipple's disease. Long-term follow-up of 88 patients. *Gastroenterology* 1985; **88**: 1867–73.

20 Ryser RJ, Locksley RM, Eng SC, *et al.* Reversal of dementia associated with Whipple's disease by trimethoprim-sulfamethoxazole, drugs that penetrate the blood-brain barrier. *Gastroenterology* 1984; **86**: 745–52.

21 Feurle GE, Junga NS, Marth T. Efficacy of ceftriaxone or meropenem as initial therapies in Whipple's disease. *Gastroenterology* 2010; **138**: 478–86.

22 Feurle GE, Moos V, Blaker H, *et al.* Intravenous ceftriaxone, followed by 12 or three months of oral treatment with trimethoprim-sulfamethoxazole in Whipple's disease. *J Infect* 2013; **66**: 263–70.

23 Feurle GE, Moos V, Schinnerling K, *et al.* The immune reconstitution inflammatory syndrome in Whipple disease: a cohort study. *Ann Intern Med* 2010; **153**: 710–17.

24 Von Herbay A, Maiwald M, Ditton HJ, Otto HF. Histology of intestinal Whipple's disease revisited. A study of 48 patients. *Virchows Arch* 1996; **429**: 335–43.

CHAPTER 50
Short-Bowel Syndrome

Alan L. Buchman
Center for Gastroenterology and Nutrition, Skokie, IL, USA

Summary

Short-bowel syndrome (SBS) is defined as malabsorption due to insufficient intestinal surface area, with an inability to sustain an adequate nutritional, electrolyte, or hydration status in the absence of specialized nutritional support. In adults, it is typically the consequence of extensive bowel resection, with loss of absorptive surface area. Over time, the intestine can adapt in order to ensure more efficient absorption. Overall, the most important aspect of the management of patients with SBS is the provision of adequate nutrition and of sufficient fluid and electrolytes to prevent dehydration. Anastomosis of the residual small bowel to the colon is the most important surgical procedure, enhancing the ability of the colon to become an energy-absorptive organ and allowing for decreased dependence on parenteral nutrition (PN). The prognosis for patients with SBS depends on the patient's age, the type and extent of bowel resection, along with the underlying disease and health of residual intestine.

Case

A 57-year-old man with atrial fibrillation develops severe abdominal pain. He is diagnosed with an acute abdomen. He undergoes an emergent exploratory laparotomy, where an embolism is found in the superior mesenteric artery, 200 cm of gangrenous small bowel is resected, and an ileostomy is created. He undergoes a second-look surgery 2 days later, and a jejunocolic anastamosis is created. Total parenteral nutrition (TPN) is initiated postoperatively and, once bowel function returns, enteral nutrition is initiated with the goal of gradually decreasing the requirement for TPN.

Definition and Epidemiology

Intestinal failure is defined as an inability to sustain an adequate nutritional, electrolyte, or hydration status in the absence of specialized nutritional support, and is often seen in patients with SBS, which typically occurs in adults with less than 200 cm of functional intestine. However, the degree of intestinal function is better described in terms of energy absorption and loss, rather than the length of residual intestine, and some patients with SBS will not have sufficient loss of functional capacity to develop intestinal failure [1]. The patients at highest risk generally have a duodenostomy or ejunoileal anastamosis with less than 35 cm of residual intestine, a jejunocolic or ileocolic anastamosis with less than 60 cm of residual intestine, or an end jejunostomy with less than 115 cm of residual intestine [2].

The incidence of SBS is difficult to assess given the lack of a national registry and prospective studies. However, based on multinational European data, the incidence and prevalence of severe SBS, necessitating long-term PN, is estimated to be between two and four cases per 1 million persons per year [1]. These numbers, however, do not reflect patients who do not require PN, and approximately 50–70% can successfully be weaned off it [3].

Pathophysiology

The major consequence of extensive bowel resection is loss of absorptive surface area, which results in malabsorption of macro- and micronutrients, electrolytes, and water [4]. The degree of malabsorption is determined by the length and function of the remaining intestine and by the specific portions of small and large intestine resected, including whether the colon remains in continuity.

The length of the small intestine is estimated at 3–8 m in the adult, and nutrient absorption is preserved until more than one-half of the small intestine is removed [5]. Nutrient absorption may take place at any level of the small intestine, but crypt morphology and microvillus enzyme and transporter activity predict a proximal to distal gradient in absorptive capacity, and as such, most macronutrients are absorbed in the proximal 100 cm [6,7].

Patients with a proximal jejunostomy have rapid gastric emptying of liquids and rapid intestinal transit, both of which can severely limit nutrient digestive and absorptive processes. In addition, these patients are net secretors of salt and fluid, as jejunal fluid secretion is stimulated by oral intake and subsequent gastric emptying, so they excrete more fluid than they ingest. On unrestricted diets, these patients cannot absorb large volumes of water and electrolytes, and at least 100 cm of intact jejunum is required to maintain a positive water and electrolyte balance in adults [8], though cases of infants surviving with nutritional autonomy from 10 cm of residual jejunum have been reported.

The intestine can adapt after bowel resection in order to ensure more efficient absorption. These changes are most pronounced in the ileum, which attains the morphologic characteristics of the jejunum, with increased villous density and height and an increase in length. Conversely, the specialized cells of the terminal ileum, in which vitamin B_{12} and intrinsic factor receptors are located, and in which bile salts are absorbed, cannot be replaced by jejunal

Practical Gastroenterology and Hepatology Board Review Toolkit, Second Edition. Edited by Nicholas J. Talley, Kenneth R. DeVault, Michael B. Wallace, Bashar A. Aqel and Keith D. Lindor.

compensation. These adaptive changes may take up to 2 years to develop fully, and depend on the presence of food and biliary/pancreatic secretions. Because of this, patients with SBS are encouraged to start oral intake as soon as possible after surgery [9]. In addition, the colon becomes an important digestive organ in those with SBS. It has a large reserve absorptive capacity for sodium and water, and preservation of even part of the colon can significantly reduce fecal electrolyte and water losses [10].

Clinical Features

Ileal resection leads to interruption of the enterohepatic circulation of bile acids, resulting in decreased hepatic bile acid secretion and altered composition of bile. The bile becomes supersaturated with cholesterol, resulting in gallstone formation. Gallbladder hypomotility in the presence of PN likely contributes to gallstone formation as well [10, 11].

Fat malabsorption due to bile acid deficiency in patients with extensive ileal resection is associated with the development of oxalate kidney stones, as the unabsorbed long-chain fatty acids compete with oxalate for calcium, and a larger amount of free oxalate is lost to the colon, where it is absorbed and excreted by the kidney. Patients whose colon is in continuity generally should receive an oxalate-restricted diet [10].

Liver disease often develops in those requiring long-term PN, with >50% found to have severe liver disease after 5 years of PN [12]. Liver failure will develop in approximately 15% of all PN-dependent patients [13].

Other complications of SBS are catheter-related complications (including infection – sepsis, exit site, and tunnel infections; catheter occlusion – thrombotic and nonthromtotic; and catheter breakage), d-lactic acidosis, renal dysfunction, metabolic bone disease, memory deficits, and other neurologic abnormalities.

Differential Diagnosis

SBS may be a congenital or acquired condition. The causes of SBS in the pediatric population can be congenital or acquired, whereas in adults SBS typically results from surgical resection of bowel. In addition, functional SBS or intestinal failure may also occur in conditions of severe malabsorption, in which the bowel length is often intact (Table 50.1).

Therapeutics

Most available data on the treatment of SBS are based on retrospective analyses of case series (Figure 50.1).

Medical Management

The most important aspects in the management of patients with SBS are provision of adequate nutrition, provision of sufficient fluid and electrolytes to prevent dehydration, and correction and prevention of acid–base disturbances. Furthermore, it is important to treat the underlying disorder, such as Crohn's disease, whenever possible [5].

Massive enterectomy is associated with gastric hypersecretion for the initial 6 months [14, 15]; these patients will benefit from acid reduction, which serves to reduce fluid losses [16–18]. High doses of oral H_2-receptor antagonists, proton pump inhibitors (PPIs), or intravenous preparations are typically necessary, due to medication malabsorption. In addition, excessive fluid losses typically require

Table 50.1 Causes of SBS and intestinal failure.

Adults	Catastrophic vascular accidents: • Superior mesenteric venous thrombosis • Superior mesenteric arterial embolism • Superior mesenteric arterial thrombosis Chronic intestinal pseudo-obstruction[a] Intestinal resection for tumor Midgut volvulus Multiple intestinal resections for Crohn's disease Radiation enteritis[a] Refractory sprue[a] Scleroderma and mixed connective-tissue disease[a] Trauma
Children	Congenital villous atrophy[a] Extensive aganglionosis[a] Gastroschisis Jejunal or ileal atresia Necrotizing enterocolitis Microvillus inclusion disease[a] Midgut volvulus

[a]Functional SBS may also occur in conditions with severe malabsorption, in which bowel length remains intact.

the use of antimotility agents, such as high doses of loperamide hydrochloride (4–16 mg/day) or diphenoxylate. If these agents are ineffective, codeine sulfate or tincture of opium is often necessary. Rarely, patients may require treatment with octreotide, which can slow intestinal transit and increase water and sodium absorption [1] (Table 50.2).

Oral rehydration solutions (ORSs) improve hydration and decrease PN fluid requirements, especially in those patients with a proximal jejunostomy or with less than 100 cm of jejunum remaining [17]. These solutions take advantage of the sodium–glucose cotransporter and the solvent drag that follows intracellular transport of sodium and water [19]. Optimal solutions have a sodium concentration of at least 90 mEq/L. The best and least expensive ORS is that recommended by the World Health Organization (WHO), which has substantially more sodium than most commercially available solutions. Patients with SBS should be advised to avoid consumption of water and to drink ORSs whenever thirsty [5].

Patients who have undergone massive enterectomy typically require PN initially. Once they are hemodynamically stable, enteral nutrition should be started as soon as possible, and advanced gradually as tolerated. When patients are able to eat, they should be encouraged to eat a regular diet (with modifications as discussed later), and to eat substantially more than was typical before the resection (hyperphagia), in order to compensate for the malabsorption. This may be accomplished by the use of multiple small meals, and is perhaps the single most important dietary intervention in reducing the need for TPN [5, 20].

The absorption of nitrogenous macronutrients is least affected by the decreased intestinal absorptive surfaced area. It has been reasoned that if dietary protein were provided in a predigested form, it would be more readily absorbed. However, in seven patients with an end-jejunostomy, energy, carbohydrate, nitrogen, fat, electrolyte, fluid, and mineral absorption, as well as stool weight, were similar regardless of whether or not a peptide-based enteral formula was provided. Based on this experience, the utility of peptide-based diets is largely without merit [21, 22].

Most intestinal dissacharidases are present in the highest concentration in the proximal small intestine, which often remains intact in patients who undergo massive enterectomy. In the absence of significant jejunal resection or documented lactase deficiency,

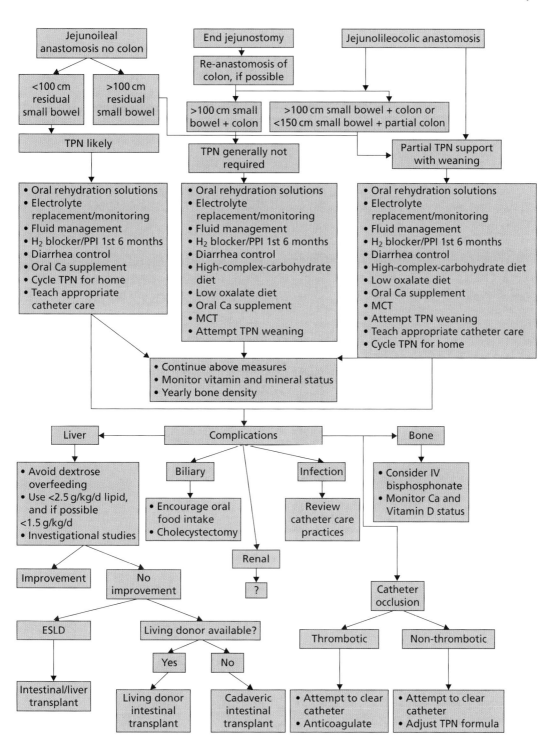

Figure 50.1 Management of SBS. TPN, total parenteral nutrition; MCT, medium-chain triglycerides; PPI, proton pump inhibitor; ESLD, end-stage liver disease. Source: Buchman 2003 [1]. Reproduced with permission of Elsevier.

lactose-containing foods should not be limited, as they are an important source of dietary calcium [23, 24].

Patients with SBS whose colon is in continuity should consume a high-complex-carbohydrate diet, as starches, non-starch polysaccharides, and soluble fiber pass undigested into the colon, where bacteria ferment them into short-chain fatty acids (SCFAs), including butyrate, proprionate, and acetate. SCFAs provide fuel for the colonocyte and significantly reduce fecal energy losses. As such, the colon becomes an important digestive organ in patients with SBS

[25, 26]. Furthermore, sodium and water absorption are stimulated by SCFAs, though decreased fecal losses have not been documented clinically [27].

Lipid digestion may be impaired, as micelle formation is limited due to ileal bile salt malabsorption. Treatment with bile salt replacement, such as ox bile or the conjugated bile acid chylosarcosine, has been reported in a few patients; it decreases fecal fat in most, but leavs fecal volume unchanged or increased [28–32]. Cholestyramine may be useful in decreasing bile salt-induced diarrhea in those with

Table 50.2 Therapeutic agents used to decrease intestinal transit and stool volume.

Agent	Dosage
Loperamide	4–6 mg four times daily
Diphenoxylate/atropine	2.5–5.0 mg four times daily
Codeine sulfate	15 mg two to four times daily
Ranitidine	300 mg twice daily
Omeprazole	40 mg twice daily
Octreotide	50–100 µg SC twice daily

SC, subcutaneous.

less than 100 cm of terminal ileum resected but should not be used in patients with more than 100 cm of ileal resection, because it can worsen steatorrhea by binding dietary lipid [33].

In those patients with their colon in continuity, a high-fat diet can lead to more diarrhea. However, this must be balanced against the fact that fat is an important energy source, given its increased energy density when compared to carbohydrates. Overall, limited data are available to support the use of low-fat diets [34].

It is important to assess the vitamin and mineral status of these patients at regular intervals. It is unusual for water-soluble vitamin deficiencies to develop, except in those with duodenostomies or proximal jejunostomies, because water-soluble vitamins are absorbed in the proximal jejunum. However, folate deficiency may develop in patients with proximal jejunal resection, and these patients should receive daily folate. In addition, vitamin B_{12} deficiency is seen in patients who have >60 cm of terminal ileum resected, and supplementation is necessary [5].

Fat-soluble vitamin deficiencies are more common, and develop as a result of decreased bile salt reabsorption and associated fat maldigestion. Cholestyramine can cause fat-soluble vitamin deficiency as well, due to its effects of binding to bile salts, and should not be used if more than 100 cm of terminal ileum has been resected as it will lead to enhanced malabsorption [33]. Vitamin A deficiency is characterized by night blindness and xerophthalmia. Vitamin D deficiency manifests as osteomalacia. Vitamin E deficiency manifests as hemolysis and various neurologic deficits. Vitamin K deficiency is uncommon in those patients with an intact colon, as 60% of vitamin K is synthesized by colonic bacteria; however, it can be seen in those without a residual colon or in those who have taken antibiotics [5].

Fecal losses of zinc and selenium can be significant, and deficiencies will develop. Zinc deficiency has been associated with growth abnormalities, delayed wound healing, and immune dysfunction. Selenium deficiency has been associated with various abnormalities, including cardiomyopathy, peripheral neuropathy, and proximal muscle weakness and pain [5].

The length of remaining bowel necessary to prevent dependence on PN is approximately 100 cm in the absence of an intact colon or 60 cm in the presence of a colon [2, 6, 35]. For those who require long-term PN, gradual attempts should be made to wean them from PN; approximately 50% can discontinue PN and resume oral intake after 1–2 years [3]. Because PN solutions are hypertonic, they are infused into a central vein. PN is typically given in a continuous fashion in the initial postoperative phase, but over time the infusions are gradually compressed into a cycled regimen (with adjustments to volume and nutritional support).

Growth factors have been studied in patients with SBS. A double-blinded, randomized, placebo-controlled trial of growth hormone in 41 PN-dependent patients showed that PN requirements in treated patients could be reduced by an additional 2 L/week over

the reduction with standard therapies [36]. In addition, treatment with a synthetic analogue of glucagon-like peptide 2 (GLP 2), an intestinotrophic agent, was shown to increase villous height, with increased fluid absorption and modest improvements in energy absorption, leading to a decrease in PN of about 2 L/week and a corresponding reduction of one-night-per-week infusion [37]. However, these effects tended to regress in most patients once the medication was discontinued [38,39].

Surgical Management

Anastamosis of the small bowel to the colon is the most important surgical procedure, enhancing the ability of the colon to become an energy-absorptive organ and allowing for decreased dependence on PN. Other surgical procedures aimed at tapering dilated, non-functional intestine are available, but they should be reserved for highly selected individuals with dilated, non-functional segments of intestine [1]. In the Bianchi procedure, the surgeon divides the dilated bowel and performs an end-to-end anastamosis, thereby doubling the bowel length [40]. In the serial transverse enteroplasty procedure (STEP), a linear staple is applied from alternating and opposite directions along the mesenteric border to incompletely divide the dilated intestine, which leads to tapering of the dilated intestine [41].

The main indication for intestinal transplantation is PN-dependent SBS complicated by progressive liver disease, and as such, intestinal transplantation is often combined with liver transplantation. If patients are referred for evaluation for transplantation prior to the development of advanced fibrosis, isolated intestinal transplantation can be carried out. These patients have a better prognosis than those requiring a combined transplant. In addition, patients with significant fluid losses and refractory dehydration despite appropriate medical management are candidates for intestinal transplantation. Survival has improved considerably since intestinal transplantation was introduced, and patients who have undergone transplantation more recently have better survival, largely due to improved surgical techniques and improved immunosuppressive regimens [42, 43]. While the short-term survival in those receiving intestinal transplantation approaches 90%, the 5-year survival is closer to 50%, which is far worse than in those requiring long-term home PN. As such, intestinal transplantation is not a replacement for home PN. Along those lines, both premature intestinal transplantation and late referral for transplantation, which often requires the addition of a liver graft, must be avoided. High-risk patients should be identified early and referred to a center where intestinal rehabilitation and transplantation are both practiced [44].

Prognosis

The prognosis for patients with SBS depends on the type and extent of bowel resection, along with the underlying disease and health of residual intestine. Patients with limited resections have an excellent prognosis, assuming careful management of their malabsorptive issues. As would be expected, patients with small bowel length <50 cm, including those with high jejunostomies and severe malabsorption, have a worse prognosis. In addition, mesenteric infarction as a cause for the bowel resection has a worse prognosis – as does radiation enteritis – when it leads to SBS. However, overall prognosis, including survival and quality of life, is improving, largely because of increasing experience with long-term TPN and means of assessing nutritional needs [3].

Take Home Points

- Short-bowel syndrome (SBS) is characterized by malabsorption due to insufficient intestinal surface area.
- SBS is usually the consequence of extensive bowel resection.
- Over time, the intestine can adapt to ensure more efficient absorption.
- Acid suppression and antimotility agents serve to decrease fluid losses.
- Oral rehydration solutions (ORSs) improve dehydration and decrease TPN fluid requirements.
- Patients should generally be encouraged to eat a regular diet, and to eat substantially more than was typical prior to the resection (hyperphagia).
- Approximately 50% of patients can discontinue total parenteral nutrition (TPN) after 2 years.
- Anastamosis of the small bowel to the colon is the most important surgical procedure, allowing the colon to become an energy-absorptive organ.
- Prognosis depends on the type and extent of bowel resection, along with the underlying disease.
- Growth-factor therapy may be useful in reducing the requirement for parenteral nutrition (PN).

References

1 Buchman AL, Scolapio J, Fryer J. AGA technical review on short bowel syndrome and intestinal transplantation. *Gastroenterology* 2003; **124**: 1111–34.
2 Carbonnel F, Cosnes J, Chevret S, *et al.* The role of anatomic factors in nutritional autonomy after extensive small bowel resection. *J Parenter Enteral Nutr* 1996; **20**: 275–80.
3 Messing B, Crenn P, Beau P, *et al.* Long-term survival and parenteral nutrition dependence in adult patients with the short bowel syndrome. *Gastroenterology* 1999; **117**: 1043–50.
4 Andersson H, Bosaeus I, Brummer RJ, *et al.* Nutritional and metabolic consequences of extensive bowel resection. *Dig Dis* 1986; **4**: 193–202.
5 Buchman AL. Etiology and initial management of short bowel syndrome. *Gastroenterology* 2006; **130** (2 Suppl. 1): S5–S15.
6 Borgstrom B, Dahlqvist A, Lundh G, *et al.* Studies of intestinal digestion and absorption in the human. *J Clin Invest* 1957; **36**: 1521–36.
7 Clarke RM. Mucosal architecture and epithelial cell production rate in the small intestine of the albino rat. *J Anat* 1970; **107**: 519–29.
8 Nightingale JM, Lennard-Jones JE, Walker ER, *et al.* Jejunal efflux in short bowel syndrome. *Lancet* 1990; **336**: 765–8.
9 Cisler JJ, Buchman AL. Intestinal adaptation in short bowel syndrome. *J Invest Med* 2005; **53**: 402–13.
10 Nightingale JM, Lennard-Jones JE, Gertner, DJ, *et al.* Colonic preservation reduces need for parenteral therapy, increases incidence of renal stones, but does not change high prevalence of gall stones in patients with a short bowel. *Gut* 1992; **33**: 1493–7.
11 Roslyn JJ, Pitt HA, Mann LL, *et al.* Gallbladder disease in patients on long-term parenteral nutrition. *Gastroenterology* 1983; **84**: 148–54.
12 Cavicchi M, Beau P, Crenn P, *et al.* Prevalence of liver disease and contributing factors in patients receiving home parenteral nutrition for permanent intestinal failure. *Ann Intern Med* 2000; **132**: 525–32.
13 Chan S, McCowen KC, Bistrian BR, *et al.* Incidence, prognosis, and etiology of end-stage liver disease in patients receiving home total parenteral nutrition. *Surgery* 1999; **126**: 28–34.
14 Windsor CW, Fejfar J, Woodward DA. Gastric secretion after massive small bowel resection. *Gut* 1969; **10**: 779–86.
15 Williams NS, Evans P, King RF. Gastric acid secretion and gastrin production in the short bowel syndrome. *Gut* 1985; **26**: 914–9.
16 Jeppesen PB, Staun M, Tjellesen, L, *et al.* Effect of intravenous ranitidine and omeprazole on intestinal absorption of water, sodium, and macronutrients in patients with intestinal resection. *Gut* 1998; **43**: 763–9.
17 Jacobsen O, Ladefoged K, Stage JG, *et al.* Effects of cimetidine on jejunostomy effluents in patients with severe short-bowel syndrome. *Scand J Gastroenterol* 1986; **21**: 824–8.
18 Nightingale JM, Walker ER, Farthing MJ, *et al.* Effect of omeprazole on intestinal output in the short bowel syndrome. *Aliment Pharmacol Ther* 1991; **5**: 405–12.
19 Fordtran JS. Stimulation of active and passive sodium absorption by sugars in the human jejunum. *J Clin Invest* 1975; **55**: 728–37.
20 Cosnes J, Gendre JP, Evard D, *et al.* Compensatory enteral hyperalimentation for management of patients with severe short bowel syndrome. *Am J Clin Nutr* 1985; **41**: 1002–9.
21 McIntyre PB, Fitchew M, Lennard-Jones JE. Patients with a high jejunostomy do not need a special diet. *Gastroenterology* 1986; **91**: 25–33.
22 Levy E, Frileux P, Sandrucci, S, *et al.* Continuous enteral nutrition during the early adaptive stage of the short bowel syndrome. *Br J Surg* 1988; **75**: 549–53.
23 Marteau P, Messing B, Arrigoni E, *et al.* Do patients with short-bowel syndrome need a lactose-free diet? *Nutrition* 1997; **13**: 13–6.
24 Arrigoni E, Marteau P, Briet F, *et al.* Tolerance and absorption of lactose from milk and yogurt during short-bowel syndrome in humans. *Am J Clin Nutr* 1994; **60**: 926–9.
25 Bond JH, Currier BE, Buchwald H, *et al.* Colonic conservation of malabsorbed carbohydrate. *Gastroenterology* 1980; **78**: 444–7.
26 Cummings JH, Gibson GR, Macfarlane GT. Quantitative estimates of fermentation in the hind gut of man. *Acta Vet Scand* 1989; **86**(Suppl.): 76–82.
27 Nordgaard I, Hansen BS, Mortensen PB. Colon as a digestive organ in patients with short bowel. *Lancet* 1994; **343**: 373–6.
28 Little KH, Schiller LR, Bilhartz LE, *et al.* Treatment of severe steatorrhea with ox bile in an ileectomy patient with residual colon. *Dig Dis Sci* 1992; **37**: 929–33.
29 Fordtran JS, Bunch F, Davis GR. Ox bile treatment of severe steatorrhea in an ileectomy-ileostomy patient. *Gastroenterology* 1982; **82**: 564–8.
30 Djurdjevic D, Popvic O, Necic D, *et al.* Ox bile treatment of severe steatorrhea in a colectomy and ileectomy patient. *Gastroenterology* 1988; **95**: 1160.
31 Heydorn S, Jeppesen PB, Mortensen PB. Bile acid replacement therapy with cholylsarcosine for short-bowel syndrome. *Scand J Gastroenterol* 1999; **34**: 818–23.
32 Kapral C, Wewalka F, Praxmarer V, *et al.* Conjugated bile acid replacement therapy in short bowel syndrome patients with a residual colon. *Z Gastroenterol* 2004; **42**: 583–9.
33 Hofmann AF, Poley JR. Role of bile acid malabsorption in pathogenesis of diarrhea and steatorrhea in patients with ileal resection. I. Response to cholestyramine or replacement of dietary long chain triglyceride by medium chain triglyceride. *Gastroenterology* 1972; **62**: 918–34.
34 Woolf GM, Miller C, Kurian R, *et al.* Diet for patients with a short bowel: high fat or high carbohydrate? *Gastroenterology* 1983; **84**: 823–8.
35 Jeppesen PB, Mortensen PB. Intestinal failure defined by measurements of intestinal energy and wet weight absorption. *Gut* 2000; **46**: 701–6.
36 Byrne TA, Wilmore DW, Iyer K, *et al.* Growth hormone, glutamine, and an optimal diet reduces parenteral nutrition in patients with short bowel syndrome: a prospective, randomized, placebo-controlled, double-blind clinical trial. *Ann Surg* 2005; **242**: 655–61.
37 Jeppesen PB, Pertkiewicz M, Messing B, *et al.* Teduglutide reduces need for parenteral support among patinets with short bowel syndrome with intestinal failure. *Gastroenterology* 2012; **143**: 1473–81.
38 Jeppesen PB, Sanguinetti EL, Buchman A, *et al.* Teduglutide (ALX-0600), a dipeptidyl peptidase IV resistant glucagon-like peptide 2 analogue, improves intestinal function in short bowel syndrome patients. *Gut* 2005; **54**: 1224–31.
39 Compher C, Gilroy R, Pertkiewicz M, *et al.* Maintenance of parenteral nutrition volume reduction, without weight loss, after stopping teduglutide in a subset of patinets with short bowel syndrome. *JPEN* 2011; **35**: 603–9.
40 Bianchi A. Intestinal loop lengthening – a technique for increasing small intestinal length. *J Pediatr Surg* 1980; **15**: 145–51.
41 Kim HB, Lee PW, Garza JW, *et al.* Serial transverse enteroplasty (STEP): a novel bowel lengthening procedure. *J Pediatr Surg* 2003; **38**: 425–9.
42 Fishbein TM, Kaufman SS, Florman SS, *et al.* Isolated intestinal transplantation: proof of clinical efficacy. *Transplantation* 2003; **76**: 636–40.
43 Lacaille F, Vass N, Sauvat, *et al.* Long-term outcome, growth and digestive function in children 2 to 18 years after intestinal transplantation. *Gut* 2008; **57**: 455–61.
44 Fryer JP. Intestinal transplantation: current status. *Gastroenterol Clin North Am* 2007; **36**: 145–59, vii.

CHAPTER 50

CHAPTER 51
Protein-Losing Gastroenteropathy

Lauren K. Schwartz[1] and Carol E. Semrad[2]
[1] Division of Gastroenterology, Mount Sinai Hospital, New York, NY, USA
[2] Gastroenterology Section, The University of Chicago, Chicago, IL, USA

Summary

Protein-losing gastroenteropathy (PLGE) is a condition characterized by excessive loss of serum proteins into the gastrointestinal (GI) tract that results in symptomatic hypoproteinemia. It is not a single condition but rather a manifestation of various disease states, both intestinal and extraintestinal, that compromise the GI mucosal barrier and/or lymphatic flow. Clinically, patients present with edema, ascites, and pericardial or pleural effusions. To make the diagnosis, excess fecal protein loss must be documented by measuring α-1-antitrypsin clearance or using nuclear scintigraphy. Further evaluation is then directed at establishing the underlying cause. Treatment goals include aggressive protein supplementation to improve nutritional status and, when possible, treatment of the underlying disease to stop protein loss.

Case

A 72-year-old man is referred for chronic diarrhea, weight loss, and edema. He has a past history of diabetes and hypertension. He began passing six to seven loose stools daily with associated gas/bloating and abdominal pain 4 years ago. He lost 36 kg (80 lb) of weight. He developed lower-extremity edema 4 months ago. On physical examination, he is well developed, his heart and lungs are normal, and his extremities have 4+ pitting edema. Outside evaluation shows low total protein and albumin levels, normal urinalysis, and negative stool studies. Esophagogastroduodenoscopy (EGD) and lower endoscopy with biopsies are unrevealing. Further evaluation shows increased fecal fat (70 g fat diet) of 15 g/day (normal <7 g/dL), increased α-1-antitrypsin level in the stool, and low vitamin B_{12} and zinc levels. Mesenteric Doppler study shows increased velocities of the celiac and superior mesenteric arteries. Video capsule endoscopy shows denuded areas, predominantly in the jejunum (Figure 51.1). Upper double-balloon enteroscopy confirms denuded mucosa in the jejunum. Biopsies reveal active jejunitis with morphology typical of ischemia (Figure 51.2). Mesenteric angiography shows no vascular lesion amendable to bypass. The impression is chronic ischemic enteritis due to small-vessel disease causing malabsorption and protein-losing enteropathy. The patient is treated with prednisone, leading to improvement in his diarrhea, serum protein levels, and edema.

Pathophysiology

Normally, a small amount of plasma proteins leaks into the intestinal lumen, where it is digested and reabsorbed for use in protein synthesis. In PLGE, up to 60% of plasma proteins are exuded into the intestinal lumen every day, overwhelming digestive and absorptive capacities and resulting in high fecal protein loss. Hypoproteinemia develops when the rate of protein loss exceeds the body's rate of protein synthesis [1,2]. Because the liver can only increase albumin synthesis by 25%, hypoalbuminemia quickly develops [3]. Reductions in other proteins with slow rates of synthesis (e.g., gamma globulins) are also common.

The two major mechanisms of PLGE are intestinal lymphatic obstruction and mucosal disease (Figure 51.3, Table 51.1). Lymphatic obstruction or impaired flow results in increased lymphatic pressure, rupture of lacteals, and protein leakage across the intestinal epithelium. Mucosal disease causes protein leakage through an ulcerated epithelial barrier or increased permeability. The molecular basis of intestinal protein leakage due to the latter is unknown. Loss of heparin sulfate and syndecan-1 proteins on intestinal epithelial cells may be responsible [4].

Etiology

Primary Intestinal Lymphangiectasia

Primary intestinal lymphangiectasia is a rare disorder characterized by dilated intestinal lacteals that leak chylous fluid into the intestinal lumen. It classically presents in childhood or young adulthood with bilateral lower-extremity edema. Most cases are sporadic, though some occur as part of a syndrome (von Recklinghausen, Turner, Noonan, Klippel–Trenauny, Hennekam, yellow-nail syndromes) [5].

Secondary Intestinal Lymphangiectasia

Secondary intestinal lymphangiectasia refers to dilated intestinal lymphatics resulting from secondary causes of impaired lymphatic flow. These causes include cardiac conditions, lymphoma, tuberculosis, hepatic venous outflow obstruction, and chemotherapy. Cardiac and hepatic causes are believed to obstruct lymphatic flow through venous congestion. The Fontan procedure, an operation for patients with a single ventricle, is also linked to venous congestion, but the underlying pathophysiology of protein loss appears more complex [6].

Practical Gastroenterology and Hepatology Board Review Toolkit, Second Edition. Edited by Nicholas J. Talley, Kenneth R. DeVault, Michael B. Wallace, Bashar A. Aqel and Keith D. Lindor.
© 2016 John Wiley & Sons, Ltd. Published 2016 by John Wiley & Sons, Ltd. Companion website: www.practicalgastrohep.com

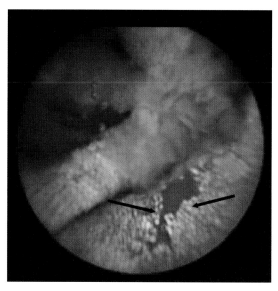

Figure 51.1 Denuded jejunal mucosa in PLGE, caused by chronic intestinal ischemia.

Mucosal Disorders with Erosions, Ulcers, or Denuded Areas

These have a clear breach in the epithelial barrier, with concurrent inflammation, which promotes protein loss. Examples include inflammatory bowel disease (IBD), intestinal ischemia (Figure 51.1), erosive gastritis, and non-steroidal anti-inflammatory drug (NSAID) enteropathy.

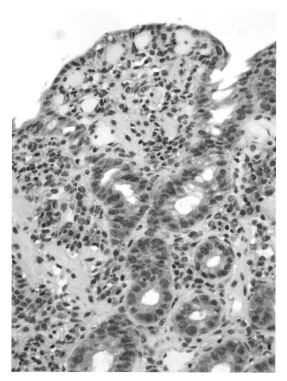

Figure 51.2 Jejunal biopsy with surface atrophy and regenerating crypts characteristic of ischemia. Source: Courtesy of Dr. Jerrold Turner.

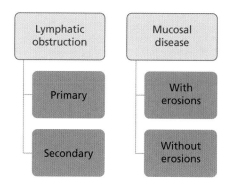

Figure 51.3 Mechanisms of PLGE.

Mucosal Disorders without Erosions

Mucosal disorders without erosions are characterized by increased epithelial permeability in the absence of macroscopic injury. Classic examples include Ménétrier's disease, celiac disease, eosinophilic gastroenteritis, and systemic lupus erythematosus (SLE).

Clinical Features

The most common presentation of PLGE is edema due to hypoproteinemia. Ascites and pleural and pericardial effusions may also occur. Low serum albumin levels are primarily responsible for loss of oncotic pressure and third-spacing of fluid. Decreased serum gamma globulin (IgM, IgA, IgG) levels are common, but generally do not lead to infectious complications. Other proteins with slow turnover rates that are often reduced include transferrin, fibrinogen, α-1-antitrypsin, and ceruloplasmin.

In those with lymphatic obstruction, chylous fluid leaks across the intestinal epithelium into the lumen, resulting in the loss of fat, fat-soluble vitamins (A, D, E, K), and lymphocytes as well as protein. Lymphopenia can result in impaired cellular immunity. Chylous effusions can also occur [5].

In patients with primary intestinal mucosal disease, abdominal bloating, diarrhea, malabsorption (fat and carbohydrate), and weight loss predominate, and decreased protein absorption may contribute to low protein levels.

Diagnosis

The diagnosis of PLGE should be suspected when a patient presents with hypoproteinemia that is not explained by decreased protein intake or absorption. The first step to making a diagnosis is a history focused on diet intake and GI symptoms. Hypoalbuminemia with a normal serum total protein level suggests impaired hepatic synthesis or renal losses (nephrotic syndrome), whereas hypoalbuminemia with a low total protein suggests fecal loss (PLGE) or malnutrition.

Tests for Intestinal Protein Loss

The most sensitive test for fecal protein loss is α-1-antitrypsin clearance. α-1-antitrypsin is a glycoprotein that functions as a protease inhibitor. It is resistant to intestinal degradation and is excreted intact in the stool, making it an ideal endogenous marker of intestinal protein loss [7, 8]. Plasma and stool concentrations of α-1-antitrypsin must be measured, as must stool volume. Stool is

Table **51.1** Causes of PLGE.

Lymphatic obstruction		Mucosal disease	
Primary	Secondary	Erosive	Non-erosive
Intestinal lymphangiectasia	**Cardiac**	**Inflammatory**	Inflammatory
Idiopathic	Constrictive pericarditis	Crohn's disease	Celiac disease
Syndrome-associated	Congestive heart failure	Ulcerative colitis	Allergic gastroenteropathy
	Tricuspid regurgitation	Behçet's disease	Eosinophilic gastroenteritis
	Congenital heart disease	Graft-versus-host disease	Collagenous colitis
	Fontan procedure		
Other congenital malformations	**Hepatobiliary**	**Esophageal and gastric**	**Gastric**
Intestinal lymphatic hypoplasia	Hepatic vein outflow	Erosive esophagitis and gastritis	Ménétrier's disease
Lymphangiomatosis	obstruction	Esophageal and gastric ulcers	Lymphocytic gastritis
	Portal hypertensive		Secretory hypertrophic gastropathy
	gastroenteropathy		*H. pylori* infection
	Infectious	**Infectious**	**Infectious**
	Mesenteric tuberculosis	*Clostridium difficile*	Bacterial overgrowth
	Whipple's disease	Invasive infectious enteritis	Tropical sprue
			Viral infection
			Parasitic infection
			Whipple's disease
	Neoplastic	**Neoplastic**	**Collagen vascular**
	Intestinal lymphoma	Lymphoma	Systemic lupus erythematosus
	Kaposi's sarcoma	Gastric cancer	Sjögren's disease
		Kaposi's sarcoma	Mixed connective-tissue disease
		Waldenstrom	
		macroglobulinemia	
	Toxic	**Toxic**	
	Chemotherapy	Non-steroidal anti-inflammatory	
	Arsenic	drugs	
		Chemotherapy	
		Radiation therapy	
	Other	**Other**	
	Mesenteric sarcoidosis	Intestinal ischemia	
	Retroperitoneal fibrosis	Amyloidosis	
	Mesenteric venous thrombosis		

collected over 1–3 days, as spot samples are unreliable. α-1-antitrypsin loss (mL/day) can be derived as follows:

$$\text{Clearance} = \frac{(\text{stool A1–AT concentration}) \times \left(\begin{array}{c}\text{stool}\\\text{volume}\end{array}\right)}{(\text{plasma A1–AT concentration})}$$

$$\text{A1–AT} = \text{α-1-antitrypsin concentration in mg/100 g dry}$$
$$\text{stool weight}$$

Normally, α-1-antitrypsin clearance is <13 mL/day. In patients with PLGE, clearance is >24 mL/day, or >56 mL/day with diarrhea [9]. Diarrhea increases protein loss, perhaps due to rapid transit or increased protein leakage. GI bleeding also elevates stool protein levels. In individuals with suspected esophageal or gastric protein loss (e.g., Ménétrier's disease), the test may not be reliable because α-1-antitrypsin is degraded at a gastric pH <3. Acid-suppressive therapy should be administered at the time of study to overcome this limitation [10, 11].

Other methods of detecting protein loss from the GI tract involve:
1 Infusing radiolabeled macromolecules (e.g., chromium-51-albumin) into the bloodstream and measuring fecal radioactivity to estimate clearance [12].
2 Carrying out nuclear scintigraphy to detect extravasation of tagged molecules (e.g., technetium-99 albumin) into the intestine [13].
The former technique is rarely used because it is costly and labor-intensive. Nuclear scintigraphy is useful in both detecting and localizing the site of protein loss. It also allows documentation of response to therapy [14].

Tests to Determine Underlying Etiology

Once PLGE is established, efforts are directed toward the identification of the underlying cause. Patient history is extremely valuable in guiding tests. EGD, push enteroscopy, or colonoscopy with biopsies is indicated in those with suspected primary GI disease. Video capsule endoscopy, computed tomographic enterography (CTE), and small-bowel series may be helpful in those with a patchy distribution of intestinal disease. In women with unexplained edema and PLGE, testing for SLE is warranted. In those with suspected cardiac disease, cardiac evaluation is indicated.

Therapy

The goals of therapy for PLGE are twofold.
1 To reverse protein loss by treating the underlying disease.
2 To improve nutritional status through protein supplementation.
Treatment to reverse protein loss varies by disease and includes both medical and surgical therapies.

Medical Therapies

- **Corticosteroids** have been effective in collagen vascular diseases, IBD, collagenous colitis, allergic eosinophilic gastroenteritis, and amyloidosis, as well as following the Fontan operation. Use of other immunomodulators, such as cyclosporine, has also been reported [15].
- **Octreotide** has been effective in Ménétrier's disease [16,17], amyloidosis [18], and intestinal lymphangiectasia [19].
- **Heparin** injections have been somewhat successful in post-Fontan PLGE [6]. Success in therapy may be related to an underlying loss of heparin sulfate on intestinal epithelial cells.

- **Antibiotics** are indicated for infectious causes of PLGE, such as *Clostridium difficile*, tuberculosis, Whipple's disease, and *Helicobacter pylori*.
- **Chemotherapy** should be directed at underlying malignancies.
- **Biologics** such as antibodies to epidermal growth factor and tumor necrosis factor (TNF)-α have been used for Ménétrier's disease and IBD, respectively.

Surgical Therapies
- **Cardiac surgery:** Definitive treatment of constrictive pericarditis entails removal of the pericardium. In post-Fontan patients, fenestration of the systemic venous pathway has been shown to reverse protein loss. Cardiac transplantation may be required for refractory PLGE in these patients.
- **Segmental intestinal resection:** Resection of diseased bowel segments reverses protein loss in Crohn's disease [20] and localized intestinal lymphangiectasia [21].
- **Gastrectomy:** Subtotal or total gastrectomy is the definitive treatment for Ménétrier's disease refractory to medical therapy.

Nutrition Support
Individuals with PLGE need to eat a high-protein diet. They may require 2–3 g/kg dry weight of protein per day (an average adult requires 0.8–1.2 g/kg protein per day). To estimate protein needs, fecal losses derived from α-1-antitrypsin clearance can be added to baseline daily requirements. Urine urea nitrogen balance can also be measured to ensure adequate protein intake. Dietary counseling by a registered dietician is recommended. High-protein foods include meat, milk, cheese, and eggs. Modular protein concentrates and oral supplements can be used to increase protein intake. In patients who require tube feeding, high-protein enteral feeds are available. Parenteral supplementation may be necessary if enteral intake fails.

In children with primary intestinal lymphangiectasia, a low-fat diet can reduce GI symptoms, promote growth, and perhaps improve hypoalbuminemia [22, 23]. The efficacy of this approach is less well established in secondary lymphangiectasia. The dietary regimen restricts long-chain triglycerides (LCTs), which are absorbed into the lymphatic circulation and may increase lymphatic pressure and promote protein loss. In contrast, medium-chain triglycerides (MCTs) are absorbed into the portal system and do not aggravate lymphatic hypertension. Effective regimens limit LCT intake to 5–10 g/day (enough to meet essential fatty acid needs) and add MCT oils to food and beverages for additional calories. A daily multivitamin plus individual supplements as needed is recommended.

Monitoring
Patients with PLGE should be monitored for protein levels and vitamin and mineral deficiencies. Fat-soluble vitamins (A, E, D, K) are of particular importance in those with lymphangiectasia because extravasated lymph fluid is rich in these vitamins. Monitor for essential fatty acid deficiency in those on a low-fat diet by measuring blood triene/tetrene ratio.

Take Home Points

Diagnosis:
- Suspect protein-losing gastroenteropathy (PLGE) when both serum total protein and albumin levels are low (hypoproteinemia).
- The α-1-antitrypsin clearance test quantifies fecal protein loss and establishes the diagnosis of PLGE.
- Endoscopy with biopsy may help determine the cause of PLGE in those with suspected mucosal disease.

Therapy:
- Treat the underlying disease to reverse intestinal protein loss.
- Provide a high-protein diet and protein-rich oral supplements or, if needed, parenteral protein to maintain nutritional status.
- Low-fat diets are effective in patients with intestinal lymphangiectasia.

References
1 Waldmann TA. Protein-losing enteropathy. *Gastroenterology* 1966; **50**: 422–43.
2 Laster L, Waldmann TA. Serum proteins and the gastrointestinal tract. *Med Ann Dist Columbia* 1965; **34**: 459–62.
3 Wochner RD, Weissman SM, Waldmann TA, *et al.* Direct measurement of the rates of synthesis of plasma proteins in control subjects and patients with gastrointestinal protein loss. *J Clin Invest* 1968; **47**: 971–82.
4 Bode L, Salvestrini C, Park PW, *et al.* Heparan sulfate and syndecan-1 are essential in maintaining murine and human intestinal epithelial barrier function. *J Clin Invest* 2008; **118**: 229–38.
5 Vignes S, Bellanger J. Primary intestinal lymphangiectasia (Waldmann's disease). *Orphanet J Rare Dis* 2008; **3**. 5.
6 Rychik J. Protein-losing enteropathy after Fontan operation. *Congenit Heart Dis* 2007; **2**: 288–300.
7 Bernier JJ, Florent C, Desmazures C, *et al.* Diagnosis of protein-losing enteropathy by gastrointestinal clearance of alpha1-antitrypsin. *Lancet* 1978; **2** (8093): 763–4.
8 Florent C, L'Hirondel C, Desmazures C, *et al.* Intestinal clearance of alpha 1-antitrypsin. A sensitive method for the detection of protein-losing enteropathy. *Gastroenterology* 1981; **81**: 777–80.
9 Strygler B, Nicar MJ, Santangelo WC, *et al.* Alpha 1-antitrypsin excretion in stool in normal subjects and in patients with gastrointestinal disorders. *Gastroenterology* 1990; **99**: 1380–7.
10 Florent C, Vidon N, Flourie B, *et al.* Gastric clearance of alpha-1-antitrypsin under cimetidine perfusion. New test to detect protein-losing gastropathy? *Dig Dis Sci* 1986; **31**: 12–15.
11 Reinhart WH, Weigand K, Kappeler M, *et al.* Comparison of gastrointestinal loss of alpha-1-antitrypsin and chromium-51-albumin in Menetrier's disease and the influence of ranitidine. *Digestion* 1983; **26**: 192–6.
12 Waldmann TA. Protein-losing enteropathy and kinetic studies of plasma protein metabolism. *Semin Nucl Med* 1972; **2**: 251–63.
13 Chiu NT, Lee BF, Hwang SJ, *et al.* Protein-losing enteropathy: diagnosis with (99m)Tc-labeled human serum albumin scintigraphy. *Radiology* 2001; **219**: 86–90.
14 Wang SJ, Tsai SC, Lan JL. Tc-99m albumin scintigraphy to monitor the effect of treatment in protein-losing gastroenteropathy. *Clin Nucl Med* 2000; **25**: 197–9.
15 Sunagawa T, Kinjo F, Gakiya I, *et al.* Successful long-term treatment with cyclosporin A in protein losing gastroenteropathy. *Intern Med* 2004; **43**: 397–9.
16 Yeaton P, Frierson HF Jr. Octreotide reduces enteral protein losses in Menetrier's disease. *Am J Gastroenterol* 1993; **88**: 95–8.
17 Green BT, Branch MS. Menetrier's disease treated with octreotide long-acting release. *Gastrointest Endosc* 2004; **60**: 1028–9.
18 Fushimi T, Takahashi Y, Kashima Y, *et al.* Severe protein losing enteropathy with intractable diarrhea due to systemic AA amyloidosis, successfully treated with corticosteroid and octreotide. *Amyloid* 2005; **12**: 48–53.
19 Filik L, Oguz P, Koksal A, *et al.* A case with intestinal lymphangiectasia successfully treated with slow-release octreotide. *Dig Liver Dis* 2004; **36**: 687–90.
20 Ferrante M, Penninckx F, De Hertogh G, *et al.* Protein-losing enteropathy in Crohn's disease. *Acta Gastroenterol Belg* 2006; **69**: 384–9.
21 Connor FL, Angelides S, Gibson M, *et al.* Successful resection of localized intestinal lymphangiectasia post-Fontan: role of (99m)technetium-dextran scintigraphy. *Pediatrics* 2003; **112**: e242–7.
22 Jeffries GH, Chapman A, Sleisenger MH. Low-fat diet in intestinal lymphangiectasia. Its effect on albumin metabolism. *N Engl J Med* 1964; **270**: 761–6.
23 Tift WL, Lloyd JK. Intestinal lymphangiectasia. Long-term results with MCT diet. *Arch Dis Child* 1975; **50**: 269–76.

CHAPTER 51

Acute Mesenteric Ischemia and Chronic Mesenteric Insufficiency

Timothy T. Nostrant

Department of Internal Medicine, University of Michigan, Ann Arbor, MI, USA

Summary

Acute mesenteric ischemia (AMI) is rare (0.1% of hospital admissions). Mortality and morbidity are high due to delayed diagnosis and treatment. Arterial obstruction secondary to embolus, thrombosis, or low blood flow states are the most common causes. Mesenteric venous thrombosis (MVT) should be suspected if the patient or family has a history of coagulation disorders, malignancy, or intra-abdominal inflammation, or if the patient is taking thrombotic medications. Early diagnosis is mandatory. Surgery should be the first step if peritoneal signs are present, and second-look surgery may be needed. Angiography is indicated if peritoneal signs are not found and angiographic treatment is anticipated.

Chronic mesenteric insufficiency (CMI) secondary to progressive atheromatous obstruction produces progressive weight loss with pain. Angiography is usually diagnostic. Surgical and angiographic treatments are available.

Case

A 62-year-old male is hospitalized with an anterior wall myocardial infarction (MI) with ejection fraction of 20%. He develops severe central abdominal pain and hypotension 2 days after admission. Physical exam of the abdomen is normal. The patient has a mild lactic acidosis and serum HCO_3 of 18 mmol/L. Plain film of the abdomen followed by computed tomography (CT) angiography reveals ileus and lack of bowel enhancement in the small bowel and right colon, with a patent superior mesenteric artery (SMA) and no MVT. Angiography reveals a marked decrease in intestinal blood flow, consistent with marked vasoconstriction. Intra-arterial papaverine resolves the vasoconstriction and the patient resolves his symptoms.

The patient develops small-bowel obstruction 3 months later, and surgery reveals a mid-small-bowel stricture.

Acute/Chronic Mesenteric Ischemia

AMI is the sudden onset of small-intestinal hypoperfusion, which can be caused by both non-obstructive and vascularobstructive effects. The most common causes of arterial obstruction are emboli and thrombosis of atherosclerotic vessels. Venous outflow obstruction is usually secondary to thrombosis or intestinal strangulation. Non-occlusive arterial hypoperfusion is usually due to splanchnic vasoconstriction caused by decreased cardiac output or severe hypoxia [1, 2].

Chronic mesenteric ischemia/insufficiency is caused by slow, progressive arterial narrowing of multiple atherosclerotic vessels and is associated with progressive pain and weight loss [3].

Vascular Anatomy/Function Mesenteric Circulation

The mesenteric vascular anatomy is shown in Figure 52.1 [4]. Extensive collateral circulation through the arc of Riolan, marginal artery of Drummond (SMA, inferior mesenteric artery (IMA)), and pancreaticoduodenal arcade (celiac, SMA) allows for transient reductions in perfusion without consequence. Prolonged reductions will cause vasoconstriction, decreased collateral flow, and potentially intestinal ischemia.

The celiac axis is responsible for arterial flow to the upper gastrointestinal (GI) tract, pancreas, liver, and spleen. The common hepatic artery usually gives rise to the gastroduodenal artery.

The SMA arises 1 cm below the celiac artery and terminates in the ileocolic artery. It supplies blood to the small intestines and colon proximal to the splenic flexure.

The inferior mesenteric artery arises 6–7 cm below the SMA and is responsible for the descending colon, sigmoid colon, and rectum.

Mesenteric Vascular Physiology

Arteriolar resistance is the major tool used to modulate intestinal blood flow, which makes up from 10 to 35% of cardiac output. Only 20% of mesenteric capillaries are open at any one time, allowing for large changes in splanchnic flow in order to meet digestive needs. Direct arteriolar smooth-muscle relaxation and indirect response to release of adenosine and other metabolites of mucosal ischemia are the major proposed mechanisms of autoregulation. The sympathetic nervous system and renin–angiotensin axis may also contribute [5]. Hypoxia causing direct release of inflammatory mediators such as nuclear factor kappa-light-chain-enhancer of activated B cells (nf-κB) and tumor necrosis factor (TNF) may induce vasoconstriction during prolonged hypoperfusion [5].

The intestine can compensate for a 75% acute reduction in flow for up to 12 hours if collateral vessels are well developed. Longer periods of ischemia are associated with vasoconstriction to

Practical Gastroenterology and Hepatology Board Review Toolkit, Second Edition. Edited by Nicholas J. Talley, Kenneth R. DeVault, Michael B. Wallace, Bashar A. Aqel and Keith D. Lindor.

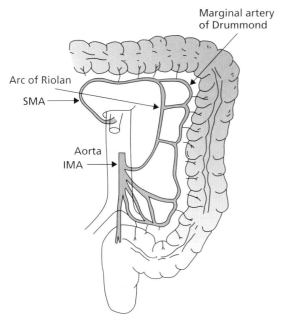

Figure 52.1 View of the small bowel and colon mesenteric vasculature. The arc of Riolan and marginal artery of Drummond are mesenteric major collaterals. Source: Rosenblum 1997 [4]. Reproduced with permission of Elsevier.

maintain peripheral arteriolar perfusion but reduce collateral flow [5, 6]. This progressive loss of intestinal flow leads to breakdown of the intestinal mucosal barrier and interaction with luminal metabolic products, including bacterial antigens, which leads to multiorgan failure and shock.

Acute Mesenteric Ischemia

The major causes of intestinal ischemia are shown in Figure 52.2 [7, 8]. The incidence of acute mesenteric ischemia is rising, likely secondary to an aging population and better cardiovascular care options for patients with severe cardiovascular disease (CVD). In younger patients, mesenteric venous insufficiency is the major cause [7].

Arterial emboli are secondary to clot dislodgement from the left atrium, left ventricle, and cardiac valves. The SMA is most vulnerable secondary to its narrow takeoff angle and large caliber. Emboli

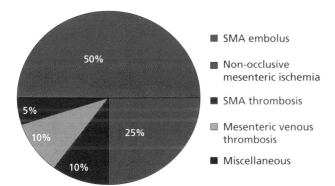

Figure 52.2 Etiologies of acute mesenteric ischemia (AMI). SMA, superior mesenteric artery.

lodge at the orifice (15%) or just distal to the takeoff of the middle colic artery (85%). Emboli are multiple, and the mid-jejunum is most vulnerable secondary to distance from collateral flow [8].

Acute thrombosis usually occurs in patients with chronic atherosclerotic mesenteric insufficiency or following abdominal trauma. Thrombosis usually occurs at the origin of multiple vessels, making revascularization difficult.

MVT is seen in patients with hypercoagulable states, portal hypertension, and inflammatory conditions such as infections, trauma, and pancreatitis. Malignancy, through either direct vascular compression or hypercoagulation, is another possibility. MVT leads to bowel-wall edema, fluid loss, systemic hypotension, arterial vasoconstriction, and ultimately submucosal hemorrhage and bowel infarction.

Inherited thrombotic disorders are found in 75% of patients with MVT, with factor V Leiden causing resistance to activated protein C in 20–40% of patients [9]. Resistance to activated protein C not related to factor V Leiden mutation accounts for 10% of cases [9]. Prothrombin gene mutations are also seen in 8–10% of patients with venous thrombosis [9, 10].

Non-occlusive Mesenteric Ischemia

Splanchnic hypoperfusion and vasoconstriction due to low-flow cardiovascular states are the mechanisms proposed. Older patients with congestive heart with or without acute MI on diuretics or digitalis are typical. Sepsis, cardiac arrhythmias, and α adrenergic agonists have been described. Younger patients using cocaine can also develop mesenteric ischemia. Cardiac surgery with long aortic clamping times may be a risk group. Prolonged vasoconstriction secondary to vasopressin and angiotensin is the major cause in cirrhosis and variceal bleeding. This form of intestinal ischemia accounts for 25% of patients today, but it had a much higher incidence before the advent of intensive care units (ICUs) and aggressive volume and vasodilatation support systems. Non-occlusive mesenteric ischemia still carries a high mortality (70%) due to diagnostic difficulties and limited treatment options in this critically ill group of patients [11].

Clinical Manifestations

Sudden-onset pain is predominant in most cases and is out of proportion to physical exam, which is in contrast to the major differential diagnoses of diverticulitis and pancreatitis. The pain is periumbilical or generalized and is associated with symptoms of sympathetic stimulation, such as anxiety, tachycardia, and peripheral vasoconstriction. Nausea and vomiting occur in up to 50% of cases. Bleeding is rare, but intense urgency with evacuation coupled with these signs should raise suspicion in patients with risk factors such as congestive heart failure (CHF), recent MI, heart arrhythmias, or coagulopathy. Hypotension and heart dysfunction may occur in patients with non-occlusive mesenteric ischemia. Severe pain lasting more than 3 hours without discernible cause in a high-risk patient mandates immediate consideration for AMI and appropriate and rapid diagnostic testing. AMI in moribund patients can present with sudden hypotension, sepsis, or coma without pain. High amylase or lipase levels without findings of pancreatitis should raise suspicion of AMI.

Diagnosis

Rapid diagnosis is essential because progression to infarction is associated with a high mortality. Intestinal viability approaches 100% if symptom duration before treatment is less than 12 hours,

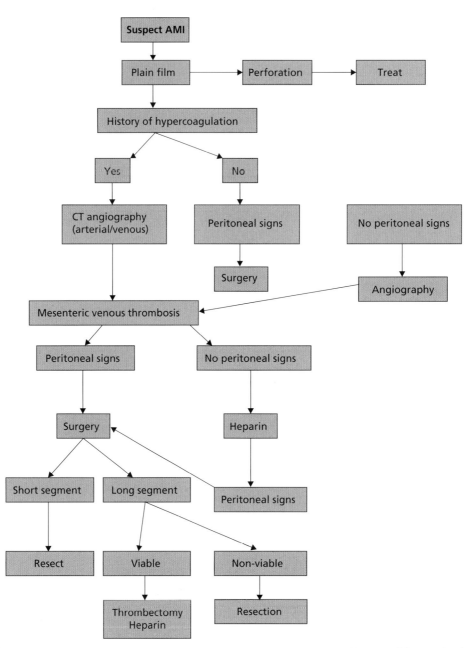

Figure 52.3 Algorithm for investigation of suspected AMI. CT, computed tomography. Source: AGA Guideline 2000 [1]. Reproduced with permission of Elsevier.

56% if it is between 12 and 24 hours, and just 18% if it is more than 24 hours [12]. Diagnostic and treatment algorithms are outlined in Figures 52.3 and 52.4 [1].

Resuscitation for hypovolemia or cardiac rhythm disturbances is preeminent. Flat plate of the abdomen to look for visceral perforation, pneumatosis, or diffuse ileus followed by contrast CT evaluation for proximal arterial occlusion or embolic disease and to exclude MVT are the first steps if peritonitis is not present and suspicion is moderate. Since emboli can lodge distal to the orifice of the SMA, proximal occlusion on CT is most likely thrombosis with or without embolic disease. Embolic disease cannot be ruled out by a normal CT exam. The presence of intramural gas, portovenous gas, and focal lack of bowel enhancement and the presence of liver/spleen infarcts on CT have a sensitivity of 64 and 92%,

respectively, but only portovenous gas sufficiently predicted transmural injury [13]. Laboratory tests such as serum lactate, amylase, and lipase, or the newer tests such as α-glutathione-S-transferase (α-GST) and intestinal fatty acid binding protein (I-FABP), take time and only have high sensitivity and specificity for intestinal ischemia when used in combination [14]. Strong clinical suspicion of mesenteric insufficiency warrants immediate angiography with vasodilators, if applicable, or immediate surgery if infarction is suspected.

Treatment Algorithms

The major cause of mortality in AMI is persistent vasoconstriction causing progressive necrosis leading to bowel infarction. This is seen in all conditions associated with AMI, but is most predominate in non-occlusive intestinal ischemia. There have been no randomized

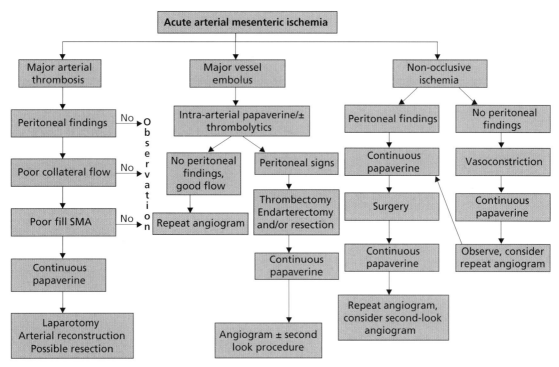

Figure 52.4 Algorithm for treatment of AMI. SMA, superior mesenteric artery. Source: AGA Guideline 2000 [1]. Reproduced with permission of Elsevier.

controlled trials (RCTs) of any single spectictherapeutic intervention. Case–control trials are not comparable due to the varying levels of ischemia and the lack of matching of comorbid conditions. Expert opinion is currently the likely basis for therapy utilization, and will continue to be so in the future. Current guideline algorithms are given in Figures 52.3 and 52.4. Mesenteric angiography for immediate diagnosis and intravenous vasodilation has been the major cause of mortality decline in the last 30 years (from 70 to 45%) (Figure 52.5). The major benefit is in arterial causes of AMI, while multidetection row CT is best for MVT (90%) [15]. The goal of treatment is to restore flow as quickly as possible. Vigorous rehydration, correction of arrhythmias, and intestinal decontamination using both oral and systemic antibiotics to decrease intestinal bacterial translocation should be started (evidence level C). Recent prospective trials

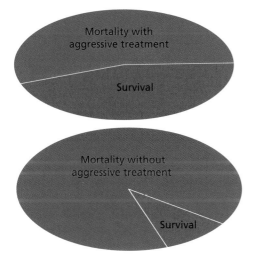

Figure 52.5 Outcome of AMI.

have shown a lower mortality and reduced multiorgan failure with antibiotic use. All vasoconstrictors should be stopped. If vasopressors are required to maintain systemic blood pressure then dobutamine, low-dose dopamine, or milrinone are preferred because of their better mesenteric perfusion. Systemic anticoagulation should be administered to prevent thrombosis formation or propagation unless active intra-abdominal bleeding or large-bowel infarction is suspected and immediate resection is anticipated. Indications for immediate surgery include persistent tenderness with sepsis, organ failure, peritonitis, and failure of radiologic endovascular procedures. Anticoagulation is typically reinstated after surgery with or without resection to prevent further thrombosis.

Therapeutic options during angiography and surgery include intra-arterial vasodilators or antithrombotic agents, angioplasty with or without intra-arterial stenting, and embolectomy, depending on the cause of AMI. Embolectomy during surgery using a balloon-tipped catheter has been the traditional treatment for mesenteric artery embolism, with angiographic embolectomy or antithrombotics reserved for high-risk surgical patients without infarction. Postoperative arterial spasm can be attenuated by intra-arterial papaverine, which can be safely infused for up to 5 days. Persistent ischemic areas should be removed during initial surgery, but a second-look surgery may need to be performed in the next 24–48 hours to resect additional ischemic or gangrenous bowel.

Acute mesenteric arterial thrombosis is treated mainly with surgical vascular reconstruction and thrombectomy, coupled with resection of non-viable segments. Survival post arterial reconstruction is associated with good patency rates and symptom-free survival (79 and 77%, respectively), but perioperative mortality can be as high as 52% [16]. Anticoagulation alone may be justified if chronic change is signaled by good collateral flow and peritoneal signs are not present.

MVT treatment is predominately medical after necrotic bowel has been resected. Heparin should be given to all patients with MVT unless the risk of bleeding is considered to be too high. Long-term warfarin following the acute event is standard.

Non-occlusive mesenteric ischemia therapy is primarily intra-arterial papaverine to prevent vasoconstriction. Repeat angiography post discontinuation of papaverine can be performed after 24 hours to verify continued resolution of vasoconstriction. Peritoneal signs warrant surgery, but delay to reanatomosis may improve survival [17].

Chronic Mesenteric Insufficiency

CMI (intestinal angina) produces symptoms of predictable postprandial pain 20–30 minutes postprandially. These symptoms usually progress over time to become continuous and are associated with fear of eating and profound weight loss. Chronic mesenteric ischemia can present with recurrent gastric ulcers and gastroparesis and should be considered in the differential diagnosis of these disorders. Chronic atherosclerotic disease is usually the cause; it involves at least two vessels in 91% and three vessels in 55% of cases. The SMA and celiac artery can be involved solely in 7 and 2%, respectively [18].

Diagnosis can be suspected by non-invasive tests and confirmed with angiography. Non-invasive tests include provocative balloon tonometry to measure postprandial mural acidosis [19], magnetic resonance imaging (MRI)/CT angiography [20], duplex ultrasonography [21], and intestinal oxygen consumption [22]. Only balloon tonometry can show mural acidosis at the time of pain and return of normal pH after pain resolves, demonstrating mesenteric ischemia as the cause of pain [23]. Large studies have not been conducted, but small studies have been promising. All other tests, including angiography, depend on exclusion of other diseases to show CMI is likely.

Percutaneous mesenteric angioplasty (PTMA) with or without stent placement and surgical revascularization are the usual choices, but RCTs are absent. Retrospective reports of surgical revascularization have shown success rates from 59 to 100% and recurrent obstruction from 0 to 26.5% [24]. Mortality is lowest and the rates are best in the most recent studies. Only case reports exist to show the value of PTMA, but experience is increasing as the population ages and comorbid illness increases [25]. If rates close in on surgical rates, PTMA may become the treatment of choice.

---

eating. Multiple vessel involvement is most common. A clinical history with mesenteric involvement of two or more vessels is required for intervention. Surgical vascular reconstruction or percutaneous transluminal mesenteric angioplasty with or without stenting is the standard treatment.

References

1 American Gastroenterological Association Medical Position Statement: guidelines on intestinal ischemia. *Gastroenterology* 2000; **118**: 951–3.

2 Wyers MC. Acute mesenteric ischemia: diagnostic approach and surgical treatment. *Semin Vasc Surg* 2010; **23**: 9–20.

3 Corcos O, Castier Y, Sibert A, *et al.* Effects of a multimodal management strategy for acute mesenteric ischemia on survival and intestinal failure. *Clin Gastroenterol Hepatol* 2013; **11**: 158–65.

4 Rosenblum GD, Boyle CM, Schwartz LB. The mesenteric circulation. Anatomy and physiology. *Surg Clin North Am* 1997; **77**: 289–306.

5 Eltzschig HK, Carmeliet P. Hypoxia and inflammation. *N Engl J Med* 2011; **364**: 656–65.

6 Dhindsa M, Sommerlad SM, DeVan AE, *et al.* Interrelationships among noninvasive measures of postischemic macro- and microvascular reactivity. *J Appl Physiol* 2008; **105**: 427–32.

7 Cappell MS. Intestinal (mesenteric) vasculopathy. I. Acute superior mesenteric arteriopathy and venopathy. *Gastroenterol Clin North Am* 1998; **27**: 783–825.

8 Arthurs ZM, Titus J, Bannazadeh M, *et al.* A comparison of endovascular revascularization with traditional therapy for the treatment of acute mesenteric ischemia. *J Vasc Surg* 2011; **53**: 698–705.

9 Amitrano L, Brancaccio V, Guardascione MA, *et al.* High prevalence of thrombophilic genotypes in patients with acute mesenteric vein thrombosis. *Am J Gastroenterol* 2001; **96**: 146–9.

10 de Visser MC, Rosendaal FR, Bertina RM. A reduced sensitivity for activated protein C in the absence of factor V Leiden increases the risk of venous thrombosis. *Blood* 1999; **93**: 1271–6.

11 Kozuch PL, Brandt LJ. Review article: diagnosis and management of mesenteric ischaemia with an emphasis on pharmacotherapy. *Aliment Pharmacol Ther* 2005; **21**: 201–15.

12 Resch TA, Acosta S, Sonesson B. Endovascular techniques in acute arterial mesenteric ischemia. *Semin Vasc Surg* 2010; **23**: 29–35.

13 Alpern MB, Glazer GM, Francis IR. Ischemic or infracted bowel: CT findings. *Radiology* 1988; **166**: 149–52.

14 Evennett NJ, Petrov MS, Mittal A, Windsor JA. Systematic review and pooled estimates for the diagnostic accuracy of serological markers for intestinal ischemia. *World J Surg* 2009; **33**: 1374–83.

15 Horton KM, Fishman EK. The current status of multidetector row CT and three-dimensional imaging of the small bowel. *Radiol Clin North Am* 2003; **41**: 199–212.

16 Kougias P, Lau D, El Sayed HF, *et al.* Determinants of mortality and treatment outcome following surgical interventions for acute mesenteric ischemia. *J Vasc Surg* 2007; **46**: 467–74.

17 Demirpolat G, Oran I, Tamsel S, *et al.* Acute mesenteric venous thrombosis. *N Engl J Med* 2001; **345**: 1683–8.

18 Tendler DA, LaMont JT. Chronic mesenteric ischemia. In: Rutgeerts P, ed. *UpToDate*. Waltham, MA: UpToDate, 2008.

19 Kolkman JJ, Groeneveld AB. Occlusive and non-occlusive gastrointestinal ischaemia: a clinical review with special emphasis on the diagnostic value of tonometry. *Scan J Gastroenterol Suppl* 1998; **225**: 3–12.

20 Meaney JF, Prince MR, Nostrant TT, Stanley JC. Gadolinium-enhanced MR angiography of visceral arteries in patients with suspected chronic mesenteric ischemia. *J Magn Reson Imaging* 1997; **7**: 171–6.

21 Gentile AT, Moneta GL, Lee RW, *et al.* Usefulness of fasting and postprandial duplex ultrasound examinations for predicting high-grade superior mesenteric artery stenosis. *Am J Surg* 1995; **169**: 476–9.

22 Moneta GL. Screening for mesenteric vascular insufficiency and follow-up of mesenteric artery bypass procedures. *Semin Vasc Surg* 2001; **14**: 186–92.

23 Boley SJ, Brandt LJ, Veith FJ, *et al.* A new provocative test for chronic mesenteric ischemia. *Am J Gastroenterol* 1991; **86**: 888–91.

24 English WP, Pearce JD, Craven TE, *et al.* Chronic visceral ischemia: symptom-free survival after open surgical repair. *Vasc Endovascular Surg* 2004; **38**: 493–503.

25 Matsumoto AH, Tegtmeyer CJ, Fitzcharles EK, *et al.* Percutaneous transluminal angioplasty of visceral arterial stenoses: results and long-term clinical follow-up. *J Vasc Interv Radiol* 1995; **6**: 165–74.

Take Home Points

- Decreased mesenteric arterial flow (thrombus, embolus) accounts for 60–70% of cases of acute mesenteric ischemia (AMI). It has a high mortality if diagnosis and treatment are delayed (70%).
- Risk factors for AMI include advanced age, atherosclerosis, low cardiac output, cardiac arrhythmias, cardiac valvular disease, recent myocardial ischemia or infarction, and mesenteric venous thrombosis (MVT). Hypercoagulation states or malignancy should be suspected in MVT.
- Mesenteric angiography with both diagnostic and treatment arms is still the gold standard, though newer imaging modalities (computed tomography (CT), Doppler ultrasonography) are gaining in use. Rapid diagnosis is still paramount.
- Intestinal vasoconstriction is the major cause of bowel infarction in all forms of AMI, and can be persistent. Vasodilator use should be frequent and may be prolonged.
- Long-term prognosis is good if the patient survives the acute event and the amount of bowel lost is small.
- Chronic mesenteric insufficiency (CMI) is caused by progressive atherosclerosis leading to postprandial pain, weight loss, and fear of

Intestinal Obstruction and Pseudo-obstruction

Magnus Halland and Purna Kashyap

Division of Gastroenterology and Hepatology, Mayo Clinic, Rochester, MN, USA

Summary

This review focuses on the diagnosis and management of intestinal mechanical obstruction and pseudo-obstruction, and in particular highlights how these conditions are differentiated. Intestinal obstruction may be partial or complete, and among those with complete obstruction, the presence of ischemia or peritonitis requires emergent surgery. Clinical recognition of intestinal pseudo-obstruction avoids unnecessary surgery and directs treatment toward symptomatic management.

Case

A 58-year-old man with no prior surgical history is evaluated in the gastroenterology clinic after three presentations to the emergency department with abdominal distension, vomiting, and pain over the past 8 months. On each occasion, a nasogastric catheter was placed, intravenous fluids were commenced, and the symptoms resolved within 48–72 hours. Computed tomography (CT) on each occasion demonstrated several dilated loops of small bowel, but no mass lesion or transition point was appreciated. He was discharged on a liquid diet, but continues to have abdominal pain and distension without vomiting. He has lost 15 lb in 12 months and has recently developed numbness in his feet.

Intestinal Obstruction

The most common causes of acute mechanical intestinal obstruction are shown in Table 53.1. They include adhesions, hernias, and malignancy. Partial bowel obstruction indicates that some intestinal contents can pass the level of blockage. Fibrous adhesions from pervious intra-abdominal surgery are the most common cause of small-bowel obstruction [1]. Acute-onset abdominal pain and vomiting is almost universally present, and obstipation (inability to pass flatus or stool) is common. Proximal intestinal obstruction is more likely to produce bilious vomiting, while more distal obstruction can rarely result in emesis of feculent material. The presence of systemic toxicity or peritoneal signs suggests vascular compromise, necessitating urgent surgical consultation for laparotomy.

Diagnosis

Consider intestinal obstruction in any patient with acute abdominal pain with vomiting. Inquire about prior intra-abdominal surgery, inflammatory bowel disease (IBD), and episodes of previous obstruction to further risk-stratify (Table 53.2). Initial laboratory testing should include a complete blood count (CBC), electrolytes, renal function, amylase, lipase, and lactate.

We recommend that patients with suspected bowel obstruction be promptly evaluated with an erect and supine plain abdominal film (Figure 53.1). An abdominal film can quickly identify patients who may need immediate surgery, such as those with pneumoperitoneum. The negative predictive value (NPV) of a normal abdominal film is imperfect and therefore cross-sectional imaging with CT radiography is often performed. This often confirms the diagnosis, but also helps identify underlying causes and complications [2, 3]. If both these tests are negative but the clinical index of suspicion remains high, further evaluation is required. Imaging of the small bowel using radiography, specialized CT, or magnetic resonance (MR) enterography may be helpful. CT and MR enterography have similar sensitivity for identifying inflammatory lesions and causes of bowel obstruction, but MR enterography may be considered in patients with previous CT scans due to the lack of ionizing radiation [4]. However, in patients with claustrophobia or implanted metal devices, it may not be feasible (Table 53.3). Video-capsule endoscopy is contraindicated in this setting, as is enteroclysis, where the small bowel is insufflated with air and contrast medium via a nasojejunal tube.

Management

Initial management of a patient with intestinal obstruction focuses on resuscitation with intravenous fluids and correction of electrolyte disturbances. Placement of a nasogastric tube is warranted in virtually all patients. Early involvement of a surgical team is crucial. Between 60 and 90% of cases of partial bowel obstruction due to adhesion resolve with conservative management [5–7], but close clinical management with serial assessment of abdominal signs is needed. In cases where peritonism and/or systemic toxicity develop, surgery is usually indicated; palliation should be considered in nonsurgical candidates.

The next priority is to establish the etiology. Plain abdominal imaging rarely reveals the diagnosis, except in cases of sigmoid volvulus and radiolucent foreign bodies. The presence of air in the rectum is unusual in cases of complete small-bowel obstruction. In general, small-bowel loops >3 cm diameter and >6 cm colonic diameter (10 cm for cecum) indicate abnormally dilated bowel (Figures 53.2–53.9). However, if the bowel is fluid-filled, as is the case

Practical Gastroenterology and Hepatology Board Review Toolkit, Second Edition. Edited by Nicholas J. Talley, Kenneth R. DeVault, Michael B. Wallace, Bashar A. Aqel and Keith D. Lindor.
© 2016 John Wiley & Sons, Ltd. Published 2016 by John Wiley & Sons, Ltd. Companion website: www.practicalgastrohep.com

Table 53.1 Causes of mechanical bowel obstruction.

Common causes	Adhesions
	Hernias
	Tumor
	Adenocarcinoma
	Lymphoma
	Metastatic tumor
	Crohn's disease
	Foreign body
	Volvulus
Uncommon causes	Intussusception
	Tumor
	Lipoma
	Meckel diverticulum
	Bezoars
	Gallstone
	Diverticular abscess
	Radiation strictures
	NSAID-induced strictures
	Retained medical devices (video-capsule endoscopy devices)

NSAID, non-steroidal anti-inflammatory drug.

Table 53.2 Making a diagnosis of mechanical bowel obstruction.

Directed history and physical examination	Duration of symptoms
	Prior abdominal or pelvic surgery
	Prior abdominal radiation
	Character of pain
	Character of emesis
	Last bowel movement or passage of flatus
	Vital signs, including checking for orthostasis
	Presence or absence of bowel sounds
	Presence of distension
	Presence of abdominal tenderness
	Presence of peritonitis

in closed-loop syndromes, dilated bowel may not be appreciated radiologically. CT is more likely to define the location and cause of intestinal obstruction. Furthermore, signs of complications such as abscesses, masses, or strangulation can be detected [8]. The addition of oral and intravenous contrast is now virtually routine. Features of strangulation include thickening of the bowel wall, pneumatosis intestinalis (gas in the bowel wall), lack of contrast enhancement of the bowel, and mesenteric inflammatory changes. In some cases, the clinical scenario dictates that the patient's need for immediate laparotomy takes priority over cross-sectional imaging to define a preoperative diagnosis.

Further Diagnostic Imaging
To further evaluate suspected small-bowel disease, a CT or MR enterography can be considered in inconclusive cases. Magnetic resonance imaging (MRI) lacks ionizing radiation but requires prolonged and repeated breath-holding. Enteroclysis is a technique whereby the proximal small bowel is catheterized with a nasojejunal tube and rapidly distended. Images are then obtained via either CT or MRI; both techniques are contraindicated in the setting of suspected acute bowel obstruction, but can be helpful in patients with recurrent or chronic symptoms of partial bowel obstruction.

Complications and Recurrence
Untreated complete intestinal obstruction is generally not survivable. After open surgical correction, most patients will develop fibrous adhesions (up to 90%), and in 10–15% of patients this will lead to recurrent intestinal obstruction several years later [9]. Once symptomatic recurrence occurs as a result of adhesions, there is increased chance of further episodes (10–30%) [10].

Laparoscopic surgery is associated with a reduced incidence of bowel obstruction compared to open laparotomy [1]. Adhesions barrier substances (such as Seprafilm) have been shown to reduce adhesion formation, but robust outcome data from prospective randomized trials are lacking [11, 12].

Large Bowel Obstruction
Obstruction of the large bowel is less common than that of the small bowel, and the most common cause is primary colonic cancer. Other causes include colonic volvulus (sigmoid or cecal), non-malignant strictures (diverticular, ischemic, radiation-induced),

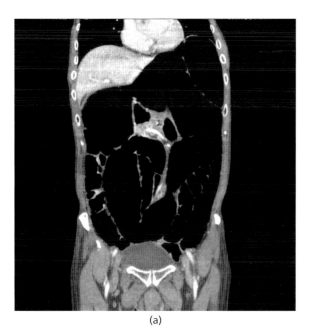

(a)

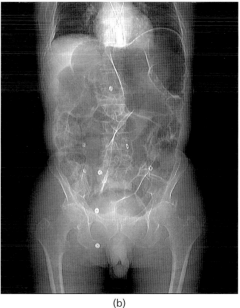

(b)

Figure 53.1 Plain abdominal radiographs of a patient with acute colonic pseudo-obstruction. Note the marked colonic dilatation.

Table 53.3 Second-line diagnostic for bowel obstruction.

Test	Radiation exposure	IV contrast	Pros	Cons
Small-bowel radiography	Yes	No	Highly sensitive for identifying presence of obstruction Better at diagnosing closed-loop syndromes	Less specific for identifying etiology Radiation exposure
CT radiography	Yes	Yes	Identifies etiology of obstruction Especially helpful in IBD Identifies presence of ischemia Shortest time to diagnosis	Radiation exposure IV contrast
MR radiography	No	Yes	No radiation exposure Highly sensitive for identifying obstruction	Limited availability in community centers Lower specificity as to etiology Contraindicated in many patients with implanted metal devices, pacemakers, neurostimulators May not be an option for patients with claustrophobia

IV, intravenous; CT, computed tomography; IBD, inflammatory bowel disease; MR, magnetic resonance.

fecal impaction, and rarely IBD. Unlike in small-bowel obstruction, vomiting is a late sign. Associated features of weight loss, iron deficiency, and rectal bleeding may be present. Colonic volvulus has a more sudden presentation, and can often be appreciated on plain abdominal radiology. The main differential diagnosis is colonic pseudo-obstruction (paralytic ileus), which commonly occurs postoperatively. Placement of a nasogastric tube is indicated in patients with nausea and vomiting, but is unlikely to help resolve the obstruction. As with small-bowel obstruction, peritoneal findings and/or imaging results suggesting perforation or ischemia require urgent surgical intervention. Optimal management depends on the cause, but except in the case of obstruction caused by sigmoid volvulus, which may be treated with a rectal tube or endoscopic decompression, surgical intervention is frequently required [13]. Cecal volvulus most commonly requires segmental resection. Fecal impaction as a cause of obstruction may be treated therapeutically by water-soluble contrast enema. In the setting of a distal (and possibly proximal) malignant partial colonic obstruction, endoscopic placement of a stent may temporarily relieve obstruction and prevent the need

for emergent surgery. Thus, bowel preparation can be administered, and semi-elective surgery has a greater chance of allowing a primary anastomosis rather than colostomy [14, 15].

Intestinal Pseudo-obstruction

Chronic Intestinal Pseudo-obstruction

Chronic intestinal pseudo-obstruction (CIPO) is rare: a recent epidemiological study suggested that the prevalence is 1 in 100 000, with no significant gender differences [16]. The condition is characterized by chronic or recurrent episodes of intestinal obstruction where a demonstrable mechanical obstructive lesion is absent. Unusual causes of obstruction, including retroperitoneal carcinomatosis and fibrosis, as well as partial bowel obstruction, must be excluded. The most common symptoms are abdominal pain, bloating, and distention. Constipation is often present, though some patients may have diarrhea caused by overflow or small-bowel bacterial overgrowth. Vomiting is only present in one-third of patients.

CHAPTER 53

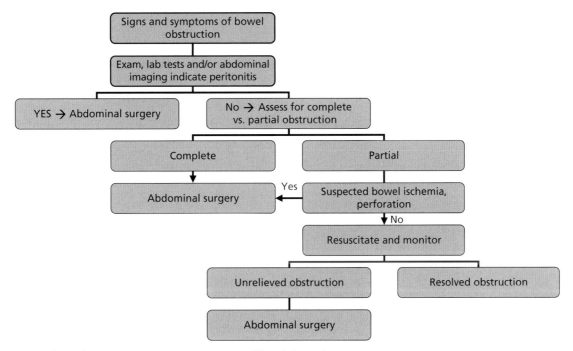

Figure 53.2 Algorithm outlining a management strategy in suspected bowel obstruction.

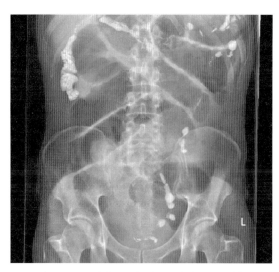

Figure 53.3 Plain, supine abdominal radiograph showing diffusely dilated small bowel. Note the presence of residual barium in a decompressed colon.

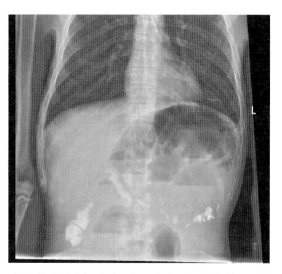

Figure 53.4 Upright abdominal radiograph showing dilated loops of small bowel and air–fluid levels in a patient with a partial small-bowel obstruction.

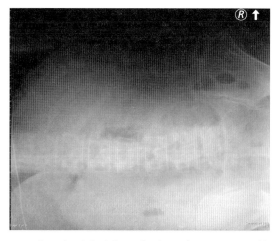

Figure 53.5 Lateral upright abdominal radiograph in a patient unable to stand. Note the presence of several air–fluid levels.

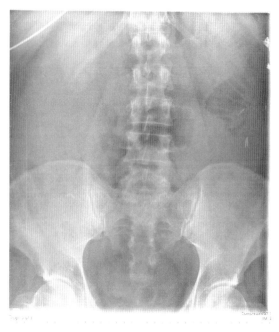

Figure 53.6 Patient presenting with recurrent episodes of abdominal pain, nausea, and vomiting. Note the presence of surgical clips and dilated loop of small bowel in the left upper quadrant.

As opposed to a single diagnostic entity, CIPO is a phenotypic expression of a disease process affecting the gut neuromuscular apparatus, including damage to the enteric nerves, smooth muscles, interstitial Cajal cells (ICCs), and immune cells. Pseudo-obstruction results when there has been significant disruption of the neural or muscular control of the gut, leading to failure of the propulsive forces of intestinal peristalsis to overcome the natural resistance to flow.

Approximately 50% of cases are deemed idiopathic (primary); a secondary cause can be identified in the other 50%. There are a variety of secondary causes, as outlined in Table 53.5; important ones to consider include paraneoplastic, diabetes mellitus, and familial/mitochondrial. Before arriving at a diagnosis, cross-sectional imaging coupled with esophagogastroduodenoscopy (EGD) is required to exclude a structural cause. Celiac disease also needs to be excluded at the time of EGD, using biopsies of the proximal small bowel. There is often a significant delay in achieving the diagnosis. No single test is "diagnostic" of CIPO, and generally the following criteria need to be present:

- **Clinical features:** Chronic symptoms of intestinal obstruction in the absence of structural obstruction.
- **Imaging features:** Dilated bowel.
- **Motility features:** Evidence of impaired small bowel or colonic motility on scintigraphy.

Furthermore, routine laboratory testing is mandatory. Thyroid-stimulating hormone (TSH), viral serology (Epstein–Barr virus (EBV), cytomegalovirus (CMV), and herpes simplex virus (HSV)), and inflammatory markers should be performed. Consider paraneoplastic CIPO in smokers and patients with significant weight loss. The most commonly associated cancers are small-cell lung cancer and carcinoid. A paraneoplastic antibody panel, including ANNA-1/anti-Hu and calcium channel antibodies, is often positive in this patient group. Full-thickness biopsy of affected segments of bowel may help differentiate between myopathic, neuropathic, and

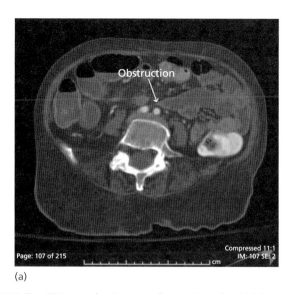

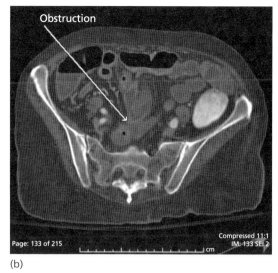

(a)   (b)

Figure 53.7 Two CT images showing areas of narrowing and multiple loops of dilated bowel. Note the presence of contrast in a non-dilated colon. At laparotomy, this patient was determined to have an internal hernia causing a partial obstruction.

other disorders and hence guide therapy. Surgery for the purpose of obtaining a biopsy alone is not recommended. Techniques for endoscopic full-thickness biopsy are not yet in routine clinical use [17].

Small-bowel manometry may be helpful in differentiating myopathic from neuropathic patterns. Unfortunately, small-bowel manometry is limited by poor specificity and is not universally available. A completely normal gastroduodenal manometry should raise serious doubt about the diagnosis of CIPO. Emerging tools for assessment of small-bowel motility includes Cine MRI and wireless motility capsules [18].

Initial management of patients with pseudo-obstruction focuses on correcting fluid, electrolyte, and nutritional deficiencies.

Inpatient management is usually required in the setting of nausea and vomiting coupled with severely dilated bowels. Acute management is similar to that of structural bowel obstruction, with nil per os status and nasogastric suctioning. Any drug with anti-motility properties should be minimized or discontinued if possible. Pro-motility agents such as metoclopramide and erythromycin are useful in the acute setting, but have little evidence to support a role in long-term care. Metoclopramide remains the only Food and Drug Administration (FDA)-approved prokinetic agent, and is often used at doses of 10 mg intravenously QID. Careful monitoring for side effects, including dystonia, is required. With long-term use, risk of depression, exacerbation of Parkinson's disease, and tardive

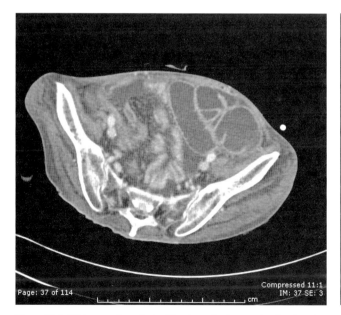

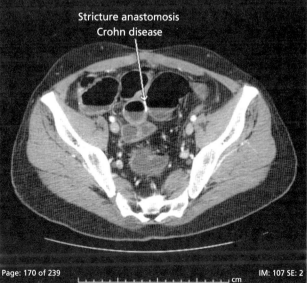

Figure 53.8 CT image of a patient with prior colonic resection for chronic ulcerative colitis presenting with nausea and vomiting. Note the dilated loops of bowel in the left pelvis compared to the decompressed loops of bowel in the right pelvis. At laparotomy, an adhesive stricture was found.

Figure 53.9 CT enterography showing a narrowed anastomosis in a patient with Crohn's disease and prior ileocolonic resection. Note the hypodense contrast in the bowel lumen compared to the higher density from IV contrast in the bowel wall. This patient was managed conservatively, without surgery.

CHAPTER 53

Table 53.4 Indications for operative intervention in bowel obstruction.

Complete bowel obstruction
Peritonitis
Evidence of ischemia
Closed loop syndrome
Failed conservative management (partial SBO)
Obstructing neoplasm

Table 53.6 Management of intestinal pseudo-obstruction.

Fluid resuscitation	
Correct electrolytes	
Antiemetics	Promethazine
	Prochlorperazine
	Ondansetron
	Granisetron
	Trimethobenzamide
	Metoclopramide
Look for and treat small bowel bacterial overgrowth	Rifaximin
	Doxycycline
	Amoxicillin/clavulinic acid
	Ciprofloxacin
	Metronidazole
Analgesia	Aim for non-narcotic control
	Tramadol
	Low-dose tricyclic antidepressants
Prokinetics	Metoclopramide
	Erythromycin
	Domperidone
	Neostigmine
	Prucalopride

dyskinesia rises. Erythromycin at a dose of 3 mg/kg promotes gastric emptying by acting on the motilin receptors, and can be used for 5–7 days in patients admitted to hospital. Tachyphylaxis makes erythromycin unsuitable for long-term use. Neostigmine can be considered among monitored inpatients. Domperidone can be used if available. Domperidone is a dopamine antagonist that does not cause the central nervous system (CNS) side effects seen with metoclopramide (except for elevation in prolactin and galactorrhea). Prucalopride, a 5-HT$_4$ agonist, is in current clinical use for constipation in irritable bowel syndrome (IBS-C). A small, randomized, double-blind crossover trial assessed its efficacy and safety among seven patients with CIPO and found it to be helpful in four at a dose of 2 mg daily [19]. An older drug with similar pharmacokinetic properties, cisapride, is highly restricted through a special-access program, due to the potential for fatal cardiac arrhythmias.

If scleroderma is a contributing cause, patients may benefit from nocturnal administration of a somatostatin analogue such as octreotide, due to promotion of migrating motor complexes [20]. Daytime administration must be avoided as it actually delays gastric emptying and small-bowel transit.

For all patients, early attention to nutrition is important; oral or enteral nutrition is preferred, though parental nutrition should be instituted if necessary. Absorption may be impaired in patients with small-bowel bacterial overgrowth. Failure of oral intake alone should not prompt transition to parenteral nutrition, as many patients in this scenario are able to tolerate slow and gentle infusions of formula via a gastrostomy or jejunostomy. Furthermore, a benefit of the venting effect of jejunostomy has been observed in some patients [21]. Patients with weight loss who are unable to tolerate oral or enteral nutrition will require parenteral nutrition. Attempts at managing abdominal pain with non-narcotic analgesia should be encouraged. Non-narcotic alternatives include

Table 53.5 Categories of intestinal pseudo-obstruction.

Neuropathic	Diabetes mellitus
	Postvagotomy
	Paraneoplastic
	Parkinson's disease
	Dysautonomia
	Hirschsprung
	Chagas
	Inflammatory neuropathies (? autoimmune)
	Familial
Myopathic	Systemic sclerosis
	Ehlers–Danlos
	Familial (including mitochrondrial myopathies)
	Inflammatory myopathies (e.g., dermatomyositis)
Mixed neuropathy/ myopathy	Amyloidosis
	Systemic sclerosis
	Radiation enteritis
Iatrogenic	Opiates
	Antipsychotics
	Antineoplastics

gabapentin, pregabalin, acetaminophen, and tramadol. Think about small bacterial overgrowth in patients with severe malabsorption, steatorrhea, vitamin B12 deficiency, and elevated serum folate. Empiric antibiotic therapy is recommended as breath-testing is unreliable among patients with CIPO and jejunal aspirates are impracticable. If possible, start with a luminally acting antibiotic such as rifaximin and treat for 7–10 days. Recurrence is common, and often cycling between antibiotics (norfloxacin, ciprofloxacin, metronidazole, amoxicillin-clavunate) with drug-free intervals is a long-term management strategy. Though autoimmune and inflammatory enteric neuropathies have been described, an efficacy of immunomodulatory therapy such as infliximab, prednisolone, and cyclophosphamide has only been observed on a case by case basis. This should only be considered in patients where full-thickness intestinal biopsy clearly demonstrates inflammation or among anti-Hu-positive patients. When a diagnosis of myenteric ganglionitis with intestinal dysmotility has been established, high-dose prednisolone (60 mg/day) with slow taper can induce remission [22]. If relapse occurs, introduction of immunomodulatory therapy should be considered, along with a repeated course of corticosteroids [23].

Despite best supportive care, up to 50% of individuals require supplemental nutrition, and a mortality of 35% over 10 years has been reported. Therefore, intestinal transplantation should be considered in severe patients in whom parenteral nutrition is unfeasible or becomes unsafe to continue. Depletion of venous access, cholestatic liver disease, and recurrent infections coupled with intestinal failure are accepted indications. Long-term outcomes of intestinal transplantation are improving, and at expert centers 1- and 5-year survival are now 90 and 70%, respectively. Unfortunately, long-term survival is suboptimal, at 40% at 10 years [24].

Enteric Dysmotility Syndromes without Visceral Dilation

Many patients are evaluated for similar symptoms to those found among patients with CIPO but lack demonstrable radiologic features of dilation. The exact pathophysiology remains unclear, but low-grade inflammatory changes have been described in cases where full-thickness biopsy has occurred [25, 26]. We do not recommend full-thickness biopsy unless it is performed opportunistically at the time of surgery for other indications. Thus, in most cases, the question as to whether these patients have a severe functional gastrointestinal (GI) disorder or a true myopathic or neuropathic disorder is somewhat unclear. A clear organic cause can be found in a minority of patients, such as those with mitochondrial neurogastrointestinal encephalopathy. Think of this condition when patients have impaired GI motility combined with ophthalmoplegia and symmetric polyneuropathies. As with CIPO, long-term prognosis is poor. A complicating factor is the use of narcotic analgesia among many patients with chronic or recurrent abdominal pain. This leads to a syndrome of opiate-induced hyperalgesia due to activation of glial cells, which is often termed "narcotic bowel syndrome." In many patients, it eventually becomes impossible to distinguish the contribution of symptoms from narcotic-induced GI hyperalgesia and decreased motility from true underlying GI pathology. An objective evaluation of GI motility can only occur if all motility-impairing medications can be stopped. The mainstay of management focuses on symptom control, including non-opiate pain-management strategies and nutritional, emotional, and psychological support.

Postoperative Ileus and Acute Colonic Pseudo-obstruction (Ogilvie Syndrome)

In clinical practice, these conditions may be difficult to distinguish, but acute colonic pseudo-obstruction is usually characterized by cecal and right-sided colonic dilation, whereas multiple fluid levels and small-bowel involvement are often found in postoperative ileus. The major risk factor for both conditions is abdominal surgery, but other surgery (orthopedic, cardiothoracic) can be associated with it. Recognized risk factors include age, use of narcotic analgesia, and electrolyte disturbances. Protective factors include minimally invasive surgery, the use of epidural analgesia, and possibly gum-chewing postoperatively [27]. The diagnosis can usually be appreciated on a plain abdominal X-ray, but CT radiography is often also performed to look for complications. The mainstay of management includes minimization of narcotic exposure, correction of electrolyte disturbances, and placement of nasogastric tubes and rectal tubes for decompression. As with mechanical bowel obstruction, the presence of fever, leucocytosis, or peritonism is an ominous sign. Neostigmine, a reversible acetylcholinesterase inhibitor, has been found to be effective in promptly reversing the obstruction among patients who have acute colonic pseudo-obstruction, but not in postoperative ileus [28]. The recommended dose is 1–2 mg IV, and as brady-arrhythmias may occur, cardiac monitoring is mandatory. Contraindications include asthma and recent myocardial infarction, and particular caution should be paid with patients already on a beta-blocker. We recommend considering neostigmine when definite evidence of colonic dilation is present and conservative management has failed. Endoscopic decompression can also be considered if conservative management fails.

Case Continued

The patient undergoes transit studies and gastroduodenal manometry. A provisional diagnosis of CIPO is made. In this case, small bowel-bacterial overgrowth caused vitamin B12 deficiency, and symptom improvement is noted following vitamin replacement and empiric antibiotic therapy.

Take Home Points

- In patients with unexplained nausea, vomiting and abdominal pain, mechanical intestinal obstruction needs to be excluded. Initial tests should include plain abdominal X-ray followed by computed tomography (CT).
- Initial resuscitation with intravenous fluids and correction of electrolytes is key.
- Early surgical referral is mandatory; virtually all patients with complete bowel obstruction or signs of peritonitis require surgery.
- Acute colonic pseudo-obstruction is common in postoperative patients, and early recognition and management are needed to prevent morbidity and mortality.
- Consider chronic intestinal pseudoobstruction in patients with obstructive features but no structural obstruction.

References

1 Gutt CN, Oniu T, Schemmer P, et al. Fewer adhesions induced by laparoscopic surgery? *Surg Endosc* 2004; **18**: 898–906.

2 Maglinte DD, Reyes BL, Harmon BH, et al. Reliability and role of plain film radiography and CT in the diagnosis of small-bowel obstruction. *AJR Am J Roentgenol* 1996; **167**: 1451–5.

3 Ha HK, Kim JS, Lee MS, et al. Differentiation of simple and strangulated small-bowel obstructions: usefulness of known CT criteria. *Radiology* 1997; **204**: 507–12.

4 Siddiki HA, Fidler JL, Fletcher JG, et al. Prospective comparison of state-of-the-art MR enterography and CT enterography in small-bowel Crohn's disease. *AJR Am J Roentgenol* 2009; **193**: 113–21.

5 Peetz DJ Jr, Gamelli RL, Pilcher DB. Intestinal intubation in acute, mechanical small-bowel obstruction. *Arch Surg* 1982; **117**: 334–6.

6 Brolin RE. Partial small bowel obstruction. *Surgery* 1984; **95**: 145–9.

7 Brolin RE, Krasna MJ, Mast BA. Use of tubes and radiographs in the management of small bowel obstruction. *Ann Surg* 1987; **206**: 126–33.

8 Mallo RD, Salem L, Lalani T, Flum DR. Computed tomography diagnosis of ischemia and complete obstruction in small bowel obstruction: a systematic review. *J Gastroint Surg* 2005; **9**: 690–4.

9 Beck DE, Opelka FG, Bailey HR, et al. Incidence of small-bowel obstruction and adhesiolysis after open colorectal and general surgery. *Dis Colon Rectum* 1999; **42**: 241–8.

10 Barkan H, Webster S, Ozeran S. Factors predicting the recurrence of adhesive small-bowel obstruction. *Am J Surg* 1995; **170**: 361–5.

11 Fazio VW, Cohen Z, Fleshman JW, et al. Reduction in adhesive small-bowel obstruction by Seprafilm adhesion barrier after intestinal resection. *Dis Colon Rectum* 2006; **49**: 1–11.

12 Oncel M, Remzi FM, Senagore AJ, et al. Comparison of a novel liquid (Adcon-P) and a sodium hyaluronate and carboxymethylcellulose membrane (Seprafilm) in postsurgical adhesion formation in a murine model. *Dis Colon Rectum* 2003; **46**: 187–91.

13 Oren D, Atamanalp SS, Aydinli B, et al. An algorithm for the management of sigmoid colon volvulus and the safety of primary resection: experience with 827 cases. *Dis Colon Rectum* 2007; **50**: 489–97.

14 Breitenstein S, Rickenbacher A, Berdajs D, et al. Systematic evaluation of surgical strategies for acute malignant left-sided colonic obstruction. *Br J Surg* 2007; **94**: 1451–60.

15 Dronamraju SS, Ramamurthy S, Kelly SB, Hayat M. Role of self-expanding metallic stents in the management of malignant obstruction of the proximal colon. *Dis Colon Rectum* 2009; **52**: 1657–61.

16 Iida H, Ohkubo H, Inamori M, et al. Epidemiology and clinical experience of chronic intestinal pseudo-obstruction in Japan: a nationwide epidemiologic survey. *J Epidemiol* 2013; **23**(4): 288–94.

17 Rajan E, Gostout CJ, Bonin EA, et al. Endoscopic full-thickness biopsy of the gastric wall with defect closure by using an endoscopic suturing device: survival porcine study. *GIE* 2012; **76**: 1014–19.

18 Ohkubo H, Kessoku T, Fuyuki A, et al. Assessment of small bowel motility in patients with chronic intestinal pseudo-obstruction using cine-MRI. *Am J Gastroenterol* 2013; **108**(7): 1130–9.

19 Emmanuel AV, Kamm MA, Roy AJ, et al. Randomised clinical trial: the efficacy of prucalopride in patients with chronic intestinal pseudo-obstruction – a double-blind, placebo-controlled, cross-over, multiple n = 1 study. *Aliment Pharmacol Ther* 2012; **35**(1): 48–55.

CHAPTER 53

20 Soudah HC, Hasler WL, Owyang C. Effect of octreotide on intestinal motility and bacterial overgrowth in scleroderma. *N Engl J Med* 1991; **325**: 1461–7.

21 Chun C, Aulakh S, Komlos F, Triadafilopoulos G. Tube to freedom: use of a venting jejunostomy in a patient with chronic intestinal pseudo-obstruction. *Dig Dis Sci* 2012; **57**(12): 3076–9.

22 De Giorgio R, Barbara G, Stanghellini V, *et al.* Clinical and morphofunctional features of idiopathic myenteric ganglionitis underlying severe intestinal motor dysfunction; a study of three cases. *Am J Gastroenterol* 2002; **97**: 2454–9.

23 Kashyap P, Farrugia G. Enteric autoantibodies and gut motility disorders. *Gastroenterol Clin North Am* 2008; **37**: 397–410.

24 Lauro A, Zanfi C, Pellegrini S, Catena F. Isolated intestinal transplant for chronic intestinal pseudo-obstruction in adults: long-term outcome. *Transplant Proc* 2013; **45**(9): 3351–5.

25 Knowles CH, Lindberg G, Panza, E. New perspectives in the diagnosis and management of enteric neuropathies. *Nat Rev Gastroenterol Hepatol* 2013; **10**(4): 206–18.

26 Lindberg G, Törnblum H, Iwarzon M, *et al.* Full-thickness biopsy findings in chronic intestinal pseudo-obstruction and enteric dysmotility. *Gut* 2009; **58**: 1084–90.

27 Chan MK, Law WL. Use of chewing gum in reducing postoperative ileus after elective colorectal resection: a systematic review. *Dis Colon Rectum* 2007; **50**(12): 2149.

28 Myrhöj T, Olsen O, Wengel B. Neostigmine in postoperative intestinal paralysis. A double-blind, clinical, controlled trial. *Dis Colon Rectum* 1988; **31**(5): 378.

PART 4

Diseases of the Colon and Rectum

54 Ulcerative Colitis, 323
Sunanda V. Kane

55 *Clostridium difficile* Infection and Pseudomembranous Colitis, 328
Byron P. Vaughn and J. Thomas Lamont

56 Colonic Ischemia, 333
Timothy T. Nostrant

57 Acute Diverticulitis, 338
Yuliya Y. Yurko and Tonia M. Young-Fadok

58 Acute Colonic Pseudo-obstruction, 343
Michael D. Saunders

59 Colonic Polyps and Colorectal Cancer, 349
John B. Kisiel, Paul J. Limburg, and Lisa A. Boardman

60 Pregnancy and Luminal Gastrointestinal Disease, 357
Sumona Saha

61 Consequences of Human Immunodeficiency Virus Infection, 363
Vera P. Luther and P. Samuel Pegram

Ulcerative Colitis

Sunanda V. Kane

Division of Gastroenterology and Hepatology, Mayo Clinic Rochester, Rochester, MN, USA

Summary

Ulcerative colitis (UC) is manifest by diffuse, continuous, and superficial inflammation that begins in the rectum and extends proximally to a variable extent in individual patients. In approximately 15% of patients with inflammatory bowel disease (IBD) confined to the colon, the pattern of inflammation is not distinguishable, necessitating the term "indeterminate colitis" or "inflammatory bowel disease unclassified" (IBD-U). Features that are helpful in discriminating between UC and Crohn's disease include: family history, smoking history, presence of perianal manifestations, aphthous ulcerations, strictures, and fistulas. Therapeutic approaches are aimed at induction and maintenance of clinical remissions. Inductive agents include aminosalicylates, corticosteroids, cyclosporine, and monoclonal antibodies targeting tumor necrosis factor (TNF). Maintenance therapies include aminosalicylates, thiopurines, and anti-TNF agents. Colectomy is an option for refractory disease.

Case

A 20-year-old male with no past medical history presents with 2 months of rectal bleeding, increasingly loose stools associated with urgency, and nocturnal bowel movements. Additionally, he describes intermittent, subjective, low-grade fevers, a 4.5 kg (10 lb) weight loss, and bilateral pain and swelling in his knees. He smokes a pack of cigarettes daily and his maternal uncle has UC. On physical exam, his abdomen is soft and non-distended, with mild, diffuse tenderness to palpation. Perianal exam reveals external skin tags with no fissure or fistula. Laboratory studies reveal mild leukocytosis with a left shift and microcytic anemia. Colonoscopy shows patchy inflammation of the entire colon with a normal terminal ileum.

Definition

UC and Crohn's disease encompass a spectrum of chronic idiopathic colitides [1]. The inflammation of UC is confined to the colon in a diffuse, continuous, and superficial (mucosal) pattern beginning at the anorectal junction and extending proximally to a distinct margin that differs among individuals. Approximately one-third of patients have disease limited to the rectum (ulcerative proctitis), one-third have disease limited to the splenic flexure (proctosigmoiditis or left-sided colitis), and one-third present with disease extending proximal to the splenic flexure up to the cecum (pancolitis). The term "indeterminate colitis" (or IBD-U) has been used to describe patients with clinical and inflammatory features that make it difficult to distinguish between classical UC and Crohn's disease [2].

Epidemiology

The incidences of UC and Crohn's disease in North America and Europe are similar, ranging from 2 to 14 cases per 100 000 population, with a prevalence of 50–200 cases per 100 000 population [3]. While IBD colitis can occur from infancy to adulthood, there is a bimodal age distribution, with the largest peak in the 2nd and 3rd decades of life and a smaller peak in the 5th and 6th decades. There is a roughly equal distribution between males and females.

Risk Factors

The primary risk factor for colitis is a family history of either UC or Crohn's disease [3]. Appendectomy at a young age appears to be protective against the development of UC, whereas cigarette smoking is the major environmental factor. Cigarette smoking is inversely associated with ("protective" against) UC but is positively associated with Crohn's disease. Within families with a history of IBD, smokers tend to develop Crohn's disease and non-smokers UC [4].

Pathophysiology

Though the immunopathologic underpinnings of IBD remain elusive, a combination of genetic disposition and triggering environmental factors is hypothesized to lead to a chronic, dysregulated, acute inflammation [5]. Currently, up to 160 genes have been identified that are associated with IBD. The penetrance appears to be higher for Crohn's disease where there is a higher concordance rate among monozygotic twins compared with dizygotic twins. While familial clustering of cases is well described, only 10–20% of patients with IBD have a positive family history.

Clinical Features

Ulcerative Colitis

Patients with UC typically experience rectal bleeding with urgency to evacuate, most commonly upon awakening or after meals. Many patients also describe increased stool frequency, nocturnal bowel

Practical Gastroenterology and Hepatology Board Review Toolkit, Second Edition. Edited by Nicholas J. Talley, Kenneth R. DeVault, Michael B. Wallace, Bashar A. Aqel and Keith D. Lindor.

movements, tenesmus, incontinence, and inability to pass gas without leakage of stool. Diarrhea is related to the extent of colonic involvement; patients with limited proctitis may describe constipation and difficulty evacuating with rectal bleeding. Patients with severe disease may present with fever, tachycardia, anorexia, and weight loss.

Indeterminate Colitis

Up to 15% of patients with IBD-colitis present with disease confined to the colon but have features precluding distinct categorization as either UC or Crohn's disease [2, 6, 7]. Patchy inflammation of the colon on endoscopy is indicative of Crohn's disease unless the colitis has been treated, in which case there may be some evidence of focal endoscopic findings.

Extraintestinal Manifestations of IBD

UC is a systemic disease that can result in inflammation of organ systems other than the gastrointestinal (GI) tract in 20–40% of patients [8]. Arthralgias and arthritis are the most common extraintestinal manifestations, affecting approximately one-quarter of patients with IBD. They are typically pauciarticular, involving larger joints and parallel disease activity. Less commonly, a polyarticular, symmetric arthritis or axial arthritis (ankylosing spondylitis, sacroiliitis) can present and progress independently of colitis [9].

Cutaneous lesions associated with colitis include erythema nodosum and pyoderma gangrenosum. Oral aphthous ulcers are fairly common but occur more often in patients with Crohn's disease. Ocular manifestations can include uveitis (iritis), scleritis, and episcleritis.

Primary sclerosing cholangitis (PSC) is another disease of nonsmokers that affects 3–4% of patients with UC or Crohn's disease. The diagnosis is usually confirmed with magnetic resonance or endoscopic cholangiography showing a classic "beads on a string" in the small bile ducts or a dominant stricture in the common hepatic or bile duct. Liver biopsy may be required in patients with involvement confined to the small intrahepatic ducts. Complications of PSC include acute cholangitis, choledocholithiasis, cholangiocarcinoma, and biliary cirrhosis.

Complications of IBD

Intestinal and systemic complications can occur in the setting of IBD-colitis [10]. Intestinal complications of UC include hemorrhage, toxic megacolon, perforation, and neoplasia.

Extraintestinal complications are related to the pathophysiology of or therapies associated with IBD-colitis. Osteopenia and osteoporosis can result from IBD itself or from chronic corticosteroid therapy, such that patients with small-bowel disease or those receiving chronic steroids should undergo bone mineral density testing and treatment for associated metabolic bone disease [11].

Anemia is common in IBD patients and is often multifactorial in etiology [12]. Iron deficiency is a common consequence of intestinal blood loss. IBD patients are at increased risk for thromboembolic events, likely attributable to chronic systemic inflammation [13].

Patients with IBD-colitis are at increased risk for colorectal carcinoma. Risk factors for neoplasia include younger age at diagnosis, long disease duration and anatomic extent, family history of colorectal cancer, severity of inflammation, and coexisting PSC [14].

Diagnosis

IBD is a clinical diagnosis that involves comprehensive integration of history, physical findings, imaging, endoscopy, and histology. Serologic studies are evolving but are not yet definitive. No single test can conclusively establish the diagnosis, and exclusion of other diseases that can mimic IBD is essential [1, 15] (Figure 54.1).

Historical Factors

Though IBD can present at any age, the classic age of onset is during the 2nd or 3rd decade of life. A family history of IBD should increase suspicion of the diagnosis in a patient with typical symptoms. Smoking increases the risk of Crohn's disease, whereas smoking cessation

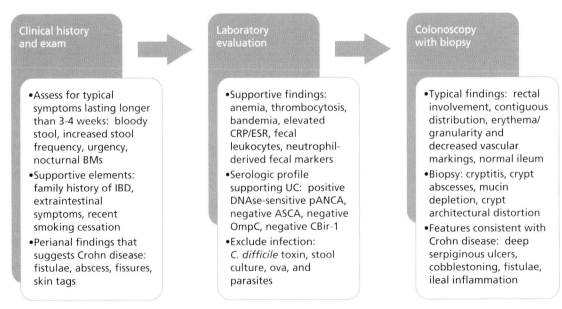

Figure 54.1 Diagnostic algorithm for UC. BM, bowel movement; IBD, inflammatory bowel disease; CRP, C-reactive protein; ESR, erythrocyte sedimentation rate; pANCA, perinuclear antineutrophil cytoplasmic antibody; ASCA, anti-*Saccharomyces cerevisiae* antibody; OmpC, antibody to *E. coli* outer membrane protein C; CBir-1, antibody to CBir1 flagellin.

is associated with onset of UC. Use of aspirin or other non-steroidal anti-inflammatory drugs (NSAIDs) is a common precipitant of disease onset or exacerbation. Additionally, many patients present after an apparent episode of infectious diarrhea or recent exposure to antibiotics [3].

Physical Examination

The physical examination is frequently unrevealing in patients with mild to moderate colitis, but those with severe or fulminant disease may demonstrate fever, tachycardia, abdominal distension, and tenderness.

Laboratory Evaluation

Laboratory studies are often normal in patients with mild disease. Anemia or electrolyte abnormalities may be present in a patient according to the chronicity and severity of symptoms. Erythrocyte sedimentation rate (ESR) and C-reactive protein (CRP) tend to parallel inflammatory activity but are not always reliable markers for individual patients [16]. In the setting of severe colitis, patients may develop hypoalbuminemia, hypokalemia, or metabolic acidosis. Stool evaluation for ova and parasites, culture, and *Clostridium difficile* toxin is important in excluding infection at the time of initial diagnosis or disease relapse. Other stool markers of intestinal inflammation (calprotectin and lactoferrin) are being explored as diagnostic or prognostic tools [17]. Serologic evaluation for presence of antibodies to nuclear or gut luminal antigens is another exciting area of investigation. However, at the time of writing, the role of these tests in diagnosis and prognosis has not been solidly established [18].

Imaging

In the setting of colitis, colonoscopy has a primary role in diagnosis; however, advances in imaging continue to evolve beyond contrast barium studies. Computed tomography (CT) and magnetic resonance imaging (MRI) provide additional information about bowel wall thickening and can better define the presence of extraintestinal complications such as abscesses or fistulas [19]. In the setting of severe colitis, patients should have supine and upright abdominal radiographs performed to evaluate for megacolon, free air, or pneumatosis.

Endoscopy

Endoscopy is essential in establishing the diagnosis of colitis, determining the anatomical distribution of involvement, excluding complicating factors in patients not responding to therapy, assessing for disease recurrence in postoperative patients, and distinguishing Crohn's disease from UC [20]. Though there are no endoscopic features that are pathognomonic for UC or for Crohn's disease, certain findings are highly suggestive [1,6]. The classic endoscopic appearance of UC includes decreased vascular markings with diffuse erythema and granularity, extending proximally from the rectum in a continuous distribution. In patients receiving rectal therapy, the rectum may appear spared. Ulceration of the ileum and visualization of fistulas during colonoscopy are diagnostic features of Crohn's disease, while pseudopolyps may be present in either UC or Crohn's disease. Wireless capsule endoscopy is not as helpful in the workup of UC as in Crohn's disease [21].

Colonoscopy also serves as the cornerstone colorectal cancer prevention strategy in this high-risk population. Consensus guidelines recommend an initial screening colonoscopy in this group beginning 8–10 years after symptom onset and then every 1–2 years. Random biopsies and biopsies targeted at suspicious lesions should be obtained, and colectomy should be considered for patients in whom dysplasia or cancer is identified [14].

Pathology

Histologic features such as crypt architectural distortion suggest chronic injury and can aid in the distinction between acute self-limited colitis and chronic idiopathic IBD [15]. Typical histologic findings in early UC include acute cryptitis, crypt abscesses, mucin depletion, and plasma cell infiltration of the lamina propria.

Differential Diagnosis

The differential diagnosis of IBD is given in Table 54.1.

Case Continued

The patient is initially started on oral mesalamine, without improvement in his symptoms. Oral corticosteroids are then initiated and the patient achieves symptomatic remission, including resolution of his joint pains and low-grade fever. He is transitioned to azathioprine (AZA) for maintenance of remission and the steroids are withdrawn over the next few months.

Therapeutics

The goals of therapy in IBD patients are to induce and maintain symptomatic remission and prevent complications of disease and therapy. The intensity used to induce remission generally dictates which maintenance strategies will be effective.

Current approaches to therapy include sequential induction to maintenance treatment according to the severity of symptoms at diagnosis [21–24] (Figure 54.2). Patients with mild UC (ambulatory

Table 54.1 Differential diagnosis of IBD.

Bacterial colitis	*Salmonella*
	Shigella
	Yersinia
	Campylobacter
	Enterohemorrhagic *E. coli*
	Enterotoxigenic *E. coli*
	Clostridium difficile
	Aeromonas
	Pleisiomonas
Viruses	Cytomegalovirus
	Herpes simplex virus
Parasites	*Entamoeba histolytica*
	Microscopic colitis
	Lymphocytic colitis
	Collagenous colitis
	Diverticular colitis
	Ischemic colitis
	Radiation enteritis/colitis
	Celiac disease
	Appendicitis
	NSAID colitis
	Neutropenic enterocolitis
	Vasculitis
	Sarcoidosis
	Amyloidosis

NSAID, non-steroidal anti-inflammatory drug.

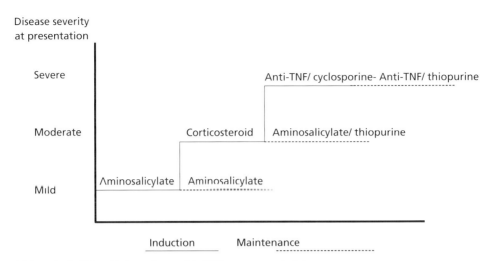

Figure 54.2 Sequential therapies for UC and indeterminate colitis. TNF, tumor necrosis factor.

patients with symptoms that do not have a major impact on quality of life, with less than four bowel movements daily, and without extraintestinal manifestations) can be treated with aminosalicylates. If symptoms completely resolve on aminosalicylates, maintenance therapy with an aminosalicylate should be continued. Patients with moderate to severe symptoms or who fail to respond to aminosalicylates are induced with corticosteroids or an anti-TNF biologic. Steroid induction more often requires maintenance therapy with a thiopurine or anti-TNF biologic, particularly if the colitis is not controlled by high-dose (e.g., 4–5 g/day) mesalamine. Patients who fail steroid induction or maintenance therapy with a thiopurine typically respond to anti-TNF induction and regularly scheduled maintenance therapy.

5-Aminosalicylates

Aminosalicylates (mesalamine, sulfasalazine, olsalazine, balsalazide) are first-line therapies for induction and remission of mild to moderate UC and, despite conflicting evidence, are often used early in the treatment algorithm for Crohn's disease [22–25]. Several oral and rectally administered preparations are available, each employing unique mechanisms for delivering 5-ASA (mesalamine) to the colon. Specific delivery mechanisms include linking 5-ASA to a carrier molecule via an azo bond that is cleaved by colonic bacteria, using moisture-dependent time-release granules that deliver 5-ASA throughout the bowel, and using pH-dependent coatings that release 5-ASA in the terminal ileum and colon [26]. Mesalamine delivered topically as an enema foam or suppository is highly effective in treating distal colitis. Side effects are rare with this class of medication, but may include interstitial nephritis, pancreatitis, hepatitis, pneumonitis, and pericarditis. Sulfasalazine is also associated with sulfa-related hypersensitivity.

Antibiotics

Antibiotics have no primary role in the treatment of UC.

Corticosteroids

Systemic corticosteroids are effective therapies in inducing remission for moderate–severe colitis and can be delivered orally or intravenously [27]. However, the unacceptable adverse effect profile of steroids precludes their long-term use as maintenance

therapies. Rectal steroids can be administered for patients with distal disease.

Thiopurine Immunosuppressants

Mercaptopurine (6-MP) and its prodrug AZA are purine analogues that interfere with nucleic acid synthesis and exhibit anti-inflammatory properties through their cytotoxic effect on inflammatory cells [27]. They are effective therapies for maintenance of remission in UC and can facilitate withdrawal of steroids in patients who are otherwise steroid-dependent. Adverse effects include allergic reactions, infection, pancreatitis, bone-marrow suppression, and hepatitis. Additionally, there is a slightly increased risk of lymphoma [28]. Bone-marrow suppression and therapeutic efficacy are related to genetic polymorphisms of the thiopurine-S-methyltransferase (TPMT) enzyme, which can be measured to allow customized dosing in order to enhance both safety and efficacy.

Cyclosporine

Intravenous cyclosporine can be used as salvage therapy to induce remission in severe UC refractory to intravenous steroids [23, 24,27]. Though it is effective for short-term induction, maintenance therapy with a thiopurine is required. Side effects include headache, tremor, paresthesias, seizures, hypertrichosis, hypertension, renal insufficiency, and opportunistic infections. The risk of pneumocystis pneumonia during cyclosporine therapy is substantial enough to warrant antimicrobial prophylaxis.

TNF-α Inhibitors

TNF-α is a proinflammatory cytokine that plays a key role in propagating the inflammatory cascade of IBD [27,29]. Monoclonal antibodies targeted against TNF to treat UC include infliximab, adalimumab, and golimumab. The efficacy and safety profiles are comparable among the available anti-TNF agents. Opportunistic infections attributable to the immunosuppressive mechanism of these medications include fungal pneumonias and tuberculosis. Consequently, patients should be properly immunized (pneumonia, tetanus, influenza, human papilloma virus (HPV)) and routinely tested for latent tuberculosis prior to initiation of an anti-TNF therapy. Other side effects include allergic reactions, infusion or injection-site reactions, delayed hypersensitivity reactions, drug-induced lupus, heart failure, and demyelinating disease.

Surgical Therapy for UC

Indications for surgery in UC include medically refractory disease, inability to wean off steroids, toxic megacolon, perforation, and confirmed dysplasia or cancer. Surgical options include proctocolectomy with permanent ileostomy or total colectomy with ileal pouch anal anastomosis. These surgeries are considered curative for UC, though half of patients can develop inflammation in the ileal pouch, necessitating antibiotics, steroids, or anti-TNF agents [30].

Take Home Points

- There are no pathognomonic markers for ulcerative colitis (UC) or Crohn's disease.
- Diagnosis is based upon endoscopy, histology, and imaging.
- Therapeutic goals include induction and maintenance of clinical remissions.
- Aminosalicylates are inductive and maintenance therapies for mild–moderate disease.
- Corticosteroids are used to induce, but not maintain, remissions.
- Anti-TNF agents can induce and maintain remissions when conventional agents fail.
- Surgical removal of the colon is usually curative for UC.

References

1 Sands BE. From symptom to diagnosis: clinical distinctions among various forms of intestinal inflammation. *Gastroenterology* 2004; **126**: 1518–32.

2 Geboes K, Colombel JF, Greenstein A, *et al.* Indeterminate colitis: a review of the concept – what's in a name? *Inflamm Bowel Dis* 2008; **14**: 850–7.

3 Loftus EV Jr. Clinical epidemiology of inflammatory bowel disease: Incidence, prevalence, and environmental influences. *Gastroenterology* 2004; **126**: 1504–17.

4 Mahid SS, Minor KS, Soto RE, *et al.* Smoking and inflammatory bowel disease: a meta-analysis. *Mayo Clin Proc* 2006; **81**: 1462–71.

5 Xavier RJ, Podolsky DK. Unravelling the pathogenesis of inflammatory bowel disease. *Nature* 2007; **448**: 427–34.

6 Tremaine WJ. Review article: Indeterminate colitis – definition, diagnosis and management. *Aliment Pharmacol Therap* 2007; **25**: 13–7.

7 Martland GT, Shepherd NA. Indeterminate colitis: definition, diagnosis, implications and a plea for nosological sanity. *Histopathology* 2007; **50**: 83–96.

8 Ardizzone S, Puttini PS, Cassinotti A, *et al.* Extraintestinal manifestations of inflammatory bowel disease. *Dig Liver Dis* 2008; **40** (Suppl. 2): S253–9.

9 Williams H, Walker D, Orchard TR. Extraintestinal manifestations of inflammatory bowel disease. *Curr Gastroenterol Rep* 2008; **10**: 597–605.

10 Marrero F, Qadeer MA, Lashner BA. Severe complications of inflammatory bowel disease. *Med Clin North Am* 2008; **92**: 671.

11 Lichtenstein GR, Sands BE, Pazianas M. Prevention and treatment of osteoporosis in inflammatory bowel disease. *Inflammat Bowel Dis* 2006; **12**: 797–813.

12 Gasche C, Berstad A, Befrits R, *et al.* Guidelines on the diagnosis and management of iron deficiency and anemia in inflammatory bowel diseases. *Inflamm Bowel Dis* 2007; **13**: 1545–53.

13 Irving PM, Pasi KJ, Rampton DS. Thrombosis and inflammatory bowel disease. *Clin Gastroenterol Hepatol* 2005; **3**: 617–28.

14 Ullman T, Odze R, Farraye FA. Diagnosis and management of dysplasia in patients with ulcerative colitis and Crohn's disease of the colon. *Inflamm Bowel Dis* 2009; **15**: 630–8.

15 Yantiss RK, Odze RD. Diagnostic difficulties in inflammatory bowel disease pathology. *Histopathology* 2006; **48**: 116–32.

16 Jones J, Loftus EV, Panaccione R, *et al.* Relationships between disease activity and serum and fecal biomarkers in patients with Crohn's disease. *Clin Gastroenterol Hepatol* 2008; **6**: 1218–24.

17 Desai D, Faubion WA, Sandborn WJ. Review article: biological activity markers in inflammatory bowel disease. *Aliment Pharmacol Ther* 2007; **25**: 247–55.

18 Vermeire S, Vermeulen N, Van Assche G, *et al.* (Auto)antibodies in inflammatory bowel diseases. *Gastroenterol Clin North Am* 2008; **37**: 429–38.

19 Bruining DH, Loftus EV. Evolving diagnostic strategies for inflammatory bowel disease. *Curr Gastroenterol Rep* 2006; **8**: 478–85.

20 Vanderheyden AD, Mitros FA. Pathologist surgeon interface in idiopathic inflammatory bowel disease. *Surg Clin North Am* 2007; **87**: 763–85.

21 Solem CA, Loftus EV, Fletcher JG, *et al.* Small-bowel imaging in Crohn's disease: a prospective, blinded, 4-way comparison trial. *Gastrointest Endosc* 2008; **68**: 255–66.

22 Lichtenstein GR, Hanauer SB, Sandborn WJ. Management of Crohn's disease in adults. *Am J Gastroenterol* 2009; **104**: 465–83.

23 Kornbluth A, Sachar DB. Ulcerative colitis practice guidelines in adults (update): American College of Gastroenterology, Practice Parameters Committee. *Am J Gastroenterol* 2004; **99**: 1371–85.

24 Travis SP, Stange EF, Lemann M, *et al.* European consensus on the diagnosis and management of ulcerative colitis: current management. *J Crohn's Colitis* 2008; **2**: 24–62.

25 Travis SP, *et al.* European evidence based consensus on the diagnosis and management of Crohn's disease: current management. *Gut* 2006; **55**(Suppl. 1): i16–35.

26 Sandborn WJ. Oral 5-ASA therapy in ulcerative colitis: what are the implications of the new formulations? *J Clin Gastroenterol* 2008; **42**: 338–44.

27 Lichtenstein GR, Abreu MT, Cohen R, *et al.* American Gastroenterological Association Institute technical review on corticosteroids, immunomodulators, and infliximab in inflammatory bowel disease. *Gastroenterology* 2006; **130**: 940–87.

28 Kandiel A, Fraser AG, Korelitz BI, *et al.* Increased risk of lymphoma among inflammatory bowel disease patients treated with azathioprine and 6-mercaptopurine. *Gut* 2005; **54**: 1121–5.

29 Clark M, Colombel JF, Feagan BC, *et al.* American Gastroenterological Association consensus development conference on the use of biologics in the treatment of inflammatory bowel disease, June 21–23, 2006. *Gastroenterology* 2007; **133**: 312–39.

30 Pardi DS, Sandborn WJ. Systematic review: The management of pouchitis. *Aliment Pharmacol Therap* 2006; **23**: 1087–96.

CHAPTER 55

Clostridium difficile Infection and Pseudomembranous Colitis

Byron P. Vaughn and J. Thomas Lamont

Beth Israel Deaconess Medical Center, Boston, MA, USA

Summary

Colonization of the colon with *Clostridium difficile* bacteria can have varying outcomes, from asymptomatic carriage to pseudomembranous colitis to fulminant colitis. The incidence and severity of this infection have increased in the last decade, probably related to the emergence of a highly toxigenic strain associated with hospital outbreaks.

Standard treatment for *C. difficile*-associated diarrhea (CDAD) includes stopping implicated antibiotics, commencing oral metronidazole, vancomycin, or fidaxomicin therapy, and correcting secondary dehydration. *C. difficile* has not developed resistance to any of the just mentioned antibiotics, so initial response to these agents exceeds 90% in clinical trials. Recurrent infection usually responds to retreatment with these antibiotics, or to pulse-tapered therapy. Additionally, novel insights into the intestinal microbiome have led to the use of fecal microbiota transplant (FMT) as a promising treatment for recurrent CDAD. Control measures to minimize the risk of hospital-acquired infections remain an important preventative strategy.

Case

A 68-year-old woman presents to the office complaining of a 2-week history of loose stool and abdominal cramps. She was treated by her primary care physician with amoxicillin for a sinus infection 1 month ago. In addition to diarrhea, she has noticed some blood mixed with her stool. She is a diabetic and takes metformin. Her last colonoscopy, 2 years ago, showed diverticula only.

Definition and Epidemiology

"*Clostridium difficile* infection" (CDI) and "CDAD" describe the development of diarrhea that occurs in patients infected with toxin-producing *Clostridium difficile* bacteria [1]. "Pseudomembranous colitis" refers to the endoscopic appearance of scattered white mucosal plaques that can appear in the colon in patients with CDI (Figure 55.1). The presence of *C. difficile* in the colon does not always imply active infection, as asymptomatic carriage has been reported in up to 14% of hospitalized adults receiving antibiotics, and up to 70% of healthy infants [2].

The incidence of CDI rose steadily from the 1970s but remained stable throughout the 1990s at 30–40 cases per 100 000. Since 2000, however, there has been a steep rise in incidence (84 per 100 000 in 2005), and the severity of the disease has also increased, particularly in elderly patients. Sporadic outbreaks associated with severe morbidity and mortality in Canada and the United States have been linked to the virulent NAP-1/027 strain, which produces large quantities of toxins (A, B, and binary toxin) and is relatively resistant to fluoroquinolones [3].

Risk factors traditionally associated with the development of CDI include current or recent antibiotic use, advanced age, hospitalization, and comorbid illnesses [4]. Inflammatory bowel disease (IBD) has recently been recognized as an additional risk factor, being present in 16% of CDI cases in one series [5]. The Centers for Disease Control and Prevention (CDC) have recently documented infection in previously healthy young adults with no hospital or antibiotic exposure [6].

Pathophysiology

Oral ingestion of *C. difficile* spores leads to the colonization of the large bowel in some patients following antibiotic exposure, which reduces the ability of the normal colonic flora to resist colonization. These spores are resistant to heat and antibiotics, and widely contaminate the hospital environment. Colitis in CDI is related to its two exotoxins (A and B), which bind to and enter colonic epithelial cells and disrupt the cellular cytoskeleton [7]. These alterations lead to apoptosis and disintegration of the epithelial barrier function. In addition, *C. difficile* toxins can activate neutrophils, stimulate monocytes and epithelial cells to release interleukin (IL) 8, and induce tumor necrosis factor (TNF)-α release by macrophages. These effects result in colonic mucosal inflammation, microulceration, and, in some patients, pseudomembrane formation. Toxin B appears to be more potent in inducing colitis than toxin A. The NAP-1/027 strain also produces a non-A/non-B binary toxin, but the role of this toxin in colitis is unclear.

Since not every colonized individual develops CDI, differences in certain host factors probably influence the outcome of infection, including:
- The binding of toxin to epithelial receptors.
- Immunoglobulin G (IgG) and A (IgA) antitoxin antibodies.
- IL-8 production by colonic inflammatory cells.

Though 50–70% of healthy infants up to age of 12 months are transiently colonized, they do not develop diarrhea, possibly due to absent colonocyte receptors for *C. difficile* toxin [8]. Hospitalized

Practical Gastroenterology and Hepatology Board Review Toolkit, Second Edition. Edited by Nicholas J. Talley, Kenneth R. DeVault, Michael B. Wallace, Bashar A. Aqel and Keith D. Lindor.
© 2016 John Wiley & Sons, Ltd. Published 2016 by John Wiley & Sons, Ltd. Companion website: www.practicalgastrohep.com

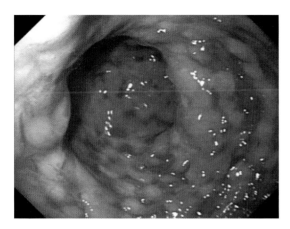

Figure 55.1 Endoscopic image of pseudomembranous colitis in patient with *Clostridium difficile* infection (CDI).

patients with asymptomatic *C. difficile* colonization have higher serum IgG antitoxin antibodies directed at toxin A than those with CDI, and high levels of these antitoxins appear to protect against recurrence in patients following initial infection [2,9,10]. Since IL-8-mediated neutrophil recruitment to the colon is central to CDI, patients with polymorphisms in the gene for this chemokine have increased susceptibility to this disease [11].

Clinical Features of *C. difficile* Infection

Patients with CDI typically develop frequent semiformed or watery diarrhea, in association with crampy abdominal pain [12]. The loose stool is usually non-bloody, and urgency or incontinence may develop in elderly patients. Peripheral edema or ascites has been observed, due to a secondary protein-losing enteropathy and hypoalbuminemia [13]. *C. difficile* is rarely invasive, but there are rare case reports of reactive arthritis after CDI or of incidental CDI of skin, blood, or bone as part of a polymicrobial infection [14,15]. In patients with an ileostomy or ileal pouch, CDI can cause ileitis with profuse stomal output.

Clinical signs of CDI are non-specific, and include low-grade fever, diffuse abdominal tenderness, and dehydration. The development of fulminant colitis or megacolon will manifest as ileus and abdominal distension, accompanied by hypotension, diffuse guarding, and rebound tenderness or rigidity if perforation occurs. Associated features include dehydration, hypokalemia, colonic hemorrhage, perforation, and sepsis [16]. Leukocytosis >15 000 cells/mm^3 is common, and CDI should always be considered in elderly patients with clinical deterioration and an elevated white count, even with minimal diarrhea.

A clinical trial used a novel score (Table 55.1) to classify disease severity with the following parameters: age, temperature, albumin, white blood cell (WBC) count, endoscopic findings, and intensive care unit (ICU) requirement [16]. A retrospective study of 1600 cases from Canada identified a number of factors associated with a higher risk of complicated CDI, which it defined as death, sepsis, megacolon, perforation, or emergency colectomy [17] (Table 55.2).

Diagnosis

The prior gold-standard test for CDI was the cell culture cytotoxin assay, but for practical and economic reasons this has been largely supplanted by DNA-based assays. Similarly, the enzyme immunoassay (EIA) for toxins A and B in stool has limited sensitivity and is not commonly used in current practice. Testing stools

Table 55.1 Criteria for the classification of *C. difficile* infection (CDI) severity. A score >2 within 48 hours is classified as "severe CDAD." Source: Adapted from Zar 2007 [16].

Factor	Points
Age >60 years	1
Temperature >38.3 °C	1
Albumin level <2.5 mg/dL	1
WBC count >15 000 cells/mm^3	1
Pseudomembranous colitis on endoscopy	2
Treatment in ICU	2

WBC, white blood cell; ICU, intensive care unit.

for either toxin alone may lead to false-negative results, as some strains produce only A or B toxin. The usefulness of diagnostic testing depends heavily on the pre-test probability of CDI; therefore, we do not recommend testing for *C. difficile* on formed stool. While repeat testing is commonly performed, there is likely little added value following an initial negative test [18–21]. A two-step algorithm involving an initial EIA test for glutamate dehydrogenase (an antigen produced constitutively by all *C. difficile* isolates) followed by toxin testing when positive can improve the diagnostic yield [22]. Stool polymerase chain reaction (PCR) for CDI is rapidly replacing other forms of diagnostic testing due to its very high sensitivity and specificity and its rapid turnaround time [23, 24]. Our practice is to order one stool PCR for a symptomatic patient. Once the patient starts treatment, stools may remain toxin-positive both during and after clinical recovery. We do not recommend repeat toxin assays to confirm elimination of toxin at the end of successful therapy, as many cured patients will be convalescent carriers.

Endoscopy (sigmoidoscopy or colonoscopy) is not required to diagnose CDI, but may be helpful in atypical presentations or when there is a high suspicion for CDI despite negative toxin assays. Endoscopic findings can range from simple erythema and friability to patchy or confluent ulcers with pseudomembranes (Figure 55.1) [25]. In some patients, the rectosigmoid may be spared, with signs of colitis only in the right or transverse colon. The risk of perforation is increased in patients with extensive ulceration or a dilated colon. In this situation, a simple examination of the rectum without air insufflation is advisable.

Case Continued

A stool sample is sent for enteric pathogen culture and *C. difficile* toxin PCR. Labs drawn show a WBC count of 15 × 10^9 and normal kidney function.

Table 55.2 Risk factors for severe/complicated *C. difficile* infection (SC-CDI) in those not infected with the hypervirulent NAP1/027 strain. Source: Modified from Pépin 2007 [17].

Risk factor	Odds ratio of SC-CDI
Age >65 years	2.1
Tube feeding within 2 months	2.0
Immunosuppression	2.7
WBC >20 × 10^9/L	3.7
Creatinine	
>100 µmol/L	2.7
>200 µmol/L	4.2

WBC, white blood cell.

CHAPTER 55

Differential Diagnosis

The differential diagnosis for patients presenting with diarrhea is long. In hospitalized patients with diarrhea, especially those treated with antibiotics, the following specific causes should be considered:

- **Antibiotic-associated osmotic diarrhea:** This occurs when antibiotics disrupt the normal bacterial metabolism of dietary carbohydrates in the colonic lumen. The subsequent accumulation of non-absorbed carbohydrates causes an osmotic diarrhea. This is usually mild and disappears with fasting or cessation of the antibiotics.
- **Infectious diarrhea:** In addition to *C. difficile*, other organisms that cause colitis during or after antibiotic use are *Staphylococcus aureus*, *Salmonella*, and *Clostridium perfringens*. *Klebsiella oxytoca* has been reported to cause an antibiotic-associated hemorrhagic colitis [26]. Rotavirus and cytomegalovirus (CMV) infection may also cause diarrhea in hospitalized patients.
- **IBD:** Patients with established or undiagnosed IBD are somewhat more likely to develop *C. difficile* than healthy age-matched patients. This may relate to frequent exposure to antibiotics or to alteration of the fecal microbiome in IBD, even without prior antibiotics. CDI in patients with IBD is associated with severe flares and increased requirement for surgery [5].

Treatment

Treatment of CDI has four main tenets, which apply to all cases of confirmed CDI:

- Discontinue the causative antibiotics (if possible).
- Initiate anti-*C. difficile* antibiotic therapy.
- Monitor for, and manage, complications.
- Initiate infection control measures.

The choice of antibiotic regimen depends on whether it is an initial infection or relapse, and on the severity of the infection itself. As noted in Table 55.1, patients aged over 65 years, those with a high WBC count, and those with an elevated creatinine are at higher risk of severe disease.

Initial CDI

Three antibiotics are available for the treatment of acute infection: metronidazole, vancomycin, and fidaxomicin. Importantly, *C. difficile* has not been reported to have resistance to any of these. For initial treatment of uncomplicated CDI, oral metronidazole 500 mg three times a day for 10–14 days is the treatment of choice. The advantages of metronidazole are its low cost and its efficacy, which was found comparable to that of vancomycin for non-severe CDI in randomized controlled trials (RCTs) [16]. The disadvantages are its side effects, including nausea and metallic taste during therapy. It is worth noting that a recent outbreak in Canada was associated with an unusually high rate (26%) of patients who failed to respond to metronidazole, but this may reflect a higher proportion of patients with severe disease due to the hypervirulent NAP-1/027 strain [27].

Vancomycin 125 mg orally four times daily is an alternative choice, but it is not effective if given intravenously (IV) as it is excreted primarily by the kidney. The disadvantages of vancomycin are its higher costs and concerns about the proliferation of vancomycin-resistant enterococci.

Fidaxomicin was recently approved for use in CDI. In a head-to-head comparison with vancomycin, both were equally effective in treating the symptoms of acute infection, but fidaxomicin had a recurrence rate of 15% versus 25% for vancomycin [30].

In severe CDI (Tables 55.1 and 55.2), oral vancomycin 125 mg four times a day is significantly more effective than metronidazole [16], and vancomycin is the drug of choice. In the presence of ileus, or in patients unable to take oral medications, vancomycin may be given via nasogastric tube or as a retention enema (500 mg four times per day) [28]. Patients with fulminant colitis require IV metronidazole (500 mg three times per day) in addition to vancomycin (500 mg four times per day), as well as review by a surgeon to consider urgent colectomy.

Recurrent CDI

Recurrence occurs in about 15–25% of successfully treated patients, and may result either from environmental reinfection with a different strain of *C. difficile* or persistence, via spores in the colon, of the same strain responsible for the initial episode. Other causes of diarrhea, such as other infections, IBD flares, or post-infectious irritable bowel syndrome (IBS), may mimic relapse of *C. difficile* (see Differential Diagnosis).

The first recurrence is usually treated with a repeat 14-day course of metronidazole or vancomycin, in the same dosage used for the initial episode, with recovery expected in about 80–90% of cases. Fidaxomicin has a lower recurrence rate in patients who have already had a recurrence, and some authorities would recommend it over metronidazole or vancomycin in this setting despite its higher cost. After the first recurrence, patients are at high risk of developing further recurrences: up to 50% in one study [29].

FMT is an emerging strategy for the treatment of recurrent CDI. While techniques for the preparation of donor stool and administration of FMT vary, duodenal infusion, colonoscopic administration, and retention enema have all been shown to be effective [33–35]. Typically, patients are treated with antibiotics to suppress *C. difficile* and are given a full-bowel lavage prior to transplantation. The benefit of FMT seems to stem from restoration of normal intestinal diversity [34,36]. While only one RCT has been undertaken to date, evidence from numerous case series supports cure rates of 80–90%, or even higher, after FMT [33, 34]. Given the high success rate of FMT for the treatment of recurrent CDI, it should be considered for the second or third recurrence. The following treatment strategies are used in patients with multiple relapses (Figure 55.2):

- Vancomycin 125mg four times daily, to eradicate remnant spores as they convert to the vegetative state in the colon [29].
- Vancomycin followed by a 4-week course of probiotics, such as *Saccharomyces boulardii*, to prevent regrowth of *C. difficile* [37].
- Vancomycin for 14 days, followed by rifaximin for 14 days [38].
- Fidaxomicin 200 mg twice daily for 10 days [32].
- Vancomycin to suppress symptoms, followed by full-bowel lavage and FMT [33, 34].

Case Continued

C. difficile PCR returns positive. The patient starts oral metronidazole 500 mg three times per day for uncomplicated, acute CDI. Her diarrhea resolves within 4 days.

A few days after she finishes the course of metronidazole, she returns to her primary care doctor with watery diarrhea and urgency. She has no features of severe disease, but a *C. difficile* PCR is again positive. She is retreated with metronidazole and improves within several days of starting therapy. She completes a full course of metronidazole therapy and has no further recurrence.

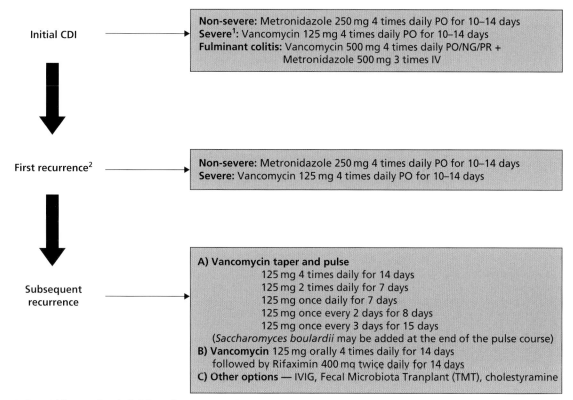

Initial CDI → **Non-severe:** Metronidazole 250 mg 4 times daily PO for 10–14 days
Severe¹: Vancomycin 125 mg 4 times daily PO for 10–14 days
Fulminant colitis: Vancomycin 500 mg 4 times daily PO/NG/PR +
Metronidazole 500 mg 3 times IV

First recurrence² → **Non-severe:** Metronidazole 250 mg 4 times daily PO for 10–14 days
Severe: Vancomycin 125 mg 4 times daily PO for 10–14 days

Subsequent recurrence → **A) Vancomycin taper and pulse**
125 mg 4 times daily for 14 days
125 mg 2 times daily for 7 days
125 mg once daily for 7 days
125 mg once every 2 days for 8 days
125 mg once every 3 days for 15 days
(*Saccharomyces boulardii* may be added at the end of the pulse course)
B) Vancomycin 125 mg orally 4 times daily for 14 days
followed by Rifaximin 400 mg twice daily for 14 days
C) Other options — IVIG, Fecal Microbiota Tranplant (TMT), cholestyramine

*1. See Table 55.1 for definition of severe CDI; **2**. non-severe recurrence*

Figure 55.2 Algorithm for the suggested management of CDI.

Prognosis

As already discussed, most patients treated for an initial episode of uncomplicated CDI are symptom-free after 7 days' treatment with metronidazole or vancomycin. Among 800 non-epidemic patients, 11% developed severe or complicated disease, with a 30-day mortality of 8% [17]. However, during the recent NAP-1/027 epidemic, the 30-day mortality attributable to CDI rose to 23% [39]. After initial treatment for non-severe disease, approximately 20% of patients develop at least one episode of recurrence, and at least half of these will proceed to further relapses of CDI.

Take Home Points

- The incidence and severity of *Clostridium difficile* infection (CDI) are increasing worldwide, partially due to the emergence of hyper-virulent strains.
- Though associated with antibiotic use in most cases, infection can also occur in otherwise healthy individuals with no known antibiotic exposure and in patients with inflammatory bowel disease (IBD) flares.
- *Clostridium difficile* toxin polymerase chain reaction (PCR) is the most accurate and rapid single test for diagnosis of CDI. If unavailable, a single test for toxin A and B or a two-step process involving enzyme immunoassay (EIA) for glutamate dehydrogenase followed by toxin testing is reasonable.
- Oral metronidazole, vancomycin, and fidaxomicin are very effective initial therapies, and should be repeated in those with a first recurrence.
- Recurrent disease follows successful initial therapy in up to 25% of cases. Fecal microbiota transplant (FMT) is an effective treatment for recurrent CDI in patients with more than three recurrences.

References

1 Kelly CP, LaMont JT. *Clostridium difficile*: more difficult than ever. *N Engl J Med* 2008; **359**: 1932–40.
2 Kyne L, Warny M, Qamar A, Kelly CP. Asymptomatic carriage of *Clostridium difficile* and serum levels of IgG antibody against toxin A. *N Engl J Med* 2000; **342**: 390–7.
3 McDonald LC, Killgore GE, Thompson A, *et al*. An epidemic, toxin gene-variant strain of *Clostridium difficile*. *N Engl J Med* 2005; **353**: 2433–41.
4 Barbut F, Petit JC. Epidemiology of *Clostridium difficile*-associated infections. *Clin Microbiol Infect* 2001; **7**: 405–10.
5 Issa M, Vijayapal A, Graham MB, *et al*. Impact of *Clostridium difficile* on inflammatory bowel disease. *Clin Gastroenterol Hepatol* 2007; **5**: 345–51.
6 Severe *Clostridium difficile*-associated disease in populations previously at low risk – four states, 2005. *Morb Mortal Wkly Rep* 2005; **54**: 1201–5.
7 Just I, Selzer J, Wilm M, *et al*. Glucosylation of Rho proteins by *Clostridium difficile* toxin B. *Nature* 1995 **8**; **375**: 500–3.
8 Eglow R, Charalabos P, Itzkowitz S, *et al*. Diminished *Clostridium difficile* toxin A sensitivity in newborn rabbit ileum is associated with decreased toxin A receptor. *J Clin Invest* 1992; **90**: 822–9.
9 Kyne L, Warny M, Qamar A, Kelly CP. Association between antibody response to toxin A and protection against recurrent *Clostridium difficile* diarrhoea. *Lancet* 2001; **357**: 189–93.
10 Leav BA, Blair B, Leney M, *et al*. Serum anti-toxin B antibody correlates with protection from recurrent *Clostridium difficile* infection (CDI). *Vaccine* 2010; **28**: 965–9.
11 Jiang Z-D, DuPont HL, Garey K, *et al*. A common polymorphism in the interleukin 8 gene promoter is associated with *Clostridium difficile* diarrhea. *Am J Gastroenterol* 2006; **101**: 1112–16.
12 Manabe YC, Vinetz JM, Moore RD, *et al*. *Clostridium difficile* colitis: an efficient clinical approach to diagnosis. *Ann Intern Med* 1995; **123**: 835–40.
13 Dansinger ML, Johnson S, Jansen PC, *et al*. Protein-losing enteropathy is associated with *Clostridium difficile* diarrhea but not with asymptomatic colonization: a prospective, case-control study. *Clin Infect Dis* 1996; **22**: 932–7.
14 Birnbaum J, Bartlett JG, Gelber AC. *Clostridium difficile*: an under-recognized cause of reactive arthritis? *Clin Rheumatol* 2008; **27**: 253–5.
15 García-Lechuz JM, Hernangómez S, Juan RS, *et al*. Extra-intestinal infections caused by *Clostridium difficile*. *Clin Microbiol Infect* 2001; **7**: 453–7.

16 Zar FA, Bakkanagari SR, Moorthi KM, Davis MB. A comparison of vancomycin and metronidazole for the treatment of *Clostridium difficile*-associated diarrhea, stratified by disease severity. *Clin Infect Dis* 2007; **45**: 302–7.

17 Pépin J, Valiquette L, Gagnon S, *et al.* Outcomes of *Clostridium difficile*-associated disease treated with metronidazole or vancomycin before and after the emergence of NAP1/027. *Am J Gastroenterol* 2007; **102**: 2781–8.

18 Planche T, Aghaizu A, Holliman R, *et al.* Diagnosis of *Clostridium difficile* infection by toxin detection kits: a systematic review. *Lancet Infect Dis* 2008; **8**: 777–84.

19 Deshpande A, Pasupuleti V, Patel P, *et al.* Repeat stool testing to diagnose *Clostridium difficile* infection using enzyme immunoassay does not increase diagnostic yield. *Clin Gastroenterol Hepatol* 2011; **9**: 665–9.

20 Mohan SS, McDermott BP, Parchuri S, Cunha BA. Lack of value of repeat stool testing for *Clostridium difficile* toxin. *Am J Med* 2006; **119**: 356.e7–8.

21 Nemat H, Khan R, Ashraf MS, *et al.* Diagnostic value of repeated enzyme immunoassays in *Clostridium difficile* infection. *Am J Gastroenterol* 2009; **104**: 2035–41.

22 Ticehurst JR, Aird DZ, Dam LM, *et al.* Effective detection of toxigenic *Clostridium difficile* by a two-step algorithm including tests for antigen and cytotoxin. *J Clin Microbiol* 2006; **44**: 1145–9.

23 Bélanger SD, Boissinot M, Clairoux N, *et al.* Rapid detection of *Clostridium difficile* in feces by real-time PCR. *J Clin Microbiol* 2003; **41**: 730–4.

24 van den Berg RJ, Bruijnesteijn van Coppenraet LS, Gerritsen H-J, *et al.* Prospective multicenter evaluation of a new immunoassay and real-time PCR for rapid diagnosis of *Clostridium difficile*-associated diarrhea in hospitalized patients. *J Clin Microbiol* 2005; **43**: 5338–40.

25 Seppälä K, Hjelt L, Sipponen P. Colonoscopy in the diagnosis of antibiotic-associated colitis. A prospective study. *Scand J Gastroenterol* 1981; **16**: 465–8.

26 Högenauer C, Langner C, Beubler E, *et al.* *Klebsiella oxytoca* as a causative organism of antibiotic-associated hemorrhagic colitis. *N Engl J Med* 2006; **355**: 2418–26.

27 Pépin J, Alary M-E, Valiquette L, *et al.* Increasing risk of relapse after treatment of *Clostridium difficile* colitis in Quebec, Canada. *Clin Infect Dis* 2005; **40**: 1591–7.

28 Apisarnthanarak A, Razavi B, Mundy LM. Adjunctive intracolonic vancomycin for severe *Clostridium difficile* colitis: case series and review of the literature. *Clin Infect Dis* 2002; **35**: 690–6.

29 McFarland LV, Elmer GW, Surawicz CM. Breaking the cycle: treatment strategies for 163 cases of recurrent *Clostridium difficile* disease. *Am J Gastroenterol* 2002; **97**: 1769–75.

30 Louie TJ, Miller MA, Mullane KM, *et al.* Fidaxomicin versus vancomycin for *Clostridium difficile* infection. *N Engl J Med* 2011; **364**: 422–31.

31 Cornely OA, Crook DW, Esposito R, *et al.* Fidaxomicin versus vancomycin for infection with *Clostridium difficile* in Europe, Canada, and the USA: a double-blind, non-inferiority, randomised controlled trial. *Lancet Infect Dis* 2012; **12**: 281–9.

32 Cornely OA, Miller MA, Louie TJ, *et al.* Treatment of first recurrence of *Clostridium difficile* infection: fidaxomicin versus vancomycin. *Clin Infect Dis* 2012; **55**(Suppl 2): S154–61.

33 Kassam Z, Lee CH, Yuan Y, Hunt RH. Fecal microbiota transplantation for *Clostridium difficile* infection: systematic review and meta-analysis. *Am J Gastroenterol* 2013; **108**: 500–8.

34 van Nood E, Vrieze A, Nieuwdorp M, *et al.* Duodenal infusion of donor feces for recurrent *Clostridium difficile*. *N Engl J Med* 2013; **368**: 407–15.

35 Hamilton MJ, Weingarden AR, Sadowsky MJ, Khoruts A. Standardized frozen preparation for transplantation of fecal microbiota for recurrent *Clostridium difficile* infection. *Am J Gastroenterol* 2012; **107**: 761–7.

36 Chang JY, Antonopoulos DA, Kalra A, *et al.* Decreased diversity of the fecal microbiome in recurrent *Clostridium difficile*-associated diarrhea. *J Infect Dis* 2008; **197**: 435–8.

37 McFarland LV, Surawicz CM, Greenberg RN, *et al.* A randomized placebo-controlled trial of *Saccharomyces boulardii* in combination with standard antibiotics for *Clostridium difficile* disease. *JAMA* 1994; **271**: 1913–8.

38 Johnson S, Schriever C, Galang M, *et al.* Interruption of recurrent *Clostridium difficile*-associated diarrhea episodes by serial therapy with vancomycin and rifaximin. *Clin Infect Dis* 2007; **44**: 846–8.

39 Pépin J, Valiquette L, Cossette B. Mortality attributable to nosocomial *Clostridium difficile*-associated disease during an epidemic caused by a hypervirulent strain in Quebec. *Can Med Assoc J* 2005; **173**: 1037–42.

CHAPTER 56
Colonic Ischemia

Timothy T. Nostrant
Department of Internal Medicine, University of Michigan, Ann Arbor, MI, USA

Summary

Colonic ischemia is increasing in incidence. Hypoperfusion and reperfusion injury are causative. The differential diagnosis is relatively small, and usually clinical history is enough to make the diagnosis. Computed tomography (CT) examination, followed by colonoscopy and biopsy if the patient is non-toxic, confirms it. Most cases resolve symptomatically in 1–2 days, with radiographic and endoscopic resolution in 10–14 days. Progression to transmural necrosis occurs in 15% of cases and manifests itself in the first few days as increasing pain, localized peritoneal findings, leukocytosis, and acidosis. Early surgery should be carried out if progression is evident. Aortic iliac reconstruction, renal transplant patients, and cardiac patients require close observation for progression because of high mortality rates. New theories about colonic ischemia are likely to come from the study of pharmacologic induced ischemia.

Case

A 62-year-old man presents with 4 hours of bilateral lower quadrant pain with recent passage of blood. He gives a history of two similar episodes that lasted 2 hours each. Physical examination shows only mild lower left abdominal tenderness and grossly bloody stool. The patient takes diuretics for hypertension and digoxin for atrial fibrillation rate control. His laboratory tests show hemoglobin of 12.5, hematocrit of 39, and white blood cell (WBC) count of 12.0. CT of the abdomen reveals mild edema of the left colon and splenic flexure with no vascular or small-bowel involvement. Unprepped colonoscopy shows multiple bluish-black blebs in the left colon, with ulcers at splenic flexure. Biopsies show acute mucosal necrosis, ghost crypt epithelial cells, and capillary hemorrhage. A diagnosis of ischemic colitis is made. The patient is treated with intravenous (IV) hydration. Diuretics and digoxin are stopped. He is well in 2 days.

Epidemiology

Colonic ischemia is the most common form of GI ischemic injury (Figure 56.1). Its course is usually mild, with spontaneous resolution. It is frequently misdiagnosed as inflammatory bowel disease (IBD) or cancer. Estimates show a crude incidence of about 7.2 cases per 100 000 patient-years [1]. Some estimates have it accounting for 1 in 5000 colonoscopies, 1 in 700 office visits, and 1 in 2000 hospital admissions, with the incidence climbing [1]. Most cases (90%) occur in patients over the age of 60, with no gender predilection [1–4].

Pathophysiology

Colonic ischemia is a result of hypoperfusion and reperfusion injury secondary to both anatomic and functional alterations in the mesenteric vasculature. Reperfusion accounts for most of the histologic and endoscopic damage, particularly when ischemia duration is short. During reperfusion, reactive oxygen species (ROS) cause tissue damage, particularly in the mucosa, since this is the most oxygen-deprived region during ischemia. Deeper layers can also be damaged if ischemia is more prolonged or more severe. These ROS perioxidate lipid membranes, causing cell lysis, ghost epithelial cells, hemorrhagic mucosal necrosis, and subsequent fibrosis, leading to radiologic and endoscopic thumbprinting, endoscopic ulcers, and deeper injury, leading in turn to pneumatosis and finally perforation of the colonic wall. Though colonic ischemia has a full course from ischemic injury to a completely normal colon that is measured in days, 15% of cases can progress to gangrene and perforation over the same period [1,3] (Figure 56.2).

Major risk factors for colonic ischemia are listed in Table 56.1. Non-occlusive ischemia is the most common form (up to 95%) and is the major reason why angiographic testing is rarely helpful. The "watershed areas" where bloodflow is minimized between the superior and inferior mesenteric artery (SMA and IMA) vascular supplies are the most common areas of involvement. The vulnerable areas are the splenic flexure and rectosigmoid junction. Left colon involvement is seen in 75% of patients, with 25% limited to the splenic flexure. Rectal involvement is rare secondary to dual vascular supply through collateralization between the IMA (mesenteric supply) and systemic circulation through hemorrhoidal vessels (iliac arteries). Right colon involvement is seen in less than 10% of cases and rarely is caused by mesenteric venous thrombosis (Figure 56.3).

Specific forms of surgery are also complicated by colonic ischemia. Aortoiliac reconstruction has an incidence of colonic ischemia of up to 7%. Many cases require surgical resection secondary to colonic gangrene. Multiple factors such as sacrificed collaterals, vascular traction, and mesenteric hematoma contribute to the injury. Renal transplantation with IMA vascular ligation is another contributor to colonic ischemia. Older patients, renal failure, fragile cardiopulmonary status, prior colonic resection with

Practical Gastroenterology and Hepatology Board Review Toolkit, Second Edition. Edited by Nicholas J. Talley, Kenneth R. DeVault, Michael B. Wallace, Bashar A. Aqel and Keith D. Lindor.

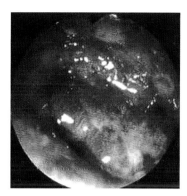

Figure 56.4 Colon ischemia: hemorrhagic phase.

The natural history is usually short-lived, since ischemia is usually short in duration. The first findings are submucosal hemorrhages secondary to arterior/capillary injury and necrosis. Thumbprinting on radiological evaluation is the typical finding, and is seen first on CT scanning and later on abdominal X-ray examination (in only 30% of cases). The endoscopic correlate of this is the hemorrhagic phase (Figure 56.4). The next finding is longitudinal ulceration, which may involve only one wall or may be circumferential. This is followed by mild mucosal scarring and then, in many cases, no abnormalities [14]. The natural history of ischemic colitis is usually less than 1 week with, complete resolution the usual end point.

Progressive disease is seen in up to 20% of patients with severe colonic ischemia. Early thumbprinting with extensive colonic ulcerations may portend a worse course, with increased mortality (29 vs. 78%). Symptoms lasting more than 24 hours with signs of systemic toxicity (high WBC count, acidosis, fever, segmental peritoneal findings) require aggressive diagnostic testing to find transmural injury or perforation and urgent surgical intervention. Risk factors for a poor prognosis include previous aortoilial reconstruction, renal transplant, previous colonic surgery, older age, comorbid metabolic illness, colonic ischemia after myocardial infarction, and isolated right-sided colitis [2].

The common differential diagnoses include diverticulitis, infections, IBD, and complicated colon cancer or radiation colitis. Typically, patients with diverticulitis will have more fever and more leukocytosis, with CT findings limited to the sigmoid colon. Splenic flexure thickening favors ischemia. Older patients have a lower incidence of IBD, but differentiation from left-side Crohn's disease can be difficult. Rapid resolution with a normal colonoscopy or a colonoscopy showing hemorrhagic necrosis predicts colonic ischemia. Infections with Shiga toxin-positive bacteria are particularly difficult, since colonoscopy can show similar findings and biopsies can show mucosal necrosis with crypt epithelial loss (ghost crypts). Antibiotic use or recent dietary indiscretion is helpful, but sporadic *C. difficile* infection is increasing, and presumably safe but actually contaminated food use (e.g., undercooked meats, contaminated vegetables, and even salad products) has been implicated in colitis causation. Cultures for enterohaemorragic *E. coli* organisms, *Shigella*, *C. difficile*, and *K. oxytoca* (so-called antibiotic-associated hemorrhagic colitis) should be taken early [15,16]. Offending drugs should be stopped, if clinically feasible. Colonic cancer is usually in the differential of colonic strictures after resolved colonic ischemia, and colonoscopy with biopsies will typically differentiate between them. Radiation colitis is a possibility in patients with prostate

cancer radiation or female genitourinary radiation treatment. The endoscopic findings will be microvascular damage with segmental ulcerations and fibrosis. Clinical history and endoscopic mucosal angiodysplasia, particularly in the rectum, will usually differentiate radiation-induced injury from uncomplicated colonic ischemia [17].

The diagnostic testing sequence depends on time from presentation, severity, and systemic toxicity. CT examination to locate disease and potential complications is the first test. Free air or severe pneumatosis requires urgent surgical evaluation. Segmental disease involving the left colon with splenic flexure or isolated right colon without CT complications mandates urgent colonoscopic evaluation if the patient has no toxicity. Endoscopic findings are highly specific, but biopsy confirmation should be done. Progressive symptoms or systemic toxicity requires CT confirmation of progression or complications.

Therapy

In most cases, early recognition, supportive therapy, and stopping potential offending substances are all that is needed (Figure 56.5). Coexisting cardiac events should be evaluated for and treated if needed. Mortality with non-gangrenous colonic ischemia is 6%. Monitoring for progression is critical. If transmural injury is suspected, antibiotics are recommended, based on animal studies showing decreased bacterial translocation (evidence level C). Cardiac function and oxygenation should be maximized (evidence level C). If progression to transmural injury occurs, prompt colonic resection with appropriate margins is recommended.

Colonic infarction has a high mortality (50–75%) due to comorbid disease. Most patients require an initial diverting colostomy with mucous fistula to assess for progressive interval damage, with second-look surgery with repeat resection if necessary (evidence level C). Aortoilial reconstruction has a high risk for transmural colonic ischemia requiring surgery.

Hypercoagulable states producing mesenteric venous thrombosis rarely cause colonic ischemia, but if it is present, anticoagulation may be required for at least 3 months, and potentially for the patient's lifetime (evidence level C).

Take Home Points

- Colonic ischemia is common and is increasing in incidence.
- Multiple common factors produce colonic ischemia, including metabolic disease, atherosclerosis, advancing population age, surgery, and certain medications
- Hypoperfusion with reperfusion injury causes ischemic injury. Reperfusion is the usual cause of radiologic and endoscopic findings.
- Most cases are non-occlusive and spontaneously resolve without sequelae. Progression is associated with increasing pain, peritoneal findings, leukocytosis, and acidosis. Surgery should be conducted early if progression is evident.
- Colonic ischemia associated with surgery, cardiac failure, or renal transplantation requires prolonged observation due to its high mortality.
- Infections, inflammatory bowel disease (IBD), and pharmacologic agents should be sought as major treatable risk factors.
- Computed tomography (CT) examination followed by colonoscopy with biopsies will usually confirm the clinical diagnosis. Angiography is rarely helpful, and barium enema is contraindicated in most cases.
- Colonic ischemia associated with pharmacologic agents is likely to shed light on pathophysiological mechanisms.

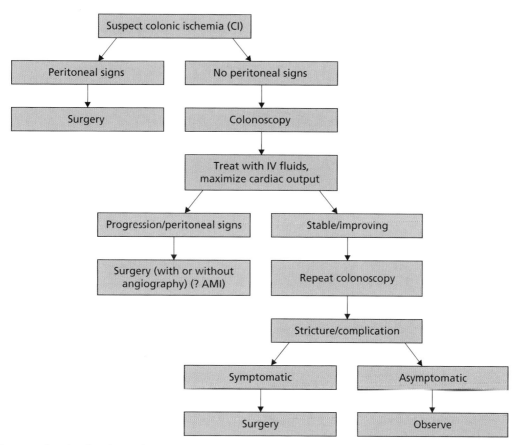

Figure 56.5 Diagnostic algorithm for colonic ischemia. IV, intravenous; AMI, acute mesenteric ischemia. Source: AGA Guideline 2000 [1]. Reproduced with permission of Elsevier.

References

1 Higgins PD, Davis KL, Laine L. Systematic review: the epidemiology of ischemic colitis. *Aliment Pharmacol Ther* 2004; **19**: 729–38.

2 Brandt LJ, Boley SJ. AGA technical review on intestinal ischemia. American Gastrointestinal Association. *Gastroenterology* 2000; **118**: 954–68.

3 Feuerstadt P, Brandt LJ. Colon ischemia: recent insights and advances. *Curr Gastroenterol Rep* 2010; **12**: 383–90.

4 O'Neill S, Yalamarthi S. Systematic review of the management of ischaemic colitis. *Colorectal Dis* 2012; **14**: e751–63.

5 Hass DJ, Kozuch P, Brandt LJ. Pharmacologically mediated colonic ischemia. *Am J Gastroenterol* 2007; **102**: 1765.

6 Longstreth GF, Yao JF. Diseases and drugs that increase risk of acute large bowel ischemia. *Clin Gastroenterol Hepatol* 2010; **8**: 49–54.

7 Chang L, Chey WD, Harris L, *et al.* Incidence of ischemic colitis and serious complications of constipation among patients using alosetron: systematic review of clinical trials and post marketing surveillance data. *Am J Gastroenterol* 2006; **101**: 1069–79.

8 Moses FM. Exercise-associated intestinal ischemia. *Curr Sports Med Rep* 2005; **4**: 91.

9 Koutroubakis IE, Sfiridaki A, Theodoropoulou A, Kouroumalis EA. Role of acquired and hereditary thrombotic risk factors in colonic ischemia of ambulatory patients. *Gastroenterology* 2001; **121**: 561.

10 Theodoropoulou A, Sfiridaki A, Oustamanolakis P, *et al.* Genetic risk factors in young patients with ischemic colitis. *Clin Gastroenterol Hepatol* 2008; **6**: 907–11.

11 West AB, Kuan S, Bennick M, Lagarde S. Glutaraldehyde colitis following endoscopy: clinical outbreak and pathological features and investigation of the outbreak. *Gastroenterology* 1995; **108**: 1250–5.

12 Greenwood DA, Brandt LJ, Reinus JF. Ischemic bowel disease in the elderly. *Gastroenterol Clin North Am* 2001; **30**: 445.

13 Park CJ, Jang MK, Shin WG, *et al.* Can we predict the development of ischemic colitis among patients with lower abdominal pain? *Dis Colon Rectum* 2007; **50**: 232–8.

14 Zuckerman GR, Prakash E, Merriman RB, *et al.* The colon single-stripe sign and its relationship to ischemic colitis. *Am J Gastroenterol* 2003; **98**: 2018.

15 Beaugerie L, Metz M, Barbut F, *et al.* Klebsiella oxytoca as an agent of antibiotic associated hemorrhagic colitis. *Clin Gastroenterol Hepatol* 2003; **1**: 370–6.

16 Dignan CR, Greenson JK. Can ischemic colitis be differentiated from C difficile colitis in biopsy specimens? *Am J Surg Pathol* 1997; **21**: 706–10.

17 Nostrant TT, Robertson JM, Lawrence TS. Radiation injury. In: Yamada T, ed. *Textbook of Gastroenterology*, 2nd edn. Philadelphia, PA: JB Lippincott, 1995: 2524–36.

CHAPTER 57

Acute Diverticulitis

Yuliya Y. Yurko[1] and Tonia M. Young-Fadok[2]

[1] Greenville Hospital System, Greenville, SC, USA
[2] Department of Surgery, Mayo Clinic College of Medicine, Mayo Clinic, Phoenix, AZ, USA

Summary

Diverticulitis occurs when diverticula in the bowel wall become inflamed. This leads to micro- or macroscopic perforation of these sac-like protrusions. Diverticulitis can be divided into complicated and uncomplicated forms, and the management differs based on the presentation. Surgical intervention is indicated in specific circumstances. This chapter summarizes the clinical manifestations and diagnosis of acute colonic diverticulitis, as well as current recommendations for medical and surgical management.

Case

A 70-year-old Caucasian woman presents to the emergency room with a 5-day history of left lower quadrant pain, fever, bloating, diarrhea, and nausea. Physical examination reveals a temperature of 38.5 °C, with localized tenderness and peritoneal signs in the left lower quadrant. Laboratory evaluation shows leukocytosis. Computed tomography (CT) scan of the abdomen and pelvis with oral and intravenous (IV) contrast demonstrates diverticulitis of the sigmoid colon with associated bowel-wall thickening and fat stranding, and with 1.0 cm intramural and 2.0 cm pericolic abscesses.

The patient is admitted and made nil per os (NPO) with IV fluid hydration. She is treated with a broad-spectrum IV antibiotic in the form of Zosyn. After 48 hours of medical management, her abdominal pain improves. She is started on clear liquids and her diet is advanced.

She undergoes colonoscopy 6 weeks later and is found to have extensive diverticulosis involving the descending and sigmoid colon, but with no evidence of malignancy. This is her fourth episode and second hospitalization with diverticulitis, and at surgical consultation sigmoid resection is recommended.

Definition and Epidemiology

"Diverticular disease of the colon" refers to the presence of sac-like protrusions of the colonic wall, generally at the site of vasa recta penetration of the circular muscle (Figure 57.1). Diverticulitis is thought to occur due to erosion of the diverticular wall by increased intraluminal pressure and/or inspissated stool particles. This progresses to inflammation and focal necrosis, ultimately leading to micro- or macroscopic perforation of the diverticulum.

Recent epidemiologic studies have shown that the prevalence of diverticular disease has increased significantly over the past century. Over the course of a lifetime, the chance of developing diverticulitis increases from 5–10% at age 40 to 30% by age 50 to 65% by age 85. There appears to be equal distribution between genders overall, but certain age groups show gender specificity (elderly women and obese young men) [1]. Geographic variation is a distinct feature of diverticulitis. Western countries have a higher prevalence (up to 45%) than the corresponding age groups of African and Asian countries (less than 0.2%). The location of disease also differs, in that left-sided diverticulitis is more common in Western countries, while right-sided diverticulitis predominates in Asian populations. Incidence appears to be related to lifestyle characteristics, as seen by the increase in prevalence of diverticulosis in those countries that have adopted a more Western diet and sedentary daily routine [2].

Pathophysiology

The etiology of diverticular disease may be linked to lifestyle factors, including, but likely not limited to, decreased dietary fiber intake, high intake of fat or red meat, lack of exercise, and obesity [3–5]. While historically patients have been advised to avoid seeds, corn, and nuts, this concept has not been proven clinically. This senior author has never seen a seed or a nut within even one of tens of thousands of diverticula!

Diverticula develop in areas of anatomic weakness of the colon wall, specifically the four points around the circumference of the colon where the vasa recta penetrate the circular muscle layer (Figure 57.1); 95% are found in the sigmoid colon [6]. While there is no hypertrophy or hyperplasia of the bowel wall in these areas, there are structural changes, including increased elastin deposition, which may decrease the resistance of the wall to intraluminal pressure [7]. Acquired diverticula are actually pulsion or "false" diverticula caused by herniation of the mucosa and muscularis mucosa through the muscle layer.

Clinical Features

Acute diverticulitis can be divided into two categories: uncomplicated and complicated. Uncomplicated cases make up 75% of diverticula and present with abdominal pain (usually in the left lower quadrant), changes in bowel habits, and nausea. The presence of pain for several days prior to seeking out medical attention often aids in the differentiation of diverticulitis from other causes of acute

Practical Gastroenterology and Hepatology Board Review Toolkit, Second Edition. Edited by Nicholas J. Talley, Kenneth R. DeVault, Michael B. Wallace, Bashar A. Aqel and Keith D. Lindor.
© 2016 John Wiley & Sons, Ltd. Published 2016 by John Wiley & Sons, Ltd. Companion website: www.practicalgastrohep.com

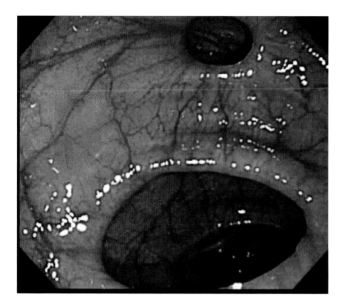

Figure 57.1 Diverticulum seen during colonoscopy, with vasa recta vessels visible.

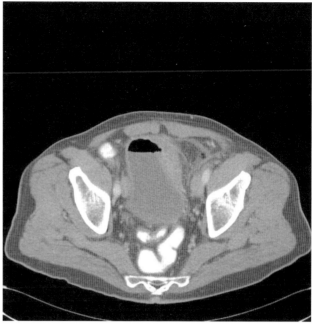

Figure 57.3 Colovesicular fistula. Air in the bladder with thickening of the bladder wall.

abdominal symptoms. Also, up to one-half of patients have had one or more previous episodes of similar pain [8].

Low-grade fever and mild leukocytosis are fairly common signs of diverticulitis, but are not always present. Other blood tests are typically normal or only mildly elevated, and sterile pyuria may be seen on urinalysis.

Diverticular bleeding typically occurs in the absence of acute diverticulitis, but a history of painless melena or bright red blood per rectum is common in patients with diverticular disease [9].

Complicated diverticulitis, with abscess, stricture, or fistula, may present in a similar fashion to uncomplicated diverticulitis.

The presence of pneumaturia, fecaluria, or pyuria is suggestive of colovesical fistula (Figures 57.2 and 57.3). A colovaginal fistula most often involves the posterior vaginal fornix in women who have had a hysterectomy. Complicated diverticulitis in the form of free perforation presents as an acute abdomen with generalized peritonitis.

The rare case of right-sided diverticulitis may present with right lower or right upper quadrant pain and can be misdiagnosed (Figure 57.4).

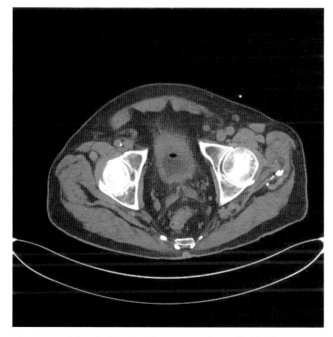

Figure 57.2 Colovesical fistula. The presence of air in the bladder is pathognomonic for this diagnosis.

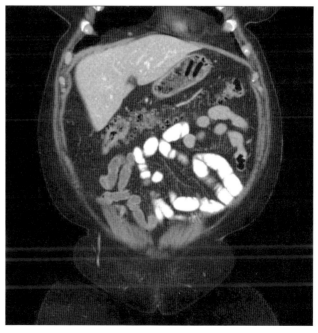

Figure 57.4 Pandiverticulosis with transverse colon diverticulitis.

CHAPTER 57

Table 57.1 Differential diagnosis of left lower quadrant abdominal pain.

Colon cancer
Acute appendicitis
Crohn's disease
Ischemic colitis
Pseudomembranous colitis
Viral gastroenteritis
Diverticular colitis
Ovarian cyst
Ovarian abscess
Ovarian torsion
Ectopic pregnancy

Diagnosis

Beside a focused history and physical examination, additional studies are necessary to confirm the diagnosis and rule out other causes of the patient's symptoms (Table 57.1). Routine abdominal and chest radiographs are commonly performed and aid in ruling out causes such as intestinal obstruction, but are otherwise non-contributory. CT of the abdomen and pelvis has become the standard for diagnosis, determining Hinchey stage and therapeutic intervention. Radiologic features of acute diverticulitis include increased soft-tissue density within pericolic fat, bowel-wall thickening, and tissue masses representing phlegmon or pericolic fluid collections representing abscesses (Figures 57.5, 57.6, and 57.7). When performed with IV and oral contrast, sensitivity and specificity are as high as 98 and 99%, respectively [10, 11].

Once the acute episode has resolved, patients should undergo elective colonoscopy (unless they have had one recently) to rule out other lesions (such as carcinoma) and make a definitive diagnosis [12]. Transabdominal high-resolution ultrasound and magnetic resonance imaging (MRI) can be used as alternative measures in patients with relative contraindication to CT, but these modalities have some disadvantages compared to CT. Barium enema plus flexible sigmoidoscopy is outdated.

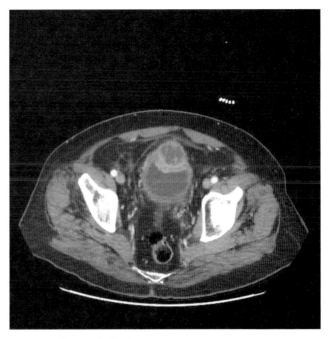

Figure 57.6 Supravesicular abscess.

Medical Management

In general, a clinically stable patient with uncomplicated diverticulitis can be managed as an outpatient [13]. They should be restricted to clear liquids and started on an antibiotic regimen to cover Gram-negatives and anaerobes (Table 57.2). If signs and symptoms improve within 48–72 hours, diet is advanced. These patients must receive explicit instruction to seek immediate medical attention if they experience an increase of abdominal pain or fever, or if they are unable to consume adequate fluids. The elderly, the immunosuppressed, those who cannot tolerate

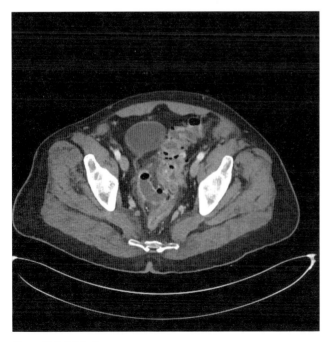

Figure 57.5 Pelvic abscess.

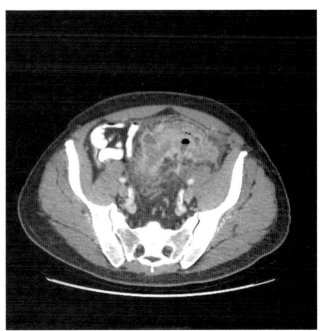

Figure 57.7 Intramural abscess.

Table 57.2 Antibiotic therapy recommendations for Gram-negative and anaerobic coverage.

First-choice therapy	
Monotherapy with a beta lactam/beta lactamase	
Ampicillin-sulbactam	3 g IV every 6 hours
Piperacillin-tazobactam	3.375 g or 4.5 g every 6 hours
Ticarcillin-clavulanate	3.1 g IV every 4 hours
Combination third-generation cephalosporin with metronidazole	
Ceftriaxone	1 g IV every 24 hours
Metronidazole	500 mg every 8 hours
Alternative regimen	
Ciproflaxin	400 mg IV every 12 hours
Metronidazole	500 mg IV every 8 hours
Levofloxacin	500 mg or 750 mg IV once a day
Metronidazole	500 mg every 8 hours
Imipenem	500 mg every 6 hours
Meropenem	1 g every 8 hours
Doripenem	500 mg every 8 hours

IV, intravenous.

Table 57.3 Indications for surgery at time of presentation in acute diverticulitis.

Peritonitis
Abscess (failed percutaneous drainage)
Obstructive symptoms
Clinical deterioration or failure to improve with medical therapy

oral hydration, those with severe comorbidities, those who fail to improve with oral antibiotic therapy within 48–72 hours, those with high fever, and those with leukocytosis should be treated in the hospital setting.

The possibility of abscess development should be explored in all patients who deteriorate or fail to improve.

Hospitalized patients are made NPO and given IV hydration. Empiric broad-spectrum IV antibiotics are directed at colonic anaerobic and Gram-negative flora, either as a single agent or as a combination of two (Table 57.2). A protective function of supplemental fiber, antispasmodics, rifaximin, and probiotics in preventing future recurrence has been studied in randomized controlled trials (RCTs) [14]. Colonoscopy should be performed following successful conservative therapy for a first attack of diverticulitis. After treatment, 30% of patients will remain asymptomatic, 30–40% will have episodic abdominal cramps without frank diverticulitis, and up to 33% will proceed to a second attack of diverticulitis. It was previously believed that prognosis became worse with a second attack [1]. Current data suggest that most patients run "true to form"; for example, if they have attacks that are manageable with oral antibiotics in the outpatient setting, subsequent attacks will likewise be manageable in the outpatient setting. In fact, 90% of patients who present with perforation have had no preceding attack, but have a factor that predisposes to this presentation. Patients at increased risk of more severe attacks include the young (under 40 years of age) and the immunosuppressed [15].

Management of Complicated Diverticulitis

Patients diagnosed with complicated diverticulitis undergo a more aggressive therapeutic regimen. Percutaneous drainage (PD) of the diverticular abscess should be performed for collections of >4 cm in the largest dimension. Antibiotic coverage is tailored once the causative organisms are identified [16–18]. The majority of patients who undergo PD of the abscess and tailored antibiotic therapies ultimately undergo elective one-stage colectomy.

If a patient has signs of peritonitis, immediate resuscitation, broad-spectrum antibiotics, and surgical exploration are performed in lieu of diagnostic studies. The mortality rate of perforated diverticulitis is 6% for purulent peritonitis and 35% for fecal peritonitis [19, 20]. Examples of appropriate antibiotics are included in Table 57.2.

Diverticular obstruction must be differentiated from carcinoma. Whenever malignancy is suspected, resection is mandatory. Obstruction due to diverticular stricture is rarely complete, and therefore, patients may undergo appropriate bowel preparation prior to surgery.

With improvement in CT technology, small diverticular abscesses not amenable to drainage can be found and treated with antibiotics. Whether these cases may be treated as uncomplicated diverticulitis is under investigation.

Surgery

Elective surgical intervention has typically been advised after a first attack of complicated diverticulitis (abscess, fistula, or stricture) or after two or more episodes of uncomplicated diverticulitis [21]. Recent data suggest that waiting for four episodes is safe in uncomplicated diverticulitis [22], particularly in the outpatient setting; this may avoid the need for operation in some patients. Tailored advice is necessary, depending on the patient's age, presentation, and comorbidities (Tables 57.3 and 57.4).

In the case of emergent surgical intervention in the patient with an acute abdomen, assessment of peritoneal contamination determines the advisability of a primary anastomosis versus a two-stage procedure. In the presence of fecal or purulent peritonitis, associated medical conditions, poor nutrition, immunosuppression, or emergency situations, two-stage procedures are indicated. The most common is a Hartmann procedure with resection of the sigmoid and creation of a colostomy and rectal stump. An alternative involves resection of the sigmoid, creation of a colorectal anastomosis, and protection with an ileostomy. This is only advised if there is minimal stool in the colon or if the ileostomy is not protective. The stomas are generally reversed after 3–6 months to allow the patient to fully recover from the emergent episode. Earlier reversal of the stoma is usually ill-advised.

Single-stage procedures are less widely touted; they include on-table washout of the proximal colon plus primary anastomosis.

Laparoscopic abdominal washout and placement of drains *without* resection is an attractive option but should be perform in highly selected group of patients (Hinchey stages II and III) [23–25]. Despite initial early enthusiasm for this approach, caution is now advised, and it should only be considered by an experienced surgeon in a setting where the patient can be closely monitored. A recent multicenter RCT in the Netherlands was halted because the patients

Table 57.4 Indications for elective operation after resolution of confirmed diverticulitis.

Abscess responding to percutaneous drainage
Fistula (colovesical, colovaginal, etc.)
Recurrent episodes
Inability to exclude carcinoma
Immunosuppression
Right-sided diverticulitis
? Young patient

randomized to the laparoscopic washout arm rather than resection and colostomy had worse results and a high reoperative rate. Intra-operative proctoscopy and air insufflation (not routine during the trial) may indicate whether a leak has sealed and washout and drains are safe.

Elective surgery after resolution of the acute episode of diverticulitis may be performed laparoscopically, and this is the approach of choice for these authors. In this instance, resection and primary anastomosis are the standard approach [26].

Take Home Points

Diagnosis:
- The diagnosis of diverticulitis is based on a focused history, physical examination, and complete blood count (CBC), with abdominal computed tomography (CT) scan used for confirmation.
- History typically includes left lower quadrant abdominal pain, fever, changes in bowel habits (obstipation, diarrhea), and nausea.
- Clinical signs may include localized or general abdominal pain with or without peritonitis, leukocytosis, pneumaturia, and fecaluria.
- The presence of abscess, peritonitis, obstruction, or fistula is classified as complicated diverticulitis.
- Colonoscopy should be performed after resolution of the acute episode to evaluate the extent of disease and rule out malignancy.
Therapy:
- Uncomplicated diverticulitis may be treated in the outpatient setting in selected circumstances and with low-risk patients.
- Inpatient treatment includes nil per os (NPO), intravenous (IV) fluids, and IV administration of broad-spectrum antibiotics to cover Gram-negatives and anaerobes.
- Complicated diverticulitis with abscess requires intervention by either percutaneous drainage (PD) of associated abscesses or (rarely, with current interventional radiology techniques) surgery.
- Complicated diverticulitis with drained abscess, microperforation with phlegmon responsive to IV antibiotics, and stricture or fistula generally require elective surgical intervention after resolution of the acute episode.
- Complicated diverticulitis with generalized peritonitis requires emergent exploration with a one- or two-stage procedure. In some situations, laparoscopic abdominal washout with drain placement may be used as a temporizing measure.
- Emergent surgical intervention commonly involves an open two-stage procedure with colostomy formation and delayed closure, but it may be done laparoscopically and with primary anastomosis in highly selected patients.

References

1 Parks TG. Natural history of diverticular disease of the colon. *Clin Gastroenterol* 1975; **4**(1): 53–69.

2 Miura S, Kodaira S, Shatari T, *et al.* Recent trends in diverticulosis of the right colon in Japan: retrospective review in a regional hospital. *Dis Colon Rectum* 2000; **43**(10): 1383–9.

3 Aldoori WH, Giovannucci EL, Rimm EB, *et al.* A prospective study of diet and the risk of symptomatic diverticular disease in men. *Am J Clin Nutr* 1994; **60**(5): 757–64.

4 Aldoori WH, Giovannucci EL, Rimm EB, *et al.* A prospective study of alcohol, smoking, caffeine, and the risk of symptomatic diverticular disease in men. *Ann Epidemiol* 1995; **5**(3): 221–8.

5 Strate LL, Liu YL, Aldoori WH, *et al.* Obesity increases the risks of diverticulitis and diverticular bleeding. *Gastroenterology* 2009; **136**(1): 115–22.

6 Rodkey GV, Welch CE. Changing patterns in the surgical treatment of diverticular disease. *Ann Surg* 1984; **200**(4): 466–78.

7 Whiteway J, Morson BC. Elastosis in diverticular disease of the sigmoid colon. *Gut* 1985; **26**(3): 258–66.

8 Konvolink CW. Acute diverticulitis under age forty. *Am J Surg* 1994; **167**(6): 562–5.

9 Meyers MA, Alonso DR, Gray GF, *et al.* Pathogenesis of bleeding colonic diverticulosis. *Gastroenterology* 1976; **71**(4): 577–83.

10 Birnbaum BA, Balthazar EJ. CT of appendicitis and diverticulitis. *Radiol Clin North Am* 1994; **32**(5): 885–98.

11 Hulnick DH, Megibow AJ, Balthazar EJ, *et al.* Computed tomography in the evaluation of diverticulitis. *Radiology* 1984; **152**(2): 491–5.

12 Baker ME. Imaging and interventional techniques in acute left-sided diverticulitis. *J Gastrointest Surg* 2008; **12**: 1314–17.

13 Alonso S, Pera M, Parés D, *et al.* Outpatient treatment of patients with uncomplicated acute diverticulitis. *Colorectal Dis* 2010; **12**: 278–82.

14 Maconi G, Barbara G, Bosetti C, *et al.* Treatment of diverticular disease of the colon and prevention of acute diverticulitis: a systematic review. *Dis Colon Rectum* 2011; **54**: 1326–38.

15 Chautems RC, Ambrosetti P, Ludwig A, *et al.* Long-term follow-up after first acute episode of sigmoid diverticulitis: is surgery mandatory?: a prospective study of 118 patients. *Dis Colon Rectum* 2002; **45**(7): 962–6.

16 Dharmarajan S, Hunt SR, Fleshman JW, Mutch MG. The efficacy of nonoperative management of acute com- plicated diverticulitis. *Dis Colon Rectum* 2011; **54**: 663–71.

17 Siewert B, Tye G, Kruskal J, *et al.* Impact of CT-guided drainage in the treatment of diverticular abscess: size matters. *AJR Am J Roentgenol* 2006; **186**: 680–6.

18 Brandt D, Gervaz P, Durmishi Y, *et al.* Percutaneous CT scan-guided drainage versus antibiotherapy alone for Hinchey II diverticulitis: a case-control study. *Dis Colon Rectum* 2006; **49**: 1533–8.

19 Nagorney DM, Adson MA, Pemberton JH. Sigmoid diverticulitis with perforation and generalized peritonitis. *Dis Colon Rectum* 1985; **28**(2): 71–5.

20 Morris CR, Harvey IM, Stebbings WS, Hart AR. Incidence of perforated diverticulitis and risk factors for death in a UK population. *Br J Surg* 2008; **95**(7): 876–81.

21 Stollman NH, Raskin JB. Diverticular disease of the colon. *J Clin Gastroenterol* 1999; **29**(3): 241–52.

22 Feingold D, Scott RS, Lee S, *et al.* Practice parameters for treatment of sigmoid diverticulitis. *Dis Colon Rectum* 2014; **57**(3): 293–4.

23 Myers E, Hurley M, O'Sullivan GC, *et al.* Laparoscopic peritoneal lavage for generalized peritonitis due to perforated diverticulitis. *Br J Surg* 2008; **95**(1): 97–101.

24 Franklin ME Jr, Portillo G, Trevino JM, *et al.* Long-term experience with the laparoscopic approach to perforated diverticulitis plus generalized peritonitis. *World J Surg* 2008; **32**(7): 1507–11.

25 Kohler L, Sauerland S, Neugebauer E. Diagnosis and treatment of diverticular disease: results of a consensus development conference. The Scientific Committee of the European Association for Endoscopic Surgery. *Surg Endosc* 1999; **13**(4): 430–6.

26 Scheidbach H, Schneider C, Rose J, *et al.* Laparoscopic approach to treatment of sigmoid diverticulitis: changes in the spectrum of indications and results of a prospective, multicenter study on 1545 patients. *Dis Colon Rectum* 2004; **47**(11): 1883–8.

CHAPTER 58

Acute Colonic Pseudo-obstruction

Michael D. Saunders

Division of Gastroenterology, University of Washington Medical Center, Seattle, WA, USA

Summary

Acute colonic pseudo-obstruction (ACPO) is a syndrome of massive dilation of the colon without mechanical obstruction that typically develops in hospitalized patients with serious underlying medical and surgical conditions. ACPO is associated with significant morbidity and mortality, and therefore requires urgent gastroenterologic evaluation. Appropriate evaluation of the markedly distended colon involves excluding mechanical obstruction and assessing for signs of ischemia and perforation. Increasing age, cecal diameter, delay in decompression, and status of the bowel significantly influence mortality. Appropriate management includes supportive therapy and selective use of neostigmine and colonoscopy for decompression. Early recognition and management are critical in minimizing complications.

Case

A 63-year-old man develops increasing abdominal distension 3 days after radical prostatectomy with bilateral lymph node dissection for prostate cancer. He passes flatus but minimal stool. His postoperative medications include morphine administered by patient-controlled analgesia. Abdominal radiographs reveal gaseous distension of the large bowel, with a cecal diameter of approximately 10 cm. He is afebrile and the leukocyte count is normal. Supportive therapy is instituted, but the patient has progressive symptoms and distension. Follow-up abdominal radiograph the next day shows persistent, marked cecal distension. Neostigmine 2 mg intravenous (IV) is administered, with prompt evacuation of flatus and stool, and resolution of colonic distension by subsequent radiograph. No adverse reactions to the infusion are noted.

Definition and Epidemiology

ACPO is characterized by massive colonic dilation with symptoms and signs of colonic obstruction without mechanical blockage [1]. ACPO is an important cause of morbidity and mortality, which can be substantial due to serious concomitant illness. Ischemia and perforation are the most feared complications of ACPO. Spontaneous perforation has been reported in 3–15% of cases, with a mortality rate estimated at 40% or higher when this occurs [2]. The clinical presentation of ACPO has been extensively documented in the literature. However, despite the accurate description of this condition, its diagnosis remains difficult and is often delayed. Early

recognition and prompt appropriate management are critical to minimizing poor outcomes. Thus, ACPO represents a true gastroenterologic emergency.

The main issues for the clinician to consider are:

1. What is the correct diagnosis?
2. Is ischemia or perforation present?
3. What is the appropriate evaluation and management?

The exact incidence of ACPO is unknown. In a retrospective series of patients undergoing orthopedic procedures reported by Norwood *et al.* [3], the incidence of ACPO was 1.3, 1.19, and 0.65% following hip replacement, spinal operation, and knee replacement, respectively. ACPO most often affects those in late middle age (mean of 60 years of age), with a slight male predominance (60%) [1]. ACPO occurs almost exclusively in hospitalized or institutionalized patients with serious underlying medical and surgical conditions. Abdominal distension usually develops over 3–7 days but can occur as rapidly as 24–48 hours. In surgical patients, symptoms and signs develop at a mean of 5 days postoperatively.

Pathophysiology

The pathogenesis of ACPO is not completely understood, but it likely results from an alteration in the autonomic regulation of colonic motor function. The parasympathetic nervous system increases contractility, whereas the sympathetic nerves decrease motility [5]. An imbalance in autonomic innervation, produced by a variety of factors, leads to excessive parasympathetic suppression or sympathetic stimulation. Because the vagal supply to the large bowel terminates at the splenic flexure and the parasympathetic innervation of the left colon originates from the sacral plexus, it has been proposed that transient parasympathetic impairment at the sacral plexus may cause atony of the distal large bowel and functional obstruction [6]. However, despite improved knowledge on the pathophysiology of colonic motility, the precise mechanisms underlying ACPO remain poorly understood.

Clinical Features

The clinical features of ACPO include abdominal distension, abdominal pain (80%), and nausea and/or vomiting (60%) [4]. Passage of flatus or stool is reported in up to 40% of patients. In one study, no significant differences were noted in the symptoms of patients with ischemic versus perforated bowel, except for a higher

Practical Gastroenterology and Hepatology Board Review Toolkit, Second Edition. Edited by Nicholas J. Talley, Kenneth R. DeVault, Michael B. Wallace, Bashar A. Aqel and Keith D. Lindor.

Table 58.1 Predisposing conditions associated with acute colonic pseudo-obstruction (ACPO): an analysis of 400 cases. Some patients had more than one associated condition. Source: Vanek 1986 [4]. Reproduced with permission of Wolters Kluwer.

Condition	Number	Percent rate
Trauma (non-operative)	45	11.3
Infection (pneumonia, sepsis most common)	40	10.0
Cardiac (myocardial infarction, heart failure)	40	10.0
Obstetrics/gynecology	39	9.8
Abdominal/pelvic surgery	37	9.3
Neurologic (Parkinson's disease, spinal cord injury, multiple sclerosis, Alzheimer's disease)	37	9.3
Orthopedic surgery	29	7.3
Miscellaneous medical conditions (metabolic, cancer, respiratory failure, renal failure)	128	32
Miscellaneous surgical conditions (urologic, thoracic, neurosurgery)	47	11.8

incidence of fever [4]. On examination, the abdomen is tympanitic, and bowel sounds are typically present. Fever, marked abdominal tenderness, and leukocytosis are more common in patients with ischemia or perforation, but also occur in those who have not developed these complications [4].

The vast majority of patients (>95%) with ACPO have it in association with a predisposing factor or clinical condition (Table 58.1). In a large retrospective series of 400 patients, the most common predisposing conditions were non-operative trauma (11%), infections (10%), and cardiac disease (10%) [4]. Cesarean section and hip surgery were the most common surgical procedures. In a retrospective analysis of 48 patients, the spine or retroperitoneum had been traumatized or manipulated in 52% [7]. Over half of the patients were receiving narcotics, and electrolyte abnormalities were present in approximately two-thirds. Thus, multiple metabolic, pharmacologic, and traumatic factors appear to alter the autonomic regulation of colonic function, resulting in pseudo-obstruction.

Diagnosis

The diagnosis of ACPO is suggested by the clinical presentation and confirmed by plain abdominal radiographs, which show varying degrees of colonic dilation (Figure 58.1). The right colon and cecum show the most marked distension, and "cutoffs" at the splenic flexure and descending colon are common. This distribution of colonic dilation may be caused by the different origins of the proximal and distal parasympathetic nerve supply to the colon. Air fluid levels and dilatation can also be seen in the small bowel.

The differential diagnosis of acute colonic distension in hospitalized or institutionalized patients includes:
- mechanical obstruction;
- toxic megacolon due to severe *Clostridium difficile* infection;
- ACPO.

The appropriate urgent evaluation of a patient with suspected ACPO therefore includes excluding mechanical obstruction and other causes of a toxic megacolon such as *Clostridium difficile*, as well as assessment for signs of peritonitis or perforation that would warrant urgent surgical intervention. The degree and duration of colonic distension should be estimated. If on plain abdominal radiographs, air is not seen throughout all colonic segments, including the rectosigmoid, then a computed tomography (CT) scan or a water-soluble contrast enema should be performed to exclude distal obstruction. Stool should be submitted for *C. difficile* toxin assay. In addition, empiric treatment for *C. difficile* while awaiting stool

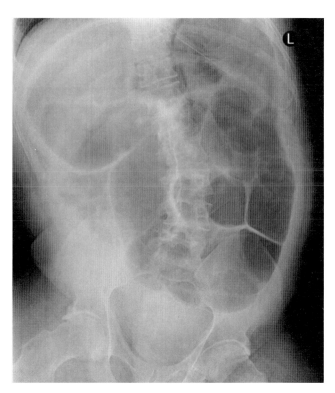

Figure 58.1 Plain abdominal radiograph of a patient with acute colonic pseudo-obstruction (ACPO), demonstrating marked colonic dilation mimicking mechanical obstruction. Varying degrees of small-intestinal dilation are evident.

results or a limited sigmoidoscopic examination assessing for the presence of pseudomembranes is reasonable if one needs an immediate diagnosis based on the severity of the patient's condition.

The assessment for ischemia or perforation includes both clinical examination and imaging studies. Fever, abdominal tenderness, and leukocytosis are more common in patients with ischemia, but also occur in those who have not developed it. Plain abdominal radiographs and CT should be assessed for evidence of free peritoneal air and pneumatosis of the bowel wall.

Therapeutics

An evidenced-based guideline for the treatment of ACPO has been published by the American Society of Gastrointestinal Endoscopy (ASGE) [8]. A proposed algorithm for its management is given in Figure 58.2. The clinical dilemma facing the clinician caring for a patient with ACPO is whether to treat them with conservative measures and close observation or to proceed with medical or endoscopic decompression of the dilated colon.

Supportive Therapy

Supportive therapy (Table 58.2) is the preferred initial management of ACPO and should be instituted in all patients [8]. Patients are given nothing by mouth. IV fluid and electrolyte imbalances are corrected. Nasogastric suction is provided to limit swallowed air from contributing further to colonic distension. Laxatives are avoided, particularly lactulose, which provides substrate for colonic bacterial fermentation, resulting in further gas production. A rectal tube should be inserted and attached to gravity drainage. Medications that can adversely affect colonic motility, such as opiates,

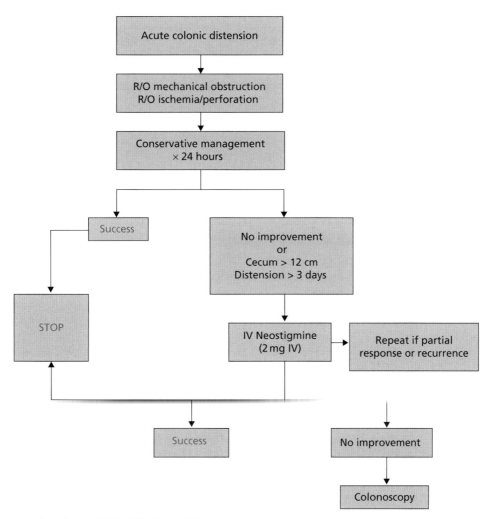

Figure 58.2 Management algorithm for ACPO. R/O, rule out; IV, intravenous.

anticholinergics, and calcium-channel antagonists, are discontinued if possible. Mobilization and ambulation of patients are encouraged, and a patient's position in bed should be changed frequently. The knee–hand position has been advocated by some to stimulate motility and promote colonic emptying [8]. Serial physical examinations and daily abdominal radiographs help closely monitor the progress of the patient. The benefits of any particular component of these supportive measures are unknown, as they have not been studied individually.

Conservative management is successful as the primary treatment in the majority of patients. Sloyer *et al.* [9] reported 25 cancer patients with ACPO (mostly non-gastrointestinal (GI) malignancies). The mean cecal diameter was 11.7 cm (range 9–18 cm). Of the 24 patients treated conservatively, 23 (96%) improved by clinical and radiologic criteria, with a median time to improvement

of 1.6 days (mean 3 days). There were no perforations or ACPO-related deaths. In another retrospective series of 151 patients, 117 (77%) had spontaneous resolution of ACPO with conservative treatment [10]. These studies demonstrate that the initial management of ACPO should be directed toward eliminating or reducing factors known to contribute to the problem.

The decision to intervene with medical therapy, colonoscopy, or surgery is dictated by the patient's clinical status. Knowing that the risk of colonic perforation is greatest with cecal diameter >12 cm [4] and when distension has been present for more than 6 days [11], patients with marked cecal distension (>10 cm) of significant duration (>4 days) and those not improving after 24–48 hours of supportive therapy are candidates for further intervention. In the absence of signs of overt peritonitis or perforation, medical therapy with neostigmine should be considered the initial therapy of choice.

Medical Therapy

Neostigmine

The only randomized, controlled therapeutic trial for ACPO involves IV neostigmine [12]. Neostigmine, a reversible acetylcholinesterase inhibitor, indirectly stimulates muscarinic receptors, thereby enhancing colonic motor activity, inducing colonic propulsion, and accelerating transit. The rationale for using

Table 58.2 Supportive therapy for ACPO.

Nothing by mouth
Correct fluid and electrolyte imbalances
Nasogastric suction
Rectal tube decompression
Limit offending medications
Frequent position changes; ambulate if possible

Table 58.3 Neostigmine for colonic decompression in patients with ACPO.

Study	Number	Design	Dose	Decompression	Recurrence
Ponec 1999 [12]	21 (neostigmine 11, placebo 10)	RCT (OL in non-responders)	2.0 mg IV over 3–5 minutes	10/11 in RCT 17/18 total	2
Huthcinson 1992 [15]	11	OL	2.5 mg IV in 1 minute	8/11	0
Stephenson 1995 [16]	12	OL	2.5 mg IV over 1–3 minutes	12/12 (two patients required two doses)	1
Turegano-Fuentes 1997 [17]	16	OL	2.5 mg IV over 60 minutes	12/16	0
Trevisani 2000 [18]	28	OL	2.5 mg IV over 3 minutes	26/28	0
Paran 2000 [19]	11	OL	2.5 mg IV over 60 minutes	10/11 (two patients required two doses)	0
Abeyta 2001 [20]	8	Retrospective	2.0 mg IV	6/8 (two patients required two doses)	0
Loftus 2002 [10]	18	Retrospective	2.0 mg IV	16/18	5
Mehta 2006 [21]	19	Prospective	2.0 mg IV	16/19	6
Total	141			123 (87%)	14 (10%)

RCT, randomized controlled trial; OL, open-label trial; IV, intravenous.

neostigmine stems from the imbalance in autonomic regulation of colonic function that is proposed to occur in ACPO. Administered intravenously, neostigmine has a rapid onset of action (1–20 minutes) and short duration (1–2 hours) [13]. The elimination half-life averages 80 minutes, but is prolonged in patients with renal insufficiency.

A randomized, double-blind, placebo-controlled trial evaluated neostigmine in patients with ACPO with a cecal diameter >10 cm and no response to 24 hours of conservative therapy [12]. Patients were randomized to receive neostigmine 2 mg or saline by IV infusion over 3–5 minutes. A clinical response was observed in 10 of 11 patients (91%) randomized to receive neostigmine, compared to 0 of 10 receiving placebo. The median time to response was 4 minutes. Eight patients not responding to initial infusion (seven placebo, one neostigmine) were administered open-label neostigmine, and all had prompt decompression. Of the 18 patients who received neostigmine, either initially or during open-label treatment, 17 (94%) had a clinical response. The recurrence of colonic distension after neostigmine decompression was low (11%). The most common side effects observed with neostigmine were mild abdominal cramping and excessive salivation. Symptomatic bradycardia requiring atropine occurred in 2 of 19 patients.

There are also several non-controlled, open-label, and retrospective series supporting the use of neostigmine in this condition [10,15–21]. Collectively, rapid decompression of colonic distension is observed in 87% of patients, with a recurrence rate of approximately 10% (Table 58.3).

Neostigmine should be given with the patient kept supine in bed, with continuous electrocardiographic (ECG) monitoring, physician assessment, and vital signs for 15–30 minutes following administration (Table 58.4). Contraindications to its use include mechanical obstruction, presence of ischemia or perforation, pregnancy, uncontrolled cardiac arrhythmias, severe active bronchospasm, and renal insufficiency (serum creatinine >3 mg/dL).

Thus, neostigmine appears to be an effective, safe, and inexpensive method of colonic decompression in ACPO. The published data support its use as the initial therapy of choice for patients not responding to conservative therapy, if there are no contraindications. In patients with only a partial response or recurrence after an initial infusion, a second dose is reasonable and often successful. If the patient fails to respond after two doses, proceeding with colonoscopic decompression is advised.

Other Pharmacologic Therapy

Administration of polyethylene glycol electrolyte solution in patients with ACPO after initial resolution may decrease the recurrence rate of colonic dilation. Sgouros et al. [23] evaluated polyethylene glycol in a randomized controlled trial (RCT) in ACPO patients who had initial resolution of colonic dilation. Therapy with polyethylene glycol resulted in a significant increase in stool and flatus output, decrease in colonic distension on radiographic measurements, and improvement in abdominal girth [23].

There are few data on strategies to prevent the development of ACPO. A recent randomized controlled clinical study evaluated whether lactulose or polyethylene glycol was effective in promoting defecation in critically ill patients [24]. The study included 308 consecutive patients with multiorgan failure. ACPO occurred in 4.1% of patients in the placebo group, 5.5% of patients in the lactulose group, and 1.0% of patients in the polyethylene glycol group. Thus, it appears that the use of polyethylene glycol to promote defecation in critically ill patients may prevent the development of ACPO, and that its use following a pseudo-obstruction episode decreases the recurrence rate.

Methynatrexone is a μ-opioid-receptor antagonist that does not cross the blood–brain barrier (BBB) [25]. There are case reports showing success with the use of methylnatrexone in colonic decompression, including in patients who previously failed or relapsed with neostigmine [25]. The use of this agent is reasonable in cases where narcotic use is a strong predisposing factor or where neostigmine is contraindicated.

Endoscopic Decompression

Procedural Aspects

Non-surgical approaches to mechanical decompression have included radiologic placement of decompression tubes, colonoscopy with or without placement of a decompression tube, and percutaneous cecostomy performed through an endoscopic or radiologic approach. Colonic decompression is the initial invasive procedure of choice for patients with marked cecal distension (>10 cm) of significant duration (>4 days) that does not improve after 24–48 hours of supportive therapy and who have contraindications to or fail neostigmine. Colonoscopy is

Table 58.4 Suggested protocol for the administration of neostigmine in ACPO.

Neostigmine 2 mg IV infusion over 3–5 minutes
Atropine available at bedside
Patient kept supine, on bedpan
Continuous ECG monitoring with vital signs for 30 minutes
Continuous physician assessment for 15–30 minutes

IV, intravenous; ECG, electrocardiogram.

Table 58.5 Recommended materials for colonoscopic decompression in ACPO.

Equipment	Comment
Colonoscope	
Olympus CF-Q160AL	Large therapeutic channel (3.8 mm)
Olympus CF-2T160C	Dual-channel (3.7 mm, 3.2 mm)
	Insertion tube outer diameter: 13.7 mm
Guidewire	
Wilson-Cook	0.035 inch, 480 cm length
	Included in decompression kit
Savary or American guidewire	Length: 210 cm
Decompression tube	
Wilson-Cook Colon	14 French
Decompression Set	Length: 175 cm
Levin tube	18 French
	Length: 80 cm

performed to prevent bowel ischemia and perforation. It should not be performed if overt peritonitis or perforation is present.

There is no well-defined standard of care regarding the use of colonoscopy in ACPO [8]. Colonoscopic decompression can be helpful in ACPO, but it is associated with a greater risk of complications, is not completely effective, and can be followed by recurrence. Oral laxatives and bowel preparations should not be administered prior to colonoscopy. Patients are often debilitated and bed-bound, making the administration of enemas impractical. Sedation is achieved using primarily benzodiazepines or propofol, titrated to patient comfort. One should limit or use only low doses of narcotic analgesics, given their deleterious effects on colonic motility.

The suggested materials needed for colonoscopic decompression are detailed in Table 58.5. The colonoscope should be advanced as far as possible. Prolonged attempts at cecal intubation are not necessary because reaching the hepatic flexure usually suffices. Air insufflation should be minimized, and the entire colon need not be examined. Gas should be aspirated and the viability of the mucosa assessed.

A tube for decompression should be placed in the right colon with the aid of a guidewire and fluoroscopic guidance. Commercial, disposable, over-the-wire colon decompression tubes are available. For example, the Wilson-Cook 14 French Colon Decompression Set includes a guiding catheter (6 French, 181 cm length), guidewire (0.035 inch, 480 cm length), and decompression catheter (14 French, 175 cm length) (Figure 58.3). The guidewire is advanced through the accessory channel of the colonoscope into the cecal pole or ascending colon. The endoscope is then removed from the patient as the guidewire is inserted, using fluoroscopy to make sure the wire tip remains in place. Following endoscope removal, the decompression tube is passed over the guidewire, using fluoroscopy to prevent loop formation and ensure tube placement into the right colon (Figure 58.4). The guidewire is removed and the tube is connected to gravity drainage.

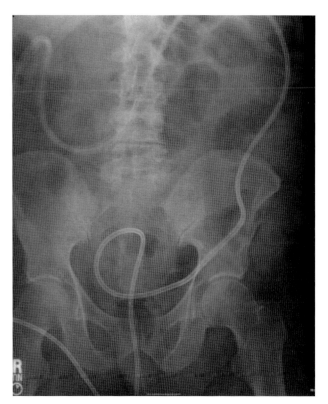

Figure 58.4 Plain abdominal radiograph of a patient with ACPO with a colonic decompression tube placed into the right colon.

Efficacy

The efficacy of colonoscopic decompression has not been established in randomized clinical trials. However, successful colonoscopic decompression has been reported in many retrospective series [7,26–29] (Table 58.6). An initial decompression colonoscopy without tube placement can be considered to be definitive therapy in less than 50% of patients [30]. To improve the therapeutic benefit, decompression tube placement at the time of colonoscopy is strongly recommended. The value of decompression tubes has not been evaluated in controlled trials, but anecdotal evidence suggests that they may lower the recurrence rate.

Safety

The complication rate of decompression colonoscopy in ACPO is approximately 1–5% [7,26–29] (Table 58.6), with perforation being the most feared adverse event, occurring in approximately 3% of cases [29].

Percutaneous Cecostomy

Percutaneous cecostomy, performed either radiologically or endoscopically, can be considered in high-surgical risk patients [31]. This approach is modeled after the percutaneous endoscopic gastrostomy pull technique. Percutaneous endoscopic cecostomy should be reserved for patients failing neostigmine and colonoscopic decompression who have no evidence of ischemia or perforation and who are felt to be at high risk for surgery.

Surgical Therapy

Surgical management is reserved for patients with signs of colonic ischemia or perforation or who fail endoscopic and pharmacologic

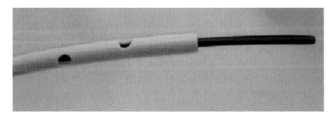

Figure 58.3 Colonic decompression tube with guidewire and side holes.

CHAPTER 58

Table 58.6 Colonoscopic decompression in ACPO.

Study	Number of patients	Successful initial decompression (%)	Overall colonoscopic success (%)	Complications (%)
Nivatvongs 1982 [25]	22	68	73	<1 (no perforations)
Strodel 1983 [26]	44	61	73	2 (1 perforation)
Bode 1984 [27]	22	68	77	4.5 (1 perforation)
Jetmore 1992 [7]	45	84	36	<1 (no perforations)
Geller 1996 [28]	41	95	88	5 (2 perforations)

efforts. Surgical intervention is associated with significant morbidity and mortality, likely related to the severity of the patient's underlying medical condition. The type of surgery performed depends on the status of the bowel. In cases of ischemic or perforated bowel, segmental or subtotal resection is indicated.

Prognosis

The outcome of ACPO is determined by multiple factors, primarily the severity of the underlying illness, but also increasing age, maximal cecal diameter, delay in decompression, and status of the bowel [4]. In the large retrospective series, no cases of perforation were seen with a cecal diameter <12 cm [4]. However, at diameters >12 cm, there was no clear relationship between the risk of ischemia or perforation and the size of the cecum. The duration and progression of colonic distension may be more important. A twofold increase in mortality occurs when cecal diameter is >14 cm, and a fivefold increase when delay in decompression is >7 days [4].

Take Home Points

- Conservative therapy is recommended as the initial preferred management for acute colonic pseudo-obstruction (ACPO).
- Potentially contributory metabolic, infectious, and pharmacologic factors should be identified and corrected.
- Active intervention is indicated for patients at risk of perforation and/or failing conservative therapy.
- Neostigmine is effective in the majority of patients.
- Colonic decompression is the initial invasive procedure of choice for patients failing or having contraindications to neostigmine.
- Surgical decompression should be reserved for patients with peritonitis or perforation.

References

1 Saunders MD. Acute colonic pseudo-obstruction. *Gastrointest Endoscopy Clin N Am* 2007; **17**: 341–60.

2 Rex DK. Colonoscopy and acute colonic pseudo-obstruction. *Gastrointest Endosc Clin N Am* 1997; **7**: 499–508.

3 Norwood MG, Lykostratis H, Garcea G, *et al.* Acute colonic pseudo-obstruction following major orthopedic surgery. *Colorect Dis* 2005; **7**: 496–9.

4 Vanek VW, Al-Salti M. Acute pseudo-obstruction of the colon (Ogilivie's syndrome). An analysis of 400 cases. *Dis Colon Rectum* 1986; **29**: 203–10.

5 De Giorgio R, Barbara G, Stanghellini V, *et al.* The pharmacologic treatment of acute colonic pseudo-obstruction. *Aliment Pharmacol Ther* 2001; **15**: 1717–27.

6 Spira IA, Rodrigues R, Wolff WI. Pseudo-obstruction of the colon. *Am J Gastroenterol* 1976; **65**: 397–408.

7 Jetmore AB, Timmcke AE, Gathright Jr BJ, *et al.* Ogilvie's syndrome: colonoscopic decompression and analysis of predisposing factors. *Dis Colon Rectum* 1992; **35**: 1135–42.

8 Eisen GM, Baron TH, Dominitz JA, *et al.* Acute colonic pseudo-obstruction. *Gastrointest Endosc* 2002; **56**: 789–92.

9 Sloyer AF, Panella VS, Demas BE, *et al.* Ogilvie's syndrome. Successful management without colonoscopy. *Dig Dis Sci* 1988; **33**: 1391–6.

10 Loftus CG, Harewood GC, Baron TH. Assessment of predictors of response to neostigmine for acute colonic pseudo-obstruction. *Am J Gastroenterol* 2002; **97**: 3118–22.

11 Johnson CD, Rice RP. The radiographic evaluation of gross cecal distention. *Am J Radiol* 1985; **145**: 1211–17.

12 Ponec RJ, Saunders MD, Kimmey MB. Neostigmine for the treatment of acute colonic pseudo-obstruction. *N Engl J Med* 1999; **341**: 137–41.

13 Aquilonius SM, Hartvig P. Clinical pharmacokinetics of cholinesterase inhibitors. *Clin Pharmacokinet* 1986; **11**: 236–49.

14 van der Spoel JI, Oudemans-van Straaten HM, Stoutenbeek CP, *et al.* Neostigmine resolves critical illness-related colonic ileus in intensive care patients with multiple organ failure – a prospective, double-blind, placebo-controlled trial. *Intensive Care Med* 2001; **27**: 822–7.

15 Hutchinson R, Griffiths C. Acute colonic pseudo-obstruction: a pharmacologic approach. *Ann R Coll Surg Engl* 1992; **74**: 364–7.

16 Stephenson BM, Morgan AR, Salaman JR, *et al.* Ogilvie's syndrome: a new approach to an old problem. *Dis Colon Rectum* 1995; **38**: 424–7.

17 Turegano-Fuentes F, Munoz-Jimenez F, Del Valle-Hernandez E, *et al.* Early resolution of Ogilvie's syndrome with intravenous neostigmine. A simple, effective treatment. *Dis Colon Rectum* 1997; **40**: 1353–7.

18 Trevisani GT, Hyman NH, Church JM. Neostigmine: safe and effective treatment for acute colonic pseudo-obstruction. *Dis Colon Rectum* 2000; **43**: 599–603.

19 Paran H, Silverberg D, Mayo A, *et al.* Treatment of acute colonic pseudo-obstruction with neostigmine. *J Am Coll Surg* 2000; **190**: 315–18.

20 Abeyta BJ, Albrecht RM, Schermer CR. Retrospective study of neostigmine for the treatment of acute colonic pseudo-obstruction. *Am Surg* 2001; **67**: 265–8.

21 Mehta R, John A, Nair P, *et al.* Factors predicting successful outcome following neostigmine therapy in acute colonic pseudo-obstruction: a prospective study. *J Gastroenterol Hepatol* 2006; **21**: 459–61.

22 Cherta I, Forne M, Quintana S, *et al.* Prolonged treatment with neostigmine for resolution of acute colonic pseudo-obstruction. *Aliment Pharmacol Ther* 2006; **23**: 1678–9.

23 Sgouros SN, Vlachogiannakos J, Vassilliadis K, *et al.* Effect of polyethylene glycol electrolyte balanced solution on patients with acute colonic-pseudo-obstruction after resolution of colonic dilation: a prospective, randomized, placebo controlled trial. *Gut* 2006; **55**: 638–42.

24 van der Spoel JI, Oudemans-van Straaten HM, Kuiper MA, *et al.* Laxation of critically ill patients with lactulose or polyethylene glycol: a two-center randomized, double-blind, placebo-controlled trial. *Crit Care Med* 2007; **35**: 2726–31.

25 Weinstock LB, Chang AC. Methylnaltrexone for treatment of acute colonic pseudo-obstruction. *J Clin Gastroenterol* 2011; **45**: 883–4.

26 Nivatvongs S, Vermeulen FD, Fang DT. Colonoscopic decompression of acute pseudo-obstruction of the colon. *Ann Surg* 1982; **196**: 598–600.

27 Strodel WE, Nostrant TT, Eckhauser FE, *et al.* Therapeutic and diagnostic colonoscopy in non-obstructive colonic dilatation. *Ann Surg* 1983; **19**: 416–21.

28 Bode WE, Beart RW, Spencer RJ, *et al.* Colonoscopic decompression for acute pseudo-obstruction of the colon (Ogilvie's syndrome): report of 22 cases and review of the literature. *Am J Surg* 1984; **147**: 243–5.

29 Geller A, Petersen BT, Gostout CJ. Endoscopic decompression for acute colonic pseudo-obstruction. *Gastrointest Endosc* 1996; **44**: 144–50.

30 Rex DK. Acute colonic pseudo-obstruction (Ogilvie's syndrome). *Gastroenterologist* 1994; **2**: 223–38.

31 Ramage JI, Baron TH. Percutaneous endoscopic cecostomy: a case series. *Gastrointest Endosc* 2003; **57**: 752–5.

CHAPTER 59
Colonic Polyps and Colorectal Cancer

John B. Kisiel, Paul J. Limburg, and Lisa A. Boardman

Division of Gastroenterology and Hepatology, Mayo Clinic, Rochester, MN, USA

Summary

Globally, more than 1 million new cases of colorectal cancer (CRC) are diagnosed each year and CRC accounts for 10% of all cancer deaths. Symptoms (hematochezia, melena, change in bowel habits, etc.) and signs (anemia, positive fecal occult blood test (FOBT), etc.) of CRC can be subtle and non-specific, but often indicate relatively advanced-stage disease. Since prognosis is inversely associated with CRC stage, early detection of premalignant adenomas or locally invasive cancers is a clinical priority. Therapy for invasive malignancy is multimodal and can involve surgery, chemotherapy, and radiation therapy. Though not universally applied, guidelines have been developed for post-therapeutic CRC surveillance to detect recurrent and metachronous lesions.

> ## Case
>
> A 42-year-old man presents to his primary care physician with a chief complaint of rectal bleeding. He is generally healthy and takes no medications. Review of his family history is significant for uterine cancer, diagnosed in his mother at the age of 32 years, and colon cancer, diagnosed in his maternal uncle at the age of 54 years.

Definition and Epidemiology

By gender, CRC incidence rates are 59.0 and 43.6 cases per 100 000 person-years for men and women, respectively [1]. Overall, CRC is the second leading cause of cancer death worldwide [2]. At the histologic level, CRC represents a variety of heterogeneous subtypes [3]. However, because adenocarcinoma represents the large majority of malignant colorectal tumors, "CRC" is used to refer to colorectal adenocarcinoma throughout the remainder of this chapter. Adenomatous polyps, also known as adenomas, are regarded as non-obligate precursor lesions for most CRCs and typically exhibit a raised, polypoid appearance at the macroscopic level. Adenoma morphology may resemble branched tubules ("tubular"), show villi arranged in a frond-like pattern ("villous"), or contain mixed features ("tubulovillous"). Large size (≥ 1 cm), high dysplasia grade, and/or villous morphology typically make up "advanced" adenomas, which are more closely related to CRC [4]. Macroscopically flat or depressed lesions, which account for approximately 10% of all adenomas, also appear to have higher malignant potential [5].

Adenoma prevalence rates are difficult to discern for average-risk adults. Available data suggest that 29–45% of asymptomatic persons in screening cohort studies may have one or more colorectal adenomas [6,7].

Hyperplastic polyps (HPPs) are characterized by increased glandular cells with relatively reduced cytoplasm, but nuclear atypia, stratification, and hyperchromatism are absent. Small, distally located HPPs do not appear to be associated with increased CRC risk, while HPPs of 1 cm or more in diameter, 30 or more in total number, and/or with mixed adenomatous features are thought to confer at least some risk elevation, particularly when coupled with a strong family history of CRC [4]. Serrated adenomas have been more recently recognized and are characterized by hyperplastic architecture with accompanying dysplastic features, such as abnormal crypt epithelium with a sawtooth pattern and nuclear atypia, supporting a premalignant phenotype. The magnitude of CRC risk associated with these serrated adenomas represents an area of active investigation [4,8].

Pathophysiology

Multiple molecular events have been linked to the sequential progression from normal mucosa to adenomatous polyp to adenocarcinoma [9] (Figure 59.1). At the genetic level, mutations in the *APC* gene (chromosome 5q) are thought to lead to disrupted cell-cycle regulation [10] and subsequent colorectal tumorigenesis. Similar *APC* mutations have been documented in familial and non-familial CRC cases [11]. Genetic alterations in *DCC*, *K-ras*, *p53*, and other growth-regulating genes have been identified in a substantial proportion of CRC cases as well [12, 13]. Cyclo-oxygenase 2 (COX-2) protein expression appears to be inducible in colorectal neoplasia, with absent or low-level concentrations in normal colorectal mucosa. Loss of DNA mismatch repair (MMR) protein expression is associated with microsatellite instability (MSI). Deficient DNA MMR protein status can be caused by germline mutation in *MLH1*, *MSH2*, *PMS1*, *PMS2*, and/or *MSH6* or by epigenetic silencing of *MLH1* and, less frequently, of *MSH2*. Among older women, approximately 20–30% of CRC cases appear to arise from methylation-induced suppression of *MLH1*, which is considered a sporadic cancer that does not confer or indicate a hereditary predisposition to CRC. Hypermethylation of other genes, including *p14* and *p16*, has been shown in 25 and 35% of non-familial CRC cases, respectively [14, 15].

Practical Gastroenterology and Hepatology Board Review Toolkit, Second Edition. Edited by Nicholas J. Talley, Kenneth R. DeVault, Michael B. Wallace, Bashar A. Aqel and Keith D. Lindor.
© 2016 John Wiley & Sons, Ltd. Published 2016 by John Wiley & Sons, Ltd. Companion website: www.practicalgastrohep.com

CHAPTER 59

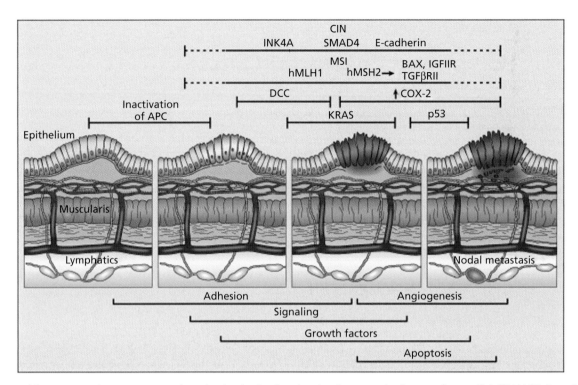

Figure 59.1 Adenoma-to-carcinoma sequence and associated molecular alterations in colon cancer development. Source: Abeloff 2008 [9]. Reproduced with permission of Elsevier.

Host Factors

CRC risk increases with advancing age, with cumulative incidence rates of 1 : 20 and 1 : 18 after age 90 years for women and men, respectively (Table 59.1). Subsite-specific CRC incidence rates also differ by gender, with the female/male rate ratio higher in the proximal (cecum, ascending and transverse, including both flexures) versus distal (descending, sigmoid, rectum) colorectum. Race/ethnicity may also contribute to CRC risk, since incidence and mortality rates are consistently higher among African-Americans relative to Caucasians [16]. However, the primary reasons for these rate differences remain incompletely defined.

Past Medical History

Prior history of colorectal adenoma(s) corresponds with a three- to sixfold increase in risk for subsequent, metachronous neoplasia [4]. Advanced adenomas (i.e., ≥1 cm diameter, high-grade dysplasia,

Table 59.1 Cumulative risk of developing CRC across 10-year age categories, by gender. Data obtained using Fast Stats: an interactive tool for access to SEER cancer statistics. Surveillance Research Program, National Cancer Institute. http://seer.cancer.gov/faststats (Accessed on April 1, 2010).

	Cumulative risk			
	Women		Men	
Age (years)	%	1 in:	%	1 in:
20	0.002	50 000	0.002	50 000
30	0.018	5556	0.016	6250
40	0.077	1299	0.079	1266
50	0.273	366	0.300	333
60	0.775	129	0.942	106
70	1.740	57	2.197	46
80	3.207	31	3.909	26
90	4.585	22	5.093	20

villous morphology) and three or more adenomas in total are associated with higher recurrence risks. Patients who have undergone prior CRC resection are prone to developing recurrent primary and second primary tumors, typically within 3 years.

Chronic ulcerative colitis (CUC) is associated with progressively increasing CRC risk, up to 2.4-fold [17]. In addition to CUC duration, colitis extent (pancolitis vs. distal colitis vs. proctitis), concomitant primary sclerosing cholangitis, and family history of CRC appear to be risk modifiers. Data regarding CRC risks for patients with Crohn's disease are more limited, but the magnitude of the association appears to be similar to that in CUC. Interestingly, recent data from Olmsted County, Minnesota show comparable CRC incidence rates between patients with inflammatory bowel disease (IBD) and a regional reference population, which the authors speculated is due to increasingly widespread use of maintenance therapy and surveillance colonoscopy [18].

Type 2 diabetes mellitus (T2DM) has been positively associated with CRC risk in multiple observational studies, presumably because insulin and/or insulin-like growth factors (IGFs) have growth-promoting effects in the colorectal mucosa [19]. Excess body weight, particularly when centrally distributed (visceral adiposity), may also increase CRC risk through an insulin-mediated mechanism. Notably, recent long-term follow-up data suggest that overall cancer mortality is reduced among morbidly obese patients who undergo bariatric surgery [20, 21].

Family History

In the United States, approximately 15–25% of all CRC cases exhibit familial clustering. Several heritable syndromes are well recognized, as discussed in this section. In the absence of a defined heritable syndrome, family history of CRC in one or more first-degree relatives increases CRC risk by about two- to fourfold [22].

Familial adenomatous polyposis (FAP) results from a mutated *APC* gene and is characterized by hundreds to thousands of colorectal adenomas, which usually develop sometime during adolescence. As many as one in five FAP patients have new-onset mutations (i.e., no known family history of polyposis). Extracolonic features of FAP include duodenal adenomas, gastric (fundic) gland hyperplasia, mandibular osteomas, and supernumerary teeth. Unless total proctocolectomy is performed, CRC is essentially universal, with a mean age at diagnosis of approximately 40 years. Attenuated FAP is associated with relatively fewer colorectal adenomas (≤100) and later onset of CRC (mean age approximately 55 years).

Lynch syndrome, synonymous with hereditary non-polyposis colorectal cancer (HNPCC) syndrome, is distinguished by germline mutations in one of the DNA MMR genes, including *MLH1*, *MSH2*, *PMS1*, *PMS2*, and *MSH6*. Germline epithelial cell adhesion molecule (*EPCAM*) gene mutations are responsible for a minority of *MSH2*-deficient, MSI Lynch syndrome cases lacking a detectable *MSH2* mutation [21, 22] and for 6.3% of all Lynch syndrome cases [23]. These mutations involve deletions at the 3′ end of *EPCAM*, leading to promoter hypermethylation and subsequent epigenetic inactivation of the downstream *MSH2* gene.

The median age for CRC diagnosis in Lynch syndrome is 46 years. Other cancer risks are also increased, including uterine, ovarian, gastric, genitourinary-tract, small-bowel, and hepatobiliary cancer. Clinical and laboratory data can be used to recognize high-risk patients and/or families [24, 25] (Table 59.2). Germline biallelic mutations in the DNA MMR genes give rise to constitutional DNA MMR deficiency (CMMRD), which is characterized by hematological and central nervous system (CNS) cancers and café-au-lait spots

in the first decade of life [26] and by an earlier age of onset for CRC than in Lynch syndrome, with an average age of 16 years (range 8–35 years) [27–30]. Muir–Torre syndrome is a Lynch syndrome variant wherein affected individuals (women/men = 1 : 2) may present with sebaceous neoplasms in addition to the cancer types previously noted. Turcot syndrome is a variant of Lynch syndrome associated with glioblastoma multiforme (GBM) with a younger age of onset and with a better prognosis than sporadic GBM.

MYH-associated polyposis (MAP) is a recently described autosomal-recessive syndrome with a colorectal adenoma burden similar to that of attenuated FAP, though patients with more than 100 adenomas have been described. Upper-gastrointestinal (GI) adenomas can be found in MAP patients, though the true incidence of these extracolonic lesions is not yet known. Biallelic mutation carriers have an 80% cumulative risk of CRC by age 70 years [31], while the CRC risk for monoallelic carriers remains incompletely defined.

Peutz–Jeghers syndrome (PJS) is characterized by multiple hamartomatous polyps scattered throughout the upper and lower GI tract. Up to 70% of PJS patients are found to have germline mutations in the *LKB1* (*STK11*) gene [32]. Other clinical features include melanin deposition around the lips, buccal mucosa, face, genitalia, hands, and feet. CRC risk is thought to be increased by foci of adenomatous epithelium within PJS polyps. Cancers of the small bowel, pancreas, biliary tree, gallbladder, breast, uterus, ovaries, and testes are also relatively more common among PJS patients. Meta-analyses of 1644 PJS cases determined that CRC was the most common PJS-associated malignancy, with a mean age at diagnosis of 43 years [33]. The cumulative risk for CRC is 3% at 40 years and 5% at 50 years [34]. The overall risk for malignancy increases with age, from 19% at age 40 up to 81% at age 70, highlighting the need for vigilant, persistent cancer screening in older patients [35].

In juvenile polyposis syndrome (JPS), mucous retention polyps can arise in the colon, stomach, and/or other parts of the GI tract, which may cause bleeding or obstruction during childhood. *SMAD4* (mothers against decapentaplegic drosophilia, homolog of 4), *BMPR1A* (bone morphogenic protein receptor 1A), and *ENG* mutations have been identified in JPS patients [36, 37]. JPS predisposes to an increased risk of young age of onset of CRC, with a median age of 42 years and a risk nearing 68% by 60 years of age [38]. An increased risk for young-onset gastric and small-bowel cancer has been reported in JPS patients [32].

Cowden syndrome is a rare autosomal-dominant genetic predisposition to hair follicle hamartomata called trichilemmomas and hamartomata of the GI tract, which gives an increased risk for thyroid, bilateral breast, and uterine cancers and CRC [39,40]. A recent review of cases reported that Cowden syndrome patients had a 16% (95% CI: 8–24%) lifetime risk of CRC, while a separate study predicted a 9% (CI 3.8–14.1%) lifetime risk [41, 42]. Hereditary mixed polyposis syndrome and serrated polyposis syndrome are two other CRC syndromes that confer an increased but not clearly defined risk for CRC [43–45]. The specific genetic defects responsible for these conditions are still to be determined.

Table 59.2 Proposed clinical criteria for the diagnosis of Lynch syndrome.

Revised International Collaborative Group–Lynch Syndrome Criteria (Amsterdam criteria II)	Revised Bethesda Guidelines for testing colorectal tumors for microsatellite instability (MSI)
There should be at least three relatives with a Lynch syndrome-associated cancer (CRC or cancer of the endometrium, small bowel, ureter, or renal pelvis) One should be a first-degree relative of the other two At least one should be diagnosed before age 50 At least two successive generations should be affected FAP should be excluded in the CRC case(s), if any Tumors should be verified by pathological examination	Tumors from individuals should be tested for MSI in the following situations: • CRC diagnosed in a patient who is less than 50 years of age • Presence of synchronous, metachronous colorectal, or other Lynch syndrome-associated tumors,[a] regardless of age • CRC with the MSI-H[b] histology[c] diagnosed in a patient who is less than 60 years of age • CRC diagnosed in one or more first-degree relatives with a Lynch syndrome-related tumor, with one of the cancers being diagnosed at under age 50 years • CRC diagnosed in two or more first- or second-degree relatives with Lynch syndrome-related tumors, regardless of age

CRC, colorectal cancer; FAP, familial adenomatous polyposis; MSI-H, microsatellite instability – high.
[a]Lynch syndrome-related tumors include colorectal, endometrial, stomach, ovarian, pancreas, ureter and renal pelvis, renal cell, breast, biliary tract, and brain (usually glioblastoma, as seen in Turcot syndrome) tumors, sebaceous gland adenomas and keratoacanthomas in Muir–Torre syndrome, and carcinoma of the small bowel.
[b]Refers to changes in two or more of the five National Cancer Institute-recommended panels of microsatellite markers.
[c]Presence of tumor-infiltrating lymphocytes, Crohn-like lymphocytic reaction, mucinous/signet-ring differentiation, or medullary growth pattern.

Young-Onset CRC

CRC is classified as being of young onset if it is diagnosed at ≤50 years of age. Between 2 and 8% of all CRCs arise at or before 50 years of age [46], and though rates of CRC for adults >50 years old are declining, the incidence of young-onset CRC is increasing [1]. Between 1992 and 2005, the rate of increase of young-onset CRC was 1.5%/year for men and 1.6%/year for women [47]. Though young-onset CRCs are often diagnosed at an advanced stage, they do not necessarily carry a poorer prognosis when compared stage to stage with older CRC cases, and may have better overall survival [48, 49]. The majority of young-onset CRCs are not explained by known hereditary CRC syndromes.

Environmental Exposures

Differences in CRC incidence, prevalence, and mortality rates by global region [50] support the hypothesis that colorectal carcinogenesis is influenced by environmental factors. Though numerous exposure agents have been associated with increased CRC risk, risk-factor modification is not generally incorporated into CRC prevention guidelines. A "Westernized" diet (high fat, low fiber, low fruit and vegetable intake) can stimulate tumor formation in animal models. Tobacco smoke contains a number of potential carcinogens, including polycyclic aromatic hydrocarbons (PAHs), nitrosamines, and aromatic amines. Cigarette smoking has been linked to a two- to threefold increase in CRC risk, most noticeably after a prolonged latency period of at least 3 decades. Emerging data suggest that cigarette smoking may be differentially associated with CRCs that exhibit MSI [51]. Colonic microflora can generate procarcinogenic metabolites [52, 53]. While no specific bacterial organisms have been convincingly established as CRC risk factors, further investigation in this area will likely be informative.

Prevention

Early detection remains the cornerstone of CRC risk reduction. Average-risk screening should begin at age 50 years, though recent national guidelines differ slightly with respect to specifically endorsed test options and the age at which to consider discontinuing screening [54, 55]. For high-risk patients, earlier, more frequent screening and surveillance is typically recommended, as discussed in greater detail in Chapter 43. Chemoprevention – the use of chemical compounds to interrupt carcinogenesis – may serve as a complementary CRC prevention strategy. Non-steroidal anti-inflammatory drugs (NSAIDs), selective COX-2 inhibitors, difluoromethylornithine (DFMO), calcium, and other compounds have been investigated as candidate CRC chemoprevention agents, but their clinical application has been limited by unacceptable toxicity [56] and/or insufficient efficacy in trials reported to date.

Clinical Features

CRC signs and symptoms are rather non-specific and are influenced by tumor size, stage, anatomic subsite, and distribution of distant metastases, when present. Patients with late-stage CRCs tend to exhibit more obvious signs and symptoms than those with early-stage tumors. General clinical features of CRC include hematochezia, melena, anemia, abdominal pain, change in bowel habits, involuntary weight loss, nausea, vomiting, and fatigue. CRCs arising from the proximal colon tend to be associated with occult bleeding and iron deficiency, whereas cancers originating in the distal colon or rectum may produce narrow-caliber stools, fecal urgency, and overt bleeding. About one in five CRC patients presents with distant metastases, manifested by hepatosplenomegaly, palpable lymphadenopathy (i.e., left supraclavicular nodes), or other signs and symptoms referable to the affected organ site(s).

Table 59.3 TNM classification scheme for tumor staging.

Primary tumor (T)	Regional lymph nodes (N)	Distant metastases (M)
T0 No evidence of primary tumor	N0 No regional lymph node metastases	M0 No distant metastases
T1 Tumor invades submucosa	N1 Metastases in 1–3 regional lymph nodes	M1 Distant metastases
T2 Tumor invades muscularis propria	N2 Metastases in ≥4 regional lymph nodes	
T3 Tumor invades through muscularis propria		
T4 Tumor invades surrounding organs or structures		

Diagnosis

Colonoscopy is the test of choice for diagnostic evaluation of the lower GI tract, since macroscopic assessment, mucosal sampling, and, when needed, therapeutic intervention (i.e., polypectomy) can be performed during a single procedure. Computed tomography (CT) colonography can serve as a useful adjunct to colonoscopy when technical challenges, obstructing lesions, concomitant medications (such as anticoagulants), or other factors do not permit complete diagnostic evaluation. Since synchronous cancers may be found in approximately 5% of all CRC cases [57], full structural assessment is required. Once the CRC diagnosis is established, preoperative staging with abdominopelvic CT and chest CT (chest CT particularly important in rectal cancer) is recommended to exclude distant metastases. For rectal cancers, endorectal ultrasound is helpful in determining the depth of mural invasion and the extent of regional lymph node involvement. Magnetic resonance imaging (MRI) of the pelvis may be used as an alternative or adjunct to endorectal ultrasound for further characterization of the tumor circumference and of the relationship of the tumor to the peritoneal reflection. Measurement of carcinoembryonic antigen (CEA) may provide additional prognostic information [58], though this test is not universally recommended. Definitive CRC stage is determined from the surgical resection specimen, using the TNM classification system (Table 59.3).

Case Continued

The patient undergoes diagnostic colonoscopy, with findings of a 2.5 cm sessile mass in the ascending colon and a 1.5 cm pedunculated polyp in the rectum. Biopsy samples are interpreted as showing invasive adenocarcinoma (with tumor-infiltrating lymphocytes and a Crohn-like lymphocytic reaction) and tubulovillous adenoma: low-grade dysplasia from the proximal and distal lesions, respectively.

Differential Diagnosis

Due to the non-specific nature of CRC-related signs and symptoms, formulation of an efficient differential diagnosis can be challenging. Given the relatively high CRC incidence rate among the general population, colonoscopy should be incorporated into the diagnostic algorithm for any of the common clinical features cited in this chapter. Atypical CRC subtypes are discussed elsewhere (see Chapter 31). Malignant tumors that can metastasize to the colorectum include breast, ovary, prostate, lung, and stomach cancers. Lymphomas and malignant melanomas may originate from or spread to

Table 59.4 Standard treatment recommendations for CRC, by presenting stage. Data obtained from O'Connell 2004 [77] and Jessup 1998 [76].

Presenting stage	TNM classification	Colon cancer		Rectal cancer	
		Standard treatment	5-year survival (%)	Standard treatment	5-year survival (%)
Stage I	T1 N0 M0 T2 N0 M0	Surgical resection	93	Surgical resection	72
Stage II	T3 N0 M0 T4 N0 M0	Surgical resection; consider adjuvant chemotherapy if pathologic features suggest high recurrence risk	72–85	Neoadjuvant chemo/radiation therapy + surgical resection + adjuvant chemo/radiation therapy	52
Stage III	Any T N1 M0 Any T N2 M0	Surgical resection with adjuvant chemotherapy	44–83	Neoadjuvant chemo/radiation therapy + surgical resection + adjuvant chemo/radiation therapy	37
Stage IV	Any T Any N M1	Chemotherapy and/or symptomatic care; consider potentially curative treatment for isolated liver or lung metastases	8	Chemotherapy and/or symptomatic care; consider potentially curative treatment for isolated liver or lung metastases	4

the colorectum. Benign lesions such as endometriosis, Crohn's disease, and solitary rectal ulcer syndrome can also mimic CRC, but these diagnoses are readily distinguishable by histology.

Therapeutics

CRC treatment is determined largely by TMN stage and may include surgical intervention, chemotherapy, and/or radiation therapy (Table 59.4). Surgical resection is generally the mainstay of CRC therapy, unless contraindicated by tumor stage, patient comorbidities, or other factors. At least 12 regional lymph nodes should be removed along with the primary tumor for definitive pathologic staging. Anastomotic site recurrence rates for all CRC are 2–4%, but may be as much as 10 times higher for rectal cancers, due to differences in surgical technique and/or tumor biology [59]. Resection of isolated liver and lung metastases appears to improve the survival rate for some patients [60, 61].

Postoperative (also known as "adjuvant") chemotherapy is routinely recommended for stage III CRCs and may be considered for select stage II CRCs [62], using one of several combination regimens, including 5-fluorouracil (5-FU), leucovorin, and oxaliplatin (collectively referred to as FOLFOX). In a large, randomized controlled trial (RCT) of subjects with stage II or III CRC, adjuvant FOLFOX therapy improved the 3-year disease-free survival rate from 72.9 to 78.2% [63]. On average, treating 19 patients with FOLFOX instead of 5-FU and leucovorin would prevent one additional CRC recurrence at 3 years. However, the added benefit of oxaliplatin is counterbalanced by possible drug-induced toxicities, such as peripheral neuropathy.

An array of chemotherapy options exists for patients with metastatic CRC (Table 59.5) [62]. First-line combination therapy with either FOLFOX or FOLFIRI (substituting irinotectan for oxaliplatin) appears to provide a response rate (defined as a composite of either complete disappearance of all detectable

Table 59.5 CRC chemotherapeutic agents. Source: Asmis 2008 [62]. Reproduced with permission of Elsevier.

Agent	Mechanism of action	Indications	Common toxicities
5-fluorouracil (5-FU)	Blocks the enzyme thymidylate synthase, which is essential for DNA synthesis	Multiple uses in combination with other agents in the adjuvant (postoperative) and palliative settings	Nausea, diarrhea MyelosuppressionFatigue
Capecitabine	Blocks thymidylate synthase (orally administered prodrug converted to 5-FU)	Multiple uses in combination with other agents in the adjuvant (postoperative) and metastatic setting	Nausea, diarrhea Myelosuppression Fatigue Palmar–plantar syndrome (hand–foot syndrome)
Oxaliplatin	Inhibits DNA replication and transcription by forming inter- and intrastrand DNA adducts/crosslinks	Used in combination with 5-FU, LV (FOLFOX) in the adjuvant (postoperative) and metastatic setting	Peripheral neuropathy Nausea, diarrhea Fatigue Myelosuppression Hypersensitivity
Irinotecan	Inhibits topoisomerase I, an enzyme that facilitates the uncoiling and recoiling of DNA during replication	Used alone or in combination with 5-FU, LV (FOLFIRI) in the metastatic setting	Cholinergic (acute diarrhea) Nausea, late diarrhea Fatigue Myelosuppression Alopecia
Bevacizumab	Monoclonal antibody that binds to the VEGF ligand	Used in combination with either FOLFOX or FOLFIRI in the metastatic setting	Hypertension Arterial thrombotic events Impaired wound healing GI perforation
Cetuximab	Monoclonal antibody to EGFR (chimeric) that blocks the ligand-binding site	Used with irinotecan or as a single agent in the metastatic setting	Acneform rash Hypersensitivity Hypomagnesemia Fatigue
Panitumumab	Monoclonal antibody to EGFR (fully humanized) that blocks the ligand-binding site	Used as a single agent in the metastatic setting	Acneform rash Hypomagnesemia Fatigue

LV, leucovorin; VEGF, vascular endothelial growth factor; GI, gastrointestinal; EGFR, epidermal growth factor receptor.

disease or a decrease in tumor size by RECIST criteria) of 31–56%, with a median progression-free survival of 7–8 months [64,65].

Molecular classification of CRC tumor DNA has been developed to direct treatment based upon the genetic phenotype of the cancer. The epidermal growth factor receptor (EGFR)-specific monoclonal antibody cetuximab, which is a mainstay of treatment for metastatic CRC with wild-type KRAS [66,67], has failed to show significant benefit in the adjuvant setting, irrespective of KRAS genotype [68]. Further benefits might be achieved by adding a biologic agent such as bevacizumab.

External-beam radiation therapy combined with systemic chemotherapy is used to treat locally advanced (T3, T4, and/or node-positive) rectal cancers. In a landmark study from 1985, the Gastrointestinal Tumor Study Group found a 33% recurrence rate among patients with locally advanced, surgically treated rectal cancer who received postoperative combination chemotherapy and radiation therapy, compared to a 55% recurrence rate for patients treated with surgery alone, after 80 months of follow-up [69]. The number needed to treat (NNT) with adjuvant combination therapy in order to prevent one additional recurrence was five in this cohort. Subsequent large trials have further defined the benefits of radiation therapy for the treatment of locally advanced rectal cancer [70–73], with preoperative (also known as "neoadjuvant") chemoradiotherapy to downsize the tumor now considered standard of care [74]. Most patients who receive neoadjuvant chemoradiation therapy are also candidates for adjuvant chemotherapy. For recurrent rectal cancers, long-term survival can be achieved for some patients using surgical resection, intraoperative radiation therapy, and adjuvant chemoradiation therapy [75].

Patients who develop bowel obstruction or other complications of locally advanced or metastatic disease may benefit from palliative chemotherapy or radiation therapy. Palliation through mechanical stenting and decompression techniques is also feasible, as discussed in Chapter 44.

Case Continued

The patient undergoes a colon cancer staging evaluation, including CT scan of the abdomen, pelvis and chest, which shows no signs of distant metastases. Based on the patient's age, family history, and cancer histology, Lynch syndrome is strongly suspected. Further testing of the tumor specimen reveals that the ascending colon cancer exhibits the MSI-high (microsatellite instability – high) phenotype. The patient is referred for genetic counseling, and a germline mutation is detected in *MLH1*.

Prognosis

CRC stage at diagnosis is a strong predictor of survival (Table 59.4) [76,77]. After definitive treatment, the presence of residual tumor, lymphovascular invasion, and elevated CEA level is a robust predictor of worsened prognosis. Additional important prognostic factors include tumor grade and residual tumor after neoadjuvant therapy. Newer methods of histologic and molecular prognostication are under active research.

Though prognosis for limited-stage disease is excellent, patients with a history of CRC are at increased risk for recurrent primary and/or second primary tumors. Guidelines for post-CRC treatment surveillance [59] are discussed in Chapter 43.

Take Home Points

- Colorectal cancer (CRC) is the fourth most common incident and second most common fatal cancer in the United States.
- Most, if not all, CRCs are preceded by macroscopically identifiable dysplastic lesions (adenomas) that can be detected and removed through effective screening.
- Personal history (colorectal adenomas, inflammatory bowel disease (IBD), diabetes mellitus) and family history (with or without a defined heritable syndrome) can affect CRC risk.
- Environmental factors such as diet, obesity, and smoking also appear to adversely affect colorectal carcinogenesis.
- CRC signs and symptoms are non-specific and influenced by tumor site, and typically signify more advanced-stage disease. Colonoscopy is the diagnostic test of choice.
- Preoperative staging evaluation is performed to define local invasion, regional lymph node involvement, and distant metastases. Common tests include chest X-ray, computed tomography (CT) scan of the abdomen and pelvis, and endoscopic ultrasound (EUS) and/or pelvic magnetic resonance imaging (MRI) (rectal cancers).
- Surgical resection is the primary treatment modality. Adjuvant chemotherapy should be recommended for patients with stage III, and some stage II, colon cancers. Neoadjuvant and adjuvant chemoradiation therapy are typically recommended for stage II and III rectal cancer patients.
- CRC prognosis is inversely associated with pathologic stage.

References

1 Edwards BK, Ward E, Kohler BA, *et al.* Annual report to the nation on the status of cancer, 1975–2006, featuring colorectal cancer trends and impact of interventions (risk factors, screening, and treatment) to reduce future rates. *Cancer* 2010; **116**: 544–73.

2 American Cancer Society. Cancer facts and statistics. Available from: http://www.cancer.org/research/cancerfactsstatistics/index (last accessed February 15, 2016).

3 Jass JR, Sobin LH, Watanabe H. The World Health Organization's histologic classification of gastrointestinal tumors. *A commentary on the second edition. Cancer* 1990; **66**: 2162–7.

4 Winawer SJ, Zauber AG, Fletcher RH, *et al.* Guidelines for colonoscopy surveillance after polypectomy: a consensus update by the US Multi-Society Task Force on Colorectal Cancer and the American Cancer Society. *Gastroenterology* 2006; **130**: 1872–85.

5 Soetikno RM, Kaltenbach T, Rouse RV, *et al.* Prevalence of nonpolypoid (flat and depressed) colorectal neoplasms in asymptomatic and symptomatic adults. *JAMA* 2008; **299**: 1027–35.

6 Winawer SJ, Zauber AG, O'Brien MJ, *et al.* Randomized comparison of surveillance intervals after colonoscopic removal of newly diagnosed adenomatous polyps. *The National Polyp Study Workgroup. N Engl J Med* 1993; **328**: 901–6.

7 Pickhardt PJ, Choi JR, Hwang I, *et al.* Computed tomographic virtual colonoscopy to screen for colorectal neoplasia in asymptomatic adults. *N Engl J Med* 2003; **349**: 2191–200.

8 Cappell MS. Pathophysiology, clinical presentation, and management of colon cancer. *Gastroenterol Clin North Am* 2008; **37**: 1–24.

9 Abeloff MD. *Abeloff's Clinical Oncology*, 2nd edn. Philadelphia, PA: Churchill Livingstone/Elsevier, 2008.

10 Bodmer WF, Bailey CJ, Bodmer J, *et al.* Localization of the gene for familial adenomatous polyposis on chromosome 5. *Nature* 1987; **328**: 614–16.

11 Suraweera N, Duval A, Reperant M, *et al.* Evaluation of tumor microsatellite instability using five quasimonomorphic mononucleotide repeats and pentaplex PCR. *Gastroenterology* 2002; **123**: 1804–11.

12 Vogelstein B, Fearon ER, Hamilton SR, *et al.* Genetic alterations during colorectal-tumor development. *N Engl J Med* 1988; **319**: 525–32.

13 Robbins DH, Itzkowitz SH. The molecular and genetic basis of colon cancer. *Med Clin North Am* 2002; **86**: 1467–95.

14 Burri N, Shaw P, Bouzourene H, *et al.* Methylation silencing and mutations of the p14ARF and p16INK4a genes in colon cancer. *Lab Invest* 2001; **81**: 217–29.

15 Shannon BA, Iacopetta BJ. Methylation of the hMLH1, p16, and MDR1 genes in colorectal carcinoma: associations with clinicopathological features. *Cancer Lett* 2001; **167**: 91–7.

16 Cheng X, Chen VW, Steele B, *et al.* Subsite-specific incidence rate and stage of disease in colorectal cancer by race, gender, and age group in the United States, 1992–1997. *Cancer* 2001; **92**: 2547–54.

17 Jess T, Rungoe C, Peyrin-Biroulet L. Risk of colorectal cancer in patients with ulcerative colitis: a meta-analysis of population-based cohort studies. *Clin Gastroenterol Hepatol* 2012; **10**: 639–45.

18 Jess T, Loftus EV Jr., Velayos FS, *et al.* Risk of intestinal cancer in inflammatory bowel disease: a population-based study from Olmsted County, Minnesota. *Gastroenterology* 2006; **130**: 1039–46.

19 Giovannucci E. Modifiable risk factors for colon cancer. *Gastroenterol Clin North Am* 2002; **31**: 925–43.

20 Sjoblom T, Jones S, Wood LD, *et al.* The consensus coding sequences of human breast and colorectal cancers. *Science* 2006; **314**: 268–74.

21 Adams TD, Gress RE, Smith SC, *et al.* Long-term mortality after gastric bypass surgery. *N Engl J Med* 2007; **357**: 753–61.

22 Butterworth AS, Higgins JP, Pharoah P. Relative and absolute risk of colorectal cancer for individuals with a family history: a meta-analysis. *Eur J Cancer* 2006; **42**: 216–27.

23 Niessen RC, Hofstra RM, Westers H, *et al.* Germline hypermethylation of MLH1 and EPCAM deletions are a frequent cause of Lynch syndrome. *Genes Chromosomes Cancer* 2009; **48**: 737–44.

24 Vasen HF, Watson P, Mecklin JP, Lynch HT. New clinical criteria for hereditary nonpolyposis colorectal cancer (HNPCC, Lynch syndrome) proposed by the International Collaborative group on HNPCC. *Gastroenterology* 1999; **116**: 1453–6.

25 Umar A, Boland CR, Terdiman JP, *et al.* Revised Bethesda Guidelines for hereditary nonpolyposis colorectal cancer (Lynch syndrome) and microsatellite instability. *J Natl Cancer Instit* 2004; **96**: 261–8.

26 Bandipalliam P. Syndrome of early onset colon cancers, hematologic malignancies & features of neurofibromatosis in HNPCC families with homozygous mismatch repair gene mutations. *Fam Cancer* 2005; **4**: 323–33.

27 Gallinger S, Aronson M, Shayan K, *et al.* Gastrointestinal cancers and neurofibromatosis type 1 features in children with a germline homozygous MLH1 mutation. *Gastroenterology* 2004; **126**: 576–85.

28 Jackson CC, Holter S, Pollett A, *et al.* Cafe-au-lait macules and pediatric malignancy caused by biallelic mutations in the DNA mismatch repair (MMR) gene PMS2. *Pediatr Blood Cancer* 2008; **50**: 1268–70.

29 Trimbath JD, Petersen GM, Erdman SH, *et al.* Cafe-au-lait spots and early onset colorectal neoplasia: a variant of HNPCC? *Fam Cancer* 2001; **1**: 101–5.

30 Wimmer K, Etzler J. Constitutional mismatch repair-deficiency syndrome: have we so far seen only the tip of an iceberg? *Hum Genet* 2008; **124**: 105–22.

31 Jenkins MA, Croitoru ME, Monga N, *et al.* Risk of colorectal cancer in monoallelic and biallelic carriers of MYH mutations: a population-based case-family study. *Cancer Epidemiol Biomarkers Prev* 2006; **15**: 312–14.

32 Kastrinos F, Syngal S. Inherited colorectal cancer syndromes. *Cancer J* 2011; **17**: 405–15.

33 van Lier MG, Wagner A, Mathus-Vliegen EM, *et al.* High cancer risk in Peutz-Jeghers syndrome: a systematic review and surveillance recommendations. *Am J Gastroenterol* 2010; **105**: 1258–64, author reply 1265.

34 Mehenni H, Resta N, Park JG, *et al.* Cancer risks in LKB1 germline mutation carriers. *Gut* 2006; **55**: 984–90.

35 Lim W, Olschwang S, Keller JJ, *et al.* Relative frequency and morphology of cancers in STK11 mutation carriers. *Gastroenterology* 2004; **126**: 1788–94.

36 Howe JR, Roth S, Ringold JC, *et al.* Mutations in the SMAD4/DPC4 gene in juvenile polyposis. *Science* 1998; **280**: 1086–8.

37 Sweet K, Willis J, Zhou XP, *et al.* Molecular classification of patients with unexplained hamartomatous and hyperplastic polyposis. *JAMA* 2005; **294**: 2465–73.

38 Jass JR, Williams CB, Bussey HJ, *et al.* Juvenile polyposis – a precancerous condition. *Histopathology* 1988; **13**: 619–30.

39 Patnaik MM, Raza SS, Khambatta S, *et al.* Oncophenotypic review and clinical correlates of phosphatase and tensin homolog on chromosome 10 hamartoma tumor syndrome. *J Clin Oncol* 2010; **28**: e767–8.

40 Hobert JA, Eng C. PTEN hamartoma tumor syndrome: an overview. *Genet Med* 2009; **11**: 687–94.

41 Riegert-Johnson DL, Gleeson FC, Roberts M, *et al.* Cancer and Lhermitte-Duclos disease are common in Cowden syndrome patients. *Hered Cancer Clin Pract* 2010; **8**: 6.

42 Tan MH, Mester JL, Ngeow J, *et al.* Lifetime cancer risks in individuals with germline PTEN mutations. *Clin Cancer Res* 2012; **18**: 400–7.

43 Whitelaw SC, Murday VA, Tomlinson IP, *et al.* Clinical and molecular features of the hereditary mixed polyposis syndrome. *Gastroenterology* 1997; **112**: 327–34.

44 Boparai KS, Reitsma JB, Lemmens V, *et al.* Increased colorectal cancer risk in first-degree relatives of patients with hyperplastic polyposis syndrome. *Gut* 2010; **59**: 1222–5.

45 Win AK, Walters RJ, Buchanan DD, *et al.* Cancer risks for relatives of patients with serrated polyposis. *Am J Gastroenterol* 2012; **107**: 770–8.

46 Boyle P, Ferlay J. Cancer incidence and mortality in Europe, 2004. *Ann Oncol* 2005; **16**: 481–8.

47 Siegel RL, Jemal A, Ward EM. Increase in incidence of colorectal cancer among young men and women in the United States. *Cancer Epidemiol Biomarkers Prev* 2009; **18**: 1695–8.

48 Quah HM, Joseph R, Schrag D, *et al.* Young age influences treatment but not outcome of colon cancer. *Ann Surg Oncol* 2007; **14**: 2759–65.

49 O'Connell JB, Maggard MA, Liu JH, *et al.* Do young colon cancer patients have worse outcomes? *World J Surg* 2004; **28**: 558–62.

50 Kamangar F, Dores GM, Anderson WF. Patterns of cancer incidence, mortality, and prevalence across five continents: defining priorities to reduce cancer disparities in different geographic regions of the world. *J Clin Oncol* 2006; **24**: 2137–50.

51 Neugut AI, Terry MB. Cigarette smoking and microsatellite instability: causal pathway or marker-defined subset of colon tumors? *J Natl Cancer Instit* 2000; **92**: 1791–3.

52 Hope ME, Hold GL, Kain R, *et al.* Sporadic colorectal cancer – role of the commensal microbiota. *FEMS Microbiol Lett* 2005; **244**: 1–7.

53 Wang X, Huycke MM. Extracellular superoxide production by *Enterococcus faecalis* promotes chromosomal instability in mammalian cells. *Gastroenterology* 2007; **132**: 551–61.

54 Levin B, Lieberman DA, McFarland B, *et al.* Screening and surveillance for the early detection of colorectal cancer and adenomatous polyps, 2008: a joint guideline from the American Cancer Society, the US Multi-Society Task Force on Colorectal Cancer, and the American College of Radiology. *Gastroenterology* 2008; **134**: 1570–95.

55 US Preventative Services Task Force. Screening for colorectal cancer: US Preventive Services Task Force recommendation statement. *Ann Intern Med* 2008; **149**: 627–37.

56 Psaty BM, Potter JD. Risks and benefits of celecoxib to prevent recurrent adenomas. *N Engl J Med* 2006; **355**: 950–2.

57 Langevin JM, Nivatvongs S. The true incidence of synchronous cancer of the large bowel. A prospective study. *Am J Surg* 1984; **147**: 330–3.

58 Locker GY, Hamilton S, Harris J, *et al.* ASCO 2006 update of recommendations for the use of tumor markers in gastrointestinal cancer. *J Clin Oncol* 2006; **24**: 5313–27.

59 Rex DK, Kahi CJ, Levin B, *et al.* Guidelines for colonoscopy surveillance after cancer resection: a consensus update by the American Cancer Society and the US Multi-Society Task Force on Colorectal Cancer. *Gastroenterology* 2006; **130**: 1865–71.

60 Simmonds PC, Primrose JN, Colquitt JL, *et al.* Surgical resection of hepatic metastases from colorectal cancer: a systematic review of published studies. *Br J Cancer* 2006; **94**: 982–99.

61 Yedibela S, Klein P, Feuchter K, *et al.* Surgical management of pulmonary metastases from colorectal cancer in 153 patients. *Ann Surg Oncol* 2006; **13**: 1538–44.

62 Asmis TR, Saltz L. Systemic therapy for colon cancer. *Gastroenterol Clin North Am* 2008; **37**: 287–95, ix.

63 Andre T, Boni C, Mounedji-Boudiaf L, *et al.* Oxaliplatin, fluorouracil, and leucovorin as adjuvant treatment for colon cancer. *N Engl J Med* 2004; **350**: 2343–51.

64 Tournigand C, Andre T, Achille E, *et al.* FOLFIRI followed by FOLFOX6 or the reverse sequence in advanced colorectal cancer: a randomized GERCOR study. *J Clin Oncol* 2004; **22**: 229–37.

65 Colucci G, Gebbia V, Paoletti G, *et al.* Phase III randomized trial of FOLFIRI versus FOLFOX4 in the treatment of advanced colorectal cancer: a multicenter study of the Gruppo Oncologico Dell'Italia Meridionale. *J Clin Oncol* 2005; **23**: 4866–75.

66 Cunningham D, Humblet Y, Siena S, *et al.* Cetuximab monotherapy and cetuximab plus irinotecan in irinotecan-refractory metastatic colorectal cancer. *N Engl J Med* 2004; **351**: 337–45.

67 De Roock W, Piessevaux H, De Schutter J, *et al.* KRAS wild-type state predicts survival and is associated with early radiological response in metastatic colorectal cancer treated with cetuximab. *Ann Oncol* 2008; **19**: 508–15.

68 Ogino S, Meyerhardt JA, Irahara N, *et al.* KRAS mutation in stage III colon cancer and clinical outcome following intergroup trial CALGB 89803. *Clin Cancer Res* 2009; **15**: 7322–9.

69 Gastrointestinal Tumor Study Group. Prolongation of the disease-free interval in surgically treated rectal carcinoma. *N Engl J Med* 1985; **312**: 1465–72.

70 Fisher B, Wolmark N, Rockette H, *et al.* Postoperative adjuvant chemotherapy or radiation therapy for rectal cancer: results from NSABP protocol R-01. *J Natl Cancer Instit* 1988; **80**: 21–9.

71 Krook JE, Moertel CG, Gunderson LL, *et al.* Effective surgical adjuvant therapy for high-risk rectal carcinoma. *N Engl J Med* 1991; **324**: 709–15.

72 Kapiteijn E, Marijnen CA, Nagtegaal ID, *et al.* Preoperative radiotherapy combined with total mesorectal excision for resectable rectal cancer. *N Engl J Med* 2001; **345**: 638–46.

73 Robertson JM. The role of radiation therapy for colorectal cancer. *Gastroenterol Clin North Am* 2008; **37**: 269–85, ix.

74 Van Cutsem EJ, Oliveira J. Colon cancer: ESMO clinical recommendations for diagnosis, adjuvant treatment and follow-up. *Ann Oncol* 2008; **19**(Suppl. 2): ii29–30.

75 Hahnloser D, Haddock MG, Nelson H. Intraoperative radiotherapy in the multimodality approach to colorectal cancer. *Surg Oncol Clin N Am* 2003; **12**: 993–1013, ix.

76 Jessup JM, Stewart AK, Menck HR. The National Cancer Data Base report on patterns of care for adenocarcinoma of the rectum, 1985–95. *Cancer* 1998; **83**: 2408–18.

77 O'Connell JB, Maggard MA, Ko CY. Colon cancer survival rates with the new American Joint Committee on Cancer sixth edition staging. *J Natl Cancer Instit* 2004; **96**: 1420–5.

CHAPTER 60

Pregnancy and Luminal Gastrointestinal Disease

Sumona Saha

Division of Gastroenterology and Hepatology, University of Wisconsin School of Medicine and Public Health, Madison, WI, USA

Summary

The gastrointestinal (GI) tract is altered during pregnancy, largely due to the inhibitory effects of progesterone on smooth-muscle motility and changes in anatomy caused by the growing uterus. This poses a unique medical stress to the GI tract and is a period of development for new or exacerbation of existing GI disorders. Diagnosis and management of common conditions pose special challenges for the clinician caring for the pregnant patient, due to the difficulty of balancing efficacy of therapy with safety for both the mother and fetus.

The Food and Drug Administration (FDA) pregnancy risk classification provides some guidance regarding medication safety in pregnancy, but it is often misunderstood to be a grading system rather than a shorthand classification system for the data that are available [1].

Esophagus and Stomach

Gastroesophageal Reflux Disease

Gastroesophageal reflux disease (GERD) is common in pregnancy. Heartburn is experienced by 30–50% of pregnant women, though the incidence may be as high as 80% [2]. Risk factors for heartburn in pregnancy include increasing gestational age, multigravidity, high pre-pregnancy body mass index (BMI), excessive pregnancy weight gain, and a history of heartburn, as well as maternal age, smoking, race, and sleep-disordered breathing [3].

The cause of GERD in pregnancy is likely related to estrogen- and progesterone-mediated decreases in lower esophageal sphincter (LES) pressure. This begins in the second and third trimesters and resolves quickly after delivery [4]. Increased intra-abdominal pressure caused by the enlarging uterus [5], abnormal esophageal peristalsis [6], and delayed gastric emptying [7] may also contribute to the development of GERD.

Lifestyle modification is the first line of treatment. Patients who fail conservative measures should be treated with antacids and alginic acid. Aluminum-, magnesium-, and calcium-based antacids have no FDA classification and are generally considered safe in pregnancy. See Table 60.1 for treatment details.

Peptic Ulcer Disease

The incidence of peptic ulcer disease (PUD) appears decreased in pregnancy [8, 9], though the incidence estimate is based on case reports and retrospective studies as diagnostic tests are often avoided during gestation, so it may be underestimated [10]. Esophagogastroduodenoscopy (EGD) is the test of choice when there is concern for complicated PUD.

Patients found to have *Helicobacter pylori* infection should generally be treated after pregnancy and lactation are completed [11].

Nausea and Vomiting of Pregnancy and Hyperemesis Gravidarum

Nausea and vomiting of pregnancy (NVP) is one of the most common GI disorders of pregnancy, affecting 70–80% of pregnant women [12]. Most cases of NVP resolve after the first trimester, but up to 10% of women have symptoms beyond 22 weeks [13]. Women with severe NVP may have hyperemesis gravidarum (HG), a condition associated with fluid, electrolyte, and acid–base imbalance, nutritional deficiency, and weight loss [14]. HG is commonly defined as the occurrence of more than three episodes of vomiting per day with associated ketonuria and weight loss of more than 3 kg or 5% of body weight [15].

Risk factors for NVP and HG include younger maternal age, primigravida status, low educational achievement, non-smoking status, obesity, and multiple gestations [16,17]. NVP in a prior pregnancy may also be a risk factor for its development in subsequent ones [18].

Human chorionic gonadotropin (hCG) is thought to play a major role [19] in NVP, though the relationship between serum hCG levels in the first trimester and the frequency or intensity of nausea and vomiting has not been found to be consistently positive [20].

On physical exam, most women with NVP have normal vital signs and a benign physical exam, while those with HG may demonstrate evidence of dehydration and orthostasis. Women with suspected HG should be evaluated for muscle wasting and weakness, peripheral neuropathy, and altered mental status. Laboratory abnormalities in women with HG may include increased serum blood urea nitrogen, creatinine, and hematocrit, as well as ketonuria and increased urine-specific gravity. In addition, patients may also exhibit hypochloremic metabolic alkalosis or metabolic acidosis with severe volume contraction [21]. Vitamin and mineral deficiencies, such as vitamin B1 (thiamine), iron, calcium, and folate, are also possible [22]. Liver enzymes are abnormal in up to 50% of hospitalized patients with HG [22], with alanine aminotransferase levels generally greater than those of aspartate aminotransferase. Serum amylase and lipase elevation are seen in 10–15% of women

Practical Gastroenterology and Hepatology Board Review Toolkit, Second Edition. Edited by Nicholas J. Talley, Kenneth R. DeVault, Michael B. Wallace, Bashar A. Aqel and Keith D. Lindor.

Table 60.1 Drugs used for GI disease in pregnancy.

Drug	FDA pregnancy category	Dosing	Recommendations in pregnancy
GERD and PUD			
Aluminum-based antacids	N/A		Can cause constipation
Magnesium-based antacids	N/A		Avoid in late pregnancy, as may arrest labor and precipitate seizures; can cause diarrhea
Calcium-based antacids	N/A		Safe
Sucralfate	B	1 g 1 hour before meals and at bedtime	Safe and effective
Bismuth subsalicylate	C		In humans, chronic salicylate use is linked to congenital defects and premature closure of ductus arteriosus *in utero*
H$_2$RA	B	Dosing according to retail brand	Excellent safety profile in humans
PPIs	B/C	Dosing according to retail brand	Considered safe in pregnancy
			Category B, except for omeprazole, which is category C
			Reserve for refractory patients
Nausea and vomiting of pregnancy			
Vitamin B$_6$	A	10–25 mg three times daily	Effective in two small studies
Antihistamines			
Doxylamine/B6	A	12.5 mg twice daily	Recently reintroduced to the US market
Antiemetics			
Prochlorperazine	C	5–10 mg three times daily	Effective but may cause excessive sedation
Promethazine	C	12.5–25.0 mg four times daily	Effective but may cause excessive sedation
Metoclopramide	B	10–20 mg four times daily	Avoid long-term, high-dose use due to risk of tardive dyskinesia
Ondansetron	B	4–8 mg three times daily	Widely used in clinical practice, but data showing efficacy are lacking
Constipation/diarrhea/IBS			
Laxatives			
Polyethylene glycol	C	17 g daily	Preferred laxative in pregnancy
Lactulose	B	15–30 mL up to four times daily	Can cause bloating, flatulence, and cramping and exacerbate nausea
Senna	C	2–4 tablets daily to twice daily	Acceptable for short-term use
Bisacodyl	B	5–15 mg as needed	Use limited because of induced cramping
Mineral oil	–		Contraindicated, as can decrease maternal absorption of fat-soluble vitamins, leading to neonatal hypoprothrombinemia and hemorrhage
Castor oil	–		Contraindicated, as may induce uterine contractions
Antidiarrheals			
Loperamide	B	2–4 mg after each unformed stool	Preferred antidiarrheal in preganncy
Diphenoxylate with atropine sulfate	C	1–2 tablets four times daily	Not recommended, due to possible teratogenicity
Abdominal pain			
Dicyclomine	B		Not recommended for routine use in pregnancy
Hyoscyamine	C		Not recommended for routine use in pregnancy
Tricyclic antidepressants	C/D	Dose differs according to retail brand	Limit use to patients with severe symptoms
SSRIs	C/D	Dose differs according to retail brand	Paroxetine class D, others C
			Limit use to patients with severe symptoms
IBD			
5 aminosalicylic acid (5-ASA)	B/C	Dose differs according to retail brand	Sulfasalazine, mesalamine, mesalamine MMX, and balsalazide are category B and can be safely used rectally and orally
			Olsalazine is category C
			Folate supplementation (1 mg BID) is recommended for sulfasalazine
Corticosteroids	C	Variable	May increase the risk of orofacial clefts with first-trimester use
Budesonide	C	9 mg daily	Probably safe, but no controlled studies in pregnancy
6-mercaptopurine/azathioprine	D	Up to 1.5 mg/kg/2.5 mg/kg	Probably safe for continued use in pregnancy
			Avoid starting *de novo* in pregnancy
Cyclosporine	C	Weight-based IV/oral form	Growth retardation, but may be disease causality
Methotrexate	–		Contraindicated in pregnancy, due to teratogenicity
Thalidomide	–		Contraindicated in pregnancy, due to teratogenicity
Infliximab	B	5 mg/kg IV	Likely low risk in pregnancy
		Induction at 0, 2, and 4 weeks	
		Maintenance every 8–10 weeks	
Adalimumab	B	Induction: 160 mg SC week 0, 80 mg SC week 2	Likely low risk in pregnancy
		Maintenance: 40 mg SC every other week	
Certolizumab	B	Induction: 400 mg SC at 0, 2, and 4 weeks	Likely low risk in pregnancy
		Maintenance: 400 mg SC monthly	May have lowest rate of transplancental transfer of the anti-TNF agents
Natalizumab	C	300 mg IV every 4 weeks	No data on safety in human pregnancy
Vedolizumab	B	Induction: 300 mg IV at 0, 2, and 6 weeks	No data on safety in human pregnancy
		Maintenance: 300 mg IV every 8 weeks	
Metronidazole	B	250–500 mg oral/IV 3 times daily	Safe
Fluoroquinolones	C	250–500 mg twice daily	Avoid long-term use
Rifaximin	C	550 mg twice daily	Probably safe, as not absorbed

GERD, gastroesophageal reflux disease; PUD, peptic ulcer disease; H$_2$RA, histamine receptor agonist; PPI, proton pump inhibitor; IBS, irritable bowel syndrome; IBD, inflammatory bowel disease; SSRI, selective serotonin reuptake inhibitor; IV, intravenous; TNF, tumor necrosis factor.

with HG [21]. Finally, thyroid-stimulating hormone (TSH) levels may be low in NVP and HG, due to crossreaction between the alpha-subunit of hCG and the TSH receptor.

NVP is associated with a favorable fetal outcome. A meta-analysis of 11 studies found a decreased risk of miscarriage (common odds ratio = 0.36, 95% CI: 0.32–0.42), without consistent associations of perinatal mortality, in women with NVP [23].

HG is associated with adverse outcomes in both newborn and mother, with an increased risk of low pregnancy weight gain, low birth weight, small size for gestational age, preterm birth, congenital malformations, and poor 5-minute Apgar scores [24, 25].

Treatments for NVP and HG range from simple dietary modifications to drug therapy and total parenteral nutrition (TPN). Severity of symptoms and maternal weight loss should be used to determine the aggressiveness of treatment. Women should be advised to eat several small, bland, low-fat meals throughout the day. Small volumes of salty liquids, such as electrolyte-replacement sport beverages, are also advised. Women who cannot tolerate the smell of hot foods should be recommended to eat cold foods [26]. Ginger is the only non-pharmacologic intervention recommended by the American College of Obstetricians and Gynecologists (ACOG) [27]. Ginger is believed to help improve NVP by stimulating GI-tract motility and the flow of saliva, bile, and gastric secretions.

Women with symptoms unresponsive to dietary modification and pharmacologic treatment require additional support with intravenous (IV) fluid therapy, enteral nutrition, or parenteral nutrition to prevent fetal intrauterine growth restriction, maternal dehydration, and malnutrition.

See Table 60.1 for details of pharmacologic options.

Small Intestine and Colon

Irritable Bowel Syndrome

Despite the prevalence of irritable bowel syndrome (IBS) among reproductive-aged women, only a few studies of IBS in pregnancy exist. One study found moderately increased risks for miscarriage (OR 1.21, 95% CI: 1.13–1.30) and ectopic pregnancy (OR 1.28%, 95% CI: 1.06–1.55) in women with IBS diagnosed before pregnancy, suggesting the need for high-quality prenatal care for this population [28].

Constipation

Up to 40% of pregnant women experience constipation in pregnancy [29]. Low stool frequency (fewer than three bowel movements per week), hard stools, and/or difficulties on evacuation are good clinical criteria for constipation in pregnancy [30].

Constipation in pregnancy is largely attributed to decreased colonic motility due to high levels of progesterone [31]. Other factors which may contribute include lower levels of motilin [31], decreased oral intake of food and fluid due to nausea and vomiting, psychological stress, iron supplementation, and mechanical pressure on the rectosigmoid colon from the enlarging uterus [32].

Education and reassurance about normal bowel habits in pregnancy are important in the initial management. First-line therapy should include increased physical activity, avoidance of constipating foods and supplements such as those containing iron and calcium, and increased fluid and fiber intake. Patients failing these measures should be offered stool-bulking agents. Wheat bran is highly effective, but often causes abdominal bloating or flatulence. Soluble fiber, such as pectin, psyllium, and oat bran, causes fecal

water retention, while non-soluble fiber, such as methylcellulose, enhances fecal bulk.

See Table 60.1 for a summary of constipation drugs used in pregnancy.

Diarrhea

The prevalence of diarrhea in pregnancy is largely unknown. The causes are essentially the same as for the non-pregnant population: infection, medications, functional diarrhea, malabsorption, inflammatory bowel disease (IBD), and endocrine disorders such as hyperthyroidism and adrenal insufficiency. In the case of bacterial infection, the common etiologies are *Campylobacter*, *Shigella*, *E. coli*, and *Salmonella* [31]. Severe symptoms, such as bloody stool, fever, and abdominal pain, should raise concern over bacterial infections that are detrimental to maternal and fetal health, and should trigger an immediate workup. *Campylobacter* infection can cause intrauterine infection, abortion, stillbirth, or early neonatal death. In the newborn, it may cause neonatal sepsis or enteritis [33]. *Salmonella* and *Shigella* have been associated with poor pregnancy outcomes [34, 35]. In the absence of alarm symptoms, treatment of uncomplicated diarrhea is supportive. Symptoms lasting longer than 7 days warrant further evaluation.

Treatment should begin with conservative management, including oral rehydration, correction of electrolyte abnormalities, and dietary modification. Bismuth subsalicylate, as found in Kaopectate and Pepto-Bismol, and alosetron (FDA category B) should be avoided [36].

Abdominal Pain

Tricyclic Antidepressants

Tricyclic antidepressants are only recommended for use in pregnancy in women with severe GI symptoms of IBS [37].

Selective Serotonin Reuptake Inhibitors

Selective serotonin reuptake inhibitors (SSRIs; generally FDA category C) are usually considered safe in pregnancy [38]. Use of paroxetine (FDA category D) had been discouraged, due to reports of higher rates of cardiovascular defects in fetuses; however, recent data have not found any increased fetal risk with use in early pregnancy [39]. Use for the treatment of IBS in pregnancy should be limited to those with severe symptoms.

Antispasmodics

Studies examining the efficacy of antispasmodics in pregnancy have not been conducted. Dicyclomine (FDA category B) has been associated with congenital anomalies when used in combination with doxylamine; however, findings of teratogenicity have not been consistent [37]. Hyoscyamine (FDA category C) has not been well studied in pregnancy. Routine use of either drug in pregnancy is not recommended.

Inflammatory Bowel Disease

Infertility rates for men and women with IBD range from 5 to 14%, which is comparable to the general population [40,41]. Certain subgroups of patients, however, have much higher rates of infertility, including those who have undergone colectomy with ileal pouch construction and complex pelvic IBD surgeries, in whom infertility rates may be as high as 48% [41]. Infertility after surgery is likely caused by impaired tubal function due to adhesion formation after deep pelvic dissection. Ileorectal anastomosis and laparoscopic

CHAPTER 60

restorative proctocolectomy may have improved postoperative conception rates compared to standard open colectomy with ileal pouch anal anastomosis (IPAA) [42, 43].

Fertility in men is decreased by sulfasalazine use, which reversibly decreases sperm count, impairs motility, and alters morphology [44]. Methotrexate may also impact male fertility by causing oligospermia [45]. Impaired fertility has been described in some men who have undergone IPAA, due to retrograde ejaculation and erectile dysfunction [46], though pouch surgery has been found to improve male sexual function [47].

Effect of Pregnancy on IBD

Pregnancy has not been shown to increase the risk of flares in women with IBD [48, 49]. The chance of having a flare in pregnancy is the same as in non-pregnant women: approximately 33% per year. The course of IBD activity in one pregnancy is not predictive of activity in subsequent pregnancies. The most important predictor of IBD course in pregnancy is the level of disease activity at the time of conception [50]. It is strongly recommended that disease be in remission before conceiving. Women should be counseled to continue medications and not resume smoking after delivery, to reduce the risk of flaring during pregnancy and postpartum.

Effect of IBD on Pregnancy

Women appear to be at increased risk for preterm birth, low birth weight, and cesarean section [51]. Congenital malformation rates have not been shown to be higher in most studies [52, 53].

Whether active disease at conception and/or during pregnancy increases the risk of adverse outcome or simply having IBD increases risk is not clear. Several recent studies have found the increased risk of adverse events in women with IBD to be independent of disease activity [54, 55]. Nevertheless, to minimize the negative sequelae of active disease, such as malnutrition and increased risk of thrombosis, it is recommended that disease be aggressively managed in pregnancy.

Treatment of IBD in pregnancy is essentially the same as in the non-pregnant state, as active disease poses a greater risk to the pregnancy than does therapy. See Table 60.1 for medications used in IBD.

Celiac Disease

Celiac disease may increase the risk of female infertility. Some studies using serological screening have found significantly higher rates of celiac disease among women with unexplained infertility compared with the general population [56, 57] though data are conflicting [58, 59]. Whether a gluten-free diet improves fertility is currently unknown, as studies have shown varied results [60–62].

Maternal celiac disease may increase the risk of intrauterine growth restriction, low birth weight, and preterm delivery, so it is widely recommended that conception be deferred until the patient is in clinical remission to minimize the effects of poor nutritional status on pregnancy outcomes.

Acute Abdominal Pain

Abdominal pain in pregnancy poses a clinical challenge, given the differential is broad and includes obstetric and non-obstetric causes. The presentation of common conditions may be altered, leading to difficulty in diagnosis. Non-obstetric causes of acute abdominal pain can be divided broadly into four categories: GI, genitourinary, vascular, and other (see Table 60.2). Some of the more common GI causes of abdominal pain in pregnancy are discussed in this section.

Table 60.2 Causes of acute abdominal pain in pregnancy. Source: Mehta 2010 [60]. Reproduced with permission of Wiley.

Obstetric	Non-obstetric
Ruptured of rectus abdominis muscle	GI
Acute fatty liver of pregnancy	• Appendicitis
Ectopic pregnancy	• Pancreatitis
Pre-eclampsia/HELLP syndrome	• PUD
Placental abruption	• Cholecystitis
Pelvic vein thrombosis	• Intestinal obstruction
Chorioamnionitis	• Bowel perforation
Placental precreta	Genitourinary
Uterine rupture	• Cystitis
Torsion of pedunculated myoma	• Pyelonephritis
Torsion of the pregnant uterus	• Ovarian cyst rupture
Septic abortion with peritonitis	• Adnexal torsion
Red degeneration of myoma	• Nephrolithiasis
	Vascular
	• Superior mesenteric artery syndrome
	• Mesenteric venous thrombosis
	• Ruptured visceral artery aneurysm

GI, gastrointestinal; HELLP, hemolysis, elevated liver function, and low platelets; PUD, peptic ulcer disease.

Appendicitis

Appendicitis is the most common cause of acute abdomen in pregnancy [63]. Though the incidence of appendicitis is the same in the pregnant woman as in the non-pregnant woman, rates of perforation are higher. The diagnosis of appendicitis can be difficult, as anatomic changes caused by the gravid uterus may lead to atypical presentations; by the second trimester, the uterus displaces the appendix to the right upper quadrant, and thus patients with acute appendicitis may present with pain in the right lower quadrant, right upper quadrant, or periumbilical area, depending on gestational age [64]. In late pregnancy, rebound tenderness and guarding may be absent, due to separation of the visceral from the parietal peritoneum [65].

Graded compression ultrasound is recommended as the initial diagnostic test. Magnetic resonance imaging (MRI) without gadolinium should be performed over computed tomography (CT) when ultrasound is negative or non-diagnostic, unless contraindicated or not available [66].

Gallstone Disease

The incidence of gallstones is increased in pregnancy, due to increased bile lithogenicity and decreased gallbladder motility [67, 68]. Most women remain asymptomatic [69].

For women with uncomplicated biliary colic, the management is initially supportive, with pain control and fasting to decrease the release of cholecystokinin. Subsequent episodes tend to be more severe, and surgical intervention is appropriate when conservative therapy fails, preferably in the second trimester [70].

Acute cholecystitis is the second most common surgical condition in pregnancy [71]. Though medical therapy with bowel rest, nasogastric suctioning (if necessary), IV fluid rehydration, and antibiotics has historically been preferred, especially for patients in the first and third trimesters, recent data suggest that laparoscopic cholecystectomy can be performed safely in all trimesters [72].

Pancreatitis

Pancreatitis in pregnancy has an estimated incidence rate of 1 in 1000 to 1 in 10 000 pregnancies [73–76]. Most acute cases are attributable to gallstones. Non-biliary causes of pancreatitis, in particular alcohol and hyperlipidemia, have been associated with worse outcomes [150]. Fetal risks from pancreatitis include preterm labor, prematurity, and fetal demise [77]. Most patients can be managed conservatively with bowel rest, pain control, IV hydration, and nutritional support.

Intestinal Obstruction

Bowel obstruction most often occurs in the third trimester and postpartum, but can also occur when the uterus enters the abdomen in the 4th and 5th months. The most common cause of bowel obstruction is adhesions from prior abdominal surgery, including C-sections, followed by volvulus [78, 79]. Volvulus can occur in all regions of the small and large intestine, but most commonly involves the sigmoid colon [80].

Take Home Points

- Luminal gastrointestinal (GI) disease can develop *de novo* during pregnancy, can be unique to pregnancy, or can be an exacerbation of a pre-existing condition.
- Hormonal and mechanical changes predispose the pregnant woman to nausea and vomiting of pregnancy (NVP), heartburn, constipation, and gallstone formation.
- The differential for the acute abdomen in pregnancy is broad, as it includes obstetric and non-obstetric causes.
- Treatment should be guided by the principle "healthy mother, healthy baby," taking into consideration potential risks to mother and fetus.

References

1 Powrie R. Principles for drug prescribing in pregnancy. In Rosene-Montella K, Kelly E, Barbour LA, Lee RV, eds. *Medical Care of the Pregnant Patient*, 2nd edn. Philadelphia, PA: ACP, 2008.

2 Richter JE. Gastroesophageal reflux disease during pregnancy. *Gastroenterol Clin North Am* 2003; **32**: 235–61.

3 Habr F, Raker C, Lin C, *et al.* Predictors of gastroesophageal reflux symptoms in pregnant women screened for sleep disordered breathing: a secondary analysis. *Clin Res Hepatol Gastroenterol* 2013; **37**: 93–9.

4 Richter JE. Review article: the management of heartburn in pregnancy. *Aliment Pharmacol Ther* 2005; **22**: 749–57.

5 Van Thiel DH, Wald A. Evidence refuting a role for increased abdominal pressure in the pathogenesis of the heartburn associated with pregnancy. *Am J Obstet Gynecol* 1981; **140**: 420–2.

6 Leite LP, Johnston BT, Barrett J, *et al.* Ineffective esophageal motility (IEM): the primary finding in patients with nonspecific esophageal motility disorder. *Dig Dis Sci* 1997; **42**: 1859–65.

7 McCallum RW, Berkowitz DM, Lerner E. Gastric emptying in patients with gastroesophageal reflux. *Gastroenterology* 1981; **90**: 285–91.

8 Cunningham FG, Gant NF, Leveno KJ, *et al.* Gastrointestinal disorders. In: Cunningham FG, Gant NF, Leveno KJ, *et al.*, eds. *William's Obstetrics*. New York: McGraw-Hill, 2001: 1273–306.

9 Hess LW, Morrison JC, Hess DB. General medical disorders during pregnancy. In: DeCherney AH, Pernoll ML, eds. *Current Obstetric and Gynecologic Diagnosis and Treatment*. Norwalk, CT: Appleton & Lange, 1994.

10 Cappell MS. Gastric and duodenal ulcers during pregnancy. *Gastroenterol Clin North Am* 2003; **32**: 263–308.

11 Mahadevan U, Kane SV. American Gastroenterological Association Institute technical review on the use of gastrointestinal medications in pregnancy. *Gastroenterology* 2006; **131**: 283–311.

12 O'Brien B, Zhou Q. Variables related to nausea and vomiting during pregnancy. *Birth* 1995; **22**: 93–100.

13 Lacroix R, Eason E, Melzack R. Nausea and vomiting during pregnancy: a prospective study of its frequency, intensity, and patterns of change. *Am J Obstet Gynecol* 2000; **182**: 931–7.

14 Verberg MFG, Gillott DJ, Al-Fardan N, *et al.* Hyperemesis gravidarm, a literature review. *Hum Reprod Update* 2005; **11**: 527–39.

15 Golberg D, Szilagyi A, Graves L. Hyperemesis gravidarum and *Helicobacter pylori* infection: a systemic review. *Obstet Gynecol* 2007; **110**: 695–703.

16 Klebanoff MA, Koslowe PA, Kaslow R, *et al.* Epidemiology of vomiting in early pregnancy. *Obstet Gynecol* 1985; **66**: 612–16.

17 Brandes JM. First trimester nausea and vomiting as related to outcome of pregnancy. *Obstet Gynecol* 1967; **30**: 427–31.

18 Gadsby R, Barnie-Adshead A, Jagger C. Pregnancy nausea related to women's obstretic and personal histories. *Gynecol Obstet Invest* 1997; **43**: 108–11.

19 Niebyl JR. Nausea and vomiting in pregnancy. *N Engl J Med* 2010; **363**: 1544–50.

20 Soules MR, Hughs CL, Garcia JA, *et al.* Nausea and vomiting of pregnancy: role of human chorionic gonadotropin and 17-hydroxyprogesterone. *Obstet Gynecol* 1980; **55**: 696.

21 Goodwin TM. Hyperemesis gravidarum. *Obstet Gynecol Clin N Am* 2008; **35**: 401–17.

22 Wallstedt A, Riely CA, Shaver D, *et al.* Prevalence and characteristics of liver dysfunction in hyperemesis gravidarum. *Clin Res* 1990; **38**: 970A.

23 Weigel RM, Weigel MM. Nausea and vomiting of early pregnancy and pregnancy outcome. A meta-analytical review. *Br J Obstet Gynecol* 1989; **96**: 1312–18.

24 Dodds L, Fell DB, Joseph KS, *et al.* Outcome of pregnancies complicated by hyperemesis gravidarum. *Obstet Gynecol* 2006; **107**: 285–92.

25 Kallen B. Hyperemesis gravidarum during pregnancy and delivery outcome: a registry study. *Eur J Obstet Gynecol Reprod Biol* 1987; **26**: 291.

26 Jueckstock JK, Kaestner R, Mylonas I. Managing hyperemesis gravidarum: a multimodal challenge. *BMC Medicine* 2010; **8**: 46.

27 American College of Obstetrics and Gynecology. ACOG (American College of Obstetrics and Gynecology) practice bulletin: nausea and vomiting of pregnancy. *Obstet Gynecol* 2004; **103**: 803–14.

28 Khashan AS, Quigley FM, McNamee R, *et al.* Increased risk of miscarriage and ectopic pregnancy among women with irritable bowel syndrome. *Clin Gastroenterol Hepatol* 2012; **10**(8): 902–9.

29 Anderson AS. Dietary factors in the aetiology and treatment of constipation during pregnancy. *Br J Obstet Gynaecol* 1986; **93**: 245–9.

30 Cullen G, O'Donoghue D. Constipation and pregnancy. *Best Pract Res Clin Gastroenterol* 2007; **21**(5): 807–18.

31 Wald A. Constipation, diarrhea, and symptomatic hemorrhoids during pregnancy. *Gastroenterol Clin North Am* 2003; **32**: 309–22, vii.

32 Mehta N, Saha S, Chien EKS, *et al.* Disorders of the gastrointestinal tract in pregnancy. In: Powrie RO, Greene MF, Camann W, eds. *DeSwiet's Medical Disorders in Obstetric Practice*, 5th edn. Oxford: Wiley-Blackwell, 2010.

33 Simor AE, Ferro S. *Campylobacter jejuni* infection occurring during pregnancy. *Eur J Clin Microbiol Infect Dis* 1990; **9**: 142–4.

34 Rebarber A, Star Hampton B, Lewis V, Bender S. Shigellosis complicating preterm premature rupture of membranes resulting in congenital infection and preterm delivery. *Obstet Gynecol* 2002; **100**: 1063–5.

35 Scialli AR, Rarick TL. Salmonella sepsis and second-trimester pregnancy loss. *Obstet Gynecol* 1992; **79**: 820–1.

36 Shapiro S, Siskind V, Monson RR, *et al.* Perinatal mortality and birth-weight in relation to aspirin taken during pregnancy. *Lancet* 1976; **1**: 1375–6.

37 Hasler WL. The irritable bowel syndrome during pregnancy. *Gastroenterol Clin North Am* 2003; **32**: 385–406, viii.

38 Ericson A, Kallen B, Wiholm B. Delivery outcome after the use of antidepressants in early pregnancy. *Eur J Clin Pharmacol* 1999; **55**(7): 503–8.

39 Einarson A, Pistelli A, DeSantis M, *et al.* Evaluation of the risk of congenital cardiovascular defects associated with use of paroxetine during pregnancy. *Am J Psychiatry* 2008; **165**: 777.

40 Mahadevan U. Fertility and pregnancy in the patient with inflammatory bowel disease. *Gut* 2006; **55**: 1198–206.

41 Waljee A, Waljee J, Morris AM. Threefold increased risk of infertility: a meta-analysis of infertility after ileal pouch anal anastomosis in ulcerative colitis. *Gut* 2006; **55**(11): 1575–80.

42 Mortier PE, Gambiez L, Karoui M *et al.* Colectomy with ileorectal anastomosis preserves female fertility in ulcerative colitis. *Gastroenterol Clin* 2006; **30**(4): 594–7.

43 Bartel, SA, D'Hoore A, Cuesta MA, *et al.* Significantly increased pregnancy rates after laparoscopic restorative proctocolectomy: a cross-sectional study. *Ann Surg* 2012; **256**(6): 1045–8.

44 Heetun ZS, Byrnes C, Neary P, O'Morain C. Review article: Reproduction in the patient with inflammatory bowel disease. *Aliment Pharmacol Ther* 2007; **26**(4): 513–33.

45 French AE, Koren G. Effect of methotrexate on male fertility. *Can Fam Physician* 2003; **49**: 577–8.

46 Tianen N, Maitikanen N, Hiltunen KM. Ileal J-pouch–anal anastomosis, sexual dysfunction, and fertility. *Scand J Gastroenterol* 1999; **34**: 185–8.

47 Gorgun E, Remzi FH, Montague DK, *et al.* Male sexual function improves after ileal pouch anal anastamosis. *Colorectal Dis* 2005; **7**: 545–50.

48 Nielsen OH, Andreasson B, Bondesen S, *et al.* Pregnancy in Crohn's disease. *Scand J Gastroenterol* 1984; **19**: 724–32.

49 Nielsen OH, Andreasson B, Bondesen S, *et al.* Pregnancy in ulcerative colitis. *Scand J Gastroenterol* 1983; **18**: 735–42.

50 Miller JP. Inflammatory bowel disease in pregnancy: a review. *J Roy Soc Med* 1986; **79**: 221–5.

51 Cornish J, Tan E, Teare J, *et al.* A meta-analysis on the influence of inflammatory bowel disease on pregnancy. *Gut* 2007; **56**: 830–7.

52 Norgard B, Puho E, Pedersen L, *et al.* Risk of congenital abnormalities in children born to women with ulcerative colitis: a population-based, case-control study. *Am J Gastroenterol* 2003; **98**(9): 2006–10.

53 Dominitz JA, Young JC, Boyko EJ. Outcomes of infants born tomothers with inflammatory bowel disease: a population-based cohort study. *Am J Gastroenterol* 2002; **97**: 641–8.

54 Mahadevan U, Sandborn W, Li DK. Pregnancy outcomes in women with inflammatory bowel disease: a population based cohort study. *Gastroenterology* 2007; **113**: 1106–12.

55 Norgard B, Hundborg HH, Jacobsen BA, *et al.* Disease activity in pregnant women with Crohn's disease and birth outcomes: a regional Danish cohort study. *Am J Gastroenterol* 2007; **102**: 1947–54.

56 Collin P, Vilska S, Heinonen PK, *et al.* Infertility and coeliac disease. *Gut* 1996; **39**: 382–4.

57 Meloni GF, Dessole S, Vargiu N, *et al.* The prevalence of coeliac disease in infertility. *Hum Reprod* 1999; **14**: 2759–61.

58 Shamaly H, Mahameed A, Sharony A, Shamir R. Infertility and celiac disease: do we need more than one serological marker? *Acta Obstet Gynecol Scand* 2004; **83**: 1184–8.

59 Kolho KL, Tiitinen A, Tulppala M, *et al.* Screening for coeliac disease in women with a history of recurrent miscarriage or infertility. *Br J Obstet Gynaecol* 1999; **106**: 171–3.

60 Sher KS, Mayberry JF. Female fertility, obstetric and gynaecological history in coeliac disease: a case control study. *Acta Paediatr Suppl* 1996; **412**: 76–7.

61 Ferguson R, Holmes GK, Cooke WT. Coeliac disease: fertility and pregnancy. *Scand J Gastroenterol* 1982; **17**(1): 65–8.

62 Rujner J. Age at menarche in girls with celiac disease. *Ginekol Pol* 1999; **70**(5): 359–62.

63 Parangi S, Levine D, Henry A, *et al.* Surgical gastrointestinal disorders during pregnancy. *Am J Surg* 2007; **193**: 223–32.

64 Weingold AB. Appendicitis in pregnancy. *Clin Obstet Gynecol* 1983; **26**: 801–9.

65 Tracey M, Fletcher HS. Appendicitis in pregnancy. *Am Surg* 2000; **66**: 555–9.

66 Patel SJ, Reede, DL, Katz DS, *et al.* Imaging the pregnant patient for nonobstetric conditions: algorithms and radiation dose considerations 1. *Radiographics* 2007; **27**: 1705–22.

67 Braverman DZ, Johnson ML, Kern F. Effects of pregnancy and contraceptive steroids on gallbladder function. *N Engl J Med* 1980; **302**: 362–4.

68 Van Bodegraven AA, Böhmer CJM, Manoliu RA, *et al.* Gallbladder contents and fasting gallbladder volumes during and after pregnancy. *Scand J Gastroenterol* 1998; **33**(9): 993–7.

69 Maringhini A, Ciambra M, Baccelliere P, *et al.* Biliary sludge and gallstones in pregnancy: incidence, risk factors, and natural history. *Ann Intern Med* 1993; **119**(2): 116.

70 Lu EJ, Curet MJ, El-Sayed YY, *et al.* Medical versus surgical management of biliary tract disease in pregnancy. *Am J Surg* 2004; **188**: 755–9.

71 Sharp, Howard T. The acute abdomen during pregnancy. *Clin Obstet Gynecol* 2002; **45**(2): 405–13.

72 Date RS, Kaushal M, Ramesh A. A review of the management of gallstone disease and its complications in pregnancy. *Am J Surg* 2008; **196**: 599–608.

73 Eddy JJ, Gideonsen MD, Song JY, *et al.* Pancreatitis in pregnancy: a 10 year retrospective of 15 midwest hospitals. *Obstet Gynecol* 2008; **112**(5): 1075.

74 Pitchumoni CS, Yegneswaran B. Acute pancreatitis in pregnancy. *World J Gastroenterol* 2009; **15**(45): 5641.

75 Igbinosa O, Poddar S, Pitchumoni C. Pregnancy associated pancreatitis revisited. *Clin Res Hepatol Gastroenterol* 2013; **37**(2): 177–81.

76 Wells R, Wolf J. Gastrointestinal disease in pregnancy. In: Brandt LJ, ed. *Clinical Practice of Gastroenterology*. Philadelphia, PA: Churchill Livingstone, 1998: 1586–97.

77 Ducarme G, Maire F, Chatel P, *et al.* Acute pancreatitis during pregnancy: a review. *J Perinatol* 2013; **34**(2): 87–94.

78 Connolly MM, Unti JA, Nora PF. Bowel obstruction in pregnancy. *Surg Clin North Am* 1995; **75**: 101–13.

79 Perdue PW, Johnson HW Jr., Stafford PW. Intestinal obstruction complicating pregnancy. *Am J Surg* 1992; **164**: 384–8.

80 Montes H, Wolf J. Cecal volvulus in pregnancy. *Am J Gastroenterol* 1999; **94**: 2554.

CHAPTER 61

Consequences of Human Immunodeficiency Virus Infection

Vera P. Luther and P. Samuel Pegram

Department of Internal Medicine, Wake Forest University School of Medicine, Winston-Salem, NC, USA

Summary

Human immunodeficiency virus (HIV) infected individuals can develop gastrointestinal (GI) disorders throughout the course of HIV infection. Recent studies have demonstrated that HIV infection involves the GI tract (including the colon and rectum) from early infection with depletion of gut-associated lymphoid tissue (GALT), throughout chronic infection (when GALT may not be fully restored even with adequate antiretroviral therapy), and into full-blown acquired immunodeficiency syndrome (AIDS). HIV itself can result in a unique enteropathy. The associated progressive immunodeficiency which occurs in untreated HIV-infected patients can allow fulminant reactivation of usually benign, latent infections (e.g., cytomegalovirus (CMV) colitis or chronic, severe perirectal herpes simplex type 2 (HSV-2) infection) or the transformation of a ubiquitous pathogen into a malignant, invasive agent (e.g., *Mycobacterium avium* complex). Many sexually-transmitted infections may be more severe and more varied in presentation in HIV-infected patients, and their therapy may be more complex. These patients are also at increased risk for certain malignancies of the colon (especially Kaposi sarcoma) and rectum (human papillovirus-associated intraepithelial neoplasia).

Case

A 26-year-old gay male was diagnosed with HIV infection 5 years ago. His CD4 nadir was 140 cells/m^3 2 years after diagnosis, but he has been on antiretroviral therapy for 3 years with excellent adherence (last CD4 = 480 cells/mm^3 and HIV RNA undetectable). In addition to HIV infection, he has a history of syphilis (adequately treated with appropriate rapid plasma reagin (RPR) response), gonorrhea on two occasions (oral and rectal), and past hepatitis A and B. His glycoprotein G herpes simplex-2 serology was negative. He is otherwise healthy. Despite multiple prevention interventions by physicians and social workers, he continues to episodically have unprotected, receptive oral and anal intercourse. He attends clinic complaining of painful, blood-tinged bowel movements for 5 days associated with a low-grade fever and malaise. He denies recent travel, foreign body exposure, animal contact, or similar prior symptoms. On general physical examination the only abnormalities were mild perianal ulcerations and several tender inguinal lymph nodes; on anoscopy, there were diffuse, painful, and shallow ulcerations with overlying bloody exudates throughout the visualized anorectal field. The following studies were ordered: darkfield examination, syphilis serology, gonococcal and chlamydial DNA probes, viral culture (primarily for herpes simplex viruses in light of his good immune status), repeat glycoprotein G herpes simplex serology, *Clostridium difficile* toxin assay, and routine stool culture. Within 24 h his HSV-2 culture was positive; all other studies were negative including HSV-2 serology. The patient was treated with valacyclovir 1 g three times per day for 10 days then placed on 500 mg twice per day for prophylaxis of anogenital herpes. Follow-up serologies 8 weeks later demonstrated glycoprotein G HSV-2 seroconversion— thus, the patient had primary HSV-2 anoproctitis.

Definition and Epidemiology

Patients with HIV infection can experience a wide array of colonic and rectal problems. Most problems are infectious in etiology, especially as the untreated patient becomes more and more CD4 T-cell lymphopenic. The gut-associated lymphoid tissue (GALT) is the largest lymphoid organ infected by HIV. Pathologic changes, both structural and immunological, occur in the gut from the very onset of HIV infection [1, 2]. Within weeks of primary infection there is an acute depletion of CD4+ T lymphocytes in the GI tract which then leads to a cascade of events, including microbial translocation, systemic immune activation, chronic HIV replication, and immune destruction, and finally advanced AIDS with its associated opportunistic infections and malignancies [3–6].

Pathogenesis

CD4 T lymphocytes in the GI tract are rapidly and radically depleted in acute human HIV infection [7, 8]. The mechanism(s) by which this GALT depletion occurs is gradually being unraveled [1,9]. There appear to be both direct and indirect systems involved. HIV preferentially replicates in activated memory CD4 T cells (which represent a majority of CD4 lymphocytes in the gut), and up to 30 to 60% of CD4 T cells are infected within 2 weeks of infection of the host.

Early HIV infection and depletion of GALT result in a damaged mucosal barrier and loss of mucosal immunity. This can lead to HIV-induced enteropathy manifested as diarrhea, increased

Practical Gastroenterology and Hepatology Board Review Toolkit, Second Edition. Edited by Nicholas J. Talley, Kenneth R. DeVault, Michael B. Wallace, Bashar A. Aqel and Keith D. Lindor.
© 2016 John Wiley & Sons, Ltd. Published 2016 by John Wiley & Sons, Ltd. Companion website: www.practicalgastrohep.com

GI inflammation and permeability, and malabsorption (particularly of bile acids and vitamin B$_{12}$). This occurs in the absence of enteropathogens. Histologically, there is damage to the GI epithelial layer and inflammatory infiltrates of lymphocytes [10, 11].

A second consequence of GALT depletion is microbial translocation [12]. Microbial translocation leads to increased levels of plasma lipopolysaccharide (LPS) in patients chronically infected with HIV compared with uninfected patients. LPS is a potent immunostimulatory factor which can add to the systemic immune activation accompanying chronic HIV infection. Over time there is a slow but continuous decrease in gut CD4 T cells, resulting in a progressive decline in the production of these cells from the central memory pool [13, 14].

The goal of combination antiretroviral therapy (cART) is to decrease the plasma HIV RNA to undetectable levels. This is typically followed by a gradual increase in plasma CD4 T lymphocytes. Although it has been demonstrated that rectal HIV is decreased with cART, the restoration of intestinal CD4 T cells in chronically HIV-infected patients is substantially delayed and incomplete [15, 16]. There is some evidence that by initiating cART early in HIV infection near complete restoration of the mucosal immune system can be achieved.

Clinical Features

The consequences of HIV infection affecting the colon and rectum are variable depending on the causative etiology, the patient's degree of immunocompromise, and the portion of the GI system involved. In general, the diseases of the colon and rectum in HIV-infected patients can be categorized into those that cause enterocolitis and those that cause proctitis. These two processes have distinct clinical characteristics and distinct causative organisms. The disease entities of enteritis, colitis, and enterocolitis are characterized by inflammation of the small intestine, colon, or both. Clinical manifestations include diarrhea, abdominal cramps, and bloating. Patients who engage in sexual practices involving direct or indirect oral–anal contact are at higher risk for developing these illnesses. Anorectal disease is seen most commonly in patients who engage in receptive anal intercourse. Perirectal abscesses, anal fistulae, perianal herpes simplex virus infections, aphthous ulcerations, and infectious proctitis may occur in these patients.

Enterocolitis

While some pathogens cause relatively distinct clinical manifestations, there is significant overlap in clinical features between the various causes of diarrhea. Therefore, when evaluating patients with HIV infection and enterocolitis, it is often useful to classify the illness into syndromes characterized by watery diarrhea and those that cause an inflammatory diarrhea. Important causes of watery diarrhea in HIV-infected patients include: rotavirus, norovirus, *Vibrio* spp., enterotoxigenic *Escherichia coli* (ETEC), enteroaggregative *E. coli* (EAEC), enteropathogenic *E. coli* (EPEC), *Giardia lamblia*, *Cryptosporidium parvum*, *Isospora belli*, *Cyclospora cayetanensis*, and microsporidia [17,18]. Of note, *Cryptosporidium* is the most common protozoa identified in HIV-infected patients [19]. The clinical syndrome is characterized by watery diarrhea and may be accompanied by nausea, vomiting, myalgias, arthralgias, abdominal pain, and chills. If a fever is present, it is generally mild. Leukocytes and blood are notably absent from the stool. Chronic diarrhea may ensue [20].

Important causes of inflammatory diarrhea (dysentery) in HIV-infected patients include: *Shigella* spp., *Salmonella* spp., *Yersinia* spp., *Campylobacter* spp., enteroinvasive *E. coli* (EIEC), enterohemorrhagic *E. coli* (EHEC), and *Entamoeba histolytica* [17,18]. This diarrheal syndrome is caused by invasive organisms and is characterized by fever and the presence of blood, mucus, and leukocytes in the stool. Vomiting, tenesmus, and abdominal cramping may also be present. The onset of fever and diarrhea are often acute. Bacteremia is common with *Shigella* spp., *Salmonella* spp., and *Campylobacter* spp. Infections due to these organisms in HIV-infected individuals may be recurrent and severe [21]. Toxic megacolon has been described in association with *Shigella* spp. *Salmonella* enterocolitis occurs more commonly in HIV-infected patients than in the general population, and a diagnosis of *Salmonella* bacteremia in an HIV-infected individual meets the Centers for Disease Control (CDC) definition of AIDS [21, 22]. Infections due to *Salmonella* spp. may present with fever alone and no localizing symptoms [21].

Cytomegalovirus (CMV) is an important cause of diarrhea in severely immunocompromised HIV-infected individuals and the clinical manifestations of colonic infection due to CMV are widely variable. Patients may be asymptomatic or experience any combination of crampy abdominal pain, diarrhea, hematochezia, urgency, tenesmus, weight loss, or fevers [23, 24]. CMV is the most common viral cause of diarrhea and chronic diarrhea in AIDS patients with multiple negative stool studies [25]. Simultaneous involvement of the esophagus, stomach, or small bowel may be present as well. Bleeding or perforation may result from diffuse, ulcerating involvement of the intestine. Appendicitis due to CMV has been described [23]. Of note, concomitant CMV retinitis may be present, and all patients should undergo ophthalmologic evaluation at the time of diagnosis. CMV reactivation occurs only with advanced HIV infection (CD4 <50 cells/mm^3) [26, 27].

HIV-infected individuals who develop *Clostridium difficile*-associated diarrhea (CDAD) are prone to experience more severe clinical symptoms, relapse, or chronic disease. Toxic megacolon can occur as a complication [28].

Mycobacterium avium-intracellulare complex (MAC) is the most commonly identified organism in patients with chronic diarrhea and advanced AIDS (CD4 lymphocyte counts <50 cells/mm^3) [29]. Infections may be asymptomatic, or they may be characterized by a combination of fever, night sweats, abdominal pain, malabsorption, severe weight loss, mycobacteremia, lymphadenopathy, and anemia. Involvement of the duodenum is most common and yellow mucosal nodules may be visualized on esophagogastroduodenoscopy (EGD) [29, 30].

In contrast to MAC, intestinal infection due to *Mycobacterium tuberculosis* is quite rare but is always symptomatic. Involvement of the colon or ileocecal region is most common. Fistulae, intussusceptions, perforation, peritoneal, and rectal involvement have been reported [31].

While intestinal infections due to fungi are very rare, histoplasmosis is the most commonly reported fungal infection of the GI tract in HIV-infected patients with the most highly endemic region being the Ohio and Mississippi river valleys. *Histoplasma capsulatum* usually affects the colon and is often associated with concomitant pulmonary and hepatic involvement. In addition to diarrhea and fever, patients may present with large ulcerations, mass lesions, or peritonitis [32].

The helminths *Ancylostoma duodenale* and *Strongyloides stercoralis* are very uncommon causes of diarrhea in HIV-infected patients. Clinical manifestations include abdominal pain, diarrhea, and eosinophilia [33].

Proctitis

Proctitis refers to inflammation of the rectum. Clinical manifestations include pruritis, anorectal pain, rectal bleeding, mucopurulent anal discharge, and painful defecation. Patients with severe symptoms may also experience tenesmus or constipation. Some pathogens can cause inflammation throughout segments of the colon as well (proctocolitis). These patients may experience diarrhea and abdominal cramping in addition to symptoms of proctitis.

Neisseria gonorrhoeae is the most commonly identified cause of proctitis (approximately 30%), followed by *Chlamydia trachomatis*—genital immunotypes D or K (19%). Rectal infections due to *Neisseria gonorrhoeae* are most often asymptomatic (as often as 85% of the time, according to a recent study) [34]. When symptoms occur, mild anorectal pain, mucopurulent or bloody discharge may develop 5–7 days after exposure. Rectal infections due to *Chlamydia trachomatis* are most often asymptomatic as well, but when symptoms occur, they are typically milder. Friable mucosa and mucopurulent discharge are typically seen on anoscopy, even in asymptomatic patients. In contrast to the asymptomatic or mild disease caused by immunotypes D or K, lymphogranuloma venereum (LGV) strains of *Chlamydia trachomatis* (L1, L2, or L3) often cause severe symptoms characterized by severe anorectal pain, bloody or mucopurulent discharge, ulceration, and tenesmus. A recent re-emergence of an LGV variant (L2b) has been diagnosed (and requires special specimen handling through state health departments and the CDC) in mostly HIV-infected, gay men. A characteristic presentation is a rectal ulcer with a bloody or mucoid/purulent anorectal discharge [35].

In the primary stages of syphilis, rectal infection due to *Treponema pallidum* is often asymptomatic as the initial chancre is usually painless. However, patients may experience classic symptoms of proctitis. Also, symptoms of secondary syphilis may manifest as condylomata lata lesions, which are smooth, moist-appearing, wart-like lesions and are highly contagious [36].

Perianal disease due to herpes simplex virus (HSV) infection is most often characterized by local vesicles, pustules, or ulcerations; however, involvement of the distal rectum can occur. In addition to symptoms of proctitis, inguinal lymphadenopathy may be present. Sacral nerve dysesthesias, paresthesias, urinary retention, temporary erectile dysfunction, as well as systemic symptoms such as fever, chills, malaise, headache, and meningismus have been associated with primary HSV (usually HSV-2) infection. Recurrent infections tend to be milder, and this is especially the case with HSV-1 anogenital infection [37].

Diagnosis

In patients with advanced HIV infection or AIDS, systemic disease may accompany a GI illness. This is more common with *Salmonella* spp., *Shigella* spp., *Campylobacter* spp., CMV, and MAC. In this case, identification of a pathogen outside of the gut (i.e., via appropriate blood cultures) may suggest a diagnosis in conjunction with or in lieu of a directed GI evaluation.

Initial Evaluation for Diarrhea in an HIV-infected Patient. Obtain stool specimens for bacterial culture, Clostridium difficile toxin assay, ova and parasite examination, fecal leukocyte examination, and acid-fast stain.

- If diarrhea is chronic, severe or proctitis is present:
  - Perform flexible proctosigmoidoscopy or colonoscopy with mucosal biopsy for pathology plus virologic and parisitologic evaluation
  - Culture rectal tissue for bacteria and viruses in addition to above.
- If diarrhea and weight loss persists and above evaluation is negative:
  - EGD with small bowel biopsy

Initial Evaluation for Proctitis. Perform a careful physical examination of the skin, mucous membranes, and lymph nodes in the anogenital region. This examination should include a visual inspection of the anus for fissures, ulcerations, masses and foreign bodies, followed by digital rectal examination. Anoscopy and sigmoidoscopy with mucosal biopsy should follow if the initial examination does not yield a diagnosis. Anoscopy will often reveal rectal exudate and friability of mucus membranes. Biopsies should be evaluated for neoplasm and infection. Bacterial (including gonococcal and chlamydial), viral, and fungal cultures should be obtained as well (Table 61.1).

Gonococcal and chlamydial nucleic acid amplification testing (NAATs) may be performed on urine, rectal, and pharyngeal specimens; however, they are not currently cleared by the Food and Drug Administration (FDA) for use on rectal and pharyngeal specimens [38].

Differential Diagnosis

While most GI consequences of HIV are infectious in etiology, the availability of combination antiretroviral therapy (cART) has decreased the occurrence of GI complications. Therefore, it is important to consider drug-induced or non-infectious etiologies in the differential diagnosis as well [39]. It is also important to note that in patients with advanced HIV infection or AIDS, multiple infections may be present simultaneously [40] (Table 61.2).

Therapeutics

Therapeutic management for all causes of diarrhea should include appropriate fluid and electrolyte replacement. Symptomatic therapy with antidiarrheal agents such as bismuth subsalicylate and loperamide may be used to decrease the number of stools passed per day. However, caution should be observed with the use of antimotility drugs in the treatment of invasive forms of diarrhea as the development of toxic megacolon may occur [42]. Appropriate antimicrobial therapy is generally pathogen-specific. However, if empiric therapy is necessary, ciprofloxacin 500 mg orally twice daily for 3–5 days is appropriate for adults with febrile dysenteric diarrhea. For the empiric therapy of persistent diarrhea (>14 days' duration), metronidazole 250 mg orally three times daily for 7 days may be administered to adults. For opportunistic infections due to CMV, MAC, *Cryptosporidium* and microsporidia, cART should be included in the treatment regimen [43]. Appropriate immune reconstitution is often necessary for the cure of disease caused by these pathogens.

For the empiric treatment of proctitis, ceftriaxone 125 mg IM once, plus doxycycline 100 mg orally twice daily for 7 days may be used. Fluoroquinolones should not be used in the treatment of gonococcal disease or suspected gonococcal disease due to the high rate of fluoroquinolone resistance [44] (Figure 61.1).

CHAPTER 61

Table 61.1 Diagnostic tools for specific pathogens.

Pathogen	Diagnostic tools
CMV	Viral cytopathic effect (CPE) in tissue specimens, immunostaining, *in situ* hybridization Cultures (less sensitive and specific than histopathology)
Enteric bacteria	Stool cultures, blood cultures (*Salmonella* spp., *Shigella* spp., *Campylobacter* spp.)
Clostridium difficile	Toxin assay on stool
Mycobacterium avium-intracellulare complex	Culture of mucosal biopsy specimens, acid-fast staining of biopsy specimens Acid-fast blood cultures may be positive
Histoplasmosis	Fungal smear, culture of mucosal biopsies or blood Urine or serum *Histoplasmosis* antigen assay
Cryptosporidium	Acid-fast stain of stool, small bowel or rectal biopsies; or enzyme immunoassay (EIA) of stool samples
Isospora	Acid-fast stain of stool or mucosal biopsies
Microsporidia	Gram stain or modified trichrome stain of stool or mucosal biopsies, electron microscopy
Giardia lamblia	Ova and parasite examination or stool samples or mucosal biopsies Enzyme immunoassay (EIA) of stool samples can also be used
Entamoeba histolytica	Morphologically similar to non-pathogenic *Entamoeba dispar* Enzyme-linked immunoassay (ELISA) or PCR tests are required on stool samples to distinguish the species
Neisseria gonorrhoeae	NAATs, Gram stain, culture (see comment in section Proctitis) *Chlamydia trachomatis* NAATs, Gram stain, culture (see comment in section Proctitis)
Treponema pallidum	Darkfield microscopy (rarely used in clinical practice) Physical examination and serologic tests Rapid Plasma Reagin (RPR), Venereal Disease Research Laboratories (VDRL) or toluidine red unheated serum test (TRUST) are screening tests *Treponema Pallidum* Particle Agglutination (TP-PA) assay and Fluorescent Treponemal Antibody Absorption (FTA-ABS) test are confirmatory studies
Herpes simplex virus	Viral culture, PCR testing of swabs from lesions confirm the diagnosis Serology can assist in making the diagnosis as well

NAATs, nucleic acid amplification testing.

Prognosis

The prognoses of colonic and rectal complications of HIV infection are somewhat variable since they are disease specific and dependent on the patient's degree of immunocompromise. In general, HIV-infected individuals with good immune system preservation or reconstitution (due to cART) are likely to have favorable outcomes after appropriate therapy has been administered. However, patients with prolonged immunodeficiency states are likely to experience more severe disease, persistent disease, recurrences, and treatment failures.

Take Home Points

- Patients with HIV infection frequently have infectious and non-infectious colonic and rectal problems.
- The first immunologic casualty of primary HIV infection is the gut-associated lymphoid tissue (GALT); this depletion occurs within the first several weeks of infection and remains throughout HIV infection (restoration may not be complete even with appropriate combination antiretroviral therapy).
- HIV itself can cause a unique enteropathy.

Table 61.2 Causes of enterocolitis and proctitis in HIV-infected individuals.

	Enterocolitis	Proctitis
Viruses	Rotavirus, norovirus, adenovirus, herpes simplex virus, cytomegalovirus*, astrovirus, calcivirus, picobirnavirus, HIV	Herpes simplex virus, condyloma acuminatum (human papillomavirus infection), cytomegalovirus*
Bacteria	*Salmonella* spp., *Shigella* spp., enteroadherent *E. coli* (EAEC), enterotoxigenic *E. coli* (ETEC), enteropathogenic *E. coli* (EPEC), enteroinvasive *E. coli* (EIEC), enterohemorrhagic *E. coli* (EHEC), *Campylobacter* spp., *Yersinia* spp., *Vibrio* spp., *Clostridium difficile*, *Mycobacterium tuberculosis*[†], small bowel bacterial overgrowth[†], *Aeromonas hydrophila*[†], *Mycobacterium avium complex*[*]	*Neisseria gonorrhoeae*, *Chlamydia trachomatis*, *Chlamydia trachomatis* (lymphogranuloma venereum or LGV), *Treponema pallidum*, *Shigella flexneri*[†], *Mycobacterium tuberculosis*[†]
Fungi	*Histoplasma capsulatum*[†], *Cryptococcus neoformans*[*†], *Coccidioides immitis*[†], *Penicillium marneffei*[†]	*Histoplasma capsulatum*[†]
Protozoa	*Cryptosporidium parvum*[*], *Isospora belli*[*], *Cyclospora cayetanensis*[*], microsporidia[*] (*Enterocytozoon bienusi*, *Encephalitozoon intestinalis*), *Giardia lamblia*, *Entamoeba histolytica*, *Toxoplasma gondii*[†], *Pneumocystis jirovecii*[†], *Leishmania donovani*[†]	*Entamoeba histolytica*, *Leishmania donovani*[†]
Non-infectious considerations	Neoplasms: lymphoma, Kaposi sarcoma Idiopathic: "AIDS enteropathy" Drug-induced: protease inhibitors Pancreatic disease Inflammatory bowel disease	Neoplasms: lymphoma, Kaposi sarcoma, squamous cell carcinoma[‡] Perirectal fistulae Aphthous ulcerations Foreign bodies

[*]More likely to occur in patients with CD4 lymphocyte count <100 cells/mm³.
[†]Uncommon pathogens.
[‡]Squamous cell carcinoma of the anus and rectum is more common in men who have sex with men than in any other demographic group of HIV-infected individuals. These carcinomas are the result of HPV infection, particularly with types 16 and 18. Cytologic examinations of the anal canal, comparable to Papanicolaou smears, have been recommended [41].

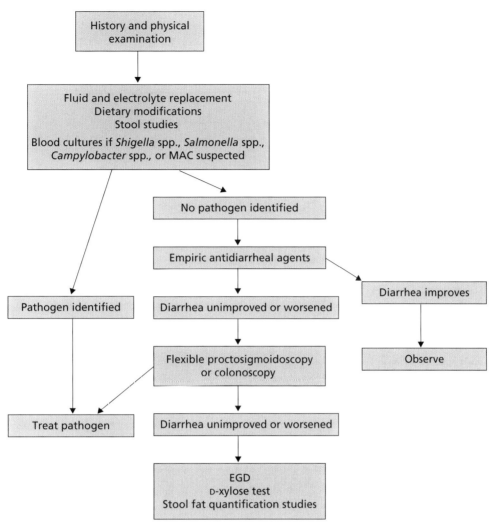

Figure 61.1 Management algorithm. MAC, *Mycobacterium avium-intracellulare* complex; EGD, esophagogastroduodenoscopy.

- With advancing CD4 lymphopenia in the untreated
- HIV-infected patient, latent organisms may reactivate to cause severe disease:
  - HSV-2 anorectal infection
  - CMV colitis.
- Common organisms may become invasive with advanced
- CD4 lymphopenia:
  - MAC infection with pan-intestinal involvement and associated mycobacteremia
  - HSV-2 primary anorectal infection
  - Cryptosporidiosis, etc.
- Genital pathogens may present atypically and be more difficult to diagnose and treat:
  - Primary (intra-anorectal chancre) and secondary (perianal condylomata lata) syphilis may be present simultaneously, and syphilis serology may be confusing with advanced HIV infection.
  - *Chlamydia trachomatis* LGV variant (L2b) can cause rectal ulcers, rectal bleeding, and mucoid/purulent anorectal discharge; diagnosis requires special specimen handling.
- HIV-associated malignancies may affect the colon and rectum:
  - Kaposi sarcoma of colon and rectum
  - HPV-associated intraepithelial neoplasia (squamous cell carcinoma) of the anorectum.

References

1 Johnson RP. How HIV guts the immune system. *N Engl J Med* 2008; **358**: 2287–9.
2 Dandekar S. Pathogenesis of HIV in the gastrointestinal tract. *Curr HIV/AIDS Rep* 2007; **4**: 10–15.
3 Chen TW, Nickle DC, Justement JS, *et al.* Persistence of HIV in gut-associated lymphoid tissue despite long-term antiretroviral therapy. *J Infect Dis* 2008; **197**: 640–2.
4 Guadalupe M, Reay E, Sandaran, *et al.* Severe CD4 depletion in gut lymphoid tissue during primary human immunodeficiency virus type 1 infection and substantial delay in restoration following highly active antiretroviral therapy. *J Virol* 2003; **77**: 11708–17.
5 Centlivre M, Sala M, Wain-Hobson S, Berkhout B. In HIV-1 pathogenesis the die is cast during primary infection. *AIDS* 2007; **21**: 1227–8.
6 van Marie G, Gill MJ, Kolodka D, *et al.* Compartmentization of the gut viral reservoir in HIV-1 infected patients. *Retrovirology* 2007; **4**: 87–92.
7 Mattapalil JJ, Douek DC, Hill B, *et al.* Massive infection and loss of memory CD4+ T cells in multiple tissues during acute SIV infection. *Nature* 2005; **434**: 1093–7.
8 Okoye A, Meyer-Schellersheim M, Brenchley JM, *et al.* Progressive CD4+ central memory T cell decline results in CD4 +effector memory insufficiency and overt disease in chronic SIV infection. *J Exp Med* 2007; **204**: 2171–85.
9 Read SW, Sereti I. HIV infection and the gut: scarred for life? *J Infect Dis* 2008; **198**: 453–5.
10 Kotler DP, Gaetz HP, Lange M, *et al.* Enteropathy associated with the acquired immunodeficiency syndrome. *Ann Intern Med* 1984; **101**: 421–8.
11 Douek DC, Picker LJ, Koup RA. T cell dynamics in HIV-1 infection. *Annu Rev Immunol* 2003; **21**: 265–304.

12 Brenchley JM, Price DA, Schacker TW, *et al.* Microbial translocation is a cause of systemic immune activation in chronic HIV infection. *Nat Med* 2006; **12**: 1365–71.

13 Giorgi JV, Lyles RH, Matud JL, *et al.* Predictive value of immunologic and virologic markers after long or short duration of HIV-1 infection. *J Acq Immun Def Synd* 2002; **29**: 346–55.

14 Brenchley JM, Schacker TW, Ruff LE, *et al.* CD4+ T cell depletion during all stages of HIV disease occurs predominantly in the gastrointestinal tract. *J Exp Med* 2004; **200**: 749–59.

15 Mehandru S, Poles MS, Tenner-Racz K, *et al.* Lack of mucosal immune reconstitution during prolonged treatment of acute and early HIV infection. *PLoS Med* 2006; **3**: e484.

16 Schacker TW, Reilly C, Bellman GJ, *et al.* Amount of lymphatic tissue fibrosis in HIV infection predicts magnitude of HAART-associated change in peripheral CD4 cell count. *AIDS* 2005; **19**: 2169–71.

17 Thom K, Forrest G. Gastrointestinal infections in immunocompromised hosts. *Curr Opin Gastroenterol* 2006; **22**: 18–23.

18 Wilcox CM, Saag MS. Gastrointestinal complications of HIV infection: changing priorities in the HAART era. *Gut* 2008; **57**: 861–70.

19 Weber R, Ledergerber B, Zbinden R, *et al.* Enteric infections and diarrhea in human immunodeficiency virus-infected persons: Prospective community-based cohort study. *Arch Intern Med* 1999; **159**: 1473.

20 Manabe YC, Clark DP, Moore RD, *et al.* Cryptosporidiosis in patients with AIDS: Correlates of disease and survival. *Clin Infect Dis* 1998; **27**: 536.

21 Angulo FJ, Swerdlow DL. Bacterial enteric infections in persons infected with human immunodeficiency virus. *Clin Infect Dis* 1995; **21** (Suppl. 1): S84–93.

22 Centers for Disease Control and Prevention (CDC). Revision of the CDC surveillance case definition for acquired immunodeficiency syndrome. *MMWR* 1987; **36**: 1–15S

23 Wilcox CM, Chalasani N, Lazenby A, *et al.* Cytomegalovirus colitis in AIDS: An endoscopic and clinical study. *Gastrointest Endosc* 1998; **48**: 58.

24 Monkemuller KE, Bussian AH, Lazenby AJ, *et al.* Special histologic stains are rarely beneficial for the evaluation of HIV-related gastrointestinal infections. *Am J Clin Pathol* 2000; **114**: 387.

25 Wilcox CM. Etiology and evaluation of diarrhea in AIDS: A global perspective at the millennium. *World J Gastroenterol* 2000; **6**: 177.

26 Chevret S, Scieux C, Garrait V, *et al.* Usefulness of the cytomegalovirus (CMV) antigenemia assay for predicting the occurrence of CMV disease and death in patients with AIDS. *Clin Infect Dis* 1999; **28**: 758.

27 Kirk O, Reiss P, Uberti-Foppa C, *et al.* Safe interruption of maintenance therapy against previous infection with four common HIV-associated opportunistic pathogens during potent antiretroviral therapy. *Ann Intern Med* 2002; **20**: 137–9.

28 Tumbarello M, Tacconelli E, Leone F, *et al.* Clostridium difficile-associated diarrhoea in patients with human immunodeficiency virus infection: a case-control study. *Eur J Gastroenterol Hepatol* 1995; **7**: 259–63.

29 Liesenfeld O, Schneider T, Schmidt W, *et al.* Culture of intestinal biopsy specimens and stool culture for detection of bacterial enteropathogens in patients infected with human immunodeficiency virus. *J Clin Microbiol* 1995; **33**: 745.

30 Horsburgh Jr CR, Gettings J, Alexander LN, *et al.* Disseminated Mycobacterium avium complex disease among patients infected with human immunodeficiency virus, 1986–2000. *Clin Infect Dis* 2001; **33**: 1938.

31 Van Altena R, Van Beckevoort D, Kersemans P, *et al.* Imaging of gastrointestinal and abdominal tuberculosis. *Eur Radiol* 2004; **14**: E103.

32 Lamps LW, Molina CP, West AB, *et al.* The pathologic spectrum of gastrointestinal and hepatic histoplasmosis. *Am J Clin Pathol* 2000; **113**: 64.

33 Cimerman S, Cimerman B, Lewi DS. Prevalence of intestinal parasitic infections in patients with acquired immunodeficiency syndrome in Brazil. *Int J Infect Dis* 1999; **3**: 203.

34 Kent CK, Chaw JK, Wong W, *et al.* Prevalence of rectal, urethral, and pharyngeal chlamydia and gonorrhea detected in 2 clinical settings among men who have sex with men: San Francisco, California, 2003. *Clin Infect Dis* 2005; **41**: 67–74.

35 Centers for Disease Control and Prevention (CDC). Lymphogranuloma venereum among men who have sex with men—Netherlands, 2003–2004. *MMWR* 2004; **53**: 985–88.

36 Mindel A, Tovey SJ, Timmins DJ, Williams P. Primary and secondary syphilis, 20 years' experience. 2. Clinical features. *Genitourin Med* 1989; **65**: 1–3.

37 Goodell SE, Quinn TC, Mkrtichian E, *et al.* Herpes simplex virus proctitis in homosexual men. Clinical, sigmoidoscopic, and histopathological features. *N Engl J Med* 1983; **308**: 868–71.

38 Young H, Manavi K, McMillan A. Evaluation of ligase chain reaction for the noncultural detection of rectal and pharyngeal gonorrhoea in men who have sex with men. *Sex Transm Infect* 2003; **79**: 484–6.

39 Call SA, Heudebert G, Saag M, *et al.* The changing etiology of chronic diarrhea in HIV-infected patients with CD4 cell counts less than 200 cells/mm³. *Am J Gastroenterol* 2000; **95**: 3142.

40 Quinn TC, Stamm WE, Goodell SE, *et al.* The polymicrobial origin of intestinal infections in homosexual men. *N Engl J Med* 1983; **309**: 576–82.

41 Panther LA, Wagner K, Proper JA, *et al.* High resolution anoscopy findings for men who have sex with men: Inaccuracy of anal cytology as a predictor of histologic highgrade anal intraepithelial neoplasia and the impact of HIV serostatus. *Clin Infect Dis* 2004; **38**: 1490.

42 King CK, Glass R, Bresee JS, Duggan C; Centers for Disease Control and Prevention. Managing acute gastroenteritis among children: oral rehydration, maintenance, and nutritional therapy. *MMWR* 2003; **52** (RR-16): 1–16.

43 Gilbert DN, Moellering RC, Eliopoulos GM, Sande MA. *The Sanford Guide to Antimicrobial Therapy*, 38th edn. Antimicrobial Therapy, Inc, USA, 2008: 15–17, 123.

44 Centers for Disease Control and Prevention (CDC). Increase in fluoroquinolone-resistant Neisseria gonorrhoeae among men who have sex with men—United States, 2003, and revised recommendations for gonorrhea treatment, 2004. *MMWR* 2004; **53**: 335–8.

PART 5

Diseases of the Pancreas

62 Acute Pancreatitis and (Peri)pancreatic Fluid Collections, 371
Santhi Swaroop Vege

63 Chronic Pancreatitis and Pancreatic Pseudocysts, 378
Pierre Hindy and Scott Tenner

64 Pancreatic Cancer and Cystic Pancreatic Neoplasms, 383
William R. Brugge

Acute Pancreatitis and (Peri)pancreatic Fluid Collections

Santhi Swaroop Vege

Division of Gastroenterology and Hepatology, Mayo Clinic, Rochester, MN, USA

Summary

Among patients with acute pancreatitis, 90% have interstitial disease and 10% have necrotizing disease. Contrast-enhanced computed tomography (CT) scan provides valuable information regarding the severity of the disease and complications, including peripancreatic fluid collections. Assessment of disease severity at admission and within the first 24 hours is of critical importance in providing optimal care. Fluid resuscitation and careful pulmonary care are also critical. The two most important markers of severity during hospitalization are persistent organ failure and (peri)pancreatic necrosis. Therapy of sterile pancreatic necrosis is medical during the first several weeks; at a later stage, when walled-off pancreas necrosis causes gastroduodenal or biliary obstruction or "persistently unwell state," intervention by a minimally invasive route for debridement may be needed. Therapy of infected pancreatic necrosis, which can be diagnosed clinically or, occasionally, by image-guided percutaneous aspiration, most often involves minimally-invasive-route debridement.

Case

A 44-year-old woman presents with severe epigastric pain requiring administration of narcotic agents. Abdominal ultrasound reveals multiple small gallstones. The common bile duct is not dilated. Serum amylase and lipase values are five times the upper limit of normal. Contrast-enhanced CT scan shows an enlarged pancreas with heterogeneous enhancement and considerable fluid around the pancreas (Figure 62.1a).

The patient is started on fluid replacement at a rate of 200 mL/h. Her hematocrit is noted to be increased from 48 to 50 and her blood urea nitrogen (BUN) from 17 to 24 mg/% 24 hours after admission. Because she shows labored respiration and deterioration of oxygenation, she is transferred to an intensive care unit (ICU), intubated with assisted ventilation, and eventually given dialysis for acute renal failure. She is also treated prophylactically with imipenem and receives total parenteral nutrition. A CT scan obtained weekly shows evolution from necrotizing pancreatitis to walled-off pancreatic and peripancreatic necrosis involving 85% of the pancreas (Figure 62.1b). She gradually improves, is extubated, and her renal function returns to normal. However, over the next several weeks, she develops abdominal pain each time she tries to consume a low-fat diet, such that her caloric intake remains unsatisfactory.

Introduction

Acute pancreatitis is an acute inflammatory condition of the pancreas [1]. At one end of the spectrum is interstitial pancreatitis, with mild edema of the pancreas associated at times with inflammation of the fat in the peripancreatic area and the development of fluid collections around the pancreas. At the other end is a more severe form of the disease, characterized by necrosis of the parenchyma, at times associated with considerable fat necrosis around the pancreas. The use of contrast-enhanced CT scan is of great help in distinguishing interstitial from necrotizing pancreatitis [2].

Definitions

Interstitial Pancreatitis

Interstitial pancreatitis is characterized by focal or diffuse enlargement of the pancreas. The parenchyma of the pancreas enhances in a homogeneous fashion when imaged by contrast-enhanced CT scan or magnetic resonance imaging (MRI) (Figure 62.2).

Pancreatic Necrosis

Pancreatic necrosis is defined by the presence of diffuse or focal areas of non-viable pancreatic parenchyma with at least 30% non-enhancement of the pancreas when imaged by contrast-enhanced CT scan or MRI. Pancreatic necrosis is usually associated with at least some peripancreatic fat necrosis [3] (Figure 62.3).

Extrapancreatic Fluid Collections

Extrapancreatic fluid collections form when pancreatic fluid extravasates out of the pancreas into the anterior pararenal space and sometimes elsewhere during acute pancreatitis. Extrapancreatic fluid collections may occur in either interstitial or necrotizing pancreatitis. In most instances, they resolve as pancreatic inflammation resolves. In some instances, however, the fluid collection persists, with two possible outcomes. In the first, when there is little in the way of peripancreatic fat necrosis, the fluid collection becomes a somewhat oval or rounded fluid-filled structure enclosed by a fibrous capsule, termed a "pancreatic pseudocyst." Pseudocysts in acute pancreatitis are rare because the simple fluid collections from which they develop usually spontaneously resolve before 4 weeks. In the second outcome, when the fluid becomes associated with substantial peripancreatic fat necrosis, the collection may persist

---

Practical Gastroenterology and Hepatology Board Review Toolkit, Second Edition. Edited by Nicholas J. Talley, Kenneth R. DeVault, Michael B. Wallace, Bashar A. Aqel and Keith D. Lindor.

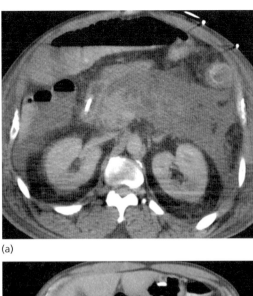

(a)

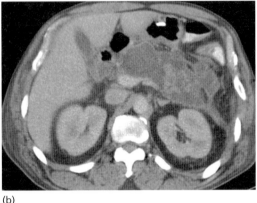

(b)

Figure 62.1 (a) Axial contrast-enhanced computed tomography (CT) image obtained in a 44-year-old female, showing subtotal necrosis of the pancreatic gland, with acute fluid collections in the anterior pararenal space. (b) Axial contrast-enhanced CT image obtained 4 weeks later, showing walled-off pancreatic and extrapancreatic necrosis.

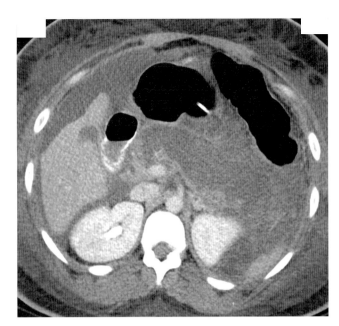

Figure 62.3 Necrotizing pancreatitis. Axial contrast-enhanced CT image obtained in a 38-year-old female, showing necrosis of the pancreatic gland with acute fluid collections in the anterior pararenal space.

indefinitely, or it may evolve into a structure enclosed by a fibrous capsule overlying the pancreas, termed "peripancreatic walled-off necrosis." The CT appearance of extrapancreatic fluid collection is of a homogeneous low-density fluid, whereas peripancreatic fat necrosis is a more heterogeneous collection, frequently containing globules of fat [4–6] (Figure 62.4).

Pancreatic Pseudocyst

A pancreatic pseudocyst is a collection of pancreatic juice enclosed by a wall of fibrous or granulation tissue. It occurs in association with acute pancreatitis, pancreatic trauma, or chronic pancreatitis. It

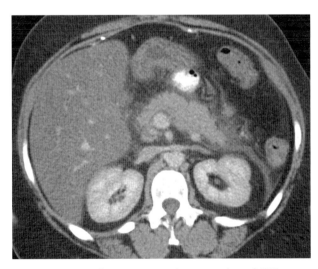

Figure 62.2 Interstitial pancreatitis. Axial contrast-enhanced CT image obtained in a 39-year-old female, showing mild swelling of the pancreatic gland but normal enhancement. Note acute fluid collections in the anterior pararenal space.

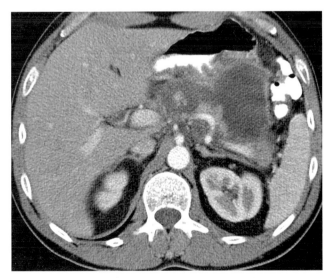

Figure 62.4 Extrapancreatic fluid collection. Axial contrast-enhanced CT image obtained in a 49-year-old male with necrotizing pancreatitis, showing pancreatic necrosis and the presence of extrapancreatic walled-off necrosis.

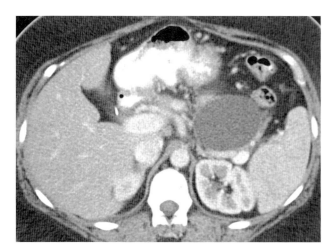

Figure 62.5 Pseudocyst. Axial contrast-enhanced CT image obtained in a 39-year-old female 6 weeks following an episode of interstitial pancreatitis, showing a 6 cm well-defined homogenous low-density fluid collection.

requires at least 4 weeks from the onset of acute pancreatitis to form a well-defined wall. Pseudocysts may gradually enlarge, stay approximately the same size, diminish, or even resolve completely. While most pseudocysts occur as a result of loculation of an extrapancreatic fluid collection, some occur as a result of pancreatic ductal disruption, leading to a localized collection of enzyme-rich pancreatic fluid that loculates close to the pancreas and, at times, at remote sites. The appearance of a pancreatic pseudocyst on CT scan is of an encapsulated, homogenous, non-enhancing, low-density fluid collection [7] (Figure 62.5).

Walled-Off Peripancreatic Necrosis

Peripancreatic necrosis evolves into a walled-off collection involving only peripancreatic tissue with sparing of the pancreatic parenchyma. It requires 3–4 weeks from the onset of pancreatitis to develop. On CT scan, it is a heterogeneous, non-enhancing, low-density structure, which may contain tiny globules of fat.

Walled-Off Pancreatic Necrosis

Walled-off pancreatic necrosis occurs when the necrosis is substantial and is confined to the pancreas. It usually takes at least 3–4 weeks to form and contains solid or semisolid pancreatic necrotic debris. On CT scan, it appears as a heterogeneous, non-enhancing, low-density structure conforming to the expected size of the pancreas and demarcated by a fibrous capsule. This entity was originally termed "central cavitary necrosis." Walled-off necrosis in the absence of walled-off peripancreatic necrosis is very uncommon.

Walled-Off Pancreatic and Peripancreatic Necrosis

This entity can be recognized 3–4 weeks after severe necrotizing pancreatitis. Walled-off pancreatic and peripancreatic necrosis involves both the pancreatic tissue that has become necrotic and peripancreatic fat which has also become necrotic. The structure that is visualized on CT scan is a somewhat ovoid or rounded, non-enhancing, low-density structure demarcated by a fibrous capsule (Figure 62.6). After a period of some additional weeks, the walled-off pancreatic and peripancreatic necrosis undergoes progressive liquefaction. On contrast-enhanced CT scan, it is difficult to distinguish the extent to which the necrosis liquefies, since the density of fluid and of necrosis as imaged on CT scan can be identical. Imaging

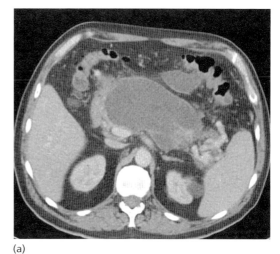

(a)

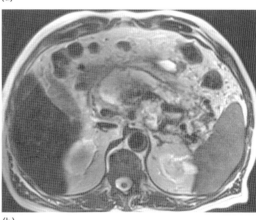

(b)

Figure 62.6 Walled-off pancreatic and peripancreatic necrosis. (a) Axial contrast-enhanced CT image obtained in a 63-year-old female with necrotizing pancreatitis, showing pancreatic necrosis and the presence of extrapancreatic walled-off necrosis. (b) Axial contrast-enhanced MRI obtained in the same patient 5 days later, better illustrating the heterogeneous appearance of the extrapancreatic necrosis.

by MRI or endoscopic ultrasound (EUS) can frequently distinguish necrotic from liquefied material [7] (Figure 62.6).

Epidemiology

Recent data show the absolute number and rate of emergency ward visits for these conditions are increasing in the United States. Hospital admissions (200 000 admissions in 2002) and direct health care costs are also increasing (annual direct costs in excess of USD2 billion) [8, 9]. In the United States, acute pancreatitis was the most common gastrointestinal (GI) hospital discharge diagnosis in 2009, with a cost of USD2.6 billion [10].

Pathophysiology

The initiating event appears to be inappropriate activation of trypsinogen to trypsin within pancreatic acinar cells. Activated trypsin then activates a variety of other proteases and phospholipase A-2, resulting in pancreatic injury. A variety of cytokines and chemokines are released from acinar cells, which attract inflammatory cells from the circulation, including macrophages and neutrophils. Inflammatory mediators from these cells intensify the

CHAPTER 62

inflammatory response within the pancreas and set in motion an amplified systemic inflammatory response that can culminate in organ failure, including refractory shock, renal failure, and respiratory failure [1].

Clinical Features

Almost all patients have severe abdominal pain lasting for many hours. The pain is frequently in the epigastrium and left upper quadrant, and may radiate to the back. The intensity of the pain rarely fluctuates and is frequently intolerable. Additional symptoms are nausea and vomiting. Physical examination is noteworthy for severe upper abdominal tenderness at times, with guarding.

The best scores/markers to predict severe acute pancreatitis at admission and at 48 hours are systemic inflammatory response syndrome (SIRS), presence of organ failure, hemoconcentration with hematocrit >44%, and an increase in APACHE II score (such as >8) [11].

The SIRS is defined by two or more of the following criteria:
- Pulse >90 bpm;
- Respirations >20/min or pCO_2 <32 mmHg;
- Rectal temperature <36 °C or >38 °C;
- White blood count (WBC) <4000 or >12 000/mm^3.

During admission, host risk factors (age, comorbidity, body mass index (BMI)), clinical risk stratification (SIRS), and response to initial therapy (e.g., persistent SIRS, BUN, creatinine) are the best means of predicting the outcome of acute pancreatitis [11]. *Patients with evidence of increased severity should be transferred to an ICU for closer monitoring, improvement in fluid resuscitation, and improvement in pulmonary care.*

It is now recognized that there are two phases in acute pancreatitis. In the early phase, lasting 7–10 days, the classification of severity is mainly clinical. The major component of this clinical classification is persistent organ failure (i.e., organ failure lasting >48 hours). The definition of organ failure is as follows:
- **Shock:** Systolic blood pressure <90 mmHg;
- **Pulmonary insufficiency:** PaO_2 ≤60 mmHg;
- **Renal failure:** Creatinine >2 mg/dL.

Recently, the modified Marshall score has been recommended for grading of organ failure [3]. In the second phase of acute pancreatitis, which takes place after 7–10 days, the classification of severity is both clinical (persistent organ failure) and morphologic (necrotizing vs. interstitial pancreatitis).

Acute Peripancreatic Fluid Collections

Acute peripancreatic fluid collections usually develop in the early phase of acute pancreatitis [3]. They are homogeneous and have no wall on CT scan. They are confined by normal fascial planes in the retroperitoneum and can be multiple. Most are asymptomatic and resolve spontaneously, without need for intervention. Rarely, they can persist beyond 4 weeks and develop a perceptible wall; in this case, they are called "pseudocysts."

Pancreatic Pseudocysts

It is now recognized that true pseudocysts following acute pancreatitis are rare [3]. On CT, they are usually found in the peripancreatic region (intrapancreatic psuedocysts are extremely rare) and contain clear fluid without any debris. The fluid is rich in amylase. The pathogenesis is usually a disruption of the main pancreatic duct or its branches, and very occasionally disconnected pancreatic duct. Intervention is rarely required for persistent symptomatic

pseudocysts after acute pancreatitis, CP, or abdominal trauma. Endoscopic transgastric or transduodenal drainage with or without transpapillary stenting is the preferred approach, over surgery. It is comparable to surgery in efficacy but superior in terms of length of hospital stay, cost, and patient satisfaction [12].

Acute Necrotic Collection

Pancreatic and/or peripancreatic necrosis classifies the acute pancreatitis as necrotizing. Patients have acute necrotic collections in the first 4–6 weeks, which can be differentiated from acute peripancreatic fluid collections by (i) possible heterogenous appearance; (ii) extension along the fascial planes, without being confined by them; and (iii) low attenuating, non-enhancing areas in the pancreas, caused by necrosis. However, it may be difficult to distinguish acute necrotic collections from acute peripancreatic fluid collections when they are purely peripancreatic, confined to a fascial plane, and contain homogenous material. MRI or abdominal ultrasound/EUS may be able to demonstrate necrotic material in such homogenous-appearing collections on CT. A large prospective study found that most acute necrotic collections are either pancreatic and peripancreatic or isolated peripancreatic (nearly equal distribution) [13]. Pure pancreatic necrotic collections without peripancreatic involvement are extremely rare.

Walled-Off Necrosis

Acute necrotic collections usually persist (unlike acute peripancreatic fluid collections) and may develop a wall after 4–6 weeks; they are called "walled-off necrosis" at that stage. Occasionally, they may be misclassified as "pseudocysts" if they appear homogenous on CT scan. As already mentioned, MRI or ultrasound (transabdominal or endoscopic) can identify the necrotic material. These collections may remain sterile or become infected. Infection usually starts 7–10 days after onset. Sterile necrosis (if symptomatic) and infected necrosis are indications for intervention after 4–6 weeks when the wall develops. It is no longer necessary to carry out fine-needle aspiration (FNA) of pancreatic or peripancreatic necrosis in order to diagnose infection [2]. Infection is most often diagnosed by clinical features like fever, chills, and leukocytosis and by worsening clinical status and the presence of gas bubbles on CT scan. It is recommended that interventions be delayed until this period to avoid mortality and morbidity [14]. Interventions should ideally be minimally invasive (endoscopic, percutaneous, laparoscopic, video-assisted retroperitoneal, or a combination). Open surgery is inferior to minimally invasive methods for debridement/necrosectomy of such collections [15].

Disconnection of the main pancreatic duct may result in pancreatic necrosis and can be diagnosed by magnetic resonance cholangiopancreatography (MRCP). This may result in persistence of walled-off necrosis, which can sometimes be managed by endoscopic reconnection of the duct with a stent, or more often by leaving the transgastric pigtail catheters in the collection for several months or by distal pancreatectomy of the excluded pancreatic tail or pancreatico-jejunostomy.

Diagnosis

The diagnosis of acute pancreatitis requires two of the following three features:
- Abdominal pain strongly suggestive of acute pancreatitis.
- Serum amylase and/or lipase at least three times the upper limit of normal.

- Characteristic findings of acute pancreatitis on imaging studies, such as contrast-enhanced CT scan.

Case Continued

The severe upper abdominal pain and markedly elevated amylase and lipase (five times the upper limit of normal) are sufficient to make a diagnosis of acute pancreatitis. CT scan is not necessary to confirm the diagnosis of acute pancreatitis and does not provide information of help in the care of the patient during the first 1–2 weeks of treatment.

The patient undergoes active treatment for multisystem organ failure. The confirmation of pancreatic necrosis based on contrast-enhanced CT scan informs the clinician that recovery will be prolonged and the patient will need nutritional support.

Differential Diagnosis

The differential diagnosis of acute pancreatitis is wide (Table 62.1). Elevations of amylase and lipase (even occasionally more than three times the upper limit of normal) may occur in at least some of these diseases.

Therapeutics

A management algorithm for acute pancreatitis is provided in Figure 62.7. Table 62.2 summarizes the evidence base.

Table 62.1 Differential diagnosis of acute pancreatitis.

Abdominal conditions	Intestinal perforation
	Intestinal obstruction
	Mesenteric vascular disease
	Biliary tract disease
	Abdominal aortic aneurysm
Thoracic conditions	Acute myocardial infarction

Interstitial Pancreatitis

The therapy of interstitial pancreatitis is supportive. Fluid resuscitation and careful monitoring of oxygen saturation are key. Organ failure occurs in less than 10% of cases and is usually transient.

Necrotizing Pancreatitis

Necrotizing pancreatitis is generally a more severe disease than interstitial pancreatitis [2, 3]. One-half of the patients who die do so in the first 7–14 days because of persistent organ failure. The other half die later from complications of the necrotizing pancreatitis, such as unresolved organ failure or development of infected necrosis. Clinical care in the first several weeks is dominated by fluid resuscitation, careful pulmonary care, and treatment of other clinical features, such as refractory shock, renal failure, and evolving pulmonary insufficiency, which may require intubation. The adequacy of fluid resuscitation should be monitored every 12 hours. If the BUN has increased during this interval, additional fluid resuscitation is required.

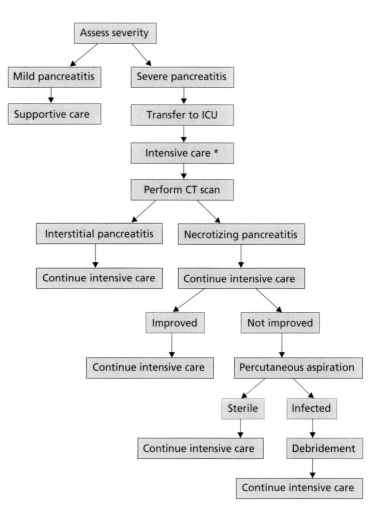

Figure 62.7 Management algorithm for treatment of acute pancreatitis. *Treat organ failure, start enteral feeding.

CHAPTER 62

Table 62.2 Evidence-based therapeutics.

Supportive care (level of evidence 3)
Transfer to an intensive care unit (ICU) (level of evidence 3)
Nutritional support: enteral feeding (level of evidence 2)
Use of prophylaxis antibiotics in necrotizing pancreatitis is not recommended (level of evidence 3)
Treatment of infected necrosis – surgical debridement (level of evidence 3)
Treatment of sterile necrosis – medical (level of evidence 3)
Role of endoscopic retrograde cholangiopancreatography (ERCP) and biliary sphincterotomy – limited (level of evidence 1)

Feeding can be oral in mild acute pancreatitis if the patients can tolerate it. In severe cases (usually clear by day 5), enteral feeding by the nasojejunal or nasogastric route is recommended for several weeks until the complications resolve and the patient can eat. If enteral feeding is not tolerated or is inadequate to meet the nutritional requirements – and only then – total parenteral nutritional (TPN) will be needed.

Nasojejunal feeding is currently thought to be safer and less expensive than TPN, but has not as yet been proven to reduce the severity of acute pancreatitis. Several recent randomized prospective placebo-controlled trials have failed to establish a benefit of prophylactic antibiotics in preventing the development of infected necrosis. The use of antibiotics should be restricted to those who have an infection, and at times during a prolonged hospitalization, a patient may require brief courses of antibiotics for well-documented infection, such as pneumonia or urinary or respiratory tract infection. Antibiotics should be discontinued once infections are properly treated. At other times, a patient may appear septic and can be placed on broad-spectrum antibiotics for a few days while appropriate cultures are obtained. If a source of infection is not discovered, the antibiotics should be discontinued.

Urgent endoscopic sphincterotomy has a role in severe biliary pancreatitis in case of documented cholangitis. It may be considered in those with dilated bile duct and with stones on imaging in the absence of cholangitis. Otherwise, it is elective before cholecystectomy in patients with biliary pancreatitis.

Case Continued

Early transfer to an ICU is required, given evidence of organ failure in need of more intensive supervision. The patient's fluid resuscitation of only 200 mL/h is clearly inadequate in view of the increased hematocrit and BUN during the first 24 hours of hospitalization. She is placed on TPN rather than nasojejunal feeding. She is also given imipenem as a prophylactic antibiotic. A biliary sphincterotomy is not performed because there is no evidence of ascending cholangitis, the patient's common bile duct is not dilated, and her liver function tests (LFTs) return to normal within 48 hours.

Because she develops severe abdominal pain each time she tries to eat, she undergoes a surgical cystojejunostomy with aspiration of the fluid and debridement of necrotic pancreatic tissue. She leaves the hospital 1 week after the surgery, receiving insulin for diabetes mellitus and pancreatic enzymes for steatorrhea.

Prognosis

Prognosis of interstitial pancreatitis is generally favorable, with mortality below 2%. Mortality is usually due to unresolved organ failure, especially in a patient with comorbidity.

Prognosis of necrotizing pancreatitis is more severe. In necrotizing pancreatitis not associated with organ failure or other complications, mortality is less than 5%. Mortality of necrotizing pancreatitis in association with multisystem organ failure is as high as 50%.

Take Home Points

- The diagnosis of acute pancreatitis requires two of the following three features: abdominal pain strongly suggestive of acute pancreatitis; serum amylase and/or lipase at least three times the upper limit of normal; and characteristic findings of acute pancreatic on imaging studies, such as contrast-enhanced computed tomography (CT) scan.
- There are two phases of acute pancreatitis. In the early phase, lasting 7–10 days, clinical classification of severity is based on persistent organ failure. In the late phase, after 7–10 days, the clinical classification of severity is persistent organ failure; morphologic classification of severity is necrotizing versus interstitial pancreatitis.
- Approximately 90% of cases of acute pancreatitis are interstitial (mortality approximately 3%), while 10% are necrotizing (overall mortality approximately 15%).
- Risk factors for severity at admission include systemic inflammatory response syndrome (SIRS), older age, comorbidity, and obesity.
- Markers of severity at admission include SIRS, organ failure, serum hematocrit, and APACHE II score.
- Severity of acute pancreatitis during hospitalization is defined primarily by persistent organ failure and peripancreatic and/or pancreatic necrosis.
- Distinction between interstitial and necrotizing pancreatitis is made by contrast-enhanced CT scan.
- There are now well-defined criteria on contrast-enhanced CT scan by which to distinguish interstitial pancreatitis, necrotizing pancreatitis, extrapancreatic fluid collections, pancreatic pseudocyst, walled-off peripancreatic necrosis, and walled-off pancreatic necrosis (with or without walled-off extrapancreatic necrosis).
- Treatment guidelines include supportive care with aggressive rehydration, transfer to the intensive care unit (ICU) for organ dysfunction, nutritional support by enteral feeding, and use of endoscopic retrograde cholangiopancreatography (ERCP) primarily for suspected ascending cholangitis.
- Antibiotics should be given only for proven infection.
- Treatment of sterile necrosis is generally non-surgical, except in the case of symptomatic walled-off necrosis.
- Treatment of infected necrosis is usually minimally invasive debridement.

Videos of interest to readers of this chapter can be found by visiting the companion website at:

http://www.practicalgastrohep.com/

62.1 Minor papillotomy in a patient with acute recurrent pancreatitis and pancreas divisum with Santorinicele.
62.2 Drainage of a pseudocyst with stents.
62.3 Endoscopic ultrasound aspiration of a cyst.

References

1 Pandol SJ, Saluja AK, Imrie CW, Banks PA. Acute pancreatitis: bench to the bedside. *Gastroenterology* 2007; **132**: 1127–51.

2 Tenner S, Baillie J, Dewitt J, Vege SS. American College of Gastroenterology guideline: management of acute pancreatitis. *Am J Gastroenterol* 2013; **108**: 1400–15.

3 Banks PA, Bollen T, Dervenis C, *et al.* Classification of acute pancreatitis – 2012: revision of the Atlanta classification and definitions by international consensus. *Gut* 2013; **62**: 102–11.

4 Lenhart DK, Balthazar EJ. MDCT of acute mild (nonnecrotizing) pancreatitis: abdominal complications and fate of fluid collections. *Am J Roentgenol* 2008; **190**: 643–9.

5 Morgan DE. Imaging of acute pancreatitis and its complications. *Clin Gastroenterol Hepatol* 2008; **6**: 1077–85.

6 van Santvoort HC, Bollen TL, Besselink MG, *et al.* Describing peripancreatic collections in severe acute pancreatitis using morphologic terms: an international interobserver agreement study. *Pancreatology* 2008; **8**: 593–9.

7 Takahashi N, Papachristou GI, Schmit GD, *et al.* CT findings of walled-off pancreatic necrosis (WOPN): differentiation from pseudocyst and prediction of outcome after endoscopic therapy. *Eur Radiol* 2008; **18**: 2522–9.

8 Fagenholz PJ, Fernandez-del Castillo C, Harris NS, *et al.* Direct medical costs of acute pancreatitis hospitalization in United States. *Pancreas* 2007; **35**: 302–7.

9 Fagenholz PJ, Fernandez-del Castillo C, Harris NS, *et al.* Increasing United States hospital admissions for acute pancreatitis 1988–2003. *Ann Epidemiol* 2007; **17**: 491–7.

10 Peery AE, Dellon ES, Lund J, *et al.* Burden of gastrointestinal diseases in the United States. 2012 update. *Gastroenterology* 2012; **143**: 1179–87.

11 Working Group IAP/APA Acute Pancreatitis Guidelines. IAP/APA evidence-based guidelines in the management of acute pancreatitis. *Pancreatology* 2013; **13**(4 Suppl. 2): e1–15.

12 Varadarajulu S, Bang JY, Sutton BS, *et al.* Equal efficacy of endoscopic and surgical cystogastrostomy for pancreatic pseudocyst drainage in a randomized trial. *Gastroenterology* 2013; **145**: 583–90.

13 Bakker OJ, van Santvoort H, Besselink MG, *et al.* Extrapancreatic necrosis without pancreatic parenchymal necrosis : a separate entity in necrotizing pancreatitis? *Gut* 2012; **18**: 143–9.

14 Freeman ML, Werner J, van Santvoort HC, *et al.* Interventions for pancreatic necrosis: summary of a multidisciplinary consensus conference. *Pancreas* 2012; **41**: 1176–94.

15 van Santvoort HC, Besselink MG, Bakker OJ, *et al.* A step-up approach or open necrosectomy for necrotizing pancreatitis. *New Engl J Med* 2010; **362**: 1491–502.

CHAPTER 62

Chronic Pancreatitis and Pancreatic Pseudocysts

Pierre Hindy and Scott Tenner

Division of Gastroenterology, Department of Medicine, State University of New York – Health Sciences Center, Brooklyn, NY, USA

Summary

Though chronic pancreatitis has a variety of clinical manifestations, patients most often present with intermittent chronic abdominal pain. The pain originates from a myriad of protean manifestations, including inflammation and increased ductal and/or parenchymal pressure. In select patients, endoscopic or surgical decompression of the pancreatic duct has been shown to decrease pain. Pancreatic duct disruption and/or increased pancreatic ductal pressure can lead to a pseudocyst formation. In patients with chronic pancreatitis, the pancreatic duct can become obstructed by fibrous scarring, inspissated protein, or stone(s), and the ongoing pancreatic secretion proximal to the obstruction leads to a saccular dilation of the duct, filled with pancreatic juice. These saccular dilatations can enlarge to become fibrous, non-epithelialized, walled-off cysts: pseudocysts. Pseudocysts can cause symptoms of pain, early satiety, nausea, vomiting, and weight loss, and can be complicated by obstruction (biliary and or enteric), hemorrhage, and infection. In the patient with chronic pancreatitis who develops symptomatic pseudocysts, a multidisciplinary approach to drain these cysts, including endoscopic, surgical, and percutaneous methods, should be considered, depending on local expertise and the character and location of the cysts.

Case

A 53-year-old male suffering from depression and a long history of chronic alcohol abuse presents to the ER with complaints of mid-abdominal pain and changes in his bowel habits. He has slowly developed loose, malodorous stools. The symptoms have been intermittently occurring over the past 5 years but now have become more persistent. He has developed insulin-dependent diabetes. Over the past year, he has developed recurrent attacks of abdominal pain. He has been told on several admissions to the hospital that he has the diagnosis of chronic pancreatitis. An endoscopic retrograde cholangiopancreaticography (ERCP) performed during the last admission demonstrated pancreatic duct stricturing and diffuse areas of ductular dilation.

A computed tomographic (CT) scan is performed, which reveals a new pseudocyst in the body of the pancreas (Figure 63.1). ERCP is performed, with placement of two transpapillary stents to promote resolution of the cysts. One stent is placed traversing the cyst in the main pancreatic duct, the other in the cyst (Figure 63.2). The patient's pain quickly resolves. Both stents are removed 2 weeks later. Pancreatic enzyme supplementation for the steatorrhea is given

(50 000 IU of lipase per meal) The diarrhea resolves over 2 weeks. The patient discontinues alcohol use, and remains well and pain-free.

Chronic Pancreatitis

Chronic pancreatitis is a syndrome of progressive, irreversible, destructive, inflammatory changes in the pancreas that results in permanent structural damage, leading to impairment of exocrine and endocrine function. Histologic changes include irregular fibrosis, acinar cell loss, islet cell loss, and inflammatory cell infiltrates.

Clinical Manifestations

The hallmark manifestations of chronic pancreatitis are abdominal pain and exocrine insufficiency. Abdominal pain is the most common presenting complaint, seen in 50–90% of patients. The pain is typically epigastric, radiates to the back, is worse after meals, and may be relieved by sitting upright or leaning forward (pancreatic position). Early in the course, the pain may be intermittent and occur in discrete attacks, but as the disease progresses, the pain becomes more continuous. Severe pain may decrease the appetite and limit food consumption, contributing to weight loss and malnutrition. Clinically significant protein and fat deficiencies do not occur until over 90% of pancreatic function is lost. Steatorrhea usually occurs prior to protein deficiencies. The clinical manifestations of fat malabsorption include loose, greasy, foul-smelling stools that are difficult to flush. Glucose intolerance occurs in chronic pancreatitis, but overt diabetes usually occurs late in the course of disease.

Diagnosis

Histology is the gold standard for the diagnosis of chronic pancreatitis; however, this is invasive and rarely performed. Therefore, the diagnosis of chronic pancreatitis is based upon a combination of clinical, radiographic, and functional findings.

The diagnosis of chronic pancreatitis is generally made by detecting calcifications in the pancreas, on either plain abdominal radiograph or CT scan. Though insensitive, the finding of pancreatic stones is quite specific. In patients with early chronic pancreatitis, the diagnosis is often difficult and is usually established by a combination of findings related to the pancreatic duct that are identified by ERCP, magnetic resonance cholangiopancreaticography (MRCP), or endoscopic ultrasonography (EUS). Early structural changes can be detected by EUS. Early functional deficiencies can be established

Practical Gastroenterology and Hepatology Board Review Toolkit, Second Edition. Edited by Nicholas J. Talley, Kenneth R. DeVault, Michael B. Wallace, Bashar A. Aqel and Keith D. Lindor.
© 2016 John Wiley & Sons, Ltd. Published 2016 by John Wiley & Sons, Ltd. Companion website: www.practicalgastrohep.com

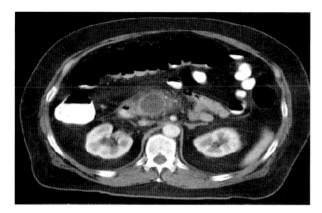

Figure 63.1 New pseudocyst in the body of the pancreas.

by a secretin stimulation test or even fecal elastase. Early in the course of chronic pancreatitis, symptoms may mask pancreatic cancer. Findings suggestive of pancreatic cancer in patients with known or suspected chronic pancreatitis include weight loss, lack of alcohol intake, and insignificant constitutional symptoms. Genetic mutations (CFTR and SPINK-1 genes) have been associated with chronic pancreatitis; however, testing for the mutation has not been recommended as it is non-diagnostic and expensive.

Treatment

Chronic pancreatitis therapy involves pain management and correction of pancreatic insufficiency. The pain associated with chronic pancreatitis, as previously described, may become continuous with the progression of the disease, and a significant change in the pain pattern should alert physicians to the development of potential serious etiologies such as peptic ulcer disease or pancreatic carcinoma.

Pain management should follow a stepwise approach. Alcohol and smoking abstinence should be considered first. Pancreatic enzymes have a limited role in the treatment of pain for chronic pancreatitis. Only one of six randomized controlled trials (RCTs) shows a statistically significant benefit, with just 52% of the pooled patient population expressing a preference for enzyme over placebo [1]. It is the opinion of the authors that pancreatic enzymes do not treat pain in patients with chronic pancreatitis, regardless of cause. Pancreatic enzymes should be reserved for use in patients manifesting malabsorption as part of the process of chronic pancreatitis. Analgesics (with opiates and/or non-steroidal anti-inflammatory drugs (NSAIDs)) should be considered next, and if patients continue to have pain, then endoscopic therapy, extracorporeal shock-wave lithotripsy, celiac nerve block, or even surgery should be considered. Surgery is usually reserved for patients who fail medical therapy. Drainage, resection, and denervation are the main surgical approaches, according to the size of the pancreatic duct and the location of disease in the pancreas.

Pancreatic insufficiency should first be treated with dietary restriction of fat intake (<20 g per day) then, if malabsorption persists, with lipase supplementation. Fat-soluble vitamins may need to be replaced, and in patients with severe weight loss, medium-chain fatty acids can be considered.

Pseudocysts

Natural History

A pancreatic pseudocyst is an amylase-rich fluid collection located within or near the pancreas. Whether in a patient with acute

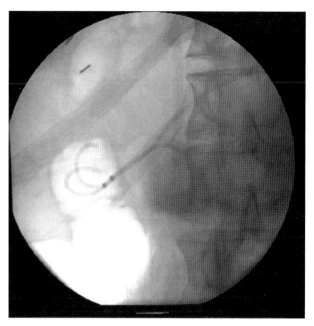

Figure 63.2 Transpapillary drainage of pseudocyst with stents in the main pancreatic duct (traversing the cyst) and in the pseudocyst.

pancreatitis or in one with chronic pancreatitis, a pseudocyst forms when there is direct leakage of pancreatic juice from an inflamed area of the gland into the parenchyma or to an adjacent space. Rarely, these cystic lesions can occur at significant distances from the pancreas, including the mediastinum and pelvis. Regardless, ductular disruption is the most important event in the formation of a pseudocyst. Ductular disruption allows this pancreatic enzyme-rich fluid to evoke an inflammatory response leading to the formation of granulation tissue and fibrosis. Over time, the cyst becomes lined by a fibrous, non-epithelialized wall.

Pancreatic pseudocysts are one of the most frequent complications in acute and chronic pancreatitis, ranging between 20 and 60% of patients [2]. Most cysts are single. The size varies from 1 to 30 cm [3].

Whereas most pseudocysts in patients with acute pancreatitis resolve spontaneously, in patients with chronic pancreatitis, many pseudocysts persist and become symptomatic. In some series, more than 90% of pseudocysts in chronic pancreatitis that are larger than 6 cm persist, and many become infected or cause pain [4, 5]. Large pseudocysts (>6 cm) and pseudocysts that failed to resolve in 6 weeks were once considered indicatons for intervention, but the management has evolved over the last decade toward a less aggressive approach. In general, asymptomatic pseudocysts do not warrant intervention. However, in patients with pseudocysts who have symptoms related to the cyst, such as pain, early satiety, and/or infection, or who have obstruction of the common bile duct or enteral tract, drainage should occur.

Diagnosis

There is a consensus that CT or magnetic resonance imaging (MRI) scanning is mandatory for planning therapy. CT imaging yields the highest sensitivity (82–100%) and specificity (98%; negative predictive value (NPV), 92–94%) and an overall accuracy of 88–94% [6]. Though the diagnosis of pseudocyst often seems simple in the setting of a cystic lesion in the pancreas associated with recent acute pancreatitis, less common cystic pathology of the pancreas often mimics pseudocysts and may lead to inappropriate interventions. Approximately 10% of pancreatic cysts are neoplastic, including mucinous cystadenomas. It is important that the clinician maintain a sense of suspicion when faced with the patient with no prior history of acute pancreatitis who is found to have a "pseudocyst." It generally takes 3–4 weeks for the fibrous non-epithelialized wall of a pseudocyst to develop. Differentiating between pseudocysts and neoplastic cysts is important in determining the method of intervention. In general, a cystic lesion can be considered a pseudocyst if the patient had an attack of acute pancreatitis more than 3–4 weeks prior or if they have a history or clinical findings consistent with chronic pancreatitis. Though cross-sectional imaging, such as CT and MRI, can provide detailed information on anatomic and morphologic characteristics of the neoplastic cysts and pseudocysts, there is a significant overlap in the morphology of these cysts. In addition to providing high-resolution images of cyst morphology, EUS also provides the opportunity for fine-needle aspiration (FNA) for fluid analysis and cytology.

EUS-guided fluid analysis can assist in differentiating cystic lesions of the pancreas. Brugge [7] showed the value of an EUS cyst fluid analysis for carcinoembryonic antigen (CEA) in guiding cyst fluid drainage. Whereas pseudocysts and serous cysts have low CEA levels, elevated pancreatic cyst CEA is associated with a mucinous cystadenoma. The Cooperative Pancreatic Cyst Study in 2004 reported on 341 patients with cystic lesions >1 cm on EUS. The major finding of this large multicenter study in favor of FNA is that when CEA is found to be >192 ng/mL in the cystic fluid, a malignant pancreatic lesion can be assumed with a sensitivity of 73% and a specificity of 84% [8].

Another complication of acute pancreatitis is pancreatic necrosis. As the pancreatic necrosis becomes walled off, the lesions appear cystic. Walled-off pancreatic necrosis (WOPN) cannot be differentiated on CT from a pancreatic pseudocyst when the cystic lesion is within the pancreatic parenchyma. Though a history of acute pancreatitis can help identify the patient with a WOPN, in an alcoholic patient, who likely has underlying chronic pancreatitis, the history may not be as helpful. EUS or MRI can assist by identifying debris within the cystic lesion; any such debris would interfere with either endoscopic or radiologic drainage.

A pseudocyst is unlikely to resolve spontaneously if: (i) it persists for more than 6 weeks; (ii) chronic pancreatitis is evident; (iii) there is a pancreatic duct anomaly (except for a communication with the pseudocyst); or (iv) the pseudocyst is surrounded by a thick wall [9]. Studying 92 patients with chronic alcoholic pancreatitis, Gouyon and colleagues [10] reported a spontaneous regression rate of 25.7%. However, pseudocysts larger than 4 cm and those localized outside the pancreas parenchyma were more associated with persistent symptoms and complications.

Symptoms

Pain in the upper abdomen is the most common symptom in patients with pseudocysts complicating chronic pancreatitis. The pathophysiology is likely related to increased intraductal and/or intraparenchymal pressure in the pancreas. Drainage procedures appear to relieve pain by a reduction of pressure within the pancreas [11]. Occasionally, the pain becomes increasingly intense, simulating that of pancreatic carcinoma. The pain may be referred to the left more than the right hypochondrium, with radiation to the back. When there is diaphragmatic involvement, the pain may be pleuritic and even felt in the shoulder. A sudden onset of pain or exacerbation of a pre-existing pain suggests hemorrhage into the cyst or

Table 63.1 Indications for drainage of a pseudocyst complicating chronic pancreatitis pain.

Weight loss and early satiety thought to be related to compression from cyst
Gastric or duodenal outlet obstruction
Infection of the pseudocyst (abscess)
Biliary obstruction

peritoneum. Small and even some moderately sized cysts may be totally asymptomatic and be discovered only incidentally.

Drainage of Pseudocysts

There are multiple non-randomized, non-blinded trials demonstrating resolution of pain in patients with chronic pancreatitis when pseudocysts are drained. Usatoff and colleagues [12] evaluated 112 patients with confirmed chronic pancreatitis who underwent open operation by drainage, resection, or a combination of both. The morbidity rate was 28%, and the mortality rate 1%. In 74% of patients, pain was relieved, and the pseudocyst recurrence rate was 3%. In general, studies have shown that patients with chronic pancreatitis suffering from pain or early satiety from an obstructive effect of a pseudocyst clearly benefit from a drainage procedure (Table 63.1). In a recent randomized controlled trial by Varadarajulu and colleagues [13] comparing endoscopic to surgical drainage, endoscopic therapy was equally effective, less costly, and associated with shorter hospital length of stay.

Medical Therapy

Medical therapy has a very limited role in the management of pancreatic pseudocysts. Though somatostatin and its octopeptide synthetic analog, octreotide, have been extensively studied, there is no evidence that a symptomatic pseudocyst can be effectively treated by using these inhibitors of pancreatic secretion alone. However, as an adjuvant treatment, octreotide and/or somatostatin may be effective [14]. In a patient who has undergone a drainage procedure for a pancreatic pseudocyst, octreotide may assist in decreasing the size and drainage, if continuous.

Pancreatic enzymes also have a limited role in the treatment of pain in patients with chronic pancreatitis, as previously mentioned.

Surgical Drainage

The indications for surgery, though generally defined, are not clearly established by evidence and are open to interpretation [15]. Typically, patients are referred to surgery late in the course of the disease, which implies that the inflammatory process can rarely be halted. The usual technical complexities of pancreatic surgery are made even more imposing by the inflammatory process, which can affect tissue planes and extend to adjacent structures and organs. Surgical treatment of pseudocysts in patients with chronic pancreatitis can include external or internal drainage (cystogastrostomy, cystduodenostomy, and cystojejunostomy) and resection. The specific methods of drainage used depend upon the maturity of the cyst wall, the location of the cyst, and whether or not cyst infection is present. In a recent series of 206 patients with chronic pancreatitis and pseudocysts treated by surgical intervention, 94% had complete pain relief or improved pain after a median follow-up of 7.3 years [2]. There was only one postoperative death. There were 10 patients (6%) who required reoperation for complications, including bleeding, fistula, and infection. Most of the patients in this series had pseudocysts in the head of the pancreas. The high rate of pain relief after resection compared to drainage may lead to fewer attacks of recurrent pain. Aside from removing the cyst, surgical therapy allows resection of the inflammatory process in the pancreas that has led to the cyst. This may have the advantage of preventing a recurrence of the cyst or development of new cysts. In general, surgeons have been performing internal drainage procedures less often and focusing more on the underlying pathology of the pancreatic duct. There is a beneficial effect to identifying the source of the cyst, the defect in the duct [15]. More versatile cystojejunostomy is preferred for giant pseudocysts (>15 cm), which are predominantly inframesocolic. In pseudocysts with coexisting chronic pancreatitis and a dilated pancreatic duct, duct drainage procedures (such as longitudinal panacreaticojejunostomy) should be preferred to cyst drainage.

Radiologic (Percutaneous) Drainage

Percutaneous drainage is typically performed using a 7–12 French pigtail catheter inserted in the pseudocyst over a needle-inserted guidewire. This guidewire can be placed by sonography, CT, or fluoroscopy. This method is not very invasive and is ideal for diagnosis, but is often ineffective due to a combination of factors, including failure to collapse the wall of the pseudocyst and failure to remove the ductal communication that feeds the pancreatic cyst the pancreatic enzyme-rich fluid. Continuous catheter drainage has more impressive results, with a low failure rate of only 16%, recurrence rate of 7%, complication rate of 18%, and mortality rate of 2% [16].

Percutaneous drainage is not preferred in the presence of a stricture of the main pancreatic duct because of the risk of a permanent external fistula. Percutaneous catheter diagnosis is less effective in multiple and loculated pseudocysts. Contraindications to percutaneous catheter diagnosis include suspicion of malignancy, intracystic hemorrhage, and presence of pancreatic ascites. Percutaneous catheter drainage should be the initial mode of treatment for high-risk patients in need of pseudocyst drainage, for patients with symptomatic or expanding immature cysts, and for patients with infected pseudocysts.

Endoscopic Drainage

An endoscopic approach to the management of pseudocysts requires careful evaluation of the patient, local expertise, and knowledge of the character and location of the pseudocyst [17]. Identifying the characteristics of the collection using transabdominal ultrasound, MRI, or, ideally, EUS, will help direct the appropriate approach, whether through endoscopy, deferring to surgical drainage, or observation, especially in minimally asymptomatic patients. In the best hands, an endoscopic approach can result in successful resolution in as much as 92% of patients with chronic pancreatitis [18].

Endoscopic cyst drainage can be performed by a transmural (transgastric/transduodenal) or transpapillary route (Figure 63.2). The transpapillary approach has been shown to be effective 85% of the time [19]. It is ideal for cysts that communicate with the main pancreatic duct. Single-step needle drainage of pancreatic pseudocysts is associated with an unacceptably high recurrence rate. Prolonged drainage with an indwelling catheter is associated with a high drainage success rate and a low recurrence rate [20].

Most pancreatic pseudocysts (>70%) communicate with the main pancreatic duct. For this reason, a transpapillary approach to drainage should be considered. If the pseudocyst communicates with the main pancreatic duct on ERCP, a 5–7 French pancreatic duct stent should be placed beyond the stricture or cyst cavity. Factors predictive of success include the presence of pancreatic duct strictures, the size of the pseudocyst (≥6 cm), the location in the body of the pancreas, and the duration of the pseudocyst (<6 months) [21]. A review of the published literature [20]

Table 63.2 General requirements for a transmural approach to drainage of pseudocysts.

Distance of pseudocyst to gastrointestinal wall <1 cm
Location judged by bulge into the lumen of upper GI tract (or EUS)
EUS location confirmed (or bulge noted)
Size >5 cm
No debris on EUS
Neoplasm ruled out
Pseudoaneurysm ruled out

GI, gastrointestinal; EUS, endoscopic ultrasonography.

shows transpapillary drainage to be a safe procedure, with low morbidity and no reported mortality. Hemorrhagic complications have occurred in less than 1% of patients and pancreatitis in 5%, and stent migration is rare.

Endoscopic transmural drainage of a pseudocyst can be performed via a transgastric or transduodenal approach, depending on the cyst's location (Table 63.2). The technique involves the endoscopic identification of the area of maximum bulge with the use of a side-viewing endoscope, needle localization of the tract for cautery, entry into the pseudocyst using a needle-knife papillotome with radiologic verification by contrast injection, and insertion of a guidewire followed by several 7–10 French stents [20]. Cystogastrostomies are especially prone to early closure if not stented, resulting in recurrence rates as high as 20%. Use of nasogastric catheter is optional.

Trevino and colleagues [22] evaluated the efficacy of combined transpapillary and transmural drainage via retrospective study of 110 patients, 36% of whom underwent simultaneous pancreatic duct stenting. Treatment success was defined by complete resolution of the pseudocyst or by a decrease in size to <2 cm with resolution of symptoms. The success rate of combined treatment was 98 versus 80% for transmural drainage alone.

Before taking a transenteric approach to cyst drainage (cystogastrostomy, cystoduodenostomy), an EUS should be performed. Though there is little evidence that this approach increases efficacy, EUS not only highlights approximate vascular structures, but also characterizes the cyst contents, which may contain debris. A biopsy of the pseudocyst wall can be obtained at the time of drainage to rule out malignancy or cystadenoma.

There are almost 1000 cases of endoscopic transmural drainage of pancreatic pseudocysts in the published literature. Technical success in achieving drainage is associated with cyst location in the head or body rather than the tail of the gland, with transmural thickness <1 cm as measured on CT scan or EUS, and with pseudocyst-complicated chronic pancreatitis as opposed to acute pancreatitis. Complications have been reported to occur in as many as 7% of cases, including perforation, sepsis, and bleeding. Antibiotic prophylaxis should be considered despite the absence of evidence that antibiotics are efficacious in the prevention of infectious complications in the drainage of pseudocysts.

Pseudocyst Recurrence

Pseudocyst recurrence is uncommon in acute pancreatitis, but more common in chronic pancreatitis. Recurrence rates do not appear to correlate with the method of drainage. Though a general recurrence rate of 15% has been reported in patients with chronic pancreatitis, higher rates tend to occur in patients with the so-called "disconnected pancreatic tail syndrome" (disconnected segments of the pancreatic duct in the proximal pancreas). Undetected stones, obstructing strictures, or recurrent stones can be a cause. A large randomized trial concluded that 0% recurrence rates were observed if stents were left for a longer period, versus 38% recurrence when the stents were removed shortly after resolution of fluid collection [23]. There are currently no randomized controlled studies comparing the various minimally invasive approaches in the management of pancreatic pseudocysts. Depending on available expertise and technology, intervention should be applied. It remains unclear whether an ERCP is necessary to document communication with the main pancreatic duct in order to attempt a transpapillary approach instead of a transmural approach. Further study will be needed to clarify the best approach to managing pseudocysts complicating chronic pancreatitis. Due to the minimal invasiveness of the approach, its reported safety, and its success rates in the literature, if expertise is available, an endoscopic approach is preferred.

Take Home Points

- The highest incidence of pancreatic pseudocysts can be found in patients with chronic pancreatitis due to alcohol abuse.
- The diagnosis of pseudocysts is most often accomplished by computed tomography (CT) scanning, endoscopic ultrasound (EUS), or endoscopic retrograde cholangiopancreaticography (ERCP); rapid progress in the improvement of diagnostic tools has enabled detection with high sensitivity and specificity.
- Different therapeutic strategies can be taken: endoscopic transpapillary or transmural drainage, percutaneous catheter drainage, or laparoscopic and/or open surgery.
- The feasibility of endoscopic drainage is highly dependent on the anatomy and topography of the pseudocyst; however, in general, endoscopic drainage provides high success and low complication rates.
- Internal drainage and pseudocyst resection are frequently used as surgical approaches with a good overall outcome, but have a somewhat higher morbidity and mortality than endoscopic intervention.

Videos of interest to readers of this chapter can be found by visiting the companion website at:

http://www.practicalgastrohep.com/

63.1 Endoscopic palliation of complete malignant colonic obstruction.

References

1 Brown A, Hughes M, Tenner S, Banks PA. Does pancreatic enzyme supplementation reduce pain in patients with chronic pancreatitis: a meta-analysis? *Am J Gastroenterol* 1997; **92**: 2032–5.

2 Schlosser W, Siech M, Beger HG. Pseudocyst treatment in chronic pancreatitis – surgical treatment of the underlying disease increases the long term success. *Dig Surg* 2005; **22**: 340–5.

3 Pitchumoni CS, Agarwal N. Pancreatic pseudocysts: when and how should drainage be performed. *Gastroenterol Clin North Am* 1999; **28**: 610–45.

4 Warshaw AL. Pancreatic cysts and pseudocysts: new rules for a new game. *Br J Surg* 1988; **76**: 533–4.

5 Bradley EL, Clements J, Gonzales A. The natural history of pancreatic pseudocysts: a unified concept of management. *Am J Surg* 1979; **137**: 135–41.

6 Aghdassi A, Mayerle J, Kraft M, *et al*. Diagnosis and treatment of pancreatic pseudocysts in chronic pancreatitis. *Pancreas* 2008; **36**: 105–12.

7 Brugge WR. Approaches to the drainage of pancreatic pseudocysts. *Curr Opin Gastroenterol* 2004; **20**: 488–92.

8 Brugge WR, Lewandrowski K, Lee-Lewandrowski E, *et al*. Diagnosis of pancreatic cystic neoplasms: a report of the Cooperative Pancreatic Cyst Study. *Gastroenterology* 2004; **126**: 1330–6.

9 Warshaw AL, Rattner DW. Timing of surgical drainage for pancreatic pseudocyst. Clinical and chemical criteria. *Ann Surg* 1985; **202**: 720–4.

10 Gouyon B, Levy P, Ruszniewski P, *et al*. Predictive factors in the outcome of pseudocysts complicating alcoholic chronic pancreatitis. *Gut* 1997; **41**: 821–5.

11 Ebbehoj N, Borly L, Bulow J, *et al*. Pancreatic tissue fluid pressure in chronic pancreatitis. Relation to pain, morphology and function. *Scand J Gastroenterol* 1990; **25**: 1046–51.

12 Usatoff V, Brancatisano R, Williamson RC. Operative treatment of pseudocysts in patients with chronic pancreatitis. *Br J Surg* 2000; **87**: 1494–9.

13 Varadarajulu S, Bang JY, Sutton BS, *et al*. Equal efficacy of endoscopic and surgical cystogastrostomy for pancreatic pseudocyst drainage in a randomized trial. *Gastroenterology* 2013; **145**(3): 583–90.

14 Gullo L, Barbara L. The treatment of pancreatic pseudocysts with octreotide. *Lancet* 1991; **338**: 540–1.

15 Bell R. Current surgical management of chronic pancreatitis. *J Gastrointest Surg* 2005; **9**: 144–54.

16 Gumaste V, Pitchumoni CS. Pancreatic pseudocyst. *Gastroenterologist* 1996; **4**: 33–43.

17 Wilcox CM. Varadarajulu S. Endoscopic therapy for chronic pancreatitis: an evidence based review. *Curr Gastroenterol Rep* 2006; **8**: 104–10.

18 Baron TH, Harewood GC, Morgan DE, *et al*. Outcome differences after endoscopic drainage of pancreatic necrosis, acute pancreatic pseudocysts, and chronic pancreatic pseudocysts. *Gastrointestinal Endoscopy* 2002; **56**: 7–17.

19 De Palma GD, Galloro G, Puzziello A, *et al*. Endoscopic drainage of pancreatic pseudocysts: a long-term follow-up study of 49 patients. *Hepatogastroenterology* 2002, **49**: 1113–15.

20 Bhattacharya D, Ammori BJ. Minimally invasive approaches to the management of pancreatic pseudocysts. *Surgical Lapro Endo Per* 2003; **13**: 141–8.

21 Catalano MF, Geenen JE, Schmalz MJ, *et al*. Treatment of pancreatic pseudocysts with ductal communication by transpapillary pancreatic duct endoprosthesis. *Gastrointest Endosc* 1995; **42**: 214–8.

22 Trevino JM, Tamhane A, Varadarajulu S. Successful stenting in ductal disruption favorably impacts treatment outcomes in patients undergoing transmural drainage of peripancreatic fluid collections. *J Gastroenterol Hepatol* 2010; **25**: 526.

23 Arvanitakis M, Delhaye M, Bali MA, *et al*. Pancreatic-fluid collections: a randomized controlled trial regarding stent removal after endoscopic transmural drainage. *Gastrointest Endosc* 2007; **65**: 609.

CHAPTER 64

Pancreatic Cancer and Cystic Pancreatic Neoplasms

William R. Brugge

Harvard Medical School and Gastrointestinal Unit, Massachusetts General Hospital, Boston, MA, USA

Pancreatic Cancer

Summary

Pancreatic cancer is the fourth most common cause of cancer death in men and women. Patients typically present at an advanced stage, with a poor prognosis. The clinical presentation may involve weight loss, abdominal discomfort, and jaundice. Painless jaundice, depression, and new-onset diabetes can suggest the diagnosis. Cross-sectional imaging has utility in diagnosis and staging. Endoscopic ultrasound (EUS) with fine-needle aspiration (FNA) is a standard approach to tissue diagnosis. Endoscopic retrograde cholangiopancreaticography (ERCP) with palliative stenting can relieve obstructive jaundice. A minority of patients are candidates for resection. Patients with metastatic disease or with contraindications to resection (e.g., invasion of the superior mesenteric artery (SMA)) may be considered for chemoradiation therapy.

Case

A 59-year-old African American man presents with a history of progressive jaundice and recent-onset depression. He is a former smoker. He has a family history of pancreatic cancer. His blood sugar is elevated. Computed tomography (CT) scan of the abdomen and pelvis reveals a 2.3 cm mass in the head of the pancreas. There is regional lymphadenopathy.

Definition and Epidemiology

The majority of pancreatic cancers result from malignant transformation of the exocrine pancreas, and more than 80% are ductal adenocarcinomas [1]. In 2013, an estimated 45 220 new cases of pancreatic cancer were diagnosed [2]. In terms of new diagnoses, pancreatic cancer is the 10th most common malignancy in men, but it does not make the top 10 in women. However, the poor prognosis makes pancreatic cancer the fourth most common cause of cancer death in both women and men [2].

Pathophysiology

Pancreatic ductal carcinoma is acquired through the accumulation of multiple genetic mutations [3]. More than 85% of ductal carcinomas have a mutation in the K-*ras* oncogene [4], and more than 90% have inactivation of the *p16* tumor-suppressor gene [5]. The major risk factors for pancreatic cancer include age, smoking, chronic pancreatitis, diabetes mellitus, male gender, and African

American race. Less commonly, hereditary syndromes may be implicated. Hereditary chronic pancreatitis caused by a mutation in the cationic trypsinogen gene accounts for a small percentage of cases [6, 7]. Cancer syndromes that increase the risk of pancreatic cancer include (in order of decreasing risk) Peutz–Jeghers syndrome (PJS), familial atypical multiple mole syndrome, *BRCA* 1 and 2 genotypes, familial adenomatous polyposis, and hereditary non-polyposis colon cancer [7].

Clinical Features

Patients with pancreatic cancer may present with abdominal or back pain, weight loss, and/or jaundice. Weight loss may be associated with diarrhea, early satiety, and/or steatorrhea. The jaundice of pancreatic cancer is classically obstructive and is characterized by an elevated direct/conjugated bilirubin, acholic (pale) stool, and dark urine. Painless jaundice is a typical presentation that can prompt concern for underlying pancreatic cancer. Atypical diabetes mellitus with new onset in an older thin adult and/or depression may be observed.

Diagnosis

Abdominal ultrasound may reveal dilatation of the biliary tree and pancreatic duct. Laboratory testing of liver function, total and direct bilirubin, amylase, lipase, and complete blood count (CBC) may direct subsequent investigations. Cross-sectional imaging may reveal a pancreatic mass, biliary or pancreatic ductal dilatation, regional or distant lymphadenopathy, metastasis, or regional invasion of vessels or duodenum (Figure 64.1). In many cases, the finding of a mass in the pancreas will prompt referral for EUS-FNA for a cytologic diagnosis and more detailed locoregional staging (Figure 64.2). ERCP can demonstrate ductal stricturing and is diagnostic in some cases with brushing and biopsy. The "double-duct sign" refers to the finding of dilatation of both the common bile duct and the pancreatic duct (Figure 64.3) and is concerning for a distal obstruction (i.e., pancreatic head mass or carcinoma of the ampulla of Vater). The tumor marker CA19-9 correlates with tumor size but is not recommended for use in screening or selecting patients for surgery. Recent studies have focused on determining epigenetic biomarkers. Circulating tumor cells may be useful in the diagnosis of pancreatic cancer but have not been sufficiently validated for routine clinical practice [8]. Positron emission tomography (PET)-CT scanning may help evaluate for distant metastasis in locally advanced disease and contribute to surgical and radiotherapeutic planning [9].

Practical Gastroenterology and Hepatology Board Review Toolkit, Second Edition. Edited by Nicholas J. Talley, Kenneth R. DeVault, Michael B. Wallace, Bashar A. Aqel and Keith D. Lindor.
© 2016 John Wiley & Sons, Ltd. Published 2016 by John Wiley & Sons, Ltd. Companion website: www.practicalgastrohep.com

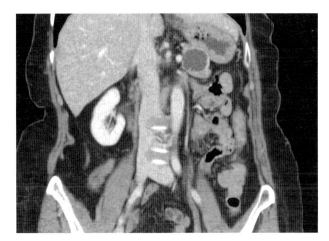

Figure 64.1 Contrast-enhanced CT scan of a pancreatic mass involving the stomach.

Case Continued

The patient is referred for EUS-FNA for tissue diagnosis and staging. The EUS reveals a 2.9 cm irregular, hypoechoic mass in the head of the pancreas. There is locoregional lymphadenopathy. The mass appears to invade the SMA. The pathologic diagnosis from the FNA is poorly differentiated adenocarcinoma.

Differential Diagnosis

See Table 64.1.

Therapeutics

Surgical resection is the only potentially curative option in the management of pancreatic cancer (Figure 64.4). Because the stage is typically advanced at presentation, surgery is only considered in a minority of cases. Approximately 20% of patients will be operative candidates at the time of diagnosis [10]. Even with appropriate patient selection and complete surgical resection, only a subset of resected patients will achieve a cure. Table 64.2 lists contraindications to surgical resection [11]. ERCP has a role in the palliation of obstructive jaundice. External beam radiation therapy with

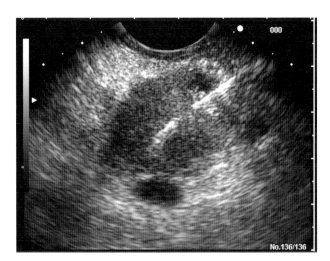

Figure 64.2 EUS-FNA of a hypoechoic pancreatic mass.

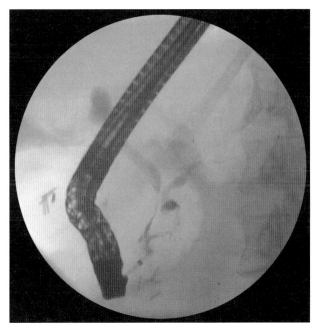

Figure 64.3 Fluoroscopic image at ERCP in a patient with metastatic cancer to the pancreas, demonstrating a classic double-duct sign. Strictures are present in both the pancreatic and bile ducts, with upstream dilatation. Incidental note is made of clips from a prior cholecystectomy.

concomitant chemotherapy (5-fluorouracil, gemcitabine, paclitaxel) is primarily used for symptom palliation, with modest improvements in mean survival. Pain pallation by EUS-guided celiac plexus neurolysis for unresectable cases is effective. EUS-guided local ablation treatments are under investigation for advanced cancers [12].

Case Continued

The patient is not a candidate for resection due to involvement of the SMA (stage T4) and is referred to oncology. Oncology recommends chemoradiation therapy for palliation of symptoms. The patient undergoes chemoradiation therapy, with initial improvement in his symptoms. His cancer progresses and he elects hospice care.

Prognosis

The prognosis for most patients with pancreatic adenocarcinoma is poor. The 5-year survival is approximately 15% for patients with presumed localized disease who undergo resection [10]. Patients who do not receive cancer-directed therapy have a 5-year survival rate of 1–5% [13]. Less common pancreatic mass lesions such as neuroendocrine tumors have a much more favorable prognosis.

Table 64.1 Differential diagnosis of mass lesions in the pancreas.

Pathologic diagnosis	Tumor type
Pancreatic adenocarcinoma	Malignant
Pancreatic neuroendocrine tumor	Malignant
Acinar cell carcinoma	Malignant
Metastatic tumor to the pancreas	Malignant
Lymphoma	Variable malignant grade
Cystic lesion of the pancreas	Benign, premalignant, or malignant
Focal pancreatitis	Benign
Autoimmune pancreatitis	Benign

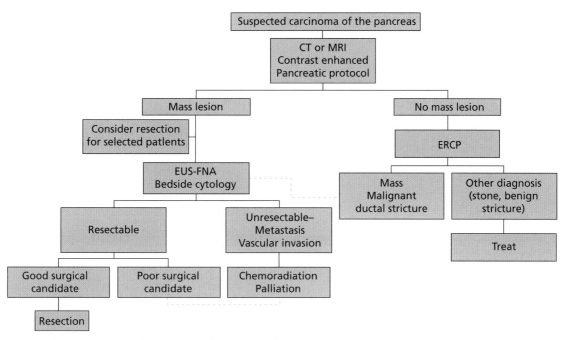

Figure 64.4 Proposed management algorithm for suspected carcinoma of the pancreas. CT, computed tomography; MRI, magnetic resonance imaging; EUS-FNA, endoscopic ultrasound-guided fine-needle aspiration; ERCP, endoscopic retrograde cholangiopancreaticography.

Table 64.2 Absolute and relative contraindications to surgical resection of pancreatic cancer. The range is represented from top (absolute) to bottom (relative) of the table. Source: Ryan 2005 [11].

Metastases to the liver, peritoneum, omentum, or any extra-abdominal site
Encasement of celiac axis, hepatic artery, or superior mesenteric artery (SMA)
Involvement of splenoportal confluence
Involvement of bowel mesentery
Involvement of superior mesenteric vein or portal vein

Take Home Points

- Pancreatic cancer has a poor prognosis; however, a subset of patients may achieve a cure.
- Painless jaundice, new-onset diabetes, and weight loss with depression are concerning.
- Cross-sectional imaging is useful for diagnosis and staging.
- The double-duct sign suggests a malignant obstruction.
- Endoscopic ultrasound-guided fine-needle aspiration (EUS-FNA) can allow a tissue diagnosis and is highly sensitive for locoregional staging.
- Surgery is the only potentially curative treatment option.

Cystic Pancreatic Neoplasms

Summary

Cystic neoplasms of the pancreas were thought to be relatively rare, but the widespread use of cross-sectional imaging has dramatically increased their identification. These cystic lesions may represent true cysts or pseudocysts and may be benign, premalignant, or malignant. Though most lesions are discovered incidentally, some patients may present with jaundice, pancreatitis, or abdominal pain. Patients with a history of alcoholism or recurrent pancreatitis have a higher pretest probability of pseudocyst. Cross-sectional imaging

and EUS with FNA are helpful in the stratification of patients by risk of malignancy. Resection is the definitive means of diagnosis and management. Management strategies such as observation are considered in older patients with comorbidities and low-risk features.

Case

A 76-year-old woman with congestive heart failure and hematuria undergoes a CT scan to rule out nephrolithiasis. A 2 cm cystic lesion is noted in the tail of the pancreas. She denies any history of pancreatitis or heavy alcohol consumption. She denies abdominal pain or discomfort. There is mild dilatation of the main pancreatic duct.

Definition and Epidemiology

While previously thought to be rare, the widespread use of cross-sectional imaging has revealed the presence of cystic lesions of the pancreas in a significant number of patients [14]. By autopsy, pancreatic cystic lesions may be found in 24% of patients [15]. Cystic lesions are more common in older patients, and the prevalence of neoplasia is related to age. The majority of cystic lesions are pseudocysts and do not have a true epithelial lining. Approximately 30% of lesions may represent true cysts with variable malignant potential.

Pathophysiology

The etiology of cystic lesions of the pancreas varies by cyst type, and the pathogenesis is not well understood. Pseudocysts are not true cystic lesions but represent extravasated pancreatic secretions and necrosis that has become walled off by neighboring structures and omentum. Serous cystadenoma is a benign multiloculated/multiseptated lesion lined by glycogen rich cells. Mucinous cystadenoma is a true cyst lined by columnar goblet cells and a stroma of ovarian-like epithelium. Intraductal papillary mucinous

CHAPTER 64

neoplasms (IPMNs) may be multiple and are characterized by ductal communication and a lining of mucin-secreting cells. They are classified as main-duct (MD) or branch-duct (BD) IPMNs according to their origin.

Clinical Features

Patients with pseudocysts generally have a history of pancreatitis, often recurrent, and may have radiographic evidence of chronic pancreatitis (gland atrophy, duct dilatation, calcification of the parenchyma, calculi in pancreatic duct). Patients with true cysts are often asymptomatic. Symptoms attributed to cystic lesions include abdominal pain, jaundice, and weight loss, and some patients may develop recurrent pancreatitis.

Diagnosis

A history of pancreatitis or longstanding heavy alcohol use increases the pre-test probability of pseudocyst. Cross-sectional imaging allows the visualization of calcifications, septa, and mural nodules, and can also suggest underlying chronic pancreatitis [16]; however, imaging alone is frequently insufficient for diagnosis. EUS provides a more sensitive examination and can be performed with FNA and aspiration of cyst fluid for amylase, carcinoembryonic antigen (CEA), cytology, and DNA analysis. High levels of CEA are the most useful marker for differentiating mucinous from non-mucinous cysts. DNA analysis of pancreatic cyst fluid demonstrates that *KRAS* mutation is highly specific (96%) for mucinous cysts [17]. Recently, molecular analysis of fluid for GNAS mutation has been

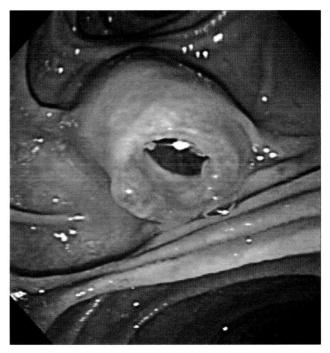

Figure 64.5 Endoscopic image of a classic fish-mouth deformity, secondary to mucin overproduction and extrusion, which is pathognomonic for intraductal papillary mucinous neoplasm (IPMN).

Table 64.3 Features and characteristics of common cystic lesions of the pancreas. Other less common cystic lesions include cystic endocrine neoplasm, ductal adenocarcinoma with cystic degeneration, lymphoepithelial cyst, and acinar cell cystadenocarcinoma.

Cyst type	Pathology	Aspirate	CEA ng/mL	Amylase	Management
Pseudocyst No true epithelial lining, walls are of adjacent structures Frequently associated with pain Look for gland atrophy, duct dilatation, calcification of the parenchyma, calculi in pancreatic duct	Develops as a result of pancreatic inflammation and necrosis, communicates with the ductal system Contains high concentrations of amylase Lining is fibrous, with granulation tissue Lacks an epithelial lining	Thin, dark, opaque, non-mucinous, with inflammatory cells	Low	High	No malignant potential Resection or endoscopic management indicated for symptoms
Mucinous cystadenoma Most common cystic neoplasm Typically occurs in middle-aged women Typically solitary 97% of cases are distal (body and tail) May be malignant at time of diagnosis	Dense mesenchymal ovarian-like stroma Lacks communication with pancreatic duct May have one or more macrocystic spaces lined by mucous secreting cells Peripheral eggshell calcification is suggestive of malignancy	Viscous, clear, variable cellularity, positive for mucin	High >200	Low	After resection, non-invasive mucinous cystadenoma – no recurrence
Serous cystadenoma Second most common cystic tumor of the pancreas Occurs in middle-aged women Typically solitary Very LOW malignant potentialCentral scar highly suggestive, but found in ~20% of cases	Typically composed of multiple, small cysts lined by glycogen-rich cuboidal epithelium Chromosomal alterations of gene for von Hippel–Lindau locus 3p25 found in majority	Less viscous, thin, clear, non-mucinous, may be bloody	Low <5	Low	Resection is curative
IPMN (side branch or main duct) Patients may have multiple cysts More common in men A dilated pancreatic duct implies MD-IPMN Mucin extrusion from widely patent ampulla (fish mouth deformity) is pathognomonic Side-branch IPMN is more common	Consists of dilated ductal segments, usually within the head of the pancreas, lined by mucous-secreting cells MD-IPMN has greater malignant potential Mural nodules and a segmental or diffuse dilatation of the pancreatic duct >15 mm are worrisome for malignancy	Viscous, clear, with mucin	High (>1000 concerning for malignancy)	High	Resection (especially for patients with nodules or symptoms) Serial imaging for high-risk patients with low-risk features

CEA, carcinoembryonic antigen; IPMN, intraductal papillary mucinous neoplasm; MD, main duct.

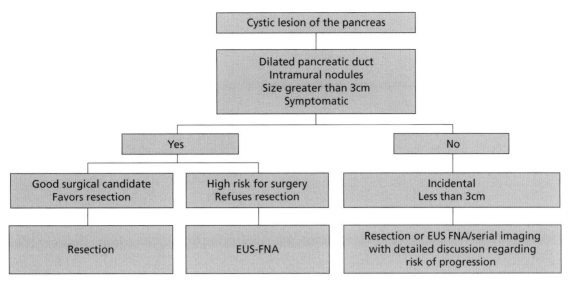

Figure 64.6 Proposed algorithm for the management of cystic lesions of the pancreas. EUS-FNA, endoscopic ultrasound-guided fine-needle aspiration.

shown to be highly specific in distinguishing BD-IPMN from other cysts. As a new technology, needle-based confocal laser endomicroscopy has also been shown to be potentially useful in distinguishing IPMN from serous cystsadenoma with a high specificity [18]. ERCP may be useful in the evaluation of IPMN, revealing a fish-mouth deformity (extrusion of mucous from a widely patent ampulla; Figure 64.5), mucinous filling defects within the pancreatogram, ductal dilatation, and/or cystic dilation of side branches. However, the use of ERCP for the diagnosis of IPMN is limited by its invasiveness and risks, and it has mostly been replaced by EUS.

For a majority of patients, surgical resection with pathologic examination is the only definitive means of diagnosis.

Differential Diagnosis
See Table 64.3.

Therapeutics
Because of the risk of malignancy, surgical resection of suspected malignant cystic neoplasms may be indicated (Figure 64.6). Resection is recommended in all surgically fit patients with MD-IPMN because of the high malignancy risk. A dilated main pancreatic duct, mural nodules, thickened enhanced cyst walls, size >3 cm, dysplasia on biopsy, and the presence of pancreatic symptoms are worrisome features for BD-IPMN and should be evaluated in order to aid in decision-making around resection and follow-up. Small, incidental pancreatic cysts may enlarge over a prolonged period, and morbidity and mortality due to these cysts are low; therefore, observation may be a safe management option in some cases [19, 20]. The decision to monitor high-risk patients with small (<2 cm) incidental cystic neoplasms should follow a discussion regarding the low risk of cancer (3.5%) but high risk of progression to malignancy (50%) [14]. Most mucinous cystic neoplasms are located in the tail of the pancreas. The risk of progression can be weighed against the risk of postoperative pancreatic fistula (29%) and mortality (0.8%) with distal pancreatectomy [21]. Surveillance can be performed with CT, magnet resonance imaging (MRI), or EUS-FNA according to cyst size stratification. Resection may be readdressed if imaging demonstrates a significant change in diameter or morphology and high-grade atypia in cyst fluid analysis.

Case Continued
The patient is referred for EUS-FNA, whcih reveals a 2 cm lesion with a mural nodule and mild main pancreatic ductal dilation. A distal pancreatectomy is performed, revealing IPMN. The patient develops a postoperative pancreatic leak but recovers and is discharged home

Prognosis
The prognosis for cystic lesions of the pancreas is much better than for pancreatic cancer. Many patients have a benign condition, and many patients with a premalignant lesion will be cured with surgical resection.

Take Home Points
- Cystic lesions of the pancreas may be benign or malignant.
- Endoscopic ultrasound-guided fine-needle aspiration (EUS–FNA) is helpful in the evaluation of cystic lesions.
- Cyst-fluid carcinoembryonic antigen (CEA) is the most useful marker for differentiation of mucinous cysts
- A fish-mouth deformity with mucin extrusion from the ampulla is pathognomonic for intraductal papillary mucinous neoplasm (IPMN).
- Peripheral eggshell calcification suggests a mucinous neoplasm.
- A multicystic lesion with a central scar indicates a serous cystadenoma.
- The risk of progression should be weighed against the risk of surgery in the management of mucinous cysts.

References
1 Wood LD, Hruban RH. Pathology and molecular genetics of pancreatic neoplasms. *Cancer J* 2012; **18**: 492–501.

2 American Cancer Society. *Cancer Facts & Figures 2013*. Atlanta, GA: American Cancer Society, 2013

3 Wolfgang CL, Herman JM, Laheru DA *et al.* Recent progress in pancreatic cancer. *CA Cancer J Clin* 2013; **63**: 318–48.

4 Chang Z, Li Z, Wang X, *et al.* Deciphering the mechanisms of tumorigenesis in human pancreatic ductal epithelial cells. *Clin Cancer Res* 2013; **19**: 549–59.

5 Botta GP, Reichert M, Reginato MJ, *et al.* ERK2-regulated TIMP1 induces hyper-proliferation of K-Ras(G12D)-transformed pancreatic ductal cells. *Neoplasia* 2013; **15**: 359–72.

6 Bartsch DK, Gress TM, Langer P. Familial pancreatic cancer – current knowledge. *Nat Rev Gastroenterol Hepatol* 2012; **9**: 445–53.

7 Rebours V, Levy P, Ruszniewski P. An overview of hereditary pancreatitis. *Dig Liver Dis* 2012; **44**(1): 8–15.

8 Herreros-Villanueva M, Gironella M, Castells A, Bujanda L. Molecular markers in pancreatic cancer diagnosis. *Clin Chim Acta* 2013; **418**: 22–9.

9 Dibble EH, Karantanis D, Mercier G, *et al.* PET/CT of cancer patients: part 1, pancreatic neoplasms. *Am J Roentgenol* 2012; **199**: 952–67.

10 Bardou M, Le Ray I. Treatment of pancreatic cancer: a narrative review of cost-effectiveness studies. *Best Pract Res Clin Gastroenterol* 2013; **27**: 881–92.

11 Ryan DP, Fernandez-del Castillo C, Willett CG, *et al.* Case records of the Massachusetts General Hospital. Case 20-2005. A 58-year-old man with locally advanced pancreatic cancer. *N Engl J Med* 2005; **352**: 2734–41.

12 Yoon WJ, Brugge WR. Endoscopic ultrasonography-guided tumor ablation. *Gastrointest Endosc Clin N Am* 2012; **22**: 359–69.

13 Kumar R, Herman JM, Wolfgang CL, Zheng L. Multidisciplinary management of pancreatic cancer. *Surg Oncol Clin N Am* 2013; **22**: 265–87.

14 Fernandez-del Castillo C, Targarona J, Thayer SP, *et al.* Incidental pancreatic cysts: clinicopathologic characteristics and comparison with symptomatic patients. *Arch Surg* 2003; **138**: 427–3, disc. 33–4.

15 Cooper CL, O'Toole SA, Kench JG. Classification, morphology and molecular pathology of premalignant lesions of the pancreas. *Pathology* 2013; **45**: 286–304.

16 Kinney T. Evidence-based imaging of pancreatic malignancies. *Surg Clin N Am* 2010; **90**: 235–49.

17 Yoon WJ, Brugge WR. Pancreatic cystic neoplasms: diagnosis and management. *Gastroenterol Clin North Am* 2012; **41**: 103–18.

18 Konda VJ, Meining A, Jamil LH, *et al.* A pilot study of in vivo identification of pancreatic cystic neoplasms with needle-based confocal laser endomicroscopy under endosonographic guidance. *Endoscopy* 2013; **45**: 1006–13.

19 Edirimanne S, Connor SJ. Incidental pancreatic cystic lesions. *World J Surg* 2008; **32**: 2028–37.

20 Garcea G, Ong SL, Rajesh A, *et al.* Cystic lesions of the pancreas. A diagnostic and management dilemma. *Pancreatology* 2008; **8**: 236–51.

21 Ferrone CR, Warshaw AL, Rattner DW, *et al.* Pancreatic fistula rates after 462 distal pancreatectomies: staplers do not decrease fistula rates. *J Gastrointest Surg* 2008; **12**: 1691–7, disc. 7–8.

PART 6

Functional Diseases of the Small and Large Intestine

65 Irritable Bowel Syndrome, 391
Elizabeth J. Videlock and Lin Chang

66 Chronic Functional Constipation and Dyssynergic Defecation, 400
Satish S.C. Rao and Yeong Yeh Lee

67 Chronic Functional Abdominal Pain, 407
Amy E. Foxx-Orenstein

68 Abdominal Bloating and Visible Distension, 412
Mark Pimentel

Irritable Bowel Syndrome

Elizabeth J. Videlock and Lin Chang

Center for Neurobiology of Stress and Resilience, Division of Digestive Diseases, David Geffen School of Medicine at UCLA, Los Angeles, CA, USA

Summary

Irritable bowel syndrome (IBS) is a prevalent chronic gastrointestinal (GI) disorder. The diagnosis is based on the presence of chronic or recurrent abdominal pain associated with altered bowel habits, though IBS is heterogenous because symptoms can vary among affected individuals. While IBS can sometimes be challenging to manage, patient care should be focused on reducing costs and improving patient satisfaction and health-related quality of life. There are frequent advances in our knowledge about the clinical presentation, pathophysiology, and treatment of IBS. This chapter reviews current theories of pathophysiology, as well as epidemiology, symptoms, comorbidities, and current and evidence-based approaches to the evaluation and treatment of IBS. Emphasis is placed on the importance of biopsychosocial aspects of care, in addition to symptom management.

Case

A 28-year-old woman is referred to a gastroenterologist by her primary care physician for evaluation and management of abdominal pain and constipation for the past year. The patient reports having intermittent abdominal pain and bloating that is associated with feeling constipated. Her constipation symptoms include hard stools, difficulty evacuating stools, and sensation of incomplete evacuation. She has a bowel movement every 1–2 days. She has had similar symptoms since college, which she associates with stress, but they used to be milder and she never sought care for them. Now her symptoms, especially the pain and bloating, make it difficult for her to concentrate on her work, and she misses work 1–2 days per month. Her sleep is sometimes disturbed, particularly when her symptoms are worse, and she feels tired during the day. She has tried increasing her fluid intake and using different over-the-counter (OTC) laxatives and fiber supplements. While these medications help to loosen her stool, she does not like taking them. The discomfort and urgency caused by the laxatives are very bothersome, and she still has pain and bloating, which are sometimes increased with the medication. She denies unintentional weight loss, blood in the stool, and a family history of colon cancer. She has annual pelvic examinations by her gynecologist, and they have been normal.

Definition and Epidemiology

IBS is a functional gastrointestinal disorder (FGID) that is characterized by abdominal pain associated with alterations in stool form and/or frequency. It is frequently diagnosed in both primary care and specialty practice [1]. While we will continue to refer to IBS as one of the FGIDs, the reader is encouraged to reconsider the traditional dichotomy between "functional" and "organic." There is a biochemical basis for all symptoms, and the complex interactions between the host and environment are affected by peripheral and central inputs. One could view IBS as multiple "organic" diseases [2]. Despite the increasing identification of distinct pathophysiology, there is not a unifying putative mechanism, and patients are grouped clinically by symptoms, so that IBS is appropriately designated as a syndrome rather than a disease.

The prevalence of IBS in population studies is around 7% [3]. Prevalence in health care-seeking populations is 10–15%, depending on the diagnostic criteria used [4]. IBS is more prevalent among women, and women are more likely to have IBS with constipation [5].

IBS accounts for significant health care costs. According to a report by the National Commission on Digestive Diseases, in 2004, there were 3.1 million ambulatory care visits with IBS noted as a diagnosis, and 52.5% listed IBS as the first diagnosis. In the same year, the indirect and direct costs of IBS totaled 1.01 billion USD [6].

Pathophysiology

Our understanding of the pathogenesis of IBS has evolved over recent years but is still far from complete. A unifying theme is that the symptoms of IBS result from dysregulation of the "brain–gut axis," which manifests as enhanced visceral perception. There is not a consensus on the underlying etiology of this dysregulation, and the disorder may represent a combination of factors. Evidence suggests that the symptom constellation of IBS may arise from several etiologies, which can differ within subgroups of patients. Figure 65.1 illustrates the range of vulnerability factors and pathophysiologic mechanisms within the brain–gut axis that can contribute to the onset and exacerbation of symptoms of IBS. Due to the fact that IBS is a multicomponent disorder with a complex pathophysiology, biomarkers

Practical Gastroenterology and Hepatology Board Review Toolkit, Second Edition. Edited by Nicholas J. Talley, Kenneth R. DeVault, Michael B. Wallace, Bashar A. Aqel and Keith D. Lindor.
© 2016 John Wiley & Sons, Ltd. Published 2016 by John Wiley & Sons, Ltd. Companion website: www.practicalgastrohep.com

VULNERABILITY OR TRIGGER FACTORS

PATHOPHYSIOLOGIC MECHANISMS IN IBS

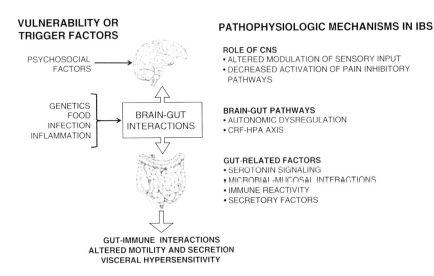

ROLE OF CNS
- ALTERED MODULATION OF SENSORY INPUT
- DECREASED ACTIVATION OF PAIN INHIBITORY PATHWAYS

BRAIN-GUT PATHWAYS
- AUTONOMIC DYSREGULATION
- CRF-HPA AXIS

GUT-RELATED FACTORS
- SEROTONIN SIGNALING
- MICROBIAL-MUCOSAL INTERACTIONS
- IMMUNE REACTIVITY
- SECRETORY FACTORS

Figure 65.1 Both "brain"- and "gut"-related mechanisms, as well as their interactions, are being explored in IBS. IBS patients show an enhanced responsiveness of this system manifesting in altered modulation of GI motility and secretion and enhanced perception of visceral events. IBS, irritable bowel syndrome; CNS, central nervous system; CRF, corticotropin-releasing factor; HPA, hypothalamic–pituitary–adrenal.

that can reliably diagnose IBS or monitor treatment response are currently lacking.

Clinical Features

GI Symptoms

The key symptom of IBS is chronic or recurrent abdominal pain and/or discomfort associated with altered bowel habits. Bowel symptoms fluctuate frequently for many patients with IBS. In one study in which participants completed stool diaries for 90 days, 78% of patients reported both loose/watery and hard/lumpy stools, with an average of three fluctuations between these extremes per month [7]. Constipation-predominant irritable bowel syndrome (IBS-C) and diarrhea-predominant irritable bowel syndrome (IBS-D) patients have different symptom profiles, with IBS-C patients reporting more overall symptoms (both lower and upper abdominal pain), and particularly bloating [8]. Pain associated with bowel movements is more common in IBS-D than IBS-C patients [7].

Extraintestinal Symptoms and Comorbid Disorders

More than half of the additional visits and costs incurred by IBS patients are for non-GI concerns [9]. Non-GI symptoms that are more common in IBS than controls include headache, back pain, fatigue, myalgia, dyspareunia, urinary frequency, and dizziness [9]. IBS patients with comorbid somatic disorders report more severe IBS symptoms and lower health-related quality of life [9]. There is a higher prevalence of psychiatric disorders in the IBS population than in controls, which is most evident in those with more severe symptoms and in tertiary referral clinics [10].

Severity

Patients with *severe* IBS have increased frequency, intensity, and persistence of symptoms and impaired health-related quality of life. They also have more psychosocial comorbidity, are more frequently seen by specialists, and undergo more diagnostic testing. In a large cross-sectional study (n = 755), the independent predictors of patient-assessed illness severity, which was determined by asking patients to rate overall severity of their IBS on a 0–20-point scale, were: abdominal pain, the belief that "something serious is wrong with body," straining with defecation, myalgias, urgency with defecation, and bloating [11].

Diagnosis

Symptom-Based Criteria

The differential diagnosis for the symptoms of IBS (Table 65.1) is very broad. However, use of the symptom-based Rome III criteria [1] and evaluation for alarm signs or symptoms, as well as exclusion of celiac disease in some populations, is sufficient to make the diagnosis of IBS. The Rome III criteria for the diagnosis of IBS were published in 2006 and are listed in Table 65.2, along with other supporting symptoms that are suggestive but not currently required for the diagnosis of IBS [1]. In a prospective study of 1848 adult patients with GI symptoms, the positive and negative likelihood ratios (95% CI) for the Rome III criteria in identifying patients without organic GI disease were 3.35 (2.97–3.79) and 0.39 (0.34–0.46), respectively [12]. While inclusion of the absence of alarm features modestly improves the positive likelihood ratio to 3.92 (2.85–5.38), it comes at the cost of an increase in the negative likelihood ratio to 0.86 (0.83–0.91) [12].

IBS is subgrouped by predominant bowel habit. Because stool form has been found to be the best predictor of predominant bowel habit in IBS, stool form rather than frequency determines bowel habit subclassification according to the Rome III criteria [1]. IBS subtypes are outlined in Table 65.3.

Table 65.1 Differential diagnosis of IBS.

IBS-C IBS-D/M	Hypothyroidism Carbohydrate maldigestion Bile acid malabsorption Chronic pancreatitis GI infection IBD Hyperthyroidism Carcinoid tumor
IBS-multiple subtypes	Celiac disease Food intolerance SIBO Enteric neuropathy or myopathy Malignancy Medication side effects Gynecologic conditions (e.g., endometriosis) Psychological conditions (e.g., depression, anxiety) Other FGIDs (e.g., functional abdominal pain syndrome, functional dyspepsia)

IBS, irritable bowel syndrome; GI, gastrointestinal; IBD, inflammatory bowel disease; SIBO, small-intestine bacterial overgrowth; FGID, functional gastrointestinal disorder.

Table 65.2 Rome III criteria and supportive symptoms. Source: Longstreth 2006 [1]. Reproduced with permission of Elsevier.

Symptom-based Rome III criteria for the diagnosis of IBS

These criteria should be filled for the last 3 months, with symptom onset at least 6 months prior to diagnosis

Recurrent abdominal pain or discomfort[a] at least 3 days per month in the last 3 months that is associated with two or more of the following:

1. Improvement with defecation
2. Onset associated with a change in frequency of stool
3. Onset associated with a change in form (appearance) of stool

Supportive symptoms (non-diagnostic)

1. Abnormal stool frequency (fewer than three bowel movements per week or more than three bowel movements per day)
2. Abnormal stool form (lumpy/hard stool or loose/watery stool)
3. Defecation straining, urgency, or a feeling of incomplete evacuation
4. Passing mucus
5. Bloating

---

[a]Discomfort means an uncomfortable sensation not described as pain.

Alarm Features

While the presence of "red flags" or alarm signs and symptoms may indicate a need for further diagnostic workup, patients with red-flag symptoms should not be excluded from the diagnosis of IBS. On average, IBS patients report the presence of at least 1.65 red-flag symptoms, but these have a low positive predictive value (PPV) for organic disease [13].

Diagnostic Testing

Historically, IBS has been a diagnosis of exclusion, but the current best evidence suggests that a battery of diagnostic tests is not necessary. The prevalence of organic disease, with the exception of celiac disease and lactose intolerance [14], in the population with symptoms of IBS (particularly in those without alarm features) is similar to that in the general population [3,15]. There is good evidence that serologic testing for celiac disease followed by endoscopic biopsy confirmation of positive results is a cost-effective strategy in North American non-constipated IBS patients [16,17].

Performing colonoscopy in patients under the age of 50 with typical symptoms of IBS and no alarm features is not recommended, as there is a low pretest probability of organic disease [3]. Additionally, a negative finding on colonoscopy is not associated with an increased sense of reassurance in patients with IBS [18]. Since the prevalence of microscopic colitis is higher in older, non-constipated patients with IBS (particularly women) [19], random biopsies are

Table 65.3 IBS subtypes by bowel habit. Source: Longstreth 2006 [1]. Reproduced with permission of Elsevier.

Subtype[a]	Percentage of stools that meet the description (over the preceding 3 months)	
	Hard or lumpy stools (Bristol type 1–2)	**Loose or watery stools (Bristol type 6–7)**
IBS with constipation (IBS-C)	≥25%	<25%
IBS with diarrhea (IBS-D)	<25%	≥25%
Mixed IBS (IBS-M)[b]	≥25%	≥25%
Unsubtyped IBS (IBS U)	<25%	<25%

[a]The word "with" is preferred to "predominant" due to symptom instability.
[b]Patients with both diarrhea and constipation that may alternate within hours or days were previously classified as IBS-A according to the Rome II criteria, but should now be referred to as IBS-M. The category of alternating IBS (IBS-A) should be reserved for patients with bowel habits that have changed over time (e.g., weeks to months).

recommended when colonoscopy is performed in patients with IBS-D [3].

Case Continued

The patient's physical examination is normal except for a mildly distended lower abdomen, which is tender to palpation without rebound. A rectal examination is normal, without paradoxical pelvic floor contraction during bear-down command. The diagnosis of IBS with constipation is discussed with the patient. She is reassured that while the symptoms can be debilitating and difficult to treat, they can be managed with appropriate care.

Therapeutics

An approach to management of IBS is outlined in Figure 65.2. Though IBS is characterized by altered stool frequency and/or consistency, the astute clinician will not assume that the patient seeks care primarily for the relief of these symptoms. Some patients fear that they have a life-threatening illness, such as colon cancer, and may find relief in receiving a positive diagnosis, reassurance, and education; these patients may not require pharmacotherapy.

Patient-Centered Care

A good health care provider–patient relationship is the cornerstone of effective care of IBS and has been shown to improve patient outcomes [20]. Elements of a good provider–patient relationship include a non-judgmental patient-centered interview, a careful and cost-effective evaluation, inquiry into the patient's understanding of the illness, patient education, and involvement of the patient in treatment decisions. As IBS is a chronic condition, it is important to assess specific reasons for the current visit, which may differ among patients (e.g., concern about cancer, worsening pain, lack of response to treatment). An intrinsic part of the clinical assessment is the psychosocial interview, which is usually quite relevant in IBS patients. Addressing psychosocial factors may improve health status and treatment response [21].

Diet

Many patients report an inconsistent symptom response to certain foods, and a 1–2-week food and symptom diary can identify potential food triggers. While most patients cannot completely control symptoms through diet alterations alone, diet-related exacerbations can be minimized. Common food triggers include high-fat foods, raw fruits and vegetables, and caffeinated beverages. Clinical trials have established that there is a group of patients who do not have celiac disease but do experience improvement in symptoms on a gluten-free diet [22]. Some patients may have symptoms related to excess fermentable oligosaccharides, disaccharides, monosaccharides, and polyols (FODMAPs). A high-FODMAP diet can result in increased gas from bacterial fermentation and can cause a laxative effect. In one trial, among patients who responded to a low-FODMAP diet, those randomized to a challenge with drinks containing fructose, fructans, or a combination were more likely to report symptom recurrence [23].

Physical Activity

Physical activity has been shown to be beneficial in chronic pain disorders such as fibromyalgia [24]. It has also been shown to improve intestinal gas transit [25]. One trial in IBS showed that 20–60

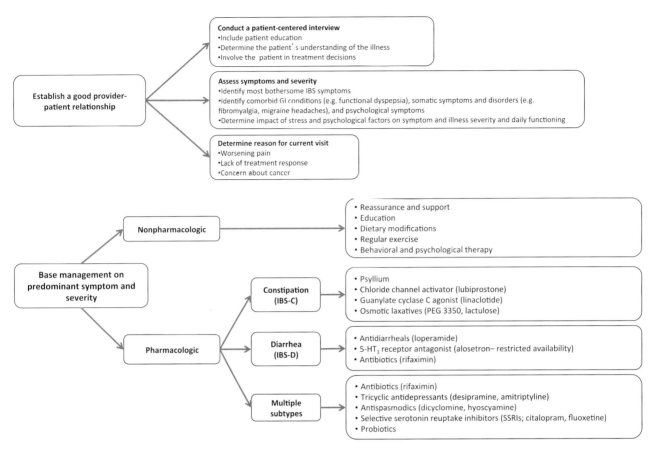

Figure 65.2 Treatment algorithm for IBS. A non-pharmacologic approach is recommended initially, and the use of medication should not preclude trials of non-pharmacologic therapies: a combination of both may be required. IBS, irritable bowel syndrome; GI, gastrointestinal.

minutes of moderate-to-vigorous activity three to five times weekly resulted in lower symptom severity after 12 weeks [26].

Therapies for IBS with Constipation

Therapies for patients with IBS-C are outlined in Table 65.4. Where available, the grade of recommendation from guidelines published by the American College of Gastroenterology (ACG) is provided [3].

Dietary Bulking Agents

Bulking agents have often been used as initial management of IBS. These include psyllium, methylcellulose, corn fiber, calcium polycarbophil, and psyllium hydrophilic mucilloid (ispaghula husk). Results from meta-analyses suggest a benefit for psyllium but not bran [27,28]. Subsequent to these analyses, there has been one high-quality trial, which did find a benefit for psyllium over placebo in IBS [29].

Table 65.4 Evidence-based pharmacological treatment of constipation.

Agent (class)	Dose	NNT (95% CI)	Grade of recommendation[a] [3]	Comment
Psyllium/ispaghula (Bulking agent)	20–25 g/day	6 (3–50)[b] pooled from six studies (n − 321)[28] 4 (2–10) for the Bijerk et al. [29] study alone (n = 178)	2C	All studies recruited patients regardless of predominant symptom
Polyethylene glycol (Osmotic laxative)	13.8 g polyethylene glycol 3350+E in 125 mL water, one to three times/day	NNT: 5 (3–28) [31]	2C	The larger trial of polyethylene glycol [31] was published after the guidelines and was not included in the evidence grading
Lubiprostone (Chloride channel activator)	8 μg twice daily	NNT for global improvement: 12 (7–44) [37]	1B	Also available in 24 μg twice daily for CIC
Linaclotide (Guanylate cyclase C agonist)	290 μg daily	NNT for composite pain and bowel symptom endpoint: 7 (5–11) [38]	NA	Also approved for the treatment of CIC at a dose of 145 μg daily

[a]See Table 65.3.
[b]To prevent one additional patient from having persistent symptoms
NNT has been recalculated where necessary, so that all are provided as the number needed to achieve a positive outcome.
NNT, number needed to treat; NA, not available; CIC, chronic idiopathic constipation.

Laxatives

Osmotic laxatives, such as polyethylene glycol or magnesium-containing products, are generally safe and well tolerated but require titration. In two trials, polyethylene glycol was effective in treating constipation symptoms in IBS-C but not abdominal pain [30, 31]. Two other osmotic laxatives, lactulose and sorbitol, may also increase stool frequency but are often associated with the side effects of bloating and/or cramping in IBS patients. The efficacy of stimulant laxatives such as senna, cascara, and bisacodyl has been better studied in chronic (functional) constipation [32] than in IBS-C, but they may be useful on an intermittent basis, though they frequently cause cramping, loose stools, and urgency.

5-HT4 Agonists

While tegaserod, a selective 5-HT4 partial agonist, is effective in improving symptoms of IBS-C [33, 34] and mixed-type irritable bowel syndrome (IBS-M) [3,35], it has been withdrawn by the Food and Drug Administration (FDA) because it increases the incidence of cardiovascular ischemic events. Prucalopride is a 5-HT4 agonist that is approved and effective in chronic constipation. It has not been studied in IBS, but there is significant overlap in the two disorders. It has no known cardiovascular effects [36].

Chloride Channel Activator

The chloride channel (ClC-2)-activator lubiprostone acts luminally to increase intestinal secretion. Lubiprostone improves global IBS symptoms, stool consistency, straining, abdominal pain/discomfort, health-related quality of life, and constipation severity [37]. The most common side effects are nausea and diarrhea [37].

Guanylate Cyclase C Agonist

Linaclotide is a minimally absorbed peptide that activates guanylate cyclase C on the luminal surface of the intestinal epithelium, resulting in increased luminal secretion. Pooled results from three high-quality trials of linaclotide in IBS-C support its efficacy in treating bowel symptoms, abdominal pain, bloating, and global IBS symptoms [38]. Linaclotide is safe and well-tolerated, with the most common adverse effect being diarrhea.

Therapies for IBS with Diarrhea

Therapies for patients with IBS-D are outlined in Table 65.5. Where available, the grade of recommendation from guidelines published by the American College of Gastroenterology (ACG) is provided [3].

Antidiarrheals

Antidiarrheal agents are frequently used in IBS with diarrheal symptoms. The only agent that has been evaluated in randomized controlled trials (RCTs) is loperamide. Though antidiarrheals can be used regularly, with doses of up to 4 mg four times daily, they are more commonly used on an as-needed basis, such as before leaving the house, a long car trip, a meal, or a stressful event.

Antibiotics

Small-intestine bacterial overgrowth (SIBO) and dysbiosis have been theorized to play a role in IBS [39]. Rifaximin is an antibiotic with low systemic absorption and broad-spectrum activity against Gram-positive and Gram-negative aerobes and anaerobes. A meta-analysis found rifaximin to be more efficacious than placebo for global IBS symptom improvement and bloating [40].

5-HT3 Antagonists

5-HT3 receptor antagonists slow gut transit and reduce visceral hypersensitivity [41, 42]. Alosetron improves abdominal pain and GI symptoms in IBS-D patients [43–47], and there is evidence for long-term efficacy [48]. Alosetron is currently available under a risk evaluation and mitigation strategy (REMS) for women with severe IBS-D. This restriction is due to the occurrence of GI-related serious adverse events, including ischemic colitis and serious complications of constipation [49]. Ramosetron is a 5-HT3 receptor antagonist that is available in Japan. In a phase II clinical trial, ramosetron was more effective than placebo for global IBS symptoms and abdominal pain and discomfort, and was not associated with ischemic colitis or serious complications of constipation [50].

Therapies for Multiple Subtypes of IBS

Therapies for patients with IBS-multiple subtypes are outlined in Table 65.6. Where available, the grade of recommendation from guidelines published by the American College of Gastroenterology (ACG) is provided [3].

Antispasmodics

Antispasmodics work by a direct effect on intestinal smooth muscle (e.g., mebeverine, papaverine, pinaverine, peppermint oil) or via their anticholinergic or antimuscarinic properties (e.g., dicyclomine, hyoscyamine, hyoscine, cimetroprium, pirenzepine). While hyoscyamine is one of the more commonly used antispasmodic agents available in the United States, it has not been studied in IBS [51]. A Cochrane Group meta-analysis found a beneficial effect of antispasmodics over placebo in improvement of abdominal pain, global assessment, and symptom score [27]. The most common

Table 65.5 Evidence-based pharmacological treatment of diarrhea.

Agent (class)	Dose	NNT (95% CI)	Grade of recommendation[a] [3]	Comment
Loperamide (Antidiarrheal)	Up to 4 mg four times daily	Studied in 2 poor-quality trials with total n = 42	2C (for reducing stool frequency and improving consistency)	
Rifaximin (Antibiotic)	550 mg three times daily for 10 days	NNT (95% CI) for adequate relief of IBS: 10 (6–16). Pooled from five studies, total n = 1733, majority non-C IBS [40]	1B (for short-term course of treatment)	Retreatment studies are ongoing
Alosetron (5-HT3 agonist)	0.5–1.0mg twice daily	8 (5–17)[b] [92]	1B for benefits outweighing risks in women with severe IBS-D	In the United States, only available under a risk-management program for women with severe IBS-D

[a] See Table 65.3.
[b] To prevent one additional patient from having persistent symptoms.
NNT, number needed to treat.

Table 65.6 Evidence-based pharmacological treatment various IBS subtypes.

Agent (class)	Dose	NNT (95% CI)	Grade of recommendation[a] [3]
Bifidobacterium infantis 35624 (Probiotic)	1×10^8 CFU daily	Improved pain and bowel symptoms in comparison to placebo (total n = 182, treatment duration 4 weeks). The same effect was not seen for a higher dose (1×10^{10} CFU), but this may be due to the properties of the formulation [65] In an 8-week trial, superior to placebo and *Lactobacillus salivarius* in treating pain and discomfort (total n for three arms = 77) [64]	2C
Other probiotics		Pooled results from 10 studies (total n = 918) reporting dichotomous outcome for pain or global symptoms, NNT: 4 (2–13) [93]	
SSRIs (e.g., fluoxetine, sertraline, paroxetine, citalopram)	10–100 mg daily	In pooled results from four studies (total n = 227), NNT for improvement of global symptoms was 3 (2–25) [27]	1B for global symptoms
TCAs (e.g. amitriptyline, imipramine, doxepin, desipramine, nortriptyline)	10–200 mg daily	In pooled results from eight studies (total n = 523), NNT for improvement of global symptoms was 4 (2–7), and in pooled results from four studies (total n = 320), NNT for improvement of abdominal pain was 4 (6–25) [27]	1B for global symptoms
Hyoscine/scopamine (Antispasmodic)	10 mg three times daily	Three trials enrolling a total of 426 patients. Outcome was global assessment of symptoms. NNT: 3 (2–25)[b] [28]	2C for short-term relief of pain/discomfort
Alverine citrate 60 mg + simethicone 300 mg (Antispasmodic)	Three times daily	Studied in one trial enrolling Rome II IBS patients (n = 409). For ≥50% decrease in abdominal pain, NNT: 8 (4–33) [52]	
Otilonium bromide (Antispasmodic)	40 mg three times daily before meals	In an RCT in Rome II IBS (total n = 339), NNT for improvement of pain frequency score by 1 point on a 0–3-point scale at week 15 compared to baseline: 7 (4–40) [53] When included in a meta-analysis for improvement in pain or symptoms (five studies, total n = 774), NNT: 5 (3–10) [28,53]	
Peppermint oil (Antispasmodic)	~200 mg three times daily	In pooled results from four trials (total n = 392), NNT for improvement in pain or global symptoms: 2 (2–3)[b] [28]	2C for short-term relief of pain/discomfort

[a]See Table 65.3.
[b]To prevent one additional patient from having persistent symptoms.
NNT, number needed to treat; CFU, colony-forming unit; SSRI, selective serotonin reuptake inhibitor; TCA, tricyclic antidepressant; IBS, irritable bowel syndrome; RCT, randomized controlled trial.

adverse effects were dry mouth, dizziness, and blurred vision [28]. Most trials included in these meta-analyses were of poor quality and did not use validated outcome measures, and the ACG Task Force concluded that "certain antispasmodics (hyoscine, cimetropium, pinaverium, and peppermint oil) may provide short-term relief of abdominal pain/discomfort in IBS (Grade 2C)" [3]. However, since publication of these guidelines, alverine citrate/simethicone and otolinium bromide have both shown efficacy in RCTs [52,53].

Probiotics

Probiotics are live organisms that, when administered in adequate quantities, confer a health benefit to the host [54]. There is evidence that they have effects that may target some of the pathophysiologic mechanisms involved in IBS, such as visceral hypersensitivity [55,56], altered motility [57–59], gut permeability [60,61], and the composition of the microbiota [62]. Probiotics have also been shown to have anti-inflammatory effects [63,64].

While many species of probiotic subjectively reduce flatulence and bloating, the only one that shows good evidence for global improvement in IBS symptoms is *B. infantis* [64,65]. Other species for which there is evidence of improvement in symptoms, particularly gas, bloating, and flatulence, are *Lactobacillus salivarius* [64], VSL# 3 (a combination of three species of *Bifidobacteria*, four species of *Lactobacilli*, and *Streptococcus salivarius* ssp. *Thermophilus*) [58], another probiotic mixture (*Lactobacillus rhamnosus* GG, *L. rhamnosus* LC705, *Bifidobacteriem breve* Bb99, and *Proprionibacterium freudenreichii* ssp. *shermanii* JS) [66], and *Bifidobacterium animalis* DN-173 010 [67].

Antidepressants

Antidepressants may work in IBS through effects on pain perception via a central modulation of visceral afferent input, GI transit, firing of primary sensory afferent nerve fibers, and treatment of comorbid psychological symptoms. Antidepressants that have been studied in IBS include tricyclic antidepressants (TCAs), selective serotonin reuptake inhibitors (SSRIs), and, to a lesser extent, serotonin-norepinephrine reuptake inhibitors (SNRIs).

The results of the systematic review and meta-analysis published by the Cochrane Group show a beneficial effect of antidepressants over placebo in improvement of abdominal pain, global assessment, and symptom score [27,68]. Based on these results, the ACG Task Force on IBS concluded that TCAs and SSRIs are more effective than placebo in relieving global IBS symptoms (Grade 1B) [3].

SSRIs are generally better tolerated than TCAs, and they are commonly used in IBS, though most trials have been small. While the benefit of SSRIs appears to be for global symptoms, their side effects include diarrhea, and so they may be more useful in patients with constipation.

Other psychotropic agents such as the SNRIs duloxetine [69] and venlafaxine [70] and the atypical antipsychotic quetiapine [71] have been studied in FGIDs in small trials, but there is not enough evidence to provide general recommendations for their use in IBS.

Non-pharmacologic Therapies

Psychological Therapies

The rationale behind psychological treatments is based on the knowledge that symptom exacerbations are triggered by stressful life events in many patients, the high prevalence of comorbid psychiatric disorders, and the influence of the brain on perception of visceral pain [72]. Cognitive behavioral therapy (CBT) is a short-term, goal-oriented form of psychotherapy that focuses on the role that maladaptive thoughts play in determining behaviors and emotional responses, which can exacerbate physical symptoms. CBT is the best-studied psychological therapy and has been assessed in IBS in 18 RCTs, the majority of which found a benefit over other interventions [72]. Gut-directed hypnotherapy is hypnosis that is directed toward relaxation and control of intestinal motility by repeated suggestion of control over symptoms, followed by ego-strengthening [72]. Hypnotherapy has been shown to be effective in IBS in multiple RCTs [73–78]. There is also evidence for the efficacy of relaxation training [79, 80] and mindfulness therapy [81].

Complementary and Alternative Medicine Approaches

Because even the most effective treatments for IBS do not help all patients, many turn to complementary and alternative medicine for relief. Furthermore, many patients prefer complementary and alternative medicine treatments because they view them as natural and time-tested. In addition, complementary and alternative medicine treatments often provide a more holistic approach and a more meaningful clinician–patient relationship than Western medicine.

Acupuncture has been a popular therapy for IBS patients. A recent Cochrane Review concluded that acupuncture was likely no better than sham acupuncture for IBS [82]. Herbal medicine is another area in which patients express interest, but only a few high-quality studies have been published. The best evidence is for Chinese herbal medicine. Bensoussan and colleagues [83] showed an improvement in symptoms and global scores over placebo for patients treated with either standard or individualized Chinese herbal medicine. Only those who received individualized treatment maintained a more sustained relief of their IBS symptoms. Other alternative and herbal medicines that have been studied are extract of artichoke [84], carmint [85], the herbal mixture STW 5 [86], and melatonin [87, 88]. Due to the limited evidence and concerns about toxicity, the ACG Task Force for IBS did not make recommendations on acupuncture or herbal therapy [3].

Case Continued

Educational materials are given to the patient. After several regular visits with her provider and following avoidance of certain food triggers and starting linaclotide, her symptoms improve, including abdominal pain, bloating, and sensation of incomplete evacuation, though she is still occasionally bothered by them. A low dose of a TCA and a probiotic are discussed as possible options if her abdominal symptoms do not continue to improve with time.

Prognosis

The prevalence of IBS in population studies remains stable over time [89]. This indicates a rate of disease disappearance in addition to onset. In a systematic review of longitudinal studies over a median follow-up period of 2 years, disappearance occurred in 12–38% of patients [90]. Symptom remission with aging is also supported by the lower disease prevalence among those over 65 years of age [91]. For the patient with IBS, strategies to prevent symptom flares include avoidance of dietary triggers and life stress and learning to manage symptoms in order to develop an increased perceived sense of control over them. Having a social support system can also be beneficial to patients, as suggested by a study that found an association between greater perceived social support and lower severity of pain and overall symptoms in a cross-sectional sample.

Take Home Points

- Irritable bowel syndrome (IBS) is a prevalent and heterogeneous disorder. Patient care should be focused on reducing costs and improving patient satisfaction and health-related quality of life.
- Diagnosis is based on symptom criteria, and diagnostic tests are not indicated in the majority of patients.
- Altered gastrointestinal (GI) motility and enhanced visceral perception due to altered brain–gut interactions are key pathophysiologic mechanisms of IBS.
- Gut transit time is often normal in IBS-C and decreased in IBS-D.
- Stool form is a better predictor of bowel habit subtype and GI transit than stool frequency in IBS.
- The most effective treatment involves a collaborative effort between patient and clinician to find the treatments that provide the greatest relief of symptoms, the best management of the illness, and the greatest improvement of daily functioning.

References

1 Longstreth GF, Thompson WG, Chey WD, *et al.* Functional bowel disorders. *Gastroenterology* 2006; **130**: 1480.

2 Camilleri M. Peripheral mechanisms in irritable bowel syndrome. *N Engl J Med* 2012; **367**: 1626.

3 Brandt LJ, Chey WD, Foxx-Orenstein AE, *et al.* An evidence-based position statement on the management of irritable bowel syndrome. *Am J Gastroenterol* 2009; **104**(Suppl. 1): S1.

4 Lovell RM, Ford AC. Global prevalence of and risk factors for irritable bowel syndrome: a meta-analysis. *Clin Gastroenterol Hepatol* 2012; **10**: 712.

5 Lovell RM, Ford AC. Effect of gender on prevalence of irritable bowel syndrome in the community: systematic review and meta-analysis. *Am J Gastroenterol* 2012; **107**: 991.

6 Everhart JE. *Functional Intestinal Disorders.* Washington, DC: US Government Printing Office: US Department of Health and Human Services, Public Health Service, National Institutes of Health, National Institute of Diabetes and Digestive and Kidney Diseases, 2008 Contract No.: NIH Publication No. 09-6443.

7 Palsson OS, Baggish JS, Turner MJ, Whitehead WE. IBS patients show frequent fluctuations between loose/watery and hard/lumpy stools: implications for treatment. *Am J Gastroenterol* 2012; **107**: 286.

8 Talley NJ, Dennis EH, Schettler-Duncan VA, *et al.* Overlapping upper and lower gastrointestinal symptoms in irritable bowel syndrome patients with constipation or diarrhea. *Am J Gastroenterol* 2003; **98**: 2454.

9 Riedl A, Schmidtmann M, Stengel A, *et al.* Somatic comorbidities of irritable bowel syndrome: a systematic analysis. *J Psychosom Res* 2008; **64**: 573.

10 Walker EA, Katon WJ, Jemelka RP, Roy-Byrne PP. Comorbidity of gastrointestinal complaints, depression, and anxiety in the epidemiologic catchment area (eca) study. *Am J Med* 1992; **92**: 26S.

11 Spiegel B, Strickland A, Naliboff BD, *et al.* Predictors of patient-assessed illness severity in irritable bowel syndrome. *Am J Gastroenterol* 2008; **103**: 2536.

12 Ford AC, Bercik P, Morgan DG, *et al.* Validation of the rome III criteria for the diagnosis of irritable bowel syndrome in secondary care. *Gastroenterology* 2013; **145**: 1262.

13 Whitehead WE, Palsson OS, Feld AD, *et al.* Utility of red flag symptom exclusions in the diagnosis of irritable bowel syndrome. *Aliment Pharmacol Ther* 2006; **24**: 137.

14 Porter CK, Cash BD, Pimentel M, *et al.* Risk of inflammatory bowel disease following a diagnosis of irritable bowel syndrome. *BMC Gastroenterol* 2012; **12**: 55.

15 Cash BD, Schoenfeld P, Chey WD. The utility of diagnostic tests in irritable bowel syndrome patients: a systematic review. *Am J Gastroenterol* 2002; **97**: 2812.

16 Mein SM, Ladabaum U. Serological testing for coeliac disease in patients with symptoms of irritable bowel syndrome: a cost-effectiveness analysis. *Aliment Pharmacol Ther* 2004; **19**: 1199.

17 Spiegel BMR, Derosa VP, Gralnek IM, *et al.* Testing for celiac sprue in irritable bowel syndrome with predominant diarrhea: a cost-effectiveness analysis. *Gastroenterology* 2004; **126**: 1721.

18 Spiegel BM, Gralnek IM, Bolus R, *et al.* Is a negative colonoscopy associated with reassurance or improved health-related quality of life in irritable bowel syndrome? *Gastrointest Endosc* 2005; **62**: 892.

19 Chey WD, Nojkov B, Rubenstein JH, *et al.* The yield of colonoscopy in patients with non-constipated irritable bowel syndrome: results from a prospective, controlled us trial. *Am J Gastroenterol* 2010; **105**: 859.

20 Stewart M, Brown JB, Donner A, *et al.* The impact of patient-centered care on outcomes. *J Fam Pract* 2000; **49**: 796.

21 Chang L, Drossman D. Optimizing patient care: the psychological interview in irritable bowel syndrome. *Clin Perspect* 2002; **5**: 336.

22 Biesiekierski JR, Newnham ED, Irving PM, *et al.* Gluten causes gastrointestinal symptoms in subjects without celiac disease: a double-blind randomized placebo-controlled trial. *Am J Gastroenterol* 2011; **106**: 508.

23 Shepherd SJ, Parker FC, Muir JG, Gibson PR. Dietary triggers of abdominal symptoms in patients with irritable bowel syndrome: randomized placebo-controlled evidence. *Clin Gastroenterol Hepatol* 2008; **6**: 765.

24 Busch AJ, Schachter CL, Overend TJ, *et al.* Exercise for fibromyalgia: a systematic review. *J Rheumatol* 2008; **35**: 1130.

25 Villoria A, Serra J, Azpiroz F, Malagelada JR. Physical activity and intestinal gas clearance in patients with bloating. *Am J Gastroenterol* 2006; **101**: 2552.

26 Johannesson E, Simren M, Strid H, *et al.* Physical activity improves symptoms in irritable bowel syndrome: a randomized controlled trial. *Am J Gastroenterol* 2011; **106**: 915.

27 Ruepert L, Quartero AO, De Wit NJ, *et al.* Bulking agents, antispasmodics and antidepressants for the treatment of irritable bowel syndrome. *Cochrane Database Syst Rev* 2011:CD003460.

28 Ford AC, Talley NJ, Spiegel BM, *et al.* Effect of fibre, antispasmodics, and peppermint oil in the treatment of irritable bowel syndrome: systematic review and meta-analysis. *BMJ* 2008; **337**: a2313.

29 Bijkerk CJ, De Wit NJ, Muris JW, *et al.* Soluble or insoluble fibre in irritable bowel syndrome in primary care? Randomised placebo controlled trial. *BMJ* 2009; **339**: b3154.

30 Khoshoo V, Armstead C, Landry L. Effect of a laxative with and without tegaserod in adolescents with constipation predominant irritable bowel syndrome. *Aliment Pharmacol Ther* 2006; **23**: 191.

31 Chapman RW, Stanghellini V, Geraint M, Halphen M. Randomized clinical trial: macrogol/peg 3350 plus electrolytes for treatment of patients with constipation associated with irritable bowel syndrome. *Am J Gastroenterol* 2013; **108**: 1508.

32 Bharucha AE, Pemberton JH, Locke GR 3rd. American gastroenterological association technical review on constipation. *Gastroenterology* 2013; **144**: 218.

33 Muller-Lissner SA, Fumagalli I, Bardhan KD, *et al.* Tegaserod, a 5-ht(4) receptor partial agonist, relieves symptoms in irritable bowel syndrome patients with abdominal pain, bloating and constipation. *Aliment Pharmacol Ther* 2001; **15**: 1655.

34 Novick J, Miner P, Krause R, *et al.* A randomized, double-blind, placebo-controlled trial of tegaserod in female patients suffering from irritable bowel syndrome with constipation. *Aliment Pharmacol Ther* 2002; **16**: 1877.

35 Chey WD, Pare P, Viegas A, *et al.* Tegaserod for female patients suffering from ibs with mixed bowel habits or constipation: a randomized controlled trial. *Am J Gastroenterol* 2008; **103**: 1217.

36 Camilleri M, Kerstens R, Rykx A, Vandeplassche L. A placebo-controlled trial of prucalopride for severe chronic constipation. *N Engl J Med* 2008; **358**: 2344.

37 Drossman DA, Chey WD, Johanson JF, *et al.* Clinical trial: lubiprostone in patients with constipation-associated irritable bowel syndrome – results of two randomized, placebo-controlled studies. *Aliment Pharmacol Ther* 2009; **29**: 329.

38 Videlock EJ, Cheng V, Cremonini F. Effects of linaclotide in patients with irritable bowel syndrome with constipation or chronic constipation: a meta-analysis. *Clin Gastroenterol Hepatol* 2013; **11**(9): 1084–92.e3.

39 Pimentel M, Chow EJ, Lin HC. Normalization of lactulose breath testing correlates with symptom improvement in irritable bowel syndrome. A double-blind, randomized, placebo-controlled study. *Am J Gastroenterol* 2003; **98**: 412.

40 Menees SB, Maneerattannaporn M, Kim HM, Chey WD. The efficacy and safety of rifaximin for the irritable bowel syndrome: a systematic review and meta-analysis. *Am J Gastroenterol* 2012; **107**: 28.

41 Delvaux M, Louvel D, Mamet JP, *et al.* Effect of alosetron on responses to colonic distension in patients with irritable bowel syndrome. *Aliment Pharmacol Ther* 1998; **12**: 849.

42 Houghton LA, Foster JM, Whorwell PJ. Alosetron, a 5-ht3 receptor antagonist, delays colonic transit in patients with irritable bowel syndrome and healthy volunteers. *Aliment Pharmacol Ther* 2000; **14**: 775.

43 Cremonini F, Nicandro JP, Atkinson V, *et al.* Randomised clinical trial: alosetron improves quality of life and reduces restriction of daily activities in women with severe diarrhoea-predominant IBS. *Aliment Pharmacol Ther* 2012; **36**: 437.

44 Chang L, Ameen VZ, Dukes GE, *et al.* A dose-ranging, phase ii study of the efficacy and safety of alosetron in men with diarrhea-predominant IBS. *Am J Gastroenterol* 2005; **100**: 115.

45 Lembo T, Wright RA, Bagby B, *et al.* Alosetron controls bowel urgency and provides global symptom improvement in women with diarrhea-predominant irritable bowel syndrome. *Am J Gastroenterol* 2001; **96**: 2662.

46 Camilleri M, Chey WY, Mayer EA, *et al.* A randomized controlled clinical trial of the serotonin type 3 receptor antagonist alosetron in women with diarrhea-predominant irritable bowel syndrome. *Arch Intern Med* 2001; **161**: 1733.

47 Camilleri M, Northcutt AR, Kong S, *et al.* Efficacy and safety of alosetron in women with irritable bowel syndrome: a randomised, placebo-controlled trial. *Lancet* 2000; **355**: 1035.

48 Chey WD, Chey WY, Heath AT, *et al.* Long-term safety and efficacy of alosetron in women with severe diarrhea-predominant irritable bowel syndrome. *Am J Gastroenterol* 2004; **99**: 2195.

49 Chang L, Chey WD, Harris L, *et al.* Incidence of ischemic colitis and serious complications of constipation among patients using alosetron: systematic review of clinical trials and post marketing surveillance data. *Am J Gastroenterol* 2006; **101**: 1069.

50 Matsueda K, Harasawa S, Hongo M, *et al.* A phase II trial of the novel serotonin type 3 receptor antagonist ramosetron in japanese male and female patients with diarrhea-predominant irritable bowel syndrome. *Digestion* 2008; **77**: 225.

51 Shaheen NJ, Robertson DJ, Crosby MA, *et al.* Hyoscyamine as a pharmacological adjunct in colonoscopy: a randomized, double blinded, placebo-controlled trial. *Am J Gastroenterol* 1999; **94**: 2905.

52 Wittmann T, Paradowski L, Ducrotte P, *et al.* Clinical trial: the efficacy of alverine citrate/simeticone combination on abdominal pain/discomfort in irritable bowel syndrome – a randomized, double-blind, placebo-controlled study. *Aliment Pharmacol Ther* 2010; **31**: 615.

53 Clave P, Acalovschi M, Triantafillidis JK, *et al.* Randomised clinical trial: otilonium bromide improves frequency of abdominal pain, severity of distention and time to relapse in patients with irritable bowel syndrome. *Aliment Pharmacol Ther* 2011; **34**: 432.

54 Guarner F, Requena T, Marcos A. Consensus statements from the workshop "probiotics and health: scientific evidence." *Nutr Hosp* 2010; **25**(5): 700.

55 Rousseaux C, Thuru X, Gelot A, et al. Lactobacillus acidophilus modulates intestinal pain and induces opioid and cannabinoid receptors. *Nat Med* 2007; **13**(1): 35–7.

56 Kamiya T, Wang L, Forsythe P, *et al.* Inhibitory effects of *Lactobacillus reuteri* on visceral pain induced by colorectal distension in sprague-dawley rats. *Gut* 2006; **55**: 191.

57 Agrawal A, Houghton LA, Morris J, *et al.* Clinical trial: the effects of a fermented milk product containing *Bifidobacterium lactis* DN-173 010 on abdominal distension and gastrointestinal transit in irritable bowel syndrome with constipation. *Aliment Pharmacol Ther* 2009; **29**: 104.

58 Kim HJ, Vazquez Roque MI, Camilleri M, *et al.* A randomized controlled trial of a probiotic combination VSL# 3 and placebo in irritable bowel syndrome with bloating. *Neurogastroenterol Motil* 2005; **17**: 687.

59 Kim HJ, Camilleri M, Mckinzie S, *et al.* A randomized controlled trial of a probiotic, VSL#3, on gut transit and symptoms in diarrhoea-predominant irritable bowel syndrome. *Aliment Pharmacol Ther* 2003; **17**: 895.

60 Zareie M, Johnson-Henry K, Jury J, *et al.* Probiotics prevent bacterial translocation and improve intestinal barrier function in rats following chronic psychological stress. *Gut* 2006; **55**: 1553.

61 Agostini S, Goubern M, Tondereau V, *et al.* A marketed fermented dairy product containing *Bifidobacterium lactis* CNCM I-2494 suppresses gut hypersensitivity and colonic barrier disruption induced by acute stress in rats. *Neurogastroenterol Motil* 2012; **24**: 376.

62 Kajander K, Myllyluoma E, Rajilic-Stojanovic M, *et al.* Clinical trial: Multispecies probiotic supplementation alleviates the symptoms of irritable bowel syndrome and stabilizes intestinal microbiota. *Aliment Pharmacol Ther* 2008; **27**: 48.

63 Mccarthy J, O'Mahony L, O'Callaghan L, *et al.* Double blind, placebo controlled trial of two probiotic strains in interleukin 10 knockout mice and mechanistic link with cytokine balance. *Gut* 2003; **52**: 975.

64 O'Mahony L, Mccarthy J, Kelly P, *et al.* Lactobacillus and bifidobacterium in irritable bowel syndrome: symptom responses and relationship to cytokine profiles. *Gastroenterology* 2005; **128**: 541.

65 Whorwell PJ, Altringer L, Morel J, *et al.* Efficacy of an encapsulated probiotic *Bifidobacterium infantis* 35624 in women with irritable bowel syndrome. *Am J Gastroenterol* 2006; **101**: 1581.

66 Kajander K, Hatakka K, Poussa T, *et al.* A probiotic mixture alleviates symptoms in irritable bowel syndrome patients: a controlled 6-month intervention. *Aliment Pharmacol Ther* 2005; **22**: 387.

67 Guyonnet D, Chassany O, Ducrotte P, *et al.* Effect of a fermented milk containing *Bifidobacterium animalis* DN-173 010 on the health-related quality of life and symptoms in irritable bowel syndrome in adults in primary care: a multicentre, randomized, double-blind, controlled trial. *Aliment Pharmacol Ther* 2007; **26**: 475.

CHAPTER 65

68 Ford AC, Talley NJ, Schoenfeld PS, *et al.* Efficacy of antidepressants and psychological therapies in irritable bowel syndrome: systematic review and meta-analysis. *Gut* 2009; **58**: 367.

69 Brennan BP, Fogarty KV, Roberts JL, *et al.* Duloxetine in the treatment of irritable bowel syndrome: an open-label pilot study. *Hum Psychopharmacol* 2009; **24**: 423.

70 Van Kerkhoven LA, Laheij RJ, Aparicio N, *et al.* Effect of the antidepressant venlafaxine in functional dyspepsia: a randomized, double-blind, placebo-controlled trial. *Clin Gastroenterol Hepatol* 2008; **6**: 746.

71 Hamner MB, Deitsch SE, Brodrick PS, *et al.* Quetiapine treatment in patients with posttraumatic stress disorder: an open trial of adjunctive therapy. *J Clin Psychopharmacol* 2003; **23**: 15.

72 Palsson OS, Whitehead WE. Psychological treatments in functional gastrointestinal disorders: a primer for the gastroenterologist. *Clin Gastroenterol Hepatol* 2013; **11**: 208.

73 Whorwell PJ, Prior A, Faragher EB. Controlled trial of hypnotherapy in the treatment of severe refractory irritable-bowel syndrome. *Lancet* 1984; **2**: 1232.

74 Lindfors P, Unge P, Arvidsson P, *et al.* Effects of gut-directed hypnotherapy on IBS in different clinical settings-results from two randomized, controlled trials. *Am J Gastroenterol* 2012; **107**: 276.

75 Forbes A, Macauley S, Chiotakakou-Faliakou E. Hypnotherapy and therapeutic audiotape: effective in previously unsuccessfully treated irritable bowel syndrome? *Int J Colorect Dis* 2000; **15**: 328.

76 Galovski TE, Blanchard EB. The treatment of irritable bowel syndrome with hypnotherapy. *Appl Psychophysiol Biofeedback* 1998; **23**: 219.

77 Palsson OS, Turner MJ, Johnson DA, *et al.* Hypnosis treatment for severe irritable bowel syndrome: investigation of mechanism and effects on symptoms. *Dig Dis Sci* 2002; **47**: 2605.

78 Roberts L, Wilson S, Singh S, *et al.* Gut-directed hypnotherapy for irritable bowel syndrome: piloting a primary care-based randomised controlled trial. *Brit J Gen Pract* 2006; **56**: 115.

79 Fernandez C, Perez M, Amigo I, Linares A. Stress and contingency management in the treatment of irritable bowel syndrome. *Stress Health* 1998; **14**: 31.

80 Van Der Veek PP, Van Rood YR, Masclee AA. Clinical trial: short- and long-term benefit of relaxation training for irritable bowel syndrome. *Aliment Pharmacol Ther* 2007; **26**: 943.

81 Gaylord SA, Palsson OS, Garland EL, *et al.* Mindfulness training reduces the severity of irritable bowel syndrome in women: results of a randomized controlled trial. *Am J Gastroenterol* 2011; **106**: 1678.

82 Manheimer E, Cheng K, Wieland LS, *et al.* Acupuncture for treatment of irritable bowel syndrome. *Cochrane Database Syst Rev* 2012(5):CD005111.

83 Bensoussan A, Talley NJ, Hing M, *et al.* Treatment of irritable bowel syndrome with chinese herbal medicine: a randomized controlled trial. *JAMA* 1998; **280**: 1585.

84 Bundy R, Walker AF, Middleton RW, *et al.* Artichoke leaf extract reduces symptoms of irritable bowel syndrome and improves quality of life in otherwise healthy volunteers suffering from concomitant dyspepsia: a subset analysis. *J Alt Complement Med* 2004; **10**: 667.

85 Vejdani R, Shalmani HR, Mir-Fattahi M, *et al.* The efficacy of an herbal medicine, carmint, on the relief of abdominal pain and bloating in patients with irritable bowel syndrome: a pilot study. *Dig Dis Sci* 2006; **51**: 1501.

86 Madisch A, Holtmann G, Plein K, Hotz J. Treatment of irritable bowel syndrome with herbal preparations: results of a double-blind, randomized, placebo-controlled, multi-centre trial. *Aliment Pharmacol Ther* 2004; **19**: 271.

87 Lu WZ, Gwee KA, Moochhalla S, Ho KY. Melatonin improves bowel symptoms in female patients with irritable bowel syndrome: a double-blind placebo-controlled study. *Aliment Pharmacol Ther* 2005; **22**: 927.

88 Song GH, Leng PH, Gwee KA, *et al.* Melatonin improves abdominal pain in irritable bowel syndrome patients who have sleep disturbances: a randomised, double blind, placebo controlled study. *Gut* 2005; **54**: 1402.

89 Olafsdottir LB, Gudjonsson H, Jonsdottir HH, Thjodleifsson B. Stability of the irritable bowel syndrome and subgroups as measured by three diagnostic criteria – a 10-year follow-up study. *Aliment Pharmacol Ther* 2010; **32**: 670.

90 El-Serag HB, Pilgrim P, Schoenfeld P. Systemic review: Natural history of irritable bowel syndrome. *Aliment Pharmacol Ther* 2004; **19**: 861.

91 Saito YA, Schoenfeld P, Locke GR 3rd. The epidemiology of irritable bowel syndrome in north america: a systematic review. *Am J Gastroenterol* 2002; **97**: 1910.

92 Ford AC, Brandt LJ, Young C, *et al.* Efficacy of 5-HT3 antagonists and 5-HT4 agonists in irritable bowel syndrome: systematic review and meta analysis. *Am J Gastroenterol* 2009; **104**: 1831.

93 Moayyedi P, Ford AC, Talley NJ, *et al.* The efficacy of probiotics in the treatment of irritable bowel syndrome: a systematic review. *Gut* 2010; **59**: 325.

CHAPTER 66

Chronic Functional Constipation and Dyssynergic Defecation

Satish S.C. Rao[1] and Yeong Yeh Lee[2]

[1] Section of Gastroenterology and Hepatology, Medical College of Georgia, Georgia Regents University, Augusta, GA, USA
[2] School of Medical Sciences, Universiti Sains Malaysia, Kubang Kerian, Kelantan, Malaysia

Summary

Chronic functional constipation is defined on the basis of symptoms alone, but dyssynergic defecation requires symptoms and physiological tests for confirmation (Rome III criteria). Exclusion of organic diseases is the first step in the evaluation of constipation. Key symptoms of constipation include straining, lumpy or hard stools, a feeling of incomplete evacuation, a sense of anorectal blockage, digital maneuvers to facilitate defecation, and fewer than three bowel movements per week. Useful investigations may include colonic transit studies, anorectal manometry, colonic manometry, dynamic magnetic resonance imaging (MRI), and electrophysiological tests. Management includes general measures, laxatives, prokinetics, and secretagogues. Biofeedback therapy is effective in patients with dyssynergic defecation. Selected refractory cases of slow-transit constipation with neuropathy may respond to surgery or sacral nerve stimulation (SNS).

Definition and Epidemiology

In the absence of alarm symptoms and apparent organic causes, most patients with constipation have a functional disorder that affects the colon and/or the anorectum. Functional constipation and dyssynergic defecation (anismus, obstructed defecation, or pelvic floor dyssynergia) are the two common subtypes, though if pain is a prominent symptom then constipation-predominant irritable bowel syndrome (IBS-C) should be considered. These three conditions overlap frequently. The Rome III criteria for functional constipation [1] and dyssynergic defecation [2] are given in Table 66.1. Note that functional constipation is defined on the basis of symptoms alone, but dyssynergic defecation requires additional physiological evaluation (Figure 66.1).

Constipation is a very common digestive symptom that affects 4 million Americans, mostly women, the elderly, and those with a lower socioeconomic status [3]. A survey of 14 407 Americans in the first National Health and Nutrition Examination Survey (NHANES) estimated that 20.8% of women and 8.0% of men reported symptoms of constipation [4], and comparable prevalence rates have been reported worldwide [5]. Constipation involves significant health care expenditure and impairment of quality of life [6].

Pathophysiology

The left colon serves as the primary conduit for transporting formed stools into the anorectum, while the right colon serves as an absorption and fermentation chamber. The rectosigmoid region senses the stool and facilitates its evacuation when socially acceptable. These functions are coordinated by neurotransmitters (including acetylcholine, nitric oxide, serotonin, and calcitonin gene-related peptide), colonic reflexes, and learned behaviors through mechanisms that are poorly understood. Problems can potentially arise at any level along the gut–brain axis (Figure 66.2).

In slow-transit constipation, the phasic motor activity exhibits significant impairment, especially in response to a meal and upon waking, even though the diurnal pattern is preserved [7]. High-amplitude propagating contractions (HAPCs) are significantly reduced, but periodic rectal motor activity (PRMA) is increased [8], indicating a reduced and retarded colonic propulsion. The colonic tone and phasic responses to a meal, derived from barostat recordings, are also reduced [9]. Neuropathy or myopathy may cause these sensorimotor disturbances in constipation [10, 11]. Constipation can be part of a more generalized form of dysmotility and pseudo-obstruction syndrome [12]. Hormonal changes may in part explain the predominance of females having this problem, but this merits more study [13]. The presence of methanogenic flora, such as *Methanobrevibacter smithii*, may predispose indirectly to constipation [14].

Pelvic-floor dyssynergia or dyssynergic defecation is most often an acquired behavioral disturbance in adulthood, but one-third of cases result from poor learning of the process of defecation during childhood [15]. Instead of relaxing the anal sphincter, there is a paradoxical contraction or involuntary spasm (anismus) during evacuation. Almost one-third of healthy subjects may exhibit this paradoxical anal contraction as well [16]. Rectal hyposensitivity, present in more than half of patients with dyssynergic defecation, occurs due to a lack of rectal stimulation or, less often, due to afferent nerve dysfunction [17].

Practical Gastroenterology and Hepatology Board Review Toolkit, Second Edition. Edited by Nicholas J. Talley, Kenneth R. DeVault, Michael B. Wallace, Bashar A. Aqel and Keith D. Lindor.
© 2016 John Wiley & Sons, Ltd. Published 2016 by John Wiley & Sons, Ltd. Companion website: www.practicalgastrohep.com

Table 66.1 Rome III criteria for functional constipation and dyssynergic defecation.

Rome III criteria for functional constipation.
Constipation must be present for the last 3 months and symptom onset must have occurred at least 6 months before diagnosis

1. Must include two or more of the following:
   a. Straining during at least 25% of defecations
   b. Lumpy or hard stools in at least 25% of defecations
   c. Sensation of incomplete evacuation following at least 25% of defecations
   d. Sensation of anorectal obstruction or blockage during at least 25% of defecations
   e. Manual maneuvers to facilitate at least 25% of defecations (e.g., digital evacuation)
   f. Fewer than three defecations per week
2. Loose stools rarely present without the use of laxatives
3. Insufficient criteria for IBS

Modified Rome III criteria for dyssynergic defecation

A. Patients must fulfill the symptom criteria for functional constipation defined above
B. Dyssynergic pattern of defecation (types 1–IV; see Figure 66.1)
C. Constipated patients must fulfill one or more of the following physiologic criteria:
   1. Inability to expel a balloon or stool-like device (e.g., fecom) within a minute
   2. Prolonged colonic transit time (more than six markers on a plain abdominal radiograph taken 120 hours after ingestion of one Sitzmarks capsule containing 24 radio-opaque markers)
   3. Inability to expel barium or >50% retention during defecography

IBS, irritable bowel syndrome.

Case 1

A 47-year-old female with no prior medical illness presents with constipation and bloating of 6 months' duration. She has a bowel movement once a week and her stools are hard and lumpy. She sometimes needs to strain, but she does not have to remove her stools with her fingers. There is no abdominal discomfort, but she feels bloated most frequently after meals. She has tried some laxatives prescribed by her primary care physician, without help. She states that her fluid and dietary fiber intake is adequate. She does not exercise much and denies any stress or psychological disturbance.

Physical examination, including digital rectal examination, is unremarkable.

Case 2

An otherwise healthy 45-year-old female with gastroesophageal reflux disease (GERD) presents with chronic constipation of 1 year's duration. She normally needs to strain during defecation. She has two or three bowel movements a week, but her stools are not always hard. Occasionally, she has fecal leakage. She seldom feels her defecation is complete, and at times she needs to use her fingers to remove the remaining stool. Her symptoms embarrass her. They seem to have gotten worse in recent months, probably in association with her recent job change, which she claims was really demanding. There is no abdominal discomfort or bloating. Laxatives do not work for her, and she denies being on any constipating drugs. She eats healthily and has plenty of fluid every day. Physical examination is unremarkable. Digital rectal examination, however, shows small hemorrhoids and a tight sphincter, especially during bearing down.

Clinical Features

Symptoms of constipation can be heterogenous, variable, subjective, and not sensitive. They include a sense of incomplete evacuation, excessive straining, digital disimpaction, infrequent (often fewer than three bowel movements/week) or hard/lumpy stool, anal blockage, abdominal discomfort, and even bloating.

It may take a trusting patient–physician relationship before patients are willing to share their more sensitive symptoms. A long history of recurring problems suggests a motility disorder, while a more recent onset – especially when accompanied by alarm features such as age ≥45, blood in stool, change in stool caliber, unintended weight loss, fever, family history of cancer, iron-deficiency anemia, rectal bleeding, vomiting, loss of appetite, and abdominal mass – suggests a colon cancer. It is important to obtain a detailed

CHAPTER 66

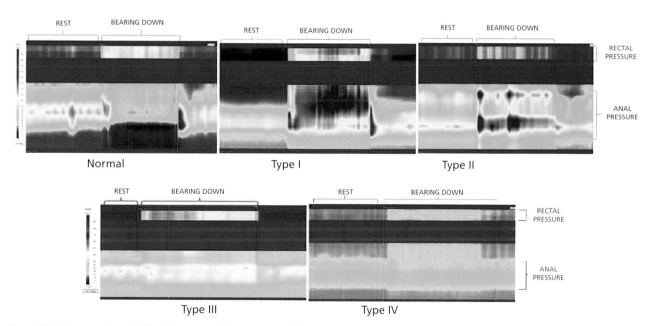

Figure 66.1 Four types (type I–IV) of dyssynergic defecation seen with high-resolution anorectal manometry, with normal finding as the comparison.

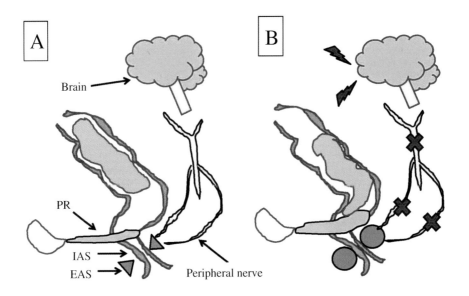

A. Normal defecation	**B. Constipation/Dyssynergic defecation**
• Normal stool perception • Normal rectal compliance • Relaxation of EAS and PR	• Rectal hyposensitivity • Abnormal rectal compliance • Paradoxical anal sphincter contraction • Poor abdominal-rectal propulsive force • Altered afferent and efferent pathway and disturbed higher cortical function

Figure 66.2 Pathological mechanisms underlying normal defecation, constipation, and dyssynergic defecation. PR, puborectalis; EAS, external anal sphincter; IAS, internal anal sphincter.

history on stool frequency, consistency, and size and on the degree of straining during evacuation. The Bristol Stool Scale is helpful in this respect. Dietary history is often poorly assessed by clinicians. It is particularly important to elicit the amount of fiber and fluid intake. Medications, including laxatives and constipating drugs, must be detailed in full, especially the type and frequency of their use. A family history of constipation can be present in one-third of patients [15]. Obstetrical, surgical, and neurological history and prior back trauma may provide important clues to the secondary etiology of constipation. Fecal incontinence can accompany constipation, especially in the elderly. A history of childhood abuse, anorexia nervosa, and psychological disturbance may point to pelvic-floor dyssynergia. Patients with dyssynergic defecation often have excessive straining for stools, incomplete sense of evacuation, and digital disimpaction; these symptoms are more common in women than men. Rectocele, rectal intussusception, and descending perineum syndrome are also frequently associated with dyssynergic defecation.

Physical signs are often absent, but detailed abdominal and neurological examination may reveal underlying systemic illnesses. There may be skin redness, tags, fissure, or hemorrhoids during the inspection of the anorectum, which will then prompt a careful digital rectal examination that also include squeeze and bearing-down maneuvers. An absence of sphincter relaxation and perineal descent is a pointer to dyssynergic defecation. Neuropathy should be suspected if the stroking of skin at four quadrants of the anorectum does not invoke any reflex contraction of the external sphincter.

Diagnosis and Differential Diagnosis

Exclusion of organic disorders is the initial step and should be prompted if the constipation is of recent onset and is accompanied by alert features. Disorders that should be considered in the differential diagnosis of constipation are shown in Table 66.2. Blood tests, endoscopy, and imaging studies are needed to exclude structural and systemic disorders. For screening purposes, complete blood count (CBC), electrolytes (potassium, calcium), glucose, and thyroid function tests (TFTs) are sufficient. Flexible sigmoidoscopy or colonoscopy is helpful in evaluating the mucosa and excluding obstructive lesions, especially cancers. A computed tomography (CT) scan of the abdomen and pelvis may be needed to evaluate any mass lesions.

Due to heterogeneity and subjectivity of symptoms, objective physiological tests are used to support the diagnosis and to determine the underlying pathophysiology. Colonic transit can be assessed with radio-opaque markers or Sitzmarks (Konsyl Pharmaceutics, Fort Worth, TX) (Table 66.1) or, more recently, with the less invasive wireless motility capsule (WMC) (SmartPill, Given Imaging, Yoqneam, Israel). WMCs have the added advantage that they can evaluate transit of other parts of the GI tract, including the small bowel and stomach, which may be delayed as part of the generalized GI dysmotility and/or intestinal pseudo-obstruction syndrome [18]. A delay in colonic transit time with Sitzmarks (six or more scattered throughout the colon) or WMCs (>59 hours) indicates slow-transit constipation [18].

Table 66.2 Causes of constipation.

Idiopathic		
Common disorders	**a.**	Inadequate water intake
	b.	Inadequate fiber intake
	c.	Overuse of coffee, tea, or alcohol
	d.	Reduced levels of exercise
	e.	Stress and other psychological disturbances
	f.	Drugs, including antidepressants, opiods, antacids, NSAIDs
	g.	Chronic laxative abuse
	h.	Dyssynergic defecation
	i.	IBS with constipation
	j.	Pregnancy
	k.	Diabetic gastroenteropathy
Less common disorders	**a.**	Normal and slow-transit constipation
	b.	IBD with stricture
	c.	Colon cancer with obstruction/strictures
	d.	Small-intestinal obstruction/stricture/lymphoma
	e.	Chronic intestinal pseudo-obstruction
	f.	Bacterial/viral and parasitic infections
	g.	Diverticular disease
	h.	Anal disorders, including fissures, hemorrhoids, and abscess
	i.	Endocrine disorders, including hypothyroidism, diabetes mellitus, hyperparathyroidism, hypercalcemia, and hypokalemia
Rare	**a.**	Neurologic disorders, including stroke, Parkinson's disease, multiple sclerosis, spinal-cord lesions or injury, Chagas' disease, and head injury
	b.	Hirschsprung's disease
	c.	Connective-tissue disorders, including scleroderma, amyloidosis, and mixed connective-tissue disease
	d.	Lead poisoning

NSAID, non-steroidal anti-inflammatory drug; IBS, irritable bowel syndrome; IBD, inflammatory bowel disease.

Patients with dyssynergic defecation may have normal or slow-transit constipation [17]. Inability to expel, a 4 cm water-filled balloon or a stool-like device such as fecom from the rectum within 1 minute is consistent with dyssynergic defecation. If anorectal manometry also reveals a dyssynergic pattern during bearing down then dyssynergic defecation is confirmed. There are four patterns of dyssynergia (first described with conventional manometry [19]), as follows:

- **Type 1:** The patient can generate an adequate pushing force (rise in intra-abdominal and intrarectal pressure), along with a paradoxical increase in the anal sphincter pressure.
- **Type 2:** The patient is unable to generate an adequate pushing force (no increase in intrarectal pressure), but can exhibit a paradoxical anal contraction.
- **Type 3:** The patient can generate an adequate pushing force (increase in intrarectal pressure), but has absent or incomplete (<20%) sphincter relaxation (i.e., no decrease in anal sphincter pressure).
- **Type 4:** The patient is unable to generate an adequate pushing force and demonstrates an absent or incomplete anal sphincter relaxation.

The availability of high-resolution (HR) and high-definition (HD) anorectal manometry allows these patterns to be more easily recognized [19] (Figure 66.1). Anorectal manometry may assist in the exclusion of Hirschsprung's disease through an absence of recto-anal inhibitory reflex (RAIR). Furthermore, rectal hyposensitivity can be shown by an increase in the volume thresholds for first sensation (≥40 mL) and desire to defecate (≥130 mL). This may be associated with an increase in the rectal compliance. HD anorectal manometry can provide both physiological and

morphological information, thereby allowing correlation between abnormal functions and anatomical abnormalities (e.g., anal sphincter defects) [19]. Defecography is rarely used and is regarded as an adjunct rather than a primary test for anorectal function. Dyssynergic defecation is suspected when there is an inability to expel or when more than 50% of the 150 mL of barium paste in the rectum is retained.

Colonic manometry is useful in determining whether patients with slow-transit constipation have neuropathy or myopathy, and can facilitate a decision for colectomy [20]. In the presence of neuropathy (absence of any two of three normal colonic motor responses, including the presence of HAPCs, meal response, and morning waking response), aggressive medical treatment often fails, and colectomy may have better clinical outcomes. Colectomy is a rather invasive procedure, and only a few centers provide it.

More complex anorectal disorders may require sophisticated imaging techniques, including 3D endoanal ultrasound and dynamic pelvic-floor MRI. Electrophysiological tests such as anal electromyography and pudendal nerve terminal motor latency (PNTML) may be useful in refractory cases, by excluding underlying neuropathy. Transcranial and transspinal magnetic stimulation offer a more comprehensive evaluation of the brain–anorectal axes. Through the assessment of transspinal motor-evoked potentials, it has been shown that patients with spinal-cord injury often have undetected lumbosacral neuropathy that explains their constipation [21].

Management

Underlying organic causes of constipation should be evaluated and treated first. Drugs that cause constipation, including antidepressants, opiods, antacids, calcium channel blockers, and non-steroidal anti-inflammatory drugs (NSAIDs), should be identified and stopped. Likewise, chronic use of laxatives that lead to habituation and dilated atonic colon must be halted. More specific evidenced-based treatments are discussed in this section. A management algorithm is given in Figure 66.3. Table 66.3 summarizes the evidence-based treatment options for functional constipation and dyssynergic defecation.

Case 1 Continued

An upper endoscopy is performed and comes back normal. Biopsies are negative for celiac disease. Duodenal aspiration for culture is sent. Screening blood results, including blood counts, potassium, calcium, and TFTs, are normal. The patient's balloon expulsion time is 15 seconds. Anorectal manometry does not suggest any dyssynergia during bearing down. Her RAIR is normal. Colonic transit time with SmartPill is 64 hours (delayed), but her colonic manometry shows a normal response to meal and on waking. She has an abnormal glucose breath test, with high methane levels. Culture from duodenal aspirate was also positive. She is placed on a course of antibiotics and linaclotide. Her symptoms are improved on follow-up.

Case 2 Continued

The patient is not able to expel the rectal balloon, even at 5 minutes. HR anorectal manometry indicates that she has type I dyssynergia during bearing down. Her RAIR is normal but she has rectal hyposensitivity (first sensation at 60 mL, desire to defecate at 200 mL)

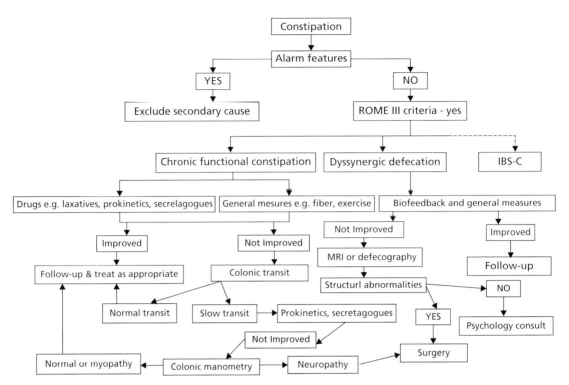

Figure 66.3 Diagnostic and management algorithm for chronic functional constipation and dyssynergic defecation. IBS-C; constipation-predominant irritable bowel syndrome, MRI; magnetic resonance imaging.

and reduced rectal compliance. Colonic transit time with SmartPill is 50 hours. She subsequently has six sessions of biofeedback therapy, which also include sensory training for her rectal hyposensitivity. Her symptoms and anorectal function are much improved after 3 months.

Table 66.3 Evidence-based management of constipation.

Treatment modalities	Prescription	Level of evidence[a]
Fluids	1.5–2.0 L/day	Level III, grade C
Dietary fiber	25 g/day	Level II, grade D [23]
Psyllium (e.g., Metamucil)	5.1 g b.i.d./day	Level II, grade B [25,27]
Methylcellulose (e.g., Celevac, Citrucel)	1.5–3 g b.i.d./day	Level III, grade C [25,27]
Lactulose (e.g., Dulphalac, Enulose)	10–20 g/15–30 mL/day	Level II, grade B [25,27]
Polyethylene glycol (e.g., Miralax)	17 g in 4–8 oz water/day	Level I, grade A [25,27]
Senna (e.g., Senokot)	15–25 mg/day	Level III, grade C [25,27]
Bisacodyl (e.g., Dulcolax)	5–15 mg/day	Level III, grade C [25,27]
Prucalopride (e.g., Resolor)	2–4 mg/day	Level I, grade A [26]
Lubiprostone (e.g., Amitiza)	24 µg b.i.d./day	Level I, grade A [27]
Linaclotide (e.g., Linzess)	145–290 µg/day	Level I, grade A [28]
Biofeedback therapy	Six 2-weekly sessions	Level I, grade A [29]
Surgery	–	Level II, grade B [25]
Sacral nerve stimulation	–	Level II, grade B [30]

[a]Level I: Good evidence. Consistent results from well-designed, well-conducted trials. Level II: Fair evidence. Results show benefit, but strength is limited by the number, quality, or consistency of the individual studies. Level III: Poor evidence. The limited number or power of the studies, or flaws in their design or conduct, render the evidence insufficient. Grade A: Good evidence in support of the use of a treatment modality. Grade B: Moderate evidence in support of the use of a treatment modality. Grade C: Poor evidence to support a recommendation for or against the use of a modality. Grade D: Moderate evidence against the use of a modality. Grade E: Good evidence to support a recommendation against the use of a modality.

Fluid, Dietary Fiber, and Exercise

Despite being generally recommended by physicians, increased fluid and dietary fiber intake have little evidence to support their claims to improve constipation. Consumption of extra fluids (isotonic or free water) alone does not result in any significant change in stool output in healthy volunteers. A beneficial effect on stool frequency can be achieved with a daily fiber intake of 25 g and fluid intake of 1.5–2.0 L/day. A systematic review of six randomized controlled trials (RCTs) showed that, compared to placebo, soluble fiber has some benefits in chronic idiopathic constipation [22], but other studies refute this claim, including the most recent report, based on dietary recall in 9375 adults in the 2005–08 NHANES [23]. Likewise, the role of exercise in gut transit time is controversial. Sedentary subjects are three times more likely to report constipation, but the effect of exercise on increasing gut transit time is inconsistent and may depend on the intensity of exercise.

Laxatives

There are many preparations of laxatives, which are generally divided into bulking agents (e.g., psyllium, methylcellulose), stool softeners (e.g., docusate), stimulants (e.g., senna, bisacodyl), osmotic laxatives (e.g., lactulose, polyethylene glycol), and enemas (e.g., phosphate). Chronic use and abuse of laxatives are common, with two-thirds of patients using them on at least a monthly basis; this may itself cause constipation, especially when patients take stimulants that result in an atonic rectum. Unfortunately, levels of dissatisfaction with laxatives are high, due to their lack of efficacy [24] and concerns about their safety. Polyethylene glycol is perhaps the exception, with strong evidence for its efficacy, even in the longer term, and a minimal risk profile, making it the laxative of choice for many practitioners today. Laxatives only relieve symptoms and do not have any effect on pathophysiology that can provide more lasting relief. As a result, the management guidelines of various societies have not made any firm recommendations to support the use of laxatives [25].

New Therapies for Functional Constipation

There are a number of new and emerging therapies that can restore colonic function, divided btween prokinetics (e.g., tegaserod, prucalopride) and secretagogues (e.g., lubiprostone, linaclotide). Prokinetics include 5-hydroxytryptamine 4 (5-HT$_4$) agonists, which can accelerate colonic transit time and gastric emptying time. Tegaserod, a partial 5-HT$_4$, has been shown to be effective in clinical trials; however, because of its coronary and cerebrovascular side effects, it has been withdrawn from the market. Newer agents with better safety profile are in development (e.g., mosapride, renzapride). Prucalopride, a dihydrobenzofurancarboxamide derivative, is a highly selective 5HT$_4$ full agonist that is available in Europe and (more recently) Asia, but currently not in the United States. A number of clinical trials have shown the efficacy of prucalopride 2 or 4 mg q.d. for 12 weeks in chronic constipation, with few adverse events despite initial concern over possible cardiac risks [25, 26]. Other new and highly selective 5HT$_4$ agonists include velusetrag and naronapride [26].

Secretagogues promote intestinal secretion, which produces softer stools and accelerates intestinal transit. Lubiprostone, a bicyclic fatty acid, acts on the type 2 chloride channels (ClC-2), leading to active secretion of chloride into the lumen, and accelerates small-bowel and colonic transit time. However, it also causes a delay in gastric emptying. RCTs have shown that, compared to placebo, lubiprostone 24 µg b.i.d. for 3 weeks is effective in improving bowel movement, stool consistency, and bloating in chronic constipation, with only minor side effects (including nausea and diarrhea) [25]. Linaclotide, another new secretagogue, is a guanylate cyclase-C (GC-C) agonist, a 14-amino-acid peptide that causes chloride and bicarbonate secretion mediated through a rise in the cyclic guanosine monophosphate. A number of RCTs have proven the efficacy and safety of linaclotide 145 µg in chronic constipation and 290 µg q.d. for 12 weeks in IBS-C [25,27].

Biofeedback Therapy for Dyssynergic Defecation

Management of dyssynergic defecation includes the standard treatment for constipation, including diet, laxatives, and pelvic-floor exercise, as well as specific treatments for neuromuscular conditioning and sensory training. Biofeedback therapy attempts to restore the normal defecation pattern through an instrument-based education program that reinforces regular behavior via repeated training. This involves diaphragmatic breathing exercises to improve the abdominal push effort and manometric-guided pelvic-floor relaxation followed by simulated defecation training. Sensory training is also performed, to improve the thresholds of stooling awareness. Intermittent inflation and deflation of the rectal balloon is used to educate patients on newer thresholds of rectal perception. On average, four to six sessions are required, with an interval of about 2 weeks. Upon completion of training, periodic reinforcement can provide good long-term outcome. RCTs have supported the effectiveness of biofeedback therapy in dyssynergic defecation, as compared to sham biofeedback or the standard therapy of diet, exercise, and laxatives. Biofeedback therapy also provides a more sustained improvement of bowel symptoms and anorectal function in the long term [28].

Refractory Cases: The Role of Surgery and Neuromodulation

Patients with slow-transit constipation of neuropathic origin are often refractory to aggressive medical treatments, and therefore surgery should be considered. Colectomy and ileostomy or ileo-rectal anastomosis are usually required, though segmental colonic resection may be considered in certain situations, especially in children. Surgery should only be considered as the last resort, and it will not be useful unless dyssynergia has been corrected. It will not relieve abdominal pain or underlying psychosocial problems. Furthermore, following colectomy, patients may develop diarrhea and/or fecal incontinence and small-bowel adhesions.

Recently, neuromodulation therapy and SNS have emerged as alternative options in refractory cases of constipation. The first sacral anterior root stimulator was implanted in 1976, to improve neurogenic bladder after spinal injury. It was later extended to improve defecation in the same group of patients. Before permanent implantation, initial testing or peripheral nerve evaluation (PNE) was performed with a temporary percutaneous lead for a screening period of 2–3 weeks in order to assess treatment response. In a recent meta-analysis of 13 studies, PNE was successful in 42–100%. Of those patients who subsequently had permanent SNS, 87% had improvement in symptoms, quality of life, and satisfaction scores [29]. Despite being effective, the exact mechanisms that underlie the success of SNS are not entirely clear. They may involve modulation of both afferent and local reflex pathways.

Take Home Points

- Exclusion of organic disorders is the first step in the evaluation of constipation. Efforts should be made to make a positive diagnosis with colorectal physiological tests.
- The Rome III criteria are used to define functional constipation (symptoms alone) and dyssynergic defecation (symptoms and physiologic tests, including expulsion tests, transit studies, anorectal manometry, and defecography).
- Colonic manometry is useful in identifying neuropathy in patients with slow-transit constipation and helps to facilitate a decision for surgery.
- General measures of management include 1.5–2.0 L fluids, 25 g daily fiber intake, exercise, and laxatives.
- Useful newer therapies include secretagogues and prokinetics (e.g., lubiprostone 24 µg b.i.d., linaclotide 145 or 290 µg q.d., prucalopride 2 or 4 mg q.d.).
- Biofeedback therapy of six 2-weekly sessions followed by periodic reinforcement is effective in relieving dyssynergic defecation.
- There is a role for surgery or sacral nerve stimulation (SNS) in selected refractory cases of constipation.

References

1 Bharucha AE, Wald A, Enck P, Rao S. Functional anorectal disorders. *Gastroenterology* 2006;**130**:1510–8.
2 Whitehead WE, Wald A, Diamant NE, *et al.* Functional disorders of the anus and rectum. *Gut* 1999;**45**(Suppl. 2): II55–9.
3 Suares NC, Ford AC. Prevalence of, and risk factors for, chronic idiopathic constipation in the community: systematic review and meta-analysis. *Am J Gastroenterol* 2011; **106**: 1582–91, quiz 1581, 1592.
4 Everhart JE, Go VL, Johannes RS, *et al.* A longitudinal survey of self-reported bowel habits in the United States. *Dig Dis Sci* 1989; **34**: 1153–62.
5 Peppas G, Alexiou VG, Mourtzoukou E, Falagas ME. Epidemiology of constipation in Europe and Oceania: a systematic review. *BMC Gastroenterol* 2008; **8**: 5.

6 Nellesen D, Yee K, Chawla A, *et al.* A systematic review of the economic and humanistic burden of illness in irritable bowel syndrome and chronic constipation. *J Manag Care Pharm* 2013; **19**: 755–64.

7 Rao SSC, Sadeghi P, Beaty J, Kavlock R. Ambulatory 24-hour colonic manometry in slow-transit constipation. *Am J Gastroenterol* 2004; **99**: 2405–16.

8 Rao SS, Sadeghi P, Batterson K, Beaty J. Altered periodic rectal motor activity: a mechanism for slow transit constipation. *Neurogastroenterol Motil* 2001; **13**: 591–8.

9 Law N-M, Bharucha AE, Zinsmeister AR. Rectal and colonic distension elicit viscerovisceral reflexes in humans. *Am J Physiol Gastrointest Liver Physiol* 2002; **283**: G384–9.

10 He CL, Burgart L, Wang L, *et al.* Decreased interstitial cell of cajal volume in patients with slow-transit constipation. *Gastroenterology* 2000; **118**: 14–21.

11 Rao SSC, Sadeghi P, Beaty J, Kavlock R. Ambulatory 24-hour colonic manometry in slow-transit constipation. *Am J Gastroenterol* 2004; **99**: 2405–16.

12 Mollen RM, Hopman WP, Kuijpers HH, Jansen JB. Abnormalities of upper gut motility in patients with slow-transit constipation. *Eur J Gastroenterol Hepatol* 1999; **11**: 701–8.

13 Preston DM, Lennard-Jones JE. Severe chronic constipation of young women: "idiopathic slow transit constipation." *Gut* 1986; **27**: 41–8.

14 Attaluri A, Jackson M, Valestin J, Rao SSC. Methanogenic flora is associated with altered colonic transit but not stool characteristics in constipation without IBS. *Am J Gastroenterol* 2010; **105**: 1407–11.

15 Rao SSC, Tuteja AK, Vellema T, *et al.* Dyssynergic defecation: demographics, symptoms, stool patterns, and quality of life. *J Clin Gastroenterol* 2004; **38**: 680–5.

16 Rao SS, Hatfield R, Soffer E, *et al.* Manometric tests of anorectal function in healthy adults. *Am J Gastroenterol* 1999; **94**: 773–83.

17 Lunniss PJ, Gladman MA, Benninga MA, Rao SS. Pathophysiology of evacuation disorders. *Neurogastroenterol Motil* 2009; **21**(Suppl. 2): 31–40.

18 Rao SSC, Camilleri M, Hasler WL, *et al.* Evaluation of gastrointestinal transit in clinical practice: position paper of the American and European Neurogastroenterology and Motility Societies. *Neurogastroenterol Motil* 2011; **23**: 8–23.

19 Lee YY, Erdogan A, Rao SSC. High resolution and high definition anorectal manometry and pressure topography: diagnostic advance or a new kid on the block? *Curr Gastroenterol Rep* 2013; **15**: 360.

20 Rao SSC, Sadeghi P, Beaty J, Kavlock R. Ambulatory 24-hour colonic manometry in slow-transit constipation. *Am J Gastroenterol* 2004; **99**: 2405–16.

21 Tantiphlachiva K, Attaluri A, Valestin J, *et al.* Translumbar and transsacral motor-evoked potentials: a novel test for spino-anorectal neuropathy in spinal cord injury. *Am J Gastroenterol* 2011; **106**: 907–14.

22 Suares NC, Ford AC. Systematic review: the effects of fibre in the management of chronic idiopathic constipation. *Aliment Pharmacol Ther* 2011; **33**: 895–901.

23 Markland AD, Palsson O, Goode PS, *et al.* Association of low dietary intake of fiber and liquids with constipation: evidence from the National Health and Nutrition Examination Survey. *Am J Gastroenterol* 2013; **108**: 796–803.

24 Remes-Troche JM, Rao SSC. Defecation disorders: neuromuscular aspects and treatment. *Curr Gastroenterol Rep* 2006; **8**: 291–9.

25 Ford AC, Suares NC. Effect of laxatives and pharmacological therapies in chronic idiopathic constipation: systematic review and meta-analysis. *Gut* 2011; **60**: 209–18.

26 Shin A, Camilleri M, Kolar G, *et al.* Systematic review with meta-analysis: highly selective 5-HT4 agonists (prucalopride, velusetrag or naronapride) in chronic constipation. *Aliment Pharmacol Ther* 2013; **39**: 239–53.

27 Videlock EJ, Cheng V, Cremonini F. Effects of linaclotide in patients with irritable bowel syndrome with constipation or chronic constipation: a meta-analysis. *Clin Gastroenterol Hepatol* 2013; **11**: 1084–92.e3, quiz e68.

28 Rao SSC, Valestin J, Brown CK, *et al.* Long-term efficacy of biofeedback therapy for dyssynergic defecation: randomized controlled trial. *Am J Gastroenterol* 2010; **105**: 890–6.

29 Thomas GP, Dudding TC, Rahbour G, *et al.* Sacral nerve stimulation for constipation. *Br J Surg* 2013; **100**: 174–81.

CHAPTER 67

Chronic Functional Abdominal Pain

Amy E. Foxx-Orenstein

Department of Internal Medicine, Mayo Clinic, Scottsdale AZ, USA

Summary

Functional abdominal pain syndrome (FAPS) is a distinct chronic gastrointestinal (GI) pain disorder characterized by constant or frequently recurring abdominal pain that is not related to food intake, defecation, or menses. It accounts for significant health care impact and has a high comorbidity with psychiatric disorders. The pain experience relates primarily to the impaired central processing of afferent signals, leading to disinhibition and severe symptoms. It is modulated by psychosocial comorbidity. The diagnosis of FAPS is symptom-based, in accord with Rome III diagnostic criteria. In the absence of alarm symptoms, an extensive workup is not required, as a cost-effective approach can be used to rule out an alternative or co-existing diagnosis. As there is no cure, effective treatment hinges on a biopsychosocial approach, with emphasis on a trusting doctor–patient relationship and negotiating reasonable treatment goals. Therapeutic options include centrally acting pharmacological agents and psychological therapies that focus more on adaptive coping than on complete cure. Antidepressants are the mainstay of pharmacotherapy, which also aims to target associated psychiatric comorbidities. A multidisciplinary approach to pain management, a patient's readiness to assume responsibility for self-care, and combination therapies can produce an augmented effect.

Case

A 45-year old female is referred to a gastroenterologist by her primary care physician for refractory abdominal pain. She describes the pain as "wrenching" and "squeezing," 9–10/10 in severity, generalized, and present nearly all the time. There does not appear to be any relation between her pain and belching, eating, defecation, or passing flatus. She has not experienced any weight loss, fever, chills, constipation, diarrhea, melena, hematochezia, nausea, or vomiting. She has had pain for years, but it has been constant over 18 months. She is on 40 mg of oxycodone four times a day for this pain. Her history is notable for depression, dysmenorrhea, and sexual abuse as a child. Surgical history includes cholecystectomy, appendectomy, hysterectomy, and an explorative laparoscopy for evaluation of dysmenorrhea. In the past 2 years, she has undergone an extensive evaluation, including colonoscopy, labwork, esophagogastroduodenoscopy (EGD), and computed tomography (CT) scan of the abdomen/pelvis, all of which are normal. She is frustrated and angry that no explanation for her pain has been found. She presents to the gastroenterology clinic after becoming offended that her primary care doctor told her that there was nothing more he could do and that he recommends that she see a psychologist or psychiatrist for further treatment.

Definition and Epidemiology

FAPS (also called "chronic idiopathic abdominal pain" or "chronic functional abdominal pain") is one of the functional abdominal disorders defined by the Rome III criteria [1] (Table 67.1). There is no cure. It is commonly associated with other painful conditions, such as fibromyalgia, and it seems to fulfill criteria for diagnosis of a somatoform pain disorder under psychiatric nosology.

No studies have focused specifically on the epidemiology of FAPS, but the prevalence in North America is reported to range from 0.5 to 2.0% [1,2]. The gender distribution is unclear. In North America, it is more common in women (1.5 : 1 female/male ratio) [3]. In one Israeli study, respondents were almost entirely women [4], but a Canadian study found no gender difference [5]. The prevalence peaks in the 4th decade of life and decreases thereafter. Due to high work absenteeism and utilization of considerable health care resources in evaluating and managing FAPS, it is associated with a significant economic burden [1,2].

Pathophysiology

No definitive neurophysiological study in FAPS has been published, but neuropathic pain induced by central sensitization is thought to be the most probable pathophysiology. The data are mostly derived from studies on patients with severe irritable bowel syndrome (IBS).

Normal gut sensitivity occurs via afferent neurons, which synapse in the dorsal horn of the spiral cord and ultimately in specialized regions of the cortex, including the medial thalamus, posterior thalamus, anterior cingulated cortex (ACC), and somatosensory cortex (SSC). Cortical modulation of sensory input originates in the ACC and results in "gating" of the dorsal horn. Individuals with functional gastrointestinal disorders (FGIDs), such as IBS and FAPS, are thought to have "turned up" central mechanisms in the brain and spinal cord, which are modulated by psychosocial and genetic factors [3]. This leads to hypersensitivity and hypervigilance, which define the patient's pain experience. It has been shown that heightened colonic sensitivity in IBS is more influenced by a psychological tendency to report pain (central component) than by a neurosensory sensitivity (peripheral component) [6]. This supports that

Practical Gastroenterology and Hepatology Board Review Toolkit, Second Edition. Edited by Nicholas J. Talley, Kenneth R. DeVault, Michael B. Wallace, Bashar A. Aqel and Keith D. Lindor.
© 2016 John Wiley & Sons, Ltd. Published 2016 by John Wiley & Sons, Ltd. Companion website: www.practicalgastrohep.com

Table 67.1 Rome III diagnostic criteria for functional abdominal pain syndrome (FAPS). Criteria are fulfilled for the last 3 months, with symptom onset at least 6 months prior to diagnosis. Source: Clouse 2006 [1]. Reproduced with permission of Elsevier.

Continuous or near-continuous abdominal pain
Does not meet criteria for IBS or other FGID
Poor symptom correlation to eating, defecation, or menses
Some loss of daily functioning due to pain
Pain is not contrived

IBS, irritable bowel syndrome; FGID, functional gastrointestinal disorder.

functional disease is associated with central dysregulation of visceral afferent input. Disinhibition of pain may relate to reduced serotonin, norepinephrine, endorphin, and other neuropeptides via the medial central nervous system (CNS) circuitry to the dorsal horn [7]. IBS has a prominent peripheral component, but as disease severity increases, the central component becomes more pronounced.

Studies of functional brain imaging in patients with IBS have found an association between disinhibition of afferent pain signals in the ACC and traumatic life events (e.g., sexual abuse), suggesting a role for past abusive experiences in development of FAPS via altered perception [8].

In contrast to IBS, where most patients have mild to moderate disease with peripheral and central input, FAPS patients fall at the severe end of the scale, with primarily central pathophysiology [3].

The frequent association of FAPS with psychiatric disorders and partial responsiveness to treatment with antidepressants suggests a prominent role of the CNS in cognitive and emotional pain modulation in this condition (Figure 67.1).

Clinical Features

Patients with FAPS usually complain of a constant, generalized pain over a large anatomical area [1, 2]. This abdominal pain may occur in the setting of other painful symptoms, suggesting a concurrent somatization disorder or perhaps overlap with other functional pain conditions such as fibromyalgia [1]. A history of physical or sexual abuse is common in patients with FAPS: as high as 30% in those attending gastroenterology clinics [9]. This history of abuse may lead to increased awareness of visceral sensation, though there is

no evidence that visceral pain thresholds are reduced in such people [1, 10].

Case Continued

When examining the patient, she is diffusely tender, but negative for hepatosplenomegaly, ascites, rebound, or masses. Before the physician lays hands on her, she squeezes her eyes shut and grimaces. Carnett test is positive.

Diagnosis

Evaluation proceeds using a clinical and psychosocial approach, with emphasis on the physical exam and observed behaviors [1, 2]. Physical examination must be thorough, and by definition will not be associated with significant abnormalities, though overlap with other medical conditions can occur. The presence of abdominal scars might prompt interrogation of symptoms preceding surgery, exposing exploratory versus therapeutic investigations.

The observation of pain behavior is also important during physical exam, as FAPS patients are likely to have an absence of autonomic arousal and to exhibit the "closed-eyes sign": eyes closed during examination, as opposed to eyes open – a fearful anticipation expression commonly seen in patients with an acute abdomen. These patients may be able to be distracted from pain during examination [2]. Abdominal wall pain should be excluded using the Carnett test, in which it increases with head raising and contraction of the rectus abdominis muscle, while visceral pain decreases. However, FAPS can also produce increased pain during abdominal wall contraction, probably due to central sensitization with viscerosomatic referral [1,2]. Psychosocial elements can also be crucial in revealing disease and illness patterns related to FAPS. Assessment of these elements is described in Table 67.2. As with other functional disorders, in the absence of alarm symptoms (i.e., unexplained weight loss, abdominal mass, bloody bowel movements, anorexia), use of diagnostic tests to exclude organic disease should not be performed routinely [11]. If the examination is negative, no further diagnostic studies are indicated.

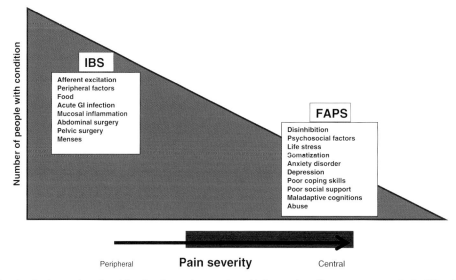

Figure 67.1 Model showing the interaction of peripheral and central processing with factors that affect symptom severity in IBS and FAPS. Source: Adapted from Sperber 2011. Reproduced with permission of Wiley.

Table 67.2 Psychosocial assessment in FAPS.

1 Life history of illness	Evaluate acute vs. chronic illness and note the presence of other chronic pain conditions
2 Reasons for seeking care now	Look for associated concerns and triggers, and worsening functional and/or psychosocial status
3 Life history of traumatic events	Assess history of abuse or of personal or family losses
4 Patient's understanding of the illness	Recognize mind–body interactions vs. looking for an organic cause
5 Impact of pain on activities and quality of life	Use to plan diagnostic and treatment decisions
6 Associated psychiatric diagnosis	Use for diagnosis and treatment of axis I and axis II psychiatric disorders
7 Role of family and culture	Recognize dysfunctional family interactions and cultural belief systems
8 Associated psychosocial impairment and available resources	Seek social networks and avoid maladaptive coping (catastrophizing)

Table 67.3 Treatment approach to FAPS.

a Establish an effective patient–physician relationship	1 Empathy
	2 Education
	3 Validation
	4 Reassurance
	5 Negotiation of treatment
	6 Setting of reasonable limits
b The treatment plan	1 Set reasonable limits
	2 Help the patient take responsibility
	3 Base treatment on symptom severity and degree of disability
	4 Prescribe medications
	5 Refer for mental health
	6 Apply specific psychological treatments
	7 Refer to a multidisciplinary pain treatment center

Differential Diagnosis

Before establishing a diagnosis of FAPS, it is important to exclude structural and metabolic GI disorders. Diagnoses to be considered include, but are not limited to, IBS, inflammatory bowel disease (IBD), pancreatitis, mesenteritis, intestinal obstruction or ischemia, ulcer disease, and abdominal wall pain. Additionally, FAPS can coexist with these disorders or any other medical condition. Features suggestive of a structural disorder include acute onset of symptoms, variable or intermittent intensity of pain, focal location of discomfort, positive diagnostic tests, response to promotility and/or anti-inflammatory agents, and improvement of symptoms with nasogastric suction or fasting.

Case Continued

The physician explains to the patient that the evaluation of her abdominal pain is consistent with FAPS, a disorder associated with abnormal perception/dysregulation of pain-control pathways. Given this diagnosis, the treatment is a combination of medication and psychotherapy, in an effort to better control her body's mechanisms of dealing with pain perception. The physician explains that total pain relief is unlikely; however, the ultimate goal will be to reach a point where her pain no longer disrupts her daily activities. She accepts the diagnosis but wants something to stop her pain right now: a medication like hydromorphone, which has worked well in the past. The physician explains that unfortunately, medications like Dilaudid are not effective for her type of pain and may cause other problems, such as narcotic bowel syndrome, which will confound her symptoms. At this time, the physician recommends starting a tricyclic antidepressant (TCA), which at low doses has an analgesic effect on the body's nervous system and therefore more directly targets the cause of her pain. She seems initially anxious at starting this type of medication, but is more amenable after understanding the rationale behind it. The physician asks her to return for a short session in 2 weeks to assess her progress, medication dosage, and any need for referral for psychotherapy.

Therapeutics

The approach to treatment of FAPS is based on a strong patient–physician relationship [1, 12, 13] (Table 67.3). It is key to demonstrate empathy, to educate the patient, to validate their illness, and to reassure them, but it is equally as important to negotiate treatment, thereby establishing reasonable limits of time and effort (Table 67.3b) [1, 2]. The focus of treatment is on management of symptoms, as opposed to targeting a cure [1, 2].

While most current pharmacotherapy recommendations for FAPS lack the support of well-designed treatment trials, they are based on extrapolation from trials of IBS and chronic pain syndromes (Table 67.4). Antidepressants are a starting point of therapy and the primary pharmacological treatment of FAPS. The rationale is that these drugs can modulate pain perception by modulating central regulatory mechanisms, and to some degree hypervigilance and visceral hypersensitivity. A recent systematic review and meta-analysis of TCAs, selective serotonin reuptake inhibitors (SSRIs), serotonin-norepinephrine reuptake inhibitors (SNRIs), and psychological therapy showed that all of these treatments were effective, with a number needed to treat (NNT) of 4 for antidepressants and psychological therapy [3,14]. While all families of antidepressants can be effective in FAPS, TCAs and duloxetine have been used successfully in chronic neuropathic pain [3]. Doses of antidepressants are generally lower than those prescribed for clinical depression [3,15].

Most analgesics offer pain relief through peripheral mechanisms and have no role in the treatment of FAPS. As FAPS is a result of abnormal central pain signaling, peripherally acting agents should have limited if any effect in providing pain relief, aside from a placebo effect [1]. Also, patients with chronic pain syndromes are prone to developing pain medication-seeking behavior, and FAPS is no exception. Thus, the use of narcotic agents for the treatment of FAPS can increase the risk of addiction and the development of the common yet under-recognized narcotic bowel syndrome [16]. In narcotic bowel syndrome, persistent use of narcotics leads to progression in the frequency, duration, and intensity of pain episodes. The criteria for diagnosing narcotic bowel syndrome are listed in Table 67.5.

Gabapentin and pregabalin are also prescribed for chronic neuropathic pain conditions. The benefit of these agents in treating visceral or central pain syndromes has not been established, but a few case reports have suggested a reduction in visceral pain [15]. As with narcotic use in FAPS, long-term treatment with benzodiazepines is not recommended, due to high abuse potential and a tendency to negatively interact with medications. Patients refractory to TCA or SSRI agents or who are already receiving high-dose therapy may profit from the addition of a different class of antidepressant in order to achieve a clinical effect by engaging different neuroreceptors. Based on clinical experience, buspirone, a non-benzodiazepine azapirone with antianxiety properties, may enhance the analgesic effect of antidepressants. Early clinical experience with low-dose (25–100 mg) quetiapine, an atypical antipsychotic agent that acts

Table 67.4 Medications for the treatment of pain in FAPS.

TCAs[a]	*Secondary amines (desipramine and nortriptyline)*	
	Starting dose	25–50 mg p.o. every night
	Escalating dose	Increase by 25 mg increments weekly, up to max. daily dose 100 mg (remember that benefit may not be seen for 6 weeks after initiation)
	Additional benefits	Tends to be better tolerated than other TCAs (tertiary amines), due to lower antihistaminic and anticholinergic effects.
	Tertiary amines (imipramine and amitriptyline)	
	Starting dose	10–25 mg
	Escalating dose	Increase by 25 mg increments weekly, up to max. daily dose 100 mg (remember that benefit may not be seen for 6 weeks after initiation)
	Additional benefits	
	Class side effects	Sedation, constipation, tachycardia, urinary retention, dry mouth, dry eyes, weight gain, hypotension, sexual dysfunction, agitation, nightmares
		May help depressive symptoms, but dose is suboptimal for treatment of major depression
	Time to action	2–6 weeks
SSRIs	*Short half-life (paroxetine)*	
	Medium half-life (citalopram, escitalopram)	
	Long half-life (fluoxetine)	
	Starting dose	10–20 mg p.o. daily
	Escalating dose	Increase by 10 mg increments, up to max. daily dose of 60 mg, if necessary
		Often, dose escalation is not necessary (as is the case with TCAs)
		Many patients find benefit at 20 mg daily
	Additional benefits	Anxiety reduction, as well as treatment of OCD, social phobia, and agoraphobia
		Treatment of associated depressive disorder, if present
	Class side effects	Insomnia, diarrhea, night sweats, weight loss, agitation, sexual dysfunction
	Time to action	3–6 weeks
SNRIs[a]	*Duloxetine*	
	Starting dose	20–30 mg p.o. daily (take with meals to reduce nausea)
	Escalating dose	Increase by 30 mg increments weekly, to a max. daily dose of 90 mg
	Additional benefits	Treatment of coexisting psychiatric disorders
		Peripheral pain modulation
		Less sexual dysfunction in comparison to SSRIs
	Venlafaxine	
	Starting dose	37.5 mg p.o. twice daily
	Escalating dose	After 1–2 weeks, increase to 50 mg p.o. twice daily
		After another 1–2 weeks, increase to 75 mg p.o. twice daily
		Continue to increase by 25 mg increments every 1–2 weeks
		Most people will require 150 mg total daily dose until benefit is seen
		Max. daily dose is 225 mg
	Additional benefits	Central antinociception at higher doses
		Treatment of coexisting psychiatric disorders
		Peripheral pain modulation
		Less sexual dysfunction in comparison to SSRIs
	Class side effects	Nausea, agitation, dizziness, fatigue, liver dysfunction
	Time to action	3–6 weeks
Augmenting agents[b]	*Buspirone*	
	Starting dose	7.5 mg p.o. twice daily
	Escalating dose	After 1–2 weeks, increase to 15 mg p.o. twice daily
		After another 1–2 weeks, increase to 30 mg p.o. twice daily
		Continue to increase in similar increments up to 30 mg p.o. twice daily
	Additional benefits	Anxiety reduction
	Quetiapine	
	Starting dose	25 mg p.o. daily
	Escalating dose	Increase by 25 mg increments every 1–2 weeks, to a max. daily dose of 100 mg
	Additional benefits	Anxiety reduction, alleviation of insomnia
	Side effect	Rare possibility of torsades de pointes and sudden death in high-risk individuals
		Side effects less likely, given the relatively low dosage compared to the 400–600 mg dose for indications of bipolar disorder and schizophrenia

[a]First-line pharmacotherapy for the treatment of functional abdominal pain includes either a TCA or an SNRI.
[b]These medications should not be used alone for the treatment of FAPS. They are intended to be used in conjunction with one of the preceding medications, in order to augment the effects of both.
TCA, tricyclic antidepressant; OCD, obsessive–compulsive disorder; SSRI, selective serotonin reuptake inhibitor; SNRI, serotonin-norepinephrine reuptake inhibitor.

on dopamine receptors, has demonstrated some benefit in treating patients with chronic pain syndromes.

Though no clinical trials have been performed to evaluate the efficacy of psychological treatment in FAPS, it is often used in a comprehensive approach to pain management, alongside pharmacotherapy and a strong physician–patient relationship. Recommendations are based on clinical studies in IBS and somatic functional symptoms [3]. Cognitive behavioral therapy (CBT) identifies maladaptive thoughts, perceptions, and behaviors and so guides the patient to develop new ways of achieving control over symptoms. It has been shown to have beneficial effects in FAPS and IBS studies [17]. Hypnotherapy has been well studied in IBS, with good short- and long-term results [18]. Interpersonal or dynamic psychotherapy and stress management techniques can be a part of a multicomponent behavioral approach to symptom management in FGIDs, but they may not be available in many centers [3].

Combination treatments involving two classes of antidepressants, addition of gabapentin or another neuropathic pain agent, or

Table 67.5 Diagnostic criteria for narcotic bowel syndrome.

Chronic or frequently recurring abdominal pain that is treated with acute high-dose or chronic narcotics and all of the following:
The pain worsens or incompletely resolves with continued or escalating dosages of narcotics
There is marked worsening of pain when the narcotic dose wanes and improvement when narcotics are reinstituted ("soar and crash")
There is a progression of the frequency, duration, and intensity of pain episodes
The nature and intensity of the pain are not explained by a current or previous GI diagnosis

combination psychological and pharmacological therapies can be effective for symptoms refractory to any one of these approaches. Other modalities may be found at a multidisciplinary pain treatment center and should be sought for more refractory patients.

Prognosis

The quality of life in patients with functional abdominal pain is generally poor. Ultimately, a patient's appreciation of factors contributing to their illness, their pain process, and their coping strategies are significant predictors of quality of life and response to treatment. Patients with a history of compound traumatic life events (e.g., emotional, sexual, or physical abuse, death, divorce) tend to have a poorer prognosis [1, 3].

Take Home Points

- Functional abdominal pain is a debilitating chronic functional pain syndrome that is not explained by a structural or metabolic disorder.
- The pain is not contrived.
- The etiology of functional abdominal pain is related to alterations in endogenous pain modulation systems, including dysfunction of cortical and peripheral pain modulation circuits.
- The diagnosis is symptom-based, with further diagnostic evaluation depending on the presence of alarm features.
- The object of treatment is management of pain by improvement of symptom control and coping skills.
- Treatment begins with a therapeutic physician–patient relationship. It includes pharmacotherapy, non-pharmacotherapy, and combination treatments aimed at improving symptom control.
- A cure is unlikely.

References

1 Clouse RE, Mayer EA, Aziz Q, *et al.* Functional abdominal pain syndrome. *Gastroenterology* 2006; **130**: 1492–7.

2 Drossman DA. Functional abdominal pain syndrome. *Clin Gastroenterol Hepatol* 2004; **2**: 353–65.

3 Sperber AD, Drosssman DA. Review article: the functional abdominal pain syndrome. *Aliment Pharmacol Ther* 2011; **33**: 514–24.

4 Sperber AD, Shvartzman P, Friger M, Fich A. Unexpectedly low prevalence rates of IBS among adult Israeli Jews. *Neurogastroenterol Motil* 2005; **17**: 207–11.

5 Thompson WG, Irvine EJ, Pare P, *et al.* Functional gastrointestinal disorders in Canada: first population-based survey using Rome II criteria with suggestions for improving the questionnaire. *Dig Dis Sci* 2002; **47**: 225–35.

6 Dorn SD, Palsson OS, Thiwan SI, *et al.* Increased colonic pain sensitivity in irritable bowel syndrome is the result of increased tendency to report pain than increased neurosensory sensitivity. *Gut* 2007; **56**: 1202–9.

7 Nozu T, Kudaira M. Altered rectal sensory response induced by balloon distention in patients with functional abdominal pain syndrome. *Biopsychosoc Med* 2009; **3**: 13.

8 Ringel Y, Drossman DA, Leserman JL, *et al.* Effect of abuse history on pain reports and brain responses to aversive visceral stimulation: an FMRI study. *Gastroenterology* 2008; **134**: 396–404.

9 Drossman DA, Talley NJ, Leserman J, *et al.* Sexual and physical abuse and gastrointestinal illness. Review and recommendations. *Ann Intern Med* 1995; **123**: 782–94.

10 Ringel Y, Whitehead WE, Toner BB, *et al.* Sexual and physical abuse are not associated with rectal hypersensitivity in patients with irritable bowel syndrome. *Gut* 2004; **53**: 838–42.

11 Cash BD, Schoenfeld P, Chey WD. The utility of diagnostic tests in irritable bowel syndrome patients: a systematic review. *Am J Gastroenterol* 2002; **97**: 2812–19.

12 Chang L, Drossman DA. Optimizing patient care: the psychosocial interview in irritable bowel syndrome. *Clin Perspect Gastroenterol* 2002; **5**: 336–41.

13 Drossman DA. Biopsychosocial issues in gastroenterology. In: Feldman M, Friedman LS, Brandt LJ, eds. *Sleisenger and Fordtran's Gastrointestinal and Liver Disease*, 9th edn. Philadelphia, PA: Elsevier, 2009.

14 Ford AC, Talley NJ, Schoenfeld PS, *et al.* Efficacy of antidepressants and psychological therapies in irritable bowel syndrome: systematic review and meta-analysis. *Gut* 2009; **58**: 367–78.

15 Grover M, Drossman DA. Psychotropic agents in functional gastrointestinal disorders. *Curr Opin Pharmacol* 2008; **8**: 715–23.

16 Drossman DA. Severe and refractory chronic abdominal pain: treatment strategies. *Clin Gastroenterol Hepatol* 2008; **6**: 978–82.

17 Drossman DA, Toner BB, Whitehead WE, *et al.* Cognitive behavioral therapy versus education and desipramine versus placebo for moderate to severe functional bowel disorders. *Gastroenterology* 2003; **12**: 19–31.

18 Gonsalkorale WM, Houghton LA, Whorwell PJ. Hypnotherapy in IBS: a large scale audit of a clinical service with examination of factors influencing responsiveness. *Am J Gastroenterol* 2001; **97**: 954–61.

CHAPTER 67

Abdominal Bloating and Visible Distension

Mark Pimentel

Cedars-Sinai Medical Center, Los Angeles, CA, USA

Summary

In the practice of gastroenterology, bloating and visible distension are two of the most common presenting complaints. Despite their high prevalence, the pathophysiology of these symptoms is not always obvious. Due to the lack of defined and effective therapy for bloating, the symptoms are often ignored in the treatment of conditions where bloating is common. Incredibly, even the Rome III criteria no longer include bloating as a subcriterion for irritable bowel syndrome (IBS) [1]. This is despite expert opinion and clinical studies suggesting that the bloating symptom is the most bothersome in IBS and functional gastrointestinal disorders (FGIDs) [2–4].

Though the treatment of bloating and distension is challenging, this set of symptoms should not be underappreciated, as an understanding of the pathophysiology and effective treatments for bloating and abdominal distension will have a great impact in patient care. This chapter addresses the epidemiology, pathophysiology, and treatment options for this constellation of symptoms.

Epidemiology

Bloating, gas, and distension are very common symptoms. In a recent study, the prevalence of bloating was seen in >15% of the US population [5]. However, there are many confounding variables in the assessment of bloating that can affect these rates, including medications (e.g., narcotics or proton pump inhibitors (PPIs)) and the sensation of bloating during menstruation in women. Since many conditions or situations can lead to bloating and distension even in normal humans (e.g., legume ingestion), bloating and distension should really be considered a symptom complex rather than a diagnosis. It is therefore important when discussing the etiology of this complex to look at underlying causes and their epidemiology.

IBS is often taken to be synonymous with bloating and distension. In a study of 100 consecutive IBS subjects from 1989, three symptoms were universal to IBS: abdominal pain, altered bowel function (both by definition), and then abdominal distension [6]. Since the epidemiology of IBS has been more thoroughly studied and IBS is the most common gastrointestinal (GI) disorder [7], the epidemiology of IBS has great bearing on the prevalence of bloating.

Bloating is known to differ considerably between the subtypes of IBS. IBS is principally divided into constipation-predominant (IBS-C) and diarrhea-predominant (IBS-D) types. Subjects with IBS-C suffer from a greater degree of bloating than those with IBS-D. In one study, bloating was seen in 75% of IBS-C subjects but in only 41% of IBS-D subjects [8].

While functional bowel diseases are commonly associated with bloating and abdominal distension, it is important to recognize that many non-functional conditions can produce these symptoms as well (Table 68.1). These include conditions such as mechanical obstruction, systemic diseases, and medications. Though bloating is known to be a symptom of such conditions, there are limited epidemiologic data to support the prevalence of each. As an example, in diabetes, studies suggest that GI complaints are common, and the most common is bloating, at 35% [9].

Patient Evaluation

When evaluating a patient with bloating, it is vital to thoroughly review their history. Medications are a common cause of bloating. Any medication that has a slowing effect on the intestinal tract or even that causes constipation has the potential to contribute to bloating. Classically, narcotics are well known to contribute to these symptoms. Drugs that contribute to fermentation (e.g., acarbose, lactulose) also have the potential to cause bloating.

Diet is extremely important in patient evaluation, including a history of probiotic use. Many dietary products can produce bloating and distension. Vegetarianism (especially veganism) causes significant bloating, due to the high-residue diet. Legumes are classically associated with bloating, and the increasing use of other non-digestible products has increased the presentation of bloating in the primary care clinic. Sucralose and alcohol sugars are commonly used in diet products such as "sugar-free gum" and beverages. These non-absorbed carbohydrates are readily fermentable and contribute to symptoms.

It is also important to rule out red-flag symptoms that can represent more sinister conditions, such as weight loss and hematochezia. When present, red-flag symptoms warrant further evaluation, including imaging or endocopy to rule out inflammatory or malignant disease. The age of the patient can also be a contributing factor, as the risk of malignancy increases with age. Given the long list of etiologic factors for bloating and distension, this chapter will focus on a few key areas.

It is beyond the scope of this chapter to outline the workup or evaluation of all causes of bloating. However, it is important to consider the wide differential diagnosis when approaching these patients, as in Table 68.1. Each condition requires special assessment and consideration.

Practical Gastroenterology and Hepatology Board Review Toolkit, Second Edition. Edited by Nicholas J. Talley, Kenneth R. DeVault, Michael B. Wallace, Bashar A. Aqel and Keith D. Lindor.
© 2016 John Wiley & Sons, Ltd. Published 2016 by John Wiley & Sons, Ltd. Companion website: www.practicalgastrohep.com

Table 68.1 Causes of bloating and abdominal distension.

Category	Condition
Functional	IBS
	Functional dyspepsia
	Pseudo-obstruction
	Constipation
	Mitochondrial myopathy
	Visceral myopathy
Systemic disorders	Diabetes
	Scleroderma
	Hypothyroidism
Mechanical	Bowel obstruction
	Post-fundoplication gas bloat
	Fistulas
	Crohn's disease with stricture
	Volvulus
	Malignancy
Malabsorption	Lactose maldigestion
	Fructose maldigestion
	Celiac disease
	Tropical sprue
	Pancreatic insufficiency
Benign/lifestyle	Vegetarianism
	High dairy consumption
Drugs	Bile acid sequestrants
	Narcotics
	PPIs
	Osmotic laxatives
	Probiotics

IBS, irritable bowel syndrome; PPI, proton pump inhibitor.

Pathophysiology of Bloating and Distension

Irrespective of the cause of bloating and distension (Table 68.1), all cases have one thing in common, which is that some condition or illness has affected the gut and led to gas accumulation or increased production. In some cases, this might be a motility disorder, in others a mechanical issue. In the intestinal tract, there is a balance between gas entry and clearance. In an average day, the human gut produces up to 8 L of gas, and a balance needs to be constantly maintained in order to prevent its accumulation.

Venting is one means of gas elimination. There are only two forms of venting in humans: the passage of flatus and belching. However, the intestinal tract is nearly 6 m long. Only the proximal and distal portions of the gut have the close proximity to the environment needed for venting to occur. In the central portions of the gut, the clearance of gas relies on three main mechanisms. The first is motility. In the human small intestine, there are specific contractions designed to cleanse the intestinal tract. Specifically, the migrating motor complex (MMC) is a three-stage event that occurs every 90 minutes during fasting and strips the intestine of gas and debris [10]. It is well known that a failure of contraction leads to bacterial accumulation and bloating [11]. The second mechanism is absorption. Most of the gases of the intestine are permeable. When a gas is absorbed, it can be eliminated through the respiratory system with carbon dioxide. The third mechanism is gas conversion, which will be discussed in a moment.

It is impossible to discuss bloating and distension without discussing the intestinal microbiome, since most of the 8 L of gas produced daily is caused by fermentation within the intestinal tract. The gut is colonized with an extraordinary number of bacteria [12]. In the event of obstruction, food residue that accumulates will quickly succumb to proliferation of microbes and increased fermentation. So, in addition to the mechanical obstruction, there is a further worsening of the situation as microbes accumulate in the areas of stasis.

In addition to swallowed air, which contains predominantly nitrogen and oxygen, gases produced by microbial fermentation include hydrogen, methane, carbon dioxide, and hydrogen sulfide [13–15]. These gases are not independent of one another. Hydrogen, for example, is used as a substrate for the production of other gases [16, 17]. Methanogenic archaea and sulfate-reducing bacteria take hydrogen and convert it to methane and hydrogen sulfide as a means of generating energy [18–20]. The stoichiometry of these reactions removes 4 mol of hydrogen to produce 1 mol of methane and 5 mol of hydrogen to produce 1 mol of hydrogen sulfide [15,21]. This conversion thus reduces the bowel gas load. In essence, it is possible that this sink for hydrogen can reduce bloating.

The complex process of fermentation can be evaluated in humans through indirect techniques such as breath-testing as part of the workup for bloating. Breath-testing has been performed to diagnose small-intestinal bacterial overgrowth for more than 20 years. The breath test measures hydrogen, methane, and carbon dioxide after a prolonged fast and in response to a carbohydrate load. A premature rise in hydrogen following intake of a non-absorbed sugar such as lactulose suggests bacterial overgrowth. While traditional breath-testing for bacterial overgrowth used hydrogen only, it is clear that methane is also very important.

Methane was previously thought to be an inert gas produced by a minority of human subjects. However, there is increasing evidence for the importance of methane in the workup of bloating. This is especially true in the context of IBS-C and chronic constipation. In a meta-analysis, methane on breath test was predictive of constipation [22]. Moreover, in a recent factor analysis examining the symptoms most associated with methane production, bloating was common [23].

While IBS may be an important condition in which bloating is common, recent work suggests that abnormalities such as bacterial overgrowth are common in IBS. This may explain the bloating caused by excessive fermentation. In a recent meta-analysis, IBS subjects were found more often to have an abnormal breath test suggestive of bacterial overgrowth than were age- and sex-matched healthy controls [24]. This has been further confirmed by culture [25, 26] and deep sequencing [27]. It has been suggested that this is due to disturbances in small-bowel motility in IBS [28].

Two additional proposed mechanisms for bloating in functional disorders are abnormal gas handling in the small bowel and visceral hyperalgesia. In a series of studies, the disposition of gases in the gut was evaluated by infusion of air directly into the small intestine. In this work, it was determined that clearance of gases infused into the small intestine was more challenging in IBS than in healthy subjects [29]. There was a greater retention of gas. Obviously, the mechanisms here are complicated, and likely include alterations in intestinal motility. Investigators found that infusion of fat into the duodenum augmented the poor gas handling in IBS [30].

Finally, visceral hyperalgesia needs some consideration as a contributing factor to symptoms of bloating and distension. Distension itself is a sensation of bloating or the perception that one is bloated. It has been suggested that some patients with bloating do not have increased intestinal gas contents but rather a greater sensitivity to a normal gas pattern [31]. Unfortunately, there is no validated clinical test to diagnose visceral hyperalgesia.

Treatment

In the treatment of bloating and distension, the ideal goal is to treat the cause (Table 68.1). In the situation where there is a

Table 68.2 Drugs/concepts that have noted beneficial effects on bloating in randomized clinical trials.

Category of drug	Intervention	Mechanism of action
Absorbants	Charcoal	Adsorbs the gas itself
	Simethicone	Destabilizes lipid membranes
Secretagogues	Linaclotide	Guanylate cyclase C agonist
	Lubiprostone	Chloride channel activator
Antibiotics	Rifaximin	Reduces fermentation
Diets	Low FODMAP	Reduces fermentation
	Lactose/fructose-free	

mechanical cause of bloating, no medical therapy will be very effective and surgery might be warranted. Simple elimination of a food item or a medication may suffice in some cases. Using a careful guided clinical and diagnostic approach, these treatable causes of bloating and distension can be diagnosed and specific treatment implemented. More commonly, however, the bloating is due to a functional disorder (IBS, bacterial overgrowth or functional constipation). In this section, the treatments will focus on the use of tactics or agents for the treatment of functional bloating and distension (Table 68.2).

Elimination Diets

As already discussed, fermentation is a source of bloating and gas in patients with functional bowel disease. Various investigators have studied diets with the intention of reducing fermentation and thus bloating. Diet studies include lactose [32] or fructose avoidance [33], gluten-free diets [34], and, more recently, the low-FODMAP diet [35]. The acronym FODMAP stands for "fermentable oligo- and disaccharides, monosaccharides, and polyols."

The goal of the low-FODMAP diet is to avoid almost all fermentable products. Examples of high-FODMAP foods include legumes, fructose, and sorbitol. In studies of IBS, the low-FODMAP diet was successful in improving symptoms, and particularly bloating, in controlled trial [36]. The challenge with this technique is that the diet is very difficult to sustain, as it is very restrictive.

Gluten restriction is another technique in vogue today. However, data do not fully support a gluten-free diet. While some studies suggest it may benefit subjects, a recent study comparing FODMAP with or without gluten demonstrated that gluten restriction was not essential to the benefits of FODMAPs [35]. Nonetheless, patients looking for relief of symptoms that physicians have challenges treating will often be led to these and other self-help behaviors.

Self-Help Therapies

In the management of bloating, self-help remedies are quite common. These include probiotics, charcoal, and simethicone-based products. Such products have varying degrees of evidence to support their effect. However, most have few or no controlled data.

Probiotics represent the introduction of live bacteria into the human host to facilitate an improvement in health. While yogurt and fermented food items have been in the human diet for centuries, their medicinal properties have only recently been suggested. As food items, they are not regulated and may only claim generically to "improve gut health." To date, there are no government regulator-approved forms of probiotics allowed to market to specific disease states.

Probiotics are both a benefit and a problem, as there are now more varieties on sale than there are functional diseases to treat, each claiming benefit to gut health. The probiotic arena is one in which

production has proceeded ahead of the science for their use. However, the scientific community is now beginning to study them in more detail. While the use of probiotics such as *Bifidobacter infantis* has demonstrated benefit in IBS [37], the benefits are modest at best, and recent data suggest they may even be harmful. In the PLACIDE trial [38], subjects receiving antibiotics for various outpatient infections were randomized to probiotic treatment or placebo after completion of the course. In this large-scale, multicenter trial, probiotics offered only one significant effect: an increase in bloating. Though this study was using one type of probiotic, it is likely that a live bacterium with need to ferment as part of its metabolism will produce bloating as a side effect. On the basis of large-scale studies such as this, while probiotics may be used by patients as self help, there is no clear evidence they lessen bloating and good evidence they may worsen it.

Antibiotics

Since an initial study demonstrated that neomycin was beneficial in improving IBS symptoms [39], and more specifically bloating, there has been growing interest in antibiotcs in IBS on the basis of changes in the microbiome. The challenge was to identify an antibiotic with ideal properties for bacterial overgrowth, including gut selectivity, good antimicrobial properties, a low resistance profile, and minimal side effects. Rifaximin met these criteria. In a series of large-scale randomized controlled studies (RCTs), rifaximin was effective in improving IBS symptoms [40]. Moreover, it was particularly effective in the reduction of bloating severity. More recently, the TARGET 3 study suggested that rifaximin was effective in up to three courses, without evidence for microbial resistance or changes in the stool microbiome based on deep sequencing [27]. Given these data, rifaximin may well be the most clear and direct of all treatments for bloating.

Prokinetics

Since one of the mechanisms of both microbiome accumulation and gas retention is reduced motor function, the use of prokinetic agents to improve bloating seems intuitive. Bloating benefits have been seen with most recent serotonin agonists, including tegaserod [41], itopride [42], mosapride [43], and prucalopride [44]. The only challenge with these products is that in some countries their use is limited. For example, none of these agents is currently available in the United States. However, most are available in Latin America and Asia. The mechanism of action here is likely a combination of motility in the intestine to improve gas clearance and venting and an increase in stool output, which lessens the intestinal fermentation potential.

Secretagogues

The secretagogues are a new class of agent that have proven efficacy in the management of constipation and IBS-C. There are two primary types of secretagogue currently available: the chloride channel activators (e.g., lubiprostone) [45] and the guanylate cyclase agonists (e.g., linaclotide) [46]. While others are emerging therapies (e.g., plecanatide), lubiprostone and linaclotide are the only currently available products.

Secretagogues work by increasing intestinal secretion into the gut, thereby improving the stool wet weight. Through different mechanisms of action, both categories of drug have the net effect of increasing chloride secretion from enterocytes. The obvious benefit of this action is the relief of constipation. However, data also suggest that it improves bloating and distenstion [46]. The mechanism of this effect is unclear, but it likely has much to do with clearance of colonic contents (fermenting material).

Take Home Points

- Gas and bloating are among the most challenging symptoms faced by patients and physicians alike.
- The causes of these symptoms are varied and require good clinical evaluation.
- While functional disorders account for the majority of cases, it is important to rule out such causes as mechanical obstruction of the bowel and malignancy. It is also important to be alert to red flags.
- The mechanism of bloating and distension in functional disorders is likely one or a combination of altered intestinal motility, aberration in microbial distribution, and visceral sensory abnormalities.
- While various treatments are used for bloating, well conducted controlled trials most notably support an antibiotic, prokinetic, and secretagogue approach to pharmacotherapy.
- Diet is an important consideration. This may be simple, such as lactose avoidance, or complicated, such as the low-FODMAP diet.

References

1 Guidelines – Rome III Diagnostic Criteria for Functional Gastrointestinal Disorders. *J Gastrointestin Liver Dis* 2006; **15**: 307–12.

2 Lembo T, Naliboff B, Munakata J, *et al.* Symptoms and visceral perception in patients with pain-predominant irritable bowel syndrome. *Am J Gastroenterol* 1999; **94**: 1320–6.

3 Neri M, Laterza F, Howell S, *et al.* Symptoms discriminate irritable bowel syndrome from organic gastrointestinal diseases and food allergy. *Eur J Gastroenterol Hepatol* 2000; **12**: 981–8.

4 Pimentel M, Talley NJ, Quigley EM, *et al.* Report from the multinational irritable bowel syndrome initiative 2012. *Gastroenterology* 2013; **144**: e1–5.

5 Jiang X, Locke GR 3rd, Choung RS, *et al.* Prevalence and risk factors for abdominal bloating and visible distention: a population-based study. *Gut* 2008; **57**: 756–63.

6 Maxton DG, Morris JA, Whorwell PJ. Ranking of symptoms by patients with the irritable bowel syndrome. *BMJ* 1989; **299**: 1138.

7 Drossman DA, Sandler RS, McKee DC, Lovitz AJ. Bowel patterns among subjects not seeking health care. Use of a questionnaire to identify a population with bowel dysfunction. *Gastroenterology* 1982; **83**: 529–34.

8 Talley NJ, Dennis EH, Schettler-Duncan VA, *et al.* Overlapping upper and lower gastrointestinal symptoms in irritable bowel syndrome patients with constipation or diarrhea. *Am J Gastroenterol* 2003; **98**: 2454–9.

9 Quan C, Talley NJ, Jones MP, *et al.* Gastrointestinal symptoms and glycemic control in diabetes mellitus: a longitudinal population study. *Eur J Gastroenterol Hepatol* 2008; **20**: 888–97.

10 Szurszewski JH. A migrating electric complex of canine small intestine. *Am J Physiol* 1969; **217**: 1757–63.

11 Vantrappen G, Janssens J, Hellemans J, Ghoos Y. The interdigestive motor complex of normal subjects and patients with bacterial overgrowth of the small intestine. *J Clin Invest* 1977; **59**: 1158–66.

12 The Gut Microbiota. *Science* 2012; **336**(6086). Special issue.

13 Strocchi A, Levitt MD. Maintaining intestinal H2 balance: credit the colonic bacteria. *Gastroenterology* 1992; **102**: 1424–6.

14 Cummings JH. Fermentation in the human large intestine: evidence and implications for health. *Lancet* 1983; **1**: 1206–9.

15 Sahakian AB, Jee SR, Pimentel M. Methane and the gastrointestinal tract. *Dig Dis Sci* 2010; **55**: 2135–43.

16 Samuel BS, Hansen EE, Manchester JK, *et al.* Genomic and metabolic adaptations of Methanobrevibacter smithii to the human gut. *Proc Nat Acad Sci USA* 2007; **104**: 10 643–8.

17 Schink B. Energetics of syntrophic cooperation in methanogenic degradation. *Microbiol Mol Biol Rev* 1997; **61**: 262–80.

18 Bauchop T, Mountfort DO. Cellulose fermentation by a rumen anaerobic fungus in both the absence and the presence of rumen methanogens. *Appl Environ Microbiol* 1981; **42**: 1103–10.

19 McKay LF, Holbrook WP, Eastwood MA. Methane and hydrogen production by human intestinal anaerobic bacteria. *Acta Pathol Microbiol Immunol Scand B* 1982; **90**: 257–60.

20 Gibson GR, Cummings JH, Macfarlane GT, *et al.* Alternative pathways for hydrogen disposal during fermentation in the human colon. *Gut* 1990; **31**: 679–83.

21 Blaut M. Metabolism of methanogens. *Antonie Van Leeuwenhoek* 1994; **66**: 187–208.

22 Kunkel D, Basseri RJ, Makhani MD, *et al.* Methane on breath testing is associated with constipation: a systematic review and meta-analysis. *Dig Dis Sci* 2011; **56**: 1612–18.

23 Makhani M, Yang J, Mirocha J, *et al.* Factor analysis demonstrates a symptom cluster related to methane and non-methane production in irritable bowel syndrome. *J Clin Gastroenterol* 2011; **45**: 40–4.

24 Shah ED, Basseri RJ, Chong K, Pimentel M. Abnormal breath testing in IBS: a meta-analysis. *Dig Dis Sci* 2010; **55**: 2441–9.

25 Posserud I, Stotzer PO, Bjornsson ES, *et al.* Small intestinal bacterial overgrowth in patients with irritable bowel syndrome. *Gut* 2007; **56**: 802–8.

26 Pyleris E, Giamarellos-Bourboulis EJ, Tzivras D, *et al.* The prevalence of overgrowth by aerobic bacteria in the small intestine by small bowel culture: relationship with irritable bowel syndrome. *Dig Dis Sci* 2012; **57**: 1321–9.

27 Pimentel M, Funari V, Giamarellos-Bourboulis EJ, *et al.* The first large scale deep sequencing of the duodenal microbiome in irritable bowel syndrome reveals striking differences compared to healthy controls. *Gastroenterology* 2013; **144**: S59.

28 Pimentel M, Soffer EE, Chow EJ, *et al.* Lower frequency of MMC is found in IBS subjects with abnormal lactulose breath test, suggesting bacterial overgrowth. *Dig Dis Sci* 2002; **47**: 2639–43.

29 Salvioli B, Serra J, Azpiroz F, *et al.* Origin of gas retention and symptoms in patients with bloating. *Gastroenterology* 2005; **128**: 574–9.

30 Villoria A, Serra J, Azpiroz F, Malagelada JR. Physical activity and intestinal gas clearance in patients with bloating. *Am J Gastroenterol* 2006; **101**: 2552–7.

31 Agrawal A, Houghton LA, Lea R, *et al.* Bloating and distention in irritable bowel syndrome: the role of visceral sensation. *Gastroenterology* 2008; **134**: 1882–9.

32 Vernia P, Di Camillo M, Marinaro V. Lactose malabsorption, irritable bowel syndrome and self-reported milk intolerance. *Dig Liver Dis* 2001; **33**: 234–9.

33 Shepherd SJ, Gibson PR. Fructose malabsorption and symptoms of irritable bowel syndrome: guidelines for effective dietary management. *J Am Diet Assoc* 2006; **106**: 1631–9.

34 Cash BD, Rubenstein JH, Young PE, *et al.* The prevalence of celiac disease among patients with nonconstipated irritable bowel syndrome is similar to controls. *Gastroenterology* 2011; **141**: 1187–93.

35 Biesiekierski JR, Peters SL, Newnham ED, *et al.* No effects of gluten in patients with self-reported non-celiac gluten sensitivity after dietary reduction of fermentable, poorly absorbed, short-chain carbohydrates. *Gastroenterology* 2013; **145**: 320–8.e1–3.

36 Halmos EP, Power VA, Shepherd SJ, *et al.* A diet low in FODMAPs reduces symptoms of irritable bowel syndrome. *Gastroenterology* 2014; **146**: 67–75.e5.

37 Whorwell PJ, Altringer L, Morel J, *et al.* Efficacy of an encapsulated probiotic Bifidobacterium infantis 35624 in women with irritable bowel syndrome. *Am J Gastroenterol* 2006; **101**: 1581–90.

38 Allen SJ, Wareham K, Wang D, *et al.* Lactobacilli and bifidobacteria in the prevention of antibiotic-associated diarrhoea and Clostridium difficile diarrhoea in older inpatients (PLACIDE): a randomised, double-blind, placebo-controlled, multicentre trial. *Lancet* 2013; **382**: 1249–57.

39 Pimentel M, Chow EJ, Lin HC. Normalization of lactulose breath testing correlates with symptom improvement in irritable bowel syndrome. a double-blind, randomized, placebo-controlled study. *Am J Gastroenterol* 2003; **98**: 412–19.

40 Pimentel M, Lembo A, Chey WD, *et al.* Rifaximin therapy for patients with irritable bowel syndrome without constipation. *N Engl J Med* 2011; **364**: 22–32.

41 Muller-Lissner SA, Fumagalli I, Bardhan KD, *et al.* Tegaserod, a 5-HT(4) receptor partial agonist, relieves symptoms in irritable bowel syndrome patients with abdominal pain, bloating and constipation. *Aliment Pharmacol Ther* 2001; **15**: 1655–66.

42 Saji S. Itopride in the treatment of dysmotility-like functional dyspepsia: a randomised placebo-controlled trial. *J Dig Endosc* 2010; **1**: 171–5.

43 Mansour NM, Ghaith O, El-Halabi M, Sharara AI. A prospective randomized trial of mosapride vs. placebo in constipation-predominant irritable bowel syndrome. *Am J Gastroenterol* 2012; **107**: 792–3.

44 Tack J, Stanghellini V, Dubois D, *et al.* Effect of prucalopride on symptoms of chronic constipation. *Neurogastroenterol Motil* 2014; **26**: 21–7.

45 Barish CF, Drossman D, Johanson JF, Ueno R. Efficacy and safety of lubiprostone in patients with chronic constipation. *Dig Dis Sci* 2009; **55**(4): 1090–7.

46 Layer P, Stanghellini V. Review article: Linaclotide for the management of irritable bowel syndrome with constipation. *Aliment Pharmacol Ther* 2014; **39**: 371–84.

CHAPTER 68

PART 7

Transplantation

69 Gastrointestinal Complications of Solid Organ and Hematopoietic Cell Transplantation, 419
   Natasha Chandok and Kymberly D.S. Watt

Gastrointestinal Complications of Solid Organ and Hematopoietic Cell Transplantation

Natasha Chandok[1] and Kymberly D.S. Watt[2]

[1] Division of Gastroenterology and Hepatology, University of Western Ontario, London, ON, Canada
[2] Division of Gastroenterology and Hepatology, William J. von Liebig Transplant Center, Mayo Clinic, Rochester, MN, USA

Summary

Solid organ transplantation (SOT) and hematopoietic cell transplantation (HCT) have dramatically improved the survival and quality of life in patients with a variety of malignancies and chronic end-organ disease. Gastrointestinal (GI) complications occur in almost 40% of solid organ recipients, and similarly account for many of the non-allograft-related adverse outcomes in the HCT population. GI disorders are frequently present prior to transplant and immunosuppression may augment symptoms. Immunosuppressive drugs also have notable GI side effects, and immunosuppression predisposes patients to infections and malignancies of the liver and GI tract. Graft-versus-host disease presents with GI manifestations and can occur following SOT but is more frequently seen after HCT. Sinusoidal obstruction syndrome (SOS), also known as veno-occlusive disease (VOD), an immunosuppression regimen-related toxicity, has been reported in SOT, but is also more often seen in the HCT population. GI complications are a prevailing source of morbidity and mortality in solid organ and bone marrow transplant recipients. The gastroenterologist should have a broad clinical approach to these complex patients with a low threshold for endoscopy as histopathology is often necessary for diagnosis and management of these patients

Case

A 56-year-old man underwent a cadaveric liver transplant 4 years ago for primary sclerosing cholangitis (PSC) and cholangiocarcinoma. He has a 12-year history of pan-ulcerative colitis, and his last surveillance colonoscopy 9 months ago showed no dysplasia and mild disease activity. Aside from mild acute rejection which was successfully treated with corticosteroids, his post-transplant course has been unremarkable. Two weeks ago, he developed a new onset of bloody diarrhea with crampy abdominal pain and intermittent fevers. He is having 10 bloody bowel movements daily, urgency and tenesmus. He has not been hospitalized nor has he received antibiotics for over a year.[1] He is on tacrolimus, alendronate, simvastatin, nifedipine, and mesalamine.

Physical exam is significant for normal vital signs and moderate tenderness in the left lower quadrant but no peritonitis. Laboratory studies show a leukocytosis and thrombocytosis of 1.5 times the upper limit of normal, therapeutic tacrolimus level, and normal liver function and transaminases. Stool cultures and stool for *C. difficile* toxin are pending. A colonoscopy is performed showing pan-colitis with deep ulcerations. Multiple biopsies were performed.

Introduction

Solid organ transplantation (SOT) and hematopoietic cell transplantation (HCT) are complex treatments which have dramatically improved the survival and quality of life in patients with a variety of malignancies and organ failures. The celebrated success of transplantation is in large part due to the effectiveness of immunosuppressive medications in extending graft survival, but this success is not without a heavy price.

GI complications occur in almost 40% of solid organ recipients, and similarly account for most of the non-allograft-related adverse outcomes in the HCT population [1, 2]. GI disorders are frequently present prior to transplant and immunosuppression may augment symptoms. Immunosuppressive drugs also have notable GI side effects, and immunosuppression predisposes patients to infections and malignancies of the liver and GI tract.

In comparison to SOT, patients with HCT are at greater risk for organ toxicities and severe infections because the preparation for HCT requires aggressive myeloablative therapy or immunosuppression. As such, HCT patients are also much more susceptible to graft-versus-host disease (GVHD). In addition, sinusoidal obstruction syndrome (SOS), also known as veno-occlusive disease (VOD), an immunosuppression regimen-related toxicity, has been reported in SOT, but is more often seen in the HCT population [3].

In this chapter, we will review the important GI complications that impact transplant recipients. These complications include infections, malignancies, adverse drug events, and generalized GI disorders. We will also highlight the salient features of GVHD and SOS.

Infections in the GI System Following SOT or HCT

Infections, sometimes life-threatening, are common in patients following a solid organ or bone marrow transplant, and they

Practical Gastroenterology and Hepatology Board Review Toolkit, Second Edition. Edited by Nicholas J. Talley, Kenneth R. DeVault, Michael B. Wallace, Bashar A. Aqel and Keith D. Lindor.

Table 69.1 Common causes of diarrhea post transplant.

Infection	*Clostridium difficile*
	Campylobacter, Salmonella, Shigella, E. coli Yersinia, Vibrio parahemolyticus
	Bacterial overgrowth
	Cytomegalovirus
	Rotavirus, Adenovirus, Norwalk virus
	Giardia
	Cryptosporidium, Cyclospora
	Entamoeba histolytica
Medication	Antibiotics
	Mycophenolate mofetil
	Sirolimus
	Cyclosporine
	Tacrolimus
Other	Ischemia
	IBD, celiac, IBS recurrence
	Graft-versus-host disease
	Post-transplant lymphoproliferative disease
	Overflow diarrhea
	Colorectal cancer

IBD, inflammatory bowel disease; IBS, irritable bowel syndrome.

can present with various GI manifestations (Table 69.1). The risk of infection depends on the surgery performed, the level of the immunosuppression, the use of antibiotic medications, infectious exposures, and prophylactic measures used to prevent infection [1,4].

The infectious etiologies can be categorized by the time from transplantation—perioperative, early (1 to 6 months), and late (beyond 6 months) [1]. Early in the perioperative period, infections can be derived from pre-existing pathogens in the recipient, donor-derived infections, or infections as a consequence of the transplant operation. During the first 6 months, viral and opportunistic infections prevail, although the epidemiology of infections in this period has changed considerably with the use of routine chemoprophylaxis for opportunistic microbes [4]. After 6 months, if there is good graft function, the infections in the post-transplant host are generally community-acquired, although opportunistic infections can occur at any time, particularly when chemoprophylaxis has stopped. Risk factors for infections, particularly opportunistic ones, include poor graft function, hospitalizations, and more intense immunosuppression. Frequently, it is clinically challenging to diagnose infections in patients who are immunocompromised because these patients may not mount a typical response with fever and leukocytosis. GI symptoms are sometimes the only clinical clue to an underlying infection. Broadly speaking, a therapeutic strategy for treating infections in the post-transplant setting involves potent antimicrobial medications in conjunction with reducing immunosuppressive medications.

Viral Infections

The most significant viruses infecting the transplant patient are cytomegalovirus (CMV), herpes virus (HSV) and Epstein–Barr virus (EBV), and all can produce a variety of GI symptoms.

CMV is the most common viral infection causing symptoms after any transplant. CMV should be high on the differential diagnosis for any patient at all stages post-transplantation, particularly if the patient is not receiving CMV prophylaxis. Although CMV infection in the immunocompetent host is pervasive and usually asymptomatic, transplant patients typically present with constitutional symptoms such as fever, malaise, and anorexia. CMV infection can be localized to virtually any organ, including any portion of the GI tract. The GI tract is involved in up to one-third of patients

with CMV [5]. GI symptoms include dysphagia, nausea, emesis, abdominal pain, diarrhea, and GI bleeding. CMV causes oral ulcers, mucositis, esophagitis, gastritis, duodenitis, small intestinal enteritis, colitis, and even bowel perforation on rare occasion. CMV hepatitis, usually more severe in liver transplant recipients, requires a liver biopsy to confirm the diagnosis as it can be easily mistaken for rejection.

After a transplant, CMV infection can originate from infected leukocytes within the allograft transplanted into the CMV naive recipient, cause super-infection in a CMV-positive recipient, or be reactivated by immunosuppression [1]. The risk for CMV not only depends on the severity of immunosuppression and the CMV status of the recipient prior to transplant, but also on the type of solid organ transplanted [6]. It is more common in patients with small bowel, pancreas, and lung transplantation than liver, heart, and kidney recipients [6]. The diagnosis of CMV requires confirmation by polymerase chain reaction (PCR) of CMV DNA and/or biopsy confirmation of the involved organ.

Lowance and colleagues have demonstrated that routine anti-CMV therapy has reduced the occurrence of CMV in transplant recipients [7] and thus prophylaxis is usually prescribed for the initial 3 months after transplant. CMV prophylaxis should be restarted whenever rejection of allograft is being treated, particularly if antilymphocyte drugs are used. CMV is treated with gancyclovir or valgancyclovir (dosed according to renal function), with duration dependent on end-organ involvement.

HSV is the second most common viral infection seen following transplantation and, like CMV, it has many GI manifestations. HSV can be re-activated from the latent phase during intense immunosuppression, as occurs during the first month after transplantation. HSV in the immunocompromised host usually presents as oral ulcers and odynophagia or anorectal/genitourinary ulcers, but it can involve the intestine and liver in patients not on acyclovir. Transplant patients with odynophagia or dysphagia should be evaluated with an endoscopy to determine the etiology. Oral infection from HSV can be treated with oral acyclovir, but disseminated infection requires intravenous treatment.

Other herpesviruses—EBV, varicella zoster virus (VZV), and human herpesvirus 6 or 7 (HHV-6 or 7)—are less common than CMV and HSV following transplantation. EBV is nearly ubiquitous, affecting more than 90% of the human population. EBV persists in memory B cells [8]. With immunosuppression, transplant patients develop faulty T-cell immunity and cannot contain the growth of EBV in B-cells laden with the virus. EBV, in addition to producing an infectious mononucleosis picture with adenopathy and fever, can have a variety of GI manifestations. EBV can cause oral hairy leukoplakia, a pale adherent lesion on lateral aspect of the tongue, as well as numerous malignancies. EBV-associated lymphoproliferative disorder is the most significant of these malignancies, and it will be discussed later in the chapter.

Hepatitis C virus (HCV) and hepatitis B virus (HBV), common indications for liver transplantation, are notable co-morbid diseases in other transplant patients, particularly in kidney and pancreas transplant recipients, occurring in 10-15% [1]. These patients have a much higher liver-related mortality than matched controls [9]. Treatment with antiviral medications for hepatitis B is warranted in most cases to prevent liver disease progression. Treatment of hepatitis C may be attempted prior to transplant of non-liver organs, if the side-effect profile is tolerable and no clear organ-specific contraindication exists. Anti-HCV therapy can be attempted after transplantation but requires diligent follow-up because of the significant side effects in the already immunosuppressed patient. This therapy is also associated with a risk for allograft rejection which can be minimized by careful immunosuppression monitoring.

Fungal Infections

The most common fungal infection in the transplant population is candidiasis, most notably affecting the oral cavity and esophagus. Common GI presentations include dysphagia, odynophagia, gastroesophageal reflux disease (GERD), and, rarely, GI bleeding. *Candida* is usually seen in the first 6 months after transplantation, with increased risk associated with high-dose steroids or antibiotic use. Endoscopy reveals superficial erosions, ulcers, white nodules or plaques, and the diagnosis is confirmed by histopathology and fungal cultures. *Candida* is usually treated with topical nystatin or oral fluconazole. In cases of resistance, caspofungin, posaconazole, or voriconazole can be given.

Hepatosplenic candidiasis occurs only in HCT patients and should be considered in the HCT patient with high fever and right or left upper quadrant pain, nausea, and vomiting. The frequency of this complication is decreased with prophylactic use of antifungal agents.

Parasitic Infections

Immunosuppressed transplant patients are at risk for protozoal infections with organisms such as *Microsporidium, Cryptosporidium, Isospora belli,* and *Giardia lamblia.* These parasitic infections usually cause diarrhea, and the diagnosis can be established with stool testing for ova and parasites. Microscopic examination of small bowel or colonic biopsies may be necessary to document organisms such as *Cryptosporidium.*

Treatment of parasitic infections involves antimicrobial drugs and a reduction in immunosuppression. Interestingly, cyclosporine possesses antihelminthic properties that may suppress the parasite *Strongyloides stercoralis.*

Bacterial Infections

Infectious diarrhea is also the most common GI presentation of a variety of bacterial organisms. Notable examples of these bacteria include *Clostridium difficile, Yersinia enterocolitica, Campylobacter jejuni, Salmonella,* and *Listeria monocytogenes.* Half of transplant patients getting antibiotics acquire *Clostridium difficile* colitis, so the clinician should maintain a high index of suspicion for this entity.

GI Malignancies after SOT and HCT

Transplant outcomes in the United States continue to improve, with the 1-year survival better than 85% and the 3-year survival better than 75% in solid organ recipients [10]. With longer life expectancy, post-transplant malignancies are an important cause of morbidity and mortality, with increased probability of GI malignancy over longer follow-up duration. The overall risk of malignancy following SOT is elevated compared with the general population. Epidemiological studies reveal that the length of exposure to immunosuppressive therapy and the intensity of the regimen are clearly related to the post-transplant risk of malignancy. Immunosuppression facilitates post-transplant malignancy by impairing cancer surveillance mechanisms and creating an environment for oncogenic viruses to thrive. Immunosuppressive medications, such as calcineurin inhibitors, could also play a role, having

pro-oncogenic effects [11], where other agents such as sirolimus are thought to have anti-proliferative properties. Once cancer has established, aggressive immunosuppression can result in increased proliferation of the tumor with worse clinical outcomes [11].

Transplant patients are at risk for tumors of infectious origin as well. Examples of oncogenic infections causing malignancies that may involve the GI tract include EBV causing lymphoproliferative diseases; HHV8 causing Kaposi sarcoma; HCV and HBV causing HCC; and *Helicobacter pylori* causing gastric cancer. EBV is also linked to nasopharyngeal and oral cancer, and transplant recipients have a sixfold higher risk for oral cancer. Anal cancer, linked to HPV, also occurs at a 10 to 20-fold higher frequency in transplant recipients [1]. A large retrospective study of 73 076 patients with heart and kidney transplant found a small increased risk for colon cancer, but a curious reduction in the incidence of rectal cancer [12]. Patients who drink alcohol to excess or smoke cigarettes are at higher risk of oral/pharyngeal and GI malignancies in the transplant population, more so than in the general population.

Malignancies following HCT can be categorized as early (less than 1 year after HCT) and late (occurring beyond 1 year after HCT). Early malignancies include acute leukemia, myelodysplastic syndrome (MDS), and PTLD. Late malignancies include a variety of solid tumors.

Post-transplant Lymphoproliferative Disorder

Post-transplant lymphoproliferative disorder (PTLD) is a well known complication of chronic immunosuppression in solid organ and bone marrow transplant recipients. Aside from skin and cervical cancer, PTLD is one of the most common malignancies after transplant [13]. PTLD can involve the GI tract because the gut is endowed with an abundance of lymphoid tissue. The overall incidence of PTLD is approximately 1-3% in recipients of HCT and SOT, 30 to 50 times higher than in the general population, with a recent trend toward increased frequency [14, 15]. There is some variability with the incidence based on the type of solid organ transplant, with the highest occurrence seen in intestinal or multiorgan transplant at 11-33% [16]. The intensity of the immunosuppressive regimen is directly associated with the risk for PTLD.

The pathogenesis is partly related to B-cell proliferation induced by EBV, but EBV-negative disease can also occur. In the majority of cases, PTLD cells are of host origin. Patients are at higher risk for PTLD if they receive T-cell-depleted or HLA mismatched bone marrow, antilymphocyte antibodies, have CMV, or get primary EBV after transplantation. Transplant recipients without previous exposure to EBV are at increased risk (which is why younger children tend to be at highest risk).

Patients with PTLD can present with symptoms of infectious mononucleosis or localized lymphoproliferation involving a variety of organs. GI involvement may cause obstruction, bleeding, or perforation. A biopsy is needed for a definitive diagnosis. An early detection strategy—a rise in the titer of EBV DNA after periodic measurements—should trigger a reduction in immunosuppression and careful surveillance. Imaging modalities with CT scan and positron emission tomography (PET scan) aid in the diagnosis and staging of disease.

The treatment of PTLD is partly based on the histopathologic characteristics of the tumor. Reduction of immunosuppressive drugs is the first line therapy for all PTLD, and may be all that is required in less advanced disease. There may be a potential role for antiviral treatment in the management of EBV-associated lymphoproliferation [8]. Rituximab, an anti CD20 (B cell) antibody, in

CHAPTER 69

conjunction with reduction of immunosuppression is evolving into the standard of care for many of these patients. Monoclonal disease not responding to therapy may require more intensive chemotherapy regimens. Surgical removal or irradiation of localized lymphoproliferative tumors in the GI tract may occasionally be considered.

GI Adverse Drug Events

After transplantation, recipients are exposed to a number of immunosuppressive agents to help ensure graft survival. Several of these medications have significant GI side effects.

Cyclosporine, a calcineurin inhibitor derived from a fungus, causes gingival hyperplasia by inducing collagenolytic activity in gums [1]. Gingival hyperplasia may necessitate a substitution with tacrolimus or sirolimus. Tacrolimus, another calcineurin inhibitor, as well as cyclosporine, can cause nausea, abdominal pain, diarrhea, anorexia, and weight loss. The side effects appear dose dependent. At high levels, both cyclosporine and tacrolimus can cause cholestasis and cyclosporine increases cholesterol saturation in bile, a potential risk for gall stone formation.

Sirolimus blocks IL-2 receptor signal activation of T and B lymphocytes. It can produce a dose-dependent elevation in serum aminotransferases. A black box warning exists in the liver transplant setting for association with hepatic artery thrombosis. Specific GI side effects include mouth ulceration, incisional hernias (impairs wound healing), and diarrhea.

Mycophenolate mofetil (MMF) is an immunosuppressive agent often used in combination with a calcineurin inhibitor and prednisone. It inhibits inosine monophosphate dehydrogenase, impairing purine synthesis and proliferation of B and T lymphocytes. MMF has a number of GI side effects, including oral ulcerations, nausea, vomiting, and diarrhea. Dose reduction often improves symptoms.

Myeloablative conditioning therapy, used in HCT candidates to prevent the recipient from rejecting donor hematopoietic cells and for tumor cell ablation, makes most patients nauseated and anorexic. They can also get debilitating mucositis.

General GI Complications

Mucositis is a significant problem after HCT, and it is the most common complication of myeloablative preparative regimens [2]. Severe mucositis involves extensive oral and esophageal ulceration which can take many months to heal. Patients can develop excruciating pain with swallowing, nausea, cramping, and diarrhea. Patients may even require TPN for nutritional support in severe cases. For the majority, mucositis is self-limited. A recombinant human keratinocyte growth factor, palifermin, reduces the incidence of oral mucositis after autologous transplantation [17].

Pill-induced esophagitis is another common cause of morbidity in the transplant population. Antibiotics, anti-virals, potassium tablets, bisphosphonates, and non-steroidal anti-inflammatory drugs (NSAIDs) are among the most common medications causing esophagitis. The incidence of pill-induced esophageal injury can be reduced by instructing patients to remain upright for at least 30 min following their pills and to consume plenty of water with ingested tablets. Proton pump inhibitors (PPI) can be useful in preventing esophageal injury.

GERD is extremely common in Western societies, with an estimated prevalence of 10 to 20% [18]. Not surprisingly, there is a high incidence of GERD following transplantation, possibly precipitated by medications and/or vagal nerve injury during the operation.

Peptic ulcer disease (PUD) is very common in the transplant population, particularly in kidney recipients [19]. In a large retrospective study from Missouri of 254 renal transplant patients who had endoscopies before and after their transplantation, 10% developed new PUD following transplant [19]. When complications of PUD arise, renal recipients can especially have dire outcomes, with 20% experiencing significant bleeding. The high incidence of *Helicobacter pylori* in patients with chronic renal failure contributes to the magnitude of this problem [19]. Fortunately, the risk for severe PUD can be reduced through active pretransplant screening endoscopies, PPI therapy, and antimicrobials to eradicate *H. pylori* [1]. A high incidence of large gastric ulcers has also been reported in liver transplant patients. Generally speaking, transplant patients should avoid NSAIDs as much for the gastric toxicities as for the renal ones.

Acute biliary tract disease is a complication in the transplant recipient, with a mortality as high as 29% in some series [1]. Following orthotopic liver transplantation (OLT), there is particular concern over hepatic artery stenosis or thrombosis as the biliary tree receives its blood supply from the hepatic artery. This can result in significant biliary complications with multiple strictures. A gradual loss of hepatic artery blood flow can cause ductopenia, and this entity can be difficult to distinguish from ductopenic rejection. Hepatic artery thrombosis (HAT) can have a variety of presentations, ranging from mildly elevated liver enzymes to fulminant liver failure in the acute setting after OLT. In the late post-OLT setting, HAT presents as biliary stricturing with cholangitis and intrahepatic abscesses. An anastomotic stricture is the most common biliary tract abnormality after OLT, and it typically develops 2–6 months after transplant, but it can occur sooner. Strictures at the duct-to-duct anastomosis can usually be fixed with endoscopic therapy, whereas strictures with choledochojejunostomies might need percutaneous or surgical repair. Acute portal vein thrombosis (PVT) can also cause hepatic ischemia and severe graft dysfunction if it occurs early.

Another potentially life-threatening GI complication after transplant is colonic perforation, which has an incidence after transplantation of 1–2%, and a mortality rate of 20–38% [20]. Possible etiologies to colonic perforation include diverticular disease, ischemia, and CMV colitis. Kidney transplant recipients are at particularly high risk for ischemic gut because they often possess underlying vascular disease.

Diarrhea in transplant recipients is very common, with a variety of etiologies. Many of the possible causes have already been discussed including the most common infectious etiologies, and drug side effects specific to the transplant patient. The physician should actively look for organisms such as *C. difficile*. standard bacterial infections as discussed and organisms such as *E. histolytica, Strongyloides, G. lamblia, Cryptosporidium, Clostridium,* CMV, rotavirus, and adenovirus in the right setting. Exacerbations of underlying diseases such as inflammatory bowel disease, celiac disease, or even irritable bowel syndrome (IBS) should be considered once infection is ruled out. It is important to remember post surgical issues such as overflow diarrhea from constipation (possibly narcotic related), or stasis and bacterial overgrowth in the setting of Roux limb anastomosis.

Perianal pain is also common in transplant recipients, particularly after bone marrow transplantation. The pain usually originates near the anus in granulocytopenic patients and is due to bacterial infection. There may be an abscess in the supralevator and inter-sphincteric region without being obvious on physical exam. Ideally, a perianal abscess should be drained and treated with antibiotics before HCT. HSV2 and HPV exacerbations can result in herpes flares and condylomata growth.

Special Topics

Graft-versus-host Disease (GVHD)

GVHD is a rare complication in SOT, but it is more often encountered following HCT [21–23]. Acute GVHD occurs between day 15 and 100, and chronic GVHD occurs beyond 100 days after HCT.

Both acute and chronic GVHD affect predominantly the skin, liver, and GI tract. Patients present with fevers, skin rash, and non-specific GI symptoms such as nausea, vomiting, anorexia, and diarrhea. GVHD can also affect other organs, including the kidneys and hematopoietic system.

Acute GVHD occurs in up to 50% of patients who receive allogeneic hematopoietic cell transplantation from an HLA-identical sibling despite intensive prophylaxis with immunosuppressive medications [22]. It is also common in matched unrelated donors and in haploidentical related donors. In acute GVHD, mismatches in histocompatibility between the donor and recipient lead to activation of donor T cells which cause damage to various epithelial tissues through dysregulated cytokine production and recruitment of additional effector cells. The pathogenesis of chronic GVHD is not as well understood and further research is needed in this area [23]. Risk factors for GVHD include HLA disparity, older age, donor and recipient gender discordance, previous GVHD, amount of radiation and intensity of the transplant conditioning regimen, and the use of immunosuppression such as methotrexate, cyclosporine, or tacrolimus [23, 24].

Although the skin is classically the first organ involved, the liver is the second most common organ affected. GVHD damages the bile canaliculi leading to cholestasis, and patients develop elevated conjugated bilirubin and alkaline phosphatase. The differential diagnosis to the cholestatic liver enzyme picture in the acute post HCT setting would also include SOS, infection, and drug toxicity.

GI tract involvement in GVHD can often be severe. Patients can present with extreme diarrhea of more than 10 liters per day. The stool can be watery or bloody, and patients generally require intravenous fluids, and/or blood transfusions. As diarrhea is very common after HCT, particularly from infections such as *Clostridium difficile* and CMV, diagnosing GVHD can be challenging without rectal biopsy. On biopsy, crypt cell necrosis with accumulation of degenerative material in the dead crypts is characteristic of GVHD. In severe cases, GVHD can obliterate the entire mucosa of the gut.

Patients with upper GI tract GVHD present with anorexia, dyspepsia, nausea, and vomiting. Endoscopy shows edema of the gastric antral and duodenal mucosa, and patchy erythema. Interestingly, GVHD in the upper GI tract is more responsive to immunosuppressive therapy than in other areas of the gut.

Prophylaxis for GVHD with methotrexate and cyclosporine is routinely prescribed for several months after HCT. Patients with GVHD should be managed by transplant physicians with expertise in GVHD. A variety of immunosuppressive agents can be employed, including corticosteroids, cyclosporine, tacrolimus, rapamycin, mycophenolate mofetil, and thalidomide [22, 23].

Sinusoidal Obstruction Syndrome (SOS)

SOS or veno-occlusive disease (VOD) can occur after both allogenic and autologous hematopoietic stem cell transplantation. It has also been described with the use of high dose azathioprine or with various other chemotherapeutic agents and radiation treatments for a number of malignancies. SOS is uncommonly seen after liver transplantation, mostly in the context of azathioprine use [25]. In HCT recipients, depending on the study population and diagnostic criteria used, the incidence of SOS ranges from 5 to 70%, and the overall mortality also varies from 20 to 50% [3].

In SOS, damaged sinusoidal endothelium sloughs off and obstructs the hepatic circulation, destroying centrilobular hepatocytes. A number of mediators, including 5-hydroxytryptamine, prostaglandins, leukotrienes, and free radicals contribute to endothelial damage culminating in liver cell ischemic injury and death. In the later stages of the disease, intense fibrogenesis occurs in the sinusoids, ultimately causing obliteration of the venules and chronic venous outflow obstruction.

A number of risk factors for SOS have been identified. A few of the notable risk factors include chronic liver disease, C282Y allele of the HFE gene, advanced age, hepatic metastases, previous radiation treatment to the liver, high-dose conditioning regimens, busulfan or gemtuzumab ozogamicin exposure, cyclophosphamide, and possibly infections such as CMV and HCV [3, 26].

The clinical manifestations of SOS usually surface around 7 to 10 days after transplant. The primary symptoms are weight gain and jaundice. Patients develop ascites, right upper quadrant tenderness, hepatomegaly, and conjugated hyperbilirubinemia. In severe cases, renal, cardiac, and respiratory failure can occur.

The diagnosis of SOS can be a difficult one to make, as so many other syndromes can have a similar presentation. Although the gold standard for diagnosis is a liver biopsy, this is seldom done because of potential complications of bleeding in the setting of thrombocytopenia. An ultrasound with Doppler flow will show portal hypertension late in the course.

The majority of patients with mild disease will improve over a few weeks. Unfortunately, there are no effective treatments to offer aside from supportive care, so prevention is critically important. Prevention strategies may involve the use of reduced intensity chemotherapy regimens, ursodiol, or a fibrinolytic agent such defibrotide [26].

> ### Case Continued
>
> The most likely diagnosis is either a flare of ulcerative colitis or an infection. Although a number of organisms can cause bloody diarrhea, the two most common entities are *C. difficile* and CMV Histopathology is essential to establish a diagnosis in an immunocompromised host. The clinician should avoid empiric treatment for ulcerative colitis flares as corticosteroids will exacerbate most infections.
>
> Stool for *C. difficile* toxin is negative and CMV antigenemia and PCV are strongly positive. Colonic biopsies contain severe inflammation, crypt distortion, giant cells, and intranuclear inclusion bodies, confirming CMV colitis.
>
> The patient responded to treatment with ganciclovir.

> ### Take Home Points
>
> - Gastrointestinal (GI) complications are a prevailing source of morbidity and mortality in solid organ and bone marrow transplant recipients.

- Immunosuppression predisposes patients to infections and malignancies of the liver and GI tract.
- Drugs, including immunosuppressive medications, can cause GI complications after transplant and gastroenterologists should be familiar with these medications and their side effects.
- Graft-versus-host disease and sinusoidal obstruction syndrome are more common after HCT than SOT and have significant morbidity and mortality requiring timely diagnosis and management.

References

1 Gautam A. Gastrointestinal complications following transplantation. *Surg Clin North Am* 2006; **86:** 1195–206.

2 Copelan EA. Hematopoietic stem-cell transplantation. *N Eng J Med* 2006; **354:** 1813–26.

3 Kumar S, DeLeve LD, Kamath PS, *et al.* Hepatic veno-occlusive disease (sinusoidal obstruction syndrome) after hematopoietic stem cell transplantation. *Mayo Clin Proc* 2003; **78:** 589–98.

4 Fischer SA. Infections complicating solid organ transplantation. *Surg Clin North Am* 2006; **86:** 1127–45.

5 Rubin RH. Impact of cytomegalovirus infection on organ transplant recipients. *Rev Infect Dis* 1990; **12:** S754–66.

6 Syndman DR. Infection in solid organ transplantation. *Transplant Infect Dis* 1999; **1:** 21–9.

7 Lowance D, Neumayer HH, Legendre CM, *et al.* Valacylovir for the prevention of cytomegalovirus disease after renal transplantation. International Valacylovir Cytomegalovirus Prophylaxis Transplantation Study Group. *N Engl J Med* 1999; **340:** 1462–70.

8 Cohen JI. Epstein-Barr virus infection. *N Eng J Med* 2000; **343:** 481–92.

9 Yu JTHT, Lau GKK. Treatment of hepatitis B and C following nonliver organ transplants. *Curr Hepatitis Rep* 2003; **2:** 82–7.

10 United Network for Organ Sharing, 2008. www.unos.org

11 Gutierrez-Dalmau A, Campistol JM. Immunosuppressive therapy and malignancy in organ transplant recipients. a systematic review. *Drugs* 2007; **67:** 1167–98.

12 Stewart T, Henderson R, Grayson H, *et al.* Reduced incidence of rectal cancer, compared to gastric and colonic cancer, in a population of 73,076 men and women chronically immunosuppressed. *Clin Cancer Rev* 1997; **3:** 51–5.

13 Penn, I. Cancers complicating organ transplantation. *N Engl J Med* 1990; **323:** 1767–9.

14 Andreone P, Gramenzi A, Lorenzini S, *et al.* Posttransplantation lymphoproliferative disorders. *Arch Intern Med* 2003; **163:** 1997–2004.

15 Caillard S, Lelong C, Pessione F, *et al.* Post-transplant lymphoproliferative disorders occurring after renal transplantation in adults: report of 230 cases from the French registry. *Am J Transplant* 2006; **6:** 2735–42.

16 Cockfield SM. Identifying the patient at risk for post-transplant lymphoproliferative disorder. *Transpl Infect Dis* 2001; **3.** 70–70.

17 Spielberger R, Stiff P, Bensinger W, *et al.* Palifermin for oral mucositis after intensive therapy for hematologic cancers. *N Engl J Med* 2004; **351:** 2590–8.

18 Armstrong D. Systematic review: persistence and severity in gastro-oesophageal reflux disease. *Aliment Pharmacol Ther* 2008; **28:** 841–53.

19 Reece J, Burton F, Lingle D, *et al.* Peptic ulcer disease following renal transplantation in the cyclosporine era. *Am J Surg* 1991; **162:** 558–62.

20 Stelzner M, Vlahakos DV, Milford EL, *et al.* Colonic perforations after renal transplantation. *J Am Coll Surg* 1997; **184:** 63–9.

21 Smith DM, Agura E, Netto G, *et al.* Liver transplantation associated graft-versus-host disease. *Transplantation* 2003; **75:** 118–26.

22 Couriel D, Caldera H, Champlin R, *et al.* Acute graft-versus-host disease: pathophysiology, clinical manifestations, and management. *Cancer* 2004; **101:** 1936.

23 Bhushan V, Collins RH. Chronic graft-vs-host disease. *JAMA* 2003; **290:** 2599–03.

24 Cutler C, Giri S, Jeyapalan S, *et al.* Acute and chronic graft-versus-host disease after allogeneic peripheral-blood stem-cell and bone marrow transplantation: a meta-analysis. *J Clin Oncol* 2001; **19:** 3685–91.

25 Sebagh M, Debette M, Samuel D, *et al.* "Silent" presentation of SOS after liver transplantation as part of the process of cellular rejection with endothelial predilection. *Hepatology* 1999; **30:** 1144–50.

26 Wadleigh M, Ho V, Momtaz P, Richardson P. Hepatic veno-occlusive disease: pathogenesis, diagnosis and treatment. *Curr Opin Hematol* 2003; **10:** 451–62.

SECTION IV

Liver and Biliary Tract

Editors Keith Lindor and Bashar A. Aqel

Part 1 Diagnostic Approaches in Liver Disease, 427

Part 2 Diseases of the Liver, 463

Part 3 Liver Transplantation, 599

PART 1

Diagnostic Approaches in Liver Disease

70 Approach to History-Taking and Physical Examination in Liver and Biliary Disease, 429
   David D. Douglas

71 Acute Liver Failure, 435
   Khurram Bari and Robert J. Fontana

72 Imaging of the Liver and Bile Ducts: Radiographic and Clinical Assessment of Findings, 442
   Thomas J. Byrne and Alvin C. Silva

73 Assessment of Liver Fibrosis: Liver Biopsy and Other Techniques, 450
   Sumeet K. Asrani and Jayant Talwalkar

74 Endoscopic Techniques Used in the Management of Liver and Biliary Tree Disease: ERCP and EUS, 455
   Toufic Kachaamy and Douglas Faigel

Approach to History-Taking and Physical Examination in Liver and Biliary Disease

David D. Douglas

Division of Gastroenterology and Hepatology, Mayo Clinic, Scottsdale, AZ, USA

Summary

Basic history-taking and physical examination skills help the clinician to direct the very complex, and often costly, diagnostic array with which to diagnose liver disease. The clinician needs to be attentive to changes in areas other than the abdomen that may be affected by liver disease, in order to better evaluate the ongoing disease process. Practitioners in the health care arena are increasingly asked to manage finite financial resources. Proficiency in history-taking, physical examination, and review of laboratory results is vital in determining an accurate diagnosis or efficiently directing further diagnostic testing.

Introduction

Patients with suspected liver or biliary disease rarely present with a single symptom or complaint. The clinician will more likely be sorting through multiple complaints and symptoms, while gathering corresponding or conflicting signs found during the physical examination. Even when presented with empirical data, the art is in the inspection, percussion, auscultation, and palpation and the ability to process all available data into a meaningful diagnosis. A thoughtful review of the patient's history, physical examination findings, and relevant laboratory values is typically enough to lead the examiner to a correct diagnosis.

In 1958, Dr. Franz Ingelfinger stated that the cause of jaundice can be identified in approximately 85% of patients after careful history, physical examination, and review of standard laboratory data [1]. This is still quite true today.

History-Taking

Today's physician has a myriad of diagnostic tools available: laboratory tests range from the standard to the obscure and body imaging techniques to almost the microscopic level. Indeed, information gleaned from a visual, auditory, tactile, and olfactory examination of the patient and the interpretation of the data can be considered less than definitive, given the exacting nature of the numbers and interpretive reports produced by the laboratory and radiology. There is greater security in laboratory values and images than in the art of history-taking and interpretation of findings. Furthermore, clinicians may disagree with one another about the physical findings of examination, whereas it is more difficult (though not impossible) to argue the validity of an objective laboratory value.

Careful questioning of the patient can reveal much about the onset of symptoms and is often sufficient to lead the clinician to a diagnosis. Table 70.1 lists the important historical points to review in a patient with liver disease.

During the interview portion of the history and physical, attentive questioning can uncover potential risk factors that, when correlated with associated symptoms such as fever, malaise, and weight loss, point to a definitive diagnosis. For example, patients should be questioned about recent changes in weight. Anorexia and nausea are among the first signs of liver disease, and may be extreme with muscle wasting in cirrhosis. An unexplained weight loss of 4.5 kg (10 lb) is worrisome for a neoplasm.

Jaundice

Jaundice or icterus – a yellow coloring most noticeable on the eyes, face, hands, and trunk – results from the retention and deposition of biliary pigments. Scleral icterus occurs when the serum bilirubin rises above 3.0 mg/dL in adults. The onset of jaundice is indicative of parenchymal liver diseases, such as hepatitis and cirrhosis, or of obstruction of the extrahepatic biliary tree, as in choledocholithiasis and carcinoma of the pancreas. The causes of jaundice are typically either intrahepatic or extrahepatic (Table 70.2), and less often disorders of brisk hemolysis [1].

Patient history should include questions about the onset and duration of the jaundice and whether or not it was accompanied by symptoms of anorexia, nausea, vomiting, chills, fever, itching, or weight loss. Knowing whether or not the patient associates with other people who have also developed jaundice leads the examiner to suspect a communicable disease. Jaundice accompanied by fever and chills is considered obstructive cholangitis until proven otherwise. Painless jaundice in an older patient may be the first symptom of cancer of the head of the pancreas. Prior history of inflammatory bowel disease (IBD) would suggest an association with primary sclerosing cholangitis (PSC).

Viral Hepatitis

When questioning the patient regarding risk factors for viral hepatitis, consider that the onset of symptoms may be abrupt or insidious due to the variation in incubation periods. The incubation period

Practical Gastroenterology and Hepatology Board Review Toolkit, Second Edition. Edited by Nicholas J. Talley, Kenneth R. DeVault, Michael B. Wallace, Bashar A. Aqel and Keith D. Lindor.

Table 70.1 Important historical points to review in a patient with liver disease.

General questions	Family history of liver disease, including inherited disorders Exposure to potential hepatotoxins Presence and onset of jaundice, pruritus, anorexia, or nausea Associated symptoms, such as fever, chills, acholic stool, malaise, and myalgia Symptoms of biliary colic or cholangitis (fever, chills, right upper quadrant pain) History of "colitis" or IBD (association with PSC) History of unintentional weight loss HIV status
Hepatitis exposure questions	Blood product transfusions (especially before 1990) Intravenous drug abuse Occupational needle-stick exposures Non-sterile tattoos or body piercing High-risk sexual behaviors Recent travel to endemic areas Exposure to patients with known viral hepatitis Ingestion of raw shellfish
Medication-related questions	All prescription and OTC medications All vitamins, herbal medications, dietary supplements, and recreational drugs (patients may not consider these medications)
Alcohol-related questions	Type of alcohol consumed, amount, pattern, frequency Age of onset of drinking Date of last drink Consequences of drinking (social or legal) CAGE questions

IBD, inflammatory bowel disease; PSC, primary sclerosing cholangitis; HIV, human immunodeficiency virus; OTC, over-the-counter.

for hepatitis A averages 30 days, that for hepatitis B, 12–14 weeks (minimum 6 weeks to maximum 6 months), and that for hepatitis C, 6–12 weeks. Questions related to viral hepatitis include history of blood transfusion (especially if it occurred before 1990, when serologic testing for hepatitis C became available), intravenous drug use, tattoos, and body piercing [2]. High-risk sexual practices include anal intercourse, sex with a prostitute, history of sexually transmitted infections (STIs), multiple sexual partners (more than five a year), and intercourse with a person infected with chronic viral hepatitis [1]. Taking an occupational history alerts the examiner to high-risk professions (e.g., health professionals, especially workers in renal dialysis units, operating rooms, or trauma units with exposure to intravenous drug users, or those with a history of a needle-stick injury). Risk factors for hepatitis A include travel to the endemic areas of Mexico, Latin America, and the African subcontinent, ingestion of raw contaminated shellfish, and exposure to groups of people in which clusters of hepatitis are known to occur,

Table 70.2 Common causes of jaundice.

Extrahepatic	Intrahepatic
Malignancies	Hepatocellular diseases
Pancreatic adenocarcinoma	Viral hepatitis
Cholangiocarcinoma	Alcoholic hepatitis
Gallbladder carcinoma	Autoimmune hepatitis
Chronic pancreatitis	Primary biliary cirrhosis (PBC)
Choledocholithiasis	Primary sclerosing cholangitis (PSC)
Primary sclerosing cholangitis (PSC)	Sarcoidosis
IgG4-related disease	Drug induced cholestasis
HIV cholangiopathy	Sepsis
Choledochal cysts	Total parenteral nutrition

HIV, human immunodeficiency virus.

such as outbreaks in restaurants, mental health institutions, and day care centers [1].

Drug-Induced Liver Disease

Drug-induced liver disease can mimic viral hepatitis, biliary tract obstruction, or other types of liver disease. The most common offenders are non-steroidal anti-inflammatory drugs (NSAIDs), analgesics, and antibiotics, because of their widespread use. Acetaminophen toxicity is now the most common cause of acute hepatic failure in the United States, accounting for 40% of cases [3]. Review all medications, including prescription and over-the-counter (OTC) drugs. Ask about the use of vitamins, especially vitamin A, as well as OTC supplements purchased in health food stores. Careful questioning about potentially hepatotoxic drugs or exposure to hepatotoxins may uncover a second agent that increases the toxicity of the first (e.g., acetaminophen and alcohol). Other exposure to hepatotoxins may be discovered by questioning the patient about work history and hobby interests. Exposure to certain industrial chemicals, such as carbon tetrachloride or vinyl chloride, is well known to cause liver disease.

Non-Alcoholic Fatty Liver Disease

Metabolic causes of non-alcoholic fatty liver disease (NAFLD) include obesity, diabetes mellitus, hyperlipidemia, hypothyroidism, abetalipoproteinemia, rapid weight loss, and total parenteral nutrition. Other causes include medications such as corticosteroids, amiodarone, diltiazem, tamoxifen, irinotecan, oxaliplatin, highly active antiretroviral therapy, and toxins (carbon tetrachloride and yellow phosphorus). Steatosis is a hallmark of insulin-resistance syndrome, characterized by obesity, diabetes, hypertriglyceridemia, and hypertension. In NAFLD, patients with obesity, diabetes, and advanced age have additional risk for advanced hepatic fibrosis and cirrhosis. Many patients with fatty liver disease present with mild right upper quadrant discomfort, but they are usually otherwise asymptomatic, unless they have complications of end-stage liver disease.

Alcoholic Liver Disease

Clinical findings in alcoholic liver disease can vary widely, from asymptomatic fatty liver to severe alcoholic hepatitis or cirrhosis presenting with coagulopathy, encephalopathy, and jaundice. Though chronic alcohol abuse may be denied or downplayed by many patients with alcoholic liver disease, confirming this is critical to making the diagnosis. Important questions not only to ask the patient but also to corroborate with family and friends include the type and amount of alcohol consumed, the pattern and frequency of drinking, the age of onset of alcohol use, and the date of last drink. In addition, note any psychosocial consequences of alcohol abuse, such as arrests for public intoxication or driving under the influence. Four questions that can be useful in identifying patients with excessive alcohol use form the acronym CAGE [4]:

1 Has the patient tried to **C**ut back on alcohol use?
2 Does the patient become **A**ngry when asked about his or her alcohol intake?
3 Does the patient feel **G**uilty about his or her alcohol use?
4 Does the patient need an **E**ye opener in the morning?

Two or more affirmative responses are seen in most patients with alcoholism. In contrast, over 80% of non-alcoholic patients have a negative response to all four questions, and virtually none has an affirmative response to more than two questions. The CAGE criteria have been considered to be an efficient and effective screening tool for detecting alcoholism, with a sensitivity and specificity of 0.71 and 0.90, respectively, at a cutoff of two or more affirmative responses [5].

Right Upper Quadrant Pain

The patient who presents with abdominal pain is a challenge to the physician, in that the complaint is frequently benign yet may also indicate a serious acute pathology. The initial assessment of abdominal pain will seek to exclude the presence of an acute surgical abdomen. Once that has been done, the history and physical examination can focus on the chronicity of symptoms and the location of the pain, in order to determine the correct diagnosis. Pain associated with liver and biliary disease generally occurs in the right upper quadrant of the abdomen, though it may occasionally radiate to the back, shoulder, or epigastrium.

Most often, right upper quadrant pain is related to the biliary tree, though parenchymal liver disease (e.g., hepatitis, fatty liver disease) may be a less severe cause. Hepatic pain is the result of liver enlargement and stretching of the surrounding capsule, and is less often a cause of right upper quadrant pain.

When assessing the cause of abdominal pain, consideration of more serious causes and complications must be given priority. Ascending or acute cholangitis, a potentially serious and life-threatening illness caused by stasis and infection in the biliary tract, is diagnosed by the presence of Charcot's triad of fever, jaundice, and right upper quadrant pain. It should be noted that elevations in bilirubin may be mild and not clinically detected as jaundice in the initial physical exam, so the diagnosis may need to be reconsidered if initial laboratory studies indicate an elevated bilirubin. A definitive diagnosis of ascending cholangitis may also be made if all of the following are present: evidence of an inflammatory response (abnormal white blood cell (WBC) count and elevated C-reactive protein (CRP)), abnormal liver tests, and biliary dilation. Biliary obstruction and stasis are also predisposing factors for ascending cholangitis. Other common causes are biliary calculi, benign stenosis, and malignancy [6].

Upper abdominal pain should also be considered as a possible extension of cardiac pain or as a pulmonary or pleural process. The patient history should inquire about exertional symptoms and shortness of breath. Patients suspected of an acute coronary episode should be referred for immediate evaluation. Physical examination of the chest will assess for percussion dullness, pleural rub, and abnormal breath sounds, in order to direct the physician to a non-abdominal cause for the upper abdominal pain.

Once more serious causes of right upper quadrant pain have been considered, the history can focus on risk factors for gallstone disease, a common cause.

Physical Examination

When assessing the patient with jaundice or abnormal liver tests, much is gleaned from the initial inspection, proceeding in a head-to-toe fashion. Though pieces of data are gathered in what appears to be haphazard fashion, affecting different organ systems along the way, by completion there will be enough information to develop a reasonable diagnosis.

Note the color of the patient's skin. Jaundice is most easily seen on the face, the sclera of the eyes, and the palms of the hands. Scleral icterus should be detected by examining the patient in natural daylight, if possible, because incandescent light may mask its presence. Cyanosis of the mucous membranes indicates hypoxemia, which may result from hepatopulmonary syndrome. This syndrome is caused by pulmonary microvascular vasodilation in patients with portal hypertension, resulting in dyspnea and hypoxemia that worsen in the upright position and improve when the patient is recumbent. Pallor is suggestive of anemia. When inspecting the general characteristics of the face, the presence of temporal wasting is a sign of advanced chronic liver disease or a neoplasm, whereas bulging cheeks can be caused by parotid enlargement in alcoholic liver disease. Note the presence of spider angiomas, most commonly found on the face, neck, upper anterior chest, and thorax, in the distribution of the superior vena cava. Multiple spider angiomas can signify the presence of portal hypertension. While examining the face, pause to note the patient's mental status, looking for signs of confusion, and be alert for the odor of fetor hepaticus. Inside the mouth, look for a reddened tongue (caused by vitamin B deficiencies resulting from alcoholism) or the white plaque of lichen planus (associated with hepatitis C and other liver disorders).

Patients presenting with jaundice require a thorough assessment of the heart and lungs. Cases of congestive heart failure can cause chronic passive congestion of the liver. In the neck, look for bulging neck veins caused by portopulmonary hypertension. Venous distension can be enhanced by applying gentle manual pressure to the abdomen over the liver (hepatojugular reflux). As you progress down to the arms and hands, note any additional signs of muscle wasting in the shoulders, as well as the presence of tattoos or needle tracks, which indicate a high-risk lifestyle. Skin redness and excoriation over the chest and back indicate pruritus, especially with a "butterfly distribution" at the interscapular region that is spared from redness, indicating the limits of the patient's reach when scratching. Generalized itching may be a sign of renal or hepatic disease, and can be severe in patients with primary biliary cirrhosis and PSC. Gynecomastia in men – along with sparse facial, axillary, and pubic hair – is often found in advanced liver disease.

The hands may exhibit clubbing of fingers. Clubbing, though not exclusive to liver disease, indicates liver disease and cirrhosis when combined with palmar erythema and spider nevi. When digital clubbing is due to liver or lung disease, the fingers return to normal after transplantation. Nails may be thickened, brittle, ridged, or flat in cases of liver disease. Look for changes in the nail bed, especially an increase in the size of the lunula, which gives the cirrhotic patient's nails a "half-and-half" appearance. The upper extremity tremor of asterixis indicates liver disease, though it can also be elicited in other non-hepatic causes of metabolic encephalopathy [7].

The presence of Dupuytren contracture is more a characteristic of alcoholism than of liver disease. Caused by a shortening of the palmar fascia, it causes a flexion deformity of some of the digits, giving the hand a clawlike appearance in extreme cases. Dupuytren contracture can also be seen in diabetes mellitus, reflex sympathetic dystrophy, Peyronie disease, and malignancy, though when seen in combination with parotid enlargement and gynecomastia, it invariably indicates chronic alcoholism.

The legs and feet mirror what is seen in the arms and hands, with toe clubbing, plantar erythema, and plantar fibrosis. Signs of muscle wasting that were seen in the face and shoulders will also be present in the legs, as well as sparse hair growth patterns and xanthomas on the knees. Spider nevi are not seen on the lower extremities. Petechiae are caused by thrombocytopenia and high venous pressures in the legs. Patients with hepatitis C may have lower-extremity findings of palpable purpura due to cryoglobulinemic vasculitis [2]. The feet and legs are also the site of dependent edema, the degree of which is assessed by various methods, including the amount of pitting within a range of +1 to +4, the depth of the pit, how far the pit extends upward from the feet toward the abdomen, or simply the grade of the pit on a scale of trace, mild, moderate, severe.

Examination of the Abdomen

The examination of the abdomen begins with inspection followed by auscultation, percussion, and palpation. The patient should lie flat with the abdomen fully exposed, the arms at the sides, and the legs flat. Any areas of tenderness should be assessed last, to avoid tightening of the abdominal muscles. The abdominal examination is important in determining the presence of intraperitoneal fluid (ascites); the size of solid organs such as liver and spleen can be determined on percussion. Palpation reveals the size and quality of the liver, whether it is soft, firm, hard, or irregular, and whether the left lobe is palpable across the midline: usually a sign of chronic liver disease.

Inspection

Inspect the abdomen, looking for any asymmetry, distension, or masses. An everted umbilicus is a sign of increased abdominal pressure and may be a sign of ascites, a large abdominal mass, or an umbilical hernia. The abdominal venous system is rarely observable in the normal individual; if it is visible, the drainage of bloodflow in the lower two-thirds of the abdomen is caudal, down toward the feet – drainage of the blood in a cephalad direction, toward the head, is indicative of vena caval obstruction. In patients with the portal hypertension of cirrhosis, the increased pressure is transmitted to collateral venous channels, which become dilated over time. The appearance of these dilated vessels, which appear to radiate out from the umbilicus, is known as caput medusae.

The presence of ascites is detected by observing the movement of the intra-abdominal fluid. When a patient with ascites is in the supine position, the fluid moves to the sides and results in bulging at the flanks. When the patient turns to the side, the fluid flows to the lower side, and when the patient stands, the fluid sinks into the lower abdomen. At this point in the examination, if ascites is suspected, a more thorough assessment can be made to detect its presence. A test for shifting dullness is one such measure. When a patient lies supine, free fluid in the abdomen gravitates to the flanks, and the intestines float upward. Percussion in this position reveals an area of tympany above an area of dullness. If the patient then turns on to one side, the area of dullness "shifts" to the dependent side as the gas-filled intestine floats to the top, and the uppermost area then becomes tympanic.

An additional test for ascites is the presence of a fluid wave. The examiner taps the left flank sharply with one hand, while placing the other hand against the opposite flank. In addition, a third hand belonging to either the patient or another clinician is placed with the ulnar surface along the midline of the abdomen, to stop transmission of an impulse by subcutaneous adipose tissue. If ascites is present, a fluid wave will be felt in the opposite flank. The test may give a false-positive result in patients who are obese. Both the test for shifting dullness and the fluid wave test are unreliable in detecting ascitic fluid of less than 1000 mL [1].

Auscultation

Examiners may perform auscultation before percussion or palpation to avoid altering bowel sounds, though there is no evidence that this matters. Auscultation is used to identify the presence of bruits or peritoneal friction rubs, in order to aid in the diagnosis of liver disease.

Bruits are systolic sounds created by turbulent bloodflow through diseased or compressed blood vessels. Abdominal bruits are useful in the diagnosis of renal artery stenosis and aortic aneurysm. Epigastric bruits are common in thin individuals, especially after a meal. Bruits located over the liver are associated with alcoholic hepatitis, hepatoma, hepatic artery aneurysm, hepatic arteriovenous fistula, and pancreatic cancer. A venous hum at the umbilicus is indicative of Cruveilhier–Baumgarten syndrome, which presents with splenomegaly, portal hypertension, and a patent umbilical vein [8].

Peritoneal friction rubs, like pericardial and pleural rubs, are a sign of inflammation or infection. Heard over the liver, they suggest a diagnosis of primary and metastatic malignancies, or may occur during the first 4–6 hours after liver biopsy. Rubs can occur with or without concomitant hepatomegaly. In general, rubs are nonspecific. Less than 10% of patients with known liver tumors have a rub [8].

Percussion

Percussion of the abdomen is useful in determining the size of the liver and spleen, and can determine whether ascites is present. The focus on assessing liver size is in identifying hepatomegaly, rather than in attempting to detect a small liver seen in patients with chronic cirrhosis. At the right midclavicular line, begin mid-chest at the third rib and percuss downward. The resonant tones of the chest will gradually change to dullness as the volume of the air-filled tissue of the lung overlying the liver decreases. Continue percussing downward until the dullness becomes tympanic over the colon. The lower border of liver dullness indicates where the liver edge should be palpable.

Vertical liver span is judged by liver dullness; it measures approximately 10–12 cm in men and 8–11 cm in women. Generally, a span of less than 12 cm makes hepatomegaly unlikely [8]. The difficulty in measuring liver span is in the organ's irregular shape and the fact that an accurate measurement depends on properly identifying the midclavicular line. Different clinicians will differ in their assessment of liver span despite accurate measurements, due to the variability in determining the location of the midclavicular line.

Percussion over the spleen is used to detect splenic dullness. The spleen is normally located in the left upper quadrant within the rib cage, against the posterolateral wall of the abdominal cavity. As the spleen enlarges, it remains close to the abdominal wall and the tip moves down toward the midline. As splenic enlargement is difficult to palpate, percussing an area of dullness is a useful sign. With the patient supine and breathing normally, percuss in the lowest intercostal space in the left anterior axillary line. Normal percussion gives either the resonant or the tympanic tone of the air-filled colon and stomach. A dull tone is a positive test for splenomegaly.

Certain conditions present challenges when assessing liver or spleen size by percussion. Chronic obstructive pulmonary disease (COPD) makes assessment of the upper border of the liver difficult and results in a false-positive measurement of the size of the liver. Distension of the colon obscures the lower-border liver dullness and may result in underestimation of the size of the liver: a false-negative assessment.

Palpation

Once percussion has given the examiner the approximate size and location of the liver, palpation is the next and final portion of the examination. The abdomen is palpated to further assess the size, shape, and quality of the liver. Light palpation is used first, progressing to deep palpation as abdominal muscles relax. To palpate the liver, place the right hand above the right iliac fossa and below the area of liver dullness. Press inward and upward, gradually working higher until the edge of the liver is appreciated. You may ask the patient to take a deep breath. As the diaphragm descends, the liver is brought down, which facilitates palpation of the lower edge. The normal liver edge has a firm, smooth shape – not hard – and the left lobe should not be palpable across the midline. Normally, the liver edge is sharp; a rounded edge indicates liver disease. Enlargement of the liver can be seen in acute hepatitis and chronic liver disease. A markedly enlarged liver (>10 cm below the costal margin) occurs in primary and metastatic tumors of the liver, alcoholic liver disease, severe congestive heart failure, infiltrative diseases of the liver such as amyloidosis and myelofibrosis, and chronic myelogenic leukemia.

A non-palpable liver does not rule out hepatomegaly, but it does reduce the likelihood that an enlarged liver is present. Conversely, a palpable liver is not necessarily enlarged or diseased, but it does increase the possibility of hepatomegaly [9].

If the earlier percussion gave signs of an enlarged spleen, the spleen may be palpated, though this is more difficult than palpating the liver. Normally, the spleen is not palpable. To palpate the spleen, start with the right hand above the left iliac fossa and, applying gentle pressure through curled fingers, work toward the left costal margin. If the spleen is not felt, turn the patient on to their right side and palpate the left upper quadrant as the patient takes a deep breath. The spleen may be felt as it descends during inspiration. Causes of splenomegaly include portal hypertension due to cirrhosis of the liver, hyperplasia, congestion, infection, and infiltration by tumor or myeloid elements [9].

Abnormal Liver Function Tests

For many patients, the first sign of liver disease is abnormal laboratory test results on routine screening. Though these tests give an indication of liver or biliary disease, they are usually not sensitive or specific enough to determine the exact cause or severity of liver disease, though they may suggest a category of disease, such as hepatitis, biliary obstruction, or infiltrative liver disease. Common routine screening tests include bilirubin, aminotransferases, serum alkaline phosphatase, serum albumin, prothrombin time, and platelets.

Bilirubin

Initial laboratory tests should include serum total and unconjugated bilirubin. Serum bilirubin is fractionated and classified into one of two categories: unconjugated (indirect) bilirubin or conjugated (direct) bilirubin. Identifying the type of hyperbilirubinemia points toward a particular group of diagnoses. An elevated serum bilirubin is a specific indicator of liver disease, though hemolysis is also a possible cause [10]. The test has limited sensitivity, in that patients with cirrhosis or other hepatic diseases may have normal serum bilirubin levels.

Conjugated (direct) hyperbilirubinemia is an elevation of both conjugated and unconjugated bilirubin, and results from impaired intrahepatic excretion of bilirubin or extrahepatic obstruction. Dubin–Johnson syndrome and Rotor's syndrome cause a rise in both unconjugated and conjugated serum bilirubin levels, but there is a disproportionate increase in conjugated serum bilirubin level. Extrahepatic and intrahepatic obstructions may be caused by ductular cholestasis. Tumors or strictures are also a cause of extrahepatic obstruction.

Unconjugated (indirect) serum hyperbilirubinemia may be caused by overproduction, decreased hepatic uptake, or decreased hepatic binding and conjugation. Conditions which can result in bilirubin overproduction are hemolytic anemia, hematomas

following surgery or trauma, and ineffective erythropoiesis of iron-deficiency anemia, thalassemia, or sideroblastic anemia. Decreased hepatic uptake may occur with exposure to various drugs. Other abnormalities associated with decreased hepatic binding and conjugation of bilirubin are Crigler–Najjar syndrome and Gilbert's syndrome [11].

Aminotransferases

Aspartate aminotransferase (AST, formerly serum glutamic oxaloacetic transaminase) and alanine aminotransferase (ALT, formerly serum glutamic pyruvic transaminase) are the most commonly used indicators of hepatocellular injury. Normal ranges for aminotransferases are notably higher in men than in women. ALT elevations are more specific for liver injury, while elevations in AST can also be seen in cardiac or muscle injury, as well as being released from hemolysis of red blood cells (RBCs). AST/ALT ratios above 2 can be suggestive of alcoholic liver disease. Elevations in enzyme levels are sensitive for even mild injury. Mild enzyme elevations of less than threefold are seen in fatty liver disease, drug toxicity, and chronic hepatitis. Cirrhosis, cholestatic liver diseases, and hepatic neoplasms may also show only slightly elevated liver enzymes. Slight elevations of both AST and ALT have been noted following rigorous exercise [10].

Moderately elevated enzyme levels of up to 20 times normal value may be indicative of acute or chronic hepatitis, including viral hepatitis and autoimmune, drug-induced, and alcoholic hepatitis. High levels of aminotransferases are seen in severe viral hepatitis, drug- or toxin-induced hepatic necrosis, and ischemic hepatitis due to circulatory shock. Values of >500 IU/L may occur in acute viral hepatitis. Rarely, choledocholithiasis causing brief biliary obstruction can also cause a transient impressive rise in transaminase levels, which normalize rapidly over a few days [12].

Serum Alkaline Phosphatase

Serum levels of alkaline phosphatase primarily come from the bone and liver, though they are also found in the placenta, intestine, and kidney. Normal ranges for alkaline phosphatase vary between individuals according to such factors as age, gender, weight, and (inversely) height. Isolated elevations of alkaline phosphatase are thought to be a non-specific finding, and should only be worked up further if they persist above twice the upper limits of normal. Healthy patients with an elevated alkaline phosphatase may find that it returns to normal on follow-up.

High levels of alkaline phosphatase typically indicate cholestatic disease as a result of either intrahepatic or extrahepatic obstruction of bile flow. Elevated levels in patients with cancer may indicate metastasis to the liver or bone. Increases of threefold or more indicate extrahepatic obstruction, primary biliary cirrhosis, or cholestatic drug injury. Alkaline phosphatase may be elevated in adolescents with rapid bone growth and in pregnant patients in the third trimester. Gamma-glutamyl transpeptidase (GGT) and 5′-nucleotidase are helpful in differentiating these cases from cholestatic liver disease as they are specific to liver disease and are elevated only due to hepatic etiologies. Low serum alkaline phosphatase may be seen in hypothyroidism, pernicious anemia, zinc deficiency, and congenital hypophosphatasia [11].

Serum Albumin

Serum albumin is produced by the liver, and decreased levels are often an indication of severe or prolonged liver disease, though they are less often associated with acute liver conditions. Differential diagnoses of a low serum albumin level include protein-losing enteropathy, proteinuria, catabolic states, and poor nutritional status. In cirrhosis, a low serum albumin and elevated serum globulin may be the only abnormal liver chemistry test [11].

Prothrombin Time

Most of the proteins required in blood coagulation are produced by the liver. A prolonged prothrombin time is a sign of liver dysfunction, though it lacks sensitivity. Patients with acute liver injury and mild chronic liver disease may not exhibit prolonged prothrombin time. Other causes include congenital deficiency of coagulation factors, nutritional deficiency, and malabsorption. Antibiotics can also lead to a vitamin K deficiency, through suppression of normal gut flora.

Platelets

Though not considered a liver function test (LFT), a low platelet count due to splenic sequestration can be an early surrogate marker of portal hypertension.

Take Home Points

- Despite our technological advances, history-taking is pivotal to accurate diagnostic tests.
- The physical examination should be focused on the abdomen, but, because the impact of liver disease is systemic, attention should also be given to other regions, such as the skin, fingers, muscle mass, and head and neck.
- The use of basic examination skills, such as observation, palpation, and percussion, will generally narrow the differential diagnosis before more detailed evaluation is completed.

Acknowledgements

The author thanks Sandra J. Douglas, RN, BSN, MBA for assistance with the preparation of this chapter.

References

1 Greenberger NJ. History taking and physical examination in the patient with liver disease. In: Schiff ER, Sorrell MF, Maddrey WC, eds. *Schiff's Diseases of the Liver*, 8th edn. Philadelphia, PA: Lippincott-Raven Publishers, 1999: 193–203.

2 Swartz MH. *Textbook of Physical Diagnoses: History and Examination*, 3rd edn. Philadelphia, PA: WB Saunders Co. 1998: 354–89.

3 Friedman LS. Liver, biliary tract, and pancreas. In: McPhee SJ, Papadakis MA, Tierney LM Jr., eds. *Current Medical Diagnosis and Treatment*, 46th edn. New York, NY: McGraw-Hill Medical Publishing, 2007: 664–718.

4 Ewing JA. Detecting alcoholism. The CAGE questionnaire. *JAMA* 1984; **252**: 1905–7.

5 Aertgeerts B, Buntinx F, Kester A. The value of the CAGE in screening for alcohol abuse and alcohol dependence in general clinical populations: a diagnostic meta-analysis. *J Clin Epidemiol* 2004; **57**: 30–9.

6 Yasutoshi K, Tadahiro T, Yoshifumi K, *et al.* Definitions, pathophysiology, and epidemiology of acute cholangitis and cholecystitis: Tokyo Guidelines. *J Hepatobiliary Pancreat Surg* 2007; **14**(1): 15–26.

7 Reuben A. The liver has a body – a cook's tour. *Hepatology* 2005; **41**: 408–15.

8 Naylor CD. Physical examination of the liver. *JAMA* 1994; **271**: 1859–65.

9 Talley NJ, O'Connor S. *Clinical Examination: A Systematic Guide to Physical Diagnosis*, 7th edn. Philadelphia, PA: Elsevier, 2014.

10 Zakim D, Boyer T. *Hepatology: A Textbook of Liver Disease*, 4th edn. Philadelphia, PA: Saunders, 2003: 661–82.

11 Kaplowitz N, ed. *Liver and Biliary Diseases*, 2nd edn. Baltimore, MD: Williams & Wilkins, 1996: 207–15.

12 Fortson WC, Tedesco FJ, Stames EC, Shaw CT. Marked elevation of serum transaminase activity associated with extrahepatic biliary tract disease. *J Clin Gastroenterol* 1985; 7(6): 502–5.

CHAPTER 71

Acute Liver Failure

Khurram Bari and Robert J. Fontana

Department of Internal Medicine, University of Michigan Medical School, Ann Arbor, MI, USA

Summary

Acute liver failure (ALF) is defined as severe liver injury with coagulopathy and encephalopathy that arises within 8–26 weeks of illness onset in a patient without known liver disease. This clinical syndrome is associated with high mortality in the absence of emergency liver transplantation and demands rapid, complex management decisions for optimal patient outcomes. The most common causes of ALF in the United States are acetaminophen (APAP) overdose, indeterminate ALF, idiosyncratic drug reactions, and viral hepatitis. The likelihood of spontaneous recovery depends on the etiology of ALF, encephalopathy stage, and development of multiorgan failure. N-acetylcysteine (NAC) is recommended for all patients with suspected APAP overdose, and may also be of benefit in adults with non-APAP-related ALF and early-stage encephalopathy.

Case

A 21-year-old college student presents with increasing confusion. There is little history available. She is disoriented and uncooperative, and has no focal neurologic signs. She is hemodynamically stable and afebrile. Exam is otherwise normal; there is good nutritional status. Lab results are as follows:

- Hb 10.1 g/dL
- WBC 6.400 −10 6
- Platelets 146 000 −10 6
- INR 2.6
- AST 6829 U/L
- ALT 8265 U/L
- Bilirubin 2.2/1.5 mg/dL
- Creatinine 4.7 mg/dL

Introduction

ALF most commonly occurs in previously healthy individuals without pre-existing liver disease, with an estimated annual incidence of only one to six cases per million people in Western countries [1]. A rapid determination of the etiology allows disease-specific treatments to be initiated and helps determine whether a patient is likely to recover or to require emergency liver transplantation. With recent advancements in supportive care, short-term survival rates have improved, but many ALF patients still die from complications of cerebral edema, infections, and multiorgan failure.

Definition

ALF (fulminant hepatic failure) is defined as severe acute liver dysfunction with coagulopathy (INR > 1.5) and encephalopathy developing within 8–26 weeks of illness onset in the absence of chronic liver disease. A widely used clinical classification of ALF stratifies patients based on time from initial symptom onset to encephalopathy as hyper-acute (<1 week), acute (1–4 weeks), or sub-acute (4–12 weeks) [2,3]. Patients with hyper-ALF have the highest spontaneous recovery rate, followed by ALF and then sub-ALF.

Etiology

ALF is most commonly encountered in developing countries, due to the higher incidence of viral hepatitis in the general population [3]. In Western countries, the most common cause of ALF is acetaminophen (APAP) overdose (either intentional or therapeutic misadventure), which accounts for 40–50% of patients [1,4,5]. Though patients with non-intentional APAP overdose frequently present with more advanced degrees of encephalopathy, they have a similar survival to subjects with intentional overdose (70 vs. 70%) [4]. Idiosyncratic drug-induced liver injury (DILI) and indeterminate ALF are the next most common causes of ALF. Many drugs, as well as herbal and dietary supplements, have been associated with severe liver injury; the most commonly implicated drugs leading to liver transplantation in the United States are isoniazid, propylthiouracil, phenytoin, and valproate [6].

Fulminant hepatitis A, B, and E infection is the most common cause of ALF in developing countries, but accounts for only 3% (hepatitis A) to 7% (hepatitis B) of cases in the United States [5]. Clinical outcomes are worse with fulminant HBV as compared to hepatitis A or E. Autoimmune hepatitis accounts for up to 5% of ALF cases. In pregnant women, acute fatty liver of pregnancy, eclampsia, and the hemolysis, elevated liver tests, low platelets (HELLP) syndrome are the most common causes of ALF. Severe hepatic ischemia can also lead to ALF, but outcomes are usually determined by the underlying cardiopulmonary disease [7].

Rare causes of ALF, accounting for <10% of adult cases, include Amanita mushroom poisoning, Budd–Chiari syndrome, heat stroke, herpes hepatitis, malignant infiltration of the liver (especially lymphoma, breast cancer, and melanoma), leptospirosis, and dengue fever. Fulminant Wilson's disease should be considered in young patients with ALF who frequently have low or normal serum alkaline phosphatase levels.

Practical Gastroenterology and Hepatology Board Review Toolkit, Second Edition. Edited by Nicholas J. Talley, Kenneth R. DeVault, Michael B. Wallace, Bashar A. Aqel and Keith D. Lindor.

Table 71.1 Encephalopathy grade in ALF.

Coma grade	Clinical features
I	Changes in behavior or slow mentation with minimal change in level of consciousness
II	Gross disorientation, drowsiness, asterixis, inappropriate behavior
III	Marked confusion, incoherent speech, sleeping most of the time but arousable to vocal stimuli
IV	Comatose, unresponsive to pain, decorticate or decerebrate posturing

Case Continued

Findings show ALF with:
- short history (days);
- rapid progression;
- high transaminases;
- low bilirubin;
- renal failure.

Clinical diagnosis: acetaminophen hepatotoxicity.
Specific therapy: NAC (give immediately)

Pathophysiology

Severe acute hepatic injury results in the death of hepatocytes via either necrosis or apoptosis. The release of large quantities of both pro- and anti-inflammatory cytokines can lead to vasodilation and a systemic inflammatory response syndrome (SIRS) that may progress to multi-system organ failure [8]. In addition, damage to intrahepatic macrophages in a severely injured liver can lead to reduced immune surveillance and a greater likelihood of bacterial and fungal infections.

Renal dysfunction occurs in up to 60% of patients with APAP overdose and up to 50% of patients with ALF from other etiologies. In most cases, kidney dysfunction is multifactorial, including hypoperfusion, the effect of inflammatory cytokines, superimposed infection, and the direct effect of drugs like APAP on the kidney [9]. The predominant type of kidney injury is acute tubular necrosis, but hepatorenal physiology can contribute to renal dysfunction.

The most dreaded complication of ALF is brain edema with increased intracranial pressure (ICP), which is present in at least 30% of ALF patients (Table 71.1). Risk factors for cerebral edema in ALF patients include infection, SIRS, requirement for vasopressor support, and renal replacement therapy (Figure 71.1). High circulating ammonia levels and other neurotoxins are converted to glutamine by astrocytes, which can lead to cellular swelling via osmotic and non-osmotic pathways. In addition, the blood–brain barrier (BBB) is adversely impacted by high ammonia levels, cytokines, and toxins, which, paired with increased cerebral bloodflow due to increased nitrous oxide release, can lead to a loss of intracranial autoregulation and worsening cerebral edema [10, 11].

Diagnostic Evaluation

Initial assessment of an ALF patient includes a detailed history regarding prescription and non-prescription medication use, illicit drug use, travel, sick contacts, and medical and psychiatric comorbidities (Figure 71.1). The minimum APAP dose needed to cause severe liver injury is estimated at 4–10 g, but some patients may overdose over several days. Serum acetaminophen-protein adducts are covalent adducts of APAP with a much longer half-life than the parent compound, which can be a helpful diagnostic tool [12].

Patients presenting with very high levels of serum aminotransferase levels (more than 2000 range) most frequently have APAP overdose, viral hepatitis, or ischemia (Table 71.2). A liver biopsy is generally not recommended for prognostic purposes in ALF patients, due to the potential for sampling artifact and the risk of bleeding complications. However, biopsy may prove useful when there is suspicion of a diagnosis that may preclude liver transplantation (malignancy) or when the diagnosis mandates specific therapy (herpes, autoimmune).

Case Continued

Additional tests:
- Serum acetaminophen level undetectable
- Arterial ammonia 98 mmol/L, lactate 2.1 mmol/L, pH 7.40
- Drug screen negative
- Viral markers negative
- Ceruloplasmin normal at 15 mg/dL, serum copper normal
- Pregnancy test negative
- Ultrasonogram and head computed tomography (CT) normal

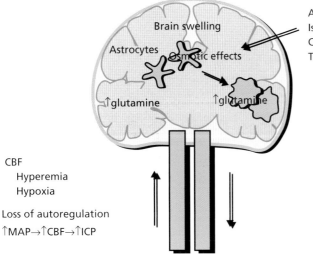

Figure 71.1 Pathophysiology of cerebral edema in ALF. In the early stages, an increase in cerebral blood flow (CBF) coupled with the impact of ammonia and other noxious stimuli (i.e., cytokines, hypoxia) on vascular endothelial cells can lead to a loss of the blood–brain barrier (BBB) and fluid accumulation in the brain. The conversion of glutamate to glutamine by astrocytes can lead to further fluid retention in the brain and worsening cerebral edema. In advanced grades of encephalopathy, a loss of intracranial autoregulation of CBF is frequently noted, which may eventually culminate in uncal herniation of the brain tissue into the foramen magnum due to the rising intracranial pressure (ICP). Source: Data provided by Will Lee, personal communication.

Table 71.2 Initial laboratory assessment of ALF.

Diagnostic testing[a]	Serum acetaminophen level (APAP-protein adducts[b]), urine tox screen
	Viral hepatitis: anti-HAV IgM, HBsAg, anti-HBc, anti-HCV, HCV-RNA, anti-HEV IgM.
	Non-hepatotrophic viruses: HSV-DNA, EBV-DNA, CMV-DNA (by PCR)
	Wilson's: ceruloplasmin, urine copper, slit lamp exam
	Autoimmune: ANA, anti-SmAb, quantitative immunoglobulin levels
	Vascular disorders: liver ultrasound with Doppler
	Ischemia: 2D cardiac echo with Doppler
	Liver histology: rarely needed (malignancy, confirm AIH)
Liver injury severity[c]	Serum AST, ALT, bilirubin (total and direct), alkaline phosphatase
	INR, factor V, fibrinogen
	Blood glucose, serum electrolytes, calcium, magnesium, phosphate
	Arterial blood gas, ammonia, lactate level
	Encephalopathy grade, Glasgow coma score, presence of vital organ failure
	Head CT scan (if comma grade 2 or higher)
	ICP monitor if grade 4 or uninterpretable neuro exam
	Blood and urine cultures daily, or if infection suspected
Liver transplantation candidacy[d]	Medical and surgical assessment of prognosis/suitability
	Psychosocial assessment (substance abuse, compliance)
	Blood group × 2
	HIV and other serologies
	Chest X-ray, EKG, 2D echocardiogram

[a]Obtain initial diagnostic testing as soon as possible after admission.
[b]Not commercially available.
[c]Obtain every 8–12 hours early on, and daily thereafter.
[d]Complete within 24 hours of intensive care unit (ICU) admission and review periodically thereafter.
HAV, hepatitis A virus; HCV, hepatitis C virus; HEV, hepatitis E virus; HSV, herpes simplex virus; EBV, Epstein–Barr virus; CMV, cytomegalovirus; PCR, polymerase chain reaction; AIH, autoimmune hepatitis; AST, aspartate transaminase; ALT, alanine transaminase; INR, international normalized ratio; CT, computed tomography; ICP, intracranial pressure; HIV, human immunodeficiency virus; EKG, electrocardiogram.

Management

The goal of supportive care is to provide the optimal environment for hepatic recovery and to prevent and treat complications of ALF while pursuing evaluation for liver transplantation [13]. Patients with poor prognostic indicators should be identified early on and referred to a liver transplantation center (Figure 71.2).

Etiology-Specific Therapies

NAC is an effective antidote for APAP overdose and is completely protective against hepatotoxicity if given within the first 8 hours after a single-time-point ingestion (Table 71.3) [14]. Any patient with ALF due to suspected APAP overdose should receive NAC promptly (irrespective of the time of ingestion). It is recommended that oral NAC be given as a loading dose of 140 mg/kg followed by 70 mg/kg every 4 hours, for 72 hours total. In subjects with nausea/vomiting or an ileus, NAC can also be given intravenously in a monitored setting (Table 71.4). Based upon the results of a double-blind, randomized controlled trial (RCT), intravenous (IV) NAC has demonstrated efficacy in adults with non-APAP-related ALF, and particularly in those with grade-1 or -2 encephalopathy [15]. However, the safety and efficacy of NAC is less well established in children with non-APAP-related ALF.

Corticosteroids are recommended for patients with severe autoimmune hepatitis, but their use should not lead to a delay in liver transplantation evaluation or listing. For pregnancy-associated disease, immediate delivery of the fetus is advisable. Subjects with

fulminant herpes simplex virus (HSV) hepatitis have a poor prognosis, and treatment with acyclovir can double the chances of spontaneous recovery. The diagnosis of mushroom poisoning depends on a history of ingestion; therapy is most effective in the first 10 hours after ingestion, and consists of gastric lavage, activated charcoal (50 g) by nasogastric tube, intravenous penicillin (1 000 000 units/kg per day in divided doses), and intravenous NAC. Entecavir should be started in patients with fulminant hepatitis B virus (HBV).

Case Continued

Initial management:
- Intravenous NAC (72 hours)
- Acid suppression, vitamin K
- Infection screen (blood, urine, chest radiograph)
- Cefotaxime and fluconazole
- Continuous venovenous hemodialysis (CVVHD)
- Propofol for severe agitation
- Elective intubation (coma grade 3) and ICP monitor
- Enteral nutrition via feeding tube
- Assessment and activation for orthotopic liver transplantation (OLT)

General Supportive Care

Monitoring of Blood Tests

After initial assessment of the etiology and severity of ALF (Table 71.2), frequent monitoring (every 8–12 hours) of hepatic and renal function, acid–base status, and blood glucose (hourly) is recommended. The factor V assay is a very sensitive marker for liver synthetic function, and changes over time can provide useful prognostic information regarding hepatic regeneration (Figure 71.2).

Nutrition

ALF patients are prone to develop hypoglycemia due to glycogen depletion and increased caloric requirements arising from their hypercatabolic state. Continuous intravenous infusion of D_{10} and D_{50} is used to prevent and treat hypoglycemia, respectively, but close monitoring is required since hyperglycemia may increase the risk of infections. Enteral nutrition with 20–25 kcal/kg per day is recommended: adequate protein (1.0–1.5 g/kg per day) should be given, with monitoring of arterial ammonia levels in those with severe hepatic dysfunction. Parenteral nutrition should only be used if tube feeding is not tolerated or is contraindicated.

Management of Infection Risk

ALF patients have enhanced susceptibility to infection due to complex immune dysfunction, the need for invasive monitoring, and indwelling catheters. Bacterial and fungal infections develop in more than 70% of ALF patients; pneumonia, urinary tract infections (UTIs), catheter-induced bacteremia, and spontaneous bacteremia, with Gram-positive cocci or enteric Gram-negative bacilli, are frequently seen. Therefore, frequent (every 24–48 hours) blood and urine culture surveillance, as well as sampling of ascites and tracheal secretions when clinically indicated, is advised.

Parenteral and enteral antibiotic prophylaxis reduces infections in ALF, but no survival benefit is seen [16]. Broad-spectrum antibiotics are widely used and are recommended in advanced coma grades, in patients with fever or other evidence of infection, and with the presence of SIRS. Antifungal agents are also frequently used to

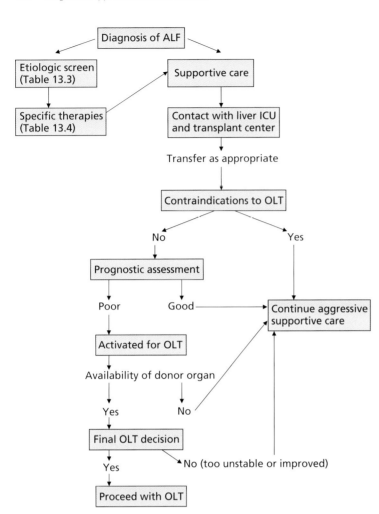

Figure 71.2 Management of ALF. A rapid determination of the etiology and severity of ALF is required so that patients with unfavorable prognostic features can be transferred to a liver transplant center. In addition, disease-specific treatments should be initiated as soon as possible, along with supportive intensive care unit (ICU) care for infectious, bleeding, and hemodynamic complications of ALF. An accurate assessment of the presence and severity of cerebral edema is critical, so that specific interventions to lower intracranial pressure (ICP) can be implemented. Despite supportive care, many ALF patients require emergency liver transplantation, with generally favorable 1-year outcomes. However, 10–20% of ALF patients listed for liver transplantation die from complications of ALF, due to the organ donor shortage [29].

Table 71.3   Treatable causes of ALF.

Cause	Therapy	Spontaneous survival with treatment
Acetaminophen overdose	NAC	~70%
Autoimmune	Corticosteroids	~50%
Herpes simplex	Acyclovir (30 mg/kg per day IV)	<25%
Hepatitis B	Entecavir or tenofovir	<25%
Amanita poisoning	Hemodialysis, benzylpenicillin (1 g/kg per day IV), and NAC	50%
Wilson's	Copper chelation	0%
Idiosyncratic DILI	Discontinuation of suspect drug	<25%
Pregnancy-related	Delivery of fetus	50%

NAC, N-acetylcysteine; IV, intravenous; DILI, drug-induced liver injury.

prevent late death from fungal infections. Fluconazole (200 mg first dose, 100 mg daily thereafter, either orally or intravenously) is safe to use in ALF and may reduce the frequency of fungal infections.

Coagulation Abnormalities and Bleeding

Hemostatic abnormalities in ALF are common and include a combination of platelet deficiency and dysfunction, as well as deficiency of anticoagulant and procoagulant proteins from both decreased hepatic synthesis and increased consumption. Interestingly, the risk of significant bleeding is less than 10%. Major sites of bleeding are the gastrointestinal (GI) tract, nasopharynx, lungs, and puncture sites. Parenteral vitamin K is given to correct any nutritional deficiency, and gastric acid suppression with a proton pump inhibitor (PPI) is advisable to reduce the risk of stress ulcers and gastric mucosal bleeding.

Platelet transfusion, fresh-frozen plasma (FFP), and cryoprecipitate are used only for active bleeding, high-risk procedures (e.g., placement of an ICP monitor), and liver transplantation. Recombinant activated factor VII (rFVIIa) may also be used prior to invasive procedures, but FFP and cryoprecipitate must be given beforehand to replete other clotting factors [17].

Table 71.4 Recommended dosing of intravenous N-acetylcysteine (NAC) in acetaminophen-overdose patients.

Day	Dose (mg/kg)	Volume of 5% dextrose (mL)	Duration of infusion (hours)
1	150	250	1
	50	500	4
	125	1000	19
2	150	1000	24
3	150	1000	24[a]

[a]Can repeat until international normalized ratio (INR) <1.5.
Oral dosing: 140 mg/kg loading dose, then 70 mg/kg every 4 hours for 72 hours.

Management of Encephalopathy Grades I and II

Encephalopathy grade I patients may be slightly disoriented without hyperreflexia and should be monitored in a quiet environment with skilled nursing. With progression to grade II, CT scan of the head to exclude any other etiology of neurologic deterioration is advised. Sedation should be avoided in early encephalopathy grades, because it prevents neurologic evaluation, but propofol or lorazepam may be needed for severe agitation. Elevation of the head of the bed to 30° helps prevent cerebral edema by improving venous return. Lactulose and rifaximin have not been shown to improve encephalopathy or survival.

Management of Encephalopathy Grades III and IV

The Glasgow Coma Scale (scale 3–15) is frequently used to assess patients with advanced encephalopathy in the intensive care unit (ICU). Tracheal intubation and mechanical ventilation are recommended in patients with grade III encephalopathy, for airway protection. A nasogastric tube should be placed to allow enteral access and to monitor for GI bleeding. Factors that increase ICP need to be avoided, including hypercapnia, neck vein compression, fluid overload, fever, hypoxia, coughing, seizures, and endotracheal suctioning. Fever is associated with poor outcome, and a core temperature of 36 °C is desirable [18].

Maintenance of hemodynamic stability and euvolemia is essential in the management of ALF. An arterial line, urinary catheter, and central line are placed, and often a pulmonary artery catheter will be needed. Initial treatment of hypotension should be intravenous fluids. Once euvolemia is achieved, vasopressors like norepinephrine and phenylephrine (if necessary) are used to maintain a mean arterial pressure (MAP) between 65 and 80 mmHg. A cerebral perfusion pressure (CPP) of >60 mmHg should be maintained (CPP = MAP − ICP). Pressor therapy increases blood pressure but may worsen oxygen delivery. Low-dose, continuous vasopressin may be used with caution as an adjunct in vasopressor-resistant hypotension. Patients with refractory hypotension despite volume resuscitation and vasopressors should be evaluated and treated for adrenal insufficiency.

Renal Support

The incidence of acute renal failure in ALF is >50%. Treatment measures include avoidance of nephrotoxic drugs, treatment of infection, provision of adequate renal perfusion, and hemodialysis. CVVHD, with less rapid fluid shifts and hemodynamic instability, is preferred over hemodialysis [19]. CVVHD should be started as soon as renal failure is suspected.

Monitoring for Raised ICP

Symptoms and physical signs of headache, vomiting, and hyperreflexia are not sensitive enough to reliably detect increases in ICP, while concomitant use of sedation and mechanical ventilation make interpretation of neurologic examination more difficult. Brain imaging may be more reliable but is not recommended, as moving patients with ALF and severe encephalopathy can exacerbate cerebral edema. Invasive continuous monitoring of ICP is the most accurate means used by most liver centers. Epidural catheters are commonly used; they have the lowest complication rate at 3.8%, with fatal hemorrhage in 1% [20]. Some centers use jugular bulb venous saturation monitoring (jugular venous oximetry) to assess cerebral oxygen delivery and consumption.

Treatment of Intracranial Hypertension

Intracranial hypertension (ICH) is defined as an ICP >20–25 mmHg for >5 minutes or a CPP <50–60 mmHg. ICH requires specific therapeutic interventions. The choice of therapy includes agents that decrease ICP either by osmotic effect (mannitol, hypertonic saline) or by decreasing cerebral blood flow (hyperventilation, hypothermia, barbiturate coma, indomethacin).

Mannitol

Osmotic diuresis with mannitol has been shown in controlled trials to correct episodes of elevated ICP and decrease cerebral edema in ALF patients; its use has also been associated with improved survival [21]. An intravenous bolus of 0.5 g/kg mannitol is the first-line therapy for raised ICP; the dose can be repeated as long as serum osmolality remains <300 mosmol/kg. Volume overload in patients with renal failure can limit the use of mannitol.

Hypertonic Saline

Hypertonic saline boluses are increasingly used as an alternative to mannitol in the treatment of ICH (30 mL of 23.4% saline or 2 mL/kg of 7.5% saline). One randomized trial showed that a continuous infusion of 30% saline with a goal serum sodium of 145–150 mmol/L resulted in a significant decrease in ICP and decreased incidence of episodes of ICH [22]. Further studies are needed to confirm the optimal level of serum sodium in ALF patients.

Hyperventilation

Hyperventilation to reduce $PaCO_2$ to 25–30 mmHg quickly decreases ICP through cerebral vasoconstriction and restores autoregulation of cerebral blood flow [23]. However, cerebral vasoconstriction can potentially worsen cerebral edema by causing cerebral hypoxia; therefore, it is safest to use it in conjunction with jugular venous saturation monitoring. Due to its short-lasting effects and concern over cerebral ischemia, hyperventilation is restricted to acute, short-term elevations of ICP.

Barbiturates

Barbiturates may also be considered when severe ICH does not respond to other measures. Pentobarbital at 3–5 mg/kg loading dose then 1–3 mg/kg every hour or thiopental at 5–10 mg/kg then 3–5 mg/kg every hour effectively decreases the cerebral metabolic rate, causes vasoconstriction, and reduces ICP. However, barbiturates can also cause myocardial depression and hypotension, requiring vasopressor support.

Hypothermia

Mild to moderate hypothermia (32–33 °C) has been shown in animals and humans to reduce ICP and normalize cerebral blood flow, possibly by preventing hyperemia or by altering brain ammonia or glucose metabolism, or through a combined effect [24]. Induction of hypothermia by a cooling blanket is a simple bedside procedure in the vasodilated state of ALF that can be continued during liver transplantation to prevent ICH. Potential side effects are increased infection, coagulation abnormalities, and cardiac dysrhythmias. Prospective studies are needed.

Seizure Management in ALF

Seizure activity may acutely elevate ICP and may cause cerebral hypoxia and thus contribute to cerebral edema. Phenytoin is the drug of choice for controlling seizure activity in ALF, and only minimal doses of benzodiazepines should be added for ongoing seizure activity. Studies of the use of prophylactic phenytoin to reduce seizure activity and brain edema have not been favorable.

Liver Support Devices

The complexity of liver metabolic, synthetic, detoxifying, and excretory functions makes application of extracorporeal hepatic support extremely challenging in ALF patients. Multiple non-biological and bioartificial liver systems have been used, with minimal success. One recent multicenter, randomized trial of an extracorporeal, porcine, hepatocyte-based, bioartificial liver in 171 patients with ALF showed the device to be safe, but overall survival was not improved [25]. More recently, a large RCT of albumin dialysis using the MARS device was completed in 102 French ALF patients; it also failed to demonstrate a therapeutic benefit [26].

Prognostic Scoring Systems

Liver transplantation has emerged as the most viable treatment option for patients with ALF and poor prognostic indicators. However, early detection of patients at substantial risk of early death remains challenging. Subject age, etiology of ALF, admission encephalopathy grade, and timing of liver transplantation all influence survival.

The King's College criteria separate patients into APAP and non-APAP groups (Table 71.5). There is acceptable specificity with survival without transplantation in patients meeting these criteria, at <15% [27]. However, the sensitivity of the criteria is low, and they may fail to identify some patients with poor outcomes. In APAP cases, addition of arterial lactate >3.5 mmol/L on admission or >3.0 mmol/L after fluid resuscitation improves the sensitivity and specificity.

Other systems, such as the Acute Physiology and Chronic Health Evaluation (APACHE) II score and the Model for End-Stage Liver Disease (MELD) score, have also been used to determine the prognosis in ALF; these scales have acceptable specificity but poor sensitivity. A recently described prognostic model called the Acute Liver Failure Study Group Index combines clinical (coma grade), laboratory (INR, serum bilirubin, phosphorus), and apoptosis markers (M30). It has an improved sensitivity of 86% but a decreased specificity of 65% [20].

Table 71.5 King's College criteria for liver transplantation in ALF.

Acetaminophen-related ALF
- Arterial pH < 7.3 (following volume resuscitation), independent of encephalopathy grade

Or
- Grade III or IV encephalopathy; and
- Prothrombin time > 100 seconds (INR > 6.0); and
- Serum creatinine >3.4 mg/dL (301 mmol/L)

Non-acetaminophen-related ALF
- PT >100 seconds (INR >6), irrespective of coma grade

Or

Any three of the following, irrespective of coma grade:
- Drug toxicity, indeterminate ALF
- Age <10 years or >40 years
- Jaundice-to-coma interval >7 days
- PT >50 seconds (INR ≥3.5)
- Serum bilirubin >17.5 mg/dL

ALF, acute liver failure; INR, international normalized ratio; PT, prothrombin time.

Case Continued

Outcome (day 2):
- ICP fluctuating: deep sedation, mannitol (1 dose)
- Temperature to 38 °C: cooling blanket to 36 °C
- Anuric: continued CVVHD
- Seizures on EEG: intravenous phenytoin
- Worsening coagulopathy and bilirubin
- Poor prognostic score
- Donor organ available: decision to proceed
- Successful OLT

Liver Transplantation

Emergency liver transplantation has become the standard of care for ALF patients with poor prognosis and failure to improve with ICU care. The ALF patient with no contraindications for liver transplantation should be evaluated and listed immediately. As per United Network of Organ Sharing (UNOS) guidelines, they are given top priority for organ allocation as a status 1A patient. The final decision about whether to proceed with liver transplantation is made based on the patient's clinical status when a donor organ is available. In the largest US study of 308 ALF patients, 135 were listed for liver transplantation and 89 (66% of listed, 29% of total cohort) received one, while 30 patients (22% of listed, 10% of total cohort) died while awaiting a graft. Another 47 patients (15%) died while not listed for liver transplantation [29].

Overall patient survival in ALF liver transplantation recipients has improved, especially with the use of low-risk grafts (whole, ABO-compatible, non-steatotic). Survival is best if recipients are <50 years and have a body mass index (BMI) <30, creatinine <2 mg/dL, and no life support [30]. After liver transplantation, 1-year survival is ~80% in ALF patients, compared to 90% in cirrhotic patients. However, ALF liver transplantation recipients have a better long-term survival than cirrhotic liver transplantation patients, in part due to their younger age [31].

Take Home Points

- Acute liver failure (ALF) is defined as severe acute liver disease with coagulopathy and encephalopathy occurring within 8–26 weeks of illness onset.
- Acetaminophen overdose (47%) is the most common cause of ALF in the United States, followed by indeterminate ALF (12%), idiosyncratic drug-induced liver injury (DILI) (11%), and viral hepatitis and other etiologies.
- N-acetylcysteine (NAC) must be given without delay to any patient with suspected APAP overdose. Other etiology-specific treatments should be used when indicated.
- The likelihood of spontaneous recovery depends on subject age, ALF etiology, and encephalopathy grade. Decisions regarding transplant candidacy must be made without delay, to allow time for procurement of a donor organ.

References

1 Bower WA, Johns M, Margolis HS, *et al.* Population-based surveillance for acute liver failure. *Am J Gastroenterol* 2007; **102**: 2459–63.

2 O'Grady JG, Schalm SW, Williams R, *et al.* Acute liver failure: redefining the syndromes. *Lancet* 1993; **342**(8866): 273–5.

3 Ichai P, Samuel D. Etiology and prognosis of fulminant hepatitis in adults. *Liver Transplant* 2008; **14**: S67–79.

4 Larson AM, Polson J, Fontana RJ, *et al*. Acetaminophen induced acute liver failure: results of a United States multicenter, prospective study. *Hepatology* 2005; **42**: 1364–72.

5 Lee WM. Etiologies of acute liver failure. *Semin Liver Dis* 2008; **28**: 142–52.

6 Fontana RJ. Acute liver failure due to drugs. *Semin Liver Dis* 2008; **28**: 175–87.

7 Taylor RM, Tujios S, Jinjuvadia A, *et al*. Short and long-term outcomes in patients with acute liver failure due to ischemic hepatitis. *Dig Dis Sci* 2012; **57**(3): 777–85.

8 Chung RT, Stravitz RT, Fontana RJ, *et al*. Pathogenesis of liver injury in acute liver failure. *Gastroenterology* 2012; **143**(3): e1–7.

9 Moore JK, Love E, Craig DG, *et al*. Acute kidney injury in acute liver failure: a review. *Expert Rev Gastroenterol Hepatol* 2013; **7**(8): 701–12.

10 Blei AT. The pathophysiology of brain edema in acute liver failure. *Neurochem Int* 2005; **47**: 71–7.

11 Jalan R, Olde Damink SWM, Hayes PC, *et al*. Pathogenesis of intracranial hypertension in acute liver failure: inflammation, ammonia and cerebral blood flow. *J Hepatol* 2004; **41**: 613–20.

12 Davern TJ, James LP, Hinson JA, *et al*. Measurement of serum acetaminophen–protein adducts in patients with acute liver failure. *Gastroenterology* 2006; **130**: 687–94.

13 Stravitz RT, Kramer AH, Davern T, *et al*. Intensive care of patients with acute liver failure: recommendations of the US acute liver failure study group. *Crit Care Med* 2007; **35**: 2498–508.

14 Smilkstein MJ, Knapp GL, Kulig KW, Rumack BH. Efficacy of oral N-acetylcysteine in the treatment of acetaminophen overdose. *N Engl J Med* 1988; **319**: 1557–62.

15 Lee WM, Hynan LS, Rossaro L, *et al*. Intravenous N-acetylcysteine improves transplant-free survival in early stage non-acetaminophen acute liver failure. *Gastroenterology* 2009; **137**: 856–64.

16 Rolando N, Gimson A, Wade J, *et al*. Prospective controlled trial of selective parenteral and enteral antimicrobial regimen in fulminant liver failure. *Hepatology* 1993; **17**: 196–201.

17 Shami VM, Caldwell SH, Hespenheide EE, *et al*. Recombinant activated factor VII for coagulopathy in fulminant hepatic failure compared with conventional therapy. *Liver Transpl* 2003; **9**(2): 138–43.

18 Jalan R, Olde Damink SWM, Deutz NEP, *et al*. Restoration of cerebral blood flow autoregulation and reactivity to carbon dioxide in acute liver failure by moderate hypothermia. *Hepatology* 2001; **34**: 50–4.

19 Davenport A, Will EJ, Davidson AM. Improved cardiovascular stability during continuous modes of renal replacement therapy in critically ill patients with acute hepatic and renal failure. *Crit Care Med* 1993; **21**: 328–38.

20 Blei AT, Olafsson S, Webster S, Levy R. Complications of intracranial pressure monitoring in fulminant hepatic failure. *Lancet* 1993; **341**: 157–8.

21 Canalese J, Gimson AES, Davis C, *et al*. Controlled trial of dexamethasone and mannitol for the cerebral oedema of fulminant hepatic failure. *Gut* 1982; **23**: 625–9.

22 Murphy N, Auzinger G, Bernal W, Wendon J. The effect of hypertonic sodium chloride on intracranial pressure in patients with acute liver failure. *Hepatology* 2002; **39**: 464–70.

23 Strauss G, Hansen BA, Knudsen GM, Larsen FS. Hyperventilation restores cerebral blood flow autoregulation in patients with acute liver failure. *J Hepatol* 1998; **28**: 199–203.

24 Jalan R, Damink SWMO, Deutz NEP, *et al*. Moderate hypothermia for uncontrolled intracranial hypertension in acute liver failure. *Lancet* 1999; **354**: 1164–8.

25 Achilles D, Brown RS Jr., Busuttil RW, *et al. Prospective, randomized, multicenter, controlled trial of a bioartificial liver in treating acute liver failure. Ann Surg* 2004; **239**: 660–70.

26 Saliba F, Camus C, Durand F, *et al*. Albumin dialysis with a noncell artificial liver support device in patients with acute liver failure: a randomized, controlled trial. *Ann Intern Med* 2013; **159**(8): 522–31.

27 O'Grady JG, Alexander GJ, Hayllar KM, Williams R. Early indicators of prognosis in fulminant hepatic failure. *Gastroenterology* 1989; **97**: 439–45.

28 Rutherford A, King LY, Hynan LS, *et al*. Development of an accurate index for predicting outcomes of patients with acute liver failure. *Gastroenterology* 2012; **143**(5): 1237–43.

29 Ostapowicz G, Fontana RJ, Schiødt FV, *et al*. Results of a prospective study of acute liver failure at 17 tertiary care centers in the United States. *Ann Intern Med* 2002; **137**(12): 947–54.

30 O'Grady JG. Postoperative issues and outcome for acute liver failure. *Liver Transplant* 2008; **14**: S97–101.

31 Bernal W, Wendon J. Liver transplantation in adults with acute liver failure. *J Hepatol* 2004; **40**: 192–7.

Imaging of the Liver and Bile Ducts: Radiographic and Clinical Assessment of Findings

Thomas J. Byrne[1] and Alvin C. Silva[2]

[1] Division of Gastroenterology and Hepatology, Mayo Clinic, Scottsdale, AZ, USA
[2] Department of Radiology, Mayo Clinic, Scottsdale, AZ, USA

Summary

Imaging of the liver and biliary tree has become a cornerstone of the hepatology practice, allowing earlier detection and more accurate staging of a host of benign and malignant conditions. Common benign entities include hemangioma, focal nodular hyperplasia (FNH), and hepatic adenoma (HA). The diagnosis of adenoma is significant due to a risk of future hemorrhage or malignant transformation. Malignant conditions include hepatocellular carcinoma (HCC) – to be suspected in the setting of cirrhosis – and cholangiocarcinoma (CCA) and metastatic tumors. A stepwise approach to the liver mass will usually lead to an accurate diagnosis. Furthermore, the capabilities of modern imaging are relatively safe, permitting a non-invasive diagnosis in a substantial percentage of cases.

Introduction

In recent decades, radiographic capabilities to assist with the diagnosis and staging of liver and biliary pathology have advanced markedly. These tools allow for highly specific benign and malignant diagnoses, in many cased obviating the need for biopsy. This chapter describes an array of radiographic hepatic and biliary findings and their clinical implications.

Liver Cysts

Hepatic cysts may be simple or complex, single or multiple, and are distinguished from mass lesions by ultrasound, computed tomography (CT), or magnetic resonance imaging (MRI). Simple liver cysts – without septations, nodules, or thickened walls – are usually asymptomatic and require no follow-up [1, 2]. Liver cysts appear to be more common in women [3]. True hepatic cysts have a lining of cuboidal epithelium and do not communicate with the biliary tree [4].

While most are asymptomatic, large liver cysts may lead to pain. Aspiration of these – sometimes with injected sclerosant (usually ethanol) – may afford relief, but recurrence is the rule [5,6]. Laparoscopic unroofing may then be considered, and offers a higher likelihood of long-term relief [7]. This also allows for histological analysis of the portion of cyst wall removed, in order to exclude biliary cystadenoma, which has malignant potential and should be considered

for total resection [2]. Cystadenoma should be considered if imaging reveals thickened walls or septae, or dilation of adjacent biliary segments. Magnetic resonance cholangiopancreatography (MRCP) may be useful when suspicion of cystadenoma exists (Figure 72.1).

Echinococcal cysts are quite rare, but can be considered in patients with cholestatic features and a history of Mediterranean or South American travel. Serologic testing for echinococcal immunoglobulin G (IgG) antibody is usually positive [2]. Surgical resection is historically the treatment of choice, but less invasive approaches involving albendazole or mebendazole prior to and following cyst aspiration can be considered [8]. Anaphylaxis remains a potential complication of procedural intervention, though pretreatment with antiparasitic agents may reduce that risk.

Patients with polycystic liver disease, including those with associated polycystic kidney disease, may present with innumerable cysts occupying the entire liver, though hepatic function is typically normal. This diagnosis is considered when more than 20 cysts of varying size are found. Selected patients may be considered for liver transplantation [9].

Hemangioma

Hemangiomas are the most common benign liver neoplasm, with up to 20% prevalence in autopsy series [10]. They have a slight female preponderance, and are usually asymptomatic. Hemangiomas are usually <5 cm in size and exist as solitary lesions in 85–90% of cases [11]. Though usually asymptomatic, larger lesions, including "giant cavernous hemangiomas," may be painful, in which case resection is an appropriate consideration [12]. Rare occasions of spontaneous or trauma-induced rupture may result in hemorrhagic shock, requiring emergent surgery or arterial embolization [11]. For exceedingly large hemangiomas, coagulopathy may occur due to ongoing spontaneous bleeding and clotting within the lesion, with resultant hypofibrinogenemia (Kasabach–Merritt syndrome) [13]. Very rare descriptions of successful liver transplantation exist for this occurrence [14].

On ultrasound, hemangiomas may appear bright, with internal bright echoes reflecting pooled liquid or clotted blood [15]. Doppler analysis may reveal blood vessels around the periphery of larger lesions [16]. The characteristic CT appearance (Figure 72.2) includes well-circumscribed borders and peripheral, nodular,

Practical Gastroenterology and Hepatology Board Review Toolkit, Second Edition. Edited by Nicholas J. Talley, Kenneth R. DeVault, Michael B. Wallace, Bashar A. Aqel and Keith D. Lindor.

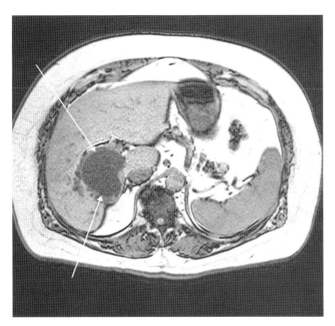

Figure 72.1 Biliary cystadenoma. MRI image demonstrates thickened cyst walls (arrows) with focal biliary dilation and displacement of a vessel.

hemangioma from metastases [18]. A confident radiographic diagnosis in an asymptomatic patient requires no follow-up if the lesion is small. Biopsy of suspected hemangioma is to be avoided except in cases of real doubt, due to bleeding risk.

Focal Nodular Hyperplasia

FNH is the second most common benign hepatic tumor. It is usually <5 cm, unencapsulated, and exists as single lesions in 80% of cases [19]. However, up to 23% of patients with FNH have multiple lesions, and FNH may also occur with hemangiomas [20]. Pathologically, FNH typically contains a central scar with abnormally arranged surrounding hepatocytes and biliary ductules. There is a strong female predominance, with at least a 6 : 1 female/male ratio, though no clear linkage between FNH and oral contraceptive (OCP) use has been demonstrated [11,21]. FNH may nonetheless increase in size in women taking OCPs [22].

On CT, FNH appears iso-attenuated to adjacent liver parenchyma prior to contrast administration. Except for the central scar, FNH shows prompt arterial phase hyperenhancement, which quickly fades on portal venous phase imaging. MRI reveals FNH to be iso- or slightly hypointense on T1 images, and iso- or mildly hyperintense on T2 images [23]. Following gadolinium contrast, FNH shows early, homogeneous, hypervascular enhancement and delayed hyperenhancement of the central scar [16]. Precontrast or dynamic contrast-enhanced MRI images using conventional magnetic resonance contrast agents may not distinguish FNH without a central scar from an uncomplicated HA. However, 1–2-hour delayed Gad-EOB-DTPA (MultiHance) imaging (or 10–20-minute delayed imaging with gadoxetate disodium (Eovist)) can reveal persistent retained enhancement of the central scar, distinguishing FNH from adenoma (Figure 72.4). In cases where the central scar is poorly seen and hepatobiliary-specific MR contrast agents

interrupted enhancement following intravenous (IV) contrast. The use of timed CT contrast allows hemangiomas to be distinguished from metastatic lesions with a sensitivity and specificity over 85% [17]. MRI shows hemangioma to have a hyperintense T2 appearance and hypointense T1 signal, distinct from surrounding normal liver, and often containing internal lobulations (Figure 72.3). MRI is the most sensitive and specific diagnostic modality for hemangioma, with one series demonstrating 100% specificity in distinguishing

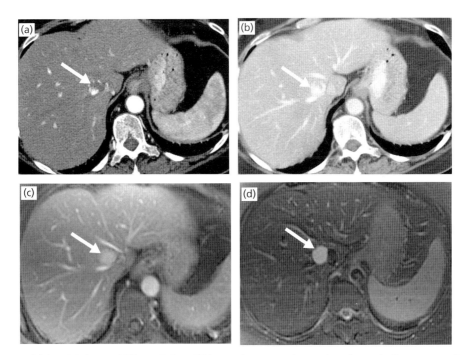

Figure 72.2 Hemangioma. (a) Arterial phase and (b) portal phase CT images demonstrate hemangioma (arrows) adjacent to a confluence of right and middle hepatic veins with inferior vena cava. (c) Delayed image showing persistent hyperenhancement relative to surrounding liver. (d) T2-weighted imaging showing hemangioma with hyperintensity approaching that of cysts.

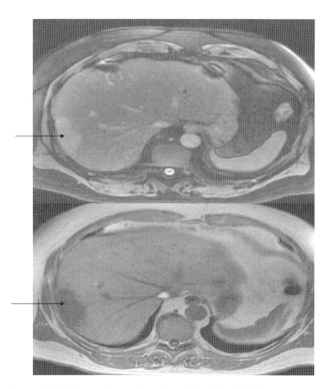

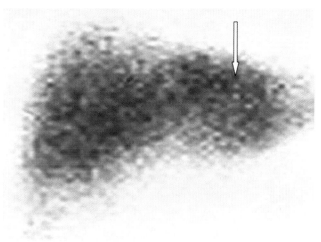

Figure 72.5 ^{99m}Tc-labeled sulfur colloid scan. Note prominent left lobe uptake (arrow) by FNH, distinguishing it from adenoma, which would have appeared as a void.

Figure 72.3 Right lobe hemangioma. Top: T2-weighted MRI image. Bottom: T1-weighted image.

slightly. The risk of rupture and bleeding is exceedingly low [16]. Because FNH may enlarge during pregnancy, resection of larger (≥5 cm) lesions, especially those on the liver surface, can be considered in select cases of contemplated pregnancy.

are unavailable or are contraindicated, scintigraphy with Tc-99m-labeled sulfur colloid may be helpful due to the presence of abundant Kupffer cells in FNH, which accumulate colloid. FNH nodules will appear hyper- or isodense to the surrounding liver, as opposed to HA, which does not usually accumulate colloid and appears as a pale "void" in the liver [24] (Figure 72.5). However, the overall accuracy of this method is relatively poor compared with CT or MRI.

FNH is usually observed, and patients can be reassured that studies have not demonstrated an increased risk of malignant transformation. Lesions may be reimaged at 6–12-month intervals for a period of 2 years to ensure stability, though size may fluctuate

Hepatic Adenoma

HA is a benign mass neoplasm consisting of proliferating hepatocytes. Kupffer cells are lacking in number compared to normal liver architecture, and especially compared to FNH, which accounts for the voided appearance of HA on sulfur colloid scan [11]. This lesion is strongly associated with the use of OCPs and androgen steroids, and certain types of glycogen storage disease [25–27]. The incidence of HA has increased in the past 4 decades, paralleling the increased use of OCPs in the same period [28–30]. HA is fed by prominent arterial vessels that course along the periphery of the lesion, which lacks a true capsule [19,25]. Accordingly, the demarcation of HA from surrounding normal liver tissue may be vague. Also, distinguishing HA from well-differentiated HCC histologically is difficult [19]. For this reason, and because of the bleeding risk, biopsy is ideally avoided, being reserved for situations where radiological impression is uncertain and tissue result will determine management. When biopsy of possible HA is performed, it should be done with imaging guidance, using an approach that places sufficient liver parenchyma between the mass and the site on the capsular surface where the needle enters the liver. With such an approach, if the lesion bleeds, there is likely to be a tamponade effect from the surrounding parenchyma. A surface adenoma approached directly – with no parenchymal tissue between it and the site of needle entry into the liver – is more likely to bleed heavily into the peritoneum.

HA is typically found incidentally in a woman of childbearing age with a significant duration of OCP usage. Lesions are usually single, but up to 30% of affected patients have multiple adenomas [11,31]. Adenomas range from 3 to 8 cm in size, though larger lesions do occur [19]. On ultrasound, HA is not easily distinguished from other benign or malignant lesions, though occasionally Doppler reveals peripheral arterial feeding vessels [16]. On CT, areas of necrosis and calcification, as well as fresh blood, may be seen [32]. Adenomas show early hypervascularity, but in a less pronounced, more heterogeneous pattern than FNH (Figure 72.6). MRI usually demonstrates

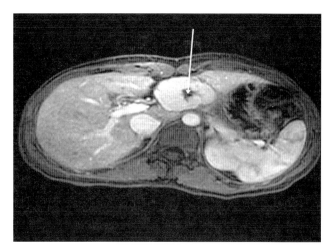

Figure 72.4 Focal nodular hyperplasia (FNH). Note slight enhancement from retained contrast on 1 hour-delayed (postgadolinium) image, with prominent central scar (arrow).

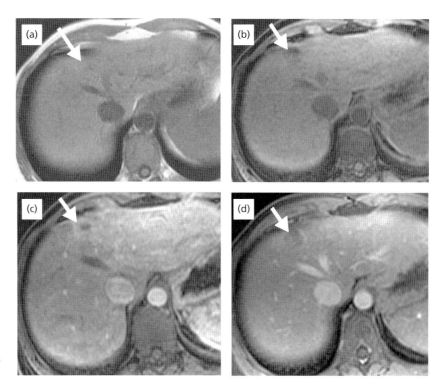

Figure 72.6 Hepatic adenoma. T1-weighted MRIs sowing medial left lobe adenoma (a) with subtle hyperintensity on in-phase sequence and (b) with progressive hypointensity on the fat-saturated sequence. (c) After contrast, the mass appears heterogeneously hypervascular on arterial phase image. (d) Delayed-phase imaging, demonstrating relative washout.

hyperintensity of HA on T2 images, with variable T1 appearance and early heterogeneous arterial enhancement following the use of gadolinium-based contrast [33].

The major clinical significance of HA is the potential for malignant transformation and spontaneous rupture with hemorrhage, rarely with hemodynamic compromise, including sudden death from massive blood loss. Pain is more likely in larger lesions, though smaller lesions that have undergone intratumoral bleeding may also cause discomfort. Radiographic or surgical evidence of intratumoral bleeding is found in up to 29% of cases [34], with higher rates for women who continue OCPs [35].

Malignant transformation appears to occur in 5–18% of cases [34,36], with most published data suggesting a risk near the middle of those parameters. Different subtypes for HA pose different risks for malignant transformation. A proposed classification system for HA subtypes, using molecular markers and immunohistochemistry [75], establishes different categories: (i) hepatocyte nuclear factor-α-inactivated HAs (lacking expression of liver-fatty acid binding protein (L-FABP), with a resultant high degree of steatosis); (ii) β-catenin-activated HAs; (iii) inflammatory HCAs with serum amyloid A (SAA) and C-reactive protein (CRP) expression; and (iv) unclassified HAs. Lesions expressing B-catenin activation are substantially more likely to undergo malignant transformation to HCC [76]. Limited data suggest MRI may permit identification of HA subtype, with one study demonstrating correct radiographic diagnosis of HA subtype in 85% of lesions, with good interobserver variability [77].

For incidentally discovered HA in a reproductive-age woman with longstanding OCP usage, elimination of OCPs is advised. Adenomas may shrink or even disappear following cessation of OCPs [37,38]. For lesions that fail to disappear completely, ongoing monitoring or resection is required due to the potential for subsequent growth after a period of initial regression, including the potential for eventual hemorrhage [39] and malignant transformation [40,41] years after OCP cessation. Management of small (<3 cm)

asymptomatic adenomas consists of serial imaging observation, though some favor resection due to the potential for growth, future bleeding, and/or malignancy. Patients should be informed of the risks of both observation and resection, and advised to avoid OCPs. Some patients elect to continue OCPs, and it should be noted that pregnancy may also stimulate adenoma growth. Because of this, stronger consideration of resection may be appropriate in the setting of contemplated pregnancy. The location of the adenoma also influences decision-making, as surface lesions raise concern of serious bleeding and hemoperitoneum. Larger adenomas, unless occurring in surgically unfit patients, should generally be resected [11,34,42]. Transarterial chemo- or bland-embolization (TACE/TABE) may be used for bleeding, or when imaging suggests impending rupture, especially if surgery is deemed high-risk [43].

Hepatic adenomatosis is characterized by multiple (more than five) adenomas. It is distinct from HAs associated with OCP use, androgen steroids, or glycogen storage disease. Some data suggest a link between hepatic adenomatosis and a form of maturity-onset diabetes of the young (MODY) [44]. The management of multiple adenomas is challenging. Liver transplantation has been successfully performed [45,46], but it is controversial given that organs are scarce and a majority of affected patients will *not* develop cancer or fatal bleeding. Some propose resection or TACE/TABE of the largest and/or most peripheral lesions [47, 48]. Observation with serial imaging has also been advocated, reserving treatment for lesions that appear to be at risk of impending rupture or that show other worrisome changes.

Nodular Regenerative Hyperplasia

Nodular regenerative hyperplasia (NRH) is a benign disorder characterized by the presence of multiple proliferative nodules of hepatocytes. The size of individual nodules ranges from a few millimeters to a few centimeters, and NRH may be indistinguishable from cirrhosis radiographically [16]. Liver biopsy reveals an absence of collagen-based fibrotic bands in NRH, and diagnosis may be aided with reticulin staining of tissue [49].

NRH is often idiopathic, but the disorder has been linked to several rheumatological and lymphoproliferative conditions, as well as inflammatory bowel disease (IBD). It appears to be more common among patients previously treated with azathioprine [50] or 6-thioguanine [51], though there is a background incidence among thiopurine-naïve IBD patients [52]. Reversibility of NRH after cessation of azathioprine has been rarely observed [53]. The condition has also been described as a cause of portal hypertension in human immunodeficiency virus (HIV) patients [54].

When NRH presents with a manifestation of portal hypertension, that event is managed in the same manner as in a patient with cirrhosis. The exception is that liver transplantation is seldom needed, given the usually preserved synthetic hepatic function. Thus, portal hypertension in NRH may be successfully managed with transjugular intrahepatic portosystemic shunts (TIPS) or surgical shunts [55]. While rare case reports exist of HCC occurring in patients with NRH, in most cases there were changes to the liver microvasculature caused by the tumor or its treatment (TACE), suggesting that NRH was the result – not the cause – of HCC [56–58]. Occasionally, patients with severe portal hypertension from NRH may experience clinical deterioration due to hepatic insufficiency. In such cases, liver transplantation is associated with favorable outcomes comparable to those for other indications [59].

Miscellaneous Benign Lesions

A host of less common liver lesions are encountered from time to time in hepatology practice. Bile duct harmartomas (also known as Meyenburg complexes) are small (<1 cm) nodules of biliary tissue isolated from the biliary tree. They are thought to result from failure of embryonic bile duct involution, and can be found incidentally on the liver surface in the surgical setting. The major clinical significance is that they may be mistaken for metastases, even though they are benign and do not require resection. Angiomyolipoma (AML) is a benign growth containing fat and smooth-muscle cells in addition to vascular tissue. It is much more commonly found in the kidney, and thus when seen radiographically in the liver it may be misdiagnosed as sarcoma [19]. Hepatic AML may be associated with pain, in which case resection is appropriate [11]. Inflammatory pseudotumor (IPT) is a rare, benign infiltrative liver process associated with fever, weight loss, and laboratory indicators of inflammation. Histologically, IPTs comprise plasma cells, lymphocytes, macrophages, and fibrous stroma [19]. The condition gets its name because it is difficult to distinguish from a malignant process

radiographically, and clinically patients may present with cachexia and other symptoms encountered in cancer. IPT may result from incomplete abscess formation or phlegmon that forms in the setting of intra-abdominal infection with portal pyemia.

Regenerative nodules (RNs) and dysplastic nodules (DNs) are masses that occur with parenchymal liver injury or a vascular insult to the liver. The primary difference is that the former is considered to be a reactive phenomenon, while the latter is a neoplasm that has strong potential for becoming HCC [25]. Radiographic distinction between the two conditions may be challenging. RNs have been described in association with biliary atresia in patients awaiting liver transplantation [60] and may generate false concern for a malignant process. The diagnosis of DN is often radiographically assigned to a mass found in a cirrhotic patient who is under surveillance for HCC, when the mass lacks either the size or the typical enhancement features of hepatoma.

Hepatocellular Carcinoma

The incidence of HCC has roughly tripled in Western nations in the past 3 decades, likely because of the hepatitis C epidemic [61]. Thus, a discovered hepatic mass in a cirrhotic patient requires prompt characterization. Furthermore, cirrhotic patients should have imaging every 6–12 months for HCC screening, as the preponderance of data indicates that screening lowers mortality [62]. Consensus imaging criteria for HCC include hypervascularity on arterial-phase views and delayed-phase "washout" with or without demonstration of peripheral enhancement (pseudocapsule) (Figure 72.7).

Other Malignant Liver and Biliary Tumors

Metastatic cancer and lymphoma remain common liver entities, and metastatic lesions are far more common than primary liver cancers [63]. Metastatic adenocarcinomas from colon, lung, breast, or pancreas are usually hypovascular, whereas metastatic neuroendocrine tumors, renal cell carcinomas (RCCs), thyroid cancers, melanomas, and sarcomas tend to be hypervascular. Both CT and MRI are useful in the detection of liver metastases, though the latter may be more sensitive [64, 65].

Cholangiocarcinoma (CCA) may involve any segment of the biliary tree, or may present as a solid intrahepatic mass. Though this is not universally accepted, due to imprecise nomenclature and imperfect assignment of diagnosis, the incidence of CCA may be increasing [66]. Because highly selected patients with hilar CCA may benefit from liver transplantation following chemoradiation [67], vigilance for this tumor is warranted in patients with primary sclerosing cholangitis (PSC), who face a lifetime risk of developing

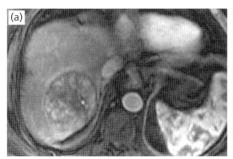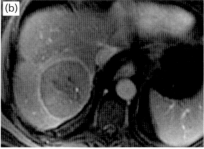

Figure 72.7 Hepatocellular carcinoma (HCC). (a) Arterial-phase contrast-enhanced MRI demonstrating heterogeneous hypervascular mass. (b) Portal-venous-phase MRI showing washout and a surrounding pseudocapsule.

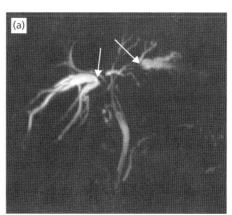

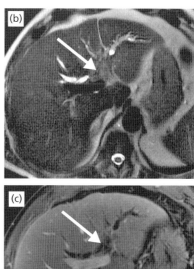

Figure 72.8 Cholangiocarcinoma (CCA). (a) MRCP image demonstrating dilated right and left biliary ducts terminating abruptly in hilum (arrows). (b) T2-weighted image of same ducts, showing ductal occlusion. (c) Contrast-enhanced image demonstrating the irregular enhancement pattern of tumor.

CCA of up to 20%. With both CT and MRI, intrahepatic CCA appears as a well-defined, lobulated mass or group of masses, with an initial peripheral rim and subsequent progressive, delayed hyperenhancement [68] (Figure 72.8). Progressive biliary dilation and increased tumor length on serial imaging help distinguish such CCAs from benign strictures [69].

Gallbladder carcinoma is the most common malignant tumor of the biliary tract [70]. On MRI, gallbladder cancers are hypointense on T1 images and heterogenously T2 hyperintense. Associated stones are sometimes found, along with hepatic invasion and/or involvement of adjacent biliary ducts. Porcelain gallbladder with circumferential gallbladder wall calcifications is sometimes seen, and is more easily identified on CT.

Cholelithiasis/Choledocholithiasis

Ultrasound (98%) is more sensitive than CT (75%) in the detection of gallstones [71]. MRCP shows gallstones to be well-defined, low-signal foci outlined by higher-intensity bile, regardless of calcium content [72] (Figure 72.9). Adenomyomatosis is a benign gallbladder condition characterized by hyperplastic changes of the gallbladder wall, with mucosal outpouching and overgrowth

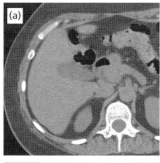

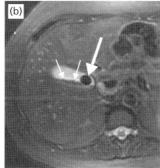

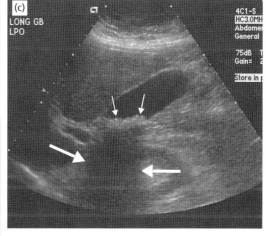

Figure 72.9 Cholelithiasis. (a) Non-enhanced CT without evidence for gallstones, as most are radio-opaque. (b) Corresponding T2-weighted MRI showing numerous small gallstones (arrowheads) and a single, larger stone (arrow). (c) Ultrasound from the same patient, demonstrating numerous, layering stones (arrows) and distal shadowing (larger arrows).

(Rokitansky–Aschoff sinuses). It can be diffuse or segmental, and should be distinguished from gallbladder carcinoma. MRI is superior to ultrasound or CT for this purpose, with diagnostic accuracy >90% for adenomyomatosis [73].

Primary Sclerosing Cholangitis

PSC involves progressive inflammation and fibrosis of a single or multiple section(s) of the biliary tree. When the disease involves a focal, high-grade narrowing of the common bile duct, a "dominant stricture" is said to be present. Dominant strictures should be scrutinized by either endoscopic retrograde cholangiopancreatography (ERCP) or repeated MRI to ensure stability, since CCA may present as a dominant stricture. On imaging, PSC appears as focal or diffuse thickening of the bile duct wall(s), with scattered areas of "skip" biliary dilation, resulting in a classic "beaded" appearance. MRCP has replaced ERCP in situations where diagnosis alone is sought, unless the patient is not a candidate for MRI.

Take Home Points

- Liver cysts and masses are common findings.
- When a liver lesion is found, accurate diagnosis can be made non-invasively in a large percentage of situations.
- Ultrasound and MRCP are superior to CT for the detection of gallstones.
- Hemangioma is the most common benign solid liver mass.
- Focal nodular hyperplasia (FNH) is a benign entity that may be distinguished radiographically from other conditions by its classic central scar and its tendency to retain hepatobiliary-specific MRI contrast on delayed images.
- Hepatic adenomas (HAs) are associated with oral contraceptive (OCP) exposure and have future bleeding and cancerous potential.
- A discovered mass in a cirrhotic patient requires evaluation for possible hepatocellular carcinoma (HCC).
- Features of HCC include arterial-phase hyperenhancement, delayed-phase washout, and a capsule/pseudocapsule.
- MRI may help identify cholangiocarcinoma (CCA), which can be treated successfully with liver transplantation in highly selected cases.

References

1 Sanfelippo PM, Beahrs OH, Weiland LH. Cystic disease of the liver. *Ann Surg* 1974; **179**: 922–5.

2 Regev A, Reddy KR, Berho M, *et al.* Large cystic lesions of the liver in adults: a 15-year experience in a tertiary center. *J Am Coll Surg* 2001; **193**: 36–45.

3 Federle MP, Brancatelli G. Imaging of benign hepatic masses. *Semin Liv Dis* 2001; **21**: 237–49.

4 vanSonnenberg E, Wroblicka JT, D'Agostino HB, *et al.* Symptomatic hepatic cysts: percutaneous drainage and sclerosis. *Radiology* 1994; **190**: 387–92.

5 Saini S, Mueller PR, Ferrucci JT Jr., *et al.* Percutaneous aspiration of hepatic cysts does not provide definitive therapy. *Am J Roentgenol* 1983; **141**: 559–60.

6 Simonetti G, Profili S, Sergiacomi GL, *et al.* Percutaneous treatment of hepatic cysts by aspiration and sclerotherapy. *Cardiovasc Intervent Radiol* 1993; **16**: 81–4.

7 Gamblin TC, Holloway SE, Heckman JT, Geller DA. Laparoscopic resection of benign hepatic cysts: a new standard. *J Am Coll Surg* 2008; **207**: 731–6.

8 Dervenis C, Delis S, Avgerinos C, *et al.* Changing concepts in the management of liver hydatid disease. *J Gastrointest Surg* 2005; **9**: 869–77.

9 Starzl TE, Reyes J, Tzakis A, *et al.* Liver transplantation for polycystic liver disease. *Arch Surg* 1990; **125**: 575–7.

10 Karhunen PJ. Benign hepatic tumours and tumour-like conditions in men. *J Clin Pathol* 1986; **39**: 183–8.

11 Trotter JF, Everson GT. Benign focal lesions of the liver. *Clin Liver Dis* 2001; **5**: 17–42, v.

12 Farges O, Daradkeh S, Bismuth H. Cavernous hemangiomas of the liver: are there any indications for resection? *World J Surg* 1995; **19**: 19–24.

13 Hoak JC, Warner ED, Cheng HF, *et al.* Hemangioma with thrombocytopenia and microangiopathic anemia (Kasabach-Merritt syndrome): an animal model. *J Lab Clin Med* 1971; **77**: 941–50.

14 Klompmaker IJ, Sloof MJ, van der Meer J, *et al.* Orthotopic liver transplantation in a patient with a giant cavernous hemangioma of the liver and Kasabach-Merritt syndrome. *Transplantation* 1989; **48**: 149–51.

15 Bree RL, Schwab RE, Glazer GM, Fink-Bennett D. The varied appearances of hepatic cavernous hemangiomas with sonography, computed tomography, magnetic resonance imaging and scintigraphy. *Radiographics* 1987; **7**: 1153–75.

16 Mortele KJ, Ros PR. Benign liver neoplasms. *Clin Liver Dis* 2002; **6**: 119–45.

17 Leslie DF, Johnson CD, Johnson CM, *et al.* Distinction between cavernous hemangiomas of the liver and hepatic metastases on CT: value of contrast enhancement patterns. *Am J Roentgenol* 1995; **164**: 625–9.

18 Kim T, Federle MP, Baron RL, *et al.* Discrimination of small hepatic hemangiomas from hypervascular malignant tumors smaller than 3cm with three-phase helical CT. *Radiology* 2001; **219**: 699–706.

19 Brunt EM. Benign tumors of the liver. *Clin Liver Dis* 2001; **5**: 1–15, v.

20 Mathieu D, Zafrani ES, Anglade MC, Dhumeaux D. Association of focal nodular hyperplasia and hepatic hemangioma. *Gastroenterology* 1989; **97**: 154–7.

21 Mathieu D, Kobeiter H, Maison P, *et al.* Oral contraceptive use and focal nodular hyperplasia of the liver. *Gastroenterology* 2000; **118**: 560–4.

22 Felix R, Langer R, Langer M, eds. Benign primary liver tumors. In: *Diagnostic Imaging in Liver Disease*. Berlin: Springer, 2005: 106.

23 Marti-Bonmati L, Casillas C, Dosda R. Enhancement characteristics of hepatic focal nodular hyperplasia and its scar by dynamic magnetic resonance imaging. *MAGMA* 2000; **10**: 200–4.

24 Buetow PC, Pantongrag-Brown L, Buck JL, *et al.* Focal nodular hyperplasia of the liver: radiologic-pathologic correlation. *Radiographics* 1996; **16**: 369–88.

25 Wanless IR. Benign liver tumors. *Clin Liver Dis* 2002; **6**: 513–26, ix.

26 Rabe T, Feldmann K, Grunwald K, Runnebaum B. Liver tumours in women on oral contraceptives. *Lancet* 1994; **344**: 1568–9.

27 Carrasco D, Prieto M, Pallardo L, *et al.* Multiple hepatic adenomas after long-term therapy with testosterone enanthate. Review of the literature. *J Hepatol* 1985; **1**: 573–8.

28 Baum JK, Bookstein JJ, Holtz F, Klein EW. Possible association between benign hepatomas and oral contraceptives. *Lancet* 1973; **2**: 926–9.

29 Rooks JB, Ory HW, Ishak KG, *et al.* Epidemiology of hepatocellular adenoma. The role of oral contraceptive use. *JAMA* 1979; **242**: 644–8.

30 Edmondson HA, Henderson B, Benton B. Liver-cell adenomas associated with use of oral contraceptives. *N Engl J Med* 1976; **294**: 470–2.

31 Ishak KG, Rabin L. Benign tumors of the liver. *Med Clin North Am* 1975; **59**: 995–1013.

32 Grazioli L, Federle MP, Brancatelli G, *et al.* Hepatic adenomas: imaging and pathologic findings. *Radiographics* 2001: **21**: 877–92, disc. 892–4.

33 Paulson EK, McClellan JS, Washington K, *et al.* Hepatic adenoma: MR characteristics and correlation with pathologic findings. *Am J Roentgenol* 1994; **163**: 113–16.

34 Cho SW, Marsh JW, Steel J, *et al.* Surgical management of hepatocellular adenoma: take it or leave it? *Ann Surg Oncol* 2008; **15**: 2795–803.

35 Shortell CK, Schwartz SI. Hepatic adenoma and focal nodular hyperplasia. *Surg Gynecol Obstet* 1991; **173**: 426–31.

36 Micchelli ST, Vivekanandan P, Boitnott JK, *et al.* Malignant transformation of hepatic adenomas. *Mod Pathol* 2008; **21**: 491–7.

37 Aseni P, Sansalone CV, Sammartino C, *et al.* Rapid disappearance of hepatic adenoma after contraceptive withdrawal. *J Clin Gastroenterol* 2001; **33**: 234–6.

38 Kawakatsu M, Vilgrain V, Erlinger S, Nahum H. Disappearance of liver cell adenoma: CT and MR imaging. *Abdom Imaging* 1997; **22**: 274–6.

39 Cheng PN, Shin JS, Lin XZ. Hepatic adenoma: an observation from asymptomatic stage to rupture. *Hepatogastroenterology* 1996; **43**: 245–8.

40 Tesluk H, Lawrie J. Hepatocellular adenoma. Its transformation to carcinoma in a user of oral contraceptives. *Arch Pathol Lab Med* 1981; **105**: 296–9.

41 Gordon SC, Reddy KR, Livingstone AS, *et al.* Resolution of a contraceptive-steroid-induced hepatic adenoma with subsequent evolution into hepatocellular carcinoma. *Ann Intern Med* 1986; **105**: 547–9.

42 Chaib E, Gama-Rodrigues J, Ribeiro MA Jr., *et al.* Hepatic adenoma. Timing for surgery. *Hepatogastroenterology* 2007; **54**: 1382–7.

43 Kim YI, Chung JW, Park JH. Feasibility of transcatheter arterial chemoembolization for hepatic adenoma. *J Vasc Interv Radiol* 2007; **18**: 862–7.

44 Greaves WO, Bhattacharya B. Hepatic adenomatosis. *Arch Pathol Lab Med* 2008; **132**: 1951–5.

45 Carreiro G, Villela-Nogueira CA, Coelho HS, *et al.* Orthotopic liver transplantation in glucose-6-phosphatase deficiency – Von Gierke disease – with multiple hepatic

adenomas and concomitant focal nodular hyperplasia. *J Pediatr Endocrinol Metab* 2007; **20**: 545–9.

46 Marino IR, Scantlebury VP, Bronsther O, *et al.* Total hepatectomy and liver transplant for hepatocellular adenomatosis and focal nodular hyperplasia. *Transpl Int* 1992; **5**(Suppl. 1): S201–5.

47 Yoshidome H, McMasters KM, Edwards MJ. Management issues regarding hepatic adenomatosis. *Am Surg* 1999; **65**: 1070–6.

48 Lee SH, Hahn ST. Treatment of multiple hepatic adenomatosis using transarterial chemoembolization: a case report. *Cardiovasc Intervent Radiol* 2004; **27**: 563–5.

49 Naber AH, Van Haelst U, Yap SH. Nodular regenerative hyperplasia of the liver: an important cause of portal hypertension in non-cirrhotic patients. *J Hepatol* 1991; **12**: 94–9.

50 Vernier-Massouille G, Cosnes J, Lemann M, *et al.* Nodular regenerative hyperplasia in patients with inflammatory bowel disease treated with azathioprine. *Gut* 2007; **56**: 1404–9.

51 Dubinsky MC, Vasiliauskas EA, Singh H, *et al.* 6-thioguanine can cause serious liver injury in inflammatory bowel disease patients. *Gastroenterology* 2003; **125**: 298–303.

52 De Boer NK, Tuynman H, Bloemena E, *et al.* Histopathology of liver biopsies from a thiopurine-naive inflammatory bowel disease cohort: prevalence of nodular regenerative hyperplasia. *Scand J Gastroenterol* 2008; **43**: 604–8.

53 Seiderer J, Zech CJ, Diebold J, *et al.* Nodular regenerative hyperplasia: a reversible entity associated with azathioprine therapy. *Eur J Gastroenterol Hepatol* 2006; **18**: 553–5.

54 Mallet V, Blanchard P, Verkarre V, *et al.* Nodular regenerative hyperplasia is a new cause of chronic liver disease in HIV-infected patients. *AIDS* 2007; **21**: 187–92.

55 Reshamwala PA, Kleiner DE, Heller T. Nodular regenerative hyperplasia: not all nodules are created equal. *Hepatology* 2006; **44**: 7–14.

56 Kataoka TR, Tsukamoto Y, Kanazawa N, *et al.* Concomitant hepatocellular carcinoma and non-Hodgkin's lymphoma in a patient with nodular regenerative hyperplasia. *Pathol Int* 2006; **56**: 279–82.

57 Nzeako UC, Goodman ZD, Ishak KG. Hepatocellular carcinoma and nodular regenerative hyperplasia: possible pathogenetic relationship. *Am J Gastroenterol* 1996; **91**: 879–84.

58 Kobayashi S, Saito K, Nakanuma Y. Nodular regenerative hyperplasia of the liver in hepatocellular carcinoma. An autopsy study. *J Clin Gastroenterol* 1993; **16**: 155–9.

59 Krasinskas AM, Eghtesad B, Kamath PS, *et al.* Liver transplantation for severe intrahepatic noncirrhotic portal hypertension. *Liver Transpl* 2005; **11**: 627–34, disc. 610–11.

60 Liang JL, Cheng YF, Concejero AM, *et al.* Macro-regenerative nodules in biliary atresia: CT/MRI findings and their pathological relations. *World J Gastroenterol* 2008; **14**: 4529–34.

61 El-Serag HB, Mason AC. Rising incidence of hepatocellular carcinoma in the United States. *N Engl J Med* 1999; **340**: 745–50.

62 El-Serag HB, Marrero JA, Rudolph L, Reddy KR. Diagnosis and treatment of hepatocellular carcinoma. *Gastroenterology* 2008; **134**: 1752–63.

63 Ros PR, Taylor HM. Malignant tumors of the liver. In: Gore RM, Levine MS, eds. *Textbook of Gastrointestinal Radiology*, 2nd edn. Philadelphia, PA: WB Saunders, 2000: 1523–68.

64 Furuhata T, Okita K, Tsuruma T, *et al.* Efficacy of SPIO-MR imaging in the diagnosis of liver metastaes from colorectal carcinomas. *Dig Surg* 2003; **20**: 321–5.

65 Bartolozzi C, Donati F, Cioni D, *et al.* Detection of colorectal liver metastases: a prospective multicenter trial comparing unenhanced MRI, MnDPDP-enhanced MRI, and spiral CT. *Eur Radiol* 2004; **14**: 14–20.

66 Welzel TM, McGlynn KA, Hsing AW, *et al.* Impact of classification of hilar cholangiocarcinomas (Klatskin tumors) on the incidence of intra- and extrahepatic cholangiocarcinoma in the United States. *J Natl Cancer Inst* 2006; **98**: 873–5.

67 Heimbach JK, Haddock MG, Alberts SR, *et al.* Transplantation for hilar cholangiocarcinoma. *Liver Transpl* 2004; **10**: S65–8.

68 Zhang Y, Uchida M, Abe T, *et al.* Intrahepatic peripheral cholangiocarcinoma: comparison of dynamic CT and dynamic MRI. *J Comput Assist Tomogr* 1999; **23**: 670–7.

69 Park MS, Kim TK, Kim KW, *et al.* Differentiation of extrahepatic bile duct cholangiocarcinoma from benign stricture: findings at MRCP versus ERCP. *Radiology* 2004; **233**: 234–40.

70 Rooholamini SA, Tehrani NS, Razavi MK, *et al.* Imaging of gallbladder carcinoma. *Radiographics* 1994; **14**: 291–306.

71 Memel DS, Balfe DM, Semelka RC. The biliary tract. In: Lee JKT, Sagel SS, Stanley RJ, Heiken JP, eds. *Computed Body Tomography with MRI Correlation*, Vol. 2, 3rd edn. Philadelphia, PA: Lippincott, 1998: 779–803.

72 Baron RL, Shuman WP, Lee SP, *et al.* MR appearance of gallstones in vitro at 1.5T: correlation with chemical composition. *Am J Roentgenol* 1989; **153**: 497–502.

73 Yoshimitsu K, Honda H, Aibe H, *et al.* Radiologic diagnosis of adenomyomatosis of the gallbladder: comparative study among MRI, CT and transabdominal US. *J Comput Assist Tomogr* 2001; **25**: 843–50.

74 Nainani N, Panesar M. Nephrogenic systemic fibrosis. *Am J Nephrol* 2009; **29**: 1–9.

75 Bioulac-Sage P, Rebouissou S, Thomas C, *et al.* Hepatocellular adenoma subtype classification using molecular markers and immunohistochemistry. *Hepatology* 2007; **46**: 740–8.

76 Bioulac-Sage P, Laumonier H, Couchy G, *et al.* Hepatocellular adenoma management and phenotypic classification: the Bourdeaux experience. *Heaptology* 2009; **50**: 481–9.

77 Ronot M, Bahrami S, Calderaro J, *et al.* Hepatocellular adenomas: accuracy of magnetic resonance imaging and liver biopsy in subtype classification. *Hepatology* 2011; **53**: 1182–91.

CHAPTER 73

Assessment of Liver Fibrosis: Liver Biopsy and Other Techniques

Sumeet K. Asrani[1] and Jayant Talwalkar[2]

[1] Baylor University Medical Center, Dallas, TX, USA
[2] Division of Gastroenterology and Hepatology, Mayo Clinic, Rochester, MN, USA

Summary

Assessment of fibrosis is crucial in the management of patients with liver disease. Liver biopsy remains the most definitive test in assessing the severity of liver disease. The most important complication of liver biopsy is bleeding, which occurs in 0.1–0.3% of patients. Recently, several non-invasive techniques by which to assess fibrosis, such as serum biomarkers and ultrasound- and magnetic resonance-based elastography, have been introduced as an alternative to liver biopsies. These techniques provide complementary information that may help reduce – though not eliminate – the need for biopsies in assessment of fibrosis.

Case

A 55-year-old man with chronic hepatitis C is evaluated for antiviral therapy and underlying cirrhosis. He does not wish to undergo a liver biopsy. He wants to know if there are other techniques by which to diagnose whether he has advanced fibrosis.

Liver Biopsy

Liver biopsies serve several roles, including diagnosis of disease and assessment of the stage of fibrosis. It is estimated that a liver biopsy, in combination with blood tests to identify causes of chronic liver disease, will provide an accurate diagnosis in about 90% of patients with unexplained liver test abnormalities.

The presence of advanced fibrosis on biopsy has implications for the initiation of disease-specific interventions (e.g., antiviral therapy) and for the introduction of screening and surveillance strategies (e.g., endoscopic evaluation of varices or interval imaging for hepatocellular carcinoma (HCC)). Assessing fibrosis is especially important in patients who may have more than one cause of liver disease (e.g., concomitant alcohol use and obesity and viral hepatitis), which may portend a faster rate of progression to cirrhosis. Liver biopsies also play an integral role in the management of patients after liver transplantation. Besides identification of other disease processes, such as acute cellular rejection, venous outflow obstruction, or infection, liver biopsies are followed in a protocol manner in several transplant centers to gauge the level of fibrosis, especially among patients with viral hepatitis. The presence of fibrosis may dictate expectant management of recurrent disease or lead to consideration of retransplantation.

Technique and Safety

A typical percutaneous liver biopsy will sample about 1/50 000 (0.002%) of the total liver mass, and therefore sampling error can be a concern. Among patients with chronic hepatitis C, up to 30% will have a difference of one histologic stage in two specimens obtained from the liver. Sampling error is probably even greater for cholestatic liver diseases, especially primary sclerosing cholangitis. It is minimized when larger specimens are obtained: the ideal biopsy specimen is about 2.5 cm long and 1.4 mm wide and contains more than six portal tracts [1].

Most percutaneous liver biopsies are performed under the guidance of imaging such as ultrasonography. The use of ultrasonography helps to avoid inadvertent biopsy of adjacent structures, such as the gallbladder, and in some studies, has shown a lower rate of complications than "blind" biopsy. In many centers, all liver biopsies are done by radiologists. The diminishing involvement of gastroenterologists in carrying out liver biopsies is illustrated by the fact that liver biopsy is no longer a requirement of gastroenterology training programs. Biopsies are usually done transthoracically, though a subcostal approach can be used (only with imaging guidance) if an approach to the left lobe is desired. At our institution, liver biopsies are done by either a radiologist or a hepatology physician assistant. We have demonstrated that a physician assistant, trained by hepatologists and using a portable ultrasound device for guidance can obtain quality liver biopsy specimens with minimal morbidity and no mortality. Light sedation with midazolam and/or fentanyl may be employed, though most patients in the authors' institution do not require sedation.

Complications and Risks of Liver Biopsy

The most common complication of liver biopsy is pain, which occurs in up to 50% of patients. Pain often radiates to the right shoulder. Analgesics are required in 10–30% of patients after percutaneous liver biopsy. Oral agents are given for analgesia, unless pain is severe, in which case parenteral opiate agents are administered.

Practical Gastroenterology and Hepatology Board Review Toolkit, Second Edition. Edited by Nicholas J. Talley, Kenneth R. DeVault, Michael B. Wallace, Bashar A. Aqel and Keith D. Lindor.
© 2016 John Wiley & Sons, Ltd. Published 2016 by John Wiley & Sons, Ltd. Companion website: www.practicalgastrohep.com

Prolonged pain may be caused by persistent bleeding or bile leak and can lead to imaging with computed tomography (CT) or ultrasonography. The most important risk of liver biopsy is serious bleeding, which occurs in 0.1–0.3% of patients. Bleeding does not usually require transfusions and generally subsides spontaneously. In rare cases, transarterial embolization or even surgery is required to stop bleeding. Patients undergoing ultrasound marking prior to liver biopsy are at lower risk of complications (0.5 vs. 2.2%). Ultrasound-guided biopsies performed in the radiology department are also associated with significantly less pain [1]. Clinically significant infection after liver biopsy is unusual unless there is concomitant biliary obstruction. Prophylaxis against infectious endocarditis is not recommended. Pneumothorax and perforation of the gallbladder or colon have become increasingly uncommon with the widespread use of ultrasound guidance. The risk of death from liver biopsy is about 0.03%.

Preprocedure Assessment and Equipment

The role of prebiopsy testing remains unclear. The utility of obtaining tests that may reflect bleeding tendency, such as platelet count of prothrombin time, is unclear. Laboratory and clinical requirements for liver biopsy vary, but a hemoglobin ≥ 8 g/dL, platelets $\geq 50 \times 10^9$/L, and prothrombin time or international normalized ratio (INR) ≤ 1.5 is often required. Bleeding time before liver biopsy is not usually performed unless the patient has a history suggestive of a bleeding disorder. The use of aspirin and non-steroidal anti-inflammatory drugs (NSAIDs) is not considered a contraindication to biopsy, though, when possible, aspirin is held for 1 week and NSAIDs for 24 hours before percutaneous liver biopsy. The use of the antiplatelet agent clopidogrel is considered a contraindication to liver biopsy and it should be stopped for at least 5 days before the procedure. Heparin is discontinued 12–24 hours prior to biopsy. Antiplatelet agents may be restarted 48–72 hours after biopsy. Warfarin may be started the day after biopsy. In patients with coagulopathy, as well as those with marked perihepatic ascites, biopsies can be obtained transvenously, usually via the right jugular vein. This technique usually produces specimens of excellent quality. If open or laparoscopic abdominal surgery is necessary for another indication, biopsies may also be obtained under direct visualization.

Absolute contraindications to percutaneous biopsy include inability to cooperate, uncorrected coagulopathy, marked ascites, and mechanical biliary obstruction with dilated intrahepatic bile ducts. Before biopsy, imaging should be obtained to exclude large masses or multiple cysts. Bleeding risk may be higher in patients with amyloidosis, diffuse hepatic malignancy, vascular lesions, and sickle cell disease; therefore, some have suggested that transjugular liver biopsy be performed when one of these is known or highly suspected. Percutaneous biopsies may be obtained in patients with hemophilia after appropriate factor replacement.

Various needles are used for percutaneous biopsy. The choice is left to the operator. In patients with cirrhosis, cutting devices, such as the Tru-Cut or Vim–Silverman needle, may give less fragmented specimens than suction devices. Biopsy with a cutting needle is often done using a spring-loaded device ("gun"), which is simpler to use than manual cutting needles. Suction devices, such as the Jamshidi, Menghini, or Klatskin needles, are simple to use and can obtain longer biopsy specimens than cutting needles.

Almost all liver biopsies are done in an outpatient setting unless the patient requires hospitalization for other reasons. Some centers advise an overnight fast, though a light breakfast which may be advantageous in patients with an intact gall bladder: a light meal before biopsy enhances emptying of the gallbladder, which can decrease the risk of gallbladder puncture. Intravenous access is established in almost all patients, though some liver transplant recipients who have undergone repeated biopsy may not need it. A preprocedure transfusion crossmatch may be performed in some centers.

Technique

Though the specifics of liver biopsy will vary according to the type of needle used and whether ultrasound guidance is employed, the overall procedure should include the following:

1 Review of the risks of biopsy with the patient and signing of a consent form. The explanation of risks should include bleeding, perforation of adjacent organs, and pain.
2 Explanation of the procedure to the patient.
3 Establishment of of intravenous access, in some patients – particularly those at highest risk for bleeding, such as inpatients.
4 Conscious sedation, if requested by the patient.
5 Identification of the site of needle entrance between the anterior and midaxillary lines, using either ultrasound guidance (preferred) or percussion.
6 Maintenance of a sterile field using a sterile drape and iodine swabs.
7 Administration of local anesthesia using 1% lidocaine. A 22-gauge spinal needle allows safe infiltration of the intercostal area and liver capsule, and minimizes the risk of bleeding due to sudden unexpected movement. The spinal needle should be inserted superior to the rib, oriented parallel to the floor, and aimed toward the contralateral shoulder (intact gallbladder) or xiphoid (absent gallbladder). When the 22 G needle reaches the liver capsule, the thoracic wall will act as a fulcrum, causing the syringe side of the needle to swing superiorly on inspiration. This gives a good measurement of depth and of the direction of approach of the liver.
8 Creation of a 3–4 mm nick in the skin. This is particularly important with suction needles, which have a duller edge than cutting needles.
9 Practice of patient breathing. Have the patient take an easy breath and hold at end-expiration, when the biopsy will be performed.
10 Performance of the biopsy. The caliber of most needles is about 1.6 cm, and the length is usually 1.6–1.8 cm.
11 Forwarding of the specimen to the pathology laboratory, with appropriate labeling. The authors' pathology department requests that the specimen be sent in formalin.

Postbiopsy Monitoring

Most complications will occur within 3 hours of biopsy. Usually, patients lie on the right lateral decubitus side, though the benefits of this position are unknown. After the biopsy, patients are observed in the liver biopsy room, with blood pressures done every 5 minutes for 15 minutes. If the patient is stable, they are transferred to an outpatient nursing unit, where they are observed for 3 hours. If they remain stable, they are dismissed. Patients undergoing testing are often asked to stay locally and discouraged from lifting significant weight for the next 24 hours. They are advised to have a traveling companion and to stay within 30 minutes of the hospital for 24 hours in case late complications occur. The major complications – bleeding and perforation of an adjacent organ – are usually heralded by abdominal pain and/or hypotension. Should such symptoms occur

CHAPTER 73

Table 73.1 Commonly used staging systems for hepatic fibrosis.

Chronic hepatitis: Batts and Ludwig	Stage 0: no fibrosis
	Stage 1: portal fibrosis
	Stage 2: periportal fibrosis
	Stage 3: septal fibrosis
	Stage 4: cirrhosis
Chronic hepatitis: Ishak	Stage 0: no fibrosis
	Stage 1: fibrous expansion of some portal areas
	Stage 2: fibrous expansion of most portal areas
	Stage 3: fibrous expansion of most portal areas with occasional portal–portal bridging
	Stage 4: fibrous expansion of portal areas with marked bridging
	Stage 5: marked bridging with occasional nodules (incomplete cirrhosis)
	Stage 6: cirrhosis
NAFLD: Clinical Research Network	Stage 0: no fibrosis
	Stage 1: perisinusoidal or periportal fibrosis
	Stage 2: both perisinusoidal and portal/periportal fibrosis
	Stage 3: bridging fibrosis
	Stage 4: cirrhosis
NAFLD: Brunt	Stage 0: no fibrosis
	Stage 1: perisinusoidal/periportal fibrosis; focally or extensively present
	Stage 2: perisinusoidal/pericellular fibrosis with focal or extensive periportal fibrosis
	Stage 3: perisinusoidal/pericellular fibrosis and portal fibrosis with focal or extensive bridging fibrosis
	Stage 4: cirrhosis

NAFLD, non-alcoholic fatty liver disease.

and persist after biopsy, cross-sectional imaging, usually with CT, should be performed.

Interpretation

The clinical pathologic correlation is of paramount importance in the interpretation of liver biopsy. The most commonly used staging systems are detailed in Table 73.1.

Alternatives to Assessment of Liver Fibrosis

Liver biopsy is considered the reference standard for staging liver fibrosis. However, it has limitations in the form of its invasive nature, cost, risk of complications, and sampling error. There is also significant inter- and intraobserver variability. As already mentioned, up to 30% of patients with chronic hepatitis C will have a difference of one histological stage in two specimens obtained from the liver. Further, pathologists may disagree on staging, especially between sequential stages. Therefore, there has been interest in exploring non-invasive methodologies.

Two major techniques are the use of serum-based biomarkers to indirectly assess liver fibrosis (biologic properties) and the use of ultrasound- and magnetic resonance imaging (MRI)-based techniques, utilizing the principles of elastography, to stage fibrosis (physical properties). Table 73.2 lists some of the advantages and disadvantages of these techniques [2]. A common theme among all techniques is the inability to accurately differentiate between moderate stages of fibrosis, though they all have excellent performance in identifying subjects with cirrhosis and normal liver parenchyma.

Serum Biomarkers

Several serum biomarkers have been studied, mostly in viral hepatitis and non-alcoholic fatty liver disease (NAFLD), and an extensive discussion is outside the scope of this chapter [2,3]. Serum biomarkers can either be liver-specific or non-liver-specific. They may either be markers of the process of fibrosis, such as those that capture elements of extracellular matrix (e.g., glycoproteins and collagens), or indirect markers, looking at alterations in hepatic function (e.g., prothombin time or platelet count). Some of the proposed combinations of biomarker panels are proprietary (e.g., Fibrotest), others combine commonly obtained lab tests (e.g., ast to platelet ratio, APRI), while still others combine patient characteristics, such as age and body mass index (BMI) (e.g., NAFLD fibrosis score). The area under a receiver operating characteristic curve (AUROC) varies, but

Table 73.2 Advantages and disadvantages of non-invasive methods of assessing liver fibrosis. Source: Adapted from Castera 2012 [2].

	Serum biomarkers	Measurement of liver stiffness		
		Transient elastography	**ARFI**	**MR elastography**
Advantages	Good reproducibility	Liver stiffness is a genuine physical property of liver tissue	Liver stiffness is a genuine physical property of liver tissue	Liver stiffness is a genuine physical property of liver tissue
	High applicability (95%)	Good reproducibility	Performance likely equivalent to that of TE	Performance may be higher than that of TE for significant fibrosis
	Low cost and wide availability (not patented)	Well validated	Region of interest smaller than that in TE, but chosen by the operator	Involves examination of the whole liver
	Well validated	High performance for cirrhosis	Can be implemented on a regular ultrasound machine	Can be implemented on a regular MRI machine
		User-friendly (rapid, results immediately available; short learning curve)	High applicability; overcomes the limitations of TE (ascites and obesity)	High applicability; overcomes the limitations of TE (ascites and obesity)
Disadvantages	Non-specific of the liver	Requires a dedicated device	Ongoing validation	Further validation warranted
	Unable to discriminate between intermediate stages of fibrosis	Region of interest cannot be chosen	Unable to discriminate between intermediate stages of fibrosis	Not applicable in case of iron overload
	Performance not as good as TE for fibrosis	Unable to discriminate between intermediate stages of fibrosis	Narrow range of values	Requires an MRI facility
	Results not immediately available	Low applicability (80%, obesity, ascites, limited operator experience)	Quality criteria not well defined	Time-consuming
	Cost and limited availability (proprietary)	False positive in case of acute hepatitis, extra-hepatic cholestasis, and congestion	Prognostic value in cirrhosis?	Costly
	Limitations in hemolysis, Gilbert's syndrome, inflammation, etc.			

is usually upwards of 0.8 for detection of cirrhosis and marginally lower for detection of significant fibrosis (stage F2 or greater). The benefits of serum markers are that they are easily repeatable, are non-invasive, can be performed in an outpatient setting, are applicable to large populations, and may have increased diagnostic accuracy when combined with complementary techniques such as transient elastography (see later). Most markers or panels, however, are less likely to discriminate between intermediate stages of fibrosis. Fibrosis may be overestimated in certain condition; for example, panels relying on bilirubin may overestimate fibrosis in patients with Gilbert's syndrome or hemolysis, while panels relying on transaminases may be overestimated by the presence of acute hepatitis.

Ultrasound-Based Elastography

Elastography is a relatively novel method by which to assess the intrinsic property of the liver parenchyma, or liver stiffness, with elevated stiffness associated with presence of advanced fibrosis. Three specific US techniques include transient elastography, acoustic radiation force impulse imaging, and shear-wave elastography [4].

Ultrasound-based transient elastography was first introduced over a decade ago. It is a single-dimension-based technique that relies on measurement of the velocity of a low-frequency (50 Hz) elastic shear wave propagating through the liver. This propagation is directly related to tissue stiffness (elastic modulus), expressed as $E = 3pv^2$, where v is the velocity and p is the density of tissue, which is assumed to be constant. Shear waves propagate faster in stiffer tissue. The volume measured is 10×40 mm long and 26–65 mm below the skin surface. Results are expressed in kilopascals and range from 2.5 to 75.0 kPa, where a normal value is approximately 5 kPa and a value above around 12–14 kPa implies cirrhosis. Accurate measurement requires at least 10 validated measurements with a success ratio greater than 60% (ratio of valid measurements to total number of measurements) and a variation of range of less than 30% of the median value. The AUROC is upwards of 0.9 for the diagnosis of cirrhosis and around 0.84 for presence of fibrosis. The sensitivity and specificity among viral hepatitis for the detection of cirrhosis are 0.83 and 0.89, respectively [2].

Acoustic radiation force impulse imaging is based on measurement of the velocity of short-duration acoustic pulses generated by mechanically exciting liver tissue using manual compression by the US probe. The shear-wave velocity is measured in a smaller region. The AUROC is also upwards of 0.93 for detection of the presence of cirrhosis. Shear-wave elastography, a newer technique, has the ability to image liver stiffness in real time and allows the operator to choose the size and location of the region of interest.

US-based techniques have the advantages of being outpatient procedures and of only taking a few minutes to perform. Transient elastography has excellent reproducibility for interobserver and intraobserver agreement. Liver stiffness may be uninterpretable, however. One limitation of this technique, mostly due to obesity, ascites, and operator experience, is incomplete examination (approximately 80% of cases). Given that the liver is in a non-elastic envelope, space-occupying abnormalities such as edema (acute hepatitis), inflammation (hepatitis B flares), cholestasis (e.g., biliary obstruction), and passive congestion may interfere with liver stiffness measurement.

Diagnosis of significant fibrosis for transient elastography and for serum biomarkers may be equivalent, especially in patients with hepatitis C. However, in the diagnosis of cirrhosis, transient elastography may be more accurate. Liver biopsy may still be preferred amongst patients with hepatitis B, given that elevated liver stiffness may reflect a flare. On the other hand, elastography may have a role in quiescent disease (e.g., inactive carriers), as it can confirm the absence of significant fibrosis. Strategies such as the combination of biomarkers and transient elastography have led to a 50% reduction in liver biopsies for diagnoses of significant fibrosis and a 70% reduction for cirrhosis. Figure 73.1 provides an algorithm for

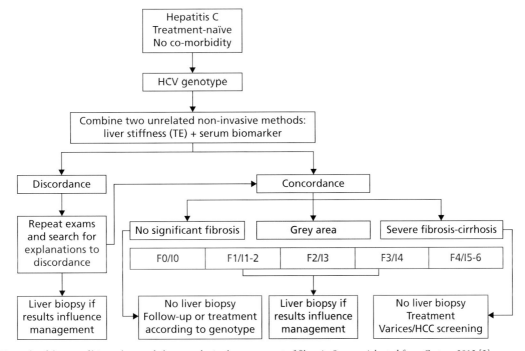

Figure 73.1 Example of the use of biomarkers and elastography in the assessment of fibrosis. Source: Adapted from Castera 2012 [2].

the evaluation of fibrosis in patients with hepatitis C virus (HCV)-related liver disease [2].

Magnetic Resonance Elastography

Magnetic resonance elastography (MRE) is an MRI-based technique used to evaluate the mechanical properties of tissue [5, 6]. Mechanical shear waves are generated within the liver and imaged using special MRI sequences; the information is then processed in order to generate quantitative maps of mechanical properties. This technology is available at several centers. It includes an active driver that transmits acoustic waves to the passive driver; the active driver sends 60 Hz acoustic vibrations through a connected 7.6 m-long plastic tube. The passive pneumatic driver is placed against the chest and upper abdomen of the patient. Measurements of liver stiffness are obtained at the scale of 0–10 kPa. Based on previous studies, normal liver stiffness ranges between 1.5 and 2.9 kPa. Cirrhosis is often seen in persons with values greater than 5.2 kPa. The reported sensitivity of distinguishing fibrotic liver from normal is 80–98%, and the specificity 90–100%. Contraindications to performing MRE include cardiac pacemakers and severe claustrophobia. MRE performs well in pediatrics patients, obese patients, and ascites, as well as post-transplant patients. Other advantages include a lower rate of incomplete examinations. MRE is performed in a supine position and in a state of fast. It allows for evaluation of morphological changes (MRI component) and provides a sense of liver stiffness across the entire liver surface, counteracting the possibility that areas of elevated stiffness or fibrosis might be patchy. Chronic inflammation may lead to higher stiffness. Acute flares of chronic viral hepatitis may also lead to elevated stiffness. Other causes of elevated stiffness include acute biliary obstruction and passive congestion due to congestive heart failure or an elevated central venous pressure [5, 6]. Studies have compared ultrasound and MRE, with one study claiming equivalence and another claiming the superiority of MRE. Such disparate results may be due to differences in patient populations and the spectrum of fibrosis stages [7, 8]. A disadvantage of MRE is poor performance characteristics in patients with high iron overload, due to signal-to-noise limitations. Examination time is also longer.

Evaluation of Portal Hypertension

The role of elastography has been examined in predicting portal hypertension and in gauging the presence of clinically significant portal hypertension. Liver stiffness measurement by transient elastography has an excellent correlation with hepatic venous pressure gradient values below a differential of −12 mmHg. Changes in liver stiffness values over time may also be predictive of decompensation. It is suggested that elevated liver stiffness values may be associated with an increased risk of HCC [9]. Recently, spleen stiffness

has been evaluated [10]. A high spleen stiffness of about 10.5 kPa is predictive of esophageal varices. There is a high correlation between spleen stiffness and hepatic venous pressure gradient measurement. MRE may be used to predict the development of decompensation [11]. There may be a role for elastography in assessing response to etiology specific therapy (e.g., antiviral therapy), with a decrease in liver stiffness being a potential surrogate for good response to treatment.

> ### Take Home Points
>
> - Liver biopsy remains the most definitive test by which to determine the amount of hepatic fibrosis.
> - The most severe complication of liver biopsy is bleeding, which occurs in 0.1–0.3% of patients.
> - Exchange of information between the clinician and the pathologist is imperative in liver biopsy interpretation, because the findings on liver biopsy are often not specific to a diagnosis.
> - Two major alternative techniques are the use of serum-based biomarkers to indirectly assess liver fibrosis (biologic properties) and the use of ultrasound- and magnetic resonance imaging (MRI)-based techniques, utilizing the principles of elastography, to stage fibrosis (physical properties).
> - Non-invasive markers are limited by their inability to distinguish between moderate cases of fibrosis.

References

1 Rockey DC, Caldwell SH, Goodman ZD, *et al.* Liver biopsy. *Hepatology* 2009; **49**: 1017–44.
2 Castera L. Noninvasive methods to assess liver disease in patients with hepatitis B or C. *Gastroenterology* 2012; **142**: 1293–302.e4.
3 Castera L, Vilgrain V, Angulo P. Noninvasive evaluation of NAFLD. *Nat Rev Gastroenterol Hepatol* 2013; **10**: 666–75.
4 Berzigotti A, Castera L. Update on ultrasound imaging of liver fibrosis. *J Hepatol* 2013; **59**: 180–2.
5 Venkatesh SK, Yin M, Ehman RL. Magnetic resonance elastography of liver: technique, analysis, and clinical applications. *J Magn Reson Imaging* 2013; **37**: 544–55.
6 Venkatesh SK, Yin M, Ehman RL. Magnetic resonance elastography of liver: clinical applications. *J Comput Assist Tomogr* 2013; **37**: 887–96.
7 Bohte AE, de Niet A, Jansen L, *et al.* Non-invasive evaluation of liver fibrosis: a comparison of ultrasound-based transient elastography and MR elastography in patients with viral hepatitis B and C. *Eur Radiol* 2014; **24**: 638–48.
8 Huwart L, Sempoux C, Vicaut E, *et al.* Magnetic resonance elastography for the noninvasive staging of liver fibrosis. *Gastroenterology* 2008; **135**: 32–40.
9 Singh S, Fujii LL, Murad MH, *et al.* Liver stiffness is associated with risk of decompensation, liver cancer, and death in patients with chronic liver diseases: a systematic review and meta-analysis. *Clin Gastroenterol Hepatol* 2013; **11**: 1573–84.e1–2, quiz e88–9.
10 Singh S, Eaton JE, Murad MH, *et al.* Accuracy of spleen stiffness measurement in detection of esophageal varices in patients with chronic liver disease: systematic review and meta-analysis. *Clin Gastroenterol Hepatol* 2014; **12**(6): 935–45.e4.
11 Asrani SK, Talwalkar JA, Kamath PS, *et al.* Role of magnetic resonance elastography in compensated and decompensated liver disease. *J Hepatol* 2014; **60**: 934–9.

Endoscopic Techniques Used in the Management of Liver and Biliary Tree Disease: ERCP and EUS

Toufic Kachaamy[1] and Douglas Faigel[2]

[1] Western Regional Medical center at Cancer Treatment Center of America, Goodyear, AZ, United States
[2] Division of Gastroenterology and Hepatology, The Mayo Clinic, Scottsdale, AZ, USA

Summary

Endoscopic ultrasound (EUS) and endoscopic retrograde cholangiopancretography (ERCP) are advanced endoscopic procedures performed by endoscopists with specialized training. They require specialized side-viewing endoscopes and real-time interpretation of ultrasound and fluoroscopic images. ERCP has evolved to be mainly a therapeutic modality, given its small but significant complication risk. EUS provides high-resolution ultrasound images of the gastrointestinal (GI) tract and surrounding organs, producing superior imaging to other modalities in certain areas such as the distal common bile duct. It is useful in patients with intermediate risk of choledocholithiasis, in obtaining diagnosis in extrinsic malignant biliary obstructions, and in the workup of ampullary tumors. ERCP is useful in the workup of intrinsic biliary strictures and for treatment of choledocholithiasis, bile leaks, and biliary obstructions, whether benign or malignant.

Equipment and Review of Technology

EUS and ERCP are considered advanced endoscopic procedures, the skills for which are usually acquired, in the United States, during a dedicated additional 4th year of training. They have evolved to be complementary to each other in the diagnosis and management of hepatobiliary diseases. They require, in addition to endoscopic skills, an advanced knowledge of anatomy and the ability to interpret ultrasound and fluoroscopic images in real time.

ERCP

ERCP is performed using a side-viewing endoscope (duodenoscope) with an elevator. The side-viewing orientation allows *en face* viewing of the duodenal papilla, and the elevator allows manipulation of a variety of tools to cannulate the bile and/or pancreatic ducts and effect therapy. ERCP is performed in a fluoroscopically equipped room. Catheters and guidewires are passed into the bile duct under endoscopic and fluoroscopic guidance. A variety of catheters, guidewires, stone extraction balloons and baskets, dilating balloons, and stents allow therapeutic interventions to be performed. In addition, small-caliber endoscopes (cholangioscopes) can be passed into the bile duct for direct visualization and sampling of biliary pathology. Because ERCP can be associated with a significant complication rate, it has become almost exclusively a therapeutic modality. Diagnostic ERCP has been largely replaced with magnetic resonance cholangiopancreatography (MRCP) and EUS, except in settings where direct intraductal tissue sampling is required, as in suspected cholangiocarcinoma.

EUS

EUS is one of the most specialized endoscopic disciplines to have evolved over the last 30 years. It combines a flexible endoscope with an ultrasound probe at the tip. This allows the acquisition of high-resolution images of areas of the body that are otherwise difficult to image. The ability of EUS to image layers of the GI tract and surrounding structures is unmatched. In addition, it allows the safe acquisition of tissue for diagnostic purposes from areas which can be difficult to access safely from the percutaneous route, either because of vascular structures or because of major intervening organs.

In general, echoendoscopes are available in two configurations: radial scanning and curvilinear array devices. The echoendoscope ultrasound transducers use a frequency of 5–20 MHz. Higher-frequency scanning allows greater resolution of details at the expense of depth of penetration. Use of Doppler technology allows imaging of blood flow within vessels, which is an important diagnostic tool and avoids vascular injury during tissue sampling. Radial echoendoscopes generate an ultrasound image perpendicular to the long axis of the endoscope and can create 360° images. This allows efficient scanning of large areas and offers images similar to those of computed tomography (CT). In contrast, linear-array echoendoscopes produce an ultrasound image in a single plane parallel to the long axis of the endoscope. This makes it possible to perform fine-needle aspiration (FNA) under real-time ultrasonographic visualization. Echoendoscopes are mostly oblique-viewing, providing images similar to those of the side-viewing duodenoscope used for ERCP. Forward-viewing echoendoscopes are also available. Echoendoscopes are stiffer and larger endoscopes than gastroscopes, which makes intubation of the esophagus slightly more difficult and less comfortable to the patient. Additionally, through the scope, ultrasound probes may be passed through the working channel of forward- or side-viewing endoscopes and used to image small GI mural lesions, or passed into the ducts during ERCP for intraductal ultrasound (IDUS).

Detailed examination of the bile duct from the ampulla to the liver hilum can be performed using radial or linear echoendoscopes.

Practical Gastroenterology and Hepatology Board Review Toolkit, Second Edition. Edited by Nicholas J. Talley, Kenneth R. DeVault, Michael B. Wallace, Bashar A. Aqel and Keith D. Lindor.

High-resolution images of the gallbladder can show sludge not previously seen on other imaging. EUS can only obtain limited views of the liver close to the GI lumen. This includes most of the left lobe and, to a much lesser extent, the right lobe of the liver. Other structures that can be examined include the pancreas, cystic duct, portal vein/confluence, spleen and splenic vessels, common hepatic artery, hepatic vein, celiac artery, aorta, and inferior vena cava.

EUS is moving toward becoming a therapeutic tool. Commonly performed therapeutic procedures include drainage of fluid collections. Other procedures, such as treatment of variceal bleeding and biliary drainage, are being performed in selected centers, but have not become standard of care due to a lack of specialized tools, training issues, and possible high complication rates. With the evolution of technology, therapeutic EUS is a promising new frontier.

How to Perform ERCP and EUS

Both ERCP and EUS can be performed with moderate sedation, but specialized centers are mostly moving toward monitored anesthesia care, especially for complicated and prolonged procedures. In certain situations, a patient is consented for both EUS and ERCP; one such example is when choledocholithiasis is suspected in patients who cannot have an MRCP. When choledocholithiasis is identified on EUS, an ERCP can be performed during the same session. Another example is the patient with malignant biliary obstruction, where EUS is used to diagnose, stage, and biopsy the tumor and then ERCP is immediately performed for stent placement. Most of the time, either EUS or ERCP is performed, based on the indication.

The duodenoscope is used for ERCP. ERCP is mostly performed in the prone position, but can be performed in the supine or left lateral position. For ERCP, the scope is positioned in the second portion of the duodenum, which requires scope advancement into the second portion and then reduction to a short position in order to obtain the desired views of the papilla. The bile duct is cannulated with a plastic catheter and guidewire. Injection of radio-opaque contrast allows the generation of cholangiograms. A variety of through-the-scope tools are available to perform sphincterotomy, stone extraction, stricture dilation, and stent insertion.

EUS is performed in the left lateral position, similar to upper endoscopy. While views are side-viewing for ERCP and oblique-viewing for EUS, they are by and large similar. Esophageal intubation with EUS is slightly more difficult than with ERCP, because of the large ultrasound probe on the tip of the echoendoscope and the stiffer nature of the scope. The EUS exam is usually done by "stations," where the echoendoscope is positioned in certain areas of the GI tract to allow specific imaging of certain body parts. The exam usually starts with positioning in the duodenal bulb, where images of the common bile duct and the head of the pancreas are seen. With fine manipulation, the entire bile duct, a portion of the right liver lobe, and the liver hilum can be examined at this station. Positioning in the proximal stomach allows examination of the body of the pancreas, left lobe of the liver, celiac area, and common hepatic artery. The gallbladder is generally visualized from the gastric antrum and duodenal bulb. A complete EUS examination requires constant scope movement to allow scanning of the areas of interest.

Like the duodenoscope, the linear echoendoscope has an elevator, which allows angulation of the needle for specific targeting of lesions. The needle, covered by a sheath, is inserted through the working channel of the linear echoendoscope and then advanced under real-time imaging into the lesion of interest. Once in the lesion, the needle is advanced back and forth to obtain tissue, which

in most cases is cytology. Tissue cores can sometimes be obtained with a core needle, but this is more technically challenging, and the success rate in obtaining tissue is dependent on multiple factors, including the location of the lesion and the configuration of the echoendoscope. The use of Doppler allows the avoidance of major vascular structures.

Role of EUS and ERCP in the Diagnosis and Management of Hepatobiliary Disease

Suspected Choledocholithiasis

Patients with choledocholithiasis usually present with abdominal pain and abnormal liver tests, with biliary pancreatitis, and less commonly with abnormal liver tests (in patients who have previously undergone cholecystectomy). The initial test is usually a transabdominal right upper quadrant ultrasound. In patients with cholelilithiasis, completely normal liver tests have a very high negative predictive value (NPV) (>95%) for choledocholithiasis. Their positive predictive value (PPV) is poor, and thus further testing is needed. Based on the results, the patient risk of having choledocholithiasis is classified as high, intermediate, or low. Patients with a common bile duct stone seen on ultrasound, clinical cholangitis, a bilirubin >4 mg/dL, or both dilated common bile duct and bilirubin between 1.8 and 4.0 mg/dL are considered high risk and should proceed directly to ERCP for therapy. Patients with either a dilated common bile duct or a bilirubin between 1.8 and 4.0 mg/dL, or with any one of age over 55 years, abnormal livers tests other than bilirubin, or gallstone pancreatitis, are at intermediate risk of having bile duct stones and require further testing. Patients with none of these risk factors are at low risk of having a common bile duct stone.

Patients in the intermediate risk group (10–50% chance) for choledocholithiasis require further testing. Testing depends on local availability and expertise. Patients who are planned to have cholecystectomy can have an intraoperative cholangiogram with possible bile duct exploration or ERCP when a stone is identified. Alternatively, an MRCP or EUS can be performed [1]. A good-quality MRCP with slices of <5 mm has a sensitivity of over 85% for common bile duct stones, is non-invasive, and does not usually require sedation. While EUS is more sensitive than MRCP for small (<6 mm) stones, it is invasive, less readily available, and requires sedation [2,3]. On EUS, a common bile duct stone is seen as a hyperechoic area with acoustic shadowing (Figure 74.1). Once a common bile duct stone is confirmed, an ERCP should be performed for therapy (Figure 74.2). Endoscopic biliary sphincterotomy, followed by balloon (Figures 74.3 and 74.4) or basket extraction, is routinely performed for treatment of choledocholithiasis. For large stones (>2 cm), additional maneuvers, such as large balloon dilation or lithotripsy, may be needed for successful removal. Large balloon dilation (>10 mm) of the biliary orifice after endoscopic biliary sphincterotomy – also known as sphincteroplasty – has been shown to be effective and safe for the removal of large common bile duct stones [4]. Lithotripsy (breaking up of stones) can be accomplished by mechanical lithotripsy (the stone is captured in a specialized large basket and crushed) or by laser or electrohydraulic lithotripsy (the stone is fragmented). Laser or electrohydraulic lithotripsy is performed under direct endoscopic visualization, by passing a cholangioscope into the bile duct. An alternative approach is to place a biliary stent in order to achieve biliary drainage, and either refer the patient to a center with more expertise or repeat the ERCP after 2 months, preparing for large stone removal. Stenting often reduces

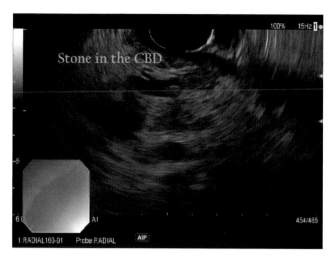

Figure 74.1 Stone in the common bile duct (CBD).

the size of the stone and may facilitate the subsequent endoscopic retrograde cholangiography (ERC) [5].

Biliary Obstructions and Strictures

Biliary obstructions can be benign, malignant, or indeterminate.

Benign Biliary Strictures

In clearly benign biliary obstruction, such as post cholecystectomy or post liver transplant, ERC is the next endoscopic procedure of choice, because of its therapeutic capabilities. For post-cholecystectomy biliary strictures, balloon dilation and endoscopic placement of multiple plastic stents, with subsequent stent exchanges as needed, is successful in over 80% of patients. The approach involves gradual dilation and placement of an increasing number of stents or of as many stents as possible [6–8]. Post-transplant biliary strictures remain the most common complication

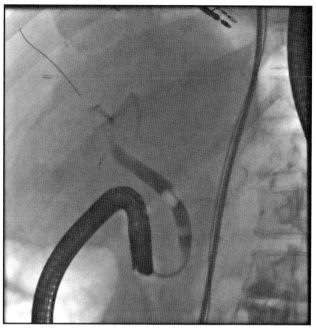

Figure 74.3 Stone sweep on ERCP.

of liver transplant. They can be anastomotic or non-anastomotic. Anastomotic strictures are very focal, narrowing at the site of the anastomosis. They are best treated with progressive placement of multiple plastic stents until stricture resolution is seen. The success rate of such an approach is 80–100%, avoiding the need for surgery [9]. Recently, the use of a single self-expanding covered metal stent has been described and reported to be effective, though stent migration occurs in around 16% of cases, leading to success rates that are less than those seen in placement of multiple plastic stents

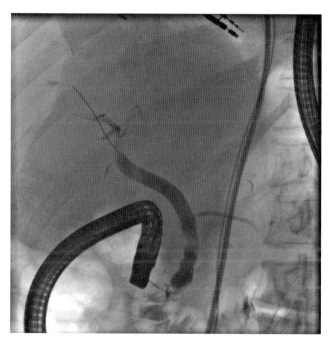

Figure 74.2 Stone on ERCP fluoro.

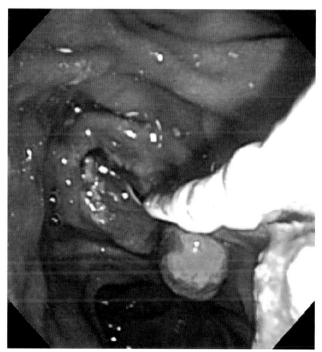

Figure 74.4 Endoscopic view of a stone.

[10]. Non-anastomotic strictures after liver transplant are usually ischemic, related to events such as hepatic artery thrombosis and prolonged hypoperfusion during surgery. They are difficult to treat, because of their non-focal nature and frequent involvement of the bifurcation or intrahepatic ducts. Endoscopic success in treating these patients is less than 50%, and often retransplantation is needed [11]. Distal biliary strictures secondary to chronic pancreatitis can be treated endoscopically, either with multiple side-by-side plastic stents with stent exchanges for over a year [12] or with placement of a self-expanding covered metal stent for over 6 months. Migration of the covered metal stent is frequent, and more success has been reported with flared-end covered metal stents and stents with anchoring devices [13, 14].

Malignant Biliary Obstructions

These often present with painless jaundice and undergo transabdominal ultrasound, CT, or MRCP as part of the initial workup. Malignant etiologies include pancreatic head masses, cholangiocarcinoma, and extrinsic compressions from metastases or malignant adenopathy.

Role of EUS

EUS can be very helpful in the differentiation between extrinsic compression and intrinsic ductal pathology in biliary strictures and in the diagnosis of obstruction due to pancreatic cancer. An extrinsic mass is typically seen as a hypoechoic lesion causing compression of the ductal system with proximal dilation. Primary biliary malignancy is usually associated with a bile duct wall thickness of >3 mm with hypoechoic changes. EUS FNA (Figure 74.5) of masses or lymph nodes that are causing compression is sensitive and specific. EUS has an estimated sensitivity of 78% (95% CI: 69–85%) and a specificity of 84% (95% CI: 78–91%) in detecting malignant biliary strictures [15]. FNA is likely to improve the sensitivity and specificity. EUS FNA of suspected cholangiocarcinoma should not be performed if the patient is a potential liver transplant candidate, as the possible risk of peritoneal seeding precludes them from transplantation. In patients with solid pancreatic lesions, EUS FNA has a sensitivity of 92% (95% CI: 91–93%) and a specificity of 96% (95% CI: 93–98%) [16]. In pancreatic head masses, EUS FNA avoids the potential seeding that can be seen with percutaneous biopsies and is thus the preferred method of tissue acquisition. In clearly resectable patients with pancreatic masses, a tissue diagnosis is not always

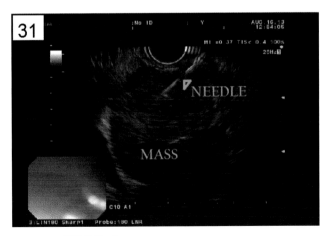

Figure 74.5 EUS FNA of a mass.

needed, and the decision to perform FNA should be made in a multidisciplinary fashion after discussion of the pros and cons with the surgical oncologist, the oncologist, and the patient. Certain findings, such as a lack of pancreatic ductal dilation, should raise suspicion of alternative diagnoses other than pancreatic cancer. Peripancreatic lymphoma can present as a pancreatic mass and is less likely to cause jaundice. Autoimmune pancreatitis can present with a pancreatic head mass causing jaundice; the treatment is steroids and non-surgical management.

Role of ERCP

The role of ERCP is both diagnostic and therapeutic in biliary obstructions.

Diagnostic

ERCP can provide tissue diagnosis with brush cytology and intraductal biopsies when the diagnosis is unclear. The addition of molecular cytologic techniques, such as fluorescent *in situ* hybridization (FISH), can improve the diagnostic yield. Obtaining tissue during ERCP, as opposed to EUS, avoids the problem related to seeding in suspected cholangiocarcinoma.

Therapeutic

Pancreatic head cancer is the most common malignant cause of distal biliary obstruction. ERCP can be therapeutic, either as a palliation preoperatively or for definitive palliation in patients who are not operative candidates. Preoperatively, the role of ERCP is limited to patients who will undergo neoadjuvant treatment before surgery or patients in whom surgery will be delayed for at least several weeks. Routine preoperative palliation of jaundice in patients who will undergo surgery in a timely manner for pancreatic head cancer has been associated with an increase in complications and should be avoided. ERCP with stent can be considered preoperatively if there is a delay. The choice of stent is currently undefined. For definitive palliation in non-surgical candidates, self-expanding metal stent (SEMS) should be used, as they are associated with fewer complications and with less need for repeated procedures as compared to plastic stents, as long as patient survival is expected to be over 3 months. Studies have not shown the patency of covered SEMS to be superior to that of uncovered SEMS. In addition, they have a higher migration rate and may be associated with an increased risk of cholecystitis, though this issue is controversial. For these reasons, and because they are more expensive, it is the authors' preference to place an uncovered SEMS for distal biliary obstructions. With the introduction of newer chemotherapeutic agents, patient with pancreatic cancer are surviving longer. The need for reintervention in these patients is encountered more frequently. The optimal management of an occluded metal stent has not been established; options include exchange for a covered stent, balloon sweep if the stent is occluded with debris, and restenting with another stent for an uncovered stent with tissue ingrowth or overgrowth.

Proximal or Hilar Obstructions

Hilar obstructions can be caused by cholangiocarcinoma, hepatocellular carcinoma, gallbladder cancer, or lymph nodes. Palliation of these patients is technically challenging, and the optimal management strategy continues to be debated. Covered metal stents should not be used because the stent occludes the contralateral duct. Uncovered metal stents are likely more effective than plastic stents, but are more difficult to treat once they obstruct. Unilateral stenting can be effective in relief of jaundice, without the added technical complication rate of bilateral stenting [17]. In the setting of cholangitis, or if unilateral stenting does not adequately relieve jaundice, bilateral stenting is needed. Bilateral uncovered SEMS in highly successful centers is associated with longer patency rates without added complications, but without improvement in survival [18]. Sometimes, percutaneous stenting is needed in these patients in addition to or instead of endoscopic stenting when endoscopic stenting is not technically feasible. Endoscopic treatment of hilar obstruction is very technically challenging and should only be attempted in centers with significant expertise in its management. Important principles to adhere to include using as little contrast as necessary to perform the procedure and avoiding injection of ducts that will not be drained. Significant preprocedure planning is needed for these patients, with a CT and or MRCP to provide a roadmap, minimize injection of contrast, and aim for drainage of the healthiest part of the liver.

Indeterminate Biliary Strictures

Indeterminate biliary strictures are strictures that cannot be clearly classified as malignant or benign after initial investigations, which typically include imaging and ERCP with tissue sampling. In these patients, if a mass or bile duct wall thickening (>3 mm) is seen, EUS FNA has a significant yield. When EUS is non-diagnostic, cholangioscopy and biopsy under vision are performed. This strategy yields a diagnosis in over 90% of patients [19]. Cholangioscopy involves direct visualization of the bile duct. The device most commonly used for cholangioscopy is the single-operator disposable SpyGlass system, which is introduced through the duodenscope accessory channel into the bile duct and has its own channel. A biopsy forceps (spybite) introduced through the cholangioscope allows sampling of tissue under direct vision.

Bile Leaks

Bile leaks occur after surgery and trauma. The most common cause is cholecystectomy, with leaks arising from either the cystic duct or the duct of Luschka: a small intrahepatic duct that runs through the gallbladder fossa. Endoscopic treatment with biliary stenting with or without biliary sphincterotomy diverts the bile from the injured area and results in resolution of the leak in 4–6 weeks in over 90% of cases [20].

Primary Sclerosing Cholangitis

Primary sclerosing cholangitis (PSC) is a progressive disease that causes fibrosis of the bile duct with resultant cirrhosis and increased risk of cholangitis and cholangiocarcinoma. Patients with PSC presenting with a dominant stricture or acute worsening in liver tests require intervention to rule out cholangiocarcinoma and attempt biochemical improvement. This is usually accomplished by ERCP with cytology and FISH. Occasionally, EUS and cholangioscopy are needed, as in indeterminate strictures (see earlier). The aim of therapeutic ERCP in PSC is dilation of dominant strictures. If stenting is performed, it should be for a few weeks only [21].

Ampullary Tumors

Ampullary adenomas can be resected endoscopically. Adenomas of less than 1 cm in size with no signs of malignancy, such as ulceration, bleeding, or induration suggestive of submucosal infiltration, can be resected without prior EUS. For all other adenomas, an EUS is recommended to check for any signs of malignancy and to assess adenoma extension into the common bile duct. Patients with malignancy or great extension into the common bile duct should be referred for surgical intervention, if their overall health allows it. Endoscopic resection is performed with a snare cautery, much like colonic polypectomy. Interventions to decrease the risk of post-ERCP pancreatitis should be performed (see later).

Occult Cholelithiasis and Microlithiasis

EUS is the most sensitive test for detecting small (<1 cm) gallstones and microlithiasis (<3 mm crystals), which are thought to be causes of recurrent pancreatitis [22, 23]. It has a role in the workup of patient with recurrent biliary colic and biliary pancreatitis and negative transabdominal ultrasound.

Sphincter of Oddi Dysfunction

Sphincter of Oddi dysfunction (SOD) is post-cholecystectomy recurrent biliary-like abdominal pain. Type 1 SOD has both biliary ductal dilation and liver test abnormalities, type 2 has either biliary dilation or liver test abnormalities, and type 3 has neither. While type 1 patients usually improve with sphincterotomy and type 2 may improve, type 3 patients appear to have worse outcomes with sphincterotomy, based on data from the National Institutes of Health (NIH)-funded EPISOD trial, which at the time of writing was only published in abstract form. These patients may benefit from EUS for detection of occult choledocholithiasis or other diagnoses.

Miscellaneous Uses of EUS

EUS imaging of the liver is limited to most of the left lobe and a part of the right lobe. This makes its utility in assessing the liver limited. EUS can detect lesions – including metastases – in these areas that are less than 1 cm and not seen on other imaging, and samples can be taken via EUS FNA. EUS can also be a cost-effective means of obtaining a liver biopsy using coring needles, if incorporated as part of the workup of liver test abnormalities, such as when biliary obstruction is suspected and ruled out [24]. It can diagnose portal biliopathy (Figure 74.2) and help with the diagnosis and management of gastric and esophageal varices. It can be used to access the biliary tree, as in EUS-guided ERC in altered anatomy or after failed ERCP. These are novel uses of EUS and are likely to be very useful in the future as tools improve and experience is gained, decreasing the risk of complications.

Complications of EUS and ERCP

EUS is a safe procedure, with overall complication rates similar to those of upper endoscopy. EUS FNA has a slightly higher risk of complications, including a <2% risk of pancreatitis with FNA of pancreatic lesions and a 1% risk of bleeding, which normally requires no intervention. Infectious complications are more common with cyst FNA, so antibiotic prophylaxis is usually given. EUS-guided biliary drainage has a 15% complication rate. Perforations of the pharynx and of the duodenal bulb may occur more commonly with EUS than with standard esophagogastroduodenoscopy (EGD), due to the inflexible metal ultrasound transducer. Other complications, such as malignant seeding and spinal cord injury from celiac plexus interventions, are rare [25].

ERCP is associated with a significant complication rate. This has led to almost complete replacement of diagnostic ERCP by MRCP and EUS. Careful attention to strict adherence to proper indications is essential to optimizing patient outcome. Complications include pancreatitis, which can be severe. The incidence of pancreatitis, especially in the severe form, can be significantly decreased by administration of rectal indomethacin or pancreatic duct stenting in those with risk factors for post-ERCP pancreatitis [26,27]. Bleeding is mostly related to sphincterotomy and is increased in patients who are anticoagulated in the first 72 hours after the procedure. Infectious complications are more common in patients with incomplete drainage, such as PSC and hilar stricture, and in immunocompromised patients, such as after liver transplantation; antibiotic prophylaxis is usually recommended. Cholecystitis occurs after metal stenting for malignant obstruction; whether it is related to tumor obstructing the cystic duct or to the type of stent used is still not clear. Other complications, such as perforation and severe cardiovascular complications, are uncommon, but can be severe [28]. Perforations on ERCP may be of the duct(s), on sphincterotomy, or at a site distal to the ampulla due to scope trauma. Perforations of the ducts or on sphincterotomy usually respond to conservative therapy with stenting, antibiotics, and nil per os. Perforations away from the ampulla and large sphincterotomy perforations may require surgery. Notably, retroperitoneal air on CT scans after sphincterotomy is not uncommon and does not by itself indicate a clinical perforation.

Take Home Points

- Endoscopic ultrasound (EUS) continues to be mostly a diagnostic modality.
- Endoscopic retrograde cholangiopancreatography (ERCP) is almost exclusively used as a therapeutic modality.
- EUS is useful in establishing a diagnosis in patient with intermediate risk of having choledocholithiasis.
- ERCP is highly successful in the removal of common bile duct stones.
- ERCP is highly successful in management of most benign biliary strictures.
- ERCP can selectively be used in preoperative palliation of malignant biliary strictures.
- ERCP is very useful in palliation of malignant biliary strictures in patients who are not resection candidates.
- A strategy of EUS followed by ERCP with cholangioscopy obtains a definitive diagnosis in the majority of indeterminate biliary strictures.
- ERCP is highly successful in treating postoperative bile leaks.
- The safety of EUS is similar to that of upper endoscopy, with a slight added risk mostly from fine-needle aspiration (FNA).
- Complication rates in ERCP can be decreased by paying attention to proper indications and by administering rectal indomethacin and placing a pancreatic duct stent in procedures where risk factors for post-ERCP pancreatitis exist.

Videos of interest to readers of this chapter can be found by visiting the companion website at:

http://www.practicalgastrohep.com/

74.1 Endoscopic removal of bile duct stones.
74.2 Placement of self-expanding metal stent for palliation of malignant biliary obstruction.
74.3 Endoscopic ultrasound of a solitary liver hypoechoic metastasis.
74.4 Mini living donor liver transplantation.
74.5 Plastic stent placement for an anastomotic biliary stricture.
74.6 Endoscopic retrograde cholangiopancreatography.

References

1 ASGE Standards of Practice Committee, Maple JT, Ben-Menachem T, et al. The role of endoscopy in the evaluation of suspected choledocholithiasis. *Gastrointest Endosc* 2010; **71**(1): 1–9.

2 Verma D, Kapadia A, Eisen GM, Adler DG. EUS vs MRCP for detection of choledocholithiasis. *Gastrointest Endosc* 2006; **64**(2): 248–54.

3 McMahon CJ. The relative roles of magnetic resonance cholangiopancreatography (MRCP) and endoscopic ultrasound in diagnosis of common bile duct calculi: a critically appraised topic. *Abdom Imaging* 2008; **33**(1): 6–9.

4 Attasaranya S, Cheon YK, Vittal H, et al. Large-diameter biliary orifice balloon dilation to aid in endoscopic bile duct stone removal: a multicenter series. *Gastrointest Endosc* 2008; **67**(7): 1046–52.

5 Horiuchi A, Nakayama Y, Kajiyama M, et al. Biliary stenting in the management of large or multiple common bile duct stones. *Gastrointest Endosc* 2010; **71**(7): 1200–3.e2.

6 Bergman JJ, Burgemeister L, Bruno MJ, et al. Long-term follow-up after biliary stent placement for postoperative bile duct stenosis. *Gastrointest Endosc* 2001; **54**(2): 154–61.

7 De Palma GD, Galloro G, Romano G, et al. Long-term follow-up after endoscopic biliary stent placement for bile duct strictures from laparoscopic cholecystectomy. *Hepatogastroenterology* 2003; **50**(53): 1229–31.

8 Costamagna G, Tringali A, Mutignani M, et al. Endotherapy of postoperative biliary strictures with multiple stents: results after more than 10 years of follow-up. *Gastrointest Endosc* 2010; **72**(3): 551–7.

9 Kao D, Zepeda-Gomez S, Tandon P, Bain VG. Managing the post-liver transplantation anastomotic biliary stricture: multiple plastic versus metal stents: a systematic review. *Gastrointest Endosc* 2013; **77**(5): 679–91.

10 Arain MA, Attam R, Freeman ML. Advances in endoscopic management of biliary tract complications after liver transplantation. *Liver Transpl* 2013; **19**(5): 482–98.

11 Verdonk RC, Buis CI, van der Jagt EJ, et al. Nonanastomotic biliary strictures after liver transplantation, part 2: Management, outcome, and risk factors for disease progression. *Liver Transpl* 2007; **13**(5): 725–32.

12 Catalano MF, Linder JD, George S, et al. Treatment of symptomatic distal common bile duct stenosis secondary to chronic pancreatitis: comparison of single vs. multiple simultaneous stents. *Gastrointest Endosc* 2004; **60**(6): 945–52.

13 Perri V, Boškoski I, Tringali A, et al. Fully covered self-expandable metal stents in biliary strictures caused by chronic pancreatitis not responding to plastic stenting: a prospective study with 2 years of follow-up. *Gastrointest Endosc* 2012; **75**(6): 1271–7.

14 Park DH, Lee SS, Lee TH, et al. Anchoring flap versus flared end, fully covered self expandable metal stents to prevent migration in patients with benign biliary strictures: a multicenter, prospective, comparative pilot study (with videos). *Gastrointest Endosc* 2011; **73**(1): 64–70.

15 Garrow D, Miller S, Sinha D, et al. Endoscopic ultrasound: a meta-analysis of test performance in suspected biliary obstruction. *Clin Gastroenterol Hepatol* 2007; **5**(5): 616–23.

16 Chen J, Yang R, Lu Y, et al. Diagnostic accuracy of endoscopic ultrasound-guided fine-needle aspiration for solid pancreatic lesion: a systematic review. *J Cancer Res Clin Oncol* 2012; **138**(9): 1433–41.

17 De Palma GD, Galloro G, Siciliano S, et al. Unilateral versus bilateral endoscopic hepatic duct drainage in patients with malignant hilar biliary obstruction: results of a prospective, randomized, and controlled study. *Gastrointest Endosc* 2001; **53**(6): 547–53.

18 Naitoh I, Ohara H, Nakazawa T, et al. Unilateral versus bilateral endoscopic metal stenting for malignant hilar biliary obstruction. *J Gastroenterol Hepatol* 2009; **24**(4): 552–7.

19 Nguyen NQ, Schoeman MN, Ruszkiewicz A. Clinical utility of EUS before cholangioscopy in the evaluation of difficult biliary strictures. *Gastrointest Endosc* 2013; **78**(6): 868–74.

20 Huang CS, Lichtenstein DR. Postcholecystectomy bile leak: what is the optimal treatment? *Gastrointest Endosc* 2005; **61**(2): 276–8.

21 McLoughlin M, Enns R. Endoscopy in the management of primary sclerosing cholangitis. *Curr Gastroenterol Rep* 2008; **10**(2): 177–85.

22 Coyle WJ, Lawson JM. Combined endoscopic ultrasound and stimulated biliary drainage in cholecystitis and microlithiasis: diagnosis and outcomes. *Gastrointest Endosc* 1996; **44**(1): 102–3.

23 Liu CL, Lo CM, Chan JK, *et al.* EUS for detection of occult cholelithiasis in patients with idiopathic pancreatitis. *Gastrointest Endosc* 2000; **51**(1): 28–32.

24 Stavropoulos SN, Im GY, Jlayer Z, *et al.* High yield of same-session EUS-guided liver biopsy by 19-gauge FNA needle in patients undergoing EUS to exclude biliary obstruction. *Gastrointest Endosc* 2012; **75**(2): 310–18.

25 ASGE Standards of Practice Committee, Early DS, Acosta RD, *et al.* Adverse events associated with EUS and EUS with FNA. *Gastrointest Endosc* 2013; **77**(6): 839–43.

26 Freeman ML. Pancreatic stents for prevention of post-endoscopic retrograde cholangiopancreatography pancreatitis. *Clin Gastroenterol Hepatol* 2007; **5**(11): 1354–65.

27 Elmunzer BJ, Scheiman JM, Lehman GA, *et al.* A randomized trial of rectal indomethacin to prevent post-ERCP pancreatitis. *N Engl J Med* 2012; **366**(15): 1414–22.

28 ASGE Standards of Practice Committee, Anderson MA, Fisher L, *et al.* Complications of ERCP. *Gastrointest Endosc* 2012; **75**(3): 467–73.

CHAPTER 74

PART 2

Diseases of the Liver

75 Acute Viral Hepatitis: Hepatitis A, Hepatitis E, and Other Viruses, 465
Iliana Doycheva and Juan F. Gallegos-Orozco

76 Chronic Hepatitis B and D, 473
Vijayan Balan, Jorge Rakela, and Rebecca Corey

77 Hepatitis C, 480
Michael Charlton and Travis Dick

78 Bacterial and Other Non-viral Infections of the Liver, 487
Maria Teresa A. Seville, Roberto L. Patron, Ann McCullough, and Shimon Kusne

79 Alcoholic Liver Disease, 498
Moira Hilscher and Vijay Shah

80 Drug-Induced Liver Injury, 503
Einar Björnsson and Naga Chalasani

81 Autoimmune Liver Diseases, 508
Justin A. Reynolds and Elizabeth J. Carey

82 Vascular Diseases of the Liver, 513
Brenda Ernst, Pierre Noel, and Bashar A. Aqel

83 Metabolic Syndrome and Non-alcoholic Fatty Liver Disease, 522
Paul Angulo

84 Hemochromatosis, Wilson's Disease, and Alpha-1-Antitrypsin Deficiency, 530
Lisa M. Glass and Rolland C. Dickson

85 Hepatic Manifestations of Systemic Diseases, 538
Stephen Crane Hauser

86 Diseases of the Biliary Tract and Gallbladder, 543
Wajeeh Salah and M. Edwyn Harrison

87 Portal Hypertension, 554
Humberto C. Gonzalez and Patrick S. Kamath

88 TIPS, 567
Santiago Cornejo and Sailendra Naidu

89 Primary Carcinoma of the Liver, 574
Renumathy Dhanasekaran, Julie K. Heimbach, and Lewis R. Roberts

90 Pregnancy and Liver Disease, 582
J. Eileen Hay

91 Pediatric Liver Disease, 587
Tamir Miloh

Acute Viral Hepatitis: Hepatitis A, Hepatitis E, and Other Viruses

Iliana Doycheva and Juan F. Gallegos-Orozco

Division of Gastroenterology, Hepatology and Nutrition, University of Utah School of Medicine, Salt Lake City, UT, USA

Summary

Infections by hepatotropic and non-hepatotropic viruses are a frequent cause of acute hepatitis. Hepatitis A and E are enterally transmitted viral infections (HAV and HEV, respectively), prevalent worldwide. The clinical spectrum ranges from asymptomatic to acute liver failure (ALF). Diagnosis of hepatitis A relies on serum anti-HAV immunoglobulin M (IgM), while that of hepatitis E requires heightened clinical suspicion and serologic or molecular confirmation. Prognosis is excellent, with spontaneous resolution in most cases. Mortality is greater in HEV than in HAV, especially in pregnant patients, in whom it is up to 25%. No specific antiviral treatment is available for HAV or HEV. Effective immunoprophylaxis for hepatitis A is widely accessible, while a safe and effective recombinant HEV vaccine has recently been tested in clinical trials. Non-hepatotropic viruses, such as herpesviruses, adenoviruses, enteroviruses, and parvovirus B-19, can cause acute hepatitis and have significant consequences in immunocompromised individuals.

Case

A healthy 20-year-old white woman presents to an acute care clinic 3 weeks after vacationing in Mexico, with a 5-day history of malaise, fatigue, low-grade fever, headache, nausea, anorexia, and dark urine. On physical examination, she is afebrile and jaundiced, and has tender hepatomegaly. There are no signs of chronic liver disease and her neurologic exam is normal. Laboratory tests reveal normal complete blood count (CBC), blood urea nitrogen (BUN), creatinine, and international normalized ratio (INR), with alanine transaminase (ALT) 3500 IU/L, aspartate transaminase (AST) 3200 IU/L, and total bilirubin 6 g/dL. Abdominal ultrasound reveals hepatomegaly with normal gallbladder, bile ducts, and spleen.

Hepatitis A

Definition and Epidemiology

Hepatitis A is an acute, self-limited, necroinflammatory viral infection of the liver. HAV is a positive-sense, single-stranded, linear RNA hepatotropic virus classified in its own genus (*Hepatovirus*) within the Picornaviridae family [1, 2]. It is primarily transmitted via the fecal–oral route.

The epidemiology of HAV varies around the world, in close relation to the overall sanitary conditions of a region. Geographical areas worldwide can be divided into high, intermediate, and low levels of endemicity. Prevalence is low among industrialized countries compared to developing nations, where the majority of subjects have been infected in early childhood. The overall age-adjusted seroprevalence of anti-HAV among US-born adults aged >19 years was 30% in 1999–2006, based on results from the National Health and Nutrition Examination Survey (NHANES). Since the introduction of HAV vaccination for all children at age 1 in 1995, the prevalence of positive HAV antibodies has increased from 8% in 1988–94 to 39% in 2007–08, based on NHANES [3].

There are 1.5 million cases per year of acute HAV reported worldwide. A steady 90% decline in the incidence of HAV in the United States has been noted over the last decade. When asymptomatic infections and under-reporting were taken into account, it was estimated that approximately 2700 new infections occurred in 2011 [4]. Rates for acute HAV declined in all age groups. The highest rate in 2011 was for persons aged 20–29 years. The incidence rate was similar among males and females [4].

Several groups are at higher risk of HAV infection: travelers from non-endemic to endemic areas; military personnel stationed in endemic regions; children, employees, and parents of children attending daycare centers; persons working with non-human primates; clients and employees of institutions for the developmentally disabled; men who have sex with other men (MSM); and intravenous drug users (IVDUs). In the United States, the most frequently identified epidemiologic risk factor for hepatitis A is international travel (reported by 15% of patients overall), especially to Mexico and Central and South America (72%), followed by sexual or household contact with hepatitis A patients (10%), MSM (9%), suspected food- or waterborne outbreak (7.5%), spending time in a daycare center (4%), and IVDU (2%); the majority of reported cases have no known risk factor (65%) [5].

Pathophysiology

HAV is transmitted almost exclusively by the fecal–oral route, and is associated with viral shedding in stool during the 2–6-week incubation period. The virus is stable at ambient temperatures and at low

Practical Gastroenterology and Hepatology Board Review Toolkit, Second Edition. Edited by Nicholas J. Talley, Kenneth R. DeVault, Michael B. Wallace, Bashar A. Aqel and Keith D. Lindor.
© 2016 John Wiley & Sons, Ltd. Published 2016 by John Wiley & Sons, Ltd. Companion website: www.practicalgastrohep.com

pH, enabling it to survive in the environment and be transmitted through contaminated food and drinking water. Three HAV genotypes have been identified, divided into subtypes A and B, but likely there is only one serotype.

Once ingested, HAV reaches the small bowel, traverses the intestinal mucosa, and gains access to the liver through the portal vein. To enter cells, HAV interacts with its cellular receptor 1, HAVCR1, a significant allergy and autoimmunity determinant in humans. Viral RNA uncoats within the hepatocyte cytoplasm, and ribosomes bind to form polysomes. Viral proteins are synthesized and virus particles are assembled and excreted back to the intestinal lumen via the biliary tract. Feces can contain up to 10^9 infectious virions per gram. Fecal shedding of the virus reaches its maximum shortly (14–21 days) before the onset of hepatocellular injury, which corresponds to the time at which the subject is most contagious. This is paralleled by extended viremia, which follows a similar pattern to fecal shedding, though at a much lower magnitude. Hepatocellular injury ensues, with a marked increase of serum aminotransferase activity. Viral antigen continues to be shed for up to 3 weeks after aminotransferase elevation, though sensitive molecular techniques can detect continued shedding of HAV RNA for many weeks. Fortunately, prolonged viral shedding is rare and has only been documented in infected premature infants. Long-term fecal viral shedding does not occur.

At present, the mechanisms responsible for hepatocellular injury in HAV infection are poorly understood. The virus does not appear to be cytopathic, suggesting that liver injury is the result of an immunopathologic response to infection in the hepatocyte, rather than to a direct viral effect. The currently accepted hypothesis is that hepatocellular injury is the result of activated human leukocyte antigen (HLA)-restricted, virus-specific, cytotoxic CD8+ lymphocytes. These cells have been shown to secrete interferon (IFN)-γ and hence stimulate the recruitment of additional, non-specific inflammatory cells to the liver [1,4]. New studies have demonstrated that CD4+ regulatory T cells (Tregs) express HAVCR1, and that the HAV–HAVCR1 interaction directly inhibits Treg function and thus reduces Treg production of TGF-β, which is necessary to recruitment of leucocytes to the inflammation site and promotion of T-cell survival. HAV also reduces liver damage by inducing the production of interleukin (IL)-22 [6].

The lack of chronic infection in hepatitis A is the result of a robust and effective response from the adaptive immune system to HAV. Neutralizing serum antibodies can be detected concurrently with early evidence of elevation of aminotransferases and liver injury. The early humoral response largely comprises IgM antibodies, which serve as the basis of serologic diagnosis, and IgG, which can be detected shortly after symptom onset. Importantly, anti-HAV IgG persists for life and confers protection against reinfection (Figure 75.1). This is the basis for passive and active immunoprophylaxis with immune globulin and vaccination, respectively [7].

Clinical Features

The clinical spectrum of HAV ranges from asymptomatic to ALF (Table 75.1), though in most patients morbidity and mortality are minimal. The presence of symptoms strongly correlates with the age of acquisition of HAV. Children younger than 6 years generally do not develop significant symptoms (jaundice <20%), while 70–80% of older children, adolescents, and adults develop jaundice [1,2].

The clinical presentation of hepatitis A may be indistinguishable from other causes of acute viral hepatitis. After an incubation period of 2–6 weeks, patients may experience non-specific

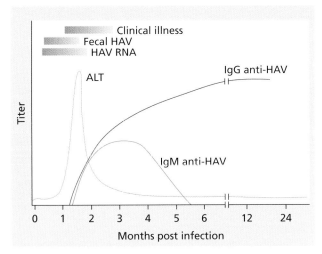

Figure 75.1 Relevant clinical, viral, and serologic events in hepatitis A. Source: Bacon 2006 [8]. Reproduced with permission of Elsevier.

prodromal symptoms, such as fatigue, malaise, low-grade fever, headache, nausea and vomiting, myalgias, arthralgias, anorexia, and weight loss. Liver-specific symptoms tend to appear later in the course, and include right upper quadrant abdominal pain, dark urine, jaundice, acholia, and pruritus. On physical exam, patients may have tender hepatomegaly, scleral icterus, and jaundice. Occasionally, patients will present with cervical lymphadenopathy and mild splenomegaly [1,2].

Complete clinical recovery is the rule, and there is no chronic infection or carrier state. The majority of patients recover within the first 8 weeks, and only rarely do laboratory abnormalities persist for up to a year [1,2] (Figure 75.1).

Other patterns of presentation include a cholestatic form, with jaundice that may persist for up to 10 weeks. Bilirubin levels may exceed 10 mg/dL in this form, and alkaline phosphatase is elevated disproportionately to aminotransferases. A relapsing form with two or more bouts of acute HAV infection, with elevation of serum aminotransferases for 3–6 weeks and remission between flares from 4 to 15 weeks, may be experience by 10–15% of patients. Relapses are entirely biochemical or are associated with mild symptoms. This form may last from 3 to 9 months. Rarely, HAV presents as ALF

Table 75.1 Relevant clinical features in hepatitis A and hepatitis E.

	HAV	HEV
Incubation period	~30 days	~40 days
Transmission	Fecal–oral	Fecal–oral, zoonotic, parenteral, vertical transmission
Person-to-person transmission	Frequent	Infrequent
Dose-dependent severity	No	Yes
Mortality	0.1–2.0% (increases with age and comorbidity; no effect of pregnancy)	1–4% (up to 25% in pregnancy)
Chronic disease	No	Yes, in immunosuppressed patients
Prevention	Immune globulin prophylaxis useful Safe and effective vaccines widely available	Immune globulin ineffective Vaccine in phase III trials

(1 in 10 000 cases) [1,2]. In a report from the US ALF group in 2008, 3% of all cases of ALF in adults were caused by hepatitis A. Hepatitis A-induced ALF had a good overall prognosis, as 58% recovered spontaneously, but 29% required liver transplantation and 13% died [9].

Extrahepatic manifestations of HAV include arthralgias, evanescent rash, and isolated cases of optic neuritis, Guillain–Barré syndrome (GBS), interstitial nephritis, and agranulocytosis. Occasionally, in genetically susceptible individuals, autoimmune hepatitis may develop following hepatitis A infection.

Case Continued

Serologic studies for viral hepatitis are remarkable for positive total anti-HAV antibodies, positive anti-HAV IgM and hepatitis B surface antibody, negative hepatitis B surface antigen, hepatitis B core IgG and IgM antibodies, and absence of anti-HCV antibodies and HEV IgG and IgM antibodies, as well as negative antinuclear antibodies and anti-smooth-muscle antibodies. Diagnosis of hepatitis A is established.

Diagnosis

There are no specific laboratory findings in hepatitis A. Patients generally have significant elevations in serum aminotransferases (500–5000 IU/L), with ALT usually higher than AST. Mild-to-moderate elevations in bilirubin can be seen, and occasionally prolonged prothrombin time and decreased serum albumin (frequently associated with ALF). Alkaline phosphatase is generally normal or only minimally elevated. Other laboratory features may include transient neutropenia, atypical lymphocytosis, and non-specific elevations of IgM and total gammaglobulin [1,2].

Hepatitis A is clinically indistinguishable from other causes of acute hepatitis; thus, the diagnosis is based on serologic testing. The presence of IgM anti-HAV antibodies establishes the diagnosis with excellent sensitivity and specificity. Anti-HAV IgM is measurable at the time symptoms develop and can be detected up to 6 months after the acute infection. A small proportion of recently vaccinated persons (8–20%) can have a transient IgM anti-HAV response. Anti-HAV IgM persists in cases of relapsing disease. Thereafter, beginning at convalescence and persisting indefinitely, anti-HAV IgG predominates and confers lifelong immunity. Thus, anti-HAV IgG serves as a marker of prior HAV infection or prior vaccination, while anti-HAV IgM serves as a marker of acute or recent infection [2,7].

Liver biopsy is rarely indicated, but when performed, the pathologic features are similar to those encountered in other forms of acute viral hepatitis, including ballooning of hepatocytes, coagulative necrosis, focal necrosis, portal expansion by mononuclear cell infiltrate, periportal inflammation, and Kupffer cell proliferation. Occasionally, cholestasis may be prominent, and interface hepatitis with or without bridging necrosis is frequently present in severe cases [1].

Differential Diagnosis

A thorough history and physical exam, together with appropriate laboratory tests, can help differentiate HAV from other causes. Useful tests include hepatitis B, C, and E serologies, antinuclear and anti-smooth-muscle antibodies, other bacterial or viral serologies if appropriate, and serum and/or urine drug levels, including acetaminophen and alcohol. In rare instances, patients may harbor more than one viral infection, such as chronic hepatitis B or C with

Table 75.2 Differential diagnosis of acute hepatitis.

Category	Specific condition
Viral hepatitis	Hepatitis A, B, C, D, and E
	Epstein–Barr virus (EBV)
	Cytomegalovirus (CMV)
	Herpes simplex
	Varicella
Bacterial infections	Leptospirosis
	Q fever
	Rocky Mountain spotted fever
	Secondary syphilis
	Typhoid fever
Systemic infections	Bacterial infections
	Tuberculosis
Parasitic infections	Liver flukes
	Toxocariasis
	Toxoplasmosis
Drugs/toxins	Acetaminophen
	Amoxicillin with clavulanic acid
	Isoniazid, rifampin
	Sulfonamides
	Fluconazole, itraconazole
	Antiseizure medications
	Oral contraceptives
	Alcohol
	Herbal supplements
Metabolic	Hyperglycemia
	Hyperthyroidism
	Wilson's disease
Autoimmune diseases	Autoimmune hepatitis
	Systemic lupus erythematosus (SLE)
Vascular	Ischemic hepatitis ("shock liver")
	Budd–Chiari syndrome
Pregnancy-related	Cholestasis of pregnancy
	HELLP syndrome
	Acute fatty liver of pregnancy
Pancreatobiliary disease	Acute cholecystitis
	Acute ascending cholangitis
	Acute pancreatitis
	Pancreatic cancer

HELLP, hemolysis, elevated liver enzymes, and low platelets.

superimposed acute hepatitis A. Occasionally, imaging studies are indicated to exclude both benign and malignant causes of obstructive jaundice [1,2] (Table 75.2).

Case Continued

The patient is prescribed acetaminophen as needed for symptom control. She is advised not to drink alcoholic beverages. Her sexual partner is contacted and is immunized with a first dose of HAV vaccine, as he has not been vaccinated in the past.

The patient recovers completely 2 weeks after initial presentation, and at a 3-month follow-up visit with her primary care physician her liver enzymes have completely normalized.

Therapeutics

Because of the self-limited nature of the disease, there is currently no specific antiviral therapy for acute hepatitis A. Treatment is generally symptomatic, and in the rare cases of ALF management is mainly supportive in an intensive care setting; only sporadically will patients require liver transplantation. Hospitalization is usually not indicated, except in the presence of significant comorbidity, inability to maintain oral intake, or when incipient liver failure is detected, especially in very young and elderly patients, as well as in subjects with underlying advanced liver disease or cirrhosis. All patients with

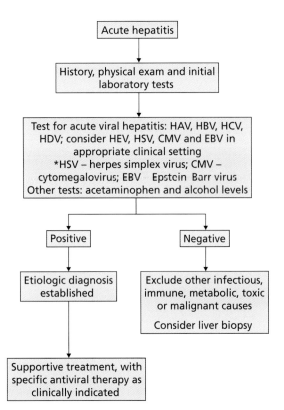

Figure 75.2 Algorithm for the management of acute viral hepatitis. HAV, HBV, HCV, HDV, HEV, hepatitis A–E virus; HSV, herpes simplex virus; CMV, cytomegalovirus; EBV, Epstein–Barr virus.

signs of ALF should be transferred to a tertiary center where liver transplant is available.

Most patients may benefit from judicious use of acetaminophen (not exceeding 2 g per day) or non-steroidal anti-inflammatory drugs (NSAIDs) for systemic symptoms. Steroids and ursodeoxycholic acid have been used in patients with the cholestatic pattern with variable success. Cholestyramine may be used in patients with severe pruritus. Time-honored interventions such as bed rest and dietary restrictions are of no significant benefit. Abstinence from alcoholic beverages seems a reasonable recommendation, albeit one without proven clinical benefit [1, 2] (Figure 75.2).

Prevention

The main measures by which to decrease the risk of HAV transmission, which are especially effective in endemic areas, include adequate sanitation, improvements in environmental hygiene, and safe water supply. Also valuable are hand-washing and special training of food handlers.

International travelers to HAV endemic areas should avoid tap water and undercooked or raw food, as well as beverages that might be contaminated with HAV. No special precautions are required for coworkers, classmates, or casual contacts of subjects infected with HAV, as spread of the disease depends on close person-to-person contact. Compliance with universal precautions in health care settings is sufficient to prevent nosocomial spread of the infection, and no further measures are required [1, 2].

There are currently excellent methods of passive and active immunization to prevent HAV infection. Before the advent of efficacious vaccines, passive immunization through transfer of anti-HAV

antibodies from immunoglobulin was the only available prophylactic measure. A dose of 0.02 mL/kg intramuscularly is 80–90% effective in preventing HAV infection for up to 5 months when administered within 2 weeks after initial exposure. Later administration may still be beneficial, as it has been demonstrated to attenuate the severity of the disease. At present, the worldwide availability of safe and effective HAV vaccines has relegated the use of immunoglobulin to postexposure prophylaxis or passive pre-exposure immunization in pregnant or lactating women and immunocompromised subjects [1, 10].

Since the mid-1990s, the US Food and Drug Administration (FDA) has licensed two formalin-inactivated HAV vaccines to be used in people aged 2 years and older, and since September 2005 in infants older than 1 year. Both commercially available vaccines (Havrix, GlaxoSmithKline; Vaqta, Merck & Co.) are highly immunogenic, with neutralizing antibodies present in 94% of subjects 4 weeks after the first dose and in almost 100% after the second dose. Immunity can last for 25 years or longer in adults and at least 14 years in children and young adults. Immunogenicity decreases in chronic liver disease (seroconversion rate 93%), immunocompromised subjects (88%), advanced cirrhosis (48%), the elderly (65%), and transplant recipients (26%) [11]. Early vaccination is recommended for all patients with chronic hepatitis B and C infection.

The recommended vaccination regimen is a two-dose schedule for both HAV vaccines, with the second dose at 6–18 months after the first. If the second dose is delayed, it can still be given without repeating the initial dose. The two vaccines have pediatric and adult formulations, are generally administered intramuscularly, and are considered interchangeable. They can be administered concomitantly with other vaccines (and even with immunoglobulin) at a different anatomic site, if immediate protection is required [10].

Twinrix is a combined vaccine containing hepatitis A and hepatitis B antigens, approved for persons 18 years and older. It contains a smaller dose of HAV, and is indicated for active immunizations only. The recommended vaccination schedule for Twinrix is 0, 1, and 6 months. An accelerated schedule can be used for pre-exposure protection, in which the three doses are given over 21 days (days 0, 7, and 21–30), with a fourth dose at 1 year.

Current recommendations on immunization and post-exposure prophylaxis to prevent hepatitis A infection are summarized in Table 75.3.

Table 75.3 Summary of current United States Advisory Committee on Immunization Practices recommendations on active and passive immunization for hepatitis A [10, 11].

Pre-exposure protection	Post-exposure prophylaxis
All children should receive HAV vaccination starting at age 1 year Persons at risk for HAV infection: • Travelers to or workers in countries with high or intermediate endemicity • Men who have sex with men (MSM) • Users of injection and non-injection illicit drugs • Persons who work with HAV-infected primates or with HAV in a research laboratory setting (occupational exposure) • Persons with clotting-factor disorders • Persons with chronic liver disease	Unvaccinated persons who have been recently exposed to HAV should receive HAV vaccination or immunoglobulin as soon as possible For healthy individuals 12 months to 40 years old, HAV vaccine is preferred For persons >40 years, immunoglobulin is preferred; vaccine may be used if immunoglobulin is not available For children ≤12 months old, immunocompromised subjects, patients with chronic liver disease, and patients for whom vaccine is contraindicated, immunoglobulin should be used

Prognosis

Prognosis for hepatitis A is excellent; most individuals recover spontaneously, without any lasting sequelae. Patients at greater risk for poor outcomes include those at the extremes of age and those with significant comorbidities, especially those with advanced liver disease or cirrhosis. About 1 out of 5 patients with HAV requires hospitalization. The hospitalization rate increases with age, from 22% among children aged younger than 5 years to 52% among persons aged 60 years or older. In 2007, the overall mortality rate was 0.03 deaths per 100 000 persons, with the highest rate among persons aged ≥75 years [4].

Hepatitis E

Definition and Epidemiology

Hepatitis E is an acute form of generally self-limited, enterally transmitted viral hepatitis. The causative agent is HEV, a spherical, non-enveloped, positive-sense, single-stranded RNA virus that is the sole member of the *Hepevirus* genus in the Hepeviridae family. The HEV genome contains three open reading frames that encode important viral proteins. There are four major genotypes, representing a single serotype. HEV1 and HEV2 are restricted to humans and are transmitted via contaminated water in developing countries, while HEV3 and HEV4 infect humans, pigs, wild boars, dears, rats, and mongooses. HEV3 and HEV4 are mainly transmitted to humans via consumption of raw or undercooked pork or venison [12,13].

Hepatitis E is the most common cause of acute viral hepatitis in developing countries. HEV1 occurs mainly in Asia, HEV2 in Africa and Mexico. HEV3 has a worldwide distribution, while HEV4 mostly occurs in South East Asia, though it has been also isolated in European pigs. Waterborne epidemics are relatively frequent and occur periodically throughout the developing world. Autochthonous HEV infections have been reported in all developed countries. Seroprevalence rates in Europe range from <5 up to 52% in southwest France. The calculated seroprevalence in the United States is 21%, with an incidence of 0.7% based on samples from NHANES 1988–94. Higher prevalence was noted between persons born outside of the United States, and specifically in Mexico. The significant difference between seroprevalences in developed countries and the growing rate of reported HEV cases in China is attributed to the variable sensitivity and specificity of the available diagnostic assays [12,14].

Pathophysiology

In endemic areas, HEV is mainly spread by fecally contaminated water. The documented forms of transmission in developed countries involve foodborne transmission, and, less commonly, transfusion of blood products and vertical transmission. The latter is associated with high neonatal mortality rate. In contrast to HAV, person-to-person transmission is uncommon [13].

After an incubation period of 2–6 weeks, elevated serum aminotransferase levels are detected; they generally remain abnormal for 1–3 months. Peak viremia occurs during the incubation period and becomes undetectable about 3 weeks after the onset of symptoms. The virus is shed in stool for an additional 2 weeks. The initial humoral response (anti-HEV IgM) is detected concomitantly with the rise in aminotransferase levels, only to decline shortly thereafter, though occasionally its persists for up to 5 months after initial

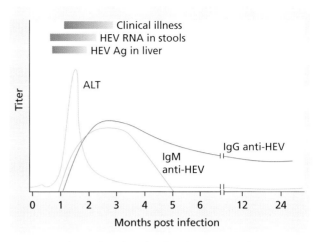

Figure 75.3 Relevant clinical, viral, and serologic events in hepatitis E. Source: Bacon 2006 [8]. Reproduced with permission of Elsevier.

infection. Anti-HEV IgG can be detected a week after the IgM response and confers lifelong immunity [12] (Figure 75.3).

HEV is a non-cytopathic virus, and the host immune response plays an important role in hepatocellular injury. However, the exact mechanism is poorly understood. T-cell proliferative response is decreased in immunocompromised patients, organ transplant recipients, and those with fulminant hepatitis E [13].

Clinical Features

The spectrum of diseases in HEV is highly variable, and the presentation is similar to that of HAV (Table 75.1). In the majority of cases, HEV is an asymptomatic or self-limiting illness that lasts 4–6 weeks. Acute icteric hepatitis is more common in elderly males and persons who drink alcohol regularly. Some patients will develop a more protracted course, characterized by significant cholestasis with persistent jaundice and pruritus, which will ultimately resolve spontaneously [12] (Figure 75.3).

HEV3 causes chronic infection, defined as persistent HEV RNA in serum or stool for 3–6 months, or more in immunocompromised patients [15]. Most solid-organ transplant (SOT) patients have no symptoms when infected with HEV, approximately 60% fail to clear the virus and develop chronic hepatitis, and 10% can progress to cirrhosis. There is no correlation between HEV RNA concentration and liver fibrosis progression. Tacrolimus-based immunosuppressive regimens, rather than cyclosporine and thrombocytopenia, are the most important predictive factor for chronic HEV [16].

Extrahepatic manifestations occur in 5% of patients infected with HEV1 or HEV3; they include GBS, Bell's palsy, acute transverse myelitis, acute meningoencephalitis, membranoproliferative or membranous glomerulonephritis, acute pancreatitis, and severe thrombocytopenia [12].

Though infrequent, ALF has been well described in hepatitis E. In some regions of the world, it accounts for a majority of viral hepatitis-related ALF, particularly among pregnant women. Additionally, patients with underlying chronic liver disease are at higher risk for decompensation, ALF, and death if infected [12].

Diagnosis

In acute infection, aminotransferase levels range between 1000 and 3000 IU/L, while in chronic infection they are typically around

300 IU/L. Tests currently available for hepatitis E are IgM and IgG anti-HEV antibodies, HEV RNA in stool or serum, and IgG avidity. The accuracy of currently available assays for IgM and IgG antibodies varies significantly, and a confirmative test using molecular techniques (rising reactivity of a specific IgG assay or positivity in immunoblot IgM assay) is usually required. The presence of anti-HEV IgG indicates recent or remote infection, while anti-HEV IgM indicates recent infection and may be found in the early phase of clinical symptoms and persist for 4–5 months. The detection of HEV RNA is consistent with current acute or chronic infection. HEV RNA in serum or stool is the diagnostic test of choice for chronic HEV in immunosuppressed patients, as seroconversion to anti-HEV antibodies is delayed or may never occur [17].

Liver biopsy is not required to diagnose hepatitis E, and there are no pathognomonic findings. Two histopathologic patterns have been described in HEV outbreaks: a cholestatic pattern, with prominent bile deposits in canaliculi and hepatocytes (58%), and a more typical hepatocellular pattern, with "ballooning," hepatocyte degeneration, and acidophilic body formation (42%). Liver biopsies in immunosuppressed patients reveal dense lymphocytic infiltration in expanded portal tracts with variable interface hepatitis and fibrosis [13, 18].

Differential Diagnosis

The differential diagnosis is given in Table 75.2. Importantly, HEV can be mistaken for drug-induced liver injury (DILI), with different studies showing 3–13% of patients initially diagnosed as DILI had acute HEV [19].

Therapeutics

Acute HEV is usually a self-limited disease. Like HAV, it requires no treatment. Patients with acute severe HEV3 infection or acute-on chronic liver disease may benefit from short-course ribavirin therapy.

Data on the treatment of chronic HEV in SOT recipients are mainly based on case reports and case series. Reduction in immunosuppression should be the first line of management of liver transplant recipients with chronic HEV. This results in viral clearance in approximately one-third of patients. Pegylated IFN-α-2a for 3–12 months should be considered if this is unsuccessful. In lung, heart, and kidney transplant recipients, treatment with IFN is contraindicated due to a high risk of rejection. Reduction of immunosuppression may not be safe in these patients. Ribavirin monotherapy for 3 months has been used instead, with a sustained virological response of up to 85%. Currently, there is no safe therapy for pregnant patients with ALF [12, 13, 20].

Prevention

Preventive measures include community-wide sanitation, personal hygiene, and clean water sources. In developed countries, avoidance of undercooked meat and shellfish and proper handling of pig feces can prevent infection.

Two vaccines have been studied in clinical trials. The first has completed phase II trial in Nepal, where it showed high immunogenicity and an efficacy of 95%. The second, HEV239, has already completed phase III trial, where it was found to be well tolerated, with an efficacy of 100%. Preliminary data in pregnant women show HEV239 is safe for both mother and fetus, but further studies are warranted [21].

Prognosis

Most immunocompetent patients with hepatitis E will have spontaneous recovery. ALF is common among pregnant patients, reaching up to 20%. Mortality rates in population surveys range between 0.1 and 0.6%; during epidemics they are 0.2–4.0%, and in pregnant women they reach 10–25%. Acute HEV in pregnancy is associated with increased rates of abortions, stillbirths, and neonatal death. Other risk factors include malnutrition, chronic liver disease, and immunosuppression [12].

Other Viruses

Other viral agents, commonly causing systemic virosis, may result in liver involvement, and must be considered in the differential diagnosis of acute hepatitis, especially when hepatitis A through E have been excluded. Clinical manifestations range from asymptomatic elevations in aminotransferases to ALF, with more prominent disease in infants and immunocompromised individuals.

Frequent offenders in this category include members of the herpesvirus family, adenoviruses, enteroviruses, and human parvovirus B-19 [22].

Herpesvirus Family

Herpesviruses are a family of large enveloped DNA viruses that infect a wide range of hosts. Herpesviruses known to infect humans include herpes simplex virus types 1 and 2 (HSV-1, -2), varicella zoster virus (VZV), cytomegalovirus (CMV), human herpesvirus types 6, 7, and 8 (HHV-6, -7, -8), and Epstein–Barr virus (EBV). Following primary infection, herpesviruses have the ability to produce latent infection for life. Reactivation can lead to recurrent disease or invasive infection and is generally triggered by host immunosuppression. Tissue damage may result from direct viral cellular injury, immune-mediated cytotoxicity, or neoplastic transformation [22, 23].

Herpes Simplex Virus

HSV infection is common and may result in a wide variety of clinical presentations, including mucocutaneous, neurologic, and visceral involvement. HSV hepatitis can occur in neonates (resulting in a high mortality rate), pregnant women, immunocompromised persons, and immunocompetent adults. In a review of the Mayo Clinic experience with ALF from 1974 to 1982, 2 of 34 cases were secondary to HSV [22].

HSV hepatitis during pregnancy is generally seen as a manifestation of primary infection and may result in ALF. Mucocutaneous lesions are absent in half of patients, and up to 25% of cases are diagnosed only at autopsy. HSV is an uncommon cause of liver disease in immunocompetent adults, but 14% of healthy individuals with acute genital herpes have mild asymptomatic elevation in aminotransferases. In immunocompromised hosts, HSV hepatitis may be the result of primary or, rarely, recurrent infection. Clinical features include fever, nausea and vomiting, abdominal pain, leukopenia, thrombocytopenia, and markedly elevated liver injury tests. Serologic diagnosis is unreliable, so liver biopsy is sometimes necessary to establish the diagnosis. Typical findings include hemorrhagic or coagulative necrosis of hepatocytes, limited mononuclear cell infiltrate, and intranuclear inclusions (Cowdry type A). Molecular confirmation is recommended. The treatment of choice is high-dose intravenous acyclovir, but valacyclovir or famciclovir may be used as a second-line therapy [23, 24].

Varicella Zoster Virus

Primary VZV infection results in varicella (chickenpox), while reactivation results in herpes zoster (shingles). Varicella in children may be accompanied by asymptomatic mild aminotransferase elevation in up to 28% of cases. In immunocompetent adults, primary infection infrequently results in severe hepatitis and occasionally ALF. Primary VZV infection in immunocompromised individuals can have devastating effects, including ALF-related mortality, which has been frequently described in SOT and hematopoietic stem cell transplant recipients, patients with acute leukemia, and patients with acquired immunodeficiency syndrome (AIDS) [23, 24].

Diagnosis relies on identification, by immunohistochemical analysis or polymerase chain reaction (PCR) techniques, of VZV within liver tissue. Viremia may be detected before clinical manifestations of infection are apparent, allowing for early diagnosis and treatment. The antiviral agent of choice is intravenous acyclovir. Prophylaxis in hematopoietic stem cell transplantation (HSCT) recipients may delay, but not prevent, disseminated herpes zoster [24].

Cytomegalovirus

CMV infection is frequent in the general population, with a seroprevalence of 70–80% among young adults. Infection in the immunocompetent host is generally asymptomatic, but can present as mononucleosis syndrome accompanied by mild elevations in liver enzymes or jaundice, which resolve spontaneously. Diagnosis of CMV hepatitis should be established with a combination of features: appropriate clinical setting, exclusion of other causes, and detection of CMV within liver tissue (viremia *per se* does not confirm the diagnosis) [22, 24].

CMV hepatitis is generally a manifestation of disseminated disease in severely immunocompromised patients, and is the most common organ-specific complication of CMV infection after liver transplantation, especially among seronegative recipients (26%). Clinical features include fever, jaundice, and significant elevation of aminotransferases, which can lead to liver dysfunction if not promptly treated [24].

Liver biopsy findings include portal mononuclear cell infiltrates, giant multinucleated cells, microscopic granulomas, multifocal necrosis, and biliary stasis. Classic "owl's eye" inclusions can be found within hepatocytes and bile duct epithelial cells [22, 24].

Ganciclovir, foscarnet, and cidofovir are antiviral agents available to treat CMV infection. Treatment may not be indicated in mild cases of CMV hepatitis in otherwise healthy individuals. High-risk liver transplant patients, defined as seronegative recipients of a graft from a CMV seropositive donor, should receive ganciclovir prophylaxis for the first few months after transplantation [23].

Epstein–Barr Virus

EBV infection has a worldwide distribution, with a prevalence of 90% in adult populations. It is generally transmitted through saliva, but parenteral and sexual transmissions have been documented. EBV has special tropism to B and T lymphocytes. Clinically, it is the most common cause of infectious mononucleosis and is the causative agent for a number of hematologic malignancies, including post-transplant lymphoproliferative disorder (PTLD) [22, 23].

Liver involvement in EBV infection is common, but generally manifests as transient and self-limited elevations in aminotransferases (80–90%) or hyperbilirubinemia (<10%) within the course of mononucleosis. Histologic findings include minimal swelling and vacuolization of hepatocytes, with lymphocytic and monocytic portal infiltration. Severe cholestasis and liver failure are uncommon in immunocompetent individuals, but have been described in patients with recent organ transplantation or with immunodeficiency from AIDS, X-linked lymphoproliferative disease (Duncan's disease), or chemotherapy. Some authors have described "chronic" hepatitis in the setting of chronic EBV infection [23, 24].

No reliable diagnostic criteria for EBV hepatitis are available, so diagnosis should be based at present on the combination of the following parameters: elevated aminotransferases, EBV serology consistent with active infection, typical histology, and demonstration of viral DNA in liver tissue. Antiviral therapy with acyclovir or ganciclovir is warranted in severe cases of EBV hepatitis, especially in immunosuppressed patients [24].

Take Home Points

- Hepatitis A virus (HAV) and hepatitis E virus (HEV) are enterally transmitted RNA viruses that share common clinical features.
- The epidemiology of hepatitis A is changing as a consequence of worldwide vaccination efforts.
- Clinical presentation of HAV and HEV are commonly indistinguishable from other forms of acute hepatitis, and a broad differential diagnosis must be considered. HEV has to be ruled out in patients with suspected drug-induced liver injury (DILI).
- Diagnosis of acute hepatitis A relies on detection of serum anti-HAV immunoglobulin M (IgM), while that of hepatitis E is based on anti-HEV IgM, rising titers of anti-HEV IgG, and/or HEV polymerase chain reaction (PCR) in serum or stool.
- The clinical course of hepatitis A is generally self-limited, with occasional atypical presentations such as cholestatic hepatitis, relapsing hepatitis, and acute liver failure (ALF).
- Genotype 3 HEV can cause chronic infection in immunosuppressed patients. The diagnosis should be established by persistent serum or stool HEV RNA using molecular methods.
- Mortality is greater in hepatitis E than in hepatitis A, especially in pregnant patients, who have a case fatality rate of up to 25%.
- Effective immunoprophylaxis for hepatitis A is widely available, while a safe and effective recombinant HEV vaccine has completed phase III clinical trials.
- Effective treatment for chronic HEV in solid-organ transplant (SOT) includes reduction of immunosuppression, ribavirin, or interferon (IFN) treatment.

References

1 Shouval D. Hepatitis A. In: Boyer TD, Manns MP, Sanyal AJ, eds. *Zakim and Boyer's Hepatology: A Textbook of Liver Disease*, 6th edn. Philadelphia, PA: Saunders Elsevier, 2012: 531–9.

2 Watson J, Sjogren MH. Hepatitis A and E. In: Schiff ER, Maddrey WC, Sorrel MF, eds. *Schiff's Diseases of the Liver*, 11th edn. Hoboken, NJ: Willey-Blackwell, 2012: 521–36.

3 Velasco-Mondragon E, Lindong I, Kamangar F. Determinants of anti-hepatitis A seroprevalence in 2- to 19-year olds in the USA using NHANES 2007–2008. *Epidemiol Infect* 2012; **140**: 417–25.

4 Centers for Disease Control and Prevention. Surveillance for viral hepatitis – United States, 2011. Available from: http://www.cdc.gov/hepatitis/Statistics/2011Surveillance/index.htm (last accessed February 15, 2016).

5 Lee WM, Squires RH, Nyberg SL, *et al.* Acute liver failure: summary of a workshop. *Hepatology* 2008; **47**: 1401–15.

6 Manangeeswaran M, Jacques J, Tami C, *et al.* Binding of hepatitis A virus to its cellular receptor 1 inhibits T-regulatory cell function in humans. *Gastroenterology* 2012; **142**: 1516–25.

7 Martin A, Lemon SM. Hepatitis A virus: from discovery to vaccines. *Hepatology* 2006; **43**: S164–72.

8 Bacon BR, O'Grady JG, DiBisceglie AM, Lake JR. *Comprehensive Clinical Hepatology*, 2nd edn. Maryland Heights, MO: Mosby, 2006.

9 Lee WM, Larson AM, Stravitz RT. AASLD position paper: the management of acute liver failure: update 2011. Available from: http://www.aasld.org/practiceguidelines/Documents/AcuteLiverFailureUpdate2011.pdf (last accessed February 15, 2016).

10 Victor JC, Monto AS, Surdina TY, *et al.* Hepatitis A vaccine versus immune globulin for postexposure prophylaxis. *N Engl J Med* 2007; **357**: 1685–94.

11 Craig AS, Schaffner W. Prevention of hepatitis A with hepatitis A vaccine. *N Engl J Med* 2004; **350**: 476–81.

12 Kamar N, Bendall R, Legrand-Abravanel F, *et al.* Hepatitis E. *Lancet* 2012; **379**: 2477–88.

13 Kamar N, Izopet J, Rostaing L. Hepatitis E virus infection. *Curr Opin Gastroenterol* 2013; **29**: 271–8.

14 Framawi MF, Johnson E, Chen S, Pannala PR. The incidence of hepatitis E virus infection in the general population of the USA. *Epidemiol Infect* 2011; **139**: 1145–50.

15 Kamar N, Rostaing L, Legrand-Abravanel F, Izopet J. How should hepatitis E virus infection be defined in organ-transplant recipients? *Am J Transplant* 2013; **13**: 1935–6.

16 Kamar N, Garrouste C, Haagsma EB, *et al.* Factors associated with chronic hepatitis in patients with hepatitis E virus infection who have received solid organ transplants. *Gastroenterology* 2011; **140**: 1481–9.

17 Aggarwal R. Diagnosis of hepatitis E. *Nat Rev Gastroenterol Hepatol* 2013; **10**: 24–33.

18 Sarin SK, Kumar M. Hepatitis E. In: Boyer TD, Manns MP, Sanyal AJ, eds. *Zakim and Boyer's Hepatology: A Textbook of Liver Disease*, 6th edn. Philadelphia, PA: Saunders Elsevier, 2012: 605–28.

19 Davern TJ, Chalasani N, Fontana RJ, *et al.* Acute hepatitis E infection accounts for some cases of suspected drug-induced liver injury. *Gastroenterology* 2011; **141**: 1665–72.

20 Unzueta A, Rakela J. Hepatitis E infection in liver transplant recipients. *Liver Transpl* 2014; **20**: 15–24.

21 Zhu FC, Zhang J, Zhang XF, *et al.* Efficacy and safety of recombinant hepatitis E vaccine in healthy adults: a large-scale randomized, double-blind placebo-controlled, phase 3 trial. *Lancet* 2010; **376**: 895–902.

22 Gallegos-Orozco JF, Rakela-Brodner J. Hepatitis viruses: not always what it seems to be. *Rev Med Chil* 2010; **138**: 1302–11.

23 Cisneros-Herreros JM, Herrero-Romero M. [Hepatitis due to herpes group viruses]. *Enferm Infecc Microbiol Clin* 2006; **24**: 392–7.

24 Biglino A, Rizzetto M. Systemic virosis producing hepatitis. In: Rodés J, Benhamou JP, Blei A, *et al.*, eds. *Textbook of Hepatology: From Basic Science to Clinical Practice*, 3rd edn. Oxford: Blackwell, 2007: 957–73.

CHAPTER 76

Chronic Hepatitis B and D

Vijayan Balan,[1] Jorge Rakela,[1] and Rebecca Corey[2]

[1]Division of Gastroenterology and Hepatology, Mayo Clinic, Scottsdale, AZ, USA
[2]Transplant Center, Mayo Clinic Hospital, Phoenix, AZ, USA

Summary

Current therapeutic options for chronic hepatitis B virus (HBV) infection are associated with effective viral suppression and high genetic resistance barrier; however, complete eradication of HBV, defined as disappearance of hepatitis B surface antigen (HBsAg) and development of antibody to HBsAg (anti-HBs), continues to be a rare event. Three leading professional associations, the American Association for the Study of Liver Disease (AASLD), the European Association for the Study of the Liver (EASL), and the Asian Pacific Association for the Study of the Liver (APASL), have developed therapeutic guidelines for the treatment of chronic HBV infection; their recommendations, though not identical, reflect significant similarities in spite of addressing diverse patient populations.

Though the prevalence of hepatitis delta virus (HDV) infection has declined in certain geographic areas of the world, parts of central and northern Europe have experienced resurgence due to population migrations. Specific treatment options for HDV infection are limited and response rates are generally poor.

Hepatitis B Virus

HBV, a member of the family Hepadnaviridae, is a small (42 nm diameter) enveloped DNA virus that can cause both acute and chronic infections. Patients with chronic HBV infection are also at increased risk for cirrhosis, hepatic decompensation, and hepatocellular carcinoma (HCC).

HBV consists of an inner protein core (HBc) surrounded by an outer lipoprotein envelope (HBs). The inner nucleocapsid or core contains the viral DNA genome, which consists of partially double-stranded DNA in a circular conformation and the virus-encoded HBV polymerase (reverse transcriptase). Despite its small size, HBV is a uniquely efficient virus that uses multiple strategies to maximize the limited coding capacity of its genome. HBV DNA contains overlapping genes that are transcribed in four different open reading frames (ORFs): S for the surface antigen (HBsAg), C for the nucleocapsid (core) (HBcAg) and "e" antigen gene (HBeAg), P for the polymerase gene, and X for the HBx gene. The four ORFs direct the transcription and translation of HBV proteins by using different start codons. As a result, the relatively small genome (approximately 3200 nucleotides) of the HBV virus is able to generate seven different proteins: polymerase protein (POL gene), core antigen, "e" antigen, large, medium, and small surface antigen proteins, and X

protein. HBV easily infects and replicates in hepatocytes, producing high levels of virus particles. Though HBV is a DNA virus, it undergoes a unique replication process utilizing an RNA intermediate. During replication, HBV uses reverse transcription to copy its DNA genome via this intermediate. However, because HBV polymerase, an error-prone enzyme, lacks the ability to proofread, mutations can occur frequently during viral replication. During HBV replication, up to 10^{11} viral particles can be produced per day [1, 2]. Thus, with an estimated polymerase error rate of approximately 1 error per 10^7 bases, the emergence of mutants is a common occurrence [1–3]. Because oral antiviral treatments target the active site of HBV polymerase activity, there has been growing interest in not only identifying, but also improving the treatment options for patients who develop HBV polymerase mutations during antiviral therapy [4].

Eight HBV genotypes, A through H, have been identified, with various geographic distributions. A multicenter study of 694 patients in the United States demonstrated the presence of genotypes A (35%) and D (10%), primarily among Caucasians and African Americans, as well as genotypes B (22%) and C (31%), with a predominance among Asian Americans [5]. Unlike in patients with chronic hepatitis C virus (HCV) infection, HBV genotype testing is not routinely performed in clinical practice. However, preliminary data suggest that the HBV genotype may have prognostic significance as well as predictive value in patients treated with interferon (IFN)- or pegylated IFN-based therapy [6, 7]. For example, patients with chronic HBV genotype B infection have a slower rate of progression to cirrhosis and lower rates of HCC compared to patients with chronic HBV genotype C infection [6, 8–12]. Caucasian patients infected with genotype A respond better to IFN therapy, with an HBeAg seroconversion of 40–50%. Asian patients with genotype B are more likely to respond to IFN therapy when compared with those with genotype C. HBV genotypes do not seem to influence therapeutic response to specific nucleo(s/t)ides. The clinical use of HBV genotypes is limited unless IFN therapy is an option, which is nowadays quite rare.

There are multiple sensitive and specific diagnostic tests by which to monitor response to vaccination, to diagnosis acute or chronic infection, to follow the natural course of HBV infection and establish the stage of infection, and to monitor response to antiviral treatment. Two HBV proteins can be detected in the serum of HBV-infected patients: HBsAg and hepatitis B "e" antigen (HBeAg). HBsAg, an antigen found on the outer lipoprotein envelope of HBV,

Practical Gastroenterology and Hepatology Board Review Toolkit, Second Edition. Edited by Nicholas J. Talley, Kenneth R. DeVault, Michael B. Wallace, Bashar A. Aqel and Keith D. Lindor.
© 2016 John Wiley & Sons, Ltd. Published 2016 by John Wiley & Sons, Ltd. Companion website: www.practicalgastrohep.com

is present in the serum of patients with active (acute or chronic) HBV infection; detectable HBsAg for more than 6 months indicates chronic HBV infection. The presence of HBeAg in a patient's serum indicates active infection with a high level of HBV replication. However, absence of HBeAg can also be seen in patients who have ongoing active viral replication, but due to a mutation in the precore or core promoter regions of the HBV genome, HBe Ag is either not or only poorly produced.

Four HBV-specific antibodies can be measured in serum. The presence of hepatitis B surface antibody (anti-HBs), an antibody against HBsAg, is present in the serum of patients who have developed immunity from vaccination or passive transfer of anti-HBs following administration of hepatitis B immune globulin, or in patients with previous HBV infection who recovered and developed immunity. Recombinant HBV vaccines contain a purified non-infectious HBsAg, and following vaccination, an anti-HBs level ≥10 IU/mL is considered protective. Hepatitis B core antibody (anti-HBc), an antibody against the HBV core antigen, is the first antibody to develop during an acute HBV infection; anti-HBc IgM appears initially, indicating recent exposure/infection, followed by anti-HBc IgG, which persists in the serum of patients following acute HBV infection or during chronic HBV infection. Notably, detection of anti-HBc total indicates current or past HBV infection and is *not* a marker of immunity. Hepatitis B "e" antibody (anti-HBe), an antibody against HBeAg, is present during the recovery phase of acute hepatitis B and among patients with chronic hepatitis B during the inactive carrier phase, when there is no active production of virions. In patients with HBeAg-positive chronic HBV infection, HBeAg seroconversion (loss of HBeAg and appearance of anti-HBe) is an important goal of antiviral therapy.

Lastly, there are several molecular assays that can detect and quantify circulating HBV DNA. HBV DNA detection and measurement are important criteria for determining whether or not a patient needs to receive antiviral therapy. For most assays, quantitative HBV DNA results are reported in IU/mL, or, alternatively, in copies accompanied by a conversion factor based on the international standard established by the World Health Organization (WHO) (1 IU of HBV is equivalent to 5.4 genome equivalents/copy) [13]. Some assays may have different conversion factors, depending upon their variability. In patients with chronic HBV infection, HBV DNA should be monitored consistently, using the same assay

in the same laboratory. In patients with detectable HBV DNA and suspected resistance to antiviral therapy, additional testing can be performed to confirm the presence of specific HBV polymerase mutations conferring genotypic resistance [14].

Natural History of Chronic HBV Infection

The natural history of chronic HBV infection is divided into four phases (Figure 76.1): (i) immune tolerance phase; (ii) immune clearance phase; (ii) inactive carrier phase; and (iv) reactivation phase [15].

The *immune tolerance phase* is the initial phase of infection in patients who acquire HBV infection early in life, and is characterized by the presence of HBeAg and high levels of serum HBV DNA [15]. Despite active viral replication during this phase, evidence of liver disease is often absent, with normal serum aminotransferase levels and minimal or no inflammation on liver histology [17]. Over time, the host immune system begins to mature, resulting in immune-mediated hepatocellular injury, which leads to the *immune clearance phase* [18, 19]. This phase is characterized by the presence of HBeAg, high or fluctuating levels of serum HBV DNA, and high or fluctuating serum aminotransferase levels, as well as active inflammation and often fibrosis on liver histology [20]. Most patients in this phase remain asymptomatic, though some present with a symptomatic flare of hepatitis mimicking acute hepatitis, or even with fulminant hepatic failure [21]. In some patients, these flares precede HBeAg seroconversion: the disappearance of HBeAg and the development of anti-HBe, which culminates in remission of hepatitis activity [22]. In contrast, patients who fail to seroconvert and remain HBeAg-positive continue to be at risk for progressive liver disease, which may result in cirrhosis and hepatic decompensation [23, 24], depending on the duration of the chronic hepatitis and the frequency and severity of flares [24, 25]. In addition, persistent HBeAg positivity in older patients (e.g., >35 years) has been linked with increased risk of HCC [15]. Thus, spontaneous HBeAg seroconversion is an important landmark in the natural history of chronic HBV infection. In most patients, HBeAg seroconversion is accompanied by stabilization of hepatitis, which leads to the *inactive carrier phase* [26]. This phase of chronic HBV infection is characterized by the absence of HBeAg and the presence of anti-HBe, normalization of alanine aminotransferase (ALT) levels, decrease

CHAPTER 76

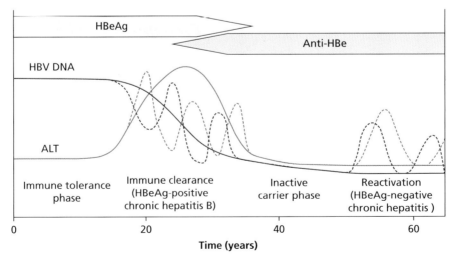

Figure 76.1 Natural course of chronic HBV infection. Source: Lok 2007 [16]. Reproduced with permission of Elsevier.

Table 76.1 Predictors of progressive liver disease in chronic hepatitis B.

	HBeAg-positive	HBeAg-negative
Underlying event	Prolonged interval before HBeAg seroconversion	Persistent viral replication
Phase-specific risk factor	Age >40 Mildly, persistently abnormal ALT Genotype (C > B)	HBV DNA persistence Abnormal ALT Precore/basal core promoter mutation
Overall risk factor	Male Alcohol Co-infection with HCV, HDV, HIV	

HBeAG, hepatitis B "e" antigen; ALT, alanine aminotransferase; HBV, hepatitis B virus; HCV, hepatitis C virus; HDV, hepatitis delta virus; HIV, human immunodeficiency virus.

in HBV DNA to low (<200 IU/mL) or undetectable levels, and, histologically, minimal to mild hepatitis. Most patients remain in this phase for many years, and often for life; this is associated with a reduced risk of subsequent complications from HBV infection [27]. In the remaining patients, hepatitis activity may return, as evidenced by the reappearance of HBV DNA and increased serum ALT (*reactivation phase*). This reactivation of hepatitis may occur with or, more commonly, without reversion to HBeAg positivity. The latter circumstance, namely resumption of hepatitis activity with HBeAg negativity and anti-HBe positivity, is described as HBeAg-negative chronic hepatitis B. Classically, this is associated with mutations in the viral genome that enable viral replication without expressing HBeAg [28]. Importantly, these patients are at risk of progressive liver disease. Because most, if not all, of these patients have gone through the HBeAg-positive chronic hepatitis phase, varying degrees of hepatic fibrosis are already present – some report cirrhosis in up to 40% of such patients [29].

The natural history of HBV infection is complex, not only because of these multiple phases in which patients may present, but also because of differences in the rate at which liver disease progresses. Table 76.1 summarizes the determinants of disease progression, ultimately leading to cirrhosis and/or HCC, in patients with chronic HBV infection.

For HBeAg-positive patients, the central factor in disease progression is the overall duration of hepatitis activity or the number of disease flares before HBeAg seroconversion. This tends to be seen in patients who remain HBeAg-positive beyond 40 years of age, those with mildly and persistently abnormal ALT without seroconversion, and those with genotype C verus genotype B [9, 30].

For patients who are HBeAg-negative, recent studies have shown that persistent viral replication is a key determinant of long-term outcome, including the development of cirrhosis and HCC. The single most important determinant in this patient population is serum HBV DNA level [31, 32]. Chen *et al.* [32] have reported that in patients with undetectable or low HBV DNA levels, the risk of developing HCC is approximately 0.1%/year. This risk increases progressively, such that in patients whose HBV DNA is greater than 1 million copies/mL, the risk of HCC is greater than 1%/year, or approximately 10% over the next 10 years. As with the risk for HCC, patients with undetectable or low-level serum HBV DNA have a low risk of cirrhosis, whereas patients who have serum DNA >1 million copies/mL may have an annual risk of cirrhosis of 2–3%/year, or approximately 25% in the next 10 years. In addition to serum HBV DNA levels, abnormal ALT and the presence of viral mutations such as precore or basal core promoter mutations have also been associated with more advanced liver disease in patients with

HBeAg-negative chronic HBV infection [33]. Finally, regardless of HBeAg status, male patients tend to have more advanced liver disease, as do patients who consume excessive alcohol and those with concomitant viral infections, such as HCV, HDV, and human immunodeficiency virus (HIV) [15].

Table 76.2 compares the recommendations given by the AASLD, EASL, and APASL [34–37]. Though these guidelines originated from different parts of the world, their criteria and recommendations are strikingly similar. The primary criteria for treatment recommendations utilized in all three guidelines include serum HBV DNA level, serum ALT level, HBeAg/anti-HBe status, the presence or absence of cirrhosis, and whether cirrhosis is compensated or decompensated. In addition, the likelihood of treatment response, potential adverse effects of treatment, risk of drug resistance, patient age, family history of HCC, pregnancy or plans for future pregnancy in female patients, cost, and patient preference should all be considered when making treatment decisions.

All three guidelines recommend starting antiviral therapy in patients with severe liver disease, such as acute liver failure, decompensated cirrhosis, or severe reactivation of chronic hepatitis B, regardless of HBV DNA and ALT levels. For patients who require liver transplantation, effective viral suppression reduces the risk of post-transplant HBV recurrence. In contrast, treatment is generally not recommended for patients with minimal disease or patients who are unlikely to achieve a sustained response to antiviral therapy, such as inactive carriers and patients in the immune-tolerant phase. However, because of the fluctuating nature of chronic HBV infection, patients who are not initially started on treatment still require routine clinical and laboratory monitoring and HCC screening. All three guidelines recommend laboratory monitoring at least every 6 months for patients in the immune-tolerant phase, or more frequently if ALT becomes elevated. In patients who are inactive carriers, AASLD guidelines recommend ALT monitoring every 3 months during the first year to confirm that the patients are inactive carriers, and ALT and HBV DNA every 6–12 months thereafter. In patients who have persistently normal ALT levels but fluctuating HBV DNA, EASL guidelines recommend monitoring ALT every 3 months and HBV DNA every 6–12 months.

In addition to laboratory monitoring, all three guidelines recommend HCC screening with either ultrasound (AASLD and EASL) or alpha fetoprotein combined with ultrasound (APASL) every 6 months for cirrhotic patients, patients with a family history of HCC, Asian men >40 years old, Asian women >50 years old, first-generation African Americans >20 years old, and all inactive HBV carriers with persistent or intermittent ALT increases and/or HBV DNA levels >2000 IU/mL.

In patients with compensated cirrhosis, the AASLD and APASL guidelines recommend antiviral therapy if serum HBV DNA level is >2000 IU/mL regardless of ALT level, whereas the EASL guidelines recommend treatment at any detectable HBV DNA level. In addition, if patients with compensated cirrhosis have increased ALT, the AASLD and APASL guidelines recommend antiviral treatment regardless of HBV DNA level.

All three guidelines agree that treatment should be initiated in non-cirrhotic patients with serum HBV DNA levels greater than 20,000 IU/mL and persistently increased ALT levels and/or histologic evidence of moderate/severe inflammation or fibrosis. In non-cirrhotic patients with HBeAg positive chronic HBV infection, an initial 3 to 6 months of observation is recommended to determine if spontaneous HBeAg seroconversion occurs. In non-cirrhotic HBeAg-negative patients with chronic HBV infection,

Table 76.2 Comparison of recommendations given by the American Association for the Study of Liver Diseases (AASLD), European Association for the Study of the Liver (EASL), and Asian Pacific Association for the Study of the Liver (APASL) [34–37]. Source: Lok 2007 [16]. Reproduced with permission of Elsevier.

	AASLD (2009)	APASL (2012)	EASL (2012)
HBV DNA cut-off level, IU/mL			
HBeAg-positive	20 000	20 000	2000
HBeAg-negative	2000–20 000	2000	2000
ALT cut-off level, U/L	30 for men, 19 for women	Traditional cut-off value of 40 U/L	Traditional cut-off value of 40 U/L
Recommendations for treatment and monitoring			
Non-cirrhotic patients			
HBeAg-positive	HBV DNA >20 000 IU/mL ALT >2× ULN Monitor for 3–6 months Treat if no spontaneous HBeAg loss Liver biopsy before treatment is optional	HBV DNA >20 000 IU/mL ALT >2× ULN Monitor for 3–6 months Treat if no spontaneous HBeAg loss Liver biopsy before treatment is optional	HBV DNA >2000 IU/mL ALT > ULN Monitor for 3–6 months Liver biopsy (or non-invasive markers of fibrosis) is recommended Treat if no spontaneous HBeAg loss and if biopsy shows moderate–severe inflammation and/or at least moderate fibrosis
	HBV DNA >20 000 IU/mL ALT ≤ 2× ULN Monitor every 3–6 months Consider biopsy in patients >40 years old, with ALT persistently 1–2× ULN, or with family history of HCC Treat if biopsy shows moderate/severe inflammation or significant fibrosis	HBV DNA >20 000 IU/mL ALT 1–2× ULN Monitor every 1–3 months Consider biopsy in patients >40 years old, with ALT persistently 1–2× ULN, or with family history of HCC Treat if biopsy shows moderate/severe inflammation or fibrosis	HBV DNA >20 000 IU/mL ALT < ULN Monitor every 3–6 months Consider biopsy in patients >30 years old, with ALT persistently 1–2× ULN, or with family history of HCC Treat if biopsy shows moderate–severe inflammation or significant fibrosis
HBeAg-negative	HBV DNA >20 000 IU/mL ALT > 2× ULN Treatment is clearly indicated, liver biopsy is optional HBV DNA 2000–20 000 IU/mL ALT 1–2× ULN Consider liver biopsy Treat if liver biopsy shows moderate/severe inflammation or significant fibrosis	HBV DNA >20 000 IU/mL ALT >2× ULN Treatment is clearly indicated, liver biopsy is optional HBV DNA >2000 IU/mL ALT 1–2× ULN Monitor ALT and HBV DNA every 1–3 months Consider liver biopsy if patient is ≥40 years old Treat if biopsy shows moderate–severe inflammation or fibrosis	HBV DNA >20 000 IU/mL ALT >2× ULN Treatment is clearly indicated, liver biopsy is optional HBV DNA >2000 IU/mL ALT > ULN Liver biopsy (or non-invasive markers of fibrosis) is recommended Treat if biopsy shows moderate–severe inflammation and/or at least moderate fibrosis
	HBV DNA ≤2000 IU/mL ALT ≤ ULN Monitor	HBV DNA ≤2000 IU/mL ALT ≤ ULN Monitor	HBV DNA ≤2000 IU/mL ALT ≤ ULN Monitor
Patients with cirrhosis			
Compensated	HBV DNA >2000 IU/mL Treat regardless of ALT level HBV DNA <2000 IU/mL Consider treatment if ALT > ULN	HBV DNA >2000 IU/mL Treat regardless of ALT level HBV DNA <2000 IU/mL Consider treatment if ALT > ULN	HBV DNA detectable Treat regardless of ALT level
Decompensated	Regardless of HBV DNA or ALT level, treat and refer for liver transplantation	Regardless of HBV DNA or ALT level, treat and refer for liver transplantation	Regardless of HBV DNA and ALT level, treat and refer for liver transplantation

HBV, hepatitis B virus; HBeAG, hepatitis B "e" antigen; ALT, alanine aminotransferase; ULN, upper limit of normal; HCC, hepatocellular carcinoma.

pretreatment observation is not required. Notably, though the overall recommendations are similar, the cut-off values of HBV DNA and ALT levels and the need for liver biopsy to determine treatment indications vary slightly among the three guidelines [37].

Recommendations for the treatment of *non-cirrhotic HBeAg-positive and HBeAg-negative patients* are summarized in Table 76.2.

Table 76.3 summarizes the antiviral agents currently used in the treatment of chronic hepatitis B. In patients identified as appropriate candidates for antiviral therapy, the primary treatment goals are to achieve sustained suppression of HBV replication and prevent progression of liver disease. Currently, there are seven treatment options approved by the US Food and Drug Administration (FDA) for chronic HBV treatment: standard IFN, pegylated interferon alfa-2a (PEG-IFN alfa-2a), lamivudine, adefovir dipivoxil, entecavir, telbivudine, and tenofovir disoproxil fumarate. A non-FDA-approved combination tablet containing a fixed dose of tenofovir and emtricitabine is also occasionally used off-label for the treatment of chronic HBV infection. Among the FDA-approved treatment options, entecavir, tenofovir, and PEG-IFN alfa-2a are considered first-line therapy by all three guidelines [34]. These

agents are not only potent but also the least prone to the development of viral resistance. Second-line agents include lamivudine, telbivudine, and adefovir [34]. Though lamivudine and telbivudine have intermediate to high potency against HBV, they are limited by the emergence of resistant HBV mutants during therapy. Adefovir is limited by its low potency, intermediate resistance profile, and potential nephrotoxicity. If an IFN-based therapy is used for treatment, PEG-IFN is preferred, due to the convenience of once-weekly injection and its improved tolerability compared to standard IFN.

Though IFN- and PEG-IFN-based therapies have the advantages of a finite duration of treatment, more durable viral response after treatment discontinuation, and a higher rate of HBeAg and HBsAg loss or seroconversion (particularly in genotype A), the benefits are not without risks. IFN/PEG-IFN therapy is costly, must be administered parenterally (by subcutaneous injection), requires frequent laboratory monitoring, is poorly tolerated due to flu-like symptoms and cytopenias, and may cause ALT flares during treatment. In order to avoid hepatic decompensation, APASL guidelines recommend avoiding IFN- or PEG-IFN-based therapy in patients with

Table 76.3 Response rates and genotypic resistance rates to approved therapies in HBeAg-positive and HBeAg-negative patients. Source: Adapted from Keeffe 2008 [38]. Reproduced with permission of Elsevier.

Treatment response parameter	Approved therapies						
	Lamivudine	Adefovir dipivoxil	Entecavir	Telbivudine	Tenofovir disoproxil fumarate	PEG-IFN[a]	PEG-IFN + lamivudine[a]
HBeAg-positive patients at week 48 or 52							
Undetectable HBV DNA level, %	36–44	13–21	67	60	76	25	69
HBeAg seroconversion, %	16–21	12–18	21	22	21	27	24
HBsAg loss, %	<1	0	2	0	3	3	3–7
Histologic improvement, %[b]	49–56	53	72	65	74	38	41
Genotypic resistance, %	27	0	0	4.4	0	0	4–11
During extended treatment[c]							
Undetectable HBV DNA level	39 (2)	39 (5)	94 (5)	79 (4)	97 (5)	19 (3.5)[c]	26 (3)[c]
HBeAg seroconversion	47 (3)	48 (5)	41 (5)	42 (4)	40 (5)	37 (3.5)[c]	25 (3)[c]
HBsAg loss	0–3 (2–3)	2 (5)	5 (2)	1.3 (2)	10 (5)	11 (3.5)[c]	15 (3)[c]
Genotypic resistance	65 (5)	42 (5)	1.2 (6)	21 (2)	0 (5)	0	NA
HBeAg-negative patients at week 48 or 52							
HBsAg loss, %	<1	0	<1	<1	0	4	3
Histologic improvement, %[b]	60–66	64–69	70	67	72	48	38
Genotypic resistance, %	23	0	0.2	2.7	0	0	1
During extended treatment[c]							
Undetectable HBV DNA level, %	6 (4)	67 (5)	NA	84 (4)	99 (5)	18 (3)[d]	13 (3)[d]
HBsAg loss, %	<1 (4)	5 (5)	NA	<1 (2)	0.3 (5)	8 (3)[d]	8 (3)[d]
Genotypic resistance, %	70–80 (5)	29 (5)	NA	8.6 (2)	0 (5)	0	NA

[a]Liver biopsy was performed at week 72 or 78, 24 weeks after stopping treatment.
[b]Histologic improvement was defined as a ≥2-point decrease in necroinflammatory score and no worsening of fibrosis score.
[c]The time point at which response was assessed in years from start of treatment is shown in parentheses.
[d]Assessment was performed while off treatment.

ALT greater than five times the upper limit of normal. Furthermore, all three guidelines recommend avoiding IFN and PEG-IFN therapy in patients with acute liver failure, decompensated cirrhosis, or severe reactivation of chronic HBV infection. Though APASL guidelines indicate that IFN or PEG-IFN can be used in carefully selected patients with compensated cirrhosis, AASLD guidelines prefer that these patients be treated with nucleo(s/t)ide analogues, due to the risk of hepatic decompensation or hepatitis flares associated with IFN or PEG-IFN.

Nucleoside (lamivudine, entecavir, telbivudine) and nucleotide (adefovir, tenofovir) analogues can be administered orally, are well tolerated, and, with the exception of adefovir, have potent antiviral activity. All of the oral nucleo(s/t)ide analogues are eliminated renally and therefore require dosage adjustment in patients with renal impairment. In general, nucleo(s/t)ide analogues are well tolerated; though tenofovir and adefovir may cause nephrotoxicity, tenofovir appears less likely to cause acute kidney injury, and in a phase III trial only 1% of patients reported increased serum creatinine after 5 years of treatment. A significant obstacle encountered with earlier nucleo(s/t)ide analogue therapy was the high rate of antiviral drug resistance during therapy. For example, resistance to lamivudine increases with duration of therapy, and has been reported in 16–32, 42, and 60–70% of patients after 1, 2, and 5 years of treatment, respectively. Newer agents (e.g., entecavir and tenofovir) have much higher barriers to resistance. Resistance rates of 1.2 and 0.0% were reported after 5 years of treatment for entecavir and tenofovir, respectively. However, it should be noted that when entecavir is used in patients with lamivudine-resistant HBV infection, resistance rates can be as high as 51% after 5 years of treatment. Determining the most appropriate duration of therapy for oral nucleo(s/t)ide analogues can be challenging because, unlike IFN or PEG-IFN, oral therapy for HBV does not have a finite duration, and discontinuation of therapy can lead to acute hepatitis exacerbations. According to the AASLD guidelines [34], the duration of nucleo(s/t)ide analogue treatment depends primarily

on HBeAg status and whether or not a patient has compensated cirrhosis. Among patients with HBeAg-positive chronic hepatitis, treatment should be continued for 6 months after HBeAg is seroconverted, HBV DNA has become undetectable, and anti-HBe has become detectable. Several studies have shown that HBeAg seroconversion accomplished by nucleo(s/t)ide analogue therapy is followed by up to 70% virologic relapse [39, 40]. Because HBeAg seroconversion induced by oral nucleo(s/t)ide analogue may not be durable, patients should be monitored closely if antiviral therapy is discontinued.

Among patients with HBeAg-negative chronic hepatitis B, treatment should be continued until the patient has become HBsAg-negative. Due to the low rates of HBsAg loss and seroconversion on oral nucleo(s/t)ide therapy, treatment is often indefinite. A recent publication from Asia reported that among patients with HBeAg-negative chronic hepatitis B who had fulfilled the stopping rule recommended by the APASL guidelines [41], which is treatment discontinuation if HBV DNA becomes undetectable for ≥6 months, there was an overall 1-year relapse rate of 45%. The authors recommended that a consolidation therapy for >64 weeks may be more appropriate [42]. Regardless of HBeAg status, HBV DNA, and ALT, patients with decompensated cirrhosis should be treated indefinitely with nucleo(s/t)ide analogue treatment.

Table 76.3 compares the potency of these anti-HBV agents, as represented by the proportion of patients with undetectable HBV DNA after 1 year of therapy in their respective registration trials [37]. It should be noted that these data are not obtained from face-to-face comparison of these agents, and they therefore must be regarded as a general comparison. Among HBeAg-positive patients, 13–76% of those in registration trials achieved undetectable HBV DNA after 1 year of therapy [43–47]. Similarly, among HBeAg-negative patients, undetectable HBV DNA was achieved in 63–93% [44, 46, 48, 49]. The percentage of HBV DNA seroconversion in this latter group is higher because, in general, HBeAg-negative patients tend to have low levels of HBV DNA before therapy.

Conclusion

The main decisions to be made by a clinician managing a patient with chronic HBV infection are (i) when to consider therapy and (ii) what agent(s) to use. The advent of potent antiviral agents with low susceptibility to resistance has revolutionized the treatment of chronic HBV infection. However, as previously mentioned, there is still some disagreement about treatment candidacy. As with medicine in general, individual patient management decisions must be based on risks and benefits of treatment; that is, on the primary benefits of antiviral therapy, include avoidance of long-term complications of HBV infection such as cirrhosis and HCC. Premature initiation of antiviral therapy may have disadvantages, including potential safety concerns in patients receiving long-term antiviral therapy. Because chronic HBV infection is often not curable and many patients may remain on suppressive antiviral therapy for decades, knowledge regarding the long-term safety of current therapies will continue to evolve… It is reassuring, however, that, to date, no significant long-term safety issues have emerged. Other important potential disadvantages of continuing long-term oral antiviral therapy are the possibility of antiviral resistance and the cumulative cost. Though the innate susceptibility to resistant mutation is lower with current first-line agents, patient compliance is a major risk factor for antiviral mutations. Patients who are exposed to intermittent antiviral courses are at higher risk of developing mutations. Non-adherence may be inadvertent or intentional, with the latter often driven by the cost. Newer antiviral agents tend to be more expensive, particularly if prescription coverage is limited; as a result, the costs associated with long-term antiviral therapy can become a significant barrier to medication adherence if patients cannot afford to pay them. The long-term cumulative expense associated with long-term antiviral therapy should be considered before embarking upon antiviral therapy that may last for decades.

Hepatitis Delta Virus

HDV is a small (26 nm diameter), defective, single-stranded, circular RNA virus [50]. There are eight genotypes (1–8) of HDV: HDV-1 is distributed worldwide, whereas HDV-2–8 are found more locally. HDV is a defective virus and can only infect and replicate within individuals who have coexisting HBV infection. The HDV RNA genome is capable of self-cleavage through a ribozyme and encodes only one structural protein, the hepatitis delta antigen (HDAg), from the antigenomic RNA. There are two forms of HDAg: a shorter (S; 22 kDa) and a longer (L; 24 kDa) form. The S form is essential for viral genomic replication. The L form participates in the assembly and formation of HDV. For complete replication and transmission, HDV depends on HBV – specifically, HBsAg. Several diagnostic tests are available for diagnosing and monitoring patients with HDV infection, including anti-HDV IgM antibody, which indicates acute infection, and anti-HDV IgG antibody, which indicates previous infection and remains positive even after viral clearance. In addition, qualitative HDV RNA can be measured in the serum of patients with active HDV replication and quantitative HDV RNA, which can be used to monitor response to antiviral therapy.

HDV infection can occur with simultaneous transmission of both HBV and HDV or via superinfection in patients who already have chronic HBV infection. Rates of HDV infection are generally more common in geographic areas where HBV is endemic, but the prevalence of HDV infection can vary and appears to be increasing in parts of central and northern Europe. In patients with acute HDV and HBV infection, clearance of HDV is dependent upon the host immune response and the ability to eradicate HBV. In patients with chronic HBV infection, clearance of HDV can only be achieved if antiviral therapy is able to eradicate HBV infection. Importantly, chronic HDV superinfection leads to more severe liver disease than chronic HBV alone, with an accelerated course of fibrosis progression, an increased risk of HCC, and early decompensation in the setting of established cirrhosis. Treatment of chronic HDV infection is particularly challenging because, unlike HBV and HCV, HDV does not have an enzymatic function (e.g., HBV polymerase) that can be used as a target for antiviral therapy. Nucleo(s/t)ide analogues are not effective at specifically reducing HDV replication. Currently, IFN and PEG-IFN are the only antiviral agents with activity against HDV infection. The current treatment recommendation is a weekly dose of PEG-IFN alfa-2b 1.5 µg/kg, or PEG-IFN alfa-2a 180 µg per week for 12 months. A sustained viral response, defined as undetectable serum HDV-RNA, can occur in approximately 20–47% of patients. Predictors of a sustained virologic response include a low HBsAg level, low HDV-RNA titers, and an elevated baseline ALT. HDV may relapse in patients if they remain HBsAg-positive [51]. Overall, current treatment options for HDV are quite limited and response rates to antiviral therapy are generally poor. However, increased understanding and ongoing research may help to identify novel agents for HDV treatment. For example, because prenylation of large HDAg is essential for viral assembly and secretion, prenylation inhibitors – drugs that can affect the interactions between the large HDV antigen and HBsAg in the HDV virion – may be useful potential treatments for HDV infection in the future.

The epidemiology of HDV infection is evolving, and there has been a significant decline of HDV in endemic areas – such as the Mediterranean basin – in association with HBV vaccination programs. However, immigration of patients with recent HDV infections to Europe has been associated with a resurgence of delta hepatitis [52]; this epidemiological change makes more pressing the need for an effective therapy for HDV.

Take Home Points

- Hepatitis B virus (HBV) genotype testing is not routinely performed in clinical practice.
- Patients with chronic HBV genotype B infection have a slower rate of progression to cirrhosis and lower rates of hepatocellular carcinoma (HCC) compared to patients with chronic HBV genotype C infection.
- HBsAg is present in the serum of patients with active (acute or chronic) HBV infection. Detectable HBsAg for more than 6 months indicates chronic HBV infection. The presence of HBeAg in a patient's serum indicates active infection with a high level of HBV replication. Absence of HBeAg can be seen in patients who have ongoing active viral replication, but in whom due to a mutation in the precore or core promoter regions of the HBV genome, HBeAg is either not or only poorly produced. Anti-HBs is present in the serum of patients who have developed immunity to vaccination or passive transfer of anti-HBs following administration of hepatitis B immune globulin and in patients with previous HBV infection who recovered and developed immunity.
- Anti-HBc is the first antibody to develop during an acute HBV infection. Detection of total anti-HBc indicates current or past HBV infection and is not a marker of immunity. Anti-HBe is present in the recovery phase of acute hepatitis B and in the inactive carrier phase of patients with chronic hepatitis B.
- Among patients with HBeAg-positive chronic hepatitis, treatment should be continued for 6 months after HBeAg has been seroconverted, HBV DNA has become undetectable, and anti-HBe has become detectable. Among patients with HBeAg-negative chronic hepatitis B, treatment should be continued until the patient has become HBsAg-negative.

- Regardless of HBeAg status, HBV DNA, and ALT, patients with decompensated cirrhosis should be treated indefinitely with nucleo(s/t)ide analogue treatment.
- Patients who are exposed to intermittent antiviral courses are at higher risk of developing mutations for 12 months.
- HDV infection can occur with simultaneous transmission of both HBV and HDV or via superinfection in patients who already have chronic HBV infection.
- PEG-IFN is the only antiviral agent with activity against HDV infection.
- Predictors of a sustained virologic response include a low HBsAg level, low HDV-RNA titers, and an elevated baseline ALT.

References

1 Coleman PF. Detecting hepatitis B surface antigen mutants. *Emerg Infect Dis* 2006; **12**: 198–203.

2 Harrison TJ. Hepatitis B virus: molecular virology and common mutants. *Semin Liver Dis* 2006; **26**: 87–96.

3 Horvat RT. Diagnostic and clinical relevance of HBV mutations. *Lab Medicine* 2011; **42**: 488–96.

4 Pawlotsky JM, Dusheiko G, Hatzakis A, *et al.* Virologic monitoring of hepatitis B virus therapy in clinical trials and practice: recommendations for a standardized approach. *Gastroenterology* 2008; **134**: 405–15.

5 Chu CJ, Keeffe EB, Han SH, *et al.* Hepatitis B virus genotypes in the United States: results of a nationwide study. *Gastroenterology* 2003; **125**: 444–51.

6 Chu CJ, Hussain M, Lok AS. Hepatitis B virus genotype B is associated with earlier HBeAg seroconversion compared with hepatitis B virus genotype C. *Gastroenterology* 2002; **122**: 1756–62.

7 Yang HI, Yeh SH, Chen PJ, *et al.* Associations between hepatitis B virus genotype and mutants and the risk of hepatocellular carcinoma. *J Natl Cancer Inst* 2008; **100**: 1134–43.

8 Chan HL, Hui AY, Wong ML, *et al.* Genotype C hepatitis B virus infection is associated with an increased risk of hepatocellular carcinoma. *Gut* 2004; **53**: 1494–8.

9 Kao JH, Wu NH, Chen PJ, *et al.* Hepatitis B genotypes and the response to interferon therapy. *J Hepatol* 2000; **33**: 998–1002.

10 Chu CM, Liaw YF. Genotype C hepatitis B virus infection is associated with a higher risk of reactivation of hepatitis B and progression to cirrhosis than genotype B: a longitudinal study of hepatitis B e antigen-positive patients with normal aminotransferase levels at baseline. *J Hepatol* 2005; **43**: 411–17.

11 Sumi H, Yokosuka O, Seki N, *et al.* Influence of hepatitis B virus genotypes on the progression of chronic type B liver disease. *Hepatology* 2003; **37**: 19–26.

12 Yu MW, Yeh SH, Chen PJ, *et al.* Hepatitis B virus genotype and DNA level and hepatocellular carcinoma: a prospective study in men. *J Natl Cancer Inst* 2005; **97**: 265–72.

13 Sorrell MF, Belongia EA, Costa J, *et al.* National Institutes of Health consensus development conference statement: management of hepatitis B. *Ann Intern Med* 2009; **150**: 104–10.

14 Lok AS, Zoulim F, Locarnini S, *et al.* Antiviral drug-resistant HBV: standardization of nomenclature and assays and recommendations for management. *Hepatology* 2007; **46**: 254–65.

15 Yim HJ, Lok AS. Natural history of chronic hepatitis B virus infection: what we knew in 1981 and what we know in 2005. *Hepatology* 2006; **43**: S173–81.

16 Lok AS. Navigating the maze of hepatitis B treatments. *Gastroenterology* 2007; **132**: 1586–94.

17 Chang MH, Hwang LY, Hsu HC, *et al.* Prospective study of asymptomatic HBsAg carrier children infected in the perinatal period: clinical and liver histologic studies. *Hepatology* 1988; **8**: 374–7.

18 Tsai SL, Chen PJ, Lai MY, *et al.* Acute exacerbations of chronic type B hepatitis are accompanied by increased T cell responses to hepatitis B core and e antigens. Implications for hepatitis B e antigen seroconversion. *J Clin Invest* 1992; **89**: 87–96.

19 Chu CM, Liaw YF. Intrahepatic distribution of hepatitis B surface and core antigens in chronic hepatitis B virus infection. Hepatocyte with cytoplasmic/membranous hepatitis B core antigen as a possible target for immune hepatocytolysis. *Gastroenterology* 1987; **92**: 220–5.

20 Liaw YF, Pao CC, Chu CM, *et al.* Changes of serum hepatitis B virus DNA in two types of clinical events preceding spontaneous hepatitis B e antigen seroconversion in chronic type B hepatitis. *Hepatology* 1987; **7**: 1–3.

21 Lok AS, Liang RH, Chiu EK, *et al.* Reactivation of hepatitis B virus replication in patients receiving cytotoxic therapy. Report of a prospective study. *Gastroenterology* 1991; **100**: 182–8.

22 Liaw YF, Chu CM, Su IJ, *et al.* Clinical and histological events preceding hepatitis B e antigen seroconversion in chronic type B hepatitis. *Gastroenterology* 1983; **84**: 216–19.

23 Fattovich G, Brollo L, Giustina G, *et al.* Natural history and prognostic factors for chronic hepatitis type B. *Gut* 1991; **32**: 294–8.

24 Liaw YF, Tai DI, Chu CM, Chen TJ. The development of cirrhosis in patients with chronic type B hepatitis: a prospective study. *Hepatology* 1988; **8**: 493–6.

25 McMahon BJ, Holck P, Bulkow L, Snowball M. Serologic and clinical outcomes of 1536 Alaska Natives chronically infected with hepatitis B virus. *Ann Intern Med* 2001; **135**: 759–68.

26 Lok AS, Heathcote EJ, Hoofnagle JH. Management of hepatitis B: 2000 – summary of a workshop. *Gastroenterology* 2001; **120**: 1828–53.

27 de Franchis R, Meucci G, Vecchi M, *et al.* The natural history of asymptomatic hepatitis B surface antigen carriers. *Ann Intern Med* 1993; **118**: 191–4.

28 Brunetto MR, Giarin MM, Oliveri F, *et al.* Wild-type and e antigen-minus hepatitis B viruses and course of chronic hepatitis. *Proc Natl Acad Sci USA* 1991; **88**: 4186–90.

29 Papatheodoridis GV, Dimou E, Dimakopoulos K, *et al.* Outcome of hepatitis B e antigen-negative chronic hepatitis B on long-term nucleos(t)ide analog therapy starting with lamivudine. *Hepatology* 2005; **42**: 121–9.

30 Yuen MF, Yuan HJ, Wong DK, *et al.* Prognostic determinants for chronic hepatitis B in Asians: therapeutic implications. *Gut* 2005; **54**: 1610–14.

31 Iloeje UH, Yang HI, Su J, *et al.* Predicting cirrhosis risk based on the level of circulating hepatitis B viral load. *Gastroenterology* 2006; **130**: 678–86.

32 Chen CJ, Yang HI, Su J, *et al.* Risk of hepatocellular carcinoma across a biological gradient of serum hepatitis B virus DNA level. *JAMA* 2006; **295**: 65–73.

33 Naoumov NV, Schneider R, Grotzinger T, *et al.* Precore mutant hepatitis B virus infection and liver disease. *Gastroenterology* 1992; **102**: 538–43.

34 Lok AS, McMahon BJ. Chronic hepatitis B: update 2009. *Hepatology* 2009; **50**: 661–2.

35 EASL. EASL clinical practice guidelines: management of chronic hepatitis B virus infection. *J Hepatol* 2012; **57**: 167–85.

36 Liaw YF, Kao JH, Piratvisuth T, *et al.* Asian-Pacific consensus statement on the management of chronic hepatitis B: a 2012 update. *Hepatol Int* 2012; **6**: 531–61.

37 Yapali S, Talaat N, Lok AS. Management of hepatitis B: our practice and how it relates to the guidelines. *Clin Gastroenterol Hepatol* 2014; **12**: 16–26.

38 Keeffe EB, Dieterich DT, Han SH, *et al.* A treatment algorithm for the management of chronic hepatitis B virus infection in the United States: 2008 update. *Clin Gastroenterol Hepatol* 2008; **6**(12): 1315–41.

39 Reijnders JGP, Perquin MJ, Zhang N, *et al.* Nucleos(t)ide analogues only induce temporary hepatitis B e antigen seroconversion in most patients with chronic hepatitis B. *Gastroenterology* 2010; **139**: 491–8.

40 Chaung KT, Ha NB, Trinh HN, *et al.* High frequency of recurrent viremia after hepatitis B e antigen seroconversion and consolidation therapy. *J Clin Gastroenterol* 2012; **46**: 865–70.

41 Liaw YF, Leung N, Kao JH, *et al.* Asian-Pacific consensus statement on the management of chronic hepatitis B: a 2008 update. *Hepatol Int* 2008; **2**: 263–83.

42 Jeng WJ, Sheen IS, Chen YC, *et al.* Off-therapy durability of response to entecavir therapy in hepatitis B e antigen-negative chronic hepatitis B patients. *Hepatology* 2013; **58**: 1888–96.

43 Chang TT, Gish RG, de Man R, *et al.* A comparison of entecavir and lamivudine for HBeAg-positive chronic hepatitis B. *N Engl J Med* 2006; **354**: 1001–10.

44 Marcellin P, Heathcote EJ, Buti M, *et al.* Tenofovir disoproxil fumarate versus adefovir dipivoxil for chronic hepatitis B. *N Engl J Med* 2008; **359**: 2442–55.

45 Lau GK, Piratvisuth T, Luo KX, *et al.* Peginterferon Alfa-2a, lamivudine, and the combination for HBeAg-positive chronic hepatitis B. *N Engl J Med* 2005; **352**: 2682–95.

46 Lai CL, Gane E, Liaw YF, *et al.* Telbivudine versus lamivudine in patients with chronic hepatitis B. *N Engl J Med* 2007; **357**: 2576–88.

47 Marcellin P, Chang TT, Lim SG, *et al.* Adefovir dipivoxil for the treatment of hepatitis B e antigen-positive chronic hepatitis B. *N Engl J Med* 2003; **348**: 808–16.

48 Lai CL, Shouval D, Lok AS, *et al.* Entecavir versus lamivudine for patients with HBeAg-negative chronic hepatitis B. *N Engl J Med* 2006; **354**: 1011–20.

49 Hadziyannis SJ, Tassopoulos NC, Heathcote EJ, *et al.* Adefovir dipivoxil for the treatment of hepatitis B e antigen-negative chronic hepatitis B. *N Engl J Med* 2003; **348**: 800–7.

50 Hughes SA, Wedemeyer H, Harrison PM. Hepatitis delta virus. *Lancet* 2011; **378**: 73–85.

51 Rizzetto M. Current management of delta hepatitis. *Liver Int* 2013; **33**(Suppl. 1): 195–7.

52 Rizzetto M. Hepatitis D: clinical features and therapy. *Dig Dis* 2010; **28**: 139–43.

CHAPTER 77

Hepatitis C

Michael Charlton[1] and Travis Dick[2]

[1] Mayo Clinic, Rochester, MN, USA
[2] Intermountain Medical Center, Murray, UT, USA

Summary

The introduction of new direct-acting antiviral (DAA) agents against hepatitis C virus (HCV) has dramatically altered the landscape of treatment for HCV. The advent of DAA therapy for HCV infection began in 2013 with approvals of sofosbuvir (a prodrug of a nucleotide analogue inhibitor of the HCV NS5B RNA-dependent RNA polymerase) and simeprevir (a NS3/4A protease inhibitors), with rapid uptake into treatment protocols. The pace of change has accelerated with subsequent approvals of ledipasvir, ombitasvir, and daclatasvir (NS5A inhibitors), the NS3/4A protease inhibitor paritaprevir, and the non-nucleoside polymerase inhibitor dasabuvir. Approvals of grazoprevir (a NS3/4A protease inhibitor) and of elbasvir and velpatasvir (NS5A inhibitors) are likely.

In order to provide health care professionals with timely guidance as new therapies become available and integrated into HCV regimens, the Infectious Diseases Society of America (IDSA) and the American Association for the Study of Liver Diseases (AASLD), in collaboration with the International Antiviral Society – USA (IAS–USA), have developed a Web-based process for the rapid formulation and dissemination of evidence-based, expert-developed recommendations for hepatitis C management. The reader is referred to the AASLD/IDSA/IAS guidelines Web site for in-depth recommendations and rationales (www.hcvguidelines.org). The AASLD/IDSA/IAS guidelines represent the work of leading authorities in the prevention, diagnosis, and treatment of hepatitis C infection. Michael Charlton is a member of the panel that developed the AASLD/IDSA/IAS guidelines. This chapter is a distillation of the most current recommendations.

Diagnosis and Evaluation

Of the ~4 million persons chronically infected with HCV in the United States, up to three-quarters are unaware that they are infected [1]. HCV is primarily transmitted through percutaneous exposure. While HCV can be transmitted from mother to infant and through non-injection drug use (e.g., snorting with a device), sexual transmission is unusual except among human immunodeficiency virus (HIV)-infected men who have unprotected sex with men. Injection of recreational drugs currently accounts for around two-thirds of acute HCV infections in the United States. Other notable risk factors for transmission of HCV include receipt of blood products before 1992, receipt of clotting factor concentrates before 1987, long-term hemodialysis, needle-stick injuries among health care workers, previous incarceration, and being tattooed. Current Centers for Disease Control and Prevention (CDC) guidelines are to offer a one-time HCV test to *all* persons born between 1945 and 1965 (referred to as the birth cohort), regardless of the presence of any other risk factor. Patients born before 1945 or after 1965 should be tested based on exposures, behaviors, and conditions that increase risk for HCV infection (Figure 77.1). HCV cannot be spread by water, food, air, hugging, coughing/sneezing, or sharing eating utensils.

Initial screening for HCV infection should be with HCV antibody (anti-HCV) [3]. A positive anti-HCV test indicates either current (active) HCV infection (acute or chronic), past infection that has resolved, or a false-positive test result [4] and should be followed by nucleic acid testing (NAT) to determine the presence of viremia (active infection). HCV RNA testing should also be considered in persons with a negative anti-HCV test who are immunocompromised (e.g., persons receiving chronic hemodialysis) or who might have been exposed to HCV within the last 6 months. A quantitative or qualitative NAT with a detection level of 25 IU/mL or lower should be used to detect HCV RNA.

Prior to the initiation of HCV therapy, quantitative HCV RNA testing is necessary to document the baseline level of viremia (i.e., viral load). Testing for HCV genotype is currently important in the selection of the most appropriate treatment regimen and should be performed in all patients for whom treatment is contemplated.

HBV and HIV co-infection have been associated with poorer prognosis in patients with HCV infection [5]. Because risk factors for these infections overlap, persons with HCV should be tested for HIV antibody and hepatitis B surface antigen (HBsAg). Because obesity and metabolic syndrome are risk factors for fibrosis progression in HCV-infected persons [6,7], HCV-infected persons who are overweight or obese should be counseled regarding strategies to reduce weight and improve insulin resistance [8]. Statins can be safely administered to patients with chronic HCV or compensated chronic liver disease, for whom cardiovascular disease (CVD) is a more common cause of mortality than liver disease [9].

A thorough physical exam (e.g., to look for stigmata of cirrhosis), routine blood tests (e.g., serum alanine transaminase, albumin, bilirubin, International Normalized Ratio (INR) levels, and complete blood cell (CBC) counts with platelets), liver imaging (e.g., ultrasound, computed tomography (CT) scan), and liver

Practical Gastroenterology and Hepatology Board Review Toolkit, Second Edition. Edited by Nicholas J. Talley, Kenneth R. DeVault, Michael B. Wallace, Bashar A. Aqel and Keith D. Lindor.
© 2016 John Wiley & Sons, Ltd. Published 2016 by John Wiley & Sons, Ltd. Companion website: www.practicalgastrohep.com

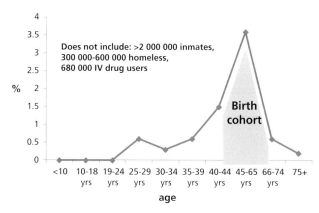

Figure 77.1 Current prevalence of HCV infection in the United States. Source: Ditah 2014 [2]. Reproduced with permission of Elsevier.

elastography should be obtained in patients diagnosed with HCV infection. Assessment of liver surface nodularity and spleen size (e.g., by liver ultrasound) is essential to determining the likelihood of cirrhosis and portal hypertension [10, 11]. The role of liver biopsies in defining the severity of disease is changing. Patients with clear evidence of cirrhosis/portal hypertension (e.g., hepatic nodularity on ultrasound) do not need liver biopsy to stage disease. While a liver biopsy can help assess the severity of liver fibrosis and inflammation andp to exclude competing causes of liver injury [12], biopsies are expensive and subject to sampling error, and carry risks of morbidity and mortality. Liver elastography can provide instant information regarding liver stiffness at the point of care, but can only reliably distinguish cirrhosis from non-cirrhosis [13]. Since persons with bridging fibrosis and cirrhosis are at increased risk of developing complications of advanced liver disease, especially hepatocellular carcinoma, they require 6–12-monthly imaging surveillance for liver cancer and 1–3-yearly screening for varices [14, 15].

When and Who to Treat

The goal of HCV therapy is to achieve a virological *cure*, often referred to as a "sustained virological response" (SVR) and defined as the continued absence of detectable HCV RNA for *at least 12 weeks* after completion of therapy. SVR at $\geq$12 weeks after the end of treatment has been shown to be durable indefinitely for >99% of patients [16, 17]. Documentation of SVR requires a quantitative or qualitative NAT with a detection level of 25 IU/mL or lower.

Benefits of SVR include a decrease in liver inflammation and a reduction in the rate of progression of liver fibrosis [18], in addition to an improved sense of well being, loss of stigma, and enhanced performance status [19]. In a study of over 3000 patients with pre- and post-treatment biopsies (biopsies separated by a mean of 20 months), about three-quarters of those who achieved an SVR had improvement in liver fibrosis [20], with cirrhosis resolving in half of these cases. SVR is also associated with a >70% reduction in the risk of liver cancer (hepatocellular carcinoma) and a 90% reduction in the risk of liver-related mortality and liver transplantation [21, 22]. Cure of HCV infection also reduces morbidity and mortality from extrahepatic manifestations of HCV infection, including cryoglobulinemic vasculitis [23], non-Hodgkin's lymphoma, and other lymphoproliferative disorders [24]. Patients achieving SVR also experience improved quality of life. For all of these reasons, HCV-infected patients should be offered antiviral therapy with the goal of achieving an SVR, preferably early in the course of their chronic

HCV infection. Current therapies for HCV infection are sufficiently safe and well tolerated that there are few absolute contraindications to treatment. Potential barriers to initiation include medical or psychiatric comorbidities, lack of acceptance of treatment (e.g., mild/early liver disease with competing priorities), and lack of access to treatment [25]. The most common barrier is lack of access.

Curing HCV infection is associated with numerous benefits, including a decrease in liver inflammation and fibrosis [18]. Of 3010 treatment-naïve HCV-infected patients with pretreatment and posttreatment biopsies (separated by a mean of 20 months), cirrhosis resolved in half of those who achieved an SVR [18]. Clinical manifestations of advanced liver disease also improved. High priority should be given to treating patients at the highest risk for liver-related complications (i.e., those with advanced fibrosis, Metavir F3 or F4), transplant recipients, patients with HIV co-infection, and patients with clinically severe extrahepatic manifestations (e.g., renal insufficiency). An algorithm for screening of more advanced liver disease is presented in Figure 77.2.

Treatment

Table 77.1 is a grid of recommended and alternative regimens for HCV treatment that are specific to HCV genotype and other factors that affect optimal choice of antiviral agents and duration of treatment, derived from seminal reports of phase 2 and 3 clinical trials [26–41]. The evidence available to inform decision-making and recommendations is evolving rapidly. There are specific considerations for persons with HIV/HCV co-infection, compensated and decompensated cirrhosis (moderate or severe hepatic impairment; CTP class B or C), post-liver-transplant HCV, and severe renal impairment, which merit detailed consideration.

Several DAA agents have recently been approved by regulatory authorities in the United States and Europe (Table 77.2). In 2013, sofosbuvir, a prodrug of a nucleotide analogue inhibitor of the HCV NS5B RNA-dependent RNA polymerase with efficacy against all HCV genotypes, was approved. Simeprevir, an inhibitor of the HCV NS3/4A protease, with efficacy against HCV genotype 1, was also approved in 2013. In 2014, ledipasvir, an inhibitor of the HCV NS5A with efficacy against genotypes 1, 3, and 4, was approved for use in fixed-dose combination with sofosbuvir. Later in the same year, a complex regimen of direct antiviral agents, referred to for brevity as the "3D combination" (reflecting the presence of three DAAs), was approved for HCV genotype 1. The 3D regimen consists of the fixed-dose combination of the NS3/4A protease inhibitor paritaprevir (boosted with the cytochrome P450 inhibitor ritonavir), coformulated with the NS5A inhibitor ombitasvir, as well the non-nucleoside polymerase inhibitor dasabuvir, with or without ribavirin. In 2015, daclatasvir (an NS5A inhibitor) was approved for treatment of HCV genotype 3 infection. Based on the results of a phase 3 clinical trial, regulatory approval of grazoprevir (GRZ, a NS3/4A protease inhibitor) and of elbasvir and velpatasvir (ELB and VEL, both NS5A inhibitors) is anticipated.

PEG-IFN has been supplanted as a routine therapy for HCV infection.

Genotype 1

As much as it has been hoped that the advent of DAAs would bring great simplification of HCV treatment, the choice of treatment for patients with HCV genotype 1 continues to vary with:
1 prior treatment experience;
2 HCV subtype (i.e., genotype 1a vs.1b);

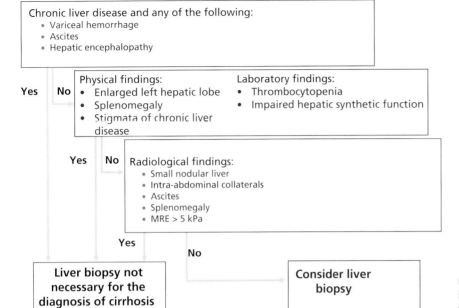

Figure 77.2 Diagnostic algorithm for investigating the presence of cirrhosis in patients with chronic liver disease.

Table 77.1 Hepatitis C virus (HCV) treatment grid.

Geno-type	Recommended Regimens	Alternative #1	Alternative #2	Other Alternatives
1	GZV + EBV × 12 weeks **if genotype 1b** **(need RAV testing for geno 1a:** **Add RBV and treat for 16 weeks if RAVs detected)** (**Not** recommend in **de**compensated cirrhosis* or liver transplant) OR: SOF + LDV** × **12 weeks**	3D (non-cirrhotic only)	SOF + DCV × **12 weeks** (non-cirrhotic only) Caveat: If compensated cirrhosis OR treatment experienced give SOF + DCV + RBV × **24 weeks** Caveat: If **de**compensated* cirrhosis, give SOF +DCV + RBV × **12** **(with RBV) −24** **(without RBV) weeks**	None
	Caveat #1 \ Caveat #2 \ If *all* of the following: \ **1.** Treatment naïve \ **2.** No cirrhosis \ **3.** HCV RNA < 6 million \ Give × **8 weeks** \ \ If *any one* of the following \ **1.** Cirrhosis (any class) \ **2.** Liver transplant \ Give SOF + LDV + RBV × **12 weeks** \ If RBV ineligible: \ SOF + LDV × **24 weeks**	Genotype 1a *OR* undifferentiated 3D + RBV × **12 weeks** \ Genotype 1b \ 3D × **12 weeks**		
2	SOF + RBV × **12 weeks** Caveat: If fibrosis stage 3-4, give SOF + RBV × **16 weeks**	SOF + DCV × **12 weeks** Caveat: If cirrhotic and RBV intolerant give SOF + DCV × **24 weeks** Caveat: If **de**compensated* cirrhosis, give SOF +DCV + RBV × **12 weeks**		None
3	SOF + DCV × **12 weeks** Caveat: If compensated cirrhosis OR SOF treatment experienced, give SOF + DCV + RBV × **24 weeks** Caveat: If **de**compensated* cirrhosis, SOF +DCV + RBV × **12 (with RBV) -24 (without RBV) weeks**	SOF + LDV + RBV × **12 weeks**	SOF + RBV × **24 weeks**	None
4	SOF + LDV × **12 weeks** Caveat: If previous SOF treatment failure, give SOF + LDV + RBV × **12 weeks**	GZV + EBV × **12 weeks** (**Not** recommend in **de**compensated cirrhosis* or liver transplant)	OBV/PTV/r + RBV × **12 weeks** (non-cirrhotic only)	SOF + RBV × **24 weeks**
5 or 6	SOF + LDV × **12 weeks** Caveat: If previous SOF treatment failure, or liver transplant give SOF + LDV + RBV × **12 weeks**	GZV + EBV + RBV × **12 weeks (Genotype 5)** GZV + EBV × **12 weeks (Genotype 6)** (**Not** recommend in **de**compensated cirrhosis* or liver transplant)	SOF + RBV × **24 weeks**	None

*Decompensated cirrhosis defined by *currently treated* hepatic encephalopathy or ascites OR Child-Pugh-Turcotte Class B or C.
**Velpatasvir is likely to replace LDV if regulatory approval is granted.
Fixed dose combination of SOF/VEL for 12 weeks is effective for patients with chronic HCV infection genotypes 1, 2, 3, 4, 5 and 6 who are treatment inexperienced and non-DAA experienced with non-cirrhotic or compensated cirrhotic stage disease.
Fixed dose combination of SOF/VEL + RBV for 12 weeks is effective for patients with decompensated cirrhosis of any genotype.

Table 77.2 Antiviral abbreviations, dosing, and notes.

Abbreviation	Drug Name	Dosing		Precautions/Notes
3D	Ombitasvir/Paritaprevir/Ritonavir plus Dasabuvir (Viekira®)	12.5/75/50 mg per tablet, take 2 tablets po qam plus 250 mg po bid		Multiple drug-drug interactions—consult pharmacist Discontinue all ethinyl estradiol prior to 3D initiation Avoid in cirrhosis
DCV	Daclatasvir	60 mg po daily Dose adjustments needed for drug interactions		Multiple drug-drug interactions—consult pharmacist
GZV/EBV	Grazoprevir/Elbasvir	100 mg/50 mg per tablet po daily		Multiple drug-drug interactions—consult pharmacist Screening for baseline elbasvir NS5A RAVs at position 28, 30, 31, and 93 should be performed in patients with HCV **genotype 1a** infection who are being considered for GZV/EBV
LDV	Ledipasvir	90 mg po daily		Should *not* be on proton pump inhibitor if possible Maximum famotidine dose 40 mg/day (If on H2 receptor antagonist, give LDV with cranberry or orange juice)
OBV/PTV/r	Ombitasvir/Paritaprevir/Ritonavir (Technivie®)	75/50 mg per tablet, take 2 tablets po qam		Multiple drug-drug interactions—consult pharmacist Discontinue all ethinyl estradiol prior to initiation Avoid in cirrhosis
RAV	Resistance associated variant			Screening for baseline elbasvir NS5A RAVs at position 28, 30, 31, and 93 should be performed in patients with HCV **genotype 1a** infection who are being considered for GZV/EBV
RBV	Ribavirin	**< 75 kg** 400 mg po qam & 600 mg po qpm	**≥ 75 kg** 600 mg po bid	Causes anemia *See also HCV Supportive Care and Renal Dosing Protocol*
SOF	Sofosbuvir	400 mg po daily		SOF discontinued in clinical trials if t-bili > 5 mg/dL

Decompensated cirrhosis defined by *currently treated* hepatic encephalopathy or ascites OR Child-Pugh-Turcotte Class B or C.

3 presence of cirrhosis;

4 viral load (to a very minor degree);

5 history of liver transplantation.

The recommendations that follow address variations in treatment based on these factors. It is highly likely that regulatory approval, if provided, of further DAAs with pangenotypic activity other than sofosbuvir (e.g., velpatasvir, ABT493 (NS3/4 protease inhibitor), and ABT530 (NS5A inhibitor)) will greatly simplify treatment algorithms.

Genotype 1a or Undifferentiated Genotype 1

There are multiple recommended treatment options for HCV genotype 1a infection (genotype 1 HCV infection that cannot be subtyped should be treated as genotype 1a infection):

1 Daily ledipasvir (90 mg)/sofosbuvir (400 mg) in fixed-dose combination for 12 weeks.

- For patients with cirrhosis, add weight-based ribavirin.
- For liver transplant recipients (fibrosis stages 0–3 and compensated cirrhosis), add weight-based ribavirin.

Table 77.3 Drugs that are contraindicated with paritaprevir/ritonavir/ombitasvir plus dasabuvir.

Drug class	Contraindicated	Comments
Alpha1-adrenoreceptor antagonists	Alfuzosin HCL	Potential for hypotension
Anticonvulsants	Carbamazepine, phenytoin, phenobarbital	Ombitasvir, paritaprevir, ritonavir, and dasabuvir exposures may decrease, leading to a potential loss of therapeutic activity of VIEKIRA PAK
Antihyperlipidemic agents	Gemfibrozil	Dasabuvir exposures increase 10-fold, which may increase the risk of QT prolongation
Antimycobacterial	Rifampin	Ombitasvir, paritaprevir, ritonavir, and dasabuvir exposures may decrease, leading to a potential loss of therapeutic activity of VIEKIRA PAK
Ergot derivatives	Ergotamine, dihydroergotamine, ergonovine, methylergonovine	Acute ergot toxicity characterized by vasospasm and tissue ischemia has been associated with coadministration of ritonavir and ergonovine, ergotamine, dihydroergotamine, or methylergonovine
Ethinyl estradiol-containing products	Ethinyl estradiol-containing medications such as combined oral contraceptives	Potential for ALT elevations
Herbal products	St. John's Wort (*Hypericum perforatum*)	Ombitasvir, paritaprevir, ritonavir, and dasabuvir exposures may decrease, leading to a potential loss of therapeutic activity of VIEKIRA PAK
HMG-CoA reductase inhibitors	Lovastatin, simvastatin	Potential for myopathy, including rhabdomyolysis
Neuroleptics	Pimozide	Potential for cardiac arrhythmias
Non-nucleoside reverse transcriptase inhibitors	Efavirenz	Coadministration of efavirenz-based regimens with paritaprevir, ritonavir plus dasabuvir is poorly tolerated and results in liver enzyme elevations
Phosphodiesterase-5 (PDE5) inhibitors	Sildenafil when dosed as REVATIO for the treatment of PAH	Increased potential for sildenafil-associated adverse events, such as visual disturbances, hypotension, priapism, and syncope
Sedatives/hypnotics	Triazolam Orally administered midazolam	Triazolam and orally administered midazolam are extensively metabolized by CYP3A4. Coadministration of triazolam or orally administered midazolam with VIEKIRA PAK may cause large increases in the concentration of these benzodiazepines. The potential exists for serious and/or life-threatening events, such as prolonged or increased sedation or respiratory depression

VIEKIRA PAK is contraindicated in patients with known hypersensitivity (e.g., toxic epidermal necrolysis (TEN) or Stevens–Johnson syndrome) to ritonavir.
ALT, alanine aminotransferase; PAH, pulmonary arterial hypertension.

CHAPTER 77

◦ Give a reduced dose of ribavirin, 600 mg/day, increased as tolerated, to liver transplant recipients with Child–Pugh–Turcotte class B or C cirrhosis.

2 Daily fixed-dose combination of paritaprevir (150 mg), ritonavir (100 mg), and ombitasvir (25 mg), plus twice-daily dosed dasabuvir (250 mg) and weight-based ribavirin (1000 mg (<75 kg) to 1200 mg (≥75 mg)) (hereafter referred to as paritaprevir/ritonavir/ombitasvir plus dasabuvir and ribavirin) for 12 weeks (paritaprevir/ritonavir/ombitasvir plus dasabuvir-containing regimens are not appropriate for patients for whom prior treatment with telaprevir or boceprevir has failed).

◦ Should *not* be used in patients with cirrhosis.

◦ Liver transplant recipients should receive 24 weeks (this combination should only be used for patients with fibrosis 0-2 following liver transplantation).

3 Daily fixed-dose combination of grazoprevir (100 mg) and elbasvir (50 mg) in fixed dose combination for 12 weeks (dosing and duration of grazoprevir based on phase 3 study results and given in anticipation of regulatory approval).

◦ *Not* recommended in *de*compensated cirrhosis or liver transplantation.

4 Daily daclatasvir (60 mg) with sofosbuvir (400 mg) for 12 weeks.

◦ Add ribavirin and treat for 24 weeks in case of *compensated* cirrhosis.

◦ Add ribavirin and treat for 12 weeks in patients with *decompensated* cirrhosis. daclatasvir/sofosbuvir/ribavirin for 12 weeks is of equal efficacy to 24 weeks in patients with decompensated cirrhosis.

5 Daily velpatasvir (100 mg)/sofosbuvir (400 mg) in fixed dose combination for 12 weeks (dosing and duration of velpatasvir based on phase 3 study results and given in anticipation of regulatory approval).

◦ Add ribavirin in case of decompensated cirrhosis.

The safety profiles of all of these recommended regimens are excellent. Most adverse events occur in ribavirin-containing arms, with discontinuation rates low even for patients with cirrhosis (approximately 2%). There are, however, some important nuances to using all three regimens.

Genotype 1b

The treatment for chronic infection with HCV genotype 1b is the same as for 1a, with the notable exception that daily fixed-dose combination of paritaprevir paritaprevir/ritonavir/ombitasvir plus dasabuvir for 12 weeks can be given *without ribavirin*.

Nuances for Ledipasvir/Sofosbuvir and Velpatasvir

The daily fixed-dose combination of ledipasvir/sofosbuvir has a critical interaction with acid-suppressing medications. Proton pump inhibitors (PPIs), for example, result in substantially decreased absorption of ledipasvir and velpatasvir. A thorough assessment of PPI use is essential prior to initiation of therapy. Acid-suppressing medications should be held for a week before and during the treatment period. For patients who require acid suppression, famotidine ≤40 mg/day or omeprazole 20 mg/day or equivalent can be provided. Ledipasvir or velpatasvir should be dosed >8 hours after famotidine, with cranberry or orange juice. Patients who are unable to wean off of higher-dose PPIs should be considered for a non-ledipasvir- or velpatasvir-containing treatment protocol.

Following the success of 12 weeks of ledipasvir/sofosbuvir in a phase 3 study of 647 treatment-naïve patients [26], a trial studied the relative efficacy of 8 versus 12 weeks of ledipasvir/sofosbuvir

[27]. Though there was no difference in SVR in the intention-to-treat analysis, relapse rates were higher in the 8-week arm (20 of 431) compared with the 12-week arm (3 of 216). *Post hoc* analyses of baseline predictors of relapse identified lower relapse rates in patients receiving 8 weeks of ledipasvir/sofosbuvir who had low baseline HCV RNA levels (<6 million IU/mL). Only 2% of patients in the study met this low viral load threshold. Thus, the *only* patients who should be considered for an 8-week course of treatment are those who are treatment-inexperienced AND non-cirrhotic AND who have an HCV RNA level of <6 million IU/mL. In practical terms, this represents a very small number of patients. In addition, the *post hoc* nature of the analysis limits confidence in abbreviating duration of therapy. The presence of cirrhosis does *not* alter the efficacy of 12 weeks of ledipasvir/sofosbuvir in treatment-naïve patients.

Postmarketing data with sofosbuvir when coadministered with amiodarone have been associated with symptomatic bradycardia and, in one case, fatal cardiac arrest. Amiodarone should be stopped for a minimum of 4 weeks prior to initiating sofosbuvir.

Nuances for Paritaprevir/Ritonavir/Ombitasvir plus Dasabuvir

The daily fixed-dose combination of paritaprevir/ritonavir/ombitasvir plus dasabuvir and ribavirin was approved by the US Food and Drug Administration (FDA) for the treatment of HCV genotype 1a infection in treatment-naïve patients based on three registration trials [28–32]. This combination comprises 10 pills divided between two doses per day. Overall, virologic failure was higher for patients with HCV genotype 1a (7 of 8) than for patients with HCV genotype 1b. Ribavirin was demonstrated to significantly enhance efficacy (as measured by SVR) in treatment-naïve, HCV genotype 1a-infected patients without cirrhosis compared to study arms without ribavirin (90 vs. 97%, respectively), due to higher rates of virologic failure (7.8 vs. 2.0%, respectively). These results confirm the need for weight-based ribavirin in patients with HCV genotype 1a. For patients with compensated (CTP class A) cirrhosis, 24 weeks of treatment with paritaprevir/ritonavir/ombitasvir plus dasabuvir and ribavirin was seen to be modestly superior to 12 weeks (88.6% in the 12-week arm versus 94.2% in the 24-week arm), primarily driven by treatment-experienced patients with cirrhosis. The difference in efficacy was enough for the FDA to approve 24 weeks for treatment-experienced patients with cirrhosis. There was no difference in SVR rates in the patients with cirrhosis who were naïve to therapy (92.2 and 92.9%, respectively) [30].

Nuances for Simeprevir and for Grazoprevir

A phase 2 clinical trial of sofosbuvir plus simeprevir was conducted in treatment-naïve and treatment-experienced patients, including those with cirrhosis [33]. The study enrolled two cohorts: cohort 1 included patients with a prior null response to peginterferon-based therapy (n = 80, Metavir F0 to F3 fibrosis), and cohort 2 included peginterferon-based therapy-responder and null-responder patients with Metavir stage F3 or F4 fibrosis (n = 87). Each cohort had 12- and 24-week treatment arms, with and without ribavirin, to address length of treatment and the role of weight-based ribavirin. The small size of the study precluded determination of a benefit of extended (24 vs. 12 weeks) therapy or the added value of ribavirin. An ongoing phase 3 study with similar design should clarify these issues. Based on this analysis, the FDA currently recommends 24 weeks for all patients with cirrhosis, regardless of treatment experience. The presence of the Q80K polymorphism does not preclude treatment with simeprevir and sofosbuvir, because the SVR rate was high in patients with HCV genotype 1a and this polymorphism (88%; 51/58).

Because of the potential for cholestasis and a signal for reversible hepatotoxicity, simeprevir should not be used in patients with jaundice or Child–Pugh–Turcotte class B or C cirrhosis.

Grazoprevir has not been used in the post-transplant setting. Based on its pharmacokinetics, important effects can be predicted for common immunosuppression agents, especially cyclosporine, of a similar sort to those for simeprevir. In the absence of real-world data regarding drug–drug interactions between grazoprevir and immunosuppressive agents, we recommend avoiding this agent in the post-transplant setting.

Genotype 2

The following are the recommended treatment options for HCV genotype 2 infection in *treatment-naïve* and *treatment-experienced* patients:

1 Daily sofosbuvir (400 mg) and weight-based ribavirin (1000 mg (<75 kg) to 1200 mg (≥75 kg)) for 12 weeks.
   ○ Extend treatment to 16 weeks in patients with cirrhosis.
2 Daily daclatasvir (60 mg) with sofosbuvir (400 mg) for 12 weeks.
   ○ Add ribavirin and treat for 24 weeks in case of *compensated* cirrhosis.
   ○ Add ribavirin and treat for 12 weeks in patients with *decompensated* cirrhosis. Daclatasvir/sofosbuvir/ribavirin for 12 weeks is of equal efficacy to 24 weeks in patients with decompensated cirrhosis.
3 Daily velpatasvir (100mg)/ sofosbuvir (400mg) in fixed dose combination for 12 weeks (dosing and duration of velpatasvir based on phase 3 study results and given in anticipation of regulatory approval).
   ○ Add ribavirin in case of decompensated cirrhosis.

In total, 201 of 214 (94%) patients with HCV genotype 2 in these trials achieved SVR with sofosbuvir plus ribavirin [34–36]. Ledipasvir does not contribute to the efficacy of treatment of genotype 2 infection. Velpatasvir (a non-structural protein 5a (NS5a) inhibitor) has pangenotypic efficacy [40, 41], providing a possible future option for patients with genotype 2 who fail to respond to sofosbuvir with ribavirin.

Genotype 3

The following are the recommended treatment options for HCV genotype 3 infection in *treatment-naïve* and *treatment experienced* patients:

1 Daily daclatasvir (60 mg) with sofosbuvir (400 mg) for 12 weeks.
   ○ Add ribavirin and treat for 24 weeks in case of *compensated* cirrhosis.
   ○ Add ribavirin and treat for 12 weeks in patients with *decompensated* cirrhosis. Daclatasvir/sofosbuvir/ribavirin for 12 weeks is of equal efficacy to 24 weeks in patients with decompensated cirrhosis.
2 Ledipasvir/sofosbuvir and weight-based ribavirin for 24 weeks for patients *with cirrhosis* who have relapsed following prior sofosbuvir treatment.

The unknown but possible risk of developing sofosbuvir and NS5a resistance suggests that patients with genotype 3 infection without cirrhosis who relapse following sofosbuvir-based therapy should wait for more potent DAA combination therapies.

Genotype 4

The following are the recommended treatment options for HCV genotype 4 infection in *treatment-naïve* patients:

1 Daily fixed-dose combination of ledipasvir (90 mg)/sofosbuvir (400 mg) for 12 weeks.
   ○ Add weight-based ribavirin id if there is prior sofosbuvir experience.
2 Daily fixed-dose combination of grazoprevir (100 mg) and elbasvir (50 mg) for 12 weeks (dosing and duration of grazoprevir based on phase 3 study results and given in anticipation of regulatory approval).
   ○ *Not* recommended in *de*compensated cirrhosis or liver transplantation.
3 Daily fixed-dose combination of paritaprevir (150 mg)/ritonavir (100 mg)/ombitasvir (25 mg) plus twice-daily dosed dasabuvir (250 mg) and weight-based ribavirin (1000 mg (<75 kg) to 1200 mg (≥75 kg)) for 12 weeks.
   ○ Non-cirrhotic patients only.
4 Daily sofosbuvir (400 mg) and weight-based ribavirin (1000 mg (<75 kg) to 1200 mg (≥75 kg)) for 24 weeks.

Though peginterferon and ribavirin for 48 weeks was the previously recommended regimen for patients with HCV genotype 4 infection, adding sofosbuvir to peginterferon and ribavirin increases response rates and markedly shortens therapy, with no apparent additional adverse effects.

Genotypes 5 and 6

There is only one recommended treatment option each for the treatment of HCV genotype 5 and 6 infection in *treatment-naïve* patients:

1 Daily sofosbuvir (400 mg) and weight-based ribavirin (1000 mg (<75 kg) to 1200 mg (≥75 kg)) plus weekly PEG-IFN for 12 weeks for treatment-naïve patients with HCV genotype 5 infection.
   ○ Weekly PEG-IFN plus weight-based ribavirin (1000 mg (<75 kg) to 1200 mg (>75 kg)) for 48 weeks is an alternative regimen for IFN-eligible, treatment-naïve patients with HCV genotype 5 infection.
2 Daily fixed-dose combination of ledipasvir (90 mg)/sofosbuvir (400 mg) for 12 weeks for treatment-naïve patients with HCV genotype 6 infection.
   ○ Daily sofosbuvir (400 mg) and weight-based ribavirin (1000 mg (<75 kg) to 1200 mg (≥75 kg)) plus weekly PEG-IFN for 12 weeks is an alternative regimen for IFN-eligible treatment-naïve patients with HCV genotype 6 infection.

Few data have been generated to help guide decision-making for patients infected with HCV genotype 5 and 6. Nonetheless, for those patients for whom immediate treatment is required, the preceding recommendations have been drawn from available data.

Nuances for Liver Transplantation

In an interim analysis of an ongoing study (TMC435HPC3016), concomitant use of simeprevir (plus daclatasvir and ribavirin) with cyclosporine at steady state resulted in an approximately sixfold increase in plasma concentrations of simeprevir compared with historical data on simeprevir in the absence of cyclosporine. This interaction may be caused by inhibition of organic anion-transporting polypeptide 1B1 (OATP1B1), p-glycoprotein (P-gp), and cytocrome P450 3A (CYP3A) by cyclosporine. Simeprevir should not be coadministered with cyclosporine. Coadministration of single-dose tacrolimus with simeprevir does not result in clinically significant changes in tacrolimus or simeprevir concentrations.

Conclusion

Putting all these data together, we have generated an algorithm by which patients with chronic hepatitis C can be treated. Though treatment of chronic hepatitis C infection has become highly effective and safe, many nuances persist. Careful consideration of patient and viral factors continues to be needed in order to achieve optimal results and, importantly, to avoid critical drug–drug interactions and treatment failures.

References

1 Smith BD, Jewett A, Burt RD. Recommendations for the identification of chronic hepatitis C virus infection among persons born during 1945–1965. *MMWR* 2012; **61**(RR-4): 1–32.

2 Ditah I, Ditah F, Devaki P, *et al.* The changing epidemiology of hepatitis C virus infection in the United States: National Health and Nutrition Examination Survey 2001 through 2010. *J Hepatol* 2014; **60**(4): 691–8.

3 Alter MJ, Seeff LB, Bacon BR, *et al.* Testing for hepatitis C virus infection should be routine for persons at increased risk for infection. *Ann Intern Med* 2004; **141**: 715–17.

4 Pawlotsky JM. Use and interpretation of virological tests for hepatitis C. *Hepatology* 2002; **36**: S65–73.

5 Thein HH, Yi Q, Dore GJ, Krahn MD. Natural history of hepatitis C virus infection in HIV-infected individuals and the impact of HIV in the era of highly active antiretroviral therapy: a meta-analysis. *AIDS* 2008; **22**: 1979–91.

6 Hourigan LF, Macdonald GA, Purdie D, *et al.* Fibrosis in chronic hepatitis C correlates significantly with body mass index and steatosis. *Hepatology* 1999; **29**: 1215–19.

7 Charlton MR, Pockros PJ, Harrison SA. Impact of obesity on treatment of chronic hepatitis C. *Hepatology* 2006; **43**(6): 1177–86.

8 Musso G, Gambino R, Cassader M, Pagano G. A meta-analysis of randomized trials for the treatment of nonalcoholic fatty liver disease. *Hepatology* 2010; **52**: 79–104.

9 Lewis JH, Mortensen ME, Zweig S, *et al.* Efficacy and safety of high-dose pravastatin in hypercholesterolemic patients with well-compensated chronic liver disease: results of a prospective, randomized, double-blind, placebo-controlled, multicenter trial. *Hepatology* 2007; **46**: 1453–63.

10 Chou R, Wasson N. Blood tests to diagnose fibrosis or cirrhosis in patients with chronic hepatitis C virus infection. *Ann Intern Med* 2013; **159**: 372.

11 Rockey DC, Bissell DM. Noninvasive measures of liver fibrosis. *Hepatology* 2006; **43**: S113–20.

12 Kleiner DE, Brunt EM, Van Natta M, *et al.* Design and validation of a histological scoring system for nonalcoholic fatty liver disease. *Hepatology* 2005; **41**: 1313–21.

13 Castera L. Noninvasive methods to assess liver disease in patients with hepatitis B or C. *Gastroenterology* 2012; **142**: 1293–302.e4.

14 Sangiovanni A, Prati GM, Fasani P, *et al.* The natural history of compensated cirrhosis due to hepatitis C virus: a 17-year cohort study of 214 patients. *Hepatology* 2006; **43**: 1303–10.

15 Fontana RJ, Sanyal AJ, Ghany MG, *et al.* Factors that determine the development and progression of gastroesophageal varices in patients with chronic hepatitis C. *Gastroenterology* 2010; **138**: 2321–31.e1–2.

16 Swain MG, Lai MY, Shiffman ML, *et al.* A sustained virologic response is durable in patients with chronic hepatitis C treated with peginterferon alfa-2a and ribavirin. *Gastroenterology* 2010; **139**: 1593–601.

17 Manns MP, Pockros PJ, Norkrans G, *et al.* Long-term clearance of hepatitis C virus following interferon alpha-2b or peginterferon alpha-2b, alone or in combination with ribavirin. *J Viral Hepat* 2013; **20**: 524–9.

18 Poynard T, McHutchison JG, Manns M, *et al.* Impact of pegylated interferon alfa-2b and ribavirin on liver fibrosis in patients with chronic hepatitis C. *Gastroenterology* 2002; **122**: 1303–13.

19 Neary MP, Cort S, Bayliss MS, Ware JE Jr. Sustained virologic response is associated with improved health-related quality of life in relapsed chronic hepatitis C patients. *Semin Liver Dis* 1999; **19**(Suppl. 1): 77–85.

20 Poynard T, McHutchison J, Manns M, *et al.* Impact of pegylated interferon alfa-2b and ribavirin on liver fibrosis in patients with chronic hepatitis C. *Gastroenterology* 2002; **122**: 1303–13.

21 Morgan TR, Ghany MG, Kim HY, *et al.* Outcome of sustained virological responders with histologically advanced chronic hepatitis C. *Hepatology* 2010; **52**: 833–44.

22 Veldt BJ, Heathcote EJ, Wedemeyer H, *et al.* Sustained virologic response and clinical outcomes in patients with chronic hepatitis C and advanced fibrosis. *Ann Intern Med* 2007; **147**: 677–84.

23 Fabrizi F, Dixit V, Messa P. Antiviral therapy of symptomatic HCV-associated mixed cryoglobulinemia: meta-analysis of clinical studies. *J Med Virol* 2013; **85**: 1019–27.

24 Gisbert JP, Garcia-Buey L, Pajares JM, Moreno-Otero R. Prevalence of hepatitis C virus infection in B-cell non-Hodgkin's lymphoma: systematic review and meta-analysis. *Gastroenterology* 2003; **125**: 1723–32.

25 Clark BT, Garcia-Tsao G, Fraenkel L. Patterns and predictors of treatment initiation and completion in patients with chronic hepatitis C virus infection. *Patient Prefer Adherence* 2012; **6**: 285–95.

26 Afdhal N, Zeuzem S, Kwo P, *et al.* Ledipasvir and sofosbuvir for untreated HCV genotype 1 infection. *N Engl J Med* 2014; **370**: 1889–98.

27 Kowdley KV, Gordon SC, Reddy KR, *et al.* Ledipasvir and sofosbuvir for 8 or 12 weeks for chronic HCV without cirrhosis. *N Engl J Med* 2014; **370**: 1879–88.

28 Kwo PY, Mantry PS, Coakley E, *et al.* An interferon-free antiviral regimen for HCV after liver transplantation. *N Engl J Med* 2014; **371**: 2375–82.

29 Ferenci P, Bernstein D, Lalezari J, *et al.* ABT-450/r-ombitasvir and dasabuvir with or without ribavirin for HCV. *N Engl J Med* 2014; **370**: 1983–92.

30 Poordad F, Hezode C, Trinh R, *et al.* ABT-450/r-ombitasvir and dasabuvir with ribavirin for hepatitis C with cirrhosis. *N Engl J Med* 2014; **370**: 1973–82.

31 Feld JJ, Kowdley KV, Coakley E, *et al.* Treatment of HCV with ABT-450/r-ombitasvir and dasabuvir with ribavirin. *N Engl J Med* 2014; **370**: 1594–603.

32 Zeuzem S, Jacobson IM, Baykal T, *et al.* Retreatment of HCV with ABT-450/r-ombitasvir and dasabuvir with ribavirin. *N Engl J Med* 2014; **370**: 1604–14.

33 Lawitz E, Sulkowski MS, Ghalib R, *et al.* Simeprevir plus sofosbuvir, with or without ribavirin, to treat chronic infection with hepatitis C virus genotype 1 in non-responders to pegylated interferon and ribavirin and treatment-naive patients: the COSMOS randomised study. *Lancet* 2014; **384**: 1756–65.

34 Lawitz E, Mangia A, Wyles D, *et al.* Sofosbuvir for previously untreated chronic hepatitis C infection. *N Engl J Med* 2013; **368**: 1878–87.

35 Jacobson IM, Gordon SC, Kowdley KV, *et al.* Sofosbuvir for hepatitis C genotype 2 or 3 in patients without treatment options. *N Engl J Med* 2013; **368**: 1867–77.

36 Zeuzem S, Dusheiko GM, Salupere R, *et al.* Sofosbuvir and ribavirin in HCV genotypes 2 and 3. *N Engl J Med* 2014; **370**: 1993–2001.

37 Sulkowski MS, Gardiner DF, Rodriguez-Torres M, *et al.* Daclatasvir plus sofosbuvir for previously treated or untreated chronic HCV infection. *N Engl J Med* 2014; **370**(3): 211–21.

38 Zeuzem S, Ghalib R, Reddy KR. Grazoprevir-elbasvir combination therapy for treatment-naive cirrhotic and noncirrhotic patients with chronic hepatitis C virus genotype 1, 4, or 6 infection: a randomized trial. *Ann Intern Med* 2015; **163**(1): 1–13.

39 Lawitz E, Gane E, Pearlman B, *et al.* Efficacy and safety of 12 weeks versus 18 weeks of treatment with grazoprevir (MK-5172) and elbasvir (MK-8742) with or without ribavirin for hepatitis C virus genotype 1 infection in previously untreated patients with cirrhosis and patients with previous null response with or without cirrhosis (C-WORTHY): a randomised, open-label phase 2 trial. *Lancet* 2015; **385**(9973): 1075–86.

40 Feld JJ, Jacobson IM, Hézode C *et al.*, Sofosbuvir and velpatasvir for HCV genotype 1, 2, 4, 5, and 6 infection. *N Engl J Med* 2015; **373**: 2599–607.

41 Curry MP, O'Leary JG, Bzowej N, *et al.* Sofosbuvir and velpatasvir for HCV in patients with decompensated cirrhosis. *N Engl J Med* 2015; **373**: 2618–28.

CHAPTER 78

Bacterial and Other Non-viral Infections of the Liver

Maria Teresa A. Seville,[1] Roberto L. Patron,[1] Ann McCullough,[2] and Shimon Kusne[1]

[1]Division of Infectious Diseases, Mayo Clinic, Scottsdale, AZ, USA
[2]Department of Laboratory Medicine and Pathology, Mayo Clinic, Scottsdale, AZ, USA

Summary

The liver parenchyma and biliary tree may be involved in infections caused by bacteria, fungi, and parasites. These occur by spread from contiguous organs or hematogenous seeding, or by toxic effects from distant infections and their treatment. The clinical presentations of these infections vary from no symptoms to hepatitis, abscess, granulomas, biliary obstruction, and liver failure. This chapter summarizes the various infections of the liver and biliary tree and their diagnosis and treatment.

Pyogenic Liver Abscess

Microbiology

The most frequently found organisms are *Escherichia coli* and *Klebsiella pneumoniae*, streptococci, and anaerobes [1–3]. *Bacteroides* spp. is the most common anaerobe [4]. *Streptococcus milleri* is also reported. It is common to grow more than one organism from an abscess aspirate, even if blood cultures yield only one pathogen [1]. There has been an increase in resistant bacteria and *Candida* spp., most likely secondary to use of biliary stents and long courses of antibiotics [5].

A unique syndrome of liver abscess secondary to a virulent *K. pneumoniae* with dissemination to the eye and central nervous system (CNS) has been reported mainly in South East Asia [6,7]. This infection is caused by capsular K1/K2 strains, which have higher resistance to phagocytosis. There is a high prevalence of diabetes in affected patients. Cases of liver abscess with hypermucoviscous *K. pneumoniae* have been reported in the United States, the majority in males of Asian origin. Over 90% of isolates were resistant to ampicillin, but multidrug-resistant isolates were uncommon [8–13].

Epidemiology

Pyogenic liver abscess is a serious infection, with an incidence of 15.0–44.9 per 100,000 patient admissions [1,14]. Earlier series showed higher prevalence in males, but more recent series report equal sex distribution [15]. Most cases occur in the 6th to 7th decades [2,15]. In one series, single and multiple abscesses occurred in 58 and 42%, respectively: 66% in the right lobe, 8% in the left lobe, and 26% in both lobes [16]. Solitary abscesses are usually located in the right lobe, whereas multiple abscesses are found in both sides [17].

Pathogenesis

Mechanisms for liver abscess formation include spread of infection from the biliary tract or the abdomen, hematogenous infection, and unclear source or cryptogenic etiology [14]. Biliary and cryptogenic etiologies are more common; up to a third of cases may be cryptogenic [18]. In the pre-antibiotic era, patients tended to be young, and the major cause was appendicitis. Patients now tend to be older and are more frequently those with benign or malignant biliary obstruction and extrahepatic malignancies [1,3,18]. Intra-abdominal diseases that may lead to liver abscess include diverticulitis, appendicitis, bowel perforation, and inflammatory bowel disease (IBD) [15]. Liver abscess can form after transarterial chemoembolization of hepatocellular carcinoma [2]. Multiple liver abscesses are associated with biliary tract disease, such as stones and cholangiocarcinoma [17]. Underlying conditions associated with liver abscess are diabetes mellitus, malignancy, and hypertension [4,14].

Clinical Features

Symptoms can be non-specific, including fever and right upper quadrant abdominal pain, often with serum alkaline phosphatase elevation [1,3,18]. Low albumin, leukocytosis, and increased alanine transaminase levels are common. The classic triad of jaundice, fever, and right upper quadrant pain is uncommon [15]. Intra-abdominal complications include rupture of the abscess into the abdomen or the biliary or gastrointestinal (GI) tract, and portal or mesenteric vein thrombosis [14]. Mortality has been reported in patients who developed sepsis, liver and multiorgan failure, and mesenteric vein thrombosis [4]. The mortality is higher with multiple liver abscesses [1,15]. Malignancy has been found to be an independent risk factor for mortality [2]. Reported mortality for cases of hypermucoviscous *K. pneumoniae* bacteremia with liver abscesses in the United States is low (10%).

Diagnosis

Radiological testing using abdominal computed tomography (CT) and ultrasonography is crucial [1] (Figure 78.1). Half of patients have a positive blood culture and three-quarters have a positive culture of aspirate of the abscess. A chest radiograph may show atelectasis, pleural effusion, or elevated right diaphragm [14,15,17].

Treatment

In general, antibiotics and abscess drainage are indicated. Duration of antibiotic treatment is not established, but some

Practical Gastroenterology and Hepatology Board Review Toolkit, Second Edition. Edited by Nicholas J. Talley, Kenneth R. DeVault, Michael B. Wallace, Bashar A. Aqel and Keith D. Lindor.

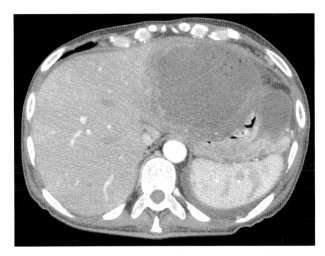

Figure 78.1 CT scan showing pyogenic liver abscess in the left lobe.

practitioners have administered intravenous antibiotics for 6 weeks or longer [2]. Choice of antibiotics is determined by culture and susceptibility results, and includes third-generation cephalosporins, cefoxitin, piperacillin–tazobactam, ampicillin–sulbactam, ciprofloxacin, levofloxacin, imipenem, and meropenem. Metronidazole is usually added to cover possible amebic abscess. Ultrasound-guided needle aspiration is useful as a diagnostic and therapeutic measure [2]. A drain is left until purulent fluid stops draining. Drainage of multiloculated or multiple abscesses is more complicated, and sometimes only the large abscess cavity can be drained [1]. Surgery may be necessary, especially with multiloculated abscesses, abscesses involving the left lobe of the liver, and abscesses accompanied by intra-abdominal disease [18]. When significant necrosis of the liver occurs, segmental hepatectomy is indicated [17].

Pylephlebitis

Septic thrombophlebitis of the portal vein or of one of its tributaries is a complication of intra-abdominal infection, and may be associated with solitary or multiple liver abscesses. In the pre-antibiotic era, it was relatively common in young individuals who had acute appendicitis. It is now a rare condition, but still carries high morbidity and mortality, mostly due to delay in diagnosis, and it should thus be considered in the right clinical setting. The most common condition associated with pylephlebitis is diverticulitis; others are malignancy, cholecystitis, abdominal and pelvic infection, pancreatitis, and hypercoagulable states [19]. Presenting symptoms may include fever, chills, abdominal pain, and distension [20].

In a review of 19 cases, 10 developed liver abscesses (8 multiple, 2 solitary) and 2 developed pulmonary embolism; the mortality rate was 32% [21]. Diagnosis was achieved by ultrasonography and CT. Bacteria involved are Gram negatives, streptococci, and anaerobes; empiric antibiotics should cover these organisms. Anticoagulation may be considered, but its indication is still under debate.

Amebic Liver Abscess

Microbiology

Entamoeba histolytica has two forms. The tetranucleated cyst is the form that is ingested and the motile trophozoite is formed in the terminal ileum or colon. *E. histolytica* can be differentiated from *E.*

dispar and *E. moshkovskii*, which are not pathogenic, by molecular techniques [22].

Epidemiology

Amebiasis is endemic in temperate and tropical climates, such as in India, Egypt, and South Africa [23]. There are 40,000–100,000 deaths from *E. histolytica* every year. In the United States, cases of amebiasis are diagnosed in immigrants and travelers to endemic countries. Infection usually results from ingestion of contaminated food or water [22]. There has been a significant increase in transmission among men who have sex with other men (MSM). A report from the United States describes only 2 of 34,000 human immunodeficiency virus (HIV)-positive individuals with invasive *E. histolytica* disease [24]. Reports from Japan, Taiwan, Korea, and Australia document significant increases in incidence in MSM [25]. This increased incidence is most likely due to anal–oral sex practices and the higher prevalence of this parasite in the Asia-Pacific countries [25].

Pathogenesis

The trophozoites attach to and then invade the colonic epithelium and then the submucosa, causing "flask-shaped ulcers" via various proteolytic enzymes and inflammatory cells; this results in diarrhea and destruction of tissue in the bowel [22]. It is believed that the trophozoites reach the liver through the portal circulation, thereby initiating the formation of an abscess.

Clinical Features

Infection with *E. histolytica* may be asymptomatic, but an estimated 4–10% of patients with asymptomatic infection will develop invasive disease each year [22]. A liver abscess is the most common extraintestinal manifestation. Patients may present with or without amebic colitis, and exposure may have occurred months or even years before presentation with a liver abscess. Symptoms and signs include diarrhea (possibly bloody), abdominal pain with right upper quadrant tenderness, hepatomegaly, fever, cough, weight loss, increased alkaline phosphatase, and leukocytosis. Usually, there is a solitary abscess in the right hepatic lobe; less common is a left lobe abscess [23]. Bacterial superinfection and sepsis may occur; these require antibiotics against gut organisms and staphylococci. Spread to neighboring structures may cause infection of the diaphragm, subdiaphragmatic area, pleura, lungs, and pericardium, causing fistulas and purulent collections [23].

Diagnosis

In the proper clinical presentation with compatible radiology, the finding of erythrocyte-containing trophozoites is diagnostic of *E. histolytica* infection [22,26]. Trophozoites may be found at the edge of the liver abscess, but usually not in the central necrotic portion (Figure 78.2). Ultrasonography and CT demonstrate a mass lesion. Serology is positive in the presence of *E. histolytica*, but not in the presence of *E. dispar*. The indirect hemagglutination (IHA) test is almost 100% positive in hepatic amebiasis [23]. In areas with a low prevalence of *E. histolytica* infection, a positive titer supports the diagnosis of an acute infection; in areas with high prevalence, a positive titer may mean previous infection rather than active current infection [27]. A fecal antigen-based enzyme-linked immunosorbent assay (ELISA) is now available for diagnosis of *E. histolytica*, with very good sensitivity and specificity [26]. A polymerase chain reaction (PCR) test is currently used as a research tool but is not available for routine clinical diagnosis.

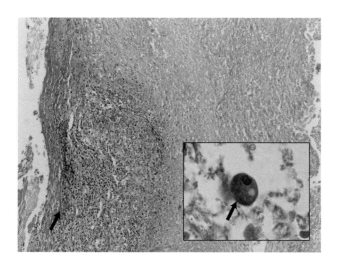

Figure 78.2 Amebic liver abscess. The wall of the abscess is on the left, with adjacent purulent inflammation. The center, though necrotic, is largely acellular. The inset shows *E. histolytica*. H&E ×200 and ×1000.

Distinguishing between a pyogenic and an amebic liver abscess may be difficult. In a review of 577 cases of liver abscess, predictive factors for pyogenic liver abscess included age >50, multiple abscesses, pulmonary findings, and an IHA titer <256 IU [27].

Treatment

Metronidazole is the cornerstone of treatment. Chloroquine, which is active against trophozoites, is added in cases with a very large abscess or multiple abscesses. Surgical drainage is rarely indicated, other than in complicated cases. Treatment with luminal agents, which include iodoquinol, paromomycin, and diloxanide, is necessary to eliminate intestinal *E. histolytica* and prevent relapse.

Acute Cholangitis

Microbiology

The usual organisms involved are *E. coli*, *Klebsiella* spp., and *Enterobacter* spp.; staphylococci and streptococci are uncommon [28]. Rarely, anaerobes such as *Bacteroides* spp. and clostridia may be present [29]; they are found more frequently in severe cases or in those who have undergone previous biliary and enteric surgery. Biliary stents may be colonized with hospital organisms that can cause infection.

Pathogenesis

Cholangitis results from biliary obstruction. Most cases occur in elderly people and are associated with cholelithiasis. When biliary obstruction occurs, it is believed that bacteria ascend the choledochus from the duodenum (or possibly from the gut through the portal circulation), colonize the bile, and cause infection. Increased pressure in the biliary tract may open the hepatocellular junctions and allow bacteria and toxins to infiltrate the general circulation [28].

Aside from cholelithiasis, other etiologies include biliary strictures, malignancy, choledochal cysts, choledochocele, and intrabiliary parasites [29]. Sometimes the cause is an occluded biliary stent [28].

Clinical Features

The median age of patients is 50–60 years. Patients may present with mild symptoms or with an acute, life-threatening illness. The Charcot triad (jaundice, fever/chills, and right upper quadrant abdominal pain) occurs in 50–100% of cases; the Reynold pentad (the Charcot triad plus hypotension and altered mental status) is much less common (<14%) [29].

Some diseases present with recurrent cholangitis, including Oriental recurrent cholangitis, acquired immunodeficiency syndrome (AIDS) cholangiopathy, and primary sclerosing cholangitis (PSC).

Oriental Recurrent Cholangitis

Oriental recurrent cholangitis is a disease of East Asia that usually affects younger individuals. The intrahepatic bile ducts form strictures, dilations, and biliary stones. The etiology remains unknown, but one possible explanation is biliary worms, specifically *Clonorchis*, *Ascaris*, and *Fasciola* spp. Patients are offered biliary procedures to dilate strictures, extract biliary stones, and place biliary stents, and sometimes segmental resection of the liver.

AIDS Cholangiopathy

AIDS cholangiopathy was first described in 1986, affecting those with a CD4 count <100. With the advent of potent antiretroviral agents, it is now rarely seen. It causes sclerosing cholangitis, mainly of the large intrahepatic bile ducts and papillary stenosis [30]. *Cryptosporidium parvum*, *Microsporidium* spp., *Cyclospora cayetanensis*, and *Mycobacterium avium* complex have been implicated in the etiology of this disease, but treatment of these infections does not affect it.

Primary Sclerosing Cholangitis

PSC is a chronic disease that causes inflammation and fibrosis of the intra- and extrahepatic bile ducts, usually affecting young and middle-aged men. Recurrent cholangitis usually starts after manipulation and surgical exploration of the biliary tract. Biliary strictures, biliary stones, and sludge are found. Ultimately, liver failure occurs, and liver transplantation may be the only solution [31].

Diagnosis

Leukocytosis, increased alkaline phosphatase and bilirubin, and mildly elevated liver transaminases are typical. Dilated bile ducts may be seen with ultrasonography and CT. Endoscopic retrograde cholangiopancreatography (ERCP) and magnetic resonance cholangiopancreatography (MRCP) may be necessary.

Treatment

The first goal in management is to stabilize the patient using intravenous fluids and antibiotics. An antibiotic with a high biliary concentration, such as piperacillin, is preferred. Blood cultures and bile cultures, if possible, should be obtained, and antibiotics adjusted based on culture and sensitivity results. Once the patient is stable, the biliary obstruction is addressed via endoscopic, percutaneous, or surgical approaches. The Tokyo Guideline for management of acute cholangitis and acute cholecystitis was recently published; it addresses the timing and modality of interventions based on severity of illness. Intravenous antibiotics and 24-hour observation prior to drainage are recommended for mild cases, while immediate or urgent drainage with appropriate antibiotics is recommended for moderate to severe cases [32].

Table 78.1 Infections that cause granulomatous hepatitis and their etiologic agents.

Infection	Infectious agent	Infection	Infectious agent
Bacterial		**Fungal**	
Tuberculosis	*Mycobacterium tuberculosis*	Candidiasis	*Candida* spp.
Atypical mycobacteria	*M. avium* complex and others	Histoplasmosis	*Histoplasma capsulatum* (Figure 78.3)
BCG infection	*M. bovis* (attenuated vaccine mycobacterium)	Cryptococcosis	*Cryptococcus neoformans*
Leprosy	*M. leprae*	Coccidioidomycosis	*Coccidioides immitis/posadasii*
Listeriosis	*Listeria monocytogenes*		
Tularemia	*Francisella tularensis*	**Viral**	
Bartonellosis	*Bartonella henselae*	CMV infection	CMV
Salmonellosis	*Salmonella* spp.	EBV infection	EBV
Brucellosis	*Brucella* spp.	Hepatitis A	HAV
Yersiniosis	*Yersinia* spp.	Hepatitis B	HBV
Whipple disease	*Tropheryma whipplei*	Hepatitis C	HCV
Psittacosis	*Chlamydia psittaci*	**Parasitic**	
Melioidosis	*Burkholderia pseudomallei*	Toxoplasmosis	*Toxoplasma gondii*
Nocardiosis	*Nocardia* spp.	Schistosomiasis	*Schistosoma* spp.
Secondary syphilis	*Treponema pallidum*	Visceral leishmaniasis	*Leishmania* spp.
Q-fever	*Coxiella burnetii*	Visceral larva migrans	*Toxocara* spp.

BCG, bacillus Calmette–Guérin; CMV, cytomegalovirus; EBV, Epstein–Barr virus; HAV, HBV, HCV, hepatitis A–C virus.

Granulomatous Hepatitis

Microbiology

Table 78.1 shows infections that cause granulomatous hepatitis (Figure 78.3). Other etiologies include autoimmune diseases, drugs, sarcoidosis (Figure 78.4), and idiopathic causes. Idiopathic granulomatous hepatitis is usually treated with steroids, but before it is assumed, a thorough investigation is needed to rule out other diagnoses.

The frequency of the etiologies of granulomatous hepatitis varies with the time period in which each study was performed. In earlier studies, hepatitis C virus (HCV) was not listed as a potential etiology. An early series from the Mayo Clinic had many idiopathic (50%) cases [33]; with improvement in diagnostic methods, the proportion of granulomatous hepatitis without a known cause has decreased. In a series from Germany [34], an infectious etiology was found in 3.4%; PCR was applied for detection of

Bartonella henselae, Listeria monocytogenes, Mycobacterium tuberculosis, M. avium, Yersinia enterocolitica, Y. pseudotuberculosis, cytomegalovirus (CMV) and Epstein–Barr virus (EBV), and *Toxoplasma gondii.*

There is also substantial variation in the distribution of etiologies of granulomatous hepatitis across countries, as noted in Table 78.2. Tuberculosis is listed in every published series, and is still an important etiology of granulomatous hepatitis.

Diagnosis

Liver biopsy demonstrates granulomas in the parenchyma. These are collections of epithelioid cells, which can include giant cells, surrounded by lymphocytes [39]. The histology of the granuloma and the surrounding tissue is important for a differential diagnosis [36]. As many as 75% of cases present with fever of unknown origin [39].

Table 78.3 shows the diagnostic methods and treatments used for bacterial infections; parasitic and fungal infections are detailed later in the chapter.

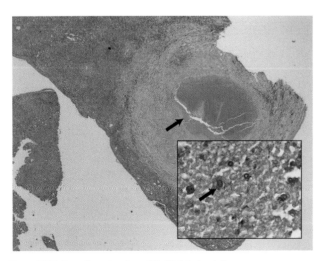

Figure 78.3 Granulomatous hepatitis. This lesion is from an immunocompromised patient with acute leukemia. There is a centrally necrotic, well-defined lesion with a granulomatous rim in the hepatic parenchyma. The inset shows fungi with budding and a thin capsule most consistent morphologically with *Histolyticum capsulatum*. Central necrosis is common in infectious granulomas. H&E ×40; periodic acid–Schiff ×400.

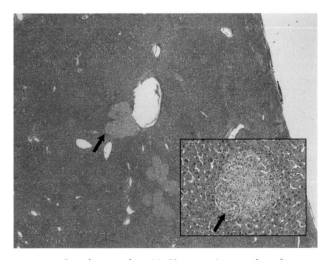

Figure 78.4 Granulomatous hepatitis. Non-caseating granuloma from sarcoidosis in liver. In contrast to many infectious granulomas, the granuloma is tightly formed, with no necrosis. H&E ×40 and ×200.

Table 78.2 Infectious etiology of granulomatous hepatitis in different countries (1990–2006).

	United States [33]	Saudi Arabia [35]	Turkey [36]	Scotland [37]	Greece [38]	Germany [34]
Years	1976–85	1990	1993–99	1991–2001	1999–2004	1996–2004
Number of cases	88	59	56	63	66	442
Mean age (years)	54.2		30	42	42	
Female/male ratio	45 : 43		30 : 26	47 : 16	51 : 15	
Sarcoidosis (%)	22		20	11.1	7.5	8.37
Autoimmune (%)				34.5	68	48.64
Hodgkin's disease (%)			1	6.3		
Drugs (%)	6	3.4	1	7.9	3	2.48
Idiopathic (%)	**50**		**19.6**	**11**	**6**	**36**
Others (%)	19	1.7		12.7	3	0.013
Infection (%)		**95**	**41**	**14.3**	**12**	**3.39**
Tuberculosis (%)	3	32.2	19.6	4.8	1.5	0.67
Brucellosis (%)		6.8	5.3			
Yersiniosis (%)						0.23
Bartonellosis (%)						0.45
Listeriosis (%)						0.67
Typhoid fever (%)		1.7	3.5			
Q-fever (%)						0.23
CMV (%)						0.45
EBV (%)			1.8			0.90
HBV (%)					3	
HCV (%)			1.8	9.5	4.5	
Schistosomiasis (%)		**54.2**			1.5	
Leishmaniasis (%)					1.5	
Hydatid cyst (%)			8.9			

CMV, cytomegalovirus; EBV, Epstein–Barr virus; HBV, HCV, hepatitis B/C virus.

Bacterial Infections of the Liver

The liver can be involved in a variety of bacterial infections, either as a result of direct liver involvement through bacteremia or contiguous spread, or through indirect effects. Common manifestations of hepatic involvement are cholestasis, jaundice, and elevations of transaminases. Some bacterial infections present as abscesses and/or granulomas. More uncommon presentations are nodular liver lesions, which can appear similar to metastatic lesions. Table 78.3 summarizes the clinical presentation, diagnosis, and treatment of selected bacterial infections.

Protozoa

Systemic protozoan infections that involve the reticuloendothelial cell system can manifest with varying degrees of hepatomegaly and fever. The pathologic changes center on Kupffer cells. *Babesia* spp., not separately discussed, may cause mild hepatomegaly and liver function abnormalities.

Malaria

Epidemiology and Organisms

Plasmodium falciparum, P. vivax, P. ovale, and *P. malariae* initially replicate in the liver after infection by the bite of an anopheline mosquito. The parasites then rupture from hepatocytes into the bloodstream to invade circulating erythrocytes, producing the malaria paroxysm.

The liver is a reservoir for *P. vivax* and *P. ovale*, which shelter there in the form of hypnozoites. Inadequate treatment of this latent phase can lead to recrudescence months to years after the eradication of the hematogenous phase.

Clinical Features

Malaria varies from indolent and asymptomatic to multisystem organ failure. The classic presentation is an acute illness characterized by paroxysms of high, spiking, often cyclical fever of 40°C or more, followed by chills, drenching sweats, rigor, and prostration/fatigue in a traveler or an immigrant from an endemic area. Patients may present with vomiting, abdominal cramps, diarrhea, and hepatosplenomegaly. Hyperbilirubinemia may be mild, due to hemolysis in milder infection, but can be more pronounced, with sepsis and organ compromise of severe infection.

A common microscopic finding of severe malaria in any vascular tissue is small-vessel thrombosis and a concentration of malarial pigments, typically seen in Kupffer cells in the liver or macrophages in the spleen.

Diagnosis

Thin and thick blood smears should be examined for the characteristic parasitic forms. Immunofluorescence and PCR-based methods can also be used to detect malarial antigens. Rapid stick- or card-type tests, based on the detection of either histidine-rich protein 2 (*P. falciparum*) or plasmodial lactate dehydrogenase (all species), can be used when microscopic examination is not available [44].

Treatment

P. falciparum infection requires prompt diagnosis and treatment. Patients can quickly develop sepsis and multiorgan failure. Those with non-falciparum malaria can usually be treated as outpatients. Atovaquone-proguanil and mefloquine are used for malaria from most areas; chloroquine can be used for infection from areas with susceptible malaria. Quinine/quinidine is used for severe complicated falciparum malaria [45]. Primaquine is added for eradication of the hepatic parasites of *P. vivax* and *P. ovale*. Pyrimethamine, artemisinin derivatives, and tetracyclines are also used. Information on malaria treatment can be obtained from the Centers for Disease Control and Prevention (CDC) Malaria Hotline (+1 770-488-7788). The World Health Organization (WHO) recommends the use of artemisinin-based combination treatment for infections from areas with endemic resistance.

Table 78.3 Bacterial infections of the liver. Source: Johannsson and Stapleton 2012 [40], Gordon 2007 [41], Mandell 2010 [42], and CDC 2013 [43].

Organism	Usual mode of transmission	Risk factor	Usual signs and symptoms	Liver manifestation	Diagnosis	Treatment
Actinomyces spp.	Endogenous flora	Poor dentition	Oral–cervical disease	Abscess	Anaerobic culture from a sterile site	Penicillin Clindamycin Tetracycline
Bartonella henselae	Inoculation	Cat scratch	Fever, papule/pustule at site of inoculation, lymphadenitis, anemia	Microabscess, Peliosis hepatis: blood-filled cystic spaces in liver	Serology Blood/tissue culture Tissue/pus PCR Warthin–Starry silver stain of tissue	Azithromycin
BCG infection	Intravesical instillation of BCG vaccine		Fever, cough, weight loss, sepsis	Granulomas	AFB culture of tissue	Isoniazid, rifampin, ethambutol
Borrelia spp.	Tick bite		Stage 1: erythema migrans, constitutional symptoms Stage 2: annular rash, meningitis, encephalitis, neuritis, atrioventricular block Stage 3: arthritis, chronic axonal polyneuropathy	Stage 2: elevated LFTs, jaundice, tender hepatosplenomegaly	Serology PCR of joint fluid	Doxycycline Amoxicillin Ceftriaxone
Brucella spp.	Direct inoculation Ingestion Inhalation	Unpasteurized dairy products, infected animal body fluids	Fever, sweats, anorexia	Hepatitis, non-caseating granulomas, abscess	Blood or tissue cultures Serology	Doxycycline + rifampin
Ehrlichiosis HME (*Ehrlichia chafeensis*) HGA (*Anaplasma phagocytophila*)	Tick bite		Fever, headache, myalgia, malaise, nausea, anorexia, vomiting, diarrhea	Elevated LFTs, hepatomegaly	HME: morulae in circulating mononuclear cells HGA: morulae in polymorphonuclear cells Serology PCR	Doxycycline
Gonorrhea (*Neisseria gonorrhoeae*)	Sexual contact		Fitz–Hugh–Curtis syndrome (acute perihepatitis), predominantly in women: fever, right upper quadrant abdominal pain, tenderness Gonococcal bacteremia: septic arthritis, dermatitis	Liver commonly involved in gonococcal bacteremia, with elevated transaminases and alkaline phosphatase Periportal inflammatory infiltrate (Fitz–Hugh–Curtis syndrome)	Blood or genital lesion culture Genital or urine nucleic acid amplificator test Violin string-like adhesions between peritoneal wall and liver capsule on laparoscopy highly suggestive	Ceftriaxone + azithromycin
Legionella spp.	Inhalation		Pneumonia, Diarrhea, hyponatremia	Elevated LFTs, hyperbilirubinemia	Detection by immunofluorescence or culture of respiratory specimens, tissue or fluid Antigenuria	Macrolides, quinolones, tetracyclines
Leprosy (*Mycobacterium leprae*)	Inhalation		Skin lesions, hypoesthesia, peripheral neuropathy	Granulomas	Fite acid-fast stain, AFB smear or PCR of tissue	Dapsone + rifampin ± clofazimine
Leptospirosis	Direct or indirect contact with urine or tissues of infected animals	Occupational animal exposure	Biphasic illness (Weil's disease): flu-like illness with cough, chest pain, abdominal pain, then defervescence; second phase with jaundice, muscle pain, renal failure, conjunctival suffusion	Jaundice	Culture of blood or CSF (first phase) or urine (second phase); serology	Severe: penicillin or ceftriaxone Mild: doxycycline
Listeria monocytogenes	Ingestion of contaminated food	Dairy or poultry products Extremes of age, pregnancy, impaired cell-mediated immunity	Fever, leukocytosis, bacteremia, meningoencephalitis	Hepatitis, microabscess, granuloma	Culture of blood, CSF, or other body fluid	Ampicillin
Melioidosis (*Burkholderia pseudomallei*)	Inhalation or inoculation through the skin	Exposure to soil and freshwater in South East Asia, especially Thailand	Pneumonia, septicemia, tonsillitis	Elevated transaminases, jaundice, microabscess, granulomas	Immunohistochemistry Culture	Ceftazidime

Disease (organism)	Transmission/source	Risk factors	Clinical presentation	Hepatic involvement	Diagnosis	Treatment
Non-tuberculous mycobacteria (*M. avium* complex, *M. kansasii*, *M. genavense*)	Environmental source (ubiquitous in environment)	AIDS, organ transplant, chronic steroids	Fever, weight loss	Elevated alkaline phosphatase, non-caseating granulomas	AFB culture or PCR of blood or bone marrow	Clarithromycin + ethambutol + rifabutin
Q-fever (*Coxiella burnetii*)	Inhalation or ingestion of contaminated raw milk	Direct or indirect contact with infected cattle, sheep, or goats	Fever, flu-like illness with pneumonitis	Acute hepatitis-like illness, isolated elevated LFTs, or FUO with granulomas (fibrin ring granuloma)	Serology, tissue or blood PCR	Tetracycline Fluoroquinolones
Rocky Mountain spotted fever (*Rickettsia rickettsii*)	Tick bite		Fever, headache, rash	Elevated ALT, jaundice, hepatomegaly	Serology	Doxycycline
Salmonella hepatitis	Ingestion	Poultry, eggs Exotic pets, especially reptiles Travel to endemic area (South East Asia, Africa) HIV Alcoholism (for severe disease)	Fever, relative bradycardia, left shift, rose spots	Alkaline phosphatase increases much higher than transaminases; hepatomegaly; typhoid nodules (lobular aggregates of Kupffer cells)	Culture of blood, bone marrow, or other sterile site, rose spots, stool, intestinal secretions	Fluoroquinolone, ceftriaxone, or azithromycin for fluoroquinolone-resistant strains
Staphylococcal/ Streptococcal toxic shock syndrome		Surgical wound infection Tampon use	Fever, mucosal hyperemia, rash, vomiting, hypotension, rapid development of multisystem organ failure	Transaminase elevation, jaundice	Culture of surgical wound, clinical/laboratory criteria	Antibiotic active against isolated organism, surgical debridement, supportive care
Syphilis (*Treponema pallidum*)	Congenital Person-to-person (sexual contact or kissing/touching active lesions)		Primary: chancre (painless, non-tender ulcer) Secondary: rash, condyloma lata, mucous patches, constitutional symptoms, generalized painless lymphadenopathy Tertiary: gummas	Congenital: hepatic gummas; Secondary: hepatitis with disproportionate alkaline phosphatase elevation Tertiary: gummas	Dark-field examination of serous transudate from moist lesions Serology: non-treponemal test (RPR or VDRL) confirmed with treponemal test (FTA-Abs, MHA-TP, syphilis IgG)	Penicillin, ceftriaxone, or doxycycline for penicillin allergic
Tuberculosis (*Mycobacterium tuberculosis*)	Airborne: inhalation of droplet nuclei	Homeless, prison inmates, persons from endemic countries, intravenous drug users	Fever, weight loss, abdominal pain, hepatomegaly	Drug-induced hepatitis due to TB drug therapy most common Granulomatous hepatitis (caseating granulomas) Hepatobiliary: nodules or abscesses with bile duct involvement (bile duct epithelial involvement or obstruction by enlarged nodes) Elevated alkaline phosphatase	AFB culture, PCR of liver biopsy	Isoniazid, rifampin, pyrazinamide, ethambutol
Tularemia (*Francisella tularensis*)	Insect bites (ticks or flies), contact with contaminated animal products	Hunting, skinning, dressing, and eating infected animals (rabbits, muskrats, beavers, squirrels)	Ulceroglandular: skin lesion (red, painful nodule which necroses to a tender nodule with raised borders) with regional tender lymphadenopathy Pneumonia	Rare liver involvement Modest transaminase elevation, jaundice, abscess	Culture of blood, sputum, pleural fluid, wound Serology, PCR	Streptomycin, gentamicin
Whipple disease (*Tropheryma whipplei*)				Rare liver involvement, hepatomegaly, transaminase elevation, granuloma	Serology, PCR	Ceftriaxone, trimethoprim–sulfamethoxazole, doxycycline

PCR, polymerase chain reaction; BCG, bacillus Calmette–Guérin; AFB, acid-fast bacillus; LFT, liver function test; HME, human monocytic ehrlich osis; HGA, human granulocytic anaplasmosis; CSF, cerebrospinal fluid; AIDS, acquired immunodeficiency syndrome; FUO, fever of unknown origin; ALT, alanine transaminase; HIV, human immunodeficiency virus; RPR, rapid plasma regain; VDRL, Venereal Disease Research Laboratory; FTA-Abs, fluorescent treponemal antibody, absorbed; MHA-TP, microhemagglutination test for *Treponema pallidum*; IgG, immunoglobulin G; TB, tuberculosis.

Leishmaniasis

Epidemiology and Organisms

Leishmania species are found worldwide and are transmitted by the bite of sand flies, which typically feed at night. Following inoculation, the organism is phagocytosed by skin macrophages. The subsequent degree of infection is determined by the cell-mediated response of the infected person.

Leishmaniasis may be asymptomatic, but frequently causes cutaneous or mucosal infections in the upper aerodigestive tract. Dissemination to the reticuloendothelial system causes visceral leishmaniasis, also known as kala-azar, in both immunocompetent and immunocompromised individuals. The most common causative organisms are *L. donovani* (eastern India, Bangladesh, and eastern Africa) and *L. infantum/L. chagasi* (southern Europe, North Africa, the Middle East, Central Asia, and South America). *Leishmania* spp. has emerged as a major pathogen in HIV/AIDS patients and an uncommon infection in military personnel returning from Middle Eastern conflicts.

Clinical Features

The incubation period is 2–8 months, with variable fever and increasing hypertrophy of the liver, spleen, and lymph nodes. Hepatosplenomegaly may be massive, and peripheral wasting, liver test abnormalities, hypoalbuminemia, hypergammaglobulinemia, and ascites can be seen. Much of the visceral leishmaniasis in South America and southern Europe is associated with HIV infection, usually in patients with a CD4 count <200/mm³. It was more common in the pre-antiretroviral era. Recurrence after treatment is common, requiring maintenance therapy in immunocompromised individuals.

Diagnosis

Demonstration of the parasite in peripheral blood smears, ascitic fluid, or biopsy of the bone marrow, spleen, or liver establishes the diagnosis. Hepatomegaly is associated with Kupffer cell hyperplasia, with numerous, small, often smudged amastigotes filling the cell. Culture of the organisms is possible in liquid media, but is not widely available. Serology is less helpful, especially in immunocompromised individuals. Newer ELISA and other tests for parasite-specific antigens, and PCR-based assays, are being developed [46].

Treatment

Sodium stibogluconate, amphotericin B, lipid-associated amphotericin B, miltefosine, paromomycin, pentamidine, and others drugs are used [47].

Toxoplasmosis

Epidemiology and Organisms

Caused by the ubiquitous *Toxoplasma gondii*, acute, congenital, ocular, and chronic syndromes of toxoplasmosis occur in both immunocompetent and immunocompromised hosts. Infection occurs through the ingestion of tissue cysts or oocysts. The organism has also been transmitted by transplantation and blood transfusion. After ingestion, the organism can disseminate through the blood. Over time, the infection is contained, but encysted organisms can persist.

Clinical Features

Acute infection in immunocompetent hosts is usually asymptomatic. Some may present with lymphadenopathy and constitutional symptoms, and rarely with hepatosplenomegaly and hepatitis. In the immunocompromised individual, any tissue shows a variable inflammatory response, characterized by cuffing mixed mononuclear inflammatory infiltrates, visible tachyzoites and cysts, and necrosis with associated phagocytes and neutrophils.

Cysts in chronic infection tend to concentrate in skeletal muscle, myocardium, and the CNS. The liver is a less common site for infection, but hepatitis is seen in disseminated infection in immunocompromised hosts. Recrudescence of latent infection in transplant recipients usually occurs within 3 months of transplantation.

Diagnosis

In immunocompetent individuals, serology is helpful. In immunocompromised ones, serology demonstrates those at risk for infection and supports the diagnosis with suggestive pathologic findings. Demonstration of the organism with compatible histologic findings, visualization of cysts in routine sections, and specific immunohistochemical confirmation of the organism are all possible. Isolation of parasites in mice or cell culture is also possible. PCR methods are available for fluid specimens [48].

Treatment

Most acute infections in immunocompetent hosts are self-limited. Treatment in immunocompromised hosts is pyrimethamine/sulfadiazine/folinic acid.

Fungi

Fungal infection of the liver is almost always a manifestation of disseminated infection in an immunocompromised host. The liver has the typical granulomatous pattern of infection seen in other organs. Focal hepatocellular disease with liver function abnormalities is expected.

The liver biopsy may demonstrate focal granulomatous lesions, and, rarely, fungal organisms may be seen [49]. *Histoplasma capsulatum* tends to favor the reticuloendothelial system in the liver with Kupffer cell hyperplasia; organisms can be seen in macrophages. *Candida* spp. cause small microabscesses with central necrosis combined with poorly defined peripheral granulomatous change; hyphae may be seen. The pattern of cryptococcosis, especially in AIDS, can vary widely, ranging from granulomatous and/or necrotic to little tissue reaction with mucinous accumulation from the capsule of *C. neoformans*. *Aspergillus* spp. in immunocompromised hosts is more necrotic than discretely granulomatous, with organisms seen at the edges of necrotic lesions, and occasional infarction due to involvement of adjacent vasculature. *Coccidioides* spp. is one of the largest fungi found in tissue, and the only one with significant internal structure, caused by its visible endospores; this infection can be seen in disseminated cases in people with a history of exposure in south-western areas of the United States.

Identification of organisms can sometimes be accomplished with hematoxylin and eosin stains or with fungal stains such as Gomori–Grocott methenamine silver (GMS), periodic acid–Schiff (PAS), and mucicarmine. Specific diagnosis can be made with culture, serology, or PCR.

Treatment is directed against the etiologic organism using amphotericin, a triazole, or echinocandin, with modification of immunosuppression where possible.

Helminths

Nematodes (roundworms), trematodes (flatworms, flukes), and cestodes (tapeworms) can cause liver disease with a variety of patterns, depending on the host response. As many species involve the liver through larval migration from the GI tract to the biliary ducts, involvement of the biliary ducts and portal areas is common.

Echinococcosis (Hydatid Disease)

Epidemiology and Organisms

Echinococcus granulosus and *E. multilocularis* are found worldwide, associated with raising livestock. Cattle and sheep are intermediate hosts, and cats and dogs are definitive hosts for adult worms. Humans acquire infection by ingesting eggs. The egg releases oncospheres, which penetrate intestinal mucosa, enter the microcirculation, and migrate to organs: typically the liver, less commonly the lungs, rarely the heart. The oncosphere becomes a cystic metacestode, which then forms daughter cysts endogenously (*E. granulosus*) or exogenously (*E. multilocularis*) in adjacent tissue. Mediterranean countries, China, and Russia have the highest prevalence rates. Northern Africa and parts of South America and Australia are endemic. There has been a recent re-emergence of echinococcosis in Israel, Central Asia, and Eastern Europe. [50]

Clinical Features

E. granulosus typically forms a unilocular asymptomatic cyst, which is usually discovered incidentally on imaging (Figure 78.5). Such cysts grow slowly, usually in the right hepatic lobe; they may reach a large size (>10 cm), and the wall may calcify. They may present as an obstructing mass (jaundice, tender hepatomegaly, palpable mass) or a rupture into adjacent tissue, with seeding of new cysts (causing pain, peritonitis, empyema, hemoptysis, and/or pulmonary symptoms, or systemic allergic reactions from the cyst contents, e.g., anaphylaxis) [51].

E. multilocularis causes more invasive, slowly progressive, and often fatal extension into liver parenchyma, termed "alveolar

hydatid disease." The less common *E. vogeli* and *E. oligarthus* cause polycystic hydatid disease.

Diagnosis

Serology confirms the diagnosis. Sharply circumscribed cysts with regular daughter orbs on imaging are diagnostic, and many calcified cysts can demonstrate the suggestive ring-like calcification. Aspiration of the cyst has been avoided traditionally, in order to decrease the likelihood of rupture, dissemination, or allergic reaction, but has been used recently for diagnosis and sterilization. Protoscolices, hooklets, or brood capsules from the interior of the cyst are diagnostic. The microscopic appearance of an intact cyst wall is pathognomonic.

Treatment

Primary treatment includes excision of the cyst, often with sterilization before surgery to avoid any complication if the cyst ruptures intraoperatively. A calcified cyst is stable and need not be removed [52]. PAIR (puncture, aspiration, injection, reaspiration) plus albendazole before and after aspiration is commonly the therapeutic approach, with good success [50]. *E. multilocularis* infections are treated with surgery and mebendazole; lifelong mebendazole is recommended for inoperable patients. Liver transplantation is a last resort.

Trematodes (Flukes)

Clonorchis sinensis, *Opisthorchis viverrini*, and *O. felineus* infect the extrahepatic and intrahepatic biliary tract, whereas *Fasciola hepatica* infects the liver parenchyma and biliary ducts [53, 54]. Relapsing bacterial cholangitis is associated with biliary tract infection by flukes.

Clonorchis and *Opisthorchis* spp. are acquired from undercooked fish. The adult flukes deposit eggs in biliary ducts. Most infections are asymptomatic. Acute complications relate to biliary obstruction, causing fever, hepatomegaly, eosinophilia, and jaundice. Late complications include gallstones (Figure 78.6), secondary bacterial infection, cirrhosis, and cholangiocarcinoma. *Metorchis bilis*, another trematode identified in human cases in the Russian territory, produces a clinical picture indistinguishable from *Opisthorchis*

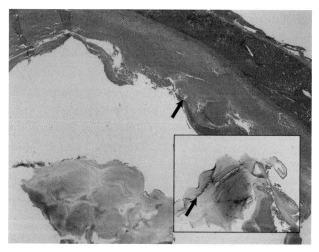

Figure 78.5 Echinococcal cyst. This 48-year-old was found to have an "incidental" liver cyst on CT and ultrasonography when being evaluated for gallbladder disease. This cyst was calcified with a thick fibrous rim. The organisms are no longer present. The unilocularity, thick fibrous rim with calcification, and layered acellular internal debris (inset) suggest the etiology. H&E ×20 and ×200.

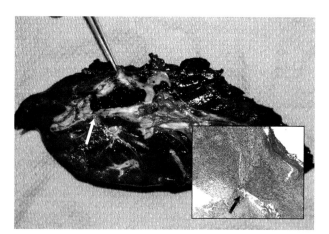

Figure 78.6 Hepatolithiasis. Liver resection from a patient with recurrent pyogenic cholangitis, showing multiple stones within large intrahepatic bile ducts. No organisms are present. The inset shows a destroyed biliary ductule with impacted stone material and dense surrounding chronic active inflammation. H&E ×200.

CHAPTER 78

[55]. Diagnosis rests on demonstration of eggs in stool or duodenal aspirate. Praziquantel is the treatment of choice.

Fasciola hepatica is acquired by ingestion of metacercariae associated with freshwater plants (e.g., watercress). It matures in the intestine, migrates though the small bowel into the peritoneal cavity, and then penetrates the liver capsule. Immature flukes reach the liver in 5–6 days and migrate through it for 5–6 weeks. Acute symptoms relate to pain from penetration of the peritoneum and hepatic capsule. After flukes establish themselves in biliary ducts, they invade the liver, causing a chronic or obstructive phase with inflammation of the biliary tract, eosinophilic microabscesses in hepatic tissue, and occasional wandering larvae, prompting ectopic subcutaneous swellings. Eosinophilia is present in all stages.

Fasciolopsis is not associated with biliary carcinoma. Diagnosis is based on finding eggs in stool. Unlike other trematodes, *Fasciola* is not sensitive to albendazole; triclabendazole is the drug of choice. ERCP may be helpful for extraction in cases of biliary obstruction.

Schistosoma spp. are an important cause of portal hypertension worldwide. Unlike other flukes, they inhabit blood vessels: typically mesenteric and portal veins. Infecting cercariae, which reside in freshwater, penetrate the skin, migrate through the blood to the lungs and liver, and continue through intestinal capillaries to the portal vein. They mature in hepatic portal venules, reproduce, and yield many eggs, disseminating to the liver. The intense reaction produced by these eggs leads to the characteristic circumscribed fibrous granuloma, Symmers (after a pathologist, Symmers, William St. Claire) fibrosis or "pipestem fibrosis," associated with *S. mansoni* and *S. mekongi* infection, causing portal hypertension (Figure 78.7). Diagnosis is made by serology or through demonstration of eggs in feces or biopsy specimens, though eggs are rare in liver biopsies. Praziquantel is effective against all organisms.

Nematodes (Roundworms)

Ascaris lumbricoides is the most common human helmintic infection and the largest human nematode. It can complete its entire life cycle in the human host, and typically resides in the small intestine. Infection is acquired by ingestion of eggs from contaminated soil.

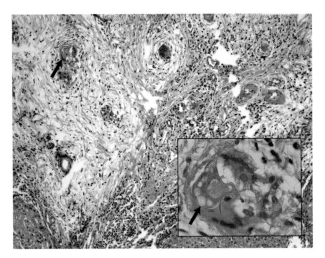

Figure 78.7 Hepatic schistosomiasis. Some intact hepatic parenchyma is visible at the extreme bottom of the photograph, but most of the liver is unidentifiable, replaced by fibrous tissue with granulomas. The inset demonstrates a granuloma, with the remains of pigmented egg and eosinophils in the upper right corner. H&E ×40 and ×400.

It causes liver, biliary, or pancreatic disease through direct obstruction of biliary ducts or the ampulla of Vater. Diagnosis is made by demonstration of eggs in stools. ERCP is utilized for extraction of the parasite, followed by albendazole or mebendazole.

The dog roundworm, *Toxocara canis*, can cause human infection when eggs are ingested from contaminated soil. The eggs hatch in the small intestine and then migrate to various organs, causing visceral larva migrans. In the liver, migrating and burrowing larvae cause nodules, characterized by eosinophilic granuloma, which may contain portions of larvae. Diagnosis rests on serology or demonstration of the larvae in tissue. The infection is self-limited. If treatment is necessary, albendazole or mebendazole may be used.

Strongyloides stercoralis rarely invades the liver when filariform larvae in hyperinfection syndrome disseminate through multiple organs.

Capillaria hepatica rarely infects the liver and causes necrotic granulomatous nodules; infection is acquired by ingestion of eggs in contaminated soil.

Take Home Points

Diagnosis:
- The classic triad of fever, right upper quadrant pain, and jaundice is uncommon in pyogenic liver abscess.
- Three-quarters of patients with granulomatous hepatitis present with fever of unknown origin.
- Previous exposures and travel history will help guide diagnosis of certain infections.
- Diagnostic methods may require testing of blood, stool, body fluid, or tissue specimens by culture, serology, special stains, or molecular methods such as polymerase chain reaction (PCR), in addition to radiological imaging.
- Cultures of the blood and abscess aspirate will usually yield the etiologic agents of a pyogenic liver abscess and guide antimicrobial therapy.
- Negative *Entamoeba histolytica* serology by indirect hemagglutination (IHA) effectively rules out amebic liver abscess.
- Collaboration among clinicians, pathologists, radiologists, and the laboratory will aid in reaching a diagnosis of infection.
- Ultrasonography and computed tomography (CT) are crucial in the diagnosis of liver abscesses.

Treatment:
- Antimicrobial therapy and drainage are necessary for most liver abscesses.
- Metronidazole is the treatment for amebic liver abscess. Luminal agents are necessary to treat intestinal amebiasis and prevent relapse.
- Treatment will depend on the etiologic agent identified.

References

1 McDonald MI, Corey GR, Gallis HA, *et al*. Single and multiple pyogenic liver abscesses. *Medicine* 1984; **63**: 291–302.

2 Wong WM, Wong BC, Hui CK, *et al*. Pyogenic liver abscess: retrospective analysis of 80 cases over a 10-year period. *J Gastroenterol Hepatol* 2002; **17**: 1001–7.

3 Rahimian J, Wilson T, Oram V, *et al*. Pyogenic liver abscess: recent trends in etiology and mortality. *Clin Infect Dis* 2004; **39**: 1654–9.

4 Perez JA, Gonzalez JJ, Baldonedo RF, *et al*. Clinical course, treatment, and multivariate analysis of risk factors for pyogenic liver abscess. *Am J Surg* 2001; **181**: 177–86.

5 Huang CJ, Pitt HA, Lipsett PA, *et al*. Pyogenic hepatic abscess: changing trends over 42 years. *Ann Surg* 1996; **223**: 600–9.

6 Fang CT, Lai SY, Yi WC, *et al*. *Klebsiella pneumoniae* genotype K1: An emerging pathogen that causes septic ocular or central nervous system complications from pyogenic liver abscess. *Clin Infect Dis* 2007; **45**: 284–93.

7 Lee, SS, Chen YS, Tsai HC, *et al.* Predictors of septic metastatic infection and mortality among patients with *Klebsiella pneumoniae* liver abscess. *Clin Infect Dis* 2008; **47**: 642–50.

8 Siu LK, Yeh KM, Lin JC, et al. Klebsiella pneumoniae liver abscess: a new invasive syndrome. *Lancet Infect Dis* 2012; **12**: 881–7.

9 McCabe R, Lambert L, Frazee B. Invasive *Klebsiella pneumonia* infections, California, USA. *Emerg Infect Dis* 2010; **16**(9): 1490–1.

10 Frazee BW, Hansen S, Lambert L. Invasive infection with hypermucoviscous *Klebsiella pneumoniae*: multiple cases presenting to a single emergency department in the United States. *Ann Emerg Med* 2008; **53**(5): 639–42.

11 Nadasky KA, Domiati-Saad R, Tribble MA. Invasive *Klebsiella pneumonia* syndrome in North America. *Clin Infect Dis* 2007; **45**; e25–8.

12 Fang FC, Sandler N, Libby SJ. Liver abscess caused by magA+ *Klebsiella pneumoniae* in North America. *J Clin Microbiol* 2005; **43**(2): 991–2.

13 Pope JV, Teich DL, Clardy P, McGillicuddy DC. *Klebsiella pneumoniae* liver abscess: an emerging problem in North America. *J Emerg Med* 2011; **41**(5): e103–5.

14 Ruiz-Hernandez JJ, Leon-Mazorra M, Conde-Martel A, *et al.* Pyogenic liver abscesses: mortality-related factors. *Eur J Gastroenterol Hepatol* 2007; **19**: 853–8.

15 Seeto RK, Rockey DC. Pyogenic liver abscess: changes in etiology, management, and outcome. *Medicine* 1996; **75**: 99–113.

16 Mohsen AH, Green ST, Read RC, *et al.* Liver abscess in adults: ten years experience in a UK centre. *Q J Med* 2002; **95**: 797–802.

17 Chou FF, Seen-Chen SM, Chen YS, *et al.* Single and multiple pyogenic liver abscesses: clinical course, etiology, and results of treatment. *World J Surg* 1997; **21**: 384–9.

18 Branum GD, Tyson GS, Branum MA, *et al.* Hepatic abscess: changes in etiology, diagnosis, and management. *Ann Surg* 1990; **212**: 655–62.

19 Nishimori H, Ezoe E, Ura H, *et al.* Septic thrombophlebitis of the portal and superior mesenteric veins as a complication of appendicitis: report of a case. *Surg Today* 2004; **34**: 173–6.

20 Chang TN, Tang L, Keller K, *et al.* Pylephlebitis, portal-mesenteric thrombosis, and multiple liver abscesses owing to perforated appendicitis. *J Ped Surg* 2001; **36**: E19–21.

21 Plemmons RM, Dooley DP, Longfield RN. Septic thrombophlebitis of the portal vein (pylephlebitis): diagnosis and management in the modern era. *Clin Infect Dis* 1995; **21**: 1114–20.

22 Stanley SL. Amoebiasis. *Lancet* 2003; **361**: 1025–34.

23 Salles JM, Moraes LA, Salles MC. Hepatic amebiasis. *Brazilian J Infect Dis* 2003; **7**: 96–110.

24 Lowther SA, Dworkin MS, Hanson DL, *et al. Entamoeba histolytica/Entamoeba dispar* infections in human immunodeficiency virus-infected patients in the United States. *Clin Infect Dis* 2000; **30**: 955–9.

25 Stark D, van Hal SJ, Matthews G, *et al.* Invasive amebiasis in men who have sex with men, Australia. *Emerg Infect Dis* 2008; **14**: 1141–3.

26 Tanyuksel M, Petro WA. Laboratory diagnosis of amebiasis. *Clin Micro Rev* 2008; **16**: 713–29.

27 Lodhi S, Sarwari AR, Salam A, *et al.* Features distinguishing amoebic from pyogenic liver abscess: a review of 577 adult cases. *Trop Med Int Health* 2004; **9**: 718–23.

28 Attasaranya S, Fogel EL, Lehman GA. Choledocholithiasis, ascending cholangitis, and gallstone pancreatitis. *Med Clin North Am* 2008; **92**: 925–60.

29 Hanau LH, Steigbigel NH. Acute (ascending) cholangitis. *Infect Dis Clin North Am* 2000; **14**: 521–46.

30 Abdalian R, Heathcote EJ. Sclerosing cholangitis: a focus on secondary causes. *Hepatology* 2006; **44**: 1063–74.

31 Silveira MG, Lindor KD. Clinical features and management of primary sclerosing cholangitis. *World J Gastroenterol* 2008; **14**: 3338–49.

32 Okamoto K, Takada T, Strasberg SM, *et al.* TG13 management bundles for acute cholangitis and cholecystitis. *J Hepatobiliary Pancreat Sci* 2013; **20**: 55–9.

33 Sartin JS, Walker RC. Granulomatous hepatitis: a retrospective review of 88 cases at the Mayo Clinic. *Mayo Clin Proc* 1991; **66**: 914–18.

34 Drebber U, Kasper HU, Ratering J, *et al.* Hepatic granulomas: histological and molecular pathological approach to differential diagnosis – a study of 442 cases. *Liver Int* 2008; **28**: 823–4.

35 Satt MB, al-Freihi H, Ibrahim EM, *et al.* Hepatic granuloma in Saudi Arabia: a clinicopathological study of 59 cases. *Am J Gastroenterol* 1990; **85**: 669–74.

36 Mert A, Ozaras R, Bilir M, *et al.* The etiology of hepatic granulomas. *J Clin Gastroenterol* 2001; **32**: 275–6.

37 Gaya DR, Thorburn D, Oien KA, *et al.* Hepatic granulomas: a 10 year single centre experience. *J Clin Pathol* 2003; **56**: 850–3.

38 Dourakis SP, Saramadou R, Alexopoulou A, *et al.* Hepatic granulomas: a 6-year experience in a single center in Greece. *Eur J Gastroenterol Hepatol* 2007; **19**: 101–4.

39 Zoutman DE, Ralph ED, Frei JV. Granulomatous hepatitis and fever of unknown origin: an 11-year experience of 23 cases with three years; follow-up. *Clin Gastroenterol* 1991; **13**: 69–75.

40 Johannsson B, Stapleton JT. Bacterial and miscellaneous infections of the liver. In: Boyer TD, Wright TL, Manns MP, eds. *Zakim and Boyer's Hepatology: A Textbook of Liver Disease*, 6th edn. Philadelphia, PA: Saunders, 2012: 656–70.

41 Gordon SC. Bacterial and systemic infections. In: Schiff ER, Sorrell MF, Maddrey WC, eds. *Schiff's Diseases of the Liver*, 10th edn. Baltimore, MD: Lippincott, Williams & Wilkins, 2007: 1379–99.

42 Mandell GL, Bennett JE, Dolin R, eds. *Mandell, Douglas and Bennett's Principles and Practice of Infectious Diseases*, 7th edn. Edinburgh: Churchill Livingstone, 2010.

43 Centers for Disease Control and Prevention. CDC Fact Sheet: gonorrhea treatment guidelines revised: guidelines to preserve last effective treatment option. July 2013. Available from: http://www.cdc.gov/std/treatment/2010/gonorrhea-treatment-guidelines-factsheet.pdf (last accessed February 15, 2016).

44 Ochola LB, Vounatsou P, Smith T, *et al.* The reliability of diagnostic techniques in the diagnosis and management of malaria in the absence of a gold standard. *Lancet Infect Dis* 2006; **6**: 582–8.

45 Laufer MK. Monitoring antimalarial drug efficacy: current challenges. *Curr Infect Dis Rep* 2009; **11**: 59–65.

46 Murray HW, Berman JD, Davies CR, Saravia NG. Advances in leishmaniasis. *Lancet* 2005; **355**: 1561–77.

47 Berman J. Current treatment approaches to leishmaniasis. *Curr Opin Infect Dis* 2003; **16**: 397–401.

48 Botterel F, Ichai P, Feray C, *et al.* Disseminated toxoplasmosis, resulting from infection of allograft, after orthotopic liver transplantation: usefulness of quantitative PCR. *J Clin Microbiol* 2002; **40**: 1648–50.

49 Lamps LW. Hepatic granulomas with an emphasis on infectious causes. *Adv Anat Pathol* 2008; **15**: 309–18.

50 Nunnari G, Pinzone MR, Gruttadauria S, *et al.* Hepatic echinococcosis: clinical and therapeutic aspects. *World J Gastroenterol* 2012; **18**(13): 1448–58.

51 McManus DP, Zhang W, Li J, Bartley PB. Echinococcosis. *Lancet* 2003; **362**: 1295–304.

52 Menezes da Silva A. Hydatid cyst of the liver: criteria for the selection of appropriate treatment. *Acta Trop* 2005; **85**: 237S.

53 Khandelwal N, Shaw J, Jain MK. Biliary parasites: diagnostic and therapeutic strategies. *Curr Treat Opt Gastroenterol* 2008; **11**: 85–95.

54 Pockros PJ, Capozza TA. Helminthic infections of the liver. *Curr Gastroenterol Rep* 2004; **6**: 287–96.

55 Mordinov VA, Yurlova NI, Ogorodova LM, Katokhin AV. *Opisthorchis felineus* and *Metorchis bilis* are the main agents of liver fluke infection of humans in Russia. *Parasitol Int* 2012; **61**: 25–31.

CHAPTER 78

CHAPTER 79

Alcoholic Liver Disease

Moira Hilscher[1] and Vijay Shah[2]

[1] Department of Internal Medicine, Mayo Clinic, Rochester, MN, USA
[2] Mayo Clinic, Rochester, MN, USA

Summary

Alcoholic liver disease (ALD) is a major driver of liver-related morbidity and mortality in the United States and worldwide. Diagnosis is made by a combination of clinical, histologic, and laboratory findings. The disease is a spectrum, ranging from fatty liver, which is generally benign, to hepatitis and cirrhosis, which can carry a poor prognosis. Though various pharmacologic therapies have been utilized, the most established treatments include supportive care, abstinence, and liver transplantation, when appropriate.

Case

A 50-year-old man is brought to the emergency room by emergency services after a syncopal episode. Some history is obtained from the patient's wife, who says that he has had a drinking problem for some years and has been feeling generally unwell for the past few days. The patient is alert and shows no signs of altered mental status or fever, but feels weak. Physical exam is significant for spider angiomas on his chest and palmar erythema. Liver edge is firm and span is increased. Spleen is palpable. No ascites or lower extremity edema is detected.

Introduction

Alcohol-associated liver disease results in a broad spectrum of histologic and clinical symptoms. Conditions such as fatty liver, alcoholic hepatitis, and alcoholic cirrhosis are induced by excessive alcohol consumption. Though fatty liver is reversible by alcohol abstinence, alcoholic hepatitis and cirrhosis are critical and potentially life-threatening manifestations of extended-duration alcohol abuse [1].

Definition and Epidemiology

As a major cause of morbidity and mortality, ALD has become a substantial health care problem for countries in the Western world, accounting for 40% of deaths from liver disease and 30% of hepatocellular carcinoma in the United States and Europe [2]. Alcoholic cirrhosis now ranks as the eighth most common cause of death in the United States [3].

Chronic alcohol abuse often results in an overlapping spectrum of histopathologic processes, ranging from steatosis (alcoholic fatty liver) and alcoholic hepatitis to cirrhosis. However, finding these entities in their isolated histopathologic state is uncommon, as they tend to overlap. Steatosis, the infiltration of liver cells with fat, develops as a short-term response to excessive alcohol consumption, occurring in 90% of heavy drinkers. In general, fatty liver is an asymptomatic, benign condition that is reversible within 4–6 weeks of abstinence. However, 5–15% of affected individuals may progress to fibrosis and cirrhosis despite abstinence.

Approximately 10–35% of people who abuse alcohol develop acute alcoholic hepatitis, characterized by necroinflammation and fibrosis as a result of hepatocellular damage. Alcoholic hepatitis also represents a spectrum of disease, which in its initial stages, like steatosis, can be reversed by abstinence. However, alcoholic hepatitis can be a serious condition; patients with severe alcoholic hepatitis have an exceptionally high short-term mortality rate and, with continued alcohol abuse, may develop cirrhosis [4]. The mortality rate of acute alcoholic hepatitis varies; it can be predicted by various quantitative scoring systems, as described later.

Pathophysiology

ALD has a multifactorial pathogenesis and can be induced by a variety of mechanisms (Figure 79.1). The two most important may be ethanol metabolism, with its generation of noxious metabolites, and genetic factors that predispose to alcohol-induced hepatic inflammation and fibrosis. Excessive ethanol consumption is the most prominent risk factor for liver injury [5,6]. Ingestion of more than 30 g of ethanol a day confers an increased risk for development of ALD and cirrhosis [7].

Metabolic Mechanisms

In the liver, alcohol is metabolized by several different enzyme systems: alcohol dehydrogenase (ADH), aldehyde dehydrogenase, and the microsomal ethanol-oxidizing system (MEOS). When blood alcohol levels are low, ADH is the predominant enzyme that metabolizes ethanol in the liver, by catalyzing the conversion of alcohol to acetaldehyde. MEOS also converts alcohol to acetaldehyde, but with two important differences: (i) the conversion is achieved with the MEOS-specific cytochrome P-450 enzyme CYP2E1; and (ii) this conversion occurs when alcohol blood levels are moderate to high. ADH oxidizes approximately 80% of ethanol and MEOS generally accounts for the remainder. These two major metabolizing pathways play a fundamental role in the development of alcohol-induced chronic liver disease [8].

Practical Gastroenterology and Hepatology Board Review Toolkit, Second Edition. Edited by Nicholas J. Talley, Kenneth R. DeVault, Michael B. Wallace, Bashar A. Aqel and Keith D. Lindor.
© 2016 John Wiley & Sons, Ltd. Published 2016 by John Wiley & Sons, Ltd. Companion website: www.practicalgastrohep.com

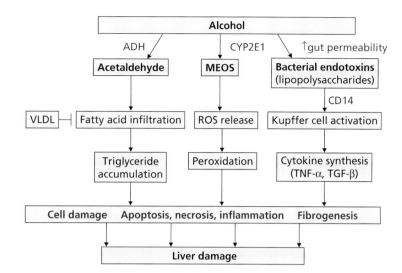

Figure 79.1 Mechanisms of alcoholic liver disease (ALD).

Acetaldehyde

Acetaldehyde is the most potent ethanol metabolite leading to liver damage. It is a reactive compound that impairs hepatocytes through the formation of protein and DNA adducts, which then induce lipid peroxidation, glutathione depletion, and mitochondrial damage.

The liver utilizes ethanol as its preferred energy source, forgoing other available fueling substrates in its presence. Ethanol metabolism operates through oxidative and non-oxidative pathways. In the first step of oxidation, ethanol is converted to acetaldehyde through the gastric isoenzyme ADH. A portion of ethanol undergoes first-pass metabolism, which disrupts intracellular pathways and alters the functional properties of the cell membranes. This allows free fatty acids (FFAs) to diffuse liberally across hepatocyte plasma membranes. Under physiologic circumstances, fatty acids undergo β-oxidation inside the hepatocyte; however, extensive ethanol metabolism alters the reduction potential of the hepatocyte and decreases mitochondrial β-oxidation of FFAs [8]. The ethanol metabolite acetaldehyde directly inhibits peroxisome proliferator-activated receptor (PPAR)-a, a transcription factor that regulates the synthesis of enzymes involved in fatty acid catabolism. Over time, this induces the accumulation of fatty acids in the liver; however, the diseased liver is increasingly unable to utilize them as energy substrates. Esters form and accumulate as triglycerides within the hepatocytes.

Oxidative Stress and MEOS

Oxidant stress is an integral factor in ethanol toxicity. The MEOS is an enzyme compound that is involved in ethanol metabolism, operating through several cytochrome P-450 isoenzymes, of which CYP2E1 is a key player. While its basal contribution to ethanol metabolism is low, chronic alcohol intake stimulates CYP2E1 expression, which fuels hepatic ethanol oxidation. Tissue-damaging reactive oxygen species (ROS) are released, which attack cellular lipids and cause peroxidation.

Genetic and Hereditary Factors

The lack of a linear relationship between quantity of alcohol consumed and the development of ALD has led to the theory of a genetically determined predisposition to ALD. Certain genetic factors may make a person more susceptible to alcohol-induced liver toxicity. In patients with ALD, gene-linked polymorphisms have

been associated with mutations in the tumor necrosis factor (TNF) promoter and in alcohol-metabolizing enzyme systems. Polymorphisms of ADH may cause reduced enzyme activity, leading to high levels of acetaldehyde, which enhance liver injury. However, to date no specific polymorphism has been definitely linked to ALD. Furthermore, genetic factors are assumed to play a role in an individual's inclination toward alcoholism.

ALD is more prevalent in men, but women are more likely to develop severe forms of the disease with less alcohol consumption. Even with weight adjustment, a similar amount of alcohol consumption results in higher blood alcohol levels in women than in men. Attempts at explaining this trend include a relative deficiency of gastric ADH in women, differences in proportions of body fat, and female hormone-related causes [9].

Clinical Features

Most patients with fatty liver are asymptomatic. Patients who have alcoholic hepatitis and cirrhosis may also be asymptomatic, but many present with non-specific symptoms, such as nausea, vomiting, weight loss, weakness, pain, fever, jaundice, and diarrhea. In the end stages of cirrhosis, symptoms of liver failure may develop.

On physical examination, 75% of patients with steatosis and alcoholic hepatitis present with hepatomegaly, regardless of the degree of liver damage. In addition, hepatic tenderness, splenomegaly, varices, and peripheral edema may occur. Among patients with more severe disease, approximately 60% present with jaundice and ascites. In the initial stages of cirrhosis, well-compensated patients may present with no abnormalities on physical examination. As the disease progresses, compensation mechanisms gradually collapse and patients present with variable degrees of hepatic failure, as well as muscle wasting, ascites, spider angiomas, portal hypertension, and, in severe cases, hepatic encephalopathy [10].

Diagnosis

A detailed drinking history should be obtained. In mild forms of liver disease, the patient often presents with no complaints. In patients with chronic alcohol problems, hepatomegaly is the most common sign of ALD. The onset of fever, jaundice, scleral icterus, or right upper quadrant tenderness is highly suggestive of liver damage as well. Other diagnostic findings that point to ALD are neutrophilic leukocytosis, thrombocytopenia, an aspartate aminotransferase (AST) : alanine aminotransferase (ALT) ratio >1, mixed hyperbilirubinemia (elevated levels of both conjugated and unconjugated bilirubinemia), hypoalbuminemia, and increased prothrombin time. High serum immunoglobin levels and low peripheral lymphocyte count are common [2]. Lab findings more indicative of alcoholic hepatitis include neutrophilic leukocytosis with left shift, AST and ALT which are mildly elevated but typically less than 400 IU/L, and an AST : ALT ratio >2 [3].

Differential Diagnosis

Alcoholic hepatitis can be difficult to distinguish from non-alcoholic steatohepatitis (NASH) histologically, but can be predicted by specific lab-based criteria. NASH occurs frequently in people with the metabolic syndrome, but also in chronic parenteral hyperalimentation-treated patients and as a side effect of certain drugs, such as estrogens and glucocorticoids. NASH is indolent in most cases, with an AST : ALT ratio <1. Differentiation between alcoholic hepatitis and NASH can be difficult in the obese patient with an unreliable alcohol history. AST : ALT ratio, body mass index (BMI), and gender are important variables in accurately differentiating patients with ALD from non-alcoholic fatty liver disease (NAFLD). These variables, weighted and combined with mean cell volume (MCV), determine the ALD/NAFLD index (ANI) (see http://www.mayoclinic.org/gi-rst/mayomodel10.html). An ANI >0 is more likely in alcoholic hepatitis patients, while a negative ANI score favors NASH [3].

Percutaneous or transjugular liver biopsy can confirm the diagnosis of alcoholic hepatitis in cases with diagnostic uncertainty or if potentially toxic or invasive therapies such as corticosteroids or transplant are being considered. Characteristic histologic features of moderate-to-severe ALD include steatosis, fibrosis, inflammation, Mallory bodies, ballooning necrosis of hepatocytes, and hemosiderin deposits [11].

Prognosis

The prognosis is largely dependent on alcohol abstinence and the degree of liver decompensation. Patients with clinically decompensated alcoholic cirrhosis have a 5-year mortality rate of 90%. The 5-year survival rate of decompensated cirrhosis patients who continue drinking is 30% at best [1]. Alcohol abstinence is the most effective way of preventing progression of ALD. Up to a certain point, already acquired pathologic liver alterations, such as steatosis, acute alcoholic hepatitis, inflammation, and mild collagen deposition, are for the most part reversible. Alcoholic steatosis has been shown to resolve completely with abstinence. However, more advanced fibrosis is less likely to resolve. Regardless, alcohol abstinence is the primary and most fundamental approach to therapy.

The severity of alcoholic hepatitis can be assessed using a prognostic index. There are several frequently applied scoring systems predictive of survival in patients with alcoholic hepatitis, each of which has unique limitations. The Maddrey Discriminant Function (MDF) is most commonly used, and is calculated by the follow equation:

DF = (4.6 × (prothrombin time (seconds) − control prothrombin time (seconds))) + serum bilirubin (mg/dL)

If DF >32, patients have a 30-day survival rate of less than 50%; when DF <32, the probability of survival in 30 days is 80–100%.

An alternative prognostic quantitative index is the Mayo End-Stage Liver Disease (MELD), a modified version of the MDF that takes into account bilirubin, International Normalized Ratio (INR), and creatinine levels:

MELD = 3.8(Ln serum bilirubin (mg/dL)) + 11.2(Ln INR) + 9.6(Ln serum creatinine (mg/dL)) + 6.4, where Ln denotes the natural logarithm.

When the MELD index is >25, the short-term survival rate is about 50% [12] (see http://www.mayoclinic.org/meld/mayomodel7/.html). American Association for the Study of Liver Diseases (AASLD) guidelines recommend a MELD score of 18 as the threshold for initiation of therapy [13].

The Glasgow Alcoholic Hepatitis Score (GAHS) employs values for age, white cell count, urea, prothrombin time ratio, and bilirubin level. Patients with a GAHS ≥9 have a 30-day survival rate of 46% and an 80-day survival rate of 40%.

The Lille score is applied to determine the response to and appropriateness of continued treatment. Its calculation employs baseline age, INR, creatinine, bilirubin, albumin, and bilirubin level after 7 days of prednisolone treatment. This score is normalized to 0, with scores closer to 1 indicative of worse prognosis. Though 0.45 was initially employed as the threshold, recent studies suggest a score of <0.56 to be indicative of benefit from prednisolone treatment and a score >0.56 to show no benefit [13]. Early change in bilirubin level (ECBL), defined as a bilirubin level that is lower at day 7 of treatment than on day 1, can also help predict patients who will benefit from corticosteroids [14].

Case Continued

The patient is subjected to blood tests, with the following results: ALT 32 IU/L, bilirubin 1.4 mg/dL, albumin 3.6 g/dL, alkaline phosphatase 100 IU/L, INR 1.6. Hepatitis serologies show no evidence of hepatitis A, B, or C. An abdominal ultrasound scan is performed, and shows an enlarged liver suggestive of fatty infiltration. The MDF score is 35.

As a supportive measure, the patient is administered intravenous fluids and vitamins. He is soon started on a course of prednisone. In addition, he receives counseling on his drinking behavior and his nutritional choices.

Management

Even in patients with severe liver cirrhosis, alcohol abstinence has been shown to be beneficial for survival. In patients who survive an episode of acute alcoholic hepatitis, abstinence is the most important factor predictive of long-term outcome [3]. Effective therapy is based on a combination of lifestyle changes and potential pharmacologic treatment (Figure 79.2). Treatment consideration is based on the extent of the alcoholic liver injury. Isolated fatty liver requires no treatment other than alcohol abstinence. For alcoholic hepatitis, a number of pharmacologic treatment options have been evaluated, but current therapy still focuses on supportive care.

Lifestyle Modification

The ultimate goal is to prevent disease progression and the possible development of decompensated cirrhosis and hepatocellular carcinoma. Lifestyle modification remains a cornerstone of therapy. People with alcohol problems are often heavy smokers as well, which may be a risk factor for progression of liver disease. Patients with end-stage liver disease have some degree of malnutrition, due to low nutrient intake and intestinal malabsorption. Nutritional deficiency

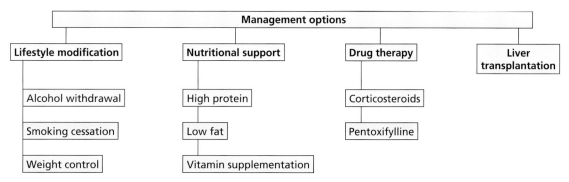

Figure 79.2 Algorithm for the management of ALD.

disrupts the integrity of the immune system and impairs the ability to respond to infection. Enteral nutrition is favored because of its lower cost and because its positive effect on gut mucosal integrity confers a decreased risk of bacterial translocation and infections [3,15]. Patients should follow a high-protein diet supplemented with vitamins B, C, and K and folic acid. Obesity is also a risk factor for the development of steatosis, alcoholic hepatitis, and cirrhosis. The approach to lifestyle modification begins with reduction of alcohol intake, smoking cessation, weight control, and nutritional supplementation.

Drug Therapy

Corticosteroids

Though both the AASLD and European Association for the Study of the Liver (EASL) guidelines recommend corticosteroids as first-line treatment for severe alcoholic hepatitis (DF ≥32), controversy persists regarding their effectiveness [13]. Examination of study results suggests that corticosteroids improve survival in patients who have hepatic encephalopathy or severe alcoholic hepatitis, with an MDF score >32 [16]. A more recent meta-analysis of individual patient data from five randomized controlled trials (RCTs) studying corticosteroid treatment for severe alcoholic hepatitis confirmed the efficacy of corticosteroids in those patients classified as complete or partial responders by the Lille model [17]. Glucocorticoids have not been well studied in those with gastrointestinal (GI) bleeding, renal failure, pancreatitis, or active infection. However, if infected patients are appropriately treated with antibiotics, their survival approaches that of non-infected patients. Typical recommended steroid courses consist of oral prednisolone 40 mg daily or parenteral methylprednisolone 32 mg daily for 4 weeks with a 4-week taper [3]. When administering glucocorticosteroids to patients with hepatic encephalopathy, a course of prednisone 40 mg daily for 30 days is recommended [9].

Pentoxifylline

Pentoxifylline (PTX) is a non-selective phosphodiesterase inhibitor that constitutes first-line therapy for alcoholic hepatitis in many centers. It is recommended by both the EASL and the AASLD as an alternative to prednisolone. Though PTX is known to reduce blood viscosity, its mechanism of action in alcoholic hepatitis is unclear [3]. While data are conflicting, several studies have reported reduced mortality in patients with severe alcoholic hepatitis treated with PTX compared with placebo [18, 19]. A reduction in the incidence of hepatorenal syndrome has also been reported in several studies [18]. Alcoholic hepatitis is characterized by elevated TNF-α levels, but this rise is blunted by treatment with PTX, which may therefore inhibit TNF-α synthesis or neutralize its receptors [3]. Observed side effects include vomiting, epigastric pain, and dyspepsia, which quickly resolve after PTX treatment is discontinued.

Anti-TNF-α

TNF-α is a major factor in the pathogenesis of alcoholic hepatitis and is associated with poor prognosis. However, anti-TNF-α agents, including infliximab and etanercept, have not shown benefit and are not recommended in treatment of alcoholic hepatitis. This may be due to the role that TNF-α plays in the stimulation of inflammatory pathways, hepatocyte growth factor, and regeneration [3,20].

Other Treatment Options

Alcohol generates significant oxidative stress, as evidenced by the detection of lipid peroxidation products in the blood of alcoholics and in livers with alcoholic changes [8]. Therefore, antioxidants have been investigated as a potential therapeutic in alcoholic hepatitis. A recent study compared treatment with corticosteroids to treatment with corticosteroids plus N-acetylcysteine (NAC) in 174 patients with alcoholic hepatitis; it found a lower mortality rate in those treated with steroids and NAC at 1 month but not at 3 or 6 months, suggesting improved short-term survival without long-term benefit [21]. Further studies are warranted before NAC in conjunction with steroids can be routinely used.

Liver Transplantation

End-stage ALD is the second most common indication for liver transplantation for chronic liver disease in the Western world [4]. However, only 5% of patients with end-stage ALD are evaluated for transplantation, the primary reasons being donor scarcity, possibility of recidivism, and the widespread perception of ALD as a self-induced affliction [4]. As a result, patients with ALD are less likely to receive a liver transplant than are patients with other forms of end-stage liver disease [22]. The 7-year survival rate after liver transplantation is an excellent 60%, and survival rates are similar among those transplanted for ALD versus other forms of end-stage liver disease. Many transplantation units demand a 6-month alcohol abstinence period before considering transplantation. Though data are limited, a few studies suggest that a 6-month pre-transplant sobriety period decreases the likelihood of recidivism post-transplant. This period also allows for potential liver recovery without continued injury from alcohol. Estimates of post-transplant recidivism for ALD vary between 11 and 49%; however, only a small fraction are reported to revert to heavy alcohol use or abuse, threatening graft viability [4].

Strict patient selection criteria remain an important component of liver transplantation. Due to controversy surrounding the 6-month abstinence period, a recent trial evaluated early liver transplantation for alcoholic hepatitis patients who failed medical therapy with glucocorticoids. This study applied stringent selection criteria, including extensive social support and no history of prior decompensating events. It confirmed a 6-month survival benefit among patients undergoing early liver transplantation after failing medical management. While long-term follow up is required, no relapse of alcoholism was observed in the 6 months post-transplant [17].

Take Home Points

- Alcoholic liver disease (ALD) encompasses a clinicohistologic spectrum (fatty liver, alcoholic hepatitis, cirrhosis).
- Metabolic and immune mechanisms, as well as hereditary factors, contribute to the pathogenesis of ALD by altering hepatocyte functioning.
- The two main alcohol-metabolizing pathways are alcohol dehydrogenase (ADH) and microsomal ethanol-oxidizing system (MEOS).
- Alcoholic fatty liver develops in response to short periods of alcohol abuse; hepatitis and cirrhosis are the results of long-term drinking.
- Accurate diagnosis of ALD is oriented by the clinical history, histology, and laboratory findings.
- Early forms of alcohol-induced liver damage can be reversed by alcohol abstinence.
- Effective treatment focuses on combining supportive measures and, in some cases, drug therapy.
- Liver transplantation is the only available long-term treatment for end-stage liver disease.

References

1 Menon KV, Gores GJ, Shah VH. Pathogenesis, diagnosis, and treatment of alcoholic liver disease. *Mayo Clin Proc* 2001; **76**(10): 1021–9.

2 Carithers R, McClain C. Alcoholic liver disease. In: Friedman LS, Brandt LJ, Sleisenger MH, eds. *Sleisenger and Fordtran's Gastrointestinal and Liver Disease*, 8th edn. Philadelphia, PA: Saunders Elsevier, 2006: 1771–92.

3 Singal AK, Kamath PS, Gores GJ, Shah VH. Alcoholic hepatitis: current challenges and future directions. *Clin Gastroenterol Hepatol* 2014; **12**(4): 555–64.

4 O'Shea RS, Dasarathy S, McCullough AJ. Alcoholic liver disease. *Hepatology* 2010; **51**(1): 307–28.

5 Maher JJ. Alcoholic steatosis and steatohepatitis. *Semin Gastrointest Dis* 2002; **13**(1): 31–9.

6 Haber PS, Warner R, Seth D, *et al.* Pathogenesis and management of alcoholic hepatitis. *J Gastroenterol Hepatol* 2003; **18**(12): 1332–44.

7 Bellentani S, Saccoccio G, Costa G, *et al.* Drinking habits as cofactors of risk for alcohol induced liver damage. The Dionysos Study Group. *Gut* 1997; **41**(6): 845–50.

8 Beier JI, McClain CJ. Mechanisms and cell signaling in alcoholic liver disease. *Biol Chem* 2010; **391**(11): 1249–64.

9 Tome S, Lucey MR. Review article: Current management of alcoholic liver disease. *Aliment Pharmacol Ther* 2004; **19**(7): 707–14.

10 Ceccanti M, Attili A, Balducci G, *et al.* Acute alcoholic hepatitis. *J Clin Gastroenterol* 2006; **40**(9): 833–41.

11 Shah VH. Alcoholic liver disease. In: Hauser SC, ed. *Mayo Clinic Gastroenterology and Hepatology Board Review*, 2nd edn. Rochester, MN: Mayo Clinic Scientific Press, 2006: 289–97.

12 Dunn W, Jamil LH, Brown LS, *et al.* MELD accurately predicts mortality in patients with alcoholic hepatitis. *Hepatology* 2005; **41**(2): 353–8.

13 Morgan TR, Chao D, Botwin G. Concepts and Controversies in the Management of Alcoholic Hepatitis. Postgraduate course presented at the American Association of the Study of Liver Diseases. 2013.

14 Mathurin P, Abdelnour M, Ramond MJ, *et al.* Early change in bilirubin levels is an important prognostic factor in severe alcoholic hepatitis treated with prednisolone. *Hepatology* 2003; **38**(6): 1363–9.

15 Singal AK, Charlton MR. Nutrition in alcoholic liver disease. *Clin Liver Dis* 2012; **16**(4): 805–26.

16 Rambaldi A, Saconato HH, Christensen E, *et al.* Systematic review: glucocorticosteroids for alcoholic hepatitis – a Cochrane Hepato-Biliary Group systematic review with meta-analyses and trial sequential analyses of randomized clinical trials. *Aliment Pharmacol Ther* 2008; **27**(12): 1167–78.

17 Mathurin P, O'Grady J, Carithers RL, *et al.* Corticosteroids improve short-term survival in patients with severe alcoholic hepatitis: meta-analysis of individual patient data. *Gut* 2011; **60**(2): 255–60.

18 Akriviadis E, Botla R, Briggs W, *et al.* Pentoxifylline improves short-term survival in severe acute alcoholic hepatitis: a double-blind, placebo-controlled trial. *Gastroenterology* 2000; **119**(6): 1637–48.

19 Whitfield K, Rambaldi A, Wetterslev J, Gluud C. Pentoxifylline for alcoholic hepatitis. *Cochrane Database Syst Rev* 2009(4):CD007339.

20 Boetticher NC, Peine CJ, Kwo P, *et al.* A randomized, double-blinded, placebo-controlled multicenter trial of etanercept in the treatment of alcoholic hepatitis. *Gastroenterology* 2008; **135**(6): 1953–60.

21 Nguyen-Khac E, Thevenot T, Piquet MA, *et al.* Glucocorticoids plus N-acetylcysteine in severe alcoholic hepatitis. *N Engl J Med* 2011; **365**(19): 1781–9.

22 Julapalli VR, Kramer JR, El-Serag HB. Evaluation for liver transplantation: adherence to AASLD referral guidelines in a large Veterans Affairs center. *Liver Transpl* 2005; **11**(11): 1370–8.

CHAPTER 80

Drug-Induced Liver Injury

Einar Björnsson[1] and Naga Chalasani[2]

[1] Division of Gastroenterology and Hepatology, Department of Medicine, The National University Hospital of Iceland, Reykjavik, Iceland
[2] Division of Gastroenterology and Hepatology, Department of Medicine, Indiana School of Medicine, Indianapolis, IN, USA

Summary

Drug-induced liver injury (DILI) is a complication of many drugs. This is not surprising, given that liver plays a central role in the metabolism of drugs. Direct toxic liver damage is associated with acetaminophen toxicity, whereas most other drugs causing liver damage have an unpredictable or *idiosyncratic* pattern of injury. Acetaminophen and other drugs are the most common causes of acute liver failure (ALF) in the United States. Physicians need to consider DILI in all patients who present with symptoms or signs of liver dysfunction. Clinically and histologically, DILI can mimic any known liver disease, and the diagnosis is one of exclusion. In patients with a high clinical suspicion of DILI, the causative drug needs to be discontinued, and patients with jaundice and/or coagulopathy must be hospitalized and in some cases considered for a liver transplantation.

Case

A 55-year-old woman presents with a few days' history of lethargy, nausea, and abdominal pain. She is originally from Iraq. She has a recent history of ulcerative colitis that is poorly controlled. Her gastroenterologist considered a tumor necrosis factor (TNF)-alpha inhibitor treatment for this, but a latent tuberculosis infection was detected and she was put on isoniazid 2 months prior to the presentation.

Due to moderate to severe upper right quadrant pain, she is admitted for surgery. Clinical examination reveals tenderness over the liver and gallbladder, and abdominal ultrasound shows sludge in the gallbladder, which has wall thickening but no dilatation of the biliary tree. Her aspartate aminotransferase (AST) is 1680, alanine aminotransferase (ALT) 1100, alkaline phosphatase 300, total bilirubin 2.0 mg/dL, and International Normalized Ratio (INR) 1.7. She undergoes laparoscopic cholecystectomy, but in the days after the operation her liver tests deteriorate and her INR increases to 5.5, and she suffers from severe lethargy. A hepatologist who is contacted recommends referral to a liver transplant center. She is put on the waiting list for a liver transplantation due to a suspicion of isoniazid-induced liver failure, but dies on the waiting list 1 week later as no graft becomes available.

Definition and Epidemiology

An adverse drug reaction (ADR) can be defined as any drug response that is unintended and noxious and occurs at the normal dose interval of the drug. "DILI," "hepatotoxicity," and "adverse liver reaction" are used interchangeably in this context. Most liver injuries due to acetaminophen are associated with overdoses of the drug, and unintentional overdose without suicidal intent is increasingly observed with acetaminophen, especially in the United States [1]. Though both intentional and unintentional acetaminophen overdose account for many cases of liver injury, most DILIs are caused by *idiosyncratic* or unexpected reactions [3]. Traditionally idiosyncratic drug reactions were not considered to be dose-dependent, but it has recently been demonstrated that drugs with a daily dose of <50 mg are very rarely associated with DILI [2]. Thus, though it is unexpected and rare, several drugs with well-documented DILI have a dose-dependent component. For most drugs, the risk of hepatotoxicity is minimal. In a retrospective study from the United Kingdom published more than 10 years ago, the highest crude incidence rates were found for chlorpromazine (1 in approximately 700 users), azathioprine and sulfasalazine (1 in 1000–1100 users), and amoxicillin-clavulanate (1 in approximately 11 000 users) [4]. A recent prospective study from Iceland revealed much higher incidence rates for DILI, with the highest risk for individual agents being 1 in 133 users for azathioprine and 1 in 148 for infliximab [4]. The risk of DILI was found to be 1 in 2350 users for amoxicilin-clavulanate [4]. Lack of systemic monitoring systems makes it very difficult to estimate the frequency of DILI, and there is no doubt that DILIs are underreported. Thus, the true incidence of idiosyncratic DILI is largely unknown. Based on retrospective data from the UK General Practice Research Database (GPRD) [4], a crude incidence rate of 2.4 cases per 100 000 inhabitants per year can be estimated. A very similar incidence was extrapolated from a Swedish study at a university hospital over a 10-year period [6]. A more reliable source of the true incidence of DILI is a careful prospective survey from the general population of a city in France [7]. All suspected cases of DILI were collected over a defined period in a defined population in a prospective fashion [7]. The incidence of DILI was found to be 13.9 cases per 100 000 inhabitants, which was at least 16 times greater than the reactions obtained through spontaneous reporting [6]. A 2-year population-based study from the whole country of Iceland demonstrated an incidence of 19 cases per 100 000 per year [5]. These results are somewhat higher than the incidence in the only other population-based study undertaken to date [7].

The likelihood of DILI is dependent on the clinical context. According to data from the US Acute Liver Failure Study Group,

Practical Gastroenterology and Hepatology Board Review Toolkit, Second Edition. Edited by Nicholas J. Talley, Kenneth R. DeVault, Michael B. Wallace, Bashar A. Aqel and Keith D. Lindor.

acetaminophen and idiosyncratic drug reactions were responsible for approximately 50% of cases of ALF [1]. DILI has been reported to occur in 2–10% of patients hospitalized for jaundice [3]. A total of 77 in 1164 (6.6%) patients in an outpatient hepatology clinic in Sweden were there because of DILI; half of these were new consults and half were being followed up after hospitalization for DILI [6]. A study from Switzerland reported an incidence of DILI in 1.4% of hospitalized patients, but DILI was not included in the diagnosis or in the physician's discharge letter in a high proportion of patients [8].

Clinical Presentation and Clinical Evaluation

Idiosyncratic DILI

Patients who suffer from DILI have a wide variety of clinical presentations. Both clinically and histologically, DILI can simulate almost all forms of acute and chronic liver injury. Thus, these patients can present with ALF with severe encephalopathy, acute hepatitis, chronic hepatitis, steatohepatitis, granulomatous hepatitis, and – though probably rare – liver cirrhosis [3,9]. Before patients develop jaundice, symptoms of liver dysfunction are usually non-specific, but lethargy and nausea are common, and sometimes severe biochemical liver test abnormalities are detected in asymptomatic individuals. A minority of patients with DILI (approximately 30%) present with symptoms suggestive of immunoallergic drug reactions with fever, rash, and eosinophilia [10,11]. In cases where histology is available, the presence of eosinophilia and centrilobular necrosis may support the role of DILI in the liver dysfunction. However, in most cases liver histology is not specific for DILI, and pathological evaluation is in many cases "compatible with" DILI.

Most idiosyncratic drug reactions occur within 1 year of starting the drug, though there are some exceptions (e.g., nitrofurantoin). Though drugs with a well-documented capacity to cause DILI can lead to a different expression in different patients, most hepatotoxic drugs have a "signature" toxicity. A hepatitic pattern is typically observed in patients with isoniazid-, disulfiram-, and diclofenac-associated hepatotoxicity, whereas cholestatic injury is seen most often with amoxicillin/clavulanate, macrolide antibiotics, and estrogens [3]. The most important initial approach to a patient with liver test abnormalities is to keep DILI in mind as a differential diagnosis. The initial evaluation should include a thorough history of drug exposure, duration of therapy, previously recognized hepatotoxicity of the implicated drug, and the severity of the reaction. Patients with jaundice (without coagulopathy) due to idiosyncratic drug reactions need to be hospitalized, as they have risk of liver failure [10,12], and those with concomitant coagulopathy should be considered for liver transplantation.

Acetaminophen

As with *idiosyncratic* drug reactions, symptoms of liver injury due to acetaminophen are non-specific. Patients with unintentional acetaminophen toxicity have typically used over-the-counter (OTC) drugs and narcotics in combination with acetaminophen, and the attending physician should be aware of the possibility of such a "therapeutic misadventure." Acetaminophen hepatotoxicity should be suspected in patients with extremely high aminotransferases and only mildly elevated bilirubin at presentation [1]. Hepatic injury typically develops 12–72 hours after suicidal intent, and liver failure 72–96 hours after ingestion. Patients with acetaminophen toxicity with encephalopathy and/or signs of kidney failure at presentation should in most cases be hospitalized in the intensive care unit (ICU), and liver transplantation assessment should be started immediately.

Diagnosis and Causality Assessment

Idiosyncratic DILI

Establishing a relationship between a drug and liver injury can be a very difficult task. As mentioned earlier, the clinical and biochemical abnormalities are usually non-specific, and there are no markers or tests to confirm the causality. Some drugs have a "signature," showing a biochemical and histological pattern typical of the drug and immunoallergic manifestation, which makes the causality assessment easier. However, given the heterogeneity of presentations, the diagnosis relies on circumstantial evidence and "guilt by association" [13]. In most cases of a strong suspicion of DILI in patients with new-onset liver disease, there is a temporal relationship between starting the suspected drug and onset of DILI. A temporal relationship between discontinuation of the drug and improvement of liver tests is also strongly suggestive of DILI. However, there are a number of pitfalls that the physician must bear in mind in the causality assessment. An important question in this context is whether the drug treatment was started before the patient developed symptoms indicative of liver disease, such as severe lethargy, nausea, and/or dark urin or pale stools. It is conceivable that the patient used the drug against symptoms associated with "hepatitis" or liver dysfunction of other etiology, for example (e.g., using a proton pump inhibitor (PPI) against abdominal discomfort or a painkiller against headache). Thus, before a drug is "accused" of being responsible for liver test abnormalities, a reasonable exclusion of other causes of liver disease should be made (see later). When available, information about the last liver tests before the implicated drug was started can be of great value.

Information about the duration of drug therapy is crucial to evaluating the time to onset of the drug reaction. For most idiosyncratic reactions, the latency period is approximately 1 week to a few months. Typically, immunoallergic reactions (fever, rash, eosinophilia) occur within a few weeks of exposure. For metabolically induced DILI, the latency period is in most cases less than 3 months. However, there are important exceptions. Patients who have been taking some drugs with well-documented hepatotoxicity, such as nitrofurantoin, diclofenac, troglitazone, and ximelagatran, with normal liver tests for months, can unexpectedly develop hepatotoxicity, which can be severe. In the best-case scenario, an important part of the causality assessment is observing a rapid biochemical and clinical improvement after discontinuation of the implicated drug, called "positive dechallenge." However, for some drugs that cause hepatotoxicity, liver injury may worsen initially for days or sometimes weeks after discontinuation. A good example is amoxicillin/clavulanate liver injury. Another is troglitazone, an agent removed from the market due to many cases of fatal hepatotoxicity, which was associated in clinical trials with liver test abnormalities that saw ALT and AST continue to rise for a period of time after discontinuation [14]. Furthermore, in patients with well-characterized DILI with a classical "signature" presenting with jaundice and/or liver failure, the condition can deteriorate despite interruption of the drug at presentation, and the patient will die if they do not undergo a liver transplantation [12].

It has been increasingly recognized that for some drugs with a clear potential of hepatotoxicity, liver tests can improve in some patients despite continuation of therapy (e.g., ximelagatran and tacrine) [14]. However, it is obvious that susceptible individuals are unable to achieve such an "adaptation" to the liver injury and may go on to develop fatal hepatotoxicity [14]. Compared with hepatocellular or hepatitic reactions, improvement in liver tests is generally slower after discontinuation of drugs leading to cholestatic reactions [15]. Information about the course of the disease after cessation is important. So too is information about previously documented drug hepatotoxicity, which may add evidence in favor of a drug etiology in the reaction.

Even if there is a strong suspicion of a drug etiology, exclusion of other causes of liver disease is *sine qua non* for establishing a diagnosis of DILI. How extensive this diagnostic workup is depends on the clinical context. Factors that may impact it include the type of liver injury, patient age, and symptomatology. With a typical cholestatic pattern, imaging plays the most important role (liver ultrasound or computed tomography (CT)), whereas in the case of hepatocellular injury, it is more important to rule out infectious etiology – though no general rule can be applied. In most cases, a reasonable examination is an abdominal ultrasound, though the information provided in typical hepatocellular (hepatitic) injury is limited. In selected cases with negative viral serologies, a polymerase chain reaction (PCR) screening may be necessary in order to exclude a very recent viral infection. History of alcohol abuse should be documented, as should recent episodes of hypotension, which can cause hepatocellular liver injury. The role of a liver biopsy in the diagnostic workup of DILI is controversial. It is a common misconception that liver histology is essential for establishing a diagnosis of a toxic etiology. As DILI has no specific histological findings, liver biopsy is of unclear value in this context. At best, histology can be compatible with DILI, and in cases of a clear-cut autoimmune hepatitis biopsy may reveal "toxic etiology compatible with DILI" even though the patient has not been exposed to a drug. Thus, a routine liver biopsy is not indicated, and if one is undertaken late in the course of the reaction, it may induce confusion among clinicians. Instruments for evaluating causality have been developed, the most common of which is the Roussel Uclaf Causality Assessment Method (RUCAM), developed by the Drug-Induced Liver Injury Network (DILIN) in the United States, though this is mainly used in research and only rarely in clinical practice [16, 17].

Acetaminophen

Many of the principles of the diagnostic workup and the causality assessment are similar in cases of acetaminophen-induced liver injury. However, blood concentration of acetaminophen can be obtained early in the course of the reaction and is an important part of the management of a patient with a suspected and confirmed acetaminophen toxicity. Later in the course, blood concentrations are not reliable. Recently, an assay has been developed for the detection of a byproduct of the toxic reaction: acetaminophen-CYS adducts, released from damaged hepatocytes, which are elevated in patients considered to have ALF of indeterminate etiology [1]. However, this assay is not yet commercially available and its validity in clinical practice needs further study.

Causative Drugs

A large number of different drugs have been associated with DILI [14]. Some have well characterized hepatotoxicity (e.g., isoniazid, phenytoin, disulfiram, amoxicillin/clavulanic acid), while in some it has only been reported in a single case report [15]. The main class of drugs reported in case series of patients with DILI has consistently been antibiotics [5–7, 12, 17], followed by non-steroidal anti-inflammatory drugs (NSAIDs). The most common antibiotics implicated have been amoxicillin/clavulanic, erythromycin, flucloxacillin, trimethoprim-sulfa, and nitrofurantoin, but antituberculous drugs such as isoniazid and rifampicin have also commonly been observed in these series [5–7, 12, 17]. In outpatients, the single most common drug implicated is diclofenac [6]. However, among patients with acute drug-induced liver failure in the United States, acetaminophen is the most common causative drug, followed by antibiotics, NSAIDs, anti-epileptics, and herbal drugs [18].

Risk Factors

Predicting the susceptibility for DILI in an individual patient is almost impossible. Obviously, if the patient has already experienced a liver injury from a particular drug, there is a great risk that this will happen again. Also, a past history of DILI from one drug has been shown to be a predictor of future DILI [9, 15]. Genetic variability in the hepatic metabolism of drugs has been considered to be the most important risk factor for DILI [3], but the clinical utility of genetic testing in this context is not known at the current time. The pathogenesis of DILI is complex and beyond the scope of this chapter. In general, increasing age appears to be a risk factor for development of DILI, but it is not entirely clear whether this reflects increased exposure to drugs in older age groups. Increasing age has been shown to be a risk factor for halothane, isoniazid, nitrofurantoin, and flucloxacillin [3]. It has also been convincingly shown that the appearance of cholestatic-type DILI is more common in old age, and hepatocellular damage seems to be inversely related to age [7, 18]. Younger age is a risk factor for certain drugs, such as valproic acid and aspirin (Reyes' syndrome) [3]. DILI has been reported to occur more often in females in some studies [5,6,12,17], but a similar preponderance between males and females has been found in others [8, 10, 19]. In a prospective study from France, similar rates of DILI were observed in males and females before the age of 50 [7]. After the age of 50, DILI became twice as high in females, suggesting an increased risk after menopause [7]. However, this has not been reproduced by other studies [5, 19]. Women have been found to be more susceptible to liver injury associated with halothane, flucloxacillin, isoniazid, nitrofurantoin, chlorpromazine, and erythromycin [3, 4, 15], whereas males have been found to have an increased risk of azathioprine-induced liver injury [3]. In a recent prospective study from Spain with more than 600 DILI cases, female sex was not found to be a predisposing factor for overall DILI [19]. The late Hyman Zimmerman, the legendary researcher of drug hepatotoxicity, observed that autoimmune hepatitis was seen almost exclusively in women [15], and this has recently been confirmed [8, 20]. Though the gender risk is unclear, females had a clear preponderance among patients with ALF due to idiosyncratic DILI undergoing a liver transplantation in the United States [18]. Females with idiosyncratic DILI also had more severe liver disease than males with idiosyncratic DILI [18].

Malnutrition and chronic alcohol abuse seem to increase the risk of liver injury due to acetaminophen [1, 15], but the role of these factors in idiosyncratic DILI is less clear. Chronic alcohol use has been reported to increase the likelihood of DILI with selected compounds, such as methotrexate, isoniazide, and halothane [15]. It is controversial whether a pre-existing liver disease makes patients more susceptible to developing DILI. Patients with non-alcoholic fatty liver disease (NAFLD) with elevated baseline levels of aminotransferases were not at an increased risk for development of hepatotoxicity while receiving treatment with statins compared to those with normal liver tests [21]. Similarly, treatment with statins in patients with hepatitis C and elevated liver tests seemed to be safe [21]. Pre-existing hepatitis B and C or co-infection has been reported to increase the risk of hepatotoxicity in human immunodeficiency virus (HIV) patients [22–24]. However, these studies did not include a control group with HIV and concomitant hepatitis B or C not treated with the implicated drug. Chronic liver disease probably has a greater effect on tolerance to and recovery from DILI than on the risk of developing DILI [15]. However, at present, there is little evidence to support the idea that cirrhotic patients experiencing DILI are at higher risk for severe outcomes, such as death from liver failure or need for liver transplantation.

Prognosis

Idiosyncratic DILI

In both large prospective and large retrospective series of unselected patients with DILI, prognosis is generally favorable [10, 12]. The prognosis is dependent on the severity of liver impairment that can develop in patients with hepatotoxicity. The prognosis of patients with drug-induced ALF accompanied by encephalopathy and coagulopathy is usually poor without transplantation, with approximately 20–50% transplant-free survival [25, 26]. Zimmerman observed that the combination of hepatocellular injury (high aminotransferases) and jaundice was associated with a poor prognosis, with a fatality rate of 10–50% for the different drugs involved [15]. This observation has been called Hy's rule and has been used by the US Food and Drug Administration (FDA) in the evaluation of drugs showing hepatotoxicity in clinical trial and cases. Fulfilling Hy's rule is considered to be a predictor of severe hepatotoxicity post-marketing. Studies from Spain and Sweden have recently confirmed these early observations and shown approximately 9–12% mortality/liver transplantation in patients with hepatocellular jaundice [10, 12]. Not only was hepatocellular liver injury due to drugs with jaundice found be a serious entity, but cholestatic-type injury was associated with 6–8% mortality/transplantation rate [10, 12]. However, in general, the prognosis in patients with hepatocellular liver injury due to drugs is worse than in those with cholestatic/mixed pattern [10, 12]. If the results of these two largest cohorts of DILI patients are combined, older age, female gender, and AST levels are independently associated with an unfavorable outcome [10, 12]. Among DILI patients prospectively collected within the United States as part of DILIN, only the presence of diabetes mellitus was an independent risk factor for severe DILI, whereas any alcohol use in the preceding months was a negative predictor of the severity of DILI [17]. The median duration between first exposure to the suspected drug was significantly longer in severe than in mild/moderate cases, in univariate but not in multivariate analysis [17]. The prognosis for drug-induced jaundice seems also to be dependent on the compound involved. In one study, mortality ranged from 40% with halothane-induced jaundice to 0% with erythromycin-induced jaundice, but the latter group was younger and had less severe liver injury [12]. Recently, the presence of both peripheral and hepatic eosinophilia in idiosyncratic liver injury has been reported to be associated with a better prognosis [11]. In another study, children with DILI due to antituberculous drugs who had hypersensitivity features had an excellent prognosis, but those without these features had considerable mortality [27]. The level of aminotransferases does not seem to be of prognostic significance in DILI [10, 12, 17]. In fact, a decrease in AST and ALT after drug discontinuation in severe DILI may not reflect improvement, but rather suggest a limited hepatic reserve and threatening ALF.

In the vast majority of cases of DILI, the patient recovers clinically, biochemically, and histologically, and a total recovery can be expected. However, chronic liver disease, including liver cirrhosis, has been reported with a suspected causative link to a number of different drugs [28]. In the first study to investigate the natural history of DILI, a high proportion of cases with persistent abnormalities was found, but these patients were identified through a histological database, indicating a selection bias [29]. A prospective follow-up with the Spanish hepatotoxicity registry revealed a chronic evolution in 5.7% of patients, and 6% of DILI patients from a single center had persistent elevated liver tests a median of 4 years after clinical recovery from DILI [28]. Patients with a cholestatic/mixed pattern of liver injury were more prone to development of chronic liver injury [30]. Recently, 6 months after enrollment in the prospective DILIN study, 14% of patients had laboratory abnormalities [17]. However, whether these patients or others reported to have a chronic evolution after DILI [28–30] will experience liver-related morbidity or mortality is not clear from these studies. A follow-up study of DILI patients from Sweden (mean follow-up 10 years) revealed that development of a clinically important liver disease after severe DILI (all patients had jaundice initially) was rare [9]. A total of 23 of 685 DILI patients who had survived acute DILI were hospitalized for liver disease during the study period, and 5 had liver-related mortality [9]. Among these, patients 5 out of 8 did not have an identifiable cause of cirrhosis, in the development of which DILI might have played a role [9]. In line with the study from the Spanish registry [30], a significantly longer duration of drug therapy prior to the detection of DILI was observed in those who developed liver-related morbidity and mortality during follow-up [9].

Acetaminophen

Prognosis is generally better in acetaminophen-induced ALF than in ALF due to other drugs, with 60–80% transplant-free survival [1, 25, 26]. In general, the presence of encephalopathy and renal impairment is predictive of an unfavorable prognosis [1]. In a recent prospective study of patients hospitalized for acetaminophen-induced liver failure in the United States, 178 patients (65%) survived, 74 (27%) died without transplantation, and 23 (8%) underwent liver transplantation [31]. Transplant-free survival rate and rate of liver transplantation were similar between those with intentional (suicide attempt) and unintentional overdose [31].

Management

Once DILI is suspected in a patient with new-onset liver disease, prompt cessation of the implicated drug(s) is usually the first step. It is obviously of crucial importance to assess the severity of the liver disease, and symptomatic patients with jaundice, encephalopathy, and/or coagulopathy should be hospitalized. Early contact should be made with a transplant center if the patient does not have an obvious contraindication for liver transplantation. Patients with suspected DILI and concomitant jaundice should be looked after carefully, and liver transplantation should be considered before they develop severe encephalopathy. In acetaminophen-induced liver failure, N-acetylcyteine (NAC) should be given immediately [1].

Other than NAC, specific treatment options for DILI are very limited. Carnitine is recommended in valproate-associated hepatotoxicity [32], and though steroids are commonly used in patients with acute liver injury caused by idiosyncratic drug reactions, their use is not supported by any controlled studies. Small cases series and case reports suggest that they may be used in patients with DILI and marked autoimmune features. The use of steroids may be justified when DILI is associated with concomitant Stevens–Johnson syndrome (SJS), as with phenytoin-induced hepatotoxicity or when autoimmune hepatitis is considered to be induced by drugs such as nitrofurantoin, halothane, minocycline, and diclofenac, though their value is unproven. Thus, patients with severe liver failure are generally hospitalized within the ICU, particularly those who reach grade III encephalopathy and/or those with renal failure. ICU treatment of renal impairment, encephalopathy, and infectious complications is beyond the scope of this chapter.

Finally, it should be pointed out that patients with DILI-related ALF should be considered for a liver transplantation early in the course of the disease. As pointed out already, patients with acetaminophen-induced liver failure generally have a better prognosis without transplantation than those with idiosyncratic drug-induced DILI ALF [25,26]. Within the US Acute Liver Failure Study Group, patients with ALF due to acetaminophen are listed less frequently than patients with other etiologies, and only 7% of patients with acetaminophen toxicity received a graft, as compared to more than 40% of idiosyncratic DILI cases [25]. Some patients in the latter category may be excluded from transplantation due to age and comorbidities, but a larger proportion of acetaminophen cases have contraindication for transplantation, due to history of substance abuse, repeated suicidal behavior, and other psychosocial issues [1].

Take Home Points

- A high suspicion of drug-induced liver injury (DILI) is mandatory in all patients presenting with liver dysfunction.
- History of a recent intake of all drugs, including over-the-counter (OTC) agents and herbal supplements, needs to be obtained.
- A diagnosis of DILI should be entertained when other diagnoses have been excluded with a reasonable doubt.
- Patients with DILI and concomitant jaundice and/or coagulopathy indicating liver failure should be watched very closely until liver tests show significant improvement.
- Patients with drug-induced ALF should be treated with N-acetylcysteine (NAC), and contact should be made with a liver transplant center early in the course of the disease.

References

1 Lee WM. Acetaminophen-related acute liver failure in the United States. *Hepatol Res* 2008; **38**: S3–8.
2 Lammert C, Einarsson S, Saha C, et al. Relationship between daily dose of oral medications and idiosyncratic drug-induced liver injury: search for signals. *Hepatology* 2008; **47**: 2003–9.
3 Larrey D. Epidemiology and individual susceptibility to adverse drug reactions affecting the liver. *Semin Liver Dis* 2002; **22**: 145–55.
4 de Abajo FJ, Montero D, Madurga M, et al. Acute and clinically relevant drug-induced liver injury: a population based case-control study. *Br J Clin Pharmacol* 2004; **58**: 71–80.
5 De Valle MB, Av Klinteberg V, Alem N, et al. Drug-induced liver injury in a Swedish University hospital out-patient hepatology clinic. *Aliment Pharmacol Ther* 2006; **24**: 1187–95.
6 Sgro C, Clinard F, Ouazir K, et al. Incidence of drug-induced hepatic injuries: a French population-based study. *Hepatology* 2002; **36**: 451–5.
7 Bjornsson ES, Bergmann OM, Bjornsson HK, et al. Incidence, presentation and outcomes in patients with drug-induced liver injury in the general population of Iceland. *Gastroenterology* 2013; **144**: 1419–25.
8 Meier Y, Cavallaro M, Roos M, et al. Incidence of drug-induced liver injury in medical inpatients. *Eur J Clin Pharmacol* 2005; **61**: 135–43.
9 Bjornsson E, Davidsdottir L. The long-term follow-up after idiosyncratic drug-induced liver injury with jaundice. *J Hepatol* 2009; **50**(3): 511–17.
10 Andrade RJ, Lucena MI, Fernandez MC, et al. Drug-induced liver injury: an analysis of 461 incidences submitted to the Spanish registry over a 10-year period. *Gastroenterology* 2005; **129**: 512–21.
11 Bjornsson E, Kalaitzakis E, Olsson R. The impact of eosinophilia and hepatic necrosis on prognosis in patients with drug-induced liver injury. *Aliment Pharmacol Ther* 2007; **25**: 1411–21.
12 Bjornsson E, Olsson R. Outcome and prognostic markers in severe drug-induced liver disease. *Hepatology* 2005; **42**: 481–9.
13 Kaplowitz N. Causality assessment versus guilt-by-association in drug hepatotoxicity. *Hepatology* 2001; **33**: 308–10.
14 Watkins PB. Idiosyncratic liver injury: challenges and approaches. *Toxicol Pathol* 2005; **33**: 1–5.
15 Zimmerman H. *Hepatotoxicity: The Adverse Effects of Drugs and Other Chemicals on the Liver.* Philadelphia, PA: Lippincott, Williams & Wilkins, 1999.
16 Danan G, Benichou C. Causality assessment of adverse reactions to drugs – I. A novel method based on the conclusions of international consensus meetings: application to drug-induced liver injuries. *J Clin Epidemiol* 1993; **46**: 1323–30.
17 Chalasani N, Fontana RJ, Bonkovsky HL, et al. Causes, clinical features, and outcomes from a prospective study of drug-induced liver injury in the United States. *Gastroenterology* 2008; **135**: 1924–34.e1–4.
18 Reuben A, Koch DG, Lee WM. Drug-induced acute liver failure: results of a US multicenter, prospective study. *Hepatology* 2010; **52**: 2065–76.
19 Lucena MI, Andrade RJ, Kaplowitz N, et al. Phneotypic characteristization of idiosyncratic drug-induced liver injury: the influence of age and gender. *Hepatology* 2009; **49**(6): 2001–9.
20 Bjornsson E, Talwalkar J, Treeprasertsuk S, et al. Drug-induced autoimmune hepatitis: clinical characteristics and prognosis. *Hepatology* 2010; **51**: 2040–8.
21 Chalasani N, Aljadhey H, Kesterson J, et al. Patients with elevated liver enzymes are not at higher risk for statin hepatotoxicity. *Gastroenterology* 2004; **126**: 1287–92.
22 Khorashadi S, Hasson NK, Cheung RC. Incidence of statin hepatotoxicity in patients with hepatitis C. *Clin Gastroenterol Hepatol* 2006; **4**: 902–7, quiz 806.
23 den Brinker M, Wit FW, Wertheim-van Dillen PM, et al. Hepatitis B and C virus co-infection and the risk for hepatotoxicity of highly active antiretroviral therapy in HIV-1 infection. *AIDS* 2000; **14**: 2895–902.
24 Bonfanti P, Landonio S, Ricci E, et al. Risk factors for hepatotoxicity in patients treated with highly active antiretroviral therapy. *J Acquir Immune Defic Syndr* 2001; **27**: 316–18.
25 Ostapowicz G, Fontana RJ, Schiodt FV, et al. Results of a prospective study of acute liver failure at 17 tertiary care centers in the United States. *Ann Intern Med* 2002; **137**: 947–54.
26 Wei G, Bergquist A, Broome U, et al. Acute liver failure in Sweden: etiology and outcome. *J Intern Med* 2007; **262**: 393–401.
27 Devarbhavi H, Karanth D, Prasanna KS, et al. Drug-induced liver injury with hypersensitivity features has a better outcome: a single-center experience of 39 children and adolescents. *Hepatology* 2011; **54**: 1344–50.
28 Bjornsson E, Kalaitzakis E, Av Klinteberg V, et al. Long-term follow-up of patients with mild to moderate drug-induced liver injury. *Aliment Pharmacol Ther* 2007; **26**: 79–85.
29 Aithal PG, Day CP. The natural history of histologically proved drug induced liver disease. *Gut* 1999; **44**: 731–5.
30 Andrade RJ, Lucena MI, Kaplowitz N, et al. Outcome of acute idiosyncratic drug-induced liver injury: long-term follow-up in a hepatotoxicity registry. *Hepatology* 2006; **44**: 1581–8.
31 Larson AM, Polson J, Fontana RJ, et al. Acetaminophen-induced acute liver failure: results of a United States multicenter, prospective study. *Hepatology* 2005; **42**: 1364–72.
32 Bjornsson E. Hepatotoxicity associated with antiepileptic drugs. *Acta Neurol Scand* 2008; **118**: 281–90.

CHAPTER 81

Autoimmune Liver Diseases

Justin A. Reynolds and Elizabeth J. Carey

Division of Gastroenterology and Hepatology, Mayo Clinic, Scottsdale, AZ, USA

Summary

Autoimmune hepatitis (AIH), primary biliary cholangitis (PBC), and celiac disease are the most common forms of autoimmune liver disease. While the pathogenesis for these disorders differs, there can be considerable overlap between them in terms of clinical presentation, biochemical markers, and histopathology. Arriving at an accurate and prompt diagnosis can help ensure disease stability and clinical remission. The purpose of this overview is to describe the clinical features, diagnosis, therapeutics, and management of these autoimmune liver disorders.

Case

A 55-year-old woman is referred for evaluation of abnormal liver enzymes of 6 months' duration. She has no prior history of liver disease, and only complains of fatigue and intermittent dry eyes. She is taking no medications. Her past medical history is unremarkable, and her family history is notable for rheumatoid arthritis and hypothyroidism. Physical examination is unremarkable, and there are no signs of chronic liver disease. Laboratory tests are notable for a normal complete blood count (CBC), International Normalized Ratio (INR), and electrolyte panel. Serum alkaline phosphatase is 430 IU/dL, aspartate aminotransferase (AST) is 205 IU/L, alanine aminotransferase (ALT) is 220 IU/L, and total bilirubin is 0.9 mg/dL. Abdominal ultrasound is negative for biliary obstruction. Further testing is negative for chronic viral hepatitis and metabolic liver disease. Serum autoantibodies are noted for titers of antinuclear antibodies (ANAs) of 1 : 160, smooth-muscle antibodies (SMAs) of 1 : 40, and antimitochondrial antibodies (AMAs) of 1 : 320, and a gamma-globulin level of 2.2 g/dL. The patient's symptoms, serum liver enzyme profile, and positive serum AMA strongly suggest a diagnosis of PBC. However, the possibility of an overlap syndrome between AIH and PBC is suggested by the higher than expected serum AST and ALT levels and positive ANA and SMA antibodies. Liver biopsy is performed, revealing histologic features of chronic non-suppurative bile duct inflammation without evidence for interface hepatitis. These findings are consistent with PBC alone.

Autoimmune Hepatitis

Definition and Epidemiology

AIH is a chronic inflammatory disorder of the liver of unknown etiology. It is characterized by a constellation of serum autoantibodies, hypergammaglobulinemia, and typical histopathology findings. Epidemiologic data on AIH in a Northern European population describe a mean incidence of 1–2 per 100 000 persons per year, with a point prevalence of 11–24 per 100 000 persons per year [1–3]. Women are nearly four times more likely to develop AIH than men, and the disease may be seen across all ethnic groups and age groups.

Pathophysiology

AIH is the result of T cell-mediated cytotoxicity, triggered by autoantigens or immunoglobulin-bound hepatocytes. This immune attack may lead to progressive necroinflammatory changes within the liver, and ultimately to fibrotic changes. Genetic predisposition for AIH has been recognized, with an increased frequency of specific major histocompatibility complex (MHC) class II DRB1 alleles (such as DRB1*0301 and DRB1*0401), which may predict response to treatment [4].

Clinical Features

The clinical presentation of AIH can be quite diverse, and ranges from asymptomatic disease to acute liver failure (ALF). The disease onset is often insidious, with a variety of non-specific complaints, such as fatigue, nausea, abdominal pain, arthralgias, jaundice, and pruritus. It may also be completely asymptomatic and diagnosed incidentally on the basis of routine laboratory work. Typically, asymptomatic patients are men. They have significantly lower serum aminotransferase levels at presentation than do symptomatic patients. However, histologic findings between the two groups, including the frequency of cirrhosis, are similar. The majority of asymptomatic patients will ultimately become symptomatic during the course of their disease [5].

Diagnosis

The diagnosis of AIH may be suspected on the basis of biochemical markers and serological tests; however, a liver biopsy is a critical prerequisite to establishing the diagnosis and beginning treatment. The diagnostic criteria for AIH and a diagnostic scoring system were established by the International Autoimmune Hepatitis Group (IAIHG) in the 1990s [6,7]. This original scoring system was developed as a research tool but may be applied in clinical cases. The revised scoring system incorporates treatment response into the aggregate score. In recent years, simplified diagnostic criteria that can identify definite and probable cases of AIH have been described [8] (Table 81.1). This version requires only four criteria for

Practical Gastroenterology and Hepatology Board Review Toolkit, Second Edition. Edited by Nicholas J. Talley, Kenneth R. DeVault, Michael B. Wallace, Bashar A. Aqel and Keith D. Lindor.
© 2016 John Wiley & Sons, Ltd. Published 2016 by John Wiley & Sons, Ltd. Companion website: www.practicalgastrohep.com

Table 81.1 Simplified diagnostic criteria for AIH. Source: Manns 2010 [10]. Reproduced with permission of Wiley.

Variable	Cutoff	Points
ANA or SMA	≥1 : 40	1
ANA or SMA	≥1 : 80	2[a]
or LKM	≥1 : 40	
or SLA	Positive	
IgG	> upper normal limit	1
	>1.10 times upper normal limit	2
Liver histology (evidence of hepatitis is a necessary condition)	Compatible with AIH	1
	Typical of AIH	2
Absence of viral hepatitis	Yes	2
		≥6: probably AIH
		≥7: definite AIH

[a]Addition of points achieved for all autoantibodies (maximum 2 points).
AIH, autoimmune hepatitis; ANA, antinuclear antibody; SMA, smooth-muscle antibody; LKM, liver–kidney microsomal antibody; SLA, soluble liver antigen; IgG, immunoglobulin G.

assessment: autoantibody titers, serum immunoglobulin G (IgG), liver histology, and exclusion of viral hepatitis. Assessment of this scoring system demonstrates excellent accuracy for diagnosing AIH in clinical practice.

Biochemical Features

Elevations in serum ALT or AST are common and may be upwards of 10 times greater than the upper normal limit. Significant elevations in serum alkaline phosphatase levels are less common in the absence of biliary injury on histology. Total bilirubin and albumin are generally normal unless advanced cirrhosis or severe inflammation is present.

Serologic Features

Serum ANA and SMA are observed together in the majority of AIH cases, and over 90% of patients with AIH will have a positive ANA, SMA, or both [9]. Serum titers greater than 1 : 40 are suggestive of AIH, whereas titers greater than 1 : 80 are more indicative of AIH. Elevated serum gamma-globulin levels (>2.0 g/dL) are also highly suggestive of AIH. In the small percentage of cases with a negative ANA and SMA and with low or normal gamma-globulin levels, a positive liver–kidney microsomal antibody (LKM) or serum perinuclear antineutrophil cytoplasmic antibody (p-ANCA) level may be suggestive.

Histologic Features

The most specific features of AIH include interface hepatitis with plasma cell infiltration and piecemeal necrosis. Eosinophils, lobular inflammation, bridging fibrosis, and cirrhosis may also be present. Rosette formation is often seen in AIH, though not exclusively. Biliary injury and/or granulomas are not commonly seen, and if present may suggest an alternative explanation of injury.

Differential Diagnosis

The differential diagnosis for AIH includes: drug-induced liver injury (DILI), with nitrofurantoin, minocycline, and isoniazid as common offenders; AMA-negative PBC; small-duct primary sclerosing cholangitis (PSC); viral hepatitis from cytomegalovirus (CMV), Epstein–Barr virus (EBV), parvovirus B19, or adenovirus; chronic hepatitis from an associated rheumatologic disorder, such as systemic lupus erythematosus (SLE); and celiac disease.

Table 81.2 Immunosuppressive treatment regimens for adults with AIH. Source: Manns 2010 [10]. Reproduced with permission of Wiley.

	Monotherapy	Combination therapy	
	Prednisone (mg/day)	Prednisone (mg/day)	Azathioprine (mg/day)
Week 1	60	30	50
Week 2	40	20	50
Week 3	30	15	50
Week 4	30	15	50
Maintenance until end point	20 and below	10	50
Reasons for preference	Cytopenia	Osteoporosis	
	Pregnancy	Brittle diabetes	
	TPMT deficiency	Obesity	
	Malignancy	Hypertension	
		Emotional lability	

AIH, autoimmune hepatitis; TPMT, thiopurine methyltransferase.

Therapeutics

Indications

Absolute indications for immunosuppressive treatment include: (i) serum AST greater than 10 times the upper normal limit; (ii) AST greater than five times the upper normal limit plus a gamma-globulin level greater than two times the upper normal limit; (iii) bridging necrosis or multiacinar necrosis seen on liver histological examination; and (iv) incapacitating symptomatic disease, including abdominal pain, fatigue, arthralgias, nausea, vomiting, and jaundice [10]. Asymptomatic disease with normal or near-normal AST and gamma-globulin levels, inactive cirrhosis, and decompensated liver disease are all contraindications to treatment.

Medical Therapy

Once the diagnosis is firmly established and liver disease is staged by biopsy, induction therapy to normalize liver tests may consist of prednisone monotherapy or combination therapy using prednisone and azathioprine (Table 81.2). Both approaches are highly efficacious, though fewer side effects are seen with the combination approach. In the United States, a fixed dose of azathioprine is usually used with the combination approach, but in Europe a weight-based dose of 1–2 mg/kg/day is more common. Maintenance therapy should be given for a minimum of 24 months, with the goal of achieving biochemical and histologic remission. Premature cessation of therapy is associated with high rates of disease relapse and may result in particularly severe flares of disease activity. While on therapy, routine monitoring of liver tests and CBCs every 3–4 months is indicated, particularly when azathioprine is given, due to the risk of hematologic toxicity. For women with AIH who are contemplating pregnancy, immunosuppressive therapy is not contraindicated. AIH flares may occur during or immediately after pregnancy, so it is unsafe to discontinue immunosuppression. Cohort studies examining the risk of teratogenicity from prednisone and azathioprine have not shown a significantly increased risk.

Treatment End Points

Remission

Complete disease remission occurs in 80% of patients within 3 years of starting therapy, but the likelihood of indefinite remission after withdrawal of therapy is only 15–20%. Thus, many physicians and patients opt to continue maintenance therapy to prevent disease relapse. If immunosuppressant withdrawal is contemplated, a

chemical markers, maintenance therapy

repeat liver biopsy should be considered to ensure complete histologic remission before proceeding. If interface hepatitis is found on biopsy despite normal biochemical markers, maintenance therapy should be continued given the high risk of relapse after treatment cessation.

Relapse Following Remission

Relapse is characterized by a minimum threefold increase in AST above upper normal limits and/or an increase in serum gammaglobulins to >2 g/dL. Other causes of a rise in liver transaminases should be excluded (e.g., DILI). The preferred management in these patients is to reinstitute therapy at induction dosing and then taper more slowly, potentially maintaining the patient on a higher dose of azathioprine. Recapturing response and preventing serial flares is important, due to a heightened risk of progression to cirrhosis and death from liver failure or requirement for liver transplantation [11].

Incomplete Response

Incomplete response to therapy is defined as prolonged therapy that has improved clinical and biochemical markers but has not induced complete remission. Approximately 10–15% of patients are classified in this manner after failing to achieve remission after 36 months of treatment. For these patients, maintaining AST levels as low as possible is the goal, but there remains an increased risk of disease progression and the development of end-stage liver disease. Alternative strategies for immunosuppression may be considered.

Treatment Failure

Treatment failure implies worsening of clinical, biochemical, and histological parameters despite conventional treatment. It occurs in less than 10% of all patients with AIH. High-dose prednisone (60 mg/day) or prednisone (30 mg/day) with high-dose azathioprine (150 mg/day) can result in improvement in the majority. Tapering to maintenance dosing should not begin until serum AST has normalized. Persistent disease activity despite aggressive treatment implies a higher risk of disease progression or drug-related side effects. The development of hepatic encephalopathy, ascites, or variceal bleeding should prompt evaluation for liver transplantation.

Alternative Therapies

Before proceeding to alternative (or salvage) therapies, treatment failure with high-dose standard induction agents should be demonstrated. Experience with alternative agents such as cyclosporine, tacrolimus, budesonide, cyclophosphamide, methotrexate, and mycophenolate mofetil has generally been small and anecdotal, and none has been incorporated into standard management algorithms. Liver transplantation is effective in patients who deteriorate despite aggressive therapy, with a 10-year patient survival of approximately 75%. While AIH can recur within the allograft, it does not commonly lead to cirrhosis or graft failure.

> ### Take Home Points
> - Autoimmune hepatitis (AIH) has a wide spectrum of presentation, ranging from an asymptomatic state to fulminant hepatic failure.
> - Typical biochemical features include serum aminotransferases over five times the upper normal limit.
> - Typical serological features include serum antinuclear antibody (ANA) or smooth-muscle antibody (SMA) at titers of 1 : 80 or higher and serum gamma-globulins exceeding 2 g/dL.

> - Interface hepatitis on liver histology is mandatory for the diagnosis.
> - Prednisone with or without azathioprine is first-line treatment.
> - Treatment should be continued for at least 24 months, and achievement of complete remission is attained in approximately 80% of patients.
> - Disease relapse can occur after cessation of treatment, or may flare while on maintenance dosing.
> - Incomplete response, treatment failure, and significant drug toxicity occur in the minority of patients.
> - Patients unresponsive to traditional therapy may have progressive liver disease ultimately requiring liver transplantation.

Primary Biliary Cholangitis

Definition and Epidemiology

PBC is a chronic, slowly progressive, cholestatic form of autoimmune liver disease that primarily affects middle-aged women. The median age of onset is at approximately 50 years, but this varies widely. PBC has a female predominance, with an 8 : 1 female-to-male ratio. The annual incidence of PBC ranges widely, from 2 to 24 cases per million individuals, while prevalence estimates range from 19 to 402 cases per million.

Pathophysiology

One highly specific feature of PBC is the involvement of AMA directed against an enzyme complex located on the inner surface of the biliary epithelial mitochondrial membrane [12]. The antibody itself is not cytotoxic, but its linkage is proposed to stimulate an autoimmune infiltrate, which causes direct biliary injury via a variety of proposed mechanisms.

Clinical Features

Many patients with PBC are asymptomatic at presentation, and are diagnosed as a result of incidental laboratory findings. The majority will eventually develop symptoms, however; the most common include fatigue, dry eyes and dry mouth (sicca syndrome), pruritus, and Raynaud's phenomenon. Other, less common features include cutaneous calcinosis, dysphagia, jaundice, and xanthelasmas.

Diagnosis

Biochemical Features

Most patients with PBC have abnormal liver tests, with an elevated serum alkaline phosphatase level being the most prominent feature (>1.5 times the upper normal limit). Mild elevations in AST and ALT may also be seen (<5 times the upper normal limit). Total bilirubin is typically normal in the absence of cirrhosis.

Serologic Features

Serum AMA is present in 90–95% of patients with PBC, at titers of 1 : 40 or above. Nearly half of PBC patients will also have a positive ANA or SMA. Serum immunoglobulins (especially IgM) may also be elevated, and other serum autoantibodies may be present, including rheumatoid factor, antithyroid antibodies, and anti-SP100 antibodies. In the small group of AMA-negative patients in whom there is an otherwise high suspicion for PBC, liver biopsy is needed to confirm.

Histologic Features

PBC is characterized by a chronic, non-suppurative cholangitis that affects septal and interlobular bile ducts. When focal lesions show intense inflammatory changes and necrosis with granuloma formation around an area of focal duct obliteration, this is referred to as a "florid duct lesion" and is considered pathognomonic for PBC. It is uncommon to find a florid duct lesion on biopsy, however, given the biopsy sample size and the patchy nature of the disease. A liver biopsy is no longer considered necessary for a diagnosis of PBC in the setting of a positive AMA and a cholestatic liver enzyme profile. Biopsy may be useful for disease staging, however, or when the diagnosis is unclear.

Overlap Syndrome with AIH

Some patients with PBC (<5%) will also have clinical and histologic features compatible with AIH. These patients are referred to as having an "overlap syndrome." Attempts have been made to establish a scoring system by which to evaluate possible overlap syndrome [7,13], but there are no large, prospective, long-term studies to indicate how best to treat it, or to guide prognosis and optimal therapy.

Therapeutics: Disease-Related Complications

Pruritus

This symptom may be quite debilitating in a certain subset of afflicted patients. Pruritus may be localized or diffuse, and is often worse at night while lying in bed. The exact cause of pruritus in PBC is unknown. Antihistamines have limited efficacy and may be negatively affected by anticholinergic side effects. Cholestyramine, a bile-acid binding resin, is frequently helpful when prescribed at an initial dose of 4 g daily (which may be titrated to a maximum of 16 g daily). This should be administered before or after breakfast, and spaced several hours from other medications so as to minimize any interference in their absorption. Sertraline (75–100 mg/day) and rifampin (150–450 mg/day) may also be effective, but patients will need to be counseled and monitored for any potential adverse reactions to these medications (rifampin can cause liver injury, hemolysis, renal impairment, and alteration of drug metabolism). Opioid antagonists such as naloxone and naltrexone may also produce some symptomatic improvement. When pruritus remains refractory to medical therapy, liver transplant is the most effective option.

Keratoconjunctivitis Sicca (Sicca Syndrome)

Secondary involvement of the salivary and lacrimal glands with inflammation in PBC patients can result in dry eyes and dry mouth. Treatment is directed toward symptomatic improvement using artificial tears and/or saliva substitutes. Cholinergic agents such as pilocarpine and cevimeline may also be helpful as oral sialogogues. General measures to improve oral hygiene and health in patients with sicca symptoms can mitigate dental caries.

Metabolic Bone Disease

Osteoporosis is commonly seen in PBC patients; the relative risk is much higher than in age- and sex-matched controls. Risk factors include age, body mass index (BMI), and stage of histologic disease. Treatment entails weight-bearing exercise, calcium supplementation (1000–1200 mg/day), vitamin D replacement, and bisphosphonates as indicated.

Fat-Soluble Vitamin Deficiency

Patients with PBC have decreased bile acid secretion, resulting in an increased risk of lipid malabsorption and, much less commonly,

Table 81.3 General monitoring for patients with PBC.

History and physical every 6–12 months.
Routine liver tests and prothrombin time every 3–6 months.
Serum vitamin A, D, and E levels in advanced liver disease.
Bone mineral density testing at diagnosis and every 2–3 years thereafter, for screening.
Screening endoscopy for esophageal varices if cirrhosis is present.
Hepatocellular carcinoma (HCC) screening with ultrasound and serum alpha-fetoprotein every 6–12 months in cirrhotic patients.

deficiencies of the fat-soluble vitamins A, D, E, and K. End-stage liver disease patients with jaundice are more likely to have vitamin deficiencies, which can lead to night blindness, osteopenia, neurological symptoms, and increased prothrombin time (with deficiencies in vitamins A, D, E, and K, respectively). Levels may be checked in cirrhotic patients and should be replaced accordingly.

Therapeutics: Primary Underlying Disease

Ursodeoxycholic Acid

Multiple randomized controlled trials (RCTs) indicate that treatment with ursodeoxycholic acid (UDCA) at a dose of 13–15 mg/kg/day will reduce cholestasis, ameliorate histologic features of PBC, and delay progression of disease as compared to placebo [14]. Some studies have even shown improved survival while on UDCA. The dose is important, as both lower (5–7 mg/kg/day) and higher (23–25 mg/kg/day) doses of UDCA have proven inferior in terms of biochemical response and cost. The vast majority of patients receiving UDCA will see improvement in liver biochemistries within 3 months, and up to 35% will have normalization of liver tests within 5 years. For those who do not achieve a complete biochemical response (defined as serum alkaline phosphatase and/or AST remaining >1.5 times the upper normal limit), contributing factors should be excluded, such as medication non-compliance, inappropriate dosing, concomitant use of cholestyramine (which interferes with UDCA absorption and must be taken at separate times), and concomitant disease such as overlap syndrome, fatty liver, autoimmune hypothyroidism, and celiac disease [15].

Liver Transplantation

Liver transplantation is the most effective therapeutic alternative for patients with end-stage liver disease due to PBC. Transplant generally improves fatigue and pruritus, though sicca symptoms persist. Bone disease initially worsens post-transplant, but eventually improves as steroids are discontinued and functional status improves. Patient and graft survival rates post-transplant are excellent, with 5-year survival rates of approximately 85%. PBC may recur in up to 25% of transplant recipients within 10 years following transplant, but this does not affect long-term patient or graft survival.

Monitoring

A guide to monitoring of patients with PBC is given in Table 81.3.

Take Home Points

- Primary biliary cholangitis (PBC) is characterized by a cholestatic liver enzyme profile, elevated serum alkaline phosphatase, and a positive antimitochondrial antibody (AMA).

CHAPTER 81

- Liver biopsy is unnecessary in establishing the diagnosis of PBC, except when AMA is negative or when doubt regarding the diagnosis is present (i.e., to rule out other diseases).
- Overlap syndrome between PBC and autoimmune hepatitis (AIH) is present in a minority of patients and should remain on the differential diagnosis lists when liver enzymes do not respond to PBC-directed therapy.
- PBC-associated symptoms include fatigue, pruritus, and sicca symptoms.
- Ursodeoxycholic acid (UDCA) at a dose of 13–15 mg/kg/day is recommended; this may improve biochemical parameters, slow progression of disease, and improve patient survival.
- Liver transplantation is a life-extending procedure for patients with end-stage liver disease due to PBC.

Celiac Disease

Definition and Epidemiology

Celiac disease is also known as gluten-sensitive enteropathy and is classically characterized by small-bowel villous atrophy, signs and symptoms of malabsorption, and improvement after withdrawal of gluten-containing foods. It may also cause chronic elevations in liver enzymes in 15–55% of newly diagnosed patients [16]. In contrast, among patients with chronic unexplained elevations in transaminases, 4–6% were subsequently diagnosed with celiac disease [17]. Celiac disease primarily occurs in patients of Northern European ancestry and has a broad spectrum of clinical manifestation, where the majority of cases are underrecognized. Recent epidemiological studies indicate a prevalence in the United States of 1 in 133 patients [18].

Clinical Features

Patients with liver injury from celiac disease do not have any direct symptomatology. They may experience gastrointestinal (GI) symptoms referable to celiac disease, such as diarrhea, steatorrhea, excess flatulence, weight loss, and dysphagia. Less commonly seen non-GI manifestations associated with celiac disease include neuropsychiatric disease, arthritis, and bone and renal disease.

Diagnosis

Biochemical Features

An elevated AST and/or ALT may occur; this is typically less than five times the upper limit of normal. Elevations in serum alkaline phosphatase and total bilirubin are uncommonly seen. The mechanism underlying these abnormalities is unknown, but two hypotheses suggest that liver damage is a result of increased intestinal permeability or chronic mucosal inflammation.

Serologic Features

Serum autoantibodies are often used to screen for suspected cases of celiac disease. Antibodies against tissue transglutaminase (anti-tTGs) are highly specific and sensitive for the diagnosis of celiac disease, but may provide a false negative in patients with IgA deficiency. Endomysial antibody assays are also highly specific, but are less widely available and more costly. Antigliadin antibody assays are no longer recommended for screening, due to a low positive predictive value (PPV).

Histologic Findings

Liver biopsy most often results in mild or non-specific findings on histology, which may include active hepatitis, steatosis, or, rarely, advanced fibrosis. Excluding a concomitant liver disease by biopsy may be a more useful indication.

Therapeutics

Treatment with a gluten-free diet results in normalization of serum transaminases in 75–95% of patients within 1 year. If abnormal liver enzymes do not improve despite gluten avoidance, an alternative etiology of liver disease should be sought. It is unknown whether severe histologic changes associated with celiac disease resolve with gluten avoidance. Liver transplantation for celiac-related liver disease is rare.

References

1 Boberg KM, Aadland E, Jahnsen J, *et al.* Incidence and prevalence of primary biliary cirrhosis, primary sclerosing cholangitis, and autoimmune hepatitis in a Norwegian population. *Scand J Gastroenterol* 1998; **33**: 99–103.

2 Werner M, Prytz H, Ohlsson B, *et al.* Epidemiology and the initial presentation of autoimmune hepatitis in Sweden: a nationwide study. *Scand J Gastroenterol* 2008; **43**: 1232–40.

3 Grønbæk L, Vilstrup H, Jepsen P. Autoimmune hepatitis in Denmark: incidence, prevalence, prognosis, and causes of death. A nationwide registry-based cohort study. *J Hepatol* 2014; **60**: 612–17.

4 Montano Loza AJ, Czaja AJ. Current therapy for autoimmune hepatitis. *Nat Clin Pract Gastroenterol Hepatol* 2007; **4**: 202–14.

5 Kogan J, Safadi R, Ashur Y, *et al.* Prognosis of symptomatic versus asymptomatic autoimmune hepatitis: a study of 68 patients. *J Clin Gastroenterol* 2002; **35**: 75–81.

6 Johnson PJ, McFarlane IG. Meeting report: International Autoimmune Hepatitis Group. *Hepatology* 1993; **18**: 998–1005.

7 Alvarez F, Berg PA, Bianchi FB, *et al.* International Autoimmune Hepatitis Group report: review of criteria for diagnosis of autoimmune hepatitis. *J Hepatol* 1999; **31**: 929–38.

8 Hennes EM, Zeniya M, Czaja AJ, *et al.* Simplified criteria for the diagnosis of autoimmune hepatitis. *Hepatology* 2008; **48**: 169–76.

9 Czaja AJ. Behavior and significance of autoantibodies in type 1 autoimmune hepatitis. *J Hepatol* 1999; **30**: 394–401.

10 Manns MP, Czaja AJ, Gorham JD, *et al.* Diagnosis and management of autoimmune hepatitis. *Hepatology* 2010; **51**: 1–31.

11 Montano-Loza AJ, Carpenter HA, Czaja AJ. Consequences of treatment withdrawal in type 1 autoimmune hepatitis. *Liver Int* 2007; **27**: 507–15.

12 Gershwin ME, Mackay IR, Sturgess A, Coppel RL. Identification and specificity of a cDNA encoding the 70 kd mitochondrial antigen recognized in primary biliary cirrhosis. *J Immunol* 1987; **138**: 3525–31.

13 Chazouillères O, Wendum D, Serfaty L, *et al.* Primary biliary cirrhosis-autoimmune hepatitis overlap syndrome: clinical features and response to therapy. *Hepatology* 1998; **28**: 296–301.

14 Lindor KD, Dickson ER, Baldus WP, *et al.* Ursodeoxycholic acid in the treatment of primary biliary cirrhosis. *Gastroenterology* 1994; **106**: 1284–90.

15 Lindor KD, Gershwin ME, Poupon R, *et al.* Primary biliary cirrhosis. *Hepatology* 2009; **50**: 291–308.

16 Abdo A, Meddings J, Swain M. Liver abnormalities in celiac disease. *Clin Gastroenterol Hepatol* 2004; **2**: 107–12.

17 Sainsbury A, Sanders DS, Ford AC. Meta-analysis: Coeliac disease and hypertransaminasaemia. *Aliment Pharmacol Ther* 2011; **34**(1): 33.

18 Fasano A, Berti I, Gerarduzzi T, *et al.* Prevalence of celiac disease in at-risk and not-at-risk groups in the United States: a large multicenter study. *Arch Intern Med* 2003; **163**(3): 286.

CHAPTER 8

CHAPTER 82

Vascular Diseases of the Liver

Brenda Ernst,[1] Pierre Noel,[1] and Bashar A. Aqel[2]

[1]Division of Hematology/Oncology, Mayo Clinic, Scottsdale, AZ, USA
[2]Division of Gastroenterology and Hepatology, Mayo Clinic, Scottsdale AZ, USA

Summary

Vascular disease of the liver can result from a number of conditions that alter the normal flow of blood within the hepatic vascular system. These diseases are usually categorized based on the location of the lesion in reference to the sinusoids.

Budd–Chiari syndrome (BCS) is post-sinusoidal, and is characterized by occlusion at the level of the hepatic veins or the suprahepatic portion of the inferior vena cava (IVC), which presents with painful hepatomegaly, ascites, and abnormal liver tests. Most cases occur in the setting of myeloproliferative disorders (MPDs) or hypercoagulable states. Diagnosis is usually established on imaging and venography, and liver biopsy is rarely needed. Treatment is determined by disease severity, underlying etiology, and duration of disease, and options include medical treatment (supportive care, diuretics, anticoagulation, thrombolysis), radiological intervention with transjugular intrahepatic portosystemic shunts (TIPS), and, rarely, surgical intervention (surgical shunts or liver transplant).

Hepatic complications of hematopoietic stem cell transplantation (HSCT) are common, including sinusoidal obstruction syndrome (SOS), acute/chronic hepatic graft-versus-host disease (HGVHD), infection, and drug-induced hepatotoxicity (DIH). SOS, characterized by rapid weight gain due to fluid retention, hyperbilirubinemia, and hepatomegaly with right upper quadrant pain, can be difficult to diagnose. Liver biopsy is the gold standard. Treatment options include tissue-type plasminogen activator with heparin, defibrotide, and antithrombin III (ATIII), and the majority of patients recover.

Budd–Chiari Syndrome

Definition and Epidemiology

BCS is a rare, heterogeneous, and potentially fatal group of disorders related to hepatic venous outflow obstruction. It is usually caused by multiple concurrent factors, including acquired and inherited thrombophilia. Venous outflow obstruction is post-sinusoidal and can occur at any level from the small hepatic veins to the suprahepatic IVC.

Though accurate estimates of incidence are lacking in Western countries, it is expected to increase, due to increased awareness and improved diagnostic methods. Prevalence was estimated to be 2.4 cases/million people based on autopsy studies in Japan [1, 2]. In Asian patients, obstruction is usually related to a thin membrane that involves the IVC at the level of the ostia draining the three major hepatic veins. In contrast, most cases reported in Western countries result from pure thrombosis of the hepatic veins. BCS can be classified according to duration, site of obstruction, and etiology (Table 82.1).

Case 1

A 40-year-old woman presents with a 2-week history of worsening right upper quadrant abdominal pain and progressive abdominal distension. Her past medical history is significant for a history of right leg deep venous thrombosis (DVT) 3 years ago, treated with 6 months of anticoagulation; she has no known history of heart disease. On exam, she appears ill, and is tachypneic but hemodynamically stable. There are no spider angiomas or scleral icterus, the heart and lung exam is normal, and she has tense ascites with tenderness over the right upper quadrant.

Pathophysiology

There is marked clinical and pathological heterogeneity among patients with BCS. This heterogeneity remains poorly understood, in part due to limitations in the assessment of hepatic hemodynamics, liver histopathology, and prothrombotic disorders [3, 4].

In general, obstruction of the hepatic venous outflow tract results in increased hepatic sinusoidal pressure and portal hypertension. The ensuing venous stasis and congestion lead to hypoxic damage to the adjacent hepatic parenchymal cells. Furthermore, the ischemic injury to the sinusoidal lining cells results in the release of free radicals, and oxidative injury to the hepatocytes ensues. These mechanisms culminate in the development of hepatocyte necrosis in the centrilobular region (zone 3) [3]. Untreated, progressive centrilobular fibrosis will progress to liver cirrhosis and will be complicated by portal hypertension, with the formation of portal venous collateral systems. The latter may lead to reduction in the hepatic sinusoidal pressure and to transient improvement in liver functions.

Etiology

Primary BCS results from an endoluminal venous pathology. Secondary BCS can result from a lesion originating outside the venous system, such as a malignant tumor (hepatocellular carcinoma (HCC), renal adenocarcinoma, adrenal adenocarcinoma, atrial myxoma), benign mass lesion (large central nodule in the

Practical Gastroenterology and Hepatology Board Review Toolkit, Second Edition. Edited by Nicholas J. Talley, Kenneth R. DeVault, Michael B. Wallace, Bashar A. Aqel and Keith D. Lindor.
© 2016 John Wiley & Sons, Ltd. Published 2016 by John Wiley & Sons, Ltd. Companion website: www.practicalgastrohep.com

Table 82.1   Classification of Budd–Chiari syndrome (BCS).

Classification according to etiology

• Primary	Hepatic venous obstruction related to endoluminal pathology (thrombosis or webs)
• Secondary	Obstruction secondary to a lesion outside the venous system (tumor, abscess)
	Flow is obstructed by invasion or compression

Classification according to site of obstruction

• Small hepatic veins	Obstruction at level of small hepatic venules that cannot be seen on venogram or Doppler ultrasound
• Large hepatic veins	Obstruction of large hepatic veins that can be seen on venogram or Doppler ultrasound
• IVC	Obstruction of IVC between the level of the hepatic veins and the right atrium
• Combined obstruction	Obstruction of hepatic veins and IVC

Classification according to disease duration

• Acute	Symptoms within 6 weeks of disease onset: 20% of patients (5% with fulminant hepatic failure
• Subacute	Symptoms over weeks to 6 months (40%)
• Chronic	Symptoms >6 months, with portal hypertension and cirrhosis (40%)

IVC, inferior vena cava.

setting of focal nodular hyperplasia), or infection (hydatid disease, parasitic cyst, abscess). An underlying etiology or risk factor that confers predisposition to the development of BCS can be identified in up to 85% of patients (Table 82.2). Multiple factors acting in combination are seen in up to 25% of patients [5].

Hematological disorders, particularly MPDs, are the most common cause of BCS, accounting for half of all cases. Most patients with an MPD at the time of presentation lack the classical diagnostic criteria of MPD. Recent advances in diagnostic tools, including the discovery of a V617F mutation in the Janus kinase 2 (JAK2) tyrosine kinase, have revolutionized the diagnosis of MPD in BCS patients in the absence of the classical criteria [6].

JAK2 tyrosine kinase mutation is a somatic point mutation that is extremely rare in healthy individuals (<1%). Several clinical studies indicate that MPD patients carrying JAK2 mutations have a higher

Table 82.2   Causes of BCS.

Common causes

Hypercoaguable states
Inherited:
• ATIII deficiency
• Protein C deficiency
• Protein S deficiency
• Factor V Leiden mutation
• Prothrombin mutation
Acquired:
• MPD
• Paroxysmal nocturnal hemoglobinuria
• Antiphospholipid syndrome
• Pregnancy
• Use of oral contraceptives

Uncommon causes

Tumor invasion:
• HCC
• Renal cell carcinoma
Miscellaneous:
• Behçet's syndrome
• IVC webs
• Trauma
• IBD
Idiopathic

ATIII, antithrombin III; MPD, myeloproliferative disorder; HCC, hepatocellular carcinoma; IVC, inferior vena cava; IBD, inflammatory bowel disease.

risk of thrombosis [7]. As a consequence of these developments, the World Health Organization (WHO) guidelines for MPD diagnosis have been revised, with JAK2 mutation screening added as a major diagnostic criterion for MPD, in conjunction with bone marrow exam. Factor V Leiden mutation, antiphospholipid syndrome, and G20210A prothrombin gene mutation are the next most common prothrombotic disorders in BCS. Acquired deficiencies can develop in the event of liver disease, liver failure, acute thrombosis, or anticoagulant therapy. The decreased levels of these coagulation inhibitors are significant only in the presence of normal or slightly reduced levels of coagulation factors. Hormonal replacement therapy, oral contraceptive pills, and pregnancy may exacerbate any of these disorders (especially in patients with heterozygous status) and lead to increased risk of BCS. Other miscellaneous causes include paroxysmal nocturnal hemoglobinuria, a rare disorder in which erythrocytes demonstrate increased susceptibility to complement-mediated hemolysis secondary to a mutation in the PIG-A gene, which can result in thrombosis, leading to BCS in 30% of patients. Paroxysmal nocturnal hemoglobinuria accounts for 5% of all BCS patients.

Clinical Manifestations

BCS typically presents with ascites (84% of patients), abdominal pain, and hepatomegaly (76%). However, 5–10% of patients can be asymptomatic when the liver sinusoids are decompressed by large intrahepatic and portosystemic shunts. The classic patient with BCS is a woman in her 3rd or 4th decade with an underlying prothrombotic disorder and taking oral contraceptive pills. The clinical presentation depends on the extent and rapidity of hepatic venous occlusion, and on whether a venous collateral circulation has developed to decompress the liver sinusoids.

The syndrome can be classified, according to presentation, into fulminant, acute, subacute, and chronic forms. Fulminant presentation is rare, occurring in only 5% of patients. It leads to hepatic dysfunction and encephalopathy within 8 weeks after development of jaundice. Acute syndrome occurs in 15% of patients and is associated with severe symptoms of short duration, including jaundice, right upper quadrant pain, hepatomegaly, and ascites. Some patients will present with variceal bleeding. Subacute presentation is common, occurring in 40% of patients. It has a more insidious onset and typically presents more than 6 months after development of thrombosis. Ascites and hepatic necrosis may be minimal, because the hepatic sinusoids are decompressed by collateral circulation. Chronic presentation is seen in approximately 40% of patients with BCS. It presents with signs and symptoms of liver cirrhosis, resulting from chronic venous congestion of the liver. Portal hypertension and esophageal varices are commonly present.

Biochemical tests of liver function are usually abnormal. The degree of abnormality varies from significant elevation (more than five times the normal level) of aminotransferases, bilirubin, and alkaline phosphatase in patients with acute and fulminant presentation, to mild elevation in patients with subacute or chronic presentation.

Case 1 Continued

Laboratory data show high alanine aminotransferase (ALT) (five times the normal level), high aspartate aminotransferase (AST) (three times the normal level), bilirubin 3 mg/dL, and International Normalized Ratio (INR) 1.5. Doppler ultrasound assessment reveals moderate ascites and thrombosis of all three hepatic veins, with extension into the IVC. The portal vein is patent. Contrast-enhanced computed tomography (CT) scan confirms these findings, without evidence of hepatic necrosis. Workup for thrombophilia confirms homozygous status for Factor V Leiden.

Diagnosis

BCS should be suspected in patients with unexplained liver dysfunction, ascites with high serum ascites–albumin gradient (SAAG >1.1) and high protein content (>2.5 g/dL), and painful hepatomegaly, particularly in patients with a known risk factor for BCS.

Advances in non-invasive vascular imaging with Doppler ultrasound, magnetic resonance imaging (MRI), and contrast-enhanced CT scanning have allowed improved diagnosis, including the recognition of asymptomatic disease. Doppler ultrasonography of the liver, with sensitivity and specificity of 85%, is the technique of choice for initial investigation when BCS is suspected. The presence of hepatic vein collaterals (spider web) is particularly useful in differentiating BCS from other liver disease. Contrast-enhanced CT scan and MRI may help to confirm the diagnosis, better identify hepatic necrosis, differentiate between acute and chronic forms of BCS, and better delineate the venous anatomy, especially when TIPS is being considered.

Advances in imaging techniques have reduced the need for liver biopsy. Biopsy is usually reserved for a small subset of patients in whom BCS is the result of isolated pure thrombosis of the small hepatic veins that cannot be seen using standard imaging techniques. Liver biopsy usually shows the classical sinusoidal dilatation around the central veins, with centrilobular necrosis (zone 3) – findings that can also be seen in patients with heart failure and constrictive pericarditis.

Case 1 Continued

The patient is started on furosemide, spironolactone, and intravenous heparin. Her symptoms and liver tests continue to worsen and she twice requires large-volume paracentesis. After evaluation, she is listed for liver transplantation. TIPS is completed on the 5th hospital day, after which liver tests stabilize and ascites becomes better controlled. Within 8 weeks, ascites resolves and bilirubin returns to normal. The patient is placed on warfarin, with a target INR of 2.5–3.0.

Therapy

Over the last few years, considerable advances have been seen in the overall understanding and practical management of primary BCS. Many of those advances have been made possible by the input of new knowledge from hematology, by technical improvement in interventional radiology, and by international collaborative efforts.

The goals of therapy are to prevent propagation of the clot, decompress the congested liver, and prevent complications related to fluid retention, malnutrition, and portal hypertension. The underlying cause of BCS should be investigated, and appropriate therapy administered. Radiological imaging is usually adequate to rule out secondary BCS.

Medical Therapy and Management of Complications

All patients with BCS should receive anticoagulation, unless contraindicated, starting with intravenous heparin and followed by warfarin with a target INR of at least 2.5, to prevent progression of thrombosis. Though there are no randomized trials confirming the therapeutic benefit of anticoagulation, several reports attribute the recent improvement in BCS outcome to its routine use. However, some, most containing small numbers of patients, document higher rates of 6-month mortality in patients receiving anticoagulation and diuretics alone.

In general, medical therapy with diuretics and anticoagulation alone should be reserved for patients without ongoing hepatic necrosis, as indicated by mild symptoms, relatively normal liver injury tests and synthetic functions, and medically controlled ascites. Patients with significant portal hypertension or evidence of synthetic dysfunction (coagulopathy, encephalopathy, or hepatorenal syndrome) should receive additional therapies [8, 9]. Patients receiving medical therapy should be monitored closely for disease progression, with regular assessment for liver functions and portal hypertension screening. Serial liver biopsies to confirm disease stability should also be considered.

Thrombolytic therapy can be used in patients with acute BCS who present within 72 hours of diagnosis (in one report, within 2 weeks of diagnosis). This treatment has had variable success, and most data are based on small case series. Treatment is usually infused into the clotted vein over 24 hours [10]. The risk of serious complications (bleeding, stroke, pulmonary embolism), combined with low efficacy, limits this treatment to patients with acute presentation with well-defined clot that is limited to hepatic veins.

In the presence of cirrhosis, varices should be assessed with endoscopy. Endoscopic eradication of varices or the use of non-selective beta-blockers to prevent bleeding is often necessary. Ascites is usually managed with diuretics or large-volume paracentesis.

Angioplasty

Short-segment obstruction or webs in the hepatic veins or the IVC are treated successfully with balloon dilation. Angioplasty can be combined with local thrombolytic therapy and stent placement to improve outcome and increase rates of long-term patency, which can be as high as 80%. Optimal anticoagulation is essential in all patients (in order to maintain patency) and frequent angiographic or Doppler assessment is recommended [3,11].

Transjugular Intrahepatic Portosystemic Shunts

The therapeutic principle of portosystemic shunting is conversion of the portal vein into an outflow tract, thereby decompressing the sinusoids. TIPS has been increasingly used for BCS in patients who have failed medical therapy (approximately two-thirds of patients), thrombolytic therapy, or endoscopic therapy for variceal bleeding, and as a bridge for liver transplantation. This approach avoids laparotomy and overcomes caudate lobe compression and occlusion of IVC, with less periprocedural mortality than surgical shunting [8,12,13].

Successful placement of TIPS can be achieved in 85–95% of patients, with few immediate complications. Long-term patency, despite routine anticoagulation, averages 30–50%. These rates have improved since the introduction and widespread use of polytetraflouroethylene (PTFE)-covered stents (67% patency rate at 1 year, compared with only 19% for non-covered stents) [14]. In some cases, portal hypertension may not progress even with stent dysfunction, possibly owing to *de novo* collateral circulation. The use of TIPS in patients who are potential candidates for liver transplant should be coordinated with the transplant team, because a poorly positioned stent (extension into the suprahepatic portion of the IVC) may create significant difficulties during the hepatectomy portion of the transplantation procedure.

Liver Transplantation

Liver transplantation may be the only option for patients with fulminant BCS or for those with decompensated liver cirrhosis who are not candidates for surgical or radiological decompression. The 5-year survival rate among patients undergoing liver transplantation is currently as high as 95%. Transplantation is indicated only for patients in whom the underlying disease that led to BCS is associated with favorable long-term prognosis [15, 16].

Appropriate patient selection is particularly important in patients with MPD. Patients with essential thrombocytosis have good long-term prognosis and should be considered for liver transplantation. Patients with polycythemia vera who have a hemoglobin >10 g/dL and a white blood cell (WBC) count <30 000/mm^3, and who do not have trisomy 8, circulating blasts, or profound hypercatabolic symptoms, have good long-term survival and are reasonable candidates for liver transplantation. Most patients have good outcome post-transplant, and use of aspirin and hydroxyurea post-transplantation is safe and effective [17]. Malignant transformation has not been reported. Though some genetic prothrombotic disorders are cured by transplantation (protein C, protein S, and antithrombin-III deficiency), thrombosis still occurs, and routine long-term anticoagulation is necessary. This is most likely related to the fact that multiple etiologic factors are present simultaneously in a patient with BCS. Careful monitoring is necessary post-transplantation, as 40% of patients have complications from anticoagulation.

Prognosis and Survival

The natural history of BCS is not well known, as most publications report on treated patients. Mortality rates are highest within the first 2 years of diagnosis and decrease over time. Retrospective studies suggest that 5-year survival rates average around 65–75%.

Several clinicopathological factors, including treatment variables, have been identified through multivariant prognostic models and found to correlate with long-term prognosis. In a large series of 237 patients, severity of encephalopathy, ascites, prothrombin time, and serum bilirubin resulted in the definition of three groups with statistically different 5-year survival rates of 89, 74, and 42% [8]. Histopathological features do not help in determining prognosis, though surgical shunt outcome may be worse in patients with advanced fibrosis. IVC obstruction has a good short-term prognosis, but long-term data are scanty. In Japan, patients with obliterative cavopathy have a 25% mortality rate over 15 years, dying from variceal bleeding, liver failure, and HCC.

Hematopoietic Stem Cell Transplantation

Definition and Epidemiology

HSCT is a commonly used treatment for hematologic and non-hematologic malignancies. More than 80% of patients will develop hepatic complications in the aftermath of HSCT [1,18]. Mortality rates from liver damage following HSCT are between 4 and 15% [19, 20].

SOS (also called hepatic veno-occlusive disease, VOD), acute or chronic HGVHD, infection, DIH, and liver dysfunction caused by the underlying malignancy are the most common reasons for liver abnormalities following HSCT [21, 22]. Among these disorders,

HGVHD accounts for 33.0–40.6% of liver dysfunction, DIH 19–30%, and post-transplantation viral hepatitis 7–15% [23, 24]. The incidence of SOS is variable, with rates between 5 and 70% in different reports [25–28]. This variability is most likely attributable to differences in the application of diagnostic criteria and reporting of mild cases [29]. A comprehensive analysis of clinical trials published between 1979 and 2007 found that SOS was reported in up to 62% (with a mean of 13.7%) of patients undergoing stem cell transplantation following myeloablative conditioning [30].

Clinicians often must evaluate liver abnormalities following HSCT. An algorithm for the assessment of patient status post-HSCT, including abdominal pain, liver biochemical abnormalities, hepatomegaly, and/or weight gain, is depicted in Figure 82.1. The first step in diagnosis, after history and physical examination, is to obtain an abdominal ultrasound or CT scan: management depends on its findings. Many patients may have no abnormal findings, in which case hepatotoxic medications should be withheld where possible, and the patient should be followed for 72 hours. If no improvement is seen within this time frame, a hepatology consultation is appropriate, to consider transjugular liver biopsy for further evaluation.

Hepatic dysfunction after HSCT is both an acute and a long-term problem, and coordination of care among multidisciplinary teams is necessary to ensure favorable outcomes for such patients. Fortunately, many treatment options exist for HGHVD, SOS, and infection. Continued research into hepatic disease processes following HSCT will undoubtedly lead to better patient selection and more effective therapies, ultimately lessening the morbidity and mortality of hepatic dysfunction in this setting. The differential diagnosis for liver dysfunction is wide, and includes HGVHD, infection, drug toxicity (Table 82.3), and SOS [32].

Case 2

A 32-year-old white female with a history of MPD complains of abdominal pain 4 days following a myeloablative, matched related-donor allogeneic HSCT. The patient was given busulfan 0.8 mg/kg (33.5 mg) IV for 4 days and cyclophosphamide 60 mg/kg (3400 mg) IV for 2 days for conditioning. She was maintained on ursodeoxycholic acid (UDCA) 300 mg orally twice daily and enoxaparin 30 mg s.c. twice daily for SOS prophylaxis.

On evaluation, she complains of severe generalized abdominal pain, rated at 10 on a scale of 1–10 pain intensity. She is not jaundiced. Abdominal examination reveals ascites with a fluid wave and generalized tenderness to palpation. The patient's weight has increased from 55.6 kg on admission to 61.6 kg.

Laboratory studies show serum AST 71 IU/L (reference range (RR): 8–43 IU/L), serum ALT 117 IU/L (RR: 7–45 U/L), serum alkaline phosphatase 120 IU/L (RR: 37–98 IU/L), serum total bilirubin 3.7 mg/dL (RR: 0.1–1.1 mg/dL), and serum direct bilirubin 2.6 mg/dL (RR: 0–0.3 mg/dL). These values were normal 5 days prior. Abdominal ultrasound reveals mild ascites, hepatosplenomegaly, unremarkable liver parenchyma, normal appearing biliary ducts, normal hepatic artery waveform, and a previously identified portal vein thrombosis, attributed to the underlying MPD.

Sinusoidal Obstruction Syndrome

Pathophysiology

SOS is triggered by endothelial injury from drug exposure or total body irradiation (TBI) used as part of a conditioning regimen [25]. Given that the sinusoidal endothelium is the initial site of injury,

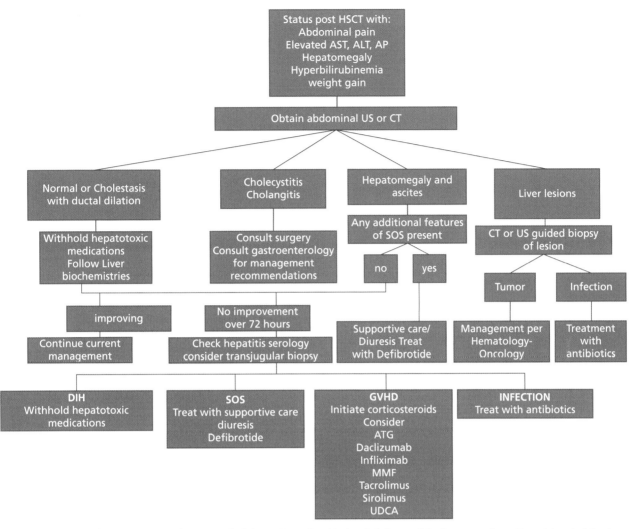

Figure 82.1 Algorithm for the assessment of patients with abdominal pain, liver biochemical abnormalities, hepatomegaly, and/or weight gain following hematopoietic stem cell transplantation (HSCT). AST, aspartate aminotransferase; ALT, alanine aminotransferase; AP, alkaline phosphatase; CT, computed tomography; US, ultrasound; GVHD, graft-versus-host disease; DIH, drug-induced hepatotoxicity; SOS, sinusoidal obstructive syndrome; ATG, antithymocyte globulin; UDCA, ursodeoxycholic acid; tPA, tissue plasminogen activator.

inducing characteristic histopathologic findings of sinusoidal obstruction, "SOS" is now used in preference to the previous "VOD" [31]. Sinusoidal endothelial cell and hepatocyte injury involving zone 3 of the hepatic acinus, triggered by intensive chemotherapy conditioning, is thought to be pivotal in the development of SOS [30,32]. Early in the course, edema causes subintimal zone thickening within sublobular venules. Erythrocyte fragments are seen in the extravascular space of Disse. Fibrin and factor VIII

are found deposited in venule walls on immunohistochemical (IHC) staining [25]. Edema results in venule lumen narrowing and increased venule resistance to bloodflow with portal hypertension. Increased venule resistance causes low-flow states, leading to hepatocyte ischemia [25]. With ongoing SOS, fibrosis forms within sinusoids, leading to destruction of sublobular venules and chronic venous outflow obstruction [33]. The histology evaluation often demonstrates dilated and congested sinusoids secondary to central vein occlusion by fibrin deposition, as depicted in Figure 82.2.

Disorders of hemostasis are believed to contribute to this process when damage to the hepatic venular and sinusoidal endothelium causes activation of the coagulation cascade [32]. Though thrombi are not commonly seen in venules on histologic examination [33], prophylaxis and treatment with anticoagulants are known to be effective for SOS, suggesting a potential role for thrombosis in the disease. Levels of protein C, protein S, ATIII, and fibrinogen are lower in patients with SOS. Levels of factor VIII, von Willebrand factor (vWF), and tissue plasminogen activator (tPA) are higher [34–36]. These findings suggest initiation of the coagulation cascade in response to endothelial injury.

Table 82.3 Drugs associated with liver toxicity following HSCT.

Busulfan
Cyclophosphamide
Cyclosporine
Fluconazole
Itraconazole
Melphalan
Methotrexate
Tacrolimus
Total parenteral nutrition
Trimethoprim–sulfamethoxazole

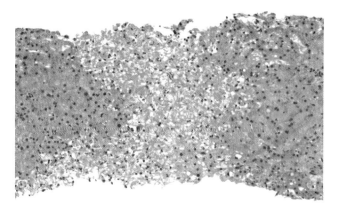

Figure 82.2 Hematoxylin and eosin stain of a liver biopsy in which the central vein is obliterated by fibrin deposition and the sinusoids are dilated and congested, consistent with SOS (20× magnification). Source: Courtesy of Dora Lam-Hamlin MD.

Clinical Features

Risk factors for SOS are listed in Table 82.4. There are four categories: risks due to pre-existing liver dysfunction, risks due to the conditioning regimen, risks related to other drugs administered, and patient/transplant type-specific risks.

Prevalence varies with the conditioning regimen, type of transplant, and diagnostic criteria applied. In the literature, the incidence of SOS varies with the composition and intensity of the conditioning regimen, from 0 (in reduced-intensity regimens) to almost 50% (when cyclophosphamide (CY) is combined with TBI) [37,38]. The highest incidence of fatal SOS is seen in CY-containing regimens. The variability of SOS reporting may be due in part to unique mechanisms within inciting agents and their application in transplant use.

Table 82.4 Risk factors for SOS.

Liver-related	Chronic viral hepatitis [32,60]
	Pre-existing liver disease (fibrosis, cirrhosis, low serum albumin) [21]
	Pretransplant elevated serum AST/ALT [41]
	Previous hepatic irradiation [21]
	Extramedullary hematopoiesis with sinusoidal fibrosis [32]
Conditioning regimen-related	Myeloablative conditioning regimen (especially high-dose busulfan and/or TBI with cyclophosphamide) [21]
	Melphalan [32]
	High-dose TBI (>14 Gy) [32]
	Concomitant sirolimus during conditioning [32]
Drug therapy-related	Acyclovir [21]
	Amphotericin B [21]
	Gemtuzumab ozogamicin (Mylotarg) [61]
	Methotrexate (for GVHD prophylaxis) [25]
	Vancomycin [21]
Transplant-related	Younger age and advanced age [25,31]
	Allogeneic HSCT > autologous HSCT [25]
	Prior HSCT [21]
	Unrelated-donor HSCT or HLA-mismatched related-donor HSCT [21]
	History of osteopetrosis, primary hemophagocytic lymphocytosis, adrenoleukodystrophy [31]

SOS, sinusoidal obstruction syndrome; AST, aspartate aminotransferase; ALT, alanine aminotransferase; TBI, total body irradiation; GVHD, graft-versus-host disease; HSCT, hematopoietic stem cell transplantation; HLA, human leukocyte antigen.

Busulfan is another component of regimens with a high frequency of SOS, and though not hepatotoxic itself, it is thought to induce necrosis through oxidative stress. When busulfan is combined with CY and sirolimus, a higher incidence of SOS is seen [38]. Higher reported rates of SOS are seen with oral busulfan than with intravenous delivery [39]. Gemtuzumab ozagamicin has caused sinusoidal injury when used to treat AML, particularly when given in close proximity to a CY-based myeloablative regimen. When patients receive combination TBI and CY, there is a clear relationship between the total dose of TBI and the development of SOS, with a frequency of severe SOS after CY/TBI >14 Gy of 20% [38]. For regimens including CY/TBI, BU/CY, and CY, carmustine, plus etoposide, the risk for developing severe SOS can be estimated using the Bearman prognostic model (which is based on height of bilirubin elevation, percentage weight gain, and time from transplant (up to day +16)) [40].

SOS is characterized by a triad of features: rapid weight gain due to fluid retention, hyperbilirubinemia, and hepatomegaly with right upper quadrant pain [41], often appearing in the 1st or 2nd week after HSCT [23,41]. SOS has been described up to 3–4 weeks after HSCT. Reports of late development are rare, though it may be unreported due to overlap of other etiologies, inducing liver dysfunction [29,41,42]. Azotemia, elevation in other liver transaminases, and thrombocytopenia are also found. Symptoms include right upper quadrant abdominal pain. Jaundice, hepatomegaly, and ascites may be found on examination.

Over one-half of patients develop multiorgan failure, including congestive heart failure (CHF), hepatorenal syndrome, and respiratory failure in some case series [21,43]. For patients surviving SOS, bilirubin values peak around 10 days following their first increase, returning to baseline [44] within an additional 10 days [28].

Diagnosis

The diagnosis of SOS is challenging due to the overlap of signs and symptoms with other conditions. A diagnosis of SOS is established by liver biopsy [25]; however, thrombocytopenia following HSCT, often refractory to platelet transfusions, may preclude the ability to obtain a liver biopsy. Thus, the diagnosis of SOS is based on clinical findings, and hepatic biopsy is not required in patients who meet the clinical criteria. Several sets of criteria for making an SOS diagnosis have been developed; all incorporate the three features of rapid weight gain due to fluid retention, hyperbilirubinemia, and hepatomegaly with right upper quadrant pain developing within 3–4 weeks of HSCT [25]. Reports of SOS occurring more than 21 days after transplant are rare [29,31]. The clinical criteria, based on the modified Seattle criteria and summarized in Table 82.5, define SOS as development of two of three clinical features within 30 days of HSCT: (i) jaundice; (ii) hepatomegaly with right upper quadrant

Table 82.5 Clinical criteria for the diagnosis of SOS.

Modified Seattle criteria [26] (Two or more must be present within 20 days of transplant)	Baltimore criteria [28] (Bilirubin >34.2 μmol/L (2 mg/dL) and two or more present within 21 days of transplant)
Bilirubin >34.2 μmol/L (2 mg/dL)	Ascites
Hepatomegaly or right upper quadrant pain	Hepatomegaly
Weight gain (>2% from pretransplant weight)	Weight gain (>5% from pretransplant weight)

pain; and (iii) ascites and/or unexplained weight gain [31]. These criteria have a specificity of 92% and sensitivity of 56% [45].

Imaging studies, such as Doppler ultrasound and MRI, aid in establishing a diagnosis of SOS by excluding other causes of hepatic dysfunction. Imaging modalities do not rule out SOS if they are unrevealing, as the diagnosis can be made on clinical criteria [31]. On ultrasound, splenomegaly, ascites, and flow within the periumbilical vein confer 100% sensitivity and 49% specificity for SOS [46]. Portal hypertension, reversal of portal flow, hepatomegaly, and thickening of the gallbladder wall may also be observed. Though less well studied for SOS, MRI may reveal hepatomegaly, thickening of the gallbladder wall, reduced portal flow, ascites, narrowing of the hepatic vein, and periportal cuffing [47]. A more recent study in patients with chemotherapy-treated colorectal metastases reported that gadotexic acid-enhanced MRI was highly specific in the diagnosis of SOS [48].

The gold standard for SOS diagnosis is liver biopsy. Hepatic biopsy can be challenging, due to the increased risk of bleeding secondary to thrombocytopenia after transplant. Percutaneous, laparoscopic, and transjugular approaches have been used. Sufficient samples are generally obtained with the transjugular approach, using contemporary methods [22,25]. This approach allows for measurement of the hepatic venous wedge pressure. A hepatic venous pressure gradient of more than 10 mmHg has 91% specificity and 60% sensitivity for SOS, with higher pressure gradients conferring a worse outcome [22]. Percutaneous liver biopsy may not be feasible, due to bleeding risk from thrombocytopenia, and laparoscopy carries the risk of a false-negative biopsy due to the patchy nature of liver involvement with SOS in early stages [25]. The current recommendation is that liver biopsies be reserved for those in whom the diagnosis is unclear and be undertaken using the transjugular approach, to reduce the risk associated with the procedure [31].

Biochemical evidence of SOS includes elevated levels of plasminogen activator inhibitor (PAI)-1 [31,49] and N-terminal peptide of type III procollagen [22] and reduced levels of ATIII and protein C [50]. The applicability of these tests to clinical decision-making remains an area for further research.

Therapy

Current management of SOS focuses on best supportive care, including management of fluid balance and avoidance of hepatotoxic agents [39]. Though there is currently no standard pharmaceutical approach, the most commonly investigated treatments for SOS are recombinant tPA with heparin, defibrotide, and ATIII. Defibrotide is approved in Europe for the treatment and prevention of SOS; in the United States, defibrotide is currently available only as an investigational new drug and under compassionate use approval from the Food and Drug Administration (FDA).

The use of tPA with heparin is based on the presence of coagulation proteins on IHC stains of liver biopsies. In a retrospective review, 10 of 42 patients treated with a median tPA dose of 60 mg over 2–4 days with a 1000 IU intravenous bolus of heparin followed by 150 IU/kg/day continuous heparin infusion experienced severe bleeding, with death from bleeding in three cases. The authors concluded that tPA with heparin should not be given to patients with severe SOS and multiorgan failure [51].

Defibrotide, a polydeoxyribonucleotide extracted from mammalian tissue, has multiple anticoagulant effects but does not lead to systemic anticoagulation. Thus, it is not associated with a bleeding risk. In study of 88 HSCT patients with severe SOS and

multiorgan failure, 36% experienced complete resolution, with 35% surviving until day +100. A decrease in serum creatinine and PAI-1 levels during therapy, younger age, autologous HSCT, and the presence of abnormal portal flow predicted better survival; busulfan conditioning and encephalopathy predicted worse survival [52]. In a phase II trial of 40 patients, 55% showed complete remission (defined as a decrease in serum total bilirubin to <34.2 μmol/L, with resolution of signs and symptoms of SOS and multiorgan failure), with 43% alive at day +100 [53]. A phase III trial examined 102 patients dosed with 6.25 mg four times a day, compared with 32 historical control patients. The day 100 complete remission rate was 24% in the treatment arm, compared to 9% in the control group (p = 0.013), with day 100 mortality rates of 62% in the treatment group and 75% in the control group (p = 0.03). Based on this study and other small studies with similar results, a dose of 25 mg/kg/day is recommended in the treatment of adults and children with SOS [31,39,54].

At least two case series have evaluated ATIII concentrate for SOS treatment. In one series, all 10 patients studied experienced improvements in thrombocytopenia, abdominal pain, ascites, and/or weight gain [55]. Though ATIII concentrate has not been evaluated in large, prospective, randomized controlled studies, its use in the setting of SOS has been considered. ATIII concentrate is given with a loading dose of 50 IU/kg every 8 hours for three doses, followed by 50 IU/kg/day for 3–12 days.

Additional treatment options for SOS include TIPS and charcoal hemofiltration. These have been reported in small numbers of patients with SOS [25]. Numerous other approaches to treatment of severe SOS have also been studied (tPA, intravenous N-acetylcysteine (NAC), human ATIII concentrate, activated protein C, prostaglandin E, prednisone, topical nitrate, vitamin E plus glutamine), but none can be recommended. Successful liver transplants for severe SOS have been completed, with the best results occurring from the transplant donor. Supportive care remains the mainstay of therapy, and should include treatment of volume overload, therapeutic paracentesis, stopping of hepatotoxic medications, treatment of underlying infections, and hemodialysis or continuous venous hemofiltration when necessary [25]. In patients with severe SOS, treatment with defibrotide at 25 mg/kg/day is recommended [31].

The only certain way to prevent fatal SOS is to avoid damaging sinusoidal endothelium. Prevention of severe sinusoidal injury should begin with an assessment of the patient at risk [38]. Table 82.4 describes the risk factors for SOS. SOS prophylaxis strategies include UDCA, defibrotide, low-molecular-weight heparin (LMWH), and low-dose continuous-infusion unfractionated heparin (UFH). Each has been evaluated in small studies. In a study of 67 patients undergoing allogeneic HSCT, patients randomized to receive UDCA had significantly lower rates of SOS compared to placebo (p = 0.03) [39,56]. In a study of defibrotide for SOS prophylaxis, 0 of 58 patients developed SOS [57]. A phase II study evaluated LMWH (dalteparin, 2500 anti-Xa IU daily from day −1 to day +30 or hospital discharge) for SOS prophylaxis in 40 patients undergoing either autologous or allogeneic HSCT; nine patients developed SOS [58]. A meta-analysis of 12 studies examining LMWH or UFH as prophylaxis for SOS (2782 patients) reported that anticoagulation did not significantly reduce the risk of SOS [59]. Heparin is not suggested as prophylaxis for SOS due to the increased risk of toxicity [31]. At these authors' institution, UDCA is preferred for SOS prophylaxis. The use of defibrotide in combination with UDCA in patients at high risk for SOS may be considered at the physician's discretion [31].

Prognosis

A majority of patients will experience resolution within 2–3 weeks, and complete recovery can occur in over 70% of patients with supportive care alone [38]. However, severe SOS is associated with a mortality of over 90% by day 100 following HSCT [27]. Death can occur in 20–50% of patients. The rate of bilirubin increase and the peak concentration are important predictors [25]. Patients with poor prognosis demonstrate early and steep rises in bilirubin, body weight, and serum ALT values >750 IU/L [38]. Death in SOS patients is usually caused by failure of other systems, such as kidney, respiratory, and cardiac failure, rather than hepatic failure. Long-term sequelae are rare, with only a small percentage of patients developing fibrosis and portal hypertension [25].

Case 2 Continued

The differential diagnosis for the patient's disorder includes SOS, acute HGVHD, infection, and DIH. The patient has no other features to suggest acute GHVD, such as diarrhea or rash. Hepatitis B and C serologies, and serologies for HSV-1 and -2, cytomegalovirus (CMV), and human immunodeficiency virus (HIV), are negative. She has been maintained on prophylactic doses of acyclovir and fluconazole during the hospital course. Therefore, acute hepatic GVHD and infection are less likely.

Several factors raise the possibility of SOS, including:
- severe abdominal pain;
- ascites;
- generalized tenderness to palpation;
- increase in weight from 55.6 kg on admission to 61.6 kg;
- elevated serum AST, ALT, alkaline phosphatase, and total and direct bilirubin.

As the decision is being made on a course of treatment for presumed SOS, the nurse reports that the patient has developed epistaxis. The bleeding is controlled with direct pressure.

The decision is made to initiate treatment with ATIII, since tPA with heparin is contraindicated in the setting of bleeding. Defibrotide is an option, but it is not readily available. The patient is given ATIII loading dose (three doses of 50 IU/kg at 8-hour intervals), followed by 3225 IU/day. UDCA is continued. Enoxaparin is discontinued due to epistaxis. The possibility of liver transplantation is discussed, but deferred, as the patient experiences stabilization of liver biochemistries and symptoms. After 7 days of treatment with ATIII plus supportive care, including aggressive diuresis, the patient's serum AST, ALT, and alkaline phosphatase normalize. Serum total bilirubin also improves, but remains elevated at 2.2 mg/dL on the day of hospital discharge.

Take Home Points

- Budd–Chiari syndrome (BCS) is more common in women, and usually presents in the 3rd or 4th decade.
- BCS should be suspected in patients with acute or chronic liver disease and one of the following:
  - Ascitic protein content >3g/dL.
  - Personal or family history of idiopathic thrombosis.
  - Platelet count >200 000, with signs of portal hypertension.
- Painful hepatomegaly, ascites, jaundice, and signs of portal hypertension are common clinical presentations of BCS.
- Non-invasive imaging with Doppler ultrasound, contrast computed tomography (CT) scan, or magnetic resonance imaging (MRI) is usually adequate to establish diagnosis. Venography and liver biopsy are rarely needed.
- Myeloproliferative disorder (MPD) and hypercoagulable disorders are among the most common causes of BCS.
- Janus kinase 2 (JAK2) mutations help to identify patients with MPD in the absence of the classical clinical presentation.
- Medical therapy with diuretics and anticoagulation is indicated for all patients, and most will require additional modalities to help control disease progression.
- Transjugular intrahepatic portosystemic shunts (TIPS) have replaced surgical shunts as the treatment of choice in patients with BCS.
- Liver transplantation is needed in 10–20% of BCS patients, and is associated with excellent 5-year survival.
- Post-transplant, most patients will require long-term anticoagulation.
- Sinusoidal obstruction syndrome (SOS), acute/chronic hepatic graft-versus-host disease (HGVHD), infection, and drug-induced hepatotoxicity (DIH) are the most common reasons for liver abnormalities following hematopoietic stem cell transplantation (HSCT).
- SOS is characterized by rapid weight gain due to fluid retention, hyperbilirubinemia, and hepatomegaly with right upper quadrant pain.
- Liver biopsy is the gold standard for SOS diagnosis.
- SOS treatment options include supportive measures and defibrotide in appropriate patients.

References

1 Okuda K. Vascular and coagulation disorders of the liver. *Semin Liver Dis* 2002; **22**(1): 1–3.
2 Okuda K. Inferior vena cava thrombosis at its hepatic portion (obliterative hepatocavopathy). *Semin Liver Dis* 2002; **22**(1): 15–26.
3 Menon KV, Shah V, Kamath PS. The Budd-Chiari syndrome. *N Engl J Med* 2004; **350**(6): 578–85.
4 Valla DC. Thrombosis and anticoagulation in liver disease. *Hepatology* 2008; **47**(4): 1384–93.
5 Zimmerman MA, Cameron AM, Ghobrial RM. Budd-Chiari syndrome. *Clin Liver Dis* 2006; **10**(2): 259–73, viii.
6 Kiladjian JJ, Cervantes F, Leebeek FW, et al. The impact of JAK2 and MPL mutations on diagnosis and prognosis of splanchnic vein thrombosis: a report on 241 cases. *Blood* 2008; **111**(10): 4922–9.
7 Primignani M, Mannucci PM. The role of thrombophilia in splanchnic vein thrombosis. *Semin Liver Dis* 2008; **28**(3): 293–301.
8 Darwish Murad S, Valla DC, de Groen PC, et al. Determinants of survival and the effect of portosystemic shunting in patients with Budd-Chiari syndrome. *Hepatology* 2004; **39**(2): 500–8.
9 Murad SD, Valla DC, de Groen PC, et al. Determinants of survival and the effect of portosystemic shunting in patients with Budd-Chiari syndrome. *Hepatology* 2004; **39**(2): 500–8.
10 Raju GS, Felver M, Olin JW, Satti SD. Thrombolysis for acute Budd-Chiari syndrome: case report and literature review. *Am J Gastroenterol* 1996; **91**(6): 1262–3.
11 Plessier A, Rautou PE, Valla DC. Management of hepatic vascular diseases. *J Hepatol* 2012; **56**(Suppl. 1): S25–38.
12 Rossle M, Olschewski M, Siegerstetter V, et al. The Budd-Chiari syndrome: outcome after treatment with the transjugular intrahepatic portosystemic shunt. *Surgery* 2004; **135**(4): 394–403.
13 Garcia-Pagan JC, Heydtmann M, Raffa S, et al. TIPS for Budd-Chiari syndrome: long-term results and prognostics factors in 124 patients. *Gastroenterology* 2008; **135**(3): 808–15.
14 Hernandez-Guerra M, Turnes J, Rubinstein P, et al. PTFE-covered stents improve TIPS patency in Budd-Chiari syndrome. *Hepatology* 2004; **40**(5): 1197–202.
15 Mentha G, Giostra E, Majno PE, et al. Liver transplantation for Budd-Chiari syndrome: a European study on 248 patients from 51 centres. *J Hepatol* 2006; **44**(3): 520–8.
16 Srinivasan P, Rela M, Prachalias A, et al. Liver transplantation for Budd-Chiari syndrome. *Transplantation* 2002; **73**(6): 973–7.

17 Melear JM, Goldstein RM, Levy MF, *et al.* Hematologic aspects of liver transplantation for Budd-Chiari syndrome with special reference to myeloproliferative disorders. *Transplantation* 2002; **74**(8): 1090–5.

18 Shuhart MC, ed. *Gastrointestinal and Hepatic Complications.* Cambridge: Blackwell Scientific, 1994.

19 Locasciulli A, Alberti A, de Bock R, *et al.* Impact of liver disease and hepatitis infections on allogeneic bone marrow transplantation in Europe: a survey from the European Bone Marrow Transplantation (EBMT) Group – Infectious Diseases Working Party. *Bone Marrow Transpl* 1994; **14**(5): 833–7.

20 Azar N, Valla D, Abdel-Samad I, *et al.* Liver dysfunction in allogeneic bone marrow transplantation recipients. *Transplantation* 1996; **62**(1): 56–61.

21 McDonald GB, Hinds MS, Fisher LD, *et al.* Veno-occlusive disease of the liver and multiorgan failure after bone marrow transplantation: a cohort study of 355 patients. *Ann Intern Med* 1993; **118**(4): 255–67.

22 Arai S, Lee LA, Vogelsang GB. A systematic approach to hepatic complications in hematopoietic stem cell transplantation. *J Hematother Stem Cell Res* 2002; **11**(2): 215–29.

23 Forbes GM, Davies JM, Herrmann RP, Collins BJ. Liver disease complicating bone marrow transplantation: a clinical audit. *J Gastroenterol Hepatol* 1995; **10**(1): 1–7.

24 Kim BK, Chung KW, Sun HS, *et al.* Liver disease during the first post-transplant year in bone marrow transplantation recipients: retrospective study. *Bone Marrow Transpl* 2000; **26**(2): 193–7.

25 Kumar S, DeLeve LD, Kamath PS, Tefferi A. Hepatic veno-occlusive disease (sinusoidal obstruction syndrome) after hematopoietic stem cell transplantation. *Mayo Clin Proc* 2003; **78**(5): 589–98.

26 Shulman HM, Hinterberger W. Hepatic veno-occlusive disease – liver toxicity syndrome after bone marrow transplantation. *Bone Marrow Transpl* 1992; **10**(3): 197–214.

27 Carreras E, Bertz H, Arcese W, *et al.* Incidence and outcome of hepatic veno-occlusive disease after blood or marrow transplantation: a prospective cohort study of the European Group for Blood and Marrow Transplantation. European Group for Blood and Marrow Transplantation Chronic Leukemia Working Party. *Blood* 1998; **92**(10): 3599–604.

28 Jones RJ, Lee KS, Beschorner WE, *et al.* Venoocclusive disease of the liver following bone marrow transplantation. *Transplantation* 1987; **44**(6): 778–83.

29 Pai RK, van Besien K, Hart J, *et al.* Clinicopathologic features of late-onset veno-occlusive disease/sinusoidal obstruction syndrome after high dose intravenous busulfan and hematopoietic cell transplant. *Leuk Lymphoma* 2012; **53**(8): 1552–7.

30 Coppell JA, Richardson PG, Soiffer R, *et al.* Hepatic veno-occlusive disease following stem cell transplantation: incidence, clinical course, and outcome. *Biol Blood Marrow Transpl* 2010; **16**(2): 157–68.

31 Dignan FL, Wynn RF, Hadzic N, *et al.* BCSH/BSBMT guideline: diagnosis and management of veno-occlusive disease (sinusoidal obstruction syndrome) following haematopoietic stem cell transplantation. *Br J Haematol* 2013; **163**(4): 444–57.

32 Tuncer HH, Rana N, Milani C, *et al.* Gastrointestinal and hepatic complications of hematopoietic stem cell transplantation. *World J Gastroenterol* 2012; **18**(16): 1851–60.

33 Shulman HM, Fisher LB, Schoch HG, *et al.* Veno-occlusive disease of the liver after marrow transplantation: histological correlates of clinical signs and symptoms. *Hepatology* 1994; **19**(5): 1171–81.

34 Lee JH, Lee KH, Kim S, *et al.* Relevance of proteins C and S, antithrombin III, von Willebrand factor, and factor VIII for the development of hepatic veno-occlusive disease in patients undergoing allogeneic bone marrow transplantation: a prospective study. *Bone Marrow Transpl* 1998; **22**(9): 883–8.

35 Vannucchi AM, Rafanelli D, Longo G, *et al.* Early hemostatic alterations following bone marrow transplantation: a prospective study. *Haematologica* 1994; **79**(6): 519–25.

36 Tanikawa S, Mori S, Ohhashi K, *et al.* Predictive markers for hepatic veno-occlusive disease after hematopoietic stem cell transplantation in adults: a prospective single center study. *Bone Marrow Transpl* 2000; **26**(8): 881–6.

37 Hogan WJ, Maris M, Storer B, *et al.* Hepatic injury after nonmyeloablative conditioning followed by allogeneic hematopoietic cell transplantation: a study of 193 patients. *Blood* 2004; **103**(1): 78–84.

38 McDonald GB. Hepatobiliary complications of hematopoietic cell transplantation, 40 years on. *Hepatology* 2010; **51**(4): 1450–60.

39 Richardson PG, Ho VT, Giralt S, *et al.* Safety and efficacy of defibrotide for the treatment of severe hepatic veno-occlusive disease. *Ther Adv Hematol* 2012; **3**(4): 253–65.

40 Bearman SI, Anderson GL, Mori M, *et al.* Venoocclusive disease of the liver: development of a model for predicting fatal outcome after marrow transplantation. *J Clin Oncol* 1993; **11**(9): 1729–36.

41 Tabbara IA, Zimmerman K, Morgan C, Nahleh Z. Allogeneic hematopoietic stem cell transplantation: complications and results. *Arch Intern Med* 2002; **162**(14): 1558–66.

42 Shah MS, Jeevangi NK, Joshi A, Khattry N. Late-onset hepatic veno-occlusive disease post autologous peripheral stem cell transplantation successfully treated with oral defibrotide. *J Cancer Res Ther* 2009; **5**(4): 312–14.

43 Vinayek R, Rakela J, eds. *Liver Disease in Hematopoietic Stem Cell Transplant Recipients.* New York, NY: Churchill Livingstone, 2000.

44 Ball LM, Egeler RM. Acute GvHD: pathogenesis and classification. *Bone Marrow Transpl* 2008; **41**(Suppl. 2): S58–64.

45 Carreras E, Granena A, Navasa M, *et al.* On the reliability of clinical criteria for the diagnosis of hepatic veno-occlusive disease. *Ann Hematol* 1993; **66**(2): 77–80.

46 Lassau N, Auperin A, Leclere J, *et al.* Prognostic value of doppler-ultrasonography in hepatic veno-occlusive disease. *Transplantation* 2002; **74**(1): 60–6.

47 van den Bosch MA, van Hoe L. MR imaging findings in two patients with hepatic veno-occlusive disease following bone marrow transplantation. *Eur Radiol* 2000; **10**(8): 1290–3.

48 Shin NY, Kim MJ, Lim JS, *et al.* Accuracy of gadoxetic acid-enhanced magnetic resonance imaging for the diagnosis of sinusoidal obstruction syndrome in patients with chemotherapy-treated colorectal liver metastases. *Eur Radiol* 2012; **22**(4): 864–71.

49 Lee JH, Lee KH, Kim S, *et al.* Plasminogen activator inhibitor-1 is an independent diagnostic marker as well as severity predictor of hepatic veno-occlusive disease after allogeneic bone marrow transplantation in adults conditioned with busulphan and cyclophosphamide. *Br J Haematol* 2002; **118**(4): 1087–94.

50 Tabbara IA, Ghazal CD, Ghazal HH. Early drop in protein C and antithrombin III is a predictor for the development of venoocclusive disease in patients undergoing hematopoietic stem cell transplantation. *J Hematother* 1996; **5**(1): 79–84.

51 Bearman SI, Lee JL, Baron AE, McDonald GB. Treatment of hepatic venocclusive disease with recombinant human tissue plasminogen activator and heparin in 42 marrow transplant patients. *Blood* 1997; **89**(5): 1501–6.

52 Richardson PG, Murakami C, Jin Z, *et al.* Multi-institutional use of defibrotide in 88 patients after stem cell transplantation with severe veno-occlusive disease and multisystem organ failure: response without significant toxicity in a high-risk population and factors predictive of outcome. *Blood* 2002; **100**(13): 4337–43.

53 Chopra R, Eaton JD, Grassi A, *et al.* Defibrotide for the treatment of hepatic veno-occlusive disease: results of the European compassionate-use study. *Br J Haematol* 2000; **111**(4): 1122–9.

54 Richardson PG, Ho VT, Cutler C, *et al.* Hepatic veno-occlusive disease after hematopoietic stem cell transplantation: novel insights to pathogenesis, current status of treatment, and future directions. *Biol Blood Marrow Transplant* 2013; **19**(1 Suppl.): S88–90.

55 Morris JD, Harris RE, Hashmi R, *et al.* Antithrombin-III for the treatment of chemotherapy-induced organ dysfunction following bone marrow transplantation. *Bone Marrow Transpl* 1997; **20**(10): 871–8.

56 Essell JH, Schroeder MT, Harman GS, *et al.* Ursodiol prophylaxis against hepatic complications of allogeneic bone marrow transplantation. A randomized, double-blind, placebo-controlled trial. *Ann Intern Med* 1998; **128**(12 Pt. 1): 975–81.

57 Dignan F, Gujral D, Ethell M, *et al.* Prophylactic defibrotide in allogeneic stem cell transplantation: minimal morbidity and zero mortality from veno-occlusive disease. *Bone Marrow Transpl* 2007; **40**(1): 79–82.

58 Forrest DL, Thompson K, Dorcas VG, *et al.* Low molecular weight heparin for the prevention of hepatic veno-occlusive disease (VOD) after hematopoietic stem cell transplantation: a prospective phase II study. *Bone Marrow Transpl* 2003; **31**(12): 1143–9.

59 Imran H, Tleyjeh IM, Zirakzadeh A, *et al.* Use of prophylactic anticoagulation and the risk of hepatic veno-occlusive disease in patients undergoing hematopoietic stem cell transplantation: a systematic review and meta-analysis. *Bone Marrow Transpl* 2006; **37**(7): 677–86.

60 Frickhofen N, Wiesneth M, Jainta C, *et al.* Hepatitis C virus infection is a risk factor for liver failure from veno-occlusive disease after bone marrow transplantation. *Blood* 1994; **83**(7): 1998–2004.

61 Giles FJ, Kantarjian HM, Kornblau SM, *et al.* Mylotarg (gemtuzumab ozogamicin) therapy is associated with hepatic venoocclusive disease in patients who have not received stem cell transplantation. *Cancer* 2001; **92**(2): 406–13.

CHAPTER 82

Metabolic Syndrome and Non-alcoholic Fatty Liver Disease

Paul Angulo

University of Kentucky Medical Center, Lexington, KY, USA

Summary

Non-alcoholic fatty liver disease (NALFD) encompasses a wide spectrum of liver injury, ranging from bland hepatic steatosis to non-alcoholic steatohepatitis (NASH). Bland steatosis follows a relatively benign clinical course, but NASH may progress to cirrhosis. NAFLD affects about one-third of the adult US population and up to 10% of adolescents and preadolescents. The demographics of NAFLD in the general population mirror those of the metabolic syndrome, which is characterized by obesity, diabetes, hypertension, and dyslipidemia. The real prevalence of NASH in the general population remains unknown, but up to 15% of patients with NASH on liver biopsy may progress to cirrhosis within 15 years. Several clinical and laboratory markers of liver injury can be used to predict the severity of NAFLD and help decide the need for a liver biopsy. Pharmacologic therapy holds promise, but lifestyle intervention with diet and increased physical activity remains the only treatment recommendation.

Case

A 38-year-old nursing student was doing well until 3 months ago, when she noticed abdominal distension associated with discomfort in the right side of her abdomen and occasional nausea. The abdominal discomfort increases with movements, bending, and breathing. Her acohol consumption is no more than 1–2 glasses of wine per week. She has not received a blood transfusion and is on no medications. She has a history of tonsillectomy and bladder augmentation surgery. She is divorced and living with her three daughters. Her weight is 80.1 kg, height 161 cm, body mass index (BMI) 30.9 kg/m², waist circumference 90 cm, and blood pressure 132/69 mmHg. Her abdomen has moderate tenderness in the right upper quadrant; the liver edge is palpable about three fingerbreadths below the costal margin and is tender. There is no palpable spleen and no ascites. The rest of the physical examination is unremarkable. Laboratory studies show total cholesterol 400 mg/dL, high-density lipoprotein (HDL) 35 mg/dL, triglycerides 522 mg/dL, fasting glucose 83 mg/dL, alanine transaminase (ALT) 64 IU/L (normal 9–29 IU/L), aspartate transaminase (AST) 58 IU/L (normal 12–31 IU/L), normal alkaline phosphatase, bilirubin, albumin, and International Normalized Ratio (INR). She is antinuclear antibody (ANA)-positive 1 : 40, anti-smooth-muscle antibody (ASMA)- and antimitochondrial antibody (AMA)-negative. She has total proteins 7.23 g/dL (normal 6.3–7.9 g/dL), γ-globulins 1.09 g/dL (normal 0.7–1.7 g/dL), negative

hepatitis serology, serum iron 118 µg/dL (normal 35–145 µg/dL), ferritin 500 µg/L (normal 20–120 µg/L), and transferrin saturation 28% (normal 14–50%). Abdominal ultrasonography and computed tomography (CT) scan show hepatomegaly with fatty infiltration of the liver.

Definition and Epidemiology

Hepatic steatosis refers to the accumulation of fat (mainly triglycerides) in hepatocytes that results from insulin resistance. NAFLD encompasses a wide range of liver pathology, with some patients presenting with steatosis and no additional features of liver injury and others presenting with nonalcoholic steatohepatitis (NASH) with or without fibrosis or cirrhosis. This range of liver pathology does not necessarily imply that individuals with steatosis are at risk for NASH or advanced fibrosis, or that those with NASH will ineludibly progress to cirrhosis. Nevertheless, some patients with NAFLD may develop cirrhosis and die from complications of portal hypertension, liver failure, and hepatocellular carcinoma (HCC) if liver transplantation is not performed. Hence, simple hepatic steatosis represents only one end of the spectrum of NAFLD. NAFLD is recognized as the most common chronic liver disease in the Western world [1].

NAFLD may be categorized as primary or secondary depending on the underlying pathogenesis (Table 83.1). Primary NAFLD occurs most commonly, and is associated with insulin-resistant states, such as obesity, type 2 diabetes, and dyslipidemia. Other conditions associated with insulin resistance, such as polycystic ovarian syndrome and hypopituitarism, have also been described in association with NAFLD. Distinction from secondary types is important, because they have different treatment and prognosis. Primary NAFLD has reached epidemic proportions in many countries around the world, as demonstrated in several population-based studies. In the United States, 34% of the population aged 30–65 years and 9.6% of the population aged 2–19 years has hepatic steatosis [2, 3]. If these figures are extrapolated to the 2014 US population, over 80 million Americans have NAFLD. The prevalence of NAFLD in the general population in the United States is about 20-fold higher than the prevalence of hepatitis C virus (HCV) infection (which affects about 4 million people) and about fourfold higher

Practical Gastroenterology and Hepatology Board Review Toolkit, Second Edition. Edited by Nicholas J. Talley, Kenneth R. DeVault, Michael B. Wallace, Bashar A. Aqel and Keith D. Lindor.
© 2016 John Wiley & Sons, Ltd. Published 2016 by John Wiley & Sons, Ltd. Companion website: www.practicalgastrohep.com

Table 83.1 Causes of non-alcoholic fatty liver disease (NAFLD).

Primary	Secondary				
	Nutritional	**Drugs**	**Metabolic**	**Toxins**	**Infections**
Obesity	Protein–calorie	Glucocorticoids	Lipodystrophy	*Amanita phalloides* mushroom	HIV
Glucose intolerance Type 2	malnutrition	Estrogens	Hypopituitarism	Phosphorus poisoning	Hepatitis C
diabetes	Rapid weight loss	Tamoxifen	Dysbetalipoproteinemia	Petrochemicals	Small-bowel diverticulosis
Hypertriglyceridemia Low	GI bypass surgery	Amiodarone	Weber–Christian disease	*Bacillus cereus* toxin	with bacterial overgrowth
HDL-cholesterol	TPN	Methotrexate			
Hypertension		Diltiazem			
		Zidovudine			
		Valproate			
		Aspirin			
		Tetracycline			
		Cocaine			

HDL, high-density lipoprotein; GI, gastrointestinal; TPN, total parental nutrition; HIV, human immunodeficiency virus.

than that of alcohol-induced liver disease (which affects about 20 million).

Pathophysiology

It is now well established that insulin resistance is the principal pathophysiologic driver of NAFLD, with adipose tissue playing a key role in the early events leading to insulin resistance. In human obesity, adipose tissue, particularly that with an intra-abdominal (visceral) location, is characterized by inflammation with an increased number of infiltrating CD14+ macrophages. Macrophages in adipose tissue correlate directly with adipose tissue mass (BMI), and even more strongly with visceral adipose tissue [4]. Weight gain is associated with the appearance of macrophages within the adipose tissue, and these changes predate the development of insulin resistance and its attendant metabolic abnormalities [5,6]. Macrophages, adipocytes, preadipocytes, and endothelial cells within the adipose tissue produce a number of adipocytokines with either pro- or anti-inflammatory effects. In insulin-resistant states, the profile of adipocytokines produced is predominantly proinflammatory, prothrombotic, and profibrogenic. A key metabolic effect of these adipocytokines is a relatively greater activity of hormone-sensitive lipase, resulting in a net increase in peripheral lipolysis and release of free fatty acids (FFAs) into the circulation. FFAs impair insulin signaling in striated muscle, decreasing the metabolic clearance of glucose. The pancreas responds to the increased glucose and FFAs by increasing insulin secretion. Over time, sustained overproduction of insulin induces injury of islet β-cells, causing a failure to produce enough insulin to maintain euglycemia and resulting in diabetes [7].

Fat accumulated in hepatocytes (steatosis) can be traced to three main sources: circulating FFAs, dietary content, and new synthesis. In patients with NAFLD on a normal diet, approximately 60% of hepatic fat derives from circulating FFAs. Peripheral insulin resistance and its resulting increase in lipolysis provide increased FFAs. Further, increased delivery of FFAs to the liver induces lipotoxicity and hepatocyte injury [8]. Hepatic steatosis leads to increased nuclear factor (NF)-κB signaling in the liver [9]. NF-κB activation then induces the production of local and systemic inflammatory mediators, such as tumor necrosis factor (TNF)-α and interleukins (IL)-6 and -1β, and the activation of Kupffer cells and macrophages within the liver. In addition, several of the proinflammatory adipocytokines induce activation of hepatic stellate cells, resulting in increased production of collagenous matrix and development of live fibrosis. Matrix production is also modulated by hepatic stellate cell apoptosis, which can be affected by cannabinoid receptor activation as well [10].

Clinical Features

A summary of the clinical features of NAFLD is given in Table 83.2.

Symptoms and Signs

Patients may complain of fatigue or malaise and a sensation of fullness or discomfort in the right upper abdomen. Hepatomegaly and acanthosis nigricans in children are common physical findings, though stigmata of chronic liver disease suggestive of cirrhosis are uncommon. The impact of NAFLD on health-related quality of life is currently being evaluated. However, several studies have found a

Table 83.2 Main clinical, laboratory, and diagnostic characteristics of NAFLD.

Clinical features	Laboratory abnormalities	Liver biopsy features	Imaging features	Exclusion of
Usually asymptomatic, sometimes mild right upper quadrant discomfort, hepatomegaly, acanthosis nigricans, "cryptogenic" cirrhosis	Elevated ALT and AST (usually less than five times normal)	Steatosis (fatty infiltration >5% hepatocytes)	Imaging indicative of fatty infiltration of the liver	Alcohol intake <140 g/week (women) or <210 g/week (men)
Often associated with features of the metabolic syndrome: hyperglycemia or type 2 diabetes, obesity, dyslipidemia (hypertriglyceridemia, low HDL-cholesterol), hypertension	Elevated alkaline phosphatase and γ-glutamyltransferase (usually less than three times normal)	Necroinflammation, typically with a zone 3 lobular distribution	(ultrasonography, CT, MRI, MRS)	Liver disease of viral, autoimmune, genetic origin; hemochromatosis
	AST : ALT ratio <1; hyperinsulinemia, hyperglycemia, and insulin resistance; dyslipidemia, elevated ferritin	Mallory bodies, hepatocyte ballooning		
		Fibrosis (perisinusoidal, perivenular, bridging, cirrhosis)		
		Portal-based injury in children (common)		

HDL, high-density lipoprotein; ALT, alanine transaminase; AST, aspartate transaminase; CT, computed tomography; MRI, magnetic resonance imaging; MRS, magnetic resonance spectroscopy.

significant detrimental impact from the several comorbidities that make up the metabolic syndrome and often cluster with NAFLD.

The most common comorbidities associated with NAFLD are the components of the metabolic syndrome, which include fasting glucose ≥100 mg/dL, central obesity with waist circumference >102 cm (40 inches) in men and >88 cm (35 inches) in women, blood pressure ≥130/85 mmHg, fasting triglyceride ≥150 mg/dL, and low HDL-cholesterol (<40 mg/dL in men, <50 mg/dL in women). The American Heart Association (AHA) and National Heart, Lung, and Blood Institute (NHLBI) require the presence of at least three of these five features to make the diagnosis of the metabolic syndrome [11], while the International Diabetes Federation (IDF) requires the presence of central obesity plus at least two of the other four components [12]. About 90% of NAFLD patients have a BMI ≥25 kg/m^2. Obesity (BMI ≥30 kg/m^2) is present in 50%, type 2 diabetes in 28%, dyslipidemia (hypertriglyceridemia, hypercholesterolemia, or low HDL-cholesterol alone or in combination) in 55%, and hypertension in 60%; almost half of all patients with NAFLD have the metabolic syndrome (i.e., at least three of the features of the metabolic syndrome) (Figure 83.1). Also, about 75% of lean patients (BMI <25 kg/m^2) with NAFLD have at least one feature of the metabolic syndrome [13].

Most patients with NAFLD and a BMI ≥35 kg/m^2 also meet the criteria for central obesity, as already defined. The presence and severity of NAFLD correlate with central obesity more strongly than does BMI, supporting the notion that fat with an intra-abdominal (visceral) location is metabolically different from fat with a more peripheral or subcutaneous location [14]. Some patients with NAFLD may have a BMI <35 kg/m^2 and still have central obesity, whereas many individuals with a high BMI do not have NAFLD. There are differences in body fat distribution among the different ethnic groups, which may be one of the factors explaining the different NAFLD prevalence among these groups in the United States, with a higher prevalence among adult Hispanic individuals (45%) as compared with white adults (33%) and African–American adults (24%). In the United States, a prevalence difference between adult men and women is found only among white people (42% men vs. 24% women) [2].

Laboratory Abnormalities

Serum liver enzyme abnormalities are often restricted to elevations of ALT and/or AST, and usually to levels below five times normal. Transaminase levels in NAFLD patients fluctuate; normal levels are present in up to 78% of patients at any one time, but levels are elevated in more than 20% of these patients if tests repeated at several points during follow-up. Alkaline phosphatase and γ-glutamyltransferase levels may be modestly elevated (generally less than three times normal) in one-third of cases, but are rarely elevated in isolation. Hyperbilirubinemia, low albumin levels, and increased INR usually indicate decompensated cirrhosis.

Serum iron tests are commonly abnormal, with elevated ferritin levels observed in up to 50% of patients and raised transferrin saturation in up to 10%. These findings may potentially lead to confusion regarding a diagnosis of hemochromatosis. Whether there is an increased prevalence of heterozygous *HFE* gene mutations among patients with NAFLD is controversial; however, their presence does not appear to be associated with increased hepatic iron or liver fibrosis. In patients with NAFLD, serum ferritin levels on their own do not allow an accurate prediction of the presence of NASH or fibrosis [15]. Serum ANAs and/or ASMAs are present in 23–36% of NAFLD patients, and may rarely indicate coexistent autoimmune liver disease. In one series of 225 NAFLD cases, 8% of autoantibody-positive patients also had coexistent features of autoimmune hepatitis on liver biopsy, but the liver biopsy features helped to exclude the diagnosis of autoimmune hepatitis in the vast majority of those with NAFLD who were ANA- and/or ASMA-positive [16]. Other laboratory abnormalities commonly seen in patients with NAFLD are hyperglycemia, hyperinsulinemia, and increased levels of triglycerides and total cholesterol and decreased levels of HDL-cholesterol.

Imaging Features

Ultrasonography, CT, and magnetic resonance imaging (MRI) can non-invasively diagnose fatty infiltration of the liver. Hepatic steatosis increases the liver echogenicity on ultrasonography, which can be contrasted against the lower echogenicity of the spleen or renal cortex. A similar pattern can be seen with diffuse fibrosis, giving rise to the term "fatty-fibrotic pattern," though the echo shadows tend to be coarser in the presence of pure fibrosis. The sensitivity and specificity of ultrasonography for detecting hepatic steatosis vary from 60 to 94% and 88 to 95%, respectively. However, the sensitivity of ultrasonography decreases with lower degrees of fatty infiltration. In the presence of ≥30% fatty infiltration, the sensitivity of ultrasonography is 80%, compared with 55% when hepatic fat content is 10–19%. Similarly, the sensitivity and specificity of ultrasonography decrease in the presence of morbid obesity to 49 and 75%, respectively [17].

On non-contrast images on CT scans, hepatic steatosis has a low attenuation and appears darker than the spleen. The sensitivity of

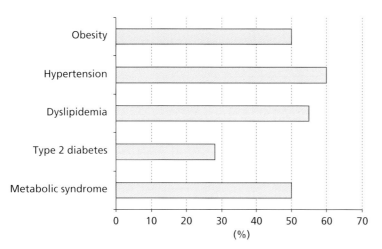

Figure 83.1 Prevalence of features of the metabolic syndrome in NAFLD [13]. Source: Data from Angulo 2007 [13].

CHAPTER 83

CT at detecting >33% hepatic steatosis is up to 93%, with a positive predictive value (PPV) of 76%. Both magnetic resonance phase-contrast imaging techniques and magnetic resonance spectroscopy (MRS) are reliable at detecting steatosis and offer good correlation with hepatic fat volume. A hepatic fat content >5% on MRS indicates the presence of steatosis [17]. However, the routine application of MRI is limited by cost and lack of availability.

Histologic Features

NAFLD is histologically indistinguishable from liver damage resulting from alcohol abuse. Liver biopsy features include steatosis, mixed inflammatory cell infiltration, hepatocyte ballooning and necrosis, glycogen nuclei, Mallory hyaline, and fibrosis [18]. The presence of steatosis alone or in combination with the other features accounts for the wide spectrum of NAFLD (Figure 83.2). Steatosis is present predominantly as macrovesicular fat, though some hepatocytes may show an admixture with microvesicular steatosis. Fatty infiltration, when mild, is typically concentrated in acinar zone 3, whereas moderate-to-severe fatty infiltration shows a more diffuse distribution. The inflammatory infiltrate usually consists of mixed neutrophils and lymphocytes, and predominates in zone 3. Ballooning degeneration of hepatocytes results from intracellular fluid accumulation and is characterized by swollen cells, typically noted in zone 3 near the steatotic hepatocytes. Mallory hyaline is found in

about half of adult patients with NAFLD and is usually located in ballooned hepatocytes in zone 3, but it is neither unique to nor specific for NAFLD. The pattern of fibrosis is one of NAFLD's characteristic features. Collagen is first laid down in the pericellular space around the central vein and in the perisinusoidal region in zone 3. In some areas, the collagen invests single cells in a pattern referred to as "chicken-wire" fibrosis, as described in alcohol-induced liver damage. This pattern of fibrosis helps to distinguish NAFLD and alcoholic liver disease (ALD) from other forms of liver disease, in which fibrosis shows an initial portal distribution.

Portal tracts are relatively spared from inflammation, though children with NAFLD may show a predominance of portal-based injury, as opposed to a lobular pericentral injury. Mallory hyaline is notably sparse or absent in children with NAFLD. In some patients at the cirrhotic stage, the features of steatosis and necroinflammatory activity are no longer present.

The histologic distinction between hepatic steatosis and NASH with high-grade inflammation and fibrosis is relatively clear; however, differentiating more subtle changes in the middle of the spectrum can be difficult. Furthermore, different histologic definitions have been used to categorize NASH. The most accepted definition of NASH requires the presence of zone 3 accentuated macrovesicular steatosis together with mild mixed lobular inflammation and hepatocellular ballooning. Though liver biopsy is the gold standard

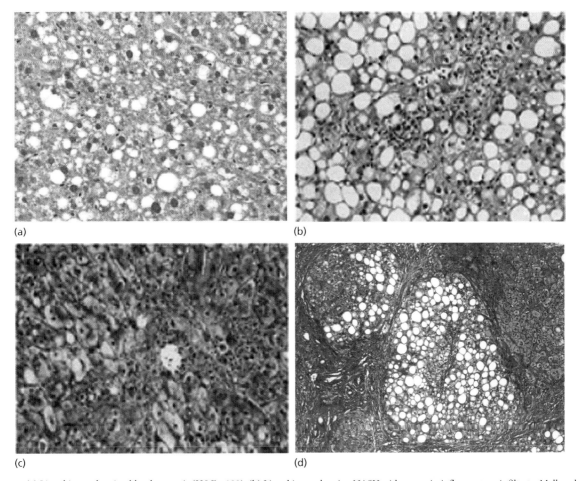

(a)

(b)

(c)

(d)

Figure 83.2 (a) Liver biopsy showing bland steatosis (H&E ×100). (b) Liver biopsy showing NASH with steatosis, inflammatory infiltrate, Mallory hyaline, and hepatocyte ballooning (H&E ×100). (c) Liver biopsy showing pericellular and perisinusoidal fibrosis in zone 3 (Masson trichrome ×400). (d) Liver biopsy showing cirrhotic-stage NAFLD (Masson trichrome ×100).

for NASH diagnosis and staging of fibrosis, sampling variability may underestimate the severity of liver injury.

Assessment of Disease Severity

Liver biopsy is the only investigation that can differentiate NASH from simple steatosis and stage the extent of fibrosis. Imaging studies such as ultrasonography, CT, and MRI are not able to distinguish between steatosis and NASH, nor can they stage the degree of hepatic fibrosis. Recently, measuring liver stiffness with ultrasound- or magnetic resonance-based elastography has been proposed as being potentially useful in the quantification of liver fibrosis in patients with a wide range of chronic liver disease [17]; however, further evaluation of these techniques in patients with NAFLD is necessary.

The potential benefits of liver biopsy must be weighed against the small risk of complications, including pain, bleeding, and death. The decision to pursue biopsy needs to be individualized and discussed with each patient. A number of clinical and laboratory features may facilitate separation of patients with simple steatosis from those with NASH, and help distinguish between those with and without advanced fibrosis. Caspase-3-generated cytokeratin (CK)-18 fragments, a marker of apoptosis measured in plasma, have been evaluated in distinguishing simple steatosis from NASH [19]. In the original study, a CK-18 value of 395 U/L had a specificity of 99.9%, a sensitivity of 85.7%, a PPV of 99.9%, and a negative predictive value (NPV) of 85.7% for the diagnosis of NASH [19]. The severity of fibrosis can also be predicted using a combination of routine clinical and laboratory variables, including older age, presence of diabetes, higher BMI, higher AST : ALT ratio, and low albumin and platelet counts [13]. These features have been combined in a numerical score named the "NAFLD Fibrosis Score" [13], which is aimed at predicting the presence or absence of advanced fibrosis in NAFLD (Table 83.3). The NAFLD Fibrosis Score has been extensively validated and is currently recommended for routine use in clinical practice.

Advanced fibrosis among NAFLD patients has been associated with levels of novel serum markers of fibrogenesis, including hyaluronic acid (HA), propeptide of type III collagen (P3NP), and the tissue inhibitor of matrix metalloproteinase-1 (TIMP-1) [20]. These serum markers have been combined in a numerical score named the "Enhanced Liver Fibrosis Panel" to predict presence and severity of liver fibrosis in NAFLD [24] (Table 83.3). This score is not yet commercially available and has not been cleared by the Food and Drug Administration (FDA); further validation is required before it can routinely be used in clinical practice.

Diagnosis

The most common clinical scenario leading to diagnosis of NAFLD is asymptomatic elevation of serum transaminase (ALT, AST)

levels not due to viral hepatitis, iron overload, or alcohol abuse. When these other liver diseases are ruled out, NAFLD is the likely cause in most cases. Transaminases, however, are elevated in only 20% of the general population with NAFLD [2]. The AST : ALT ratio is usually <1, but this increases as fibrosis advances to the cirrhotic stage. Fatty infiltration of the liver as detected by ultrasonography is also likely to be due to NAFLD in most cases. These findings by themselves are not sufficient to make a diagnosis of NAFLD, however; supportive clinical, serologic, and sometimes histologic evidence is also required. The presence of features of the metabolic syndrome increases the likelihood of NAFLD, but these features are common in the general population and not specific for the diagnosis.

The gold standard for diagnosing NAFLD is clinicopathologic correlation, based on confirmation of steatosis by liver biopsy and appropriate exclusion of other etiologies (see Table 83.2). It is important to exclude alcohol abuse as the cause of fatty liver. It is known that a minimal amount of alcohol of 20 g/day (1–2 standard drinks) in women and 30 g/day (2–3 standard drinks) in men can induce fatty liver, and these limits are commonly used to distinguish between alcoholic and non-alcoholic fatty liver. Secondary causes of NAFLD (see Table 83.1) should be ruled out because NAFLD associated with these conditions has a different course and treatment.

Differential Diagnosis

Patients with chronically elevated serum liver enzymes should have other causes excluded by clinical review and laboratory testing. The extent of laboratory evaluation should be individualized. Though 66–90% of individuals with chronically elevated liver enzymes with a negative laboratory evaluation have NAFLD, other potential diagnoses in these patients are drug-related liver injury, normal or nonspecific changes on liver biopsy, autoimmune hepatitis, chronic biliary disease, and granulomatous liver disease. A liver biopsy may be useful in diagnosing NAFLD when a potentially different diagnosis is suggested by clinical or laboratory testing. This includes the presence of autoantibodies or raised iron indices, a history of recent medication change, and the absence of detectable hepatic steatosis on cross-sectional imaging. Persistence of elevated transaminases after 3–6 months of lifestyle intervention with appropriate weight loss and control of lipids and glucose levels may also suggest another diagnosis and dictate the need for a liver biopsy.

NAFLD should be considered as a possible differential diagnosis among patients with "cryptogenic" cirrhosis. The prevalence of metabolic risk factors such as diabetes and obesity is similar among patients with cryptogenic cirrhosis and NAFLD. In addition, the prevalence rates of these risk factors are higher when compared with patients with cirrhosis of other etiologies, suggesting that NASH accounts for a substantial proportion of cases of cryptogenic

Table 83.3 Clinical and serum markers of fibrogenesis proposed as predictors of advanced (stage 3–4) fibrosis in patients with NAFLD.

Reference	n	Clinical score/serum marker	AUC	Sensitivity (%)	Specificity (%)
[13]	733	$-1.675 + 0.037 \times$ age (years) $+ 0.094 \times$ BMI (kg/m^2) $+ 1.13 \times$ IFG/diabetes (yes = 1, no = 0) $+ 0.99$ $\times$ AST : ALT ratio $-0.013 \times$ platelet ($\times 10^9$/L) $-0.66 \times$ albumin (g/dL)	0.88		
		Score < −1.455		82	77
		Score > 0.676		51	98
[20]	192	$-7.412 + (\ln(HA) \times 0.681) + (\ln(P3NP) \times 0.775) + (\ln(TIMP-1) \times 0.494)$	0.93		
		ELF = 0.3576		80	90

AUC, area under the receiver operator characteristic curve; BMI, body mass index; IFG, impaired fasting glucose; AST, aspartate transaminase; ALT, alanine transaminase; ln, logarithm negative; HA, hyaluronic acid; P3NP, propeptide of type III collagen; TIMP-1, tissue inhibitor of matrix metalloproteinase-1; ELF, enhanced liver fibrosis.

cirrhosis. Rarely, NASH is a consideration in patients with suba-cute liver failure, having been observed among individuals who have silently progressed to cirrhosis before an unknown stimulus precip-itates liver failure.

Case Continued

The clinical diagnosis of NAFLD in the patient is pretty straightforward, based on the presence of features of the metabolic syndrome (central obesity, hypertriglyceridemia, and low HDL-cholesterol), elevated transaminases (less than three times normal), confirmation of fatty infiltration of the liver on imaging studies, and a negative alcohol and medication history and negative viral serology. The presence of ANA at low titers without other laboratory features of autoimmune hepatitis, and increased ferritin with normal serum iron and transferrin saturation, are not uncommon in patients with NAFLD, as described previously. The need for a liver biopsy to confirm the diagnosis of NAFLD and stage the disease is extensively discussed with the patient, who opts to have her case reevaluated after treatment.

Table 83.4 Therapeutic options in NALF/NASH.

Lifestyle changes	Reduce weight
	Reduce total fat intake to <30% energy
	Replace saturated with unsaturated fats
	Increase fiber intake to >15 g/day
	Increase physical activity
Insulin-sensitizing agents	Metformin
	Pioglitazone
	Rosiglitazone
Antioxidants and cytoprotective agents	Vitamins E and C
	Betain
	Taurine
	NAC
	Sibilin
	Ursodeoxycholic acid
	Fibrates and statins
	Orlistat, sibutramine, phentermine
Other treatments and future areas of research	Anti-TNF-α antibodies
	Pentoxifylline
	Antifibrotic medications
	Angiotensin II receptor antagonists
	CB-1 receptor antagonists
	Caspase inhibitors

Other than ursodeoxycholic acid, none of these medications has been evaluated in well-controlled, appropriately powered, randomized trials.
NAC, N-acetylcysteine; TNF, tumor necrosis factor; CB, cannabinoid.

Prognosis

The high prevalence of NAFLD in the general population contrasts with the relatively small proportion of individuals with NAFLD who will show evidence of disease progression or develop compli-cations of end-stage liver disease. When compared to the general population of the same age and sex, NAFLD is associated with a low standardized mortality ratio of 1.34 (95% CI: 1.0003–1.7600), but significantly higher overall mortality [21]. The natural history of simple hepatic steatosis without fibrosis is relatively benign, with similar mortality on long-term follow-up to the general population of the same age and gender; the reported rate of progression to cirrhosis and liver-related mortality is less than 1% [22]. In contrast, up to 15% of patients with NASH – particularly those with fibrosis – may progress to cirrhosis within 15 years of diagnosis [22]. The presence of advanced fibrosis or cirrhosis should initiate screening for hepatocellular carcinoma and esophageal varices, with closer monitoring for disease-related complications. Histologic staging is also valuable for tracking disease progression and monitoring response to therapy. It is important to keep in mind, however, that changes in transaminase levels do not reliably correlate with histologic changes over time. In a recent long-term follow-up study, the NAFLD fibrosis score accurately separated NAFLD patients into those at low, intermediate, and high risk for the development of complications of cirrhosis and overall mortality, or for the need for liver transplantation [23].

Treatment

Treatment of NAFLD is aimed at correcting the underlying risk fac-tors and comorbid conditions, but there are no proven therapies at this point (Table 83.4).

Treatment of Associated Conditions

A large body of clinical and epidemiological data gathered over the last 3 decades indicates that obesity, type 2 diabetes melli-tus (T2DM), and dyslipidemia are major associated conditions of or predisposing factors leading to the development of NAFLD. Hence, it is reasonable to believe that the prevention or appropri-ate management of these conditions would lead to improvement

or arrest of liver disease. Weight loss, particularly if gradual, may lead to improvement in liver histology in NAFLD. However, the rate and degree of weight loss required for normalization of liver histology have not been established. Total starvation and very-low-calorie diets may cause worsening of liver histology, and thus should be avoided. The NHLBI and the National Institute of Diabetes and Digestive and Kidney Diseases (NIDDK) expert panel clini-cal guidelines for weight loss recommend that the initial target be 10% loss of baseline weight within a period of 6 months. For most, this can be achieved by losing about 0.45–0.90 kg (1–2 lb) per week. With success, further weight loss can be attempted if indicated. The panel recommends weight loss using multiple interventions and strategies, including lifestyle modification (i.e., diet modifications and increased physical activity), behavioral therapy, pharmacother-apy (i.e., orlistat, phentermine, sibutramine), and surgery, alone or in combination. The recommendation for a particular treatment modality or combination should be individualized according to BMI and the presence of concomitant risk factors and other dis-eases. The panel does not make specific recommendations for the subgroup of patients with NAFLD; however, given the lack of clini-cal trials in this area, it may be a useful and safe first step for obese patients with NAFLD. Similarly, no specific recommendations for liver test monitoring during weight loss are made, but monthly mea-surement of liver enzymes during weight loss seems appropriate.

Different dietary caloric restrictions have been used. Further studies are necessary to determine the most appropriate formula for obese and/or diabetic patients with NAFLD. In the absence of well-controlled clinical trials in patients with NAFLD, it may be tempting to recommend a heart-healthy diet, as recommended by the AHA, or a diabetic diet, as recommended by the American Diabetes Asso-ciation (ADA). Dietary supplementation with n-3 polyunsaturated and monounsaturated fatty acids may improve insulin sensitivity and prevent liver damage. Saturated fatty acids worsen insulin resis-tance, whereas dietary fiber can improve it. Nevertheless, the effect of such dietary modifications in patients with fatty liver remains to be established. Compounds with high amounts of fructose should be avoided, as several studies associate fructose with both development and worsening of NAFLD [24]. Diet to produce weight loss should always be prescribed on an individual basis, according to the patient's overall health. Patients who have obesity-related disease, such as diabetes mellitus, hyperlipidemia, or cardiovascular disease (CVD), will require close medical supervision during weight loss to adjust medication dosage as needed.

Improving insulin sensitivity with lifestyle changes or medications usually improves glucose and lipid levels in patients with diabetes and hyperlipidemia. Improving insulin sensitivity in these patients is expected to improve the liver disease, but, in many diabetic/hyperlipidemic patients with NAFLD, appropriate control of glucose and lipid levels is not always accompanied by improvement of the liver condition.

Pharmacologic Treatment

Given that achieving and maintaining appropriate weight control is a difficult task for most obese patients, the use of medications that can directly reduce the severity of liver damage independently of weight loss is a reasonable alternative. Pharmacologic therapy may also benefit patients who lack risk factors or associated conditions, such as non-obese, non-diabetic patients and those with a normal lipid profile. However, pharmacologic therapy directed specifically at the liver disease has only recently been evaluated in patients with NAFLD. Most studies have been uncontrolled and open-label and have lasted 1 year or less, and only a few have evaluated the effect of treatment on liver histology.

The results of pilot studies evaluating insulin sensitizer medications, antioxidants, lipid-lowering medications, and some hepatoprotective medications suggest that they may be of potential benefit. Medications evaluated in appropriately designed placebo-controlled trials include ursodeoxycholic acid, rosiglitazone, vitamin E, and pioglitazone. Ursodeoxycholic acid [25] and rosiglitazone [26] were not associated with a clear benefit as compared to placebo and are thus not recommended for the treatment of NAFLD. Both pioglitazone and vitamin E may improve some features of NASH, such as steatosis, inflammation, and hepatocytes ballooning, but do not have any effect on fibrosis, and thus they both are of uncertain long-term benefit [27]. Further, the well-known side effects of pioglitazone [28] and the reported higher overall mortality associated with the long-term use of vitamin E [29] preclude the use of these two medications in patients with NASH.

General Recommendations

An attempt at gradual weight loss is a useful first step in the management of patients with NAFLD, in addition to a concerted effort to maintain appropriate control of serum glucose and lipid levels. Perhaps this, along with appropriate exclusion of other liver disease, may be the only treatment recommendation for patients with pure steatosis and no evidence of necroinflammation or fibrosis, who seem to have the best prognosis within the spectrum of NAFLD. Patients with NASH, particularly those with increased fibrosis on liver biopsy, should be monitored closely, given adequate metabolic control, and offered enrollment in well-controlled clinical trials, if available. Pharmacologic therapy holds promise, but data from well-controlled clinical trials are still needed to determine not only the efficacy but also the long-term safety of the several medications available.

For those patients with cirrhotic-stage NAFLD and decompensated disease, liver transplantation is a potential life-extending therapeutic alternative, though some cirrhotic patients with NAFLD suffer from comorbid conditions that often preclude liver transplantation.

Case Continued

The patient is recommended a low-calorie, low-saturated-fat diet tailored to her preferences, plus increased physical activity, with aerobic exercise for 30–45 minutes a day at least four times a week. At her 3-month reevaluation, she has managed to lose 5 kg and her ALT and AST are within the normal range. Her total cholesterol has decreased to 290 mg/dL, and her triglyceride levels to 230 mg/dL. Treatment continues, and at her 6-month evaluation she has managed to lose a total of 9 kg ans her laboratory tests showed normal transaminases levels, a total cholesterol level of 189 mg/dL, an HDL-cholesterol level of 40 mg/dL, and a triglyceride level of 200 mg/dL.

Take Home Points

- Non-alcoholic fatty liver disease (NAFLD) affects a substantial proportion of the general population and represents the most common cause of elevated liver enzymes.
- Simple hepatic steatosis follows a relatively benign clinical course, but when steatosis or steatohepatitis is associated with increased fibrosis, the disease may progress to cirrhosis and liver cancer.
- The diagnosis of NAFLD requires exclusion of other causes of liver disease, along with confirmation of fatty infiltration of the liver on imaging studies.
- Liver biopsy is the only tool that allows grading of the several histological features of NAFLD differentiating between non-alcoholic steatohepatitis (NASH) and non-NASH. Importantly, it also allows staging of fibrosis.
- Lifestyle modification with diet and increased physical activity represents the only treatment modality with potential efficacy for patients with NAFLD.
- Pharmacologic therapy holds promise, but large, well-controlled trials are needed before any medication can be recommended.
- Ursodesocycholic acid, vitamin E, rosiglitazone, and pioglitazone are all associated with minimal clinical benefit, important side effects, or higher mortality. Therefore, none of them can be recommended for the treatment of NAFLD.

References

1 Angulo P. GI epidemiology: nonalcoholic fatty liver disease. *Aliment Pharmacol Ther* 2007; **25**: 883–9.

2 Browning JD, Szczpeniak L, Dobbins R, *et al*. Prevalence of hepatic steatosis in an urban population in the United States: impact of ethnicity. *Hepatology* 2004; **40**: 1387–95.

3 Schwimmer J, Deutsch R, Kahen T, *et al*. Prevalence of fatty liver in children and adolescents. *Pediatrics* 2006; **118**: 1388–93.

4 Weisberg SP, McCann D, Desai M, *et al*. Obesity is associated with macrophage accumulation in adipose tissue. *J Clin Invest* 2003; **112**: 1796–808.

5 Xu H, Barnes GT, Yang Q, *et al*. Chronic inflammation in fat plays a crucial role in the development of obesity related insulin resistance. *J Clin Invest* 2003; **112**: 1821–30.

6 Wisse BE. The inflammatory syndrome: the role of adipose tissue cytokines in metabolic disorders linked to obesity. *J Am Soc Nephrol* 2004; **15**: 2792–800.

7 Prentki M, Nolan CJ. Islet beta cell failure in type 2 diabetes. *J Clin Invest* 2006; **116**: 1802–12.

8 Feldstein AE, Werneburg NW, Canbay A, *et al*. Free fatty acids promote hepatic lipotoxicity by stimulating TNF-alpha expression via a lysosomal pathway. *Hepatology* 2004; **40**: 185–94.

9 Cai D, Yuan M, Frantz D, *et al*. Local and systemic insulin resistance resulting from hepatic activation of IKK-B and NK-κB. *Nat Med* 2005; **11**: 183–90.

10 Kunos G, Osei-Hyiaman D. Endocannabinoids and liver disease. IV. Endocannabinoid involvement in obesity and hepatic steatosis. *Am J Physiol Gastrointest Liver Physiol* 2008; **294**: G1101–4.

11 Grundy SM, Cleeman JI, Daniels SR, *et al.* Diagnosis and management of the metabolic syndrome. An American Heart Association/National Heart, Lung, And Blood Institute scientific statement. *Circulation* 2005; **112**: 2735–52.

12 Alberti KG, Zimmet P, Shaw J, *et al.* The metabolic syndrome – a new worldwide definition. *Lancet* 2005; **366**: 1059–62.

13 Angulo P, Hui JM, Marchesini G, *et al.* The NAFLD fibrosis score: a noninvasive system that identifies liver fibrosis in patients with NAFLD. *Hepatology* 2007; **45**: 846–54.

14 Stranges S, Dorn JM, Muti P, *et al.* Body fat distribution, relative weight, and liver enzyme levels: a population based study. *Hepatology* 2004; **39**: 754–63.

15 Angulo P, George J, Day CP, *et al.* Serum ferritin levels lack diagnostic accuracy for liver fibrosis in patients with nonalcoholic fatty liver disease. *Clin Gastroenterol Hepatol* 2104; **12**: 1163–69.

16 Adams LA, Lindor KD, Angulo P. The prevalence of autoantibodies and autoimmune hepatitis in patients with nonalcoholic fatty liver disease. *Am J Gastroenterol* 2004; **99**: 1316–20.

17 Castera L, Vilgrain V, Angulo P. Noninvasive evaluation of NAFLD. *Nat Rev Gastroenterol Hepatol* 2013; **10**: 666–75.

18 Kleiner DE, Brunt EM, Van Natta M, *et al.* Nonalcoholic Steatohepatitis Clinical Research Network. Design and validation of a histological scoring system for nonalcoholic fatty liver disease. *Hepatology* 2005; **41**: 1313–21.

19 Wieckowska A, Zein NN, Yerian LM, *et al.* In vivo assessment of liver cell apoptosis as a novel biomarker of disease severity in nonalcoholic fatty liver disease. *Hepatology* 2006; **44**: 27–33.

20 Guha IN, Parkes J, Roderick P, *et al.* Noninvasive markers of fibrosis in nonalcoholic fatty liver disease: validating the European Liver Fibrosis Panel and exploring simple markers. *Hepatology* 2008; **47**: 455–60.

21 Adams LA, Lymp JF, St Sauver J, *et al.* The natural history of nonalcoholic fatty liver disease: a population-based cohort study. *Gastroenterology* 2005; **129**: 113–21.

22 Angulo P. Long-term mortality in nonalcoholic fatty liver disease: is liver histology of any prognostic significance? *Hepatology* 2010; **51**: 373–5. Erratum in: *Hepatology* 2010; **5**: 1868.

23 Angulo P, Bugianesi E, Bjornsson ES, *et al.* Simple non-invasive systems predict long-term outcomes in patients with nonalcoholic fatty liver disease. *Gastroenterology* 2013; **145**: 782–9.

24 Vos MB, McClain CJ. Fructose takes a toll. *Hepatology* 2009; **50**: 1004–6.

25 Lindor KD, Kowdley KV, Heathcote EJ, *et al.* Ursodeoxycholic acid for treatment of nonalcoholic steatohepatitis: results of a randomized trial. *Hepatology* 2004; **39**: 770–8.

26 Ratziu V, Charlotte F, Bernhardt C, *et al.* Long-term efficacy of rosiglitazone in nonalcoholic steatohepatitis: results of the fatty liver improvement by rosiglitazone therapy (FLIRT 2) extension trial. *Hepatology* 2010; **51**: 445–53.

27 Sanyal AJ, Chalasani N, Kowdley KV, *et al.* Pioglitazone, vitamin E, or placebo for nonalcoholic steatohepatitis. *N Engl J Med* 2010; **362**: 1675–85.

28 Lincoff AM, Wolski K, Nicholls SJ, Nissen SE. Pioglitazone and risk of cardiovascular events in patient with type 2 diabetes mellitus: a meta-analysis of randomized trials. *JAMA* 2007; **298**: 1180–8.

29 Miller ER 3rd, Pastor-Barriuso R, Dalal D, *et al.* Meta-analysis: high-dosage vitamin E supplementation may increase all-cause mortality. *Ann Intern Med* 2005; **142**: 37–46.

CHAPTER 83

Hemochromatosis, Wilson's Disease, and Alpha-1-Antitrypsin Deficiency

Lisa M. Glass[1] and Rolland C. Dickson[2]

[1] Department of Internal Medicine, Division of Gastroenterology, University of Michigan Health System, Ann Arbor, MI, USA
[2] Dartmouth Hitcock Medical Center, Lebanon, NH, USA

Summary

Hemochromatosis is the most common inherited metabolic disease in Caucasians. Recent observations have clarified the molecular mechanisms and clinical penetrance of the disease. Wilson's disease is rare, but should be considered when evaluating patients with liver or neuropsychiatric disorders. Trientine is now the treatment of choice. Alpha-1-antitrypsin (A1AT) deficiency is associated with liver disease in both children and adults, and is caused by accumulation of an abnormal form of the protein in liver cells.

Case

A 58-year-old obese woman with type 2 diabetes mellitus (T2DM) is referred after an iron abnormality is noted in her sister. Testing reveals ferritin 1519 µg/mL, iron 88 µg/dL, transferrin saturation 35%, and normal aspartate aminotransferase (AST) and alanine aminotransferase (ALT).

Hereditary Hemochromatosis

Hereditary hemochromatosis is caused by genetic mutations that create excessive iron deposition in the liver, pancreas, heart, and gonads. Symptoms are initially non-specific, but end-organ damage such as cirrhosis, hepatocellular carcinoma (HCC), diabetes, and heart failure can result if untreated. Due to increased disease recognition and the advent of genetic testing, earlier diagnosis is more common than in the past [1]. There is now a risk of overdiagnosis and unnecessary intervention, given the low penetrance of the disease. Once the diagnosis is confirmed, the mainstay of treatment remains phlebotomy. Initiation prior to organ damage results in a normal life expectancy.

Epidemiology and Pathophysiology

Hereditary hemochromatosis is most commonly caused by a deficiency or dysfunction of hepcidin, the principal iron-regulatory hormone [2] (Figures 84.1 and 84.2). Hepcidin is released from the liver when total body iron is adequate. It binds to the iron transport protein, ferroportin, found on macrophages and enterocytes, which prevents release of iron from cells and iron absorption across the intestinal epithelium [1–4]. The resulting increased demand for iron leads to decreased hepcidin expression, allowing transport of iron from the gut by ferroportin and release of iron from macrophages into the circulation. The abnormal HFE protein leads to dysregulation of hepcidin–ferroportin by a mechanism that is not currently clear. Excess iron deposits in soft tissue and causes iron-induced lipid perioxidation, leading to cell injury and death, followed by Kupffer and stellate cell activation, and finally collagen deposition [3].

Hereditary hemochromatosis is primarily associated with mutations in the *HFE* gene: 80–90% are homozygous for *C282Y*, and about 5% are *C282Y/H63D* compound heterozygotes [5]. Those with only *H63D* mutations do not develop clinical iron overload, and compound heterozygotes typically develop iron overload only in the presence of another liver disease. The allelic frequency of the *C282Y* mutation in white North Americans and Northern Europeans is approximately 6–10%, making it the most common genetic disorder in this population [2,3]. About 1 : 200 to 250 Caucasians are homozygous for the *C282Y* mutation [1]; however, the penetrance of hereditary hemochromatosis is lower than previously thought, and progression to significant iron overload does not always occur [6]. A large population study found that only about 75% of patients homozygous for *C282Y* had elevated iron parameters [7], and only 28% of males and 1% of females had disease-related symptoms over 12 years [6].

The remaining 10–15% of patients with hereditary hemochromatosis have non-HFE-related disease. These include juvenile hemochromatosis, a severe form of the disease with defects in hepcidin or hemojuvelin, and mutations in the iron transporter protein ferroportin or in other proteins involved in iron metabolism, such as the transferrin receptor [3,4,8].

Clinical Features

Fatigue, abdominal pain, and arthralgias are the most common symptoms at diagnosis [9]. Liver enzyme elevation, hepatomegaly, skin hyperpigmentation, dilated and restrictive cardiomyopathies, arrhythmias, diabetes, and erectile dysfunction should also elicit consideration of hereditary hemochromatosis. Through increased awareness and family screening for hereditary hemochromatosis, 75% of patients are diagnosed by laboratory testing while asymptomatic without end-stage disease [1]. However, hereditary

Practical Gastroenterology and Hepatology Board Review Toolkit, Second Edition. Edited by Nicholas J. Talley, Kenneth R. DeVault, Michael B. Wallace, Bashar A. Aqel and Keith D. Lindor.

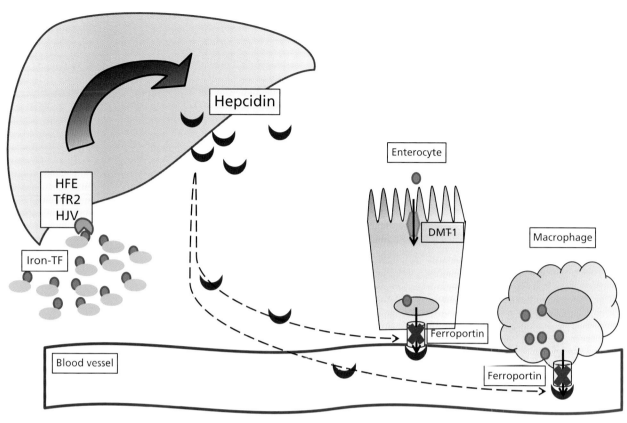

Figure 84.1 Increased hepcidin production promotes binding and internalization of ferroportin, leading to decreased iron absorption from the gut and release from macrophages. TF, transferrin; DMT-1, divalent metal transporter-1; TfR2, transferrin receptor 2; HJV, hemojuvelin.

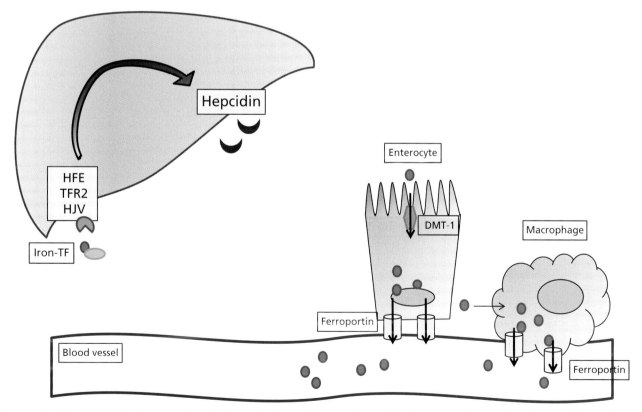

Figure 84.2 Normal physiology in states of iron deficiency. Hepcidin production is decreased, facilitating iron absorption from the gut and release from macrophages. TF, transferrin; DMT-1, divalent metal transporter-1; TfR2, transferrin receptor 2; HJV, hemojuvelin.

hemochromatosis typically causes progressive fibrosis with little or no inflammation, so up to 12% of males and 3% of females still present with cirrhosis [10, 11].

Diagnosis

Screening tests for hereditary hemochromatosis are indirect measures of iron stores, serum transferrin saturation, and ferritin (Figure 84.3) Transferrin saturation is the proportion of the iron transport protein transferrin that is saturated with iron; it first rises in the setting of iron excess. Ferritin is an iron-storage protein produced by the liver that rises as iron accumulates in tissues. Ferritin levels >300 μg/L in men and >200 μg/L in women and/or a transferrin saturation of >45% are suggestive of the diagnosis [1]. The cutoff value of transferrin saturation >45% increases the sensitivity of the screening test, but has a positive predictive value (PPV) of only about 2% [12].

Ferritin levels >1000 μg/mL are associated with an increased risk of cirrhosis (prevalence 20–45%), while the prevalence of cirrhosis with a ferritin <1000 μg/mL is less than 2% [13, 14]. Both ferritin and transferrin saturation can be elevated in the setting of acute or chronic inflammation, so timing and interpretation of testing in these settings should be considered.

HFE gene testing is recommended for any clinical features suggesting iron overload, elevation of transferrin saturation or serum ferritin, and first-degree relatives of *C282Y* homozygotes [5]. Individuals found to have *C282Y/C282Y* or *C282Y/H63D* have hereditary hemochromatosis, but their degree of iron overload should

be assessed. If the ferritin is elevated but <1000 μg/mL and the transaminases are normal, patients may proceed directly to weekly phlebotomy therapy [1]. If the ferritin is >1000 μg/mL or the liver enzymes are elevated, liver biopsy is helpful in determining hepatic iron concentration (HIC) and degree of fibrosis [1].

Patients with serum markers of iron overload without the *C282Y/C282Y* or *C282Y/H63D* genotype should undergo liver biopsy for definitive diagnosis, staging of disease, and determination of HIC. The normal limit for HIC is 1400 μg/g dry weight, while >4000 μg/L is diagnostic of the hereditary hemochromatosis phenotype. The hepatic iron index (HII), calculated by dividing the HIC by patient age, was previously used to help differentiate homozygous hereditary hemochromatosis from other causes of iron overload (>1.9 μg/g/yr vs. <1.5 μg/g/yr), but *HFE* gene testing is far more accurate [15]. When liver biopsy is not possible, magnetic resonance imaging (MRI) can provide highly accurate information regarding tissue iron content [16] and/or the degree of liver fibrosis [17].

Differential Diagnosis

Hereditary iron overload needs to be differentiated from secondary iron overload. Secondary iron overload is seen in disorders of erythropoiesis, such as β-thalassemia, and chronic liver diseases, such as chronic viral hepatitis B and C and alcoholic and non-alcoholic fatty liver disease (NAFLD). Liver biopsy and genetic testing have made differentiation more straightforward [1]. Non-HFE

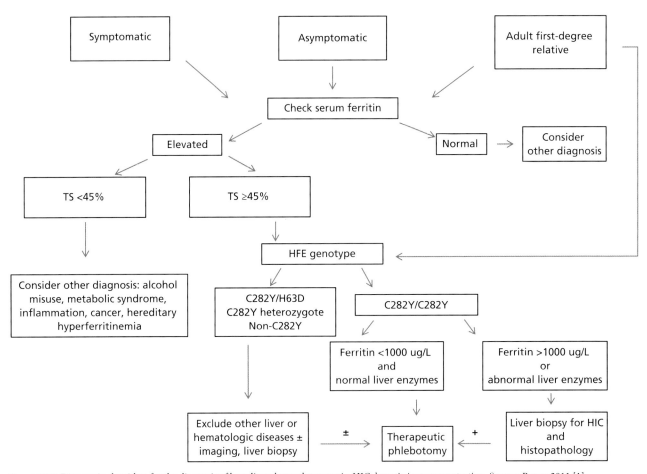

Figure 84.3 Diagnostic algorithm for the diagnosis of hereditary hemochromatosis. HIC, hepatic iron concentration. Source: Bacon 2011 [1].

hereditary hemochromatosis is also a rare possibility; it can be addressed with additional genetic testing [1].

Case Continued

Abdominal MRI shows diffuse hepatic fatty infiltration. Iron-sensitive MRI images showed mildly increased R2∗ values, corresponding to minimally increased levels of liver iron. Magnetic resonance elastography (MRE) confirms normal liver stiffness, making significant fibrosis highly unlikely. HFE testing reveals that the patient is homozygous for the *H63D* mutation. She is reassured that she has a minimal risk of developing iron-related liver disease. Weight reduction and optimization of diabetes are recommended.

Treatment

Phlebotomy remains the treatment of choice, despite the lack of placebo-controlled trials [1, 2]. A one-unit phlebotomy of 500 mL removes about 250 mg of iron. The phlebotomy requirement can be estimated from the HIC with the following equation [15]:

$$\text{Units of blood} = [(\text{HIC} - 1400)/100] \times 3.$$

Phlebotomy of 500 mL is initially performed once to twice weekly, as tolerated [1]. The serum hematocrit/hemoglobin is checked prior to each phlebotomy to allow no more than a 20% reduction in the initial value. The ferritin can be checked every 3 months during initial treatment. Phlebotomies are decreased in frequency once the ferritin level is in the normal range, and stopped once ferritin is between 50 and 100 µg/L. At that point, ferritin is checked every 2 months to gauge the rate of iron reaccumulation. This will guide maintenance phlebotomy, which is typically three to six times a year. Some patients may not reaccumulate significant iron for several years.

A trial of phlebotomy can confirm iron overload in cases where a liver biopsy is contraindicated or declined. Most individuals with normal or minimally increased amounts of tissue iron will become iron deficient after six or fewer phlebotomies [15]. If a patient can tolerate 20 phlebotomies (removal of 5 g iron) without becoming iron deficient, iron overload is confirmed.

Experimental Treatments

Deferasirox is an oral iron chelator with proven efficacy in secondary iron overload [18]. Ferritin decreased by 75% in a trial involving hereditary hemochromatosis patients, providing an alternative for patients who cannot tolerate phlebotomy due to anemia or severe heart disease. Adverse effects have included renal insufficiency, cytopenias, and elevated liver enzymes.

Erythrocytapheresis selectively removes red blood cells (RBCs) and returns plasma, allowing for greater iron removal than a standard phlebotomy session. A recent prospective trial of hereditary hemochromatosis patients showed that the target ferritin level of <50 µg/L was met with significantly fewer sessions than was standard phlebotomy (9 vs. 27, p <0.001), without a significant difference in cost [19].

Rationale

Treatment is indicated in patients with elevated ferritin levels (>300 µg/L in men and >200 µg/L in women). Patients with hereditary hemochromatosis without elevated ferritin do not require treatment and can have ferritin levels monitored annually [1].

Treatment initiated prior to end-organ damage leads to similar survival as the general population. Treatment has been shown to be of benefit even when initiated after the onset of symptoms. Fatigue, skin pigmentation, cardiomyopathy, abdominal pain, and mild hepatic fibrosis are typically improved with treatment; arthritis, diabetes, and cirrhosis are irreversible [1]. Iron depletion can improve hepatic fibrosis in 13–50% and reverse varices in close to 30% of patients [20], but patients with cirrhosis require continued HCC surveillance after de-ironing [1]. The risk of HCC in hereditary hemochromatosis cirrhotics is increased approximately 20-fold compared with the general population [21], and between 25 and 45% of premature deaths in patients with hereditary hemochromatosis are attributable to HCC [4]. The risk of HCC is greatest in men over 50 years of age. Liver transplantation is indicated for patients with hereditary hemochromatosis who develop decompensated cirrhosis or HCC [22]. Older studies show poor post-transplantation survival for patients with hereditary hemochromatosis, but a recent series suggests that the outcome may be improving, with better selection of patients and more aggressive de-ironing before transplantation [23].

Wilson's Disease

Wilson's disease is a rare (1 in 30 000 births) autosomal recessive disorder of copper transport that leads to pathologic accumulation of copper in the liver, cornea, and brain, causing hepatic, neurologic, and psychiatric disease [24–26]. The diagnosis is often difficult, and is made by a combination of clinical, laboratory, and histologic findings. Treatment with chelating agents or liver transplant has changed Wilson's disease from a universally fatal disease to one with a potentially normal life expectancy.

Pathogenesis

Wilson's disease is caused by a mutation in the *ATP7B* gene that encodes a membrane-bound copper transport protein on chromosome 13 [24–26]. This leads to (i) decreased biliary excretion of copper and (ii) decreased incorporation of copper into ceruloplasmin [24]. As bile is the only route for excess copper excretion, copper accumulates in the liver and causes acute and/or chronic liver injury. Serum ceruloplasmin is the major copper-carrying protein in the blood, accounting for 90% of circulating body copper [24]. Ceruloplasmin levels are decreased in Wilson's disease due to both decreased hepatic production and accelerated breakdown of apoceruloplasmin, the non-copper-containing form of the protein [24]. When the accumulation of copper exceeds the liver's capacity, the copper is released into the bloodstream and deposited in other organs, including the brain, kidneys, and cornea [24]. Ionic copper promotes the production of reactive oxygen species (ROS), which damage membranes – particularly the mitochondria [27].

Clinical Features

Wilson's disease typically presents at between 5 and 35 years of age, but it can present in those as young as 2 years and in those older than 70 years [24]. The severity of liver disease is quite variable at the time of diagnosis, ranging from subtle laboratory or imaging abnormalities to acute liver failure (ALF). ALF patients typically have an associated hemolytic anemia, coagulopathy unresponsive to vitamin K, and acute renal failure. Differentiating acute Wilson's disease from viral or drug-induced liver injury (DILI) is often difficult, but prompt diagnosis is critical, as mortality without liver transplant approaches 100%. AST and ALT are often modestly elevated in Wilson's disease, while alkaline phosphatase is normal or low. Many individuals remain asymptomatic while young and present later with complications of cirrhosis. Neurologic manifestations are more common as the age of presentation increases; symptoms range from subtle changes in behavior to severe extrapyramidal signs, including tremor, dysarthria, and spasticity [25]. Hemolytic anemia due to increased blood levels of ionic copper can occur either as a single acute episode or as a chronic condition [24].

Peripheral deposition of copper in Descemet's membrane of the cornea causes the characteristic gold–brown Kayser–Fleischer (KF) rings [21–26], usually requiring detection by slit-lamp examination. KF rings are present in 95% of patients with neurologic symptoms, but only 40–50% of all those presenting with liver disease [24]. KF rings are not specific for Wilson's disease, and have been found in a variety of cholestatic disorders.

Diagnosis

There are two diagnostic algorithms commonly utilized for the diagnosis of Wilson's disease. The one endorsed by the European Association for the Study of the Liver (EASL) uses a point system for laboratory/histologic findings, KF rings, neurologic symptoms, and hemolytic anemia [28]. The American Association for the Study of Liver Diseases (AASLD) algorithm begins with ceruloplasmin, KF rings, and urinary copper content, then progresses to a liver biopsy and genetic testing in selected patients [24]. Our recommended algorithm is given in Table 84.1.

Table 84.1 Diagnostic algorithm for patients with possible Wilson's disease.

Step	Test	Points	Total score	Interpretation
1	Serum ceruloplasmin: >30 mg/dL Normal 10–20 mg/dL <10 mg/dL	0 1 2 		**STOP:** diagnosis excluded **Step 2**
2	KF rings: Absent Present	0 2	≤ 3 ≥ 4	**Step 3** **STOP:** diagnosis established
3	Neurologic symptoms: points only if +KF rings Absent Mild Severe	0 1 2	≤ 3 ≥ 4	**Step 4** **STOP:** diagnosis established
4	Hemolytic anemia: Absent Present	0 1	≤ 3 ≥ 4	**Step 5** **STOP:** diagnosis established
5	Urinary Cu (in absence of acute hepatitis): Normal 1–2× ULN >2× ULN	0 1 2	0 1–3 ≥ 4	**STOP:** diagnosis unlikely **Step 6** **STOP:** diagnosis established
6	Liver Cu (in absence of cholestasis): Normal (<50 µg/g) Rhodanine + granules[a] 50–250 µg/g >5× ULN	−1 1 2	< 2 2–3 ≥ 4	**STOP:** diagnosis unlikely **Step 7** **STOP:** diagnosis established
7	Mutation analysis: No mutations detected Detected on 1 chromosome Detected on both chromosomes	0 1 4	≤2 =3 ≥4	**STOP:** diagnosis excluded **STOP:** diagnosis established

[a]Consider 24-hour urine Cu after penicillamine.
ULN, upper limit of normal.

Ceruloplasmin is the best initial screening test for Wilson's disease. Over 90% of Wilson's disease patients have low serum ceruloplasmin (<20 mg/dL). A ceruloplasmin <5 mg/dL is strong evidence of Wilson's disease; levels of 5–20 mg/dL are consistent with the diagnosis but require additional investigation, while a level >30 mg/dL virtually excludes the diagnosis. Ceruloplasmin can be elevated by acute inflammation, pregnancy, or estrogen therapy [24, 25, 29].

The diagnosis also requires demonstration of copper overload, so if KF rings are not present, an elevated 24-hour urinary copper excretion can be utilized; a level >100 µg/24 hours in symptomatic patients is usually diagnostic [24]. However, other chronic liver diseases may be associated with urinary copper excretion in this range. Results in the range 40–100 µg/24 hours are consistent with Wilson's disease but require additional testing.

The hepatic copper concentration measured in liver biopsy tissue remains the gold standard for demonstrating copper excess, but even this test can be limited by sampling error, given the marked variation in copper deposition in the cirrhotic liver [24, 25]. Values of ≥250 µg/g dry weight were present in over 90% of patients in a large retrospective series [30]. Hepatic copper levels of between 50 and 250 µg/g dry weight warrant additional testing, while a level <50 µg/g generally excludes the diagnosis. Steatosis (both micro- and macrovesicular), glycogenated hepatocyte nuclei, and hepatocyte necrosis are commonly present [25]. Cirrhosis is typically present by the 2nd decade of life and in most patients presenting with ALF.

There are two types of molecular genetic test available. Haplotype analysis of polymorphisms in genes flanking the *ATP7B* gene [24, 31] is of value in testing first-degree relatives once an index case has been clinically defined. This can identify which family members are homozygous or heterozygous [27]. Direct sequencing of the *ATP7B* gene itself can be also used to test first-degree relatives, in addition to confirming a primary diagnosis of Wilson's disease [24]. The patient's *ATP7B* gene is completely sequenced and compared with the wild type. The presence of mutations on both chromosomes is diagnostic, while a mutation on a single chromosome provides additional support for the diagnosis in the appropriate setting. The lack of mutations does not exclude the diagnosis, as more than 500 mutations have been identified thus far, and most patients are compound heterozygotes with different mutations on the two alleles [21].

Differential Diagnosis

Wilson's disease can mimic autoimmune hepatitis (AIH), with elevated immunoglobulins, anti-smooth-muscle antibody, and liver histology revealing severe piecemeal necrosis with a lymphocytic infiltrate. Therefore, Wilson's disease should be considered in patients diagnosed with AIH with an inadequate response to steroid therapy [24]. Significant steatosis with necrosis on biopsy can be misdiagnosed as fatty liver disease. Routine tests for the diagnosis of Wilson's disease are listed in Table 84.2.

Treatment

Approved medications for Wilson's disease include D-penicillamine, trientine, and zinc [24–26, 32] (Table 84.3). Trientine and penicillamine are chelating agents that promote the urinary excretion of copper, while zinc blocks copper absorption and promotes fecal excretion. Worsening of neurologic symptoms has been reported with all treatments, likely a result of mobilizing copper stores and elevating brain copper [33], but rates are highest

Table 84.2 Routine tests for the diagnosis of Wilson's disease, with common false results.

Test	Typical finding in Wilson's disease	False negative	False positive
Serum CPN	Decreased by 50% of LLN	Marked hepatic inflammation Pregnancy Estrogen therapy	Malabsorption Aceruloplasminemia Heterozygotes
24-hour urinary Cu	>100 μg	Incorrect collection Children without liver disease	Hepatocellular necrosis Cholestasis Contamination
Hepatic Cu	>250 μg/g	Regional variation in hepatic deposition	Cholestatic syndromes
KF rings	Present	Absent in: 50% of patients with *hepatic* Wilson's disease Most asymptomatic siblings	PBC

CPN, ceruloplasmin; LLN, lower limit of normal; KF ring, Kayser–Fleischer ring; PBC, primary biliary cirrhosis.

in those receiving *d*-penicillamine (10–20%). About 90% of patients with hepatic disease and 75% of those with neurologic symptoms will have improvement or stabilization in symptoms with treatment [25]. Clinical improvement, including reversal of hepatic synthetic dysfunction and jaundice, is typically seen by 6 months of treatment, but additional recovery can be seen for up to 1 year [24]. Patients who discontinue long-term medical therapy have a high likelihood of progression to acute hepatic decompensation or fulminant hepatic failure within 2–3 years [34]. Monitoring for medical compliance is critically important.

Trientine

Trientine is the preferred initial treatment for active Wilson's disease, because it is effective, has few side effects, and has a lower incidence of neurologic exacerbation than *d*-penicillamine [24]. Trientine is also a chelator of iron. The complex with iron is toxic, so iron supplementation should be avoided.

D-penicillamine

Though *d*-penicillamine is an effective anti-copper treatment, it has been largely replaced due to serious adverse effects in up to 30% of patients. Hypersensitivity reactions characterized by fever, lymphandenopathy, cytopenias, and proteinuria can occur in the first 1–3 weeks. Late reactions include nephrotoxicity (usually proteinuria) and lupus-like reactions or serious skin disorders [24].

Zinc

Zinc interferes with intestinal copper absorption by inducing enterocyte metallothionein, an endogenous chelator, and inhibiting the entry of copper into the portal circulation. It is used in initial and long-term treatment of presymptomatic patients, in maintenance, or in symptomatic patients when added to chelator therapy. Monotherapy with zinc is not advised in active liver disease, as it can induce hepatic decompensation in this settings [24, 32]. It has few side effects (mainly stomach irritation) and rarely causes neurologic deterioration.

Monitoring

Treatment with either chelating agent is monitored by measuring 24-hour urinary copper excretion. During the first phase of treatment, urinary copper excretion may be 1000–2000 μg/24 hours. Over a period of months, excretion declines as copper is removed, usually to 200–500 μg/24 hours. At this time, lowering the maintenance dose or transitioning to zinc is appropriate, with urinary monitoring every 6–12 months. Values <200 μg/24 hours can indicate non-compliance or excess copper removal. Non-adherence is supported by a serum non-ceruloplasmin-bound copper >15 μg/dL and overtreatment by a level <5 μg/dL. This value can be estimated using serum copper and ceruloplasmin. Gradual disappearance of KF rings would also confirm adequate treatment.

Therapeutic efficacy of zinc is monitored by ensuring that the urinary excretion of copper is <75 μg/day, while compliance is demonstrated by checking urinary zinc excretion.

Experimental Treatment

Ammonium tetrathiomolybdate is an experimental agent that complexes with copper either in the intestine, preventing absorption, or in the circulation, preventing cellular uptake and use [33]. In small trials, tetrathiomolybdate has been shown to control levels of free copper significantly better than trientrine, without worsening neurologic symptoms. This agent is not currently available in the United States.

Liver Transplantation

Liver transplantation is indicated for Wilson's disease patients with fulminant hepatic failure or decompensated chronic liver disease despite medical therapy [22]. There is a revised prognostic scoring system validated for children and adults with Wilson's disease presenting with ALF, which has a sensitivity, specificity, and PPV for determining the need for liver transplantation of 93, 98, and 88%, respectively [36]. Transplantation corrects the metabolic

Table 84.3 Drug treatment of Wilson's disease.

Drug	Dose	Use	Mechanism of action	Tests to monitor efficacy
Trienterine	Initial: 900–1200 mg/day, divided between 2 or 3 doses Maintenance: same	First-line therapy for active disease (+/− zinc) Side effects from *d*-penicillamine	Metal chelating agent with urinary copper excretion	Check at 1, 3, 6, 12, 18, and 24 months, then annually: 24-hour urine Cu (target 200–500 μg/day) Estimated non-ceruloplasmin- bound Cu (initial target <20 μg/dL then <10 μg/dL)
D- penicillamine (plus pyridoxine)	Initial: 1000–1500 mg/day, divided between 2–4 doses Maintenance: 750–1000 mg/day, divided between 2–4 doses	Active disease Largely replaced by trienterine, due to side effects	Metal chelating agent with urinary copper excretion	Same as trienterine
Zinc	Initial: 50 mg elemental zinc three times per day Maintenance: titrate according to efficacy monitoring	Presymptomatic Maintenance therapy	Inhibits intestinal absorption and increases fecal excretion of Cu	24-hour urine Cu (arget <75 μg/day) Estimated non-ceruloplasmin-bound Cu: <10 μg/dL

defect, and copper depletion treatment is not needed thereafter [22]. Neurologic symptoms may improve after liver transplantation, but this is unpredictable, and transplantation for neurologic indications remains controversial.

Alpha-1-Antitrypsin Deficiency

A1AT deficiency is an autosomal co-dominant disease that can lead to chronic liver disease with complications of cirrhosis and HCC in children and adults [37]. Over 100 different mutant alleles have been discovered, but mutation of the Z allele is typically associated with liver disease. ZZ allele homozygotes (PIZZ) occur in approximately 1 in 2000–5000 births in North American and Northern European populations [38]. The clinical presentation is quite variable in disease severity and patient age, a result of genetic and environmental disease modifiers. There is no treatment, except for liver transplantation in advanced liver disease.

Pathogenesis

A1AT is a protein that is produced in the liver and secreted into serum to inhibit neutrophil proteases. Liver disease results from accumulation of mutant protein in the hepatocytes, not from insufficient antiprotease function, as is the case in A1AT deficiency-associated lung disease [38, 39]. A portion of non-polymerized abnormal Z proteins are destroyed by a mechanism called endoplasmic reticulum (ER)-associated degradation. The remaining Z proteins spontaneously polymerize in the ER of the hepatocyte and cannot complete the secretory pathway [37]. The presence of these polymers can trigger cell death and lead to hepatic fibrosis and HCC. Polymerized Z proteins are more resistant to destruction than non-polymerized proteins [39], but a portion can be degraded by intracellular vacuoles in a process called autophagy. Individual variation in the efficiency of the destructive pathways may explain differences in clinical penetrance observed among ZZ homozygotes. The presence of two Z alleles is independently associated with liver disease, whereas one Z allele may increase the risk of developing liver disease from other causes [40].

Clinical Features

There is a bimodal age distribution of liver disease with A1AT deficiency. It is the most common hereditary liver disease in children, where it can present as neonatal hepatitis and cholestatic jaundice. About 80% of children with neonatal cholestasis will show no sign of chronic disease by age 18, and only 5% of patients presenting in childhood will develop life-threatening liver disease [39]. There is a second epidemiologic peak in adults, with a range in presentation from very mild and clinically insignificant disease to chronic hepatitis leading to cirrhosis and HCC [37]. A Swedish case–control study showed that adults who are homozygous for the Z allele have an 8-fold risk of developing cirrhosis and a 20-fold risk of developing HCC. Presence of the A1At heterozygote alone rarely causes liver disease. About 80–90% of adult heterozygotes with either cirrhosis or chronic hepatitis are found to have another cause of liver disease [41].

Diagnosis

Only the Z allele is associated with liver disease, so diagnosis requires determination of the serum electrophoretic A1AT phenotype, not the serum level. Liver biopsy tissue stained with periodic acid–Schiff (PAS) and treated with diastase shows the characteristic globular, red–purple intracellular inclusions, most commonly in periportal areas and at the periphery of regenerating nodules [37, 41].

Treatment

There are no specific therapies for A1AT-deficiency liver disease. Liver transplantation is indicated for those with decompensated cirrhosis or HCC. A1AT deficiency is the most common metabolic liver disease requiring transplantation in children [37]. Transplantation cures the metabolic defect: the A1AT phenotype becomes that of the donor, and liver disease does not recur [37]. Whether liver transplantation can prevent the onset or progression of lung disease is not clear [22].

Experimental Treatments

Gene therapy has been promising in mouse models, where mutant gene transcription or translation can be inhibited, while wild-type A1AT protein synthesis is generated with an exogenous mRNA [42]. There has been interest – but currently less success – in small molecules that may prevent abnormal folding of the Z protein to prevent polymerization, facilitate secretion, or promote degradation. Two medications, rapamycin and carbamazepine, have been studied in mouse models and shown to promote autophagic degradation, thereby decreasing intracellular accumulation of the abnormal protein and decreasing hepatic fibrosis [43, 44]. Enrollment for a human trial with carbamazepine is currently underway.

Take Home Points

- Hereditary hemochromatosis is most commonly caused by a deficiency or dysregulation of hepcidin, the liver-derived hormone that regulates the iron transporter ferroportin.
- Elevation of transferrin saturation or serum ferritin should be evaluated with *HFE* gene testing.
- The *C282Y/C282Y* genotype accounts for 80–90% of cases of hereditary hemochromatosis and the *C282Y/H63D* genotype for about 5%; non-HFE hemochromatosis is rare (10% of patients).
- Most cases of hereditary hemochromatosis are now discovered through laboratory testing prior to end-organ damage.
- Patients with hereditary hemochromatosis and serum ferritin >1000 ng/mL and/or elevated liver tests should undergo liver biopsy for staging.
- Phlebotomy is the best overall treatment, but oral chelation (deferasirox) is an alternative.
- Wilson's disease is caused by mutations affecting the copper transport protein ATP7B.
- Wilson's disease should be in the differential diagnosis of virtually every liver disease syndrome.
- The treatment of choice for Wilson's disease is now trientine and/or oral zinc.
- Alpha-1-antitrypsin (A1AT) deficiency can cause liver disease; partial deficiency can increase the risk of serious liver disease from other causes.
- Only the Z allele is associated with liver disease, so diagnosis requires determination of the A1AT phenotype, not the serum level.

References

1 Bacon BR, Adams PC, Kowdley KV, *et al.* Diagnosis and management of hemochromatosis: 2011 Practice Guideline by the American Association for the Study of Liver Diseases. *Hepatology* 2011; **54**: 328–43.

2 Adams PC, Barton JC. Haemochromatosis. *Lancet* 2007; **370**: 1855–60.

3 Pietrangelo A. Hereditary hemochromatosis: pathogenesis, diagnosis, and treatment. *Gastroenterology* 2010; **139**: 393–408.

4 Harrison SA, Bacon BR. Relation of hemochromatosis with hepatocellular carcinoma: epidemiology, natural history, pathophysiology, screening, treatment, and prevention. *Med Clin N Am* 2005; **89**: 391–409.

5 Olynyk JK, Trinder D, Ramm GA, *et al.* Hereditary hemochromatosis in the post-HFE era. *Hepatology* 2008; **48**: 991–1001.

6 Allen KJ, Gurrin LC, Constantine CC, *et al.* Iron-overload-related disease in HFE hereditary hemochromatosis. *N Engl J Med* 2008; **358**: 221–30.

7 Whitlock E, Garlitz B, Harris E, *et al.* Screening for hereditary hemochromatosis: a systematic review for the US Preventive Services Task Force. *Ann Intern Med* 2006; **145**: 209–23.

8 Nelson JE, Kowdley KV. Non-HFE hemochromatosis: genetics, pathogenesis, and clinical management. *Curr Gastroenterol Rep* 2005; **7**: 71–80.

9 Beutler E, Felitti V, Koziol J, *et al.* Penetrance of the 845 G to A (C282Y) HFE hereditary hemochromatosis mutation in the USA. *Lancet* 2002; **359**: 211–18.

10 Powell LW, Dixon JL, Ramm GA, *et al.* Screening for hemochromatosis in asymptomatic subjects with or without family history. *Arch Intern Med* 2006; **166**: 294–301.

11 Gleeson F, Ryan E, Barrett S, *et al.* Clinical expression of haemochromatosis in Irish C282Y homozygotes identified through family screening. *Eur J Gastroenterol Hepatol* 2004; **16**: 859–63.

12 Adams P, Zaccaro D, Moses G, *et al.* Comparison of the unsaturated iron binding capacity with transferrin saturation as a screening test to detect C282Y homozygotes for hemochromatosis in 101,168 participants in the HEIRS study. *Clin Chem* 2005; **51**: 1048–51.

13 Morrison ED, Brandhagen DJ, Phatak PD, *et al.* Serum ferritin level predicts advanced fibrosis amoing U.S. patients phenotypic hemochromatosis. *Ann Intern Med* 2003; **138**: 627–33.

14 Beaton M, Guyader D, Deugnier Y, *et al.* Noninvasive prediction of cirrhosis in C282Y-linked hemochromatosis. *Hepatology* 2002; **36**: 673–8.

15 Schrier SL, Bacon BR. Management of patients with hereditary hemochromatosis. UpToDate. Available from: http://www.uptodate.com/contents/management-of-patients-with-hereditary-hemochromatosis?source=related_link#H1 (last accessed February 15, 2016).

16 Gandon Y, Olivie D, Guyader D, *et al.* Non-invasive assessment of hepatic iron stores by MRI. *Lancet* 2004; **363**: 357–62.

17 Talwalkar JA. MR elastography for detecting hepatic fibrosis: options and considerations. *Gastroenterology* 2008; **135**: 299–302.

18 Rombout-Sestrienkona E, Neiman FH, Essers BA *et al.* Therapeutic erythrocytapheresis versus phlebotomy in the initial treatment of HFE hemochromatosis patients: results from a randomized trial. *Transfusion* 2012; **52**(3): 470–7.

19 Falize L, Guillygomarch A, Perrin M, *et al.* Reversibility of hepatic fibrosis in treated genetic hemochromatosis: a study of 36 cases. *Hepatology* 2006; **44**: 472–7.

20 Barton JC. Chelation therapy of iron overload. *Curr Gastroenterol Rep* 2007; **9**: 74–82.

21 Elmberg M, Hultcrantz R, Ekbom A, *et al.* Cancer risk in patients with hereditary hemochromatosis and in their first-degree relatives. *Gastroenterology* 2003; **125**(6): 1733.

22 Zhang KY, Tung BY, Kowdley KV. Liver transplantation for metabolic liver diseases. *Clin Liver Dis* 2007; **11**: 265–81.

23 Dar FS, Faraj W, Zaman MB, *et al.* Outcome of liver transplantation in hereditary hemochromatosis. *Transpl Int* 2009; **22**: 717–24.

24 Roberts EA, Schilsky ML. Diagnosis and treatment of Wilson disease: an update. *Hepatology* 2008; **47**: 2089–111.

25 Ala A, Walker AP, Ashkan K, *et al.* Wilson's disease. *Lancet* 2007; **369**: 397–408.

26 Ferenci P, Czlonkowska A, Stremmel W, *et al.* EASL Clinical Practice Guidelines. *J Hepatol* 2012; **56**: 671–85.

27 Ferenci P. Wilson's disease. *Clin Gastroenterol Hepatol* 2005; **3**: 726–33.

28 Ferenci P, Caca K, Loudianos G, *et al.* Diagnosis and phenotypic classification of Wilson disease. *Liver Int* 2003; **23**: 139–42.

29 Scheinberg IH, Sternlieb I. *Wilson's Disease. Major Problems in Internal Medicine*, Vol. XXIII. Philadelphia, PA: W.B. Saunders, 1984.

30 Merle U, Schaefer M, Ferenci P, Stremmel W. Clinical presentation, diagnosis and long-term outcome of Wilson's disease: a cohort study. *Gut* 2007; **56**: 115–20.

31 Thomas GR, Roberts EA, Walshe JM, Cox DW. Haplotypes and mutations in Wilson disease. *Am J Hum Genet* 1995; **56**: 1315–19.

32 Brewer GJ, Askari FK. Wilson's disease: clinical management and therapy. *J Hepatol* 2005; **42**: S13–21.

33 Brewer GJ, Askari F, Dick RB. Treatment of Wilson's disease with tetrathiomolybdate: V. Control of free copper by tetrathiomolybdate and a comparison with trientine. *Transl Res* 2009; **154**: 70–7.

34 Scheinberg IH, Jaffe ME, Sternlieb I. The use of trientine in preventing the effects of interrupting penicillamine therapy in Wilson's disease. *N Engl J Med* 1987; **317**: 209–13.

35 Brewer GJ, Dick RD, Johnson VD, *et al.* Treatment of Wilson's disease with zinc: XV. Long-term follow-up studies. *J Lab Clin Med* 1998; **132**: 264–78.

36 Dhawan A, Taylor RM, Cheeseman P, *et al.* Wilson's disease in children: 37-year experience and revised King's score for liver transplantation. *Liver Transpl* 2005; **11**(4): 441–8.

37 Fairbanks KD, Tavill AS. Liver disease in alpha 1-antitrypsin deficiency: a review. *Am J Gastroenterol* 2008; **103**: 2136–41.

38 Teckman JH, Jain A. Advances in alpha-1-antitrypsin deficiency liver disease. *Curr Gastroenterol Rep* 2014; **16**(1): 367.

39 Teckman JH. Liver disease in alpha-1-antitrypsin deficiency: current understanding and future directions. *COPD* 2013; **10**: 35–43.

40 Fink S, Schilsky ML. Inherited metabolic disease of the liver. *Curr Opin Gastroenterol* 2007; **23**: 237–43.

41 Gross JB. Metabolic diseases of the liver. In: Shearman DJC, Finlayson NDC, Camilleri M, eds. *Diseases of the Gastrointestinal Tract and Liver*. New York, NY: Churchill Livingstone, 1997: 951–85.

42 Mueller C, Tang Q, Gruntman A, *et al.* Sustained miRNA-mediated knockdown of mutant AAT with simultaneous augmentation of wild-type AAT has minimal effect on global liver miRNA profiles. *Mol Ther* 2012; **20**(3): 590–600.

43 Hidvegi T, Ewing M, Hale P, *et al.* An autophagy-enhancing drug promotes degradation of mutant alpha-1-antitrypsin Z and reduces hepatic fibrosis. *Science* 2010; **329**: 229–32.

44 Kaushal S, Annamali M, Blomenkamp K, *et al.* Rapamycin reduces intrahepatic alpha-1-antitrypsin mutant Z protein polymers and liver injury in a mouse model. *Exp Biol Med* 2010; **235**: 700–9.

CHAPTER 84

CHAPTER 85

Hepatic Manifestations of Systemic Diseases

Stephen Crane Hauser

Division of Gastroenterology and Hepatology, Mayo Clinic, Rochester, MN, USA

Summary

A wide variety of systemic diseases can affect the liver and biliary system. Many of these disorders, such as systemic congestive heart failure (CHF) and rheumatologic disorders, commonly alter liver function tests (LFTs) but rarely result in liver disease.

Cardiovascular Disorders

The liver receives nearly 30% of the total cardiac output, 65–75% via the portal venous system and 25–35% via the hepatic arterial system. More than half the oxygen supply to the liver is delivered by hepatic arterial blood. The hepatic artery also supplies the gallbladder and bile ducts. Thus, any process that substantially reduces arterial bloodflow or arterial oxygen content to the liver can result in ischemic hepatitis. The most common cardiac disorders responsible for ischemic hepatitis are acute myocardial infarction and arrhythmias. Valvular heart disease, cardiomyopathy, and pericardial tamponade (constrictive pericarditis) can also result in arterial hypotension complicated by ischemic hepatitis. Non-cardiac conditions, such as sepsis, burns, trauma, dehydration, heat stroke, hemorrhage, and peritonitis, can also cause hypotensive ischemic hepatitis. Postoperative ischemic hepatitis may occur secondary to transient perioperative ischemia, hypoxia, and other factors. Hypoxia from acute respiratory failure, pulmonary embolus, and obstructive sleep apnea can likewise result in ischemic hepatitis. Altered (diminished) portal venous bloodflow, such as portal hypertension in patients with cirrhosis, increases susceptibility to ischemic hepatitis during episodes of arterial hypotension or hypoxia. Furthermore, altered (diminished) hepatic venous outflow (i.e., CHF, Budd–Chiari syndrome) and biliary obstruction also increase an individual's risk for ischemic hepatitis with hypotension or hypoxia.

Ischemic hepatitis is usually secondary to an acute event, which may or may not be evident. By definition, ongoing hypotension, or shock, would result in multiple end-organ failure or death. Patients who recover from acute ischemia subsequently may be asymptomatic or may develop right upper quadrant pain, nausea, and vomiting. Many patients are severely ill from other consequences of hypotension or hypoxia, including, in particular, renal failure. Typically, there is a rapid rise in serum aminotransferases within 24–48 hours of the ischemic event, often to several thousand international

units per liter, with a rapid decline (40–60% per 24 hours) over the next 3–7 days back toward baseline or normal. This aminotransferase pattern can also be seen in people with acute choledocholithiasis, but the maximal levels of alanine transaminase (ALT) and aspartate transaminase (AST) more often peak in the hundreds or low thousands. Serum lactate dehydrogenase (LDH) is also elevated, often to levels greater than those of ALT. Serum bilirubin, alkaline phosphatase, and International Normalized Ratio (INR) may be modestly elevated. Mental status changes may occur, but these are due to cerebral hypotension and not hepatic encephalopathy. Liver biopsy, generally not needed to make the diagnosis, demonstrates centrilobular zone 3 necrosis and congestion with sinusoidal dilatation, rupture, and extravasation of red blood cells (RBCs). Significant inflammation and fibrosis are not present. Fulminant liver failure is rare, often fatal, and usually occurs in patients with concomitant cirrhosis or chronic CHF complicated by acute ischemic hepatitis. Prognosis is related to recovery from the acute event, with restoration of arterial blood pressure and oxygenation. There is no specific therapy for the ischemic hepatitis itself. Elective surgery and anesthesia should be avoided during episodes of ischemic hepatitis.

Congestive hepatopathy, in contrast to ischemic hepatitis, is caused by elevated right atrial pressure resulting in passive venous outflow congestion of the liver. In adults, congestive hepatopathy is one of the most common causes of mild abnormal results of liver tests. The most common cardiac causes for this condition are ischemic cardiovascular disease (CVD) and hypertensive heart disease. Valvular heart disease, cor pulmonale, and constrictive pericarditis are also commonly complicated by congestive hepatopathy. Patients may be asymptomatic or may suffer from right upper quadrant pain (hepatomegaly with stretching of the capsule), anorexia, nausea, vomiting, or diarrhea. Hepatomegaly is common (around 95%) on physical exam, along with jugular venous distension, hepatojugular reflux, splenomegaly, pleural effusion, ascites, and lower-extremity edema. Mild unconjugated hyperbilirubinemia, mild increased transaminases, mild elevation of INR, and, less often, a mild increase in alkaline phosphatase and a mild decrease in serum albumin may be seen. In patients with ascites, the serum-to-ascites albumin gradient is greater than 1.1, and the ascitic fluid protein is high (>2.5 g/dL). Histology demonstrates the classic nutmeg liver, with centrilobular zone 3 necrosis, congestion, and

Practical Gastroenterology and Hepatology Board Review Toolkit, Second Edition. Edited by Nicholas J. Talley, Kenneth R. DeVault, Michael B. Wallace, Bashar A. Aqel and Keith D. Lindor.
© 2016 John Wiley & Sons, Ltd. Published 2016 by John Wiley & Sons, Ltd. Companion website: www.practicalgastrohep.com

hemorrhage. Because this condition is often chronic, central vein fibrosis (phlebosclerosis) with extension of fibrosis into the sinusoids can occur, rarely resulting in cardiac cirrhosis. When seen, this is often secondary to chronic constrictive pericarditis or valvular heart disease (especially mitral valve disease with severe secondary tricuspid regurgitation). Zone 1 non-cirrhotic regenerative nodular hyperplasia may also be found. Even with cirrhosis, esophageal varices and other stigmata of chronic liver disease are rarely found, and the prognosis is directly related to the cardiac condition. Metabolism of certain medications, such as warfarin, may be significantly diminished in patients with congestive hepatopathy. Treatment of the underlying cardiac condition determines the prognosis.

Vascular disorders affecting the hepatic artery, portal vein, or hepatic veins can affect the liver. Hepatic infarction can occur when hepatic arterial bloodflow is compromised due to conditions acutely affecting the hepatic artery or its branches. Hepatic artery thrombosis can occur as a complication of liver transplantation, hepatobiliary surgery, aortic or hepatic artery aneurysm, intra-arterial chemotherapy and chemoembolization, radiofrequency ablation of hepatocellular carcinoma (HCC), infective endocarditis, trauma, or transjugular intrahepatic portosystemic shunt. Hypercoagulable states, vasculitis (especially polyarteritis nodosa and systemic lupus erythematosus (SLE)), tumor emboli, sickle cell crisis, toxemia of pregnancy, and cocaine use are other risk factors for hepatic infarction. Ischemic damage to the biliary system can also occur, with biliary sepsis. The most severe cases can be complicated by fulminant liver failure. Mild cases may be asymptomatic, with transient elevations in serum aminotransferase levels. Symptomatic patients may complain of nausea, vomiting, right upper quadrant pain, and fever. Serum leukocytosis and abdominal radiographic studies help make the diagnosis. Sepsis, liver abscess formation, and bile duct strictures may occur. Treatment is directed toward the underlying cause and complications.

Portal vein thrombosis as a consequence of hypercoagulable states, intra-abdominal inflammation (pancreatitis, cholecystitis, appendicitis, inflammatory bowel disease (IBD)), infection (pylephlebitis, omphalitis in children), trauma (including surgery), and stasis (cirrhosis) often results in portal hypertension, splenomegaly, and variceal bleeding. Combinations of these risk factors, especially more than one hypercoagulable state or cirrhosis plus a hypercoagulable state, greatly increase the risk of portal vein thrombosis. Hepatic encephalopathy and clinically significant ascites are much less common than cirrhosis. Uncommonly, portal biliopathy with strictures, cholangitis, and cholecystitis may occur. Extension of the thrombotic process into the superior mesenteric venous system can result in mesenteric ischemia. Hepatic artery–portal vein fistulas as a result of trauma (i.e., liver biopsy) or in patients with Osler–Weber–Rendu syndrome can cause complicated portal hypertension, biliary strictures, and hepatobiliary infection, as well as cardiac failure. Patients with Osler–Weber–Rendu syndrome also can develop hepatic artery–hepatic vein fistulas complicated by cardiac failure and portal vein–hepatic vein fistulas complicated by hepatic encephalopathy.

Disorders of hepatic venous outflow such as Budd–Chiari syndrome (secondary to hypercoagulable states, malignancies, space-occupying lesions of the liver, infections, and miscellaneous causes), membranous webs occluding the suprahepatic inferior vena cava, and sinusoidal obstruction syndrome (due to preconditioning for bone marrow transplantation, plant pyrrolizidine alkaloid poisoning, hepatic radiation, or certain medications, such as azathioprine) can result in pressure-induced hepatic necrosis and cirrhosis.

Pulmonary Disorders

Hypoxia from respiratory failure of any cause can result in ischemic hepatitis. Obstructive sleep apnea and pulmonary embolus can also be complicated by ischemic hepatitis due to hypoxia, as well as cardiac dysfunction. Alpha-1-antitrypsin (A1AT) deficiency due to the inability of the liver to export an abnormal gene product (usually the ZZ protease inhibitor type, often but not always with low serum A1AT levels) can present in the neonate (about 10%) as hepatitis or cholestasis, both of which often resolve. Later in life, it can present as chronic hepatitis, cirrhosis, cholangiocarcinoma, or HCC [1]. Liver biopsy should demonstrate portal and periportal diastase-resistant periodic acid–Schiff (PAS)-positive inclusion bodies. Interestingly, only about 10–15% of people with the ZZ protease inhibitor type develop clinically significant liver disease. Some patients, especially children, may require liver transplantation. Though serum A1AT levels normalize, it is unclear whether this benefits pulmonary disease. Up to 30% of those with cystic fibrosis develop liver disease, which can be severe in up to 5% of cases [2]. Many, however, are asymptomatic with hepatomegaly or elevated LFTs. Some patients have hepatic steatosis due to their cystic fibrosis, as well as malnutrition and other factors. Neonatal hepatitis, neonatal cholestasis, and biliary cirrhosis in childhood and early adulthood secondary to inspissated material in the small bile ducts may occur. A focal biliary cirrhosis is typical, which can progress to a generalized cirrhosis with complicated portal hypertension. This often happens before puberty. Liver biopsy can demonstrate steatosis, dilated cholangioles filled with inspissated material, and fibrosis, even in asymptomatic patients. Ultrasound, magnetic resonance cholangiography, and endoscopic retrograde cholangiopancreatography (ERCP) may help make the diagnosis. Patients with cystic fibrosis may also develop gallstones (≤12%) and nodular regenerative hyperplasia.

Renal Disorders

Autosomal dominant polycystic kidney disease (ADPKD) is associated with numerous fibrocystic disorders of the liver, including congenital hepatic fibrosis, Caroli's disease, choledochal cysts, and, more often, polycystic liver disease. Pregnancy and administration of estrogen can hasten liver cyst growth in women with ADPKD. The less common autosomal recessive polycystic kidney disease (ARPKD) can also be associated with congenital hepatic fibrosis, Caroli's disease, choledochal cysts, and cholangiocarcinoma. There are rare reports of bladder infections with urease-producing *Proteus* or *Escherichia coli* infections resulting in hyperammonemia and encephalopathy, mimicking hepatic encephalopathy in people without liver disease or portal hypertension. Stauffer's syndrome or paraneoplastic intrahepatic cholestasis with jaundice and without hepatic involvement can be seen in patients with renal cell carcinoma (RCC).

Endocrine Disorders

The liver plays a central role in the metabolism of hormones, including thyroid and adrenal hormones. Mild abnormalities of liver tests are common in patient with hyperthyroidism, especially elevated serum alkaline phosphatase and aminotransferase levels. More than mild abnormalities and even severe jaundice can be seen in people with thyroid storm [3]. Increased hepatic oxygen consumption and CHF may account for centrilobular findings of necrosis or cholestasis on liver histopathology. Hyperthyroidism (usually Graves' disease) is associated with primary biliary cirrhosis (PBC) and autoimmune hepatitis (AIH). People with hypothyroidism often have mild hepatomegaly and mild abnormalities of LFTs, especially elevated serum transaminases. Fatty liver secondary to altered lipid metabolism, mild CHF, and myopathy (creatine kinase elevation greater than AST and greater than ALT) may cause these biochemical abnormalities. Cholestasis and jaundice may be found in more severe hypothyroidism. Protein-rich ascites (>4 g/dL) can occur in the absence of liver disease, probably due to altered permeability of the peritoneum or CHF [4]. Liver histopathology may reveal centrilobular congestion and, rarely, fibrosis. Chronic autoimmune thyroiditis is associated with PBC and AIH. Hypoparathyroidism can also be associated with AIH.

Cushing's disease, due to its association with obesity, can be complicated by fatty liver or steatohepatitis, with mild elevation of LFTs, especially serum aminotransferases. Addison's disease can present with mild elevation of serum aminotransferases. Hepatomegaly may be detected in patients with acromegaly. Diabetes mellitus, especially type 2 diabetes with insulin resistance, is increasingly found (along with obesity and hyperlipidemia) as a cause of non-alcoholic fatty liver disease (NAFLD), including fatty liver, steatohepatitis, and cirrhosis. Asymptomatic elevations in serum aminotransferases and mild elevations in serum alkaline phosphatase are common in diabetic patients with NAFLD.

Rheumatologic Disorders

Many rheumatologic diseases are complicated by or associated with liver disease. In many cases, the systemic inflammation of active rheumatologic disorders is accompanied by mild, non-specific liver test abnormalities that resolve as the joint and systemic diseases resolve. Liver biopsy findings in these patients are mild and non-specific. Medications used to treat rheumatologic diseases by themselves often result in mild elevation of liver tests (i.e., non-steroidal anti-inflammatory drugs, NSAIDs). Patients with active rheumatoid arthritis (RA) often develop mild elevation of serum alkaline phosphatase and serum aminotransferases, and may have mild hepatomegaly. Liver biopsy usually demonstrates minor non-specific findings or steatosis. AIH and PBC are found in some RA patients. Nodular regenerative hyperplasia can also be seen in these patients, but is more commonly seen in the subset of more ill RA patients with Felty's syndrome (severe seropositive RA, neutropenia, and splenomegaly). Portal hypertension often occurs with complications – especially variceal bleeding – secondary to nodular regenerative hyperplasia, as well as splenomegaly. Secondary amyloidosis can be found in patients with either RA or Felty's syndrome. As in RA, patients with active SLE often develop mild aminotransferase elevation. Liver disease is rare in these patients, with the exceptions of associated AIH, PBC, and nodular regenerative hyperplasia, as well as antiphospholipid syndrome in SLE patients [5]. These patients may have anticardiolipin antibodies or lupus anticoagulant, and develop arterial vasculitis with thrombosis, resulting in hepatic infarction or Budd–Chiari syndrome, as well as portal vein thrombosis, sinusoidal obstruction syndrome, nodular regenerative hyperplasia, AIH, and pregnancy-associated HELLP syndrome (hemolysis, elevated liver enzymes, low platelet count). Active adult

Still's disease patients may have mild to moderate elevation in serum transaminases and, in rare cases, liver failure. Polymyalgia rheumatica is associated with PBC and nodular regenerative hyperplasia. Sjögren's syndrome is not infrequently associated with AIH and PBC. Scleroderma is rarely complicated by liver disease, but is associated with AIH, primary biliary hepatitis, and nodular regenerative hyperplasia. The CREST syndrome is also associated with PBC and nodular regenerative hyperplasia. Liver disease is rarely seen in patients with mixed connective-tissue disease, but there are reports of Budd–Chiari syndrome. Polymyositis/dermatomyositis is associated with PBC.

Vasculitis in disorders such as Behçet's syndrome is often associated with nodular regenerative hyperplasia. Patients with Behçet's syndrome can develop Budd–Chiari syndrome as well. Vasculitis due to polyarteritis nodosa, whether associated with hepatitis B virus infection (<10%) or not, can be complicated by liver infarction, nodular regenerative hyperplasia, biliary strictures, or acalculous cholecystitis [6]. A host of other conditions with vascular involvement, such as Churg–Straus syndrome, temporal arteritis, Takayasu arteritis, and SLE, can result in liver infarction, gallbladder necrosis, and biliary disease. The antiphospholipid syndrome, which may or may not be associated with SLE, is a hypercoagulable disorder resulting in arterial or venous thrombosis, including portal vein thrombosis and Budd–Chiari syndrome. Henoch–Schonlein purpura is a vasculitic syndrome that can involve the gallbladder, with acute acalculous cholecystitis, and the bile ducts, with ischemic necrosis and bile duct strictures.

Gastroenterologic Disorders

Celiac disease is often associated with liver disease and, in most cases, elevated LFTs [7]. Nearly half of all patients with celiac disease will have mild to moderate aminotransferase elevations. Liver biopsy in these patients usually demonstrates non-specific changes. Fatty liver may be found, but it is not clear if this is related to the elevated aminotransferases or a coincidental association. Treatment of these patients with a gluten-free diet usually results in normalization of the aminotransferases. It is useful to know that up to 9% of people with otherwise unexplained elevated aminotransferases are found to have celiac disease. Patients with celiac disease are more likely to have PBC, as well as primary sclerosing cholangitis (PSC), AIH, and nodular regenerative hyperplasia. Rare patients with celiac disease can present with severe liver disease; they may improve with institution of a gluten-free diet.

Liver disease is commonly associated with IBD. Nearly 80% of all patients with PSC have ulcerative colitis (most of the group) or colonic Crohn's disease (far fewer). Between 2 and 7% of ulcerative colitis patients develop PSC. As in celiac disease, patients with active IBD often have mild elevated aminotransferases, which may normalize with resolution of active bowel inflammation. Fatty liver, AIH, PBC, cholelithiasis (usually in patients with Crohn's disease or resection of the terminal ileum), secondary amyloidosis (more often in Crohn's disease than ulcerative colitis), and Budd–Chiari syndrome or portal vein thrombosis (hypercoagulable state) can occur in these patients. Cholangiocarcinoma complicates PSC in patients with IBD more often than in those with PSC alone.

Liver disease is rare in patients with Whipple's disease. Mild liver test abnormalities, upper abdominal pain, and hepatomegaly may be found. Liver biopsy may reveal PAS-positive macrophages and granulomas.

Hematologic Disorders

Liver involvement is common in people with hemolytic anemias. In those with sickle cell anemia, erythrocytes can sickle within the sinusoids, resulting in Kupffer cell erythrophagocytosis, dilated sinusoids, and eventually hepatic fibrosis and cirrhosis in some. Concomitant iron loading, viral hepatitis, and medications can contribute to the liver injury. Painful, thrombotic veno-occlusive crises are often accompanied by fever, hepatomegaly, and moderate elevations of serum aminotransferases and bilirubin. In a small percentage of these cases, the crisis persists and worsens with aminotransferases over 1000 IU/L and bilirubin over 15 g/dL, with hepatic infarction, liver failure coagulopathy, encephalopathy, and other end-organ failure (i.e., renal failure). In some instances, severe degrees of hepatic sequestration result in severe painful hepatomegaly and a dramatic fall in the hematocrit. People with sickle cell anemia and other hemolytic anemias also are at risk for cholelithiasis, cholecystitis, and cholangitis. Patients may also develop liver abscesses, with an increased risk of Yersinia enterocolitica infection due to iron overload. Asymptomatic patients with sickle cell anemia may have mild elevations of serum transaminases for multiple reasons, including hepatic sickling, CHF, hypoxia, medications, and viral hepatitis. Patients with hemolysis and anemia due to paroxysmal nocturnal hemoglobinuria are at risk for venous and arterial thrombosis, including Budd–Chiari syndrome, portal vein thrombosis, and splenic vein thrombosis.

Leukemias and lymphomas commonly involve the liver, with or without symptoms. Infiltration of the liver occurs in up to 50% of patients with Hodgkin's disease. Virtually all of these patients also have splenic involvement. Mild to moderate elevations of serum alkaline phosphatase and aminotransferases are more common in more advanced stages of Hodgkin's disease. Portal tract infiltration with a non-specific infiltrate is often found on liver biopsy. Reed–Sternberg cells are seen in up to 8% of cases. Surgical or laparoscopic liver biopsies are more likely to make the diagnosis than are percutaneous biopsies. Patients can develop extrahepatic obstruction due to extrahepatic bile duct involvement or secondary to infiltration of porta hepatis lymph nodes. Intrahepatic cholestasis without hepatobiliary involvement (Stauffer's syndrome) may be caused by a metabolic or paraneoplastic phenomenon or vanishing bile duct syndrome, and may improve with successful treatment of the Hodgkin's disease outside of the hepatobiliary system. Non-Hodgkin's lymphoma, like Hodgkin's disease, can be found in the liver in up to 50% of patients. Compared to primary hepatic lymphoma, secondary involvement is detectable far less often, as a mass lesion on imaging studies. Mild to moderate elevation of alkaline phosphatase and aminotransferases is not unusual. Less common presentations include extrahepatic obstruction secondary to porta hepatis nodal involvement and acute liver failure (ALF) due to diffuse hepatic infiltration. Multiple myeloma and Waldenström's macroglobulinemia can also involve the liver and spleen, with abnormal LFTs. Some of these patients develop portal hypertension with ascites and varices. Extramedullary hematopoiesis can contribute to the portal hypertension. Liver biopsy may reveal malignant infiltration of the sinusoids and portal tracts. Nearly 10% of patients with multiple myeloma also develop amyloidosis.

The majority of patients with acute leukemia have involvement of the liver. Hepatomegaly, splenomegaly, and portal hypertension are common. ALF can be a presentation of extensive hepatic infiltration. Bone marrow transplantation can be complicated by sinusoidal obstruction syndrome, graft-versus-host disease (GVHD), and numerous systemic infections that can affect the liver. Chronic leukemias also commonly involve the liver. Patients with chronic lymphocytic leukemia can develop extrahepatic obstruction due to portal hepatitis nodal involvement.

Myeloproliferative syndromes can be complicated by portal hypertension due to extramedullary hematopoiesis, as well as splenomegaly and increased portal bloodflow. Portal vein thrombosis and Budd–Chiari syndrome are often caused by myeloproliferative syndromes, which can be difficult to diagnose in their early stages in some patients. Testing for the *JAK2 V617F* mutation may help diagnose the myeloproliferative syndrome. Nodular regenerative hyperplasia can complicate many of these conditions, including myeloproliferative syndromes, Hodgkin's disease, non-Hodgkin's lymphoma, and systemic mastocytosis, all of which can infiltrate the liver.

Infiltrative Systemic Disorders

Sarcoidosis is a systemic granulomatous disorder which in the United States is much more common in African Americans than in Caucasians. By definition, multiple organ systems are involved. Pathologic involvement of the liver is frequent, occurring in over two-thirds of patients. This includes non-caseating granulomas, especially in the portal and periportal areas. Most patients are asymptomatic, with hepatomegaly in about 25% on physical examination. A similar percentage of patients will be found to have a mildly elevated serum alkaline phosphatase level and, in some cases, mildly elevated transaminases. Rarely, patients with sarcoidosis can develop cholestatic jaundice, which can be intrahepatic (with loss of intralobular bile ducts, fibrosis, and cirrhosis, in a pattern similar to PBC) or extrahepatic (with cholangiographic features similar to PSC or secondary to hilar lymphadenopathy) [8]. Granulomatous obliteration of the hepatic veins (Budd–Chiari syndrome) and involvement of the portal vein branches have been described. Portal hypertension can be multifactorial, with prehepatic (portal venous disease, nodular regenerative hyperplasia) or hepatic (cirrhosis) causes. Symptomatic cholestasis may benefit from administration of ursodeoxycholic acid. Clinically significant hepatic sarcoidosis can occur without respiratory involvement. Corticosteroid or other immunosuppressive therapy may or may not benefit those with diverse causes of cholestatic jaundice. Some may require liver transplantation [9]. Post-transplant recurrence of sarcoidosis has been reported. More controversial is the entity of isolated hepatic sarcoidosis, which occurs without involvement of other organs, unlike idiopathic granulomatous hepatitis. These patients present with fever, weight loss, and severe cholestasis (elevated alkaline phosphatase), without jaundice or complications of liver disease. Thorough evaluation to exclude other causes of granulomatous involvement of the liver (especially tuberculosis), other infections, and adverse drug reactions (ADRs) is important.

Amyloidosis is a systemic condition which, when present, usually involves the liver histologically, but causes symptoms related to the liver very infrequently. Primary amyloidosis secondary to immunoglobulin light chain or light-chain fragment deposition (AL amyloid) in the liver and other organs occurs in patients with plasma cell dyscrasias such as multiple myeloma, Waldenström's macroglobulinemia, and some B-cell malignancies. Secondary amyloidosis due to serum amyloid disposition (AA amyloid) is seen in patients with chronic inflammatory and infectious disorders, such as RA, juvenile RA, cystic fibrosis, ankylosing spondylitis, bronchiectasis, tuberculosis, familial Mediterranean fever, osteomyelitis, systemic vasculitis, and Crohn's disease. It has also been described in Hodgkin's disease, gastric cancer, and hypernephroma. The relative organ distributions and histologic patterns in the liver of primary and secondary amyloidosis overlap greatly. Hepatomegaly may occur in up to 80% of these patients, often with elevated serum alkaline phosphatase and, less often, with elevated transaminases or bilirubin. Liver biopsy, even without abnormal liver tests, usually demonstrates amyloid protein deposition in the parenchyma (sinusoidal and perisinusoidal) or in a vascular pattern (blood vessels and periportal). Immunohistochemistry and mass spectroscopy are available to diagnose different types of amyloid. There have been reports of hemorrhage and even hepatic rupture after liver biopsy in patients with systemic amyloidosis. Some patients with amyloid will have a coagulopathy. Because amyloidosis involves multiple organs, abdominal fat-pad biopsy, rectal biopsy, or duodenal biopsy (highest yield) usually makes the diagnosis. Morbidity and mortality due to amyloidosis are usually related to nonhepatic involvement. Complications of chronic liver disease, such as portal hypertension, are rare. Besides primary and secondary, other types of amyloidosis include familial amyloidosis. ATTR or type I familial amyloidosis results in systemic disease due to deposition of a liver-produced mutant transthyretin protein (prealbumin). Liver transplantation is useful in ATTR familial amyloidosis patients prior to the occurrence of advanced disease of other organs, especially neurologic dysfunction. Often, the native liver can then be transplanted into an older recipient, as systemic disease due to the transplanted liver's production of mutant transthyretin takes many years to develop.

Miscellaneous Disorders

LFT abnormalities are common in people with systemic infections [10]. A wide spectrum of extrahepatic, extrabiliary infections with diverse bacteria, fungi, and other infectious organisms release endotoxins and other bacterial cell-wall compounds that enhance the release of inflammatory cytokines. These compounds can then decrease basolateral and canalicular bile acid and organic anion transport, with mild to modest elevations in serum aminotransferases and serum alkaline phosphatase. Mild to moderate to severe (≤ 50 mg/dL) elevations of serum bilirubin may occur. Survival is dependent on the underlying disorder rather than the liver test abnormalities or liver failure (which is uncommon). Coagulopathy and pruritus are uncommon. Imaging studies to exclude structural hepatobiliary disease and to look for an extrahepatic, extrabiliary source of infection are important. Once the source of infection is identified and treated, liver test abnormalities should improve. Severe cholestasis may take weeks or even months to resolve.

A number of systemic disorders are associated with nodular regenerative hyperplasia of the liver, including many conditions associated with vasculitis, hypercoagulability, and autoimmune phenomena, as well as myeloproliferative and lymphoproliferative disorders (Table 85.1). In addition to the therapeutics directed toward portal hypertension, treatment of the underlying condition and withdrawal of offending medications (azathioprine and other chemotherapeutic agents) are critical.

Table 85.1 Systemic disorders associated with nodular regenerative hyperplasia.

Myeloproliferative disorders
Lymphoproliferative disorders
Sickle cell disease
Multiple myeloma
Hypercoagulable states
Rheumatoid arthritis (RA)
Felty's syndrome
Systemic lupus erythematosus (SLE)
Adult Still's disease
Polymyalgia rheumatica
Sjögren's syndrome
Scleroderma
CREST syndrome
Polymyositis
Behçet's syndrome
Polyarteritis nodosa
Celiac disease
Myasthenia gravis
Sarcoidosis
Cystic fibrosis

Take Home Points

- Ischemic hepatitis occurs as a result of impaired arterial bloodflow or reduced arterial oxygen content to the liver.
- Congestive hepatopathy secondary to passive venous outflow congestion of the liver is one of the most common causes of mild abnormal liver test results.
- Mild abnormalities of liver tests are common in patients with thyroid disease, adrenal disease, diabetes mellitus, rheumatologic diseases, systemic infections, and inflammatory disorders of the gastrointestinal (GI) tract.

References

1 Fairbanks KD, Tavill AS. Liver disease in alpha 1-antitrypsin deficiency: a review. *Am J Gastorenterol* 2008; **103**: 2136–41.

2 Colombo C. Liver disease in cystic fibrosis. *Curr Opin Pulm Med* 2007; **13**: 529–36.

3 Hull K, Hornstein R, Naglieri R, *et al.* Two cases of thyroid storm-associated cholestatic jaundice. *Endocr Pract* 2007; **13**: 476–80.

4 Khairy RN, Mullen KD. Hypothroidism as a mimic of liver failure in a patient with cirrhosis. *Ann Intern Med* 2007; **146**: 315–16.

5 Kaw R, Gota C, Bennett A, *et al.* Lupus-related hepatitis: complication of lupus or autoimmune association? Case report and review of the literature. *Dig Dis Sci* 2006; **51**: 813–18.

6 Ebert EC, Hagspiel KD, Nagar M, *et al.* Gastrointestinal involvement in polyarteritis nodosa. *Clin Gastroenterol Hepatol* 2008; **6**: 960–6.

7 Abdo A, Meddings J, Swain M. Liver abnormalities in celiac disease. *Clin Gastroenterol Hepatol* 2004; **2**: 107–12.

8 Kahi CJ, Saxena R, Temkit M, *et al.* Hepatobiliary disease in sarcoidosis. *Sarcoidosis Vasculitis Diffuse Lung Dis* 2006; **23**: 117–23.

9 Kennedy PTF, Zakaria N, Modani SB, *et al.* Natural history of hepatic sarcoidosis and its response to treatment. *Eur J Gastroenterol Hepatol* 2006; **18**: 721–6.

10 Chand N, Sanyal AJ. Sepsis-induced cholestasis. *Hepatology* 2007; **45**: 230–41.

11 Cremers JP, Drent M, Baughman RP, *et al.* Therapeutic approach of hepatic sarcoidosis. *Curr Opin Pulm Med* 2012; **18**: 472–82.

12 Stoller JK, Aboussouan LS. A review of alpha1-antitrypsin deficiency. *Am J Respir Crit Care Med* 2012; **185**: 246–59.

13 Behdad A, Owens SR. Systemic mastocytosis involving the gastrointestinal tract. *Arch Pathol Lab Med* 2013; **137**: 1220–3.

Diseases of the Biliary Tract and Gallbladder

Wajeeh Salah[1] and M. Edwyn Harrison[2]

[1] Mayo Clinic Health System in Eau Claire
[2] Mayo Clinic, Scottsdale, AZ, USA

Summary

Gallstone disease is common in the United States. Impacted gallstones can lead to acute cholecystitis, cholangitis, or gallstone pancreatitis. Biliary colic is a common early presenting symptom. Transabdominal ultrasound is the initial test of choice for the diagnosis of gallstone disease. Laparoscopic cholecystectomy is preferentially used to treat acute cholecystitis, while endoscopic retrograde cholangiopancreatography (ERCP) with sphincterotomy remains the gold standard for acute cholangitis. Gallbladder polyps are uncommon and are usually identified incidentally by ultrasonography. Cholecystectomy is commonly recommended for gallbladder polyps when there are findings that suggest a premalignant or malignant neoplasm.

Infection with biliary flukes, most commonly *Clonorchis sinensis* or *Opisthorchis viverrini*, is a major public health concern in endemic areas such as Asia, Eastern Europe, Africa, and Latin America. Patients infected by biliary flukes are normally asymptomatic. However, a large parasite burden can lead to mechanical obstruction of the biliary system, and multiple studies have shown a link between biliary fluke infection and cholangiocarcinoma (CCA). Antiparasitic drugs remain the treatment of choice for biliary fluke infection.

Gallbladder cancers are a rare tumor of the gastrointestinal (GI) tract, and most are discovered incidentally after an uncomplicated cholecystectomy. Endoscopic ultrasound (EUS) is the imaging modality of choice for staging of gallbladder cancers. The treatment of gallbladder cancers is usually surgical and depends on the stage of the tumor. CCA can occur anywhere along the length of the biliary tree. The most important risk factor for development of CCA is chronic inflammation of the bile ducts, most commonly due to primary sclerosing cholangitis (PSC). The diagnosis of CCA can be challenging, due to the paucicellular and heterogenous nature of the tumor and its anatomic location. Surgical resection can be an option for certain types of CCA, depending on the anatomic location and tumor stage. Patients with unresectable CCA generally have poor outcomes. However, liver transplantation may be an option for selected patients with focal disease.

PSC is a chronic disease characterized by inflammation and progressive fibrosis of the bile ducts. While cholangiography was once the gold standard for the diagnosis of PSC, magnetic resonance cholangiopancreatography (MRCP) is now recommended. Though no medical therapy has been proven to alter the course of disease in PSC, endoscopic dilation of dominant strictures is associated with a high clinical response rate. PSC remains an important etiology for liver transplantation in the United States, and excellent patient survival rates at 1 and 5 years have been reported.

Case

A 53-year-old woman with a history of hypertension who underwent cholecystectomy 20 years ago presents with 3 months of daily, right-sided, and epigastric abdominal pain that is colicky in nature. Physical examination demonstrates mild tenderness to palpation in the epigastrium and right upper quadrant. Laboratory tests, including complete blood count (CBC) and liver function tests (LFTS), are normal. Transabdominal ultrasound, abdominal computed tomography (CT) scan, and magnetic resonance imaging (MRI)/MRCP are all normal. No masses, stones, or biliary ductal dilation are seen on any of the imaging tests.

The patient continues to experience abdominal pain and is referred for an EUS, which reveals a 10.3 mm mobile, shadowing gallstone within the distal common bile duct. She is referred for an ERCP. Biliary sphincterotomy is performed and the common bile duct is swept with an extraction balloon. One 10 mm gallstone and a moderate amount of sludge are removed from the common bile duct. The patient feels well after the procedure. The abdominal pain completely resolves.

Gallstone Disease and Cholecystitis

Definition

Gallstone-related diseases are common in Western countries. The prevalence of gallstones is greater than 10% in the United States and in European countries, based on ultrasound studies [1]. Gallstone-related disease was the most common inpatient GI diagnosis, was the 14th most frequently diagnosed condition overall, and accounted for almost 800 000 office visits and an estimated 750 000 cholecystectomies in the United States during the year 2000 alone. Cholecystitis was also among the top 20 causes of GI-related deaths [2].

Presentation and Diagnosis

Uncomplicated Cholelithiasis

Symptomatic gallstones occur in a minority of patients with gallstones. Biliary colic, which is a constant rather than intermittent

Practical Gastroenterology and Hepatology Board Review Toolkit, Second Edition. Edited by Nicholas J. Talley, Kenneth R. DeVault, Michael B. Wallace, Bashar A. Aqel and Keith D. Lindor.

Table 86.1 Features of biliary colic and common complications of gallstones.

	Symptoms/signs	Lab studies	Imaging
Biliary colic	Episodic pain Poorly localized, epigastric, or right upper quadrant +/– nausea and vomiting Follows meals	Normal	Ultrasound: normal or gallstones
Acute cholecystitis	Recurrent pain similar to biliary colic, may localize to right upper quadrant May or may not relate to meals Murphy's sign Fever Palpable gallbladder (uncommon)	Leukocytosis Mild elevations in bilirubin or alkaline phosphatase, lipase, or amylase (uncommon)	Ultrasound: gallstones, thickened gallbladder wall, pericholecystic fluid, radiologic Murphy's sign HIDA: non-filling of gallbladder
Choledocholithiasis	Asymptomatic Biliary colic Cholangitis Pancreatitis	Varies with complications Elevated bilirubin, lipase/amylase, or alkaline phosphatase	Ultrasound, EUS, MRCP, ERCP: common bile duct stone and/or dilation
Cholangitis	Charcot's triad: right upper quadrant pain, jaundice, and fever One or two of these symptoms or signs, without the complete triad Reynold's pentad: Charcot's triad with hypotension and altered mental status	Leukocytosis Mild–moderate elevation in bilirubin, alkaline phosphatase, lipase, or amylase Frequent bacteremia	Ultrasound, MRCP, ERCP: common bile duct stone and/or dilation

HIDA, hepatic iminodiacetic acid scan; EUS, endoscopic ultrasound; MRCP, magnetic resonance cholangiopancreatography; ERCP, endoscopic retrograde cholangiopancreatography.

or "colicky" pain, is attributed to a gallstone obstructing the biliary neck (Table 86.1). It is classically described as an intense, persistent, epigastric or right upper quadrant pain, lasting from 15 minutes to several hours, and often associated with nausea or vomiting. It may follow a large or fatty meal. Many patients, particularly older adults, present with less classic symptoms, such as poorly localized pain with abrupt onset or relief of pain and no precipitating meal, so a high index of suspicion is important in order to recognize the symptoms prior to development of complications.

Investigation of uncomplicated cholelithiasis should start with a transabdominal ultrasound and laboratory testing, to confirm the presence of stones and assess for complications. Ultrasound is a sensitive and specific imaging study for the demonstration of stones within the gallbladder. In uncomplicated cholelithiasis, serum studies should be normal. Elevated liver tests, pancreatic enzymes, or leukocytosis may reflect choledocholithiasis or a related complication (such as acute cholecystitis). If the diagnosis is still questionable after ultrasound, a radionucleotide scan hepatic iminodiacetic acid (HIDA) scan is useful.

Acute Cholecystitis

Acute cholecystitis is the most common complication of gallstones, occurring in 20% of patients with symptomatic cholelithiasis [3]. Patients with acute cholecystitis often present with protracted, progressive biliary colic. Physical exam may reveal right upper quadrant tenderness and guarding; eventually, one might palpate an inflamed gallbladder. Murphy's sign is specific for cholecystitis. Fever and leukocytosis are commonly present. The presence of jaundice is uncommon and generally mild, and should prompt consideration of choledocholithiasis or Mirizzi's syndrome. Initial evaluation includes imaging with ultrasound, and often a HIDA scan. Ultrasound findings diagnostic of acute cholecystitis include cholelithiasis with gallbladder wall thickening, pericholecystic fluid, and a positive sonographic Murphy's sign. There is no broadly accepted diagnostic standard for acute cholecystitis. In an effort to codify the diagnosis, the 2007 Tokyo Guidelines offer three categories of diagnostic findings. One criterion from each category must be fulfilled: (i) Murphy's sign or pain/tenderness in the right upper quadrant or a right upper quadrant mass; (ii) fever, leukocytosis, or elevated C-reactive protein (CRP); (iii) confirmation by ultrasound or HIDA [4].

Treatment of Acute Cholecystitis

Laparoscopic cholecystectomy is the standard of care for patients with routine cases of acute cholecystitis. Preliminary medical management consists of intravenous (IV) hydration, with the possible addition of antibiotic therapy. Antibiotics have not generally been shown to be beneficial, but are a reasonable addition to surgical therapy if there is evidence of infection or a risk of complications from infection, as may occur in the immunocompromised or the elderly. The laparoscopic approach reduces morbidity and length of hospital stay as compared to open cholecystectomy, and has largely displaced open cholecystectomy even for most patients with more severe or complicated disease.

The timing of surgical intervention is controversial. Many surgeons argue for a "cooling off" interval to reduce the risk of technically difficult surgery that might require conversion to open cholecystectomy. A delay in surgery, however, can lead to other gallstone-related complications, such as pancreatitis, obstructive jaundice, or recurrent or chronic cholecystitis. While the controversy may persist, individual studies and meta-analyses have found no benefit from delaying surgery [5].

In patients with acute cholecystitis at high risk for surgery, such as the acutely ill, the elderly, and those with significant comorbidities (e.g., cardiac disease, severe diabetes, cirrhosis), percutaneous cholecystostomy offers an alternative to urgent surgery for decompression of the gallbladder [6]. Using ultrasound guidance, cholecystostomy can be safely performed at the bedside with a high rate of success. Cholecystotomy allows time for the patient's condition to stabilize, enabling some patients to proceed to elective surgery, which has lower mortality than emergent surgery. For patients who are not surgical candidates, percutaneous cholecystostomy has also been advocated as definitive treatment [7].

Choledocholithiasis and Cholangitis

Choledocholithiasis

Definition

Up to 15% of patients with cholelithiasis in the United States also have gallstones within the common bile duct [8]. Patients with uncomplicated ductal stones may be asymptomatic, or may present with symptoms of biliary colic. The natural history of untreated choledocholithiasis is not well delineated, but complications of choledocholithiasis include cholangitis and pancreatitis, as well as their secondary complications.

Diagnosis

There are several options for imaging of the common bile duct. Among non-invasive tests, transabdominal ultrasound is the first choice, due to its low cost and wide availability. Though its sensitivity for detecting stones in the common bile duct is only approximately 50%, that for identifying ductal dilation resulting from obstructing stones is approximately 95%. It is of limited use in obese patients or when there has been surgical manipulation of the common bile duct. Abdominal CT scan with oral contrast has a sensitivity of approximately 92% for detecting ductal stones, and is especially useful as a first test when ultrasound is not likely to be helpful [8]. ERCP, EUS, and MRCP have generally comparable sensitivities, specificities, and accuracies in diagnosing common bile duct stones [9]. More specifically, ERCP has a sensitivity of 90–95% in detecting choledocholithiasis, but its role in diagnosis is limited by its significant incidence of complications, particularly pancreatitis. It is used primarily in cases in which the probability of choledocholithiasis is high and therapy is expected. The sensitivity of EUS for detecting a ductal stone is between 94 and 98%, which matches or exceeds that of ERCP, but it is less widely available. EUS is especially useful when there is low or intermediate suspicion for a ductal stone (Figure 86.1), where it provides sensitive diagnosis without the risk inherent in ERCP. MRCP has comparable sensitivity and specificity (90–95%) to EUS, and has the added advantage of providing detailed duct anatomy [10, 11].

Treatment

After diagnosis of choledocholithiasis, ERCP with sphincterotomy and stone removal (Figure 86.2) is commonly performed, both to

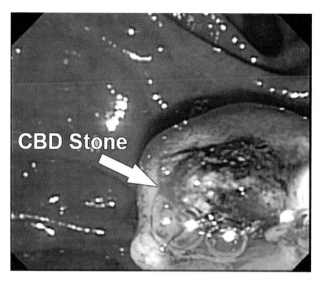

Figure 86.2 ERCP with sphincterotomy and stone removal for symptomatic choledocholithiasis.

treat symptoms and to reduce the risk of complications. Laparoscopic cholecystectomy is performed after bile duct clearance in patients who are adequate surgical candidates in order to prevent further complications of gallstone disease. Cholecystectomy is best performed during the same admission [12].

Cholangitis

Definition

Cholangitis is infection and inflammation within the biliary tract. It occurs in the setting of biliary obstruction leading to bacterial stasis and proliferation. Obstruction is most commonly caused by choledocholithiasis, but can also result from malignancy, external compression, or biliary stricture due to intrinsic biliary disease or previous surgical manipulation. Cholangitis can be rapidly fatal; it is one of a few indications for urgent ERCP or biliary surgery.

Presentation and Diagnosis

The presentation of cholangitis can range in severity from mild to life-threatening. Charcot's triad of fever, right upper quadrant pain, and jaundice is common but not universal. The additional presence of hypotension and altered sensorium, which defines Reynaud's pentad, is ominous, as it reflects spread of bacteria beyond the confines of the biliary tree. Laboratory studies in cholangitis generally show an elevated white blood cell (WBC) count and cholestatic liver test abnormalities, including elevated alkaline phosphatase, bilirubin, and gamma glutamyl tranferase, and a variable but typically mild pattern of elevated transaminases. Transabdominal ultrasound is the initial test of choice to identify bile duct dilation and stones. MRCP is useful in the stable patient when the ultrasound is not diagnostic, and may detect more subtle bile duct abnormalities or stones missed by ultrasound.

Treatment

Once the diagnosis is suspected, IV fluids should be provided, blood cultures obtained, and empiric antibiotic therapy started, and the interventional endoscopist should be alerted regarding a possible therapeutic ERCP. After initial resuscitation, the patient's clinical status should be monitored closely. If the patient shows evidence of clinical deterioration or multisystem failure (e.g., hypotension or

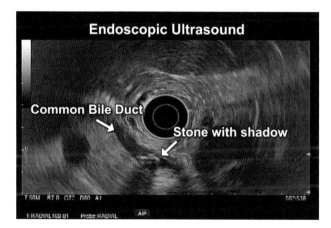

Figure 86.1 EUS image showing a shadowing gallstone within the common bile duct.

Table 86.2 Risk factors for severe cholangitis.

Historical	Advanced age
	History of smoking
Abnormal laboratory tests	Hyperbilirubinemia
	Marked leukocytosis
	Prolonged PT
	Hypoalbuminemia
	Hyperglycemia
CT findings	Papillitis
	Hepatic parenchymal changes
	Markedly inhomogeneous enhancement of the liver on arterial phase
	Periampullary diverticulum

PT, prothrombin time; CT, computed tomography.

confusion), or if there is no significant improvement in symptoms or hemodynamics over the subsequent 6–12 hours, then urgent ERCP is obligatory. ERCP may also be performed urgently for patients with risk factors for development of severe cholangitis (Table 86.2), because these patients frequently develop worsening clinical status [13–16].

Techniques for biliary decompression at ERCP include sphincterotomy, stone extraction, and placement of biliary stents. In cases of cholangitis due to malignant biliary obstruction, a metal stent can be placed for longer-term drainage and decompression. Cultures of biliary fluid should be performed routinely if blood culture results are not yet available. Percutaneous transhepatic biliary decompression can be performed if ERCP is not feasible, but surgical decompression should be avoided because of its high rate of mortality in acute cholangitis. The vast majority of patients will respond to fluids and antibiotics, so ERCP can be performed electively. The patient with cholangitis and intact gallbladder should then undergo elective cholecystectomy, because the risk of recurrent gallstone disease is high [17].

Gallbladder Polyps

Definition

A gallbladder polyp is any elevated lesion of the mucosal wall of the gallbladder, which encompasses a range of lesions including both true polyps and pseudopolyps. While usually incidental findings, polyps are potentially significant, because some can be confused with gallstones and others have malignant potential. One large, retrospective study in a Western population estimated that gallbladder polyps occur in approximately 4% of adults, based upon ultrasound findings [18]. In patients with PSC, gallbladder polyps have potentially greater clinical significance: they occur with prevalence similar to that of the general population, but have a potentially greater likelihood of malignancy [19]. Gallbladder polyps are most simply classified as either benign or malignant. The most common type of gallbladder polyp is the cholesterol polyp, a benign non-neoplastic polyp that makes up approximately 60% of all gallbladder polyps. Malignancies are relatively uncommon, accounting for less than 10% of gallbladder polyps, and are primarily adenocarcinomas. Inflammatory polyps, adenomas, hyperplastic polyps, and other miscellaneous growths make up the remainder of gallbladder polyps.

Presentation and Diagnosis

Gallbladder polyps are usually asymptomatic, and are commonly diagnosed incidentally by transabdominal ultrasound. Ultrasound is often the only test required for their evaluation: it has superior sensitivity for detection of gallbladder polyps than ERCP, CT, or oral cholecystography [20], and also differentiates polyps from stones in most cases. EUS has shown promise as an adjunct to transabdominal ultrasound in differentiating benign from malignant polyps [21].

Cholesterol Polyps

Cholesterol polyps are not neoplasms, but rather accretions of cholesterol-containing residue. Cholesterol polyps usually occur in a diffuse pattern, lining the entire gallbladder wall up to the cystic duct, which gives the epithelium a characteristic "strawberry gallbladder" appearance on gross pathologic examination. Other times, the accretions accumulate in a heaped-up pattern, forming pseudopolyps [22]. Gallbladder pseudopolyps may be difficult to distinguish from adenocarcinoma on ultrasound. One feature that helps distinguish pseudopolyps from adenomas and adenocarcinomas is that their echogenicity tends to be high, while that of the other lesions tends to be lower, similar to that of the liver [23].

Gallbladder Adenomas

Gallbladder adenomas occur infrequently and are the only form of gallbladder neoplasm with malignant potential. An adenoma–carcinoma sequence has been demonstrated, but it is not known how frequently gallbladder adenomas progress to cancer. On ultrasound, gallbladder adenomas are commonly solitary, pedunculated polyps ranging in size from 5 to 20 mm, and they are often diagnosed concurrently with gallstones. When small, these adenomas tend to be echogenic and homogenous in appearance, but they become less echogenic and more heterogeneous as they increase in size. Large gallbladder adenomas can therefore be confused with malignancies.

Carcinomatous Gallbladder

Carcinomatous gallbladder polyps are the most common type of gallbladder malignancy. Carcinomatous polyps may be diagnosed as true polyps in a small minority of cases, when they are detected incidentally during evaluation for symptomatic gallstones. In these cases, carcinomatous polyps can present in a variety of forms, including sessile, pedunculated, and raised polyps of varying sizes [24]. However, carcinomatous polyps are usually identified after they have transformed into a polypoid mass, and often after development of metastases.

Adenomyomatoses of the Gallbladder

Adenomyomatoses of the gallbladder are a group of hyperplastic epithelial growths which extend into the muscularis. They are not true adenomas, but may represent premalignant lesions. Their overall prevalence is unknown, but they occur more commonly in women than in men. Adenomyomatoses may appear polypoid, and focal areas of hyperplasia may span over 10 mm in length, making them difficult to distinguish from a neoplasm. Identification of a characteristic "V"-shaped or "comet-tail" shadow, created by reflection of the ultrasound waves off the hyperplastic wall, can help support a diagnosis of an adenomyoma, but definitive exclusion of malignancy may require surgical resection [22].

Malignancy Risk

In assessing risk of malignancy, larger gallbladder polyps are at higher risk of malignant conversion. Polyps >10 mm should be considered suspicious for malignancy, and polyps >18 mm are usually

Table 86.3 Management of gallbladder polyps.

Cholecystectomy (laparoscopic)	1. 10–18 mm polyp
	2. <10 mm polyp
	  • symptomatic
	  • growth on imaging
	3. Polyp of any size
	  • sessile
	  • solitary
	  • with PSC
	  • with cholelithiasis

Cholecystectomy (open)	Polyp >18 mm
Observation with serial imaging	Asymptomatic polyp <10 mm

invasive malignancies [20]. However, smaller polyps are not necessarily benign. Carcinomatous polyps as small as 6 mm have been reported [25], and sessile carcinomatous polyps <10 mm in size can be quite aggressive [26]. Other risk factors for malignant conversion of polyps have been recognized, including patient age >50 years, concurrent gallstones or PSC, and possibly the solitary polyp.

Treatment

Cholecystectomy is commonly recommended for gallbladder polyps when there are findings that suggest a premalignant or malignant neoplasm, or when gallstones are identified concurrently, because of the difficulty of detecting carcinomatous polyps with adjacent stones by ultrasound. Laparoscopic cholecystectomy is recommended if the polyps are large (>10 mm), symptomatic, or sessile. For polyps >18 mm, open surgery is recommended: the polyp is highly likely to be a locally invasive malignancy, and should be staged preoperatively with CT or EUS [20]. There are no clear guidelines regarding management of small, asymptomatic polyps <10 mm in size; they should be followed with serial ultrasound every 6–12 months, and cholecystectomy should be offered for those that enlarge over time (Table 86.3).

Biliary Flukes

Definition

Infection of the biliary tree by liver flukes such as *C. sinensis* and *O. viverrini* continues to be a major public health concern in endemic areas. Patients in Asia, Eastern Europe, Africa, and Latin America are at the highest risk for infection with biliary parasites [27]. Infection by *Clonorchis* or *Opisthorchis* flukes in humans occurs when the parasitic larvae are ingested, typically by eating raw freshwater fish. The larvae then journey through the small intestine and into the biliary tract. The flukes can reside in the biliary tract for up to 20 years.

Presentation

Most patients infected with these parasites are asymptomatic. When the parasites multiply and the burden becomes substantial, mechanical obstruction can develop. Patients can present with jaundice, cholangitis, or even CCA in cases of long-standing infection. They can also develop inflammatory reactions, adenomatous hyperplasia, and periductal fibrosis.

Diagnosis

Imaging of infected patients can show biliary ductal dilation or thickening of the walls of the bile duct. Ultrasound, CT, and MRI scans typically show diffuse biliary dilation of the small intrahepatic bile ducts. In cases of severe infection, clusters of flukes may show up as non-shadowing echogenic foci on ultrasound, as bile duct casts on CT, or as multiple small extended filling defects on cholangiogram [28]. Anti-parasitic drugs such as praziquantel are the treatment of choice for biliary fluke infection, and overall cure rates remain high.

Cholangiocarcinoma

Multiple studies have shown a link between biliary fluke infection and CCA. The chronic inflammatory changes and adenomatous hyperplasia of the biliary epithelium associated with biliary fluke infection (*C. sinensis* and *O. viverrini* in particular) may lead to CCA. One study from Korea indicates that as many as 80% of patients with intrahepatic and extrahepatic CCA have evidence of infection with *C. sinensis* [29]. The incidence of CCA is rising, and its diagnosis is commonly achieved at late stages of the disease, which limits the benefit of conventional therapy. A recent study examined new molecular profiling techniques that may be beneficial in developing more individualized and targeted therapies for liver fluke-associated CCA [30].

Cancer of the Gallbladder and Biliary Tree

Definition

Cancer of the gallbladder is a rare tumor of the GI tract. Though rare, it is the most common cancer of the biliary tree. The most common histologic type of gallbladder cancer is adenocarcinoma. Other rare cell types include papillary, mucinous, clear-cell, signet-ring cell, adenosquamous, squamous cell, and small-cell carcinoma. The incidence of gallbladder cancer varies across race, gender, and geography. The most important risk factor is the presence of cholelithiasis [31]. Bacterial infections with *Salmonella* and *Helicobacter* species have also been associated with gallbladder cancer [32]. The mechanism of carcinogenesis is an increase in the conversion of primary bile acids to secondary bile acids – compounds that are known carcinogens – provoked by the involved bacteria [33].

Presentation

Most gallbladder cancers are discovered incidentally after an uncomplicated cholecystectomy. Patients with gallbladder cancer may present with intermittent right upper quadrant pain similar to biliary colic. More advanced cases of gallbladder cancer can present with jaundice, weight loss, cachexia, and obstruction from local invasion of the duodenum.

Diagnosis

Imaging studies can readily detect gallbladder cancer. Ultrasound is widely available and is the best initial study for patients presenting with symptoms suggestive of gallbladder disease. Ultrasound findings suggestive of malignancy include asymmetric gallbladder wall thickening, a polypoid lesion projecting into the gallbladder lumen, and a mass invading the liver parenchyma or surrounding structures [34, 35]. In cases where gallbladder carcinoma is of clinical concern, color Doppler ultrasound can be used to determine blood-flow within the mass, a feature highly suggestive of malignancy, and to determine the presence of vascular invasion of the primary tumor [36]. Recent studies have shown that EUS with fine-needle aspiration (FNA) of a thickened gallbladder wall may have a useful role to play in the diagnosis of gallbladder cancers [37].

CHAPTER 86

Table 86.4 TNM classification and staging of gallbladder cancer. Source: American Joint Committee on Cancer, 2002. Reproduced with permission of Springer Science+Business Media.

Primary tumor stage (T)	
TX	Primary tumor cannot be assessed
T0	No evidence of primary tumor
Tis	Carcinoma in situ
T1a	Tumor invades lamina propria
T1b	Tumor invades muscle layer
T2	Tumor invades perimuscular connective tissue; no extension beyond serosa or into liver
T3	Tumor perforates the serosa (visceral peritoneum) and/or directly invades the liver and/or other adjacent organ or structure (e.g., stomach, duodenum, colon, extrahepatic bile duct, etc.)
T4	Tumor invades the main portal vein or hepatic artery, or invades multiple extrahepatic organs or structures

Regional lymph nodes (N)	
NX	Regional lymph nodes cannot be accessed
N0	No regional lymph node metastases
N1	Regional lymph node metastases (e.g., hilar, celiac, duodenal, peripancreatic, SMA)

Distant metastases (M)	
MX	Distant metastases cannot be accessed
M0	No distant metastases
M1	Distant metastases

Stage grouping	T	N	M
Stage 0	Tis	N0	M0
Stage IA	T1	N0	M0
Stage IB	T2	N0	M0
Stage IIA	T3	N0	M0
Stage IIB	T1	N1	M0
	T2	N1	M0
	T3	N1	M0
Stage III	T4	Any N	M0
Stage IV	Any T	Any N	M1

SMA, superior mesenteric artery.

Other imaging studies, such as CT, magnetic resonance angiography (MRA), and MRCP, can be useful in obtaining more information in patients with more advanced gallbladder cancer. These tests can be helpful in determining vascular invasion, nodal disease, hepatic, vascular, or bile duct invasion, and distant metastases.

Staging

EUS is currently the test of choice for staging gallbladder cancer [38]. The American Joint Committee on Cancer (AJCC) TNM classification and staging are shown in Table 86.4. The tumor (T) classification is based on depth of gallbladder wall invasion, local vascular invasion, or invasion into surrounding structures. Local lymph node (N) involvement may include the hilar (cystic duct, common bile duct, hepatic artery, and portal vein), celiac artery, periduodenal, peripancreatic, or superior mesenteric artery (SMA) lymph nodes. Other lymph node sites are considered distant metastases. Direct extension of the gallbladder carcinoma into the liver or adjacent organs is not considered metastatic (M) disease.

Surgical Therapy

The extent of surgical therapy strongly depends on the T stage of the tumor, the proximity of the tumor to critical vascular and biliary structures, and the presence of metastatic disease. Early-stage tumors (T1a) are often found incidentally in a cholecystomy specimen and are usually cured with cholecystectomy alone. T1b tumors can have regional lymph node metastases, and patients may benefit from adequate staging when subjected to lymphadenectomy [39]. T2 tumors usually require resection of the gallbladder bed (liver

segments IVB and V) and regional lymphadenectomy. The right hepatic artery, portal vein, and right bile duct lie in close proximity to the gallbladder fossa, and involvement of these structures requires a right hepatectomy. Involvement of the cystic duct stump with tumor also requires radical resection of the common bile duct and reconstruction of bilioenteric continuity with a Roux-en-Y choledochojejunostomy. The 5-year survival after liver resection of T2 gallbladder carcinoma is approximately 55%.

Cholangiocarcinoma

Definition

CCAs are cancers that occur anywhere along the length of the biliary tree. These tumors can arise from the peripheral bile ducts (intrahepatic CCA), the right, left, and common hepatic ducts (hilar CCA or Klatskin tumors), or the distal common bile duct. Based on the Surveillance, Epidemiology, and End Results (SEER) Program database, the incidence of intrahepatic CCA has increased from 0.32 per 100 000 persons in 1975–79 to 0.85 per 100 000 persons in 1995–99 [40]. Similarly, the incidence of extrahepatic CCA has decreased from 1.08 per 100 000 persons in 1979 to 0.82 per 100 000 persons in 1998. Given these data, approximately 5000 cases of CCA are diagnosed annually in the United States, with approximately half arising in the extrahepatic bile ducts and half in the intrahepatic ducts.

Risk Factors

Though several risk factors have been associated with the development of CCA, most cases remain sporadic. The most important risk factor involves chronic inflammation of the bile duct epithelium. PSC is one of the main causes of chronic inflammation of the bile duct and accounts for approximately one-third of CCA cases. The annual risk of CCA in a patient with PSC is 0.6–1.5%, which is 100-fold higher than the rate observed in the general population [41,42]. In Asia, a common risk factor for CCA is infection with the liver flukes O. viverrini and C. sinensis. Chronic inflammation from these organisms is thought to occur when their eggs are deposited into the biliary tree.

Presentation

Obstructive jaundice is the most common presenting symptom in CCA. Patients may present with complaints such as darkening of the urine, yellow discoloration of the skin, sclera, and mucous membranes and pruritus. Constitutional symptoms such as weight loss and fatigue may also be present in more advanced CCA.

Diagnosis

The diagnosis of CCA can be very challenging, due to the paucicellular and heterogenous nature of the tumor and its anatomic location. A multimodal diagnostic approach and a high clinical suspicion are needed. Imaging studies, typically ultrasound, are the initial diagnostic tests of choice in patients presenting with obstructive jaundice. They can show dilation of the intrahepatic bile ducts, determine the presence of intrahepatic metastases, and demonstrate occlusion of the hepatic arteries and portal vein or enlargement of lymph nodes.

The next test is usually a CT of the chest, abdomen, and pelvis and/or an EUS. CT and EUS can provide information regarding local invasion, relationship of the tumor to the hilar vessels, atrophy of the liver, regional and distant lymph node metastases, and distant metastases. This can be useful in determining surgical respectability.

ERCP is often performed at this juncture to investigate the extent of bile duct involvement and to provide biliary drainage. ERCP provides important information about the distal extent of the tumor along the bile duct and allows biopsy or brushing of the bile ducts in order to obtain histologic or cytologic material to support the diagnosis of CCA. A biliary stent may be inserted to alleviate obstruction or treat cholangitis. Often, the proximal (intrahepatic) extent of the tumor is not well appreciated by ERCP, and patients must undergo a percutaneous transhepatic cholangiogram (PTC). PTC may also be necessary for drainage prior to a major hepatic resection.

MRI is being used more extensively now because of its ability not only to obtain information similar to that from CT, but also to assess the vasculature using MRA/magnetic resonance venography (MRV) and the biliary tree using MRCP. Unfortunately, with current technology, the spatial resolution of MRCP is far less than that of direct cholangiography in terms of determining resectability. Angiography is infrequently obtained in this era.

Staging

TNM staging is used (see Table 86.4). The tumor (T) classification is based on extent of bile duct penetration, local vascular invasion, or invasion into surrounding structures. Local lymph node (N1) involvement generally includes the hilar (cystic duct, common bile duct, hepatic artery, and portal vein) lymph nodes alone. Other lymph node sites are generally considered metastatic disease. Metastatic disease (M1) includes distant lesions, satellite lesions within the liver parenchyma, and involvement of non-local lymph nodes.

Chemotherapy

The most common chemotherapeutic drugs for CCA are 5-flurouracil and gemcitabine. Both have been tested in combination with a variety of other drugs, including cisplatin, oxaliplatin, and paclitaxel. No studies were randomized, and most were either statistically underpowered or based on case reports. All demonstrated poor response rates. Currently, there is no randomized evidence showing a clear survival benefit for a specific chemotherapeutic regimen.

Resection and Outcomes

The resectability of CCA is predicated on the exclusion of extrahepatic and non-locoregional lymph node metastases. Laparoscopy is generally used to exclude peritoneal disease. Any obviously enlarged N2-level lymph nodes (e.g., peripancreatic, periduodenal, periportal, celiac, or SMA lymph nodes) are excised to rule out metastases. It is important to determine the extent of vascular invasion early in the course of resection of the tumor.

The extent of resection required for hilar CCA is determined by the anatomic involvement of the bile ducts with the tumor. The Bismuth–Corlette classification is used to guide resection. Resection of Bismuth–Corlette type 1 CCA (2 cm below the hepatic duct confluence) requires only resection of the extrahepatic biliary tree, the gallbladder, and regional lymph nodes. The surgical management of Bismuth–Corlette type 2 CCA (2 cm from the hepatic duct confluence) is similar to that of type 1, but may require removal of a portion of the caudate lobe or segment IVA due to their proximity to the hepatic hilus. Type 3a (involving the hepatic duct confluence and the right bile duct) and 3b (involving the hepatic duct confluence and the left bile duct) CCAs are best addressed with resection of the extrahepatic biliary tree and gallbladder, hepatic lobectomy, and regional lymphadenectomy. In all cases, bilioenteric continuity

is restored with a hepaticojejunostomy. Type IV CCA (tumor extension to the right and left biliary radicals, or multifocal tumors) is rarely resectable by conventional means.

In general, the outcome for patients with unresectable CCA is poor: 5% or less survival at 5 years. In an early report by Nakeeb *et al.* [43], the rate of major hepatic resection was only 14% and the 5-year survival was 11% [43]. Since that time, improvements in 5-year survival have paralleled the increased utilization of major hepatic resection. In most contemporary series, 75–100% of patients undergo major hepatectomy (more than four segments resected, usually via a formal lobectomy) and 5-year survivals range from 25 to 48% [44]. Morbidity in these series varies from 27 to 76%, and mortality from 0 to 12%. Recent reports have described a combination of extended hepatic resection (generally right trisegmentectomy) and concomitant vascular reconstruction (of the remnant left portal vein) [45]. Complete tumor excision (R0 resection) was achieved in 65% of patients treated with extended resection, and the 5-year survival in these patients was 57%.

Transplantation

CCA was initially thought to be an ideal indication for liver transplantation, because the procedure's radicality could address oncologic problems such as bilateral or diffuse hepatic duct involvement, invasion of the hepatic vasculature, and damaged hepatic parenchyma against predisposing diseases such as PSC. However, several different groups utilizing only liver transplantation have reported 0–47% 5-year survival, with recurrence rates of 50–80%. As these results are not significantly different from those for hepatic resection, and given the scarcity of donor livers, interest in liver transplantation for CCA has waned.

Several groups have reported encouraging results using radiation therapy for unresectable CCA or neoadjuvant therapy prior to hepatic resection. Based on these findings, a protocol was developed at the Mayo Clinic for neoadjuvant chemoradiotherapy followed by liver transplantation for CCA that is either unresectable or arising in the setting of PSC. The success of this protocol is attributable to patient selection, neoadjuvant therapy with external beam radiation and intrabiliary radiation, and operative staging of all patients prior to liver transplantation to exclude those with lymph node metastases or extrahepatic spread. Early results were encouraging and demonstrated proof of concept [46]: 25 patients were enrolled, with 7 eliminated due to metastatic disease or death during neoadjuvant treatment; of the 18 remaining, 6 had metastases at their staging laparotomy; at 44 months' follow-up, patient survival was 100%, with only one recurrence. A more recent analysis examined 71 patients enrolled over an 11-year period and compared them to 54 patients with CCA who were explored for possible surgical resection [47]: 9 patients had disease progression or could not complete the neoadjuvant treatment, 14 had positive staging operations, and 38 finally underwent liver transplantation. Of the 54 patients explored for surgical resection, 28 had unresectable disease. Five-year survival after liver transplantation was 82%, compared to 21% after resection. There were significant differences between the two groups (e.g., patient age and incidence of PSC), but this does not diminish the fact that the liver transplant patients had superior outcomes despite having more advanced disease. The most recent data from the Mayo Clinic show 80% 5-year survival after transplantation for patients with hilar CCA arising in PSC and 60% survival for those with *de novo* CCA.

Widespread application of liver transplantation for CCA has been limited by organ allocation policies and the prioritization given to deceased-donor transplantation. Fortunately, the United Network for Organ Sharing (UNOS) has recently addressed these problems and provided guidelines on granting requests for Model for End-Stage Liver Disease (MELD) score adjustments (see Chapter 96). Transplantation for patients with potentially resectable disease is highly controversial. Patients with *de novo* CCA have not fared as well as those with underlying PSC, and their survival after transplantation is only modestly better than that after resection. A randomized controlled trial (RCT) has been proposed to definitively address these issues, but it will be very difficult to carry out.

Primary Sclerosing Cholangitis

Definition
PSC is a chronic, idiopathic disease characterized by inflammation and progressive biliary fibrosis leading to strictures of the intrahepatic and extrahepatic bile ducts.

Epidemiology
PSC generally affects patients with a mean age of 40 years, and 62–72% of all affected patients are men [48]. Annual incidence of PSC is estimated to be 1 per 100 000 persons [49]. Among European and North American populations, an estimated 70–80% of patients with PSC have inflammatory bowel disease (IBD). Conversely, about 2–4% of patients with IBD have or develop PSC [50].

Pathophysiology
Cellular immune abnormalities, including CD4 lymphocyte recognition of antigens expressed on biliary epithelia, are hypothesized to initiate histologic injury. The strong association between PSC and IBD suggests an underlying infectious etiology, though compelling data have not been presented. An increased frequency of human leukocyte antigen (HLA) alleles A1, B8, and DR3 is observed in PSC but remains non-specific for disease susceptibility. A number of non-major histocompatibility complex (MHC) candidate genes may also influence susceptibility to clinical disease from PSC.

Clinical Features
A history of IBD and elevated serum liver biochemistries often prompts investigations to exclude PSC. Asymptomatic patients now represent 40–60% of all patients in observational studies [51].

Diagnosis
Elevations in serum alkaline phosphatase values are the biochemical hallmark of PSC, with values 3–10-fold the upper limit of normal in most cases [52]. Serum alanine and aspartate aminotransferase levels are usually two- threefold above normal, while total bilirubin levels may be normal in 60% of individuals at diagnosis [51]. Higher levels of total bilirubin are worrisome for advanced disease, superimposed choledocholithiasis, or malignancy. Cholangiography is the gold standard for diagnosis in PSC, characterized by segmental bile duct fibrosis with saccular dilation of normal intervening areas, resulting in the characteristic "beads on a string" appearance (Figure 86.3). MRCP has been increasingly utilized, with an overall diagnostic accuracy rate of 90% reported (Figure 86.4) [53]. Cholelithiasis is noted in up to 20% of individuals with PSC, with the majority being asymptomatic [52].

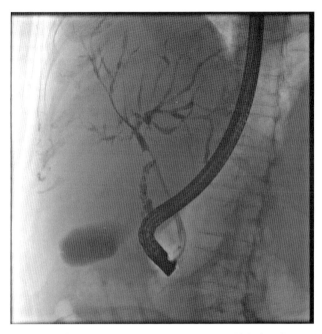

Figure 86.3 Cholangiogram in PSC, showing segmental bile duct fibrosis with saccular dilation of normal intervening areas, resulting in the characteristic "beads on a string" appearance.

Histologic Features
Liver biopsy is required for assessment of the stage of histologic disease, but is not essential for making a diagnosis of PSC unless cholangiography is normal. Periductal fibrosis with inflammation, bile duct proliferation, and ductopenia constitute the main histologic findings. Fibro-obliterative cholangiopathy, the pathologic hallmark of PSC, is uncommonly observed. The histologic classification of PSC is based on four stages and is similar to that of other chronic liver diseases [52].

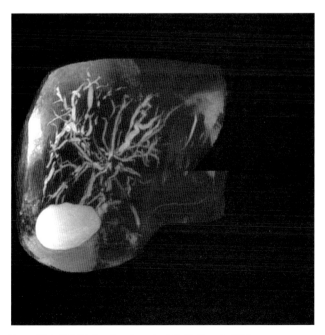

Figure 86.4 MRCP showing characteristic findings in PSC.

Therapeutics

Disease-Related Complications

Choledocholithiasis is reported at frequencies of around 5–15%, with the majority of calculi involving both central and peripheral bile ducts [52]. Endoscopic or percutaneous methods of providing biliary decompression and stone extraction have been successful. Biliary surgery, including stone extraction and bilioenteric anastomosis, may be considered when non-operative approaches have been ineffective in patients with early-stage PSC.

Dominant strictures occur in 5–10% of patients with PSC [52]. Clinical manifestations include a sudden asymptomatic increase in serum alkaline phosphatase and/or bilirubin, progressive jaundice, and bacterial cholangitis. Following empiric broad-spectrum IV antibiotic therapy, endoscopic or percutaneous therapy with balloon dilation of identified stenoses can provide significant clinical improvement. The efficacy and safety of dilation of strictures followed by placement of endoscopic stents versus balloon dilation alone has not been determined in a controlled trial setting to date. In all patients with dominant strictures, endoscopic brushings and biopsy are required to exclude malignancy.

Peristomal variceal bleeding occurs among subjects with IBD who have undergone proctocolectomy with ileostomy formation. Newer surgical techniques, including ileal pouch–anal anastomosis, are indicated to prevent this complication. Beta-adrenergic blockers and endoscopic sclerotherapy are not associated with long-term efficacy, while transjugular intrahepatic portosystemic shunts (TIPS) can be effective in treating refractory bleeding.

Several large studies have supported the association between colorectal neoplasia and PSC [54]. For invasive carcinoma or high-grade dysplasia, surgical colectomy is the treatment of choice. Patients with low-grade or indefinite histology for dysplasia may be followed with heightened endoscopic surveillance and biopsy protocols. Ursodeoxycholic acid (UDCA) cannot currently be recommended for chemoprevention, given the absence of a prospective controlled trial.

PSC and CCA

Patients with PSC have a 100-fold higher risk of developing CCA as compared to the general population [50]. The lifetime risk of CCA in patients with PSC is estimated to be between 5 and 10% [50, 55, 56]. Risk factors for CCA in PSC remain poorly understood. A serum carbohydrate antigen 19-9 (CA 19-9) level greater 130 IU/mL has a sensitivity of 79% and specificity of 98% [50]. However, this has not been shown to increase the detection of early-stage or localized cancer. Cross-sectional imaging can be helpful when a periductal mass is located in patients suspected to have CCA.

In patients with PSC who have a dominant stricture, an ERCP should be performed, along with biopsy and brush cytology of identified dominant strictures. While the sensitivity of brush cytology is low (between 18 and 40%) [57], recent studies have shown that fluorescent *in situ* hybridization (FISH) may increase the yield of conventional cytology. If a polysomy is found by FISH, the sensitivity and specificity for a diagnosis of CCA are 41 and 98%, respectively [58].

Therapeutic options for CCA in PSC are limited. Systemic chemotherapy and radiation for patients with advanced disease provide a limited survival advantage. In a protocol for highly selected patients with unresectable localized CCA, a 5-year actuarial survival rate greater than 70% after liver transplantation has been reported [59].

Medical, Endoscopic, and Surgical Treatment

No medical therapy has been proven to alter the course of disease in PSC. D-penicillamine, colchicine, corticosteroids, azathioprine, cyclosporine, and methotrexate are not considered effective treatments. RCTs have not identified a survival benefit with UDCA at a dose of 13–15 mg/kg/day [52]. Two RCTs of higher-dose UDCA also failed to identify clinical and survival benefits when compared to placebo [60, 61]. Novel therapies, including oral nicotine, pirfenidone, pentoxifylline, silymarin, mycophenolate mofetil, and tacrolimus, have not been associated with clinical benefit in patients with PSC.

The use of endoscopic dilation with sphincterotomy with or without stenting is associated with clinical response rates in 60–90% of patients. However, stent placement is associated with a markedly high risk of complications such as bacterial cholangitis when compared with balloon dilation alone [52, 62].

Surgical resection has been performed among precirrhotic individuals with extrahepatic biliary strictures refractory to endoscopic/percutaneous therapy. A number of concerns exist, however, with regard to the long-term consequences of surgical therapy. For patients requiring liver transplantation, a prior history of operative bile duct resection has been associated with longer procedure times, greater intraoperative blood loss, and increased risks for subsequent biliary complications [63, 64].

PSC remains an important etiology for liver transplantation in the United States. Excellent patient survival rates of 90–97% at 1 year and 83–88% at 5 years are reported [65]. Within 10 years following liver transplantation, recurrence rates of PSC have been reported to be between 30 and 50% [66]. In patients with PSC, the occurrence of perihilar CCA is a specific indication for liver transplantation. One multicenter analysis of patients who underwent liver transplantation for CCA showed recurrence-free survival rates of 65% [67].

Take Home Points

- Most patients with gallstones are asymptomatic.
- Ultrasonography is the initial diagnostic imaging test of choice for evaluation of cholelithiasis and cholecystitis.
- Laparoscopic cholecystectomy is the preferred therapy for the management of symptomatic cholelithiasis and cholecystitis.
- Endoscopic retrograde cholangiopancreatography (ERCP) is the preferred therapy for the management of acute cholangitis.
- Larger gallbladder polyps are at higher risk of malignant conversion, and laparoscopic cholecystectomy is recommended for gallbladder polyps >10 mm.
- Biliary fluke infection in humans is most often caused by *Clonorchis sinensis* and *Opisthorchis viverrini*, and most patients are asymptomatic. The treatment of choice for biliary fluke infection is antiparasitic drugs.
- Biliary fluke infection increases the risk of cholangiocarcinoma (CCA).
- CCA can occur anywhere along the length of the biliary tree. The most common presenting symptom is obstructive jaundice.
- The diagnosis of CCA can be very challenging and may require multiple radiologic and endoscopic studies.
- The prognosis for non-resectable CCA is generally poor, but liver transplantation may be an option, with good outcomes for selected cases.
- Gallbladder cancer is a rare tumor. Endoscopic ultrasound (EUS) is the test of choice for staging.
- A history of inflammatory bowel disease (IBD) and elevated serum liver biochemistries should prompt evaluation for primary sclerosing cholangitis (PSC).

CHAPTER 86

- Cholangiography is the gold standard for diagnosis in PSC. The cholangiogram can show a characteristic "beads on a string" appearance due to segmental bile duct fibrosis with saccular dilation of normal intervening areas.
- ERCP with endoscopic dilation, with or without stenting, is associated with good clinical response rates in selected patients with PSC.
- Liver transplantation is an option for patients with advanced PSC and is associated with excellent 1- and 5-year survival rates.

References

1 Kratzer W, Mason RA, Kachele V. Prevalence of gallstones in sonographic surveys worldwide. *J Clin Ultrasound* 1999; **27**(1): 1–7.

2 Russo MW, Wei JT, Thiny MT, *et al.* Digestive and liver diseases statistics, 2004. *Gastroenterology* 2004; **126**(5): 1448–53.

3 Carter HR, Cox RL, Polk HC Jr. Operative therapy for cholecystitis and cholelithiasis: trends over three decades. *Am Surg* 1987; **53**(10): 565–8.

4 Hirota M, Takada T, Kawarada Y, *et al.* Diagnostic criteria and severity assessment of acute cholecystitis: Tokyo Guidelines. *J Hepatobiliary Pancreat Surg* 2007; **14**(1): 78–82.

5 Gurusamy KS, Samraj K. Early versus delayed laparoscopic cholecystectomy for acute cholecystitis. *Cochrane Database Syst Rev* 2006(**6**):CD005440.

6 Yamashita Y, Takada T, Kawarada Y, *et al.* Surgical treatment of patients with acute cholecystitis: Tokyo Guidelines. *J Hepatobiliary Pancreat Surg* 2007; **14**(1): 91–7.

7 Griniatsos J, Petrou A, Pappas P, *et al.* Percutaneous cholecystostomy without interval cholecystectomy as definitive treatment of acute cholecystitis in elderly and critically ill patients. *South Med J* 2008; **101**(6): 586–90.

8 Attasaranya S, Fogel EL, Lehman GA. Choledocholithiasis, ascending cholangitis, and gallstone pancreatitis. *Med Clin North Am* 2008; **92**(4): 925–60, x.

9 Anon. NIH state-of-the-science statement on endoscopic retrograde cholangiopancreatography (ERCP) for diagnosis and therapy. *NIH Consens State Sci Statements* 2002; **19**(1): 1–26.

10 Guarise A, Baltieri S, Mainardi P, Faccioli N. Diagnostic accuracy of MRCP in choledocholithiasis. *Radiol Med* 2005; **109**(3): 239–51.

11 Mandelia A, Gupta AK, Verma DK, Sharma S. The value of magnetic resonance cholangio-pancreatography (MRCP) in the detection of choledocholithiasis. *J Clin Diagn Res* 2013; **7**(9): 1941–5.

12 Reinders JS, Goud A, Timmer R. Early laparoscopic cholecystectomy improves outcomes after endoscopic sphincterotomy for choledochocystolithiasis. *Gastroenterology* 2010; **138**(7): 2315–20.

13 Rosing DK, De Virgilio C, Nguyen AT, *et al.* Cholangitis: analysis of admission prognostic indicators and outcomes. *Am Surg* 2007; **73**(10): 949–54.

14 Tsujino T, Sugita R, Yoshida H, *et al.* Risk factors for acute suppurative cholangitis caused by bile duct stones. *Eur J Gastroenterol Hepatol* 2007; **19**(7): 585–8.

15 Hui CK, Lai KC, Yuen MF, *et al.* Acute cholangitis – predictive factors for emergency ERCP. *Aliment Pharmacol Ther* 2001; **15**(10): 1633–7.

16 Lee NK, Kim S, Lee JW, *et al.* Discrimination of suppurative cholangitis from non-suppurative cholangitis with computed tomography (CT). *Eur J Radiol* 2009; **69**(3): 528–35.

17 Boerma D, Rauws EA, Keulemans YC, *et al.* Wait-and-see policy or laparoscopic cholecystectomy after endoscopic sphincterotomy for bile-duct stones: a randomised trial. *Lancet* 2002; **360**(9335): 761–5.

18 Jorgensen T, Jensen KH. Polyps in the gallbladder. A prevalence study. *Scand J Gastroenterol* 1990; **25**(3): 281–6.

19 Karlsen TH, Schrumpf E, Boberg KM. Gallbladder polyps in primary sclerosing cholangitis: not so benign. *Curr Opin Gastroenterol* 2008; **24**(3): 395–9.

20 Yang HL, Sun YG, Wang Z. Polypoid lesions of the gallbladder: diagnosis and indications for surgery. *Br J Surg* 1992; **79**(3): 227–9.

21 Sugiyama M, Atomi Y, Yamato T. Endoscopic ultrasonography for differential diagnosis of polypoid gall bladder lesions: analysis in surgical and follow up series. *Gut* 2000; **16**(2): 250–4.

22 Owen CC, Bilhartz LE. Gallbladder polyps, cholesterolosis, adenomyomatosis, and acute acalculous cholecystitis. *Semin Gastrointest Dis* 2003; **14**(4): 178–88.

23 Kubota K, Bandai Y, Noie T, *et al.* How should polypoid lesions of the gallbladder be treated in the era of laparoscopic cholecystectomy? *Surgery* 1995; **117**(5): 481–7.

24 Levy AD, Murakata LA, Abbott RM, Rohrmann CA Jr. From the archives of the AFIP. Benign tumors and tumorlike lesions of the gallbladder and extrahepatic

25 Zielinski MD, Atwell TD, Davis PW, *et al.* Comparison of surgically resected polypoid lesions of the gallbladder to their pre-operative ultrasound characteristics. *J Gastrointest Surg* 2009; **13**(1): 19–25.

26 Ishikawa O, Ohhigashi H, Imaoka S, *et al.* The difference in malignancy between pedunculated and sessile polypoid lesions of the gallbladder. *Am J Gastroenterol* 1989; **84**(11): 1386–90.

27 Marcos LA, Terashima A, Gotuzzo E. Update on hepatobiliary flukes: fascioliasis, opisthorchiasis and clonorchiasis. *Curr Opin Infect Dis* 2008; **21**(5): 523–30.

28 Lim JH, Kim SY, Park CM. Parasitic diseases of the biliary tract. *Am J Roentgenol* 2007; **188**(6): 1596–603.

29 Choi D, Lim JH, Lee KT, *et al.* Cholangiocarcinoma and *Clonorchis sinensis* infection: a case-control study in Korea. *J Hepatol* 2006; **44**: 1066–73.

30 Vaeteewootacharn K, Seubwai W, Bhudhisawasdi V, *et al.* Potential targeted therapy for liver fluke associated cholangiocarcinoma. *J Hepatobiliary Pancreat Sci* 2014; **21**(6): 362–70.

31 Maringhini A, Moreau JA, Melton LJ 3rd, *et al.* Gallstones, gallbladder cancer, and other gastrointestinal malignancies. An epidemiologic study in Rochester, Minnesota. *Ann Intern Med* 1987; **107**: 30–5.

32 Nath G, Singh H, Shukla VK. Chronic typhoid carriage and carcinoma of the gallbladder. *Eur J Cancer Prev* 1997; **6**: 557–9.

33 Sharma V, Chauhan VS, Nath G, *et al.* Role of bile bacteria in gallbladder carcinoma. *Hepatogastroenterology* 2007; **54**(78): 1622–5.

34 Soiva M, Aro K, Pamilo M, *et al.* Ultrasonography in carcinoma of the gallbladder. *Acta Radiol* 1987; **28**: 711–14.

35 Kumar A, Aggarwal S, Berry M, *et al.* Ultrasonography of carcinoma of the gallbladder: an analysis of 80 cases. *J Clin Ultrasound* 1990; **18**: 715–20.

36 Li D, Dong BW, Wu YL, Yan K. Image-directed and color Doppler studies of gallbladder tumors. *J Clin Ultrasound* 1994; **22**: 551–5.

37 Ogura T, Kurisu Y, Masuda D, *et al.* Can endoscopic ultrasound-guided fine needle aspiration offer clinical benefit for thick-walled gallbladders? *Dig Dis Sci* 2014; **59**(8): 1917–24.

38 Kim HJ, Lee SK, Jang JW, *et al.* Diagnostic role of endoscopic ultrasonography-guided fine needle aspiration of gallbladder lesions. *Hepatogastroenterology* 2012; **59**(118): 1691–5.

39 You DD, Lee HG, Paik KY, *et al.* What is an adequate extent of resection for T1 gallbladder cancers? *Ann Surg* 2008; **247**: 835–8.

40 Shaib Y, El-Serag HB. The epidemiology of cholangiocarcinoma. *Semin Liver Dis* 2004; **24**: 115–25.

41 Burak K, Angulo P, Pasha TM, *et al.* Incidence and risk factors for cholangiocarcinoma in primary sclerosing cholangitis. *Am J Gastroenterol* 2004; **99**: 523–6.

42 Bergquist A, Ekbom A, Olsson R, *et al.* Hepatic and extrahepatic malignancies in primary sclerosing cholangitis. *J Hepatol* 2002; **36**: 321–7.

43 Nakeeb A, Pitt HA, Sohn TA. Cholangiocarcinoma: a spectrum of intrahepatic, perihilar and distal tumors. *Ann Surg* 1996; **224**: 463–75.

44 Nagorney DM, Kendrick ML. Hepatic resection in the treatment of hilar cholangiocarcinoma. *Adv Surg* 2006; **40**: 159–71.

45 Neuhaus P, Jonas S, Bechstein WO, *et al.* Extended resections for hilar cholangiocarcinoma. *Ann Surg* 1999; **230**: 808–19.

46 De Vreede I, Steers J, Burch P, *et al.* Prolonged disease-free survival after orthotopic liver transplantation plus adjuvant chemoirradiation for cholangiocarcinoma. *Liver Transpl* 2000; **6**: 309–16.

47 Rea DJ, Heimbach JK, Rosen CB, *et al.* Liver transplantation with neoadjuvant chemoradiation is more effective than resection for hilar cholangiocarcinoma. *Ann Surg* 2005; **242**: 451–61.

48 Mendes F, Lindor KD. Primary sclerosing cholangitis: overview and update. *Nat Rev Gastroenterol Hepatol* 2010; **7**: 611–19.

49 Molodecky NA, Kareemi H, Parab R, *et al.* Incidence of primary sclerosing cholangitis: a systematic review and meta-analysis. *Hepatology* 2011; **53**: 1590–9.

50 Singh S, Talwalkar JA. Primary sclerosing cholangitis: diagnosis, prognosis, and management. *Clin Gastroenterol Hepatol* 2013; **11**(8): 898–907.

51 Bambha K, Kim WR, Talwalkar J, *et al.* Incidence, clinical spectrum, and outcomes of primary sclerosing cholangitis in a United States community. *Gastroenterology* 2003; **125**: 1364–9.

52 Talwalkar JA, Lindor KD. Primary sclerosing cholangitis. *Inflamm Bowel Dis* 2005; **11**: 62–72.

53 Berstad AE, Aabakken L, Smith HJ, *et al.* Diagnostic accuracy of magnetic resonance and endoscopic retrograde cholangiography in primary sclerosing cholangitis. *Clin Gastroenterol Hepatol* 2006; **4**: 514–20.

54 Claessen MM, Vleggaar FP, Tytgat KM, *et al.* High lifetime risk of cancer in primary sclerosing cholangitis. *J Hepatol* 2009; **50**: 158–64.

55 Razumilava N, Gores GJ, Lindor KD. Cancer surveillance in patients with primary sclerosing cholangitis. *Hepatology* 2011; **54**: 1842–52.

56 Claessen MM, Vleggaar FP, Tytgat KM, *et al.* High lifetime risk of cancer in primary sclerosing cholangitis. *J Hepatol* 2009; **50**: 158–64.

57 Claessen MM, Vleggaar FP, Tytgat KM, *et al.* High lifetime risk of cancer in primary sclerosing cholangitis. *J Hepatol* 2009; **50**: 158–64.

58 Moreno Luna LE, Kipp B, Halling KC, *et al.* Advanced cytologic techniques for the detection of malignant pancreatobiliary strictures. *Gastroenterology* 2006; **131**: 1064–72.

59 Heimbach JK. Successful liver transplantation for hilar cholangocarcinoma. *Curr Opin Gastroenterol* 2008; **24**: 384–8.

60 Silveira MG, Lindor KD. High dose ursodeoxycholic acid for the treatment of primary sclerosing cholangitis. *J Hepatol* 2008; **48**(5): 692–4.

61 Olsson R, Boberg KM, de Muckadell OS, *et al.* High-dose ursodeoxycholic acid in primary sclerosing cholangitis: a 5-year multicenter, randomized, controlled study. *Gastroenterology* 2005; **129**(5): 1464–72.

62 Kaya M, Petersen BT, Angulo P, *et al.* Balloon dilation compared to stenting of dominant strictures in primary sclerosing cholangitis. *Am J Gastroenterol* 2001; **96**: 1059–66.

63 Cameron JL, Pitt HA, Zinner MJ, *et al.* Resection of hepatic duct bifurcation and transhepatic stenting for sclerosing cholangitis. *Ann Surg* 1988; **207**: 614–22.

64 Graziadei IW, Wiesner RH, Marotta PJ, *et al.* Long-term results of patients undergoing liver transplantation for primary sclerosing cholangitis. *Hepatology* 1999; **30**: 1121–7.

65 Fosby B, Karlsen TH, Melum E. Recurrence and rejection in liver transplantation for primary sclerosing cholangitis. *World J Gastroenterol* 2012; **18**: 1–15.

66 Darwish Murad S, Kim WR, Harnois DM, *et al.* Efficacy of neo-adjuvant chemoradiation, followed by liver transplantation, for perihilar cholangiocarcinoma at 12 US centers. *Gastroenterology* 2012; **143**: 88–98.e3, quiz e14.

CHAPTER 86

Portal Hypertension

Humberto C. Gonzalez and Patrick S.Kamath

Division of Gastroenterology and Hepatology, Mayo Clinic, Rochester, MN, USA

Summary

Clinical manifestations of portal hypertension include varices, ascites, spontaneous bacterial peritonitis (SBP), hepatorenal syndrome (HRS), hepatic encephalopathy, and hepatopulmonary syndrome (HPS). Detailed management for each condition is reviewed in this chapter.

Introduction

Portal hypertension results from an increase in the product of portal resistance and portal bloodflow. An increase in portal resistance may be caused by fibrosis and nodularity of the cirrhotic liver, or by intrahepatic vasoconstriction, which results largely from low levels of nitric oxide (NO), a vasodilator, and high levels of endothelin-1, a vasoconstrictor. Increased portal bloodflow in cirrhosis is a result of splanchnic and systemic dilation, effected by NO [1]. Depending on the site of increased resistance, portal hypertension is classified as presinusoidal, sinusoidal, or postsinusoidal.

Portal hypertension is defined as an increase in hepatic sinusoidal pressure to ≥ 6 mmHg. The most common cause of portal hypertension in the Western world is cirrhosis. Cirrhosis is a histological diagnosis (liver biopsy is not needed if the diagnosis is clinically evident). The major complications of portal hypertension include variceal bleeding, ascites and hepatic encephalopathy. In this setting, cirrhosis is associated with a median survival of less than 2 years.

Other common causes of portal hypertension include schistosomiasis (in the developing world) and extrahepatic portal vein thrombosis. Portal hypertension may be idiopathic, especially in patients from India and Japan. Other rarer causes of portal hypertension include splanchnic arteriovenous fistula, Budd–Chiari syndrome, polycystic liver disease, nodular regenerative hyperplasia of the liver, congenital hepatic fibrosis, myeloproliferative disorders, hepatic sarcoidosis, and hereditary hemorrhagic telangiectasia.

Diagnosis of Portal Hypertension

Portal venous pressure is measured either directly by portal venography or indirectly by the hepatic vein pressure gradient (HVPG). The HVPG is the difference between the wedged hepatic venous pressure (WHVP) and the free hepatic vein pressure (FHVP). As the HVPG is a measure of the hepatic sinusoidal pressure, in presinusoidal causes of portal hypertension, such as portal vein thrombosis, the HVPG is normal.

Ultrasonography

Changes of portal hypertension noted on ultrasonography include splenomegaly, reversal of flow in the portal vein, and portosystemic collateral bloodflow. Ultrasonography can also demonstrate ascites, and thrombosis in the portal or splenic vein.

Computed Tomography

The cirrhotic configuration of the liver, splenomegaly, portosystemic collaterals, and ascites may be demonstrated. Computed tomography (CT) can differentiate between submucosal and serosal surface varices [2], but is not yet recommended as a screening modality for esophageal varices.

Magnetic Resonance Imaging

Magnetic resonance imaging (MRI) provides an excellent view of the vascularity of the liver and the flow through the portal and azygous veins, but is still an investigational tool in the detection of esophageal varices. Magnetic resonance elastography (MRE) can measure hepatic stiffness, with values >4.9 suggesting advanced fibrosis. Portal hypertension is associated with increasing hepatic stiffness.

Varices

Varices are dilated and tortuous veins that develop in an effort to decompress the elevated hepatic sinusoidal pressure.

Case 1

A 62-year-old man presents to the emergency room (ER) at 6:00 am with complaints of vomiting blood 1 hour ago. He denies any retching or abdominal pain. His last bowel movement was last night, and was softer than his usual and dark in color.

He has a past history of alcohol consumption of up to six cans of beer a day for 30 years, but he quit 6 months ago. He also has multiple tattoos, some of which he got when he was in East Asia. He denies ever being ill in the past, and in fact does not even have a primary care physician.

On examination, he is afebrile, pulse 95, blood pressure 90/48. He appears mildly anxious. Skin examination reveals scleral icterus and multiple spider nevi on the front and back of the chest. Heart and lung examinations reveal no abnormality. He has no palpable hepatomegaly. However, the tip of the spleen is palpable 2 cm below the costal margin. There is dullness to percussion in both flanks.

In the ER, he has another emesis, and dark-red blood is noted in the pan.

Practical Gastroenterology and Hepatology Board Review Toolkit, Second Edition. Edited by Nicholas J. Talley, Kenneth R. DeVault, Michael B. Wallace, Bashar A. Aqel and Keith D. Lindor.

Pathophysiology

Portal hypertension results in the formation of portosystemic collaterals and dilation of pre-existing collaterals. Flow in these collaterals is away from the liver into the systemic circulation. The gastroesophageal area is the main site of collateral formation [3]. At the gastroesophageal junction, there are longitudinal veins in the submucosa that drain into the short and left gastric veins. The fundus of the stomach drains into the splenic veins via the short gastric veins. Splenic vein thrombosis can cause isolated gastric fundal varices. At the umbilicus, the vestigial umbilical vein (systemic) communicates with the left portal vein (portal). The varices at the umbilicus are characteristically described as "caput medusae." In the rectum, the collaterals are between the inferior mesenteric vein (portal) and the pudendal vein (systemic).

Portal pressure must be at least 10 mmHg for gastroesophageal varices to develop, and at least 12 mmHg for varices to bleed. Increased wall tension, a risk factor for bleeding in varices [4], depends on the pressure within the varix (increased with higher bloodflow through the varix), the size of the varix (larger varices are more likely to bleed), and wall thickness. Varices in the lower third of the esophagus are more likely to bleed because of the limited soft-tissue support.

Clinical Features

Variceal bleeding must be considered if a patient presents with gastrointestinal (GI) bleeding and features of chronic liver disease. Bleeding from gastric and/or esophageal varices manifests as hematemesis, hematochezia, or melena. The hematemesis is classically effortless, with vomiting of dark-red blood. Portal hypertensive gastropathy (PHG) and gastric antral vascular ectasia (GAVE) manifest more commonly with anemia.

Detection of Varices: Esophagogastroduodenoscopy

All patients with cirrhosis should be screened for varices with an esophagogastroduodenoscopy (EGD). Varices are graded during withdrawal of the endoscope with the esophagus maximally inflated after deflating the stomach. Medium/large varices are >5 mm in diameter and small varices are <5 mm in diameter. The presence or absence of red signs on varices should be noted. Patients without varices develop them at a rate 8% per year. Patient with evidence of small varices develop large varices at a rate of 8% a year [5].

Treatment

Management of esophageal varices includes prevention of the initial bleed (primary prophylaxis), control of acute variceal bleeding, and prevention of rebleeding (secondary prophylaxis).

Non-selective β-blockers and endoscopic band ligation (endoscopic variceal legation, EVL) are the most common strategies used to treat varices. Other therapies include sclerotherapy, transjugular intrahepatic portosystemic shunts (TIPS), and surgical shunts.

β-blockers must be non-selective (e.g., propranolol or nadolol). $β_1$-receptor blockade decreases the cardiac output; $β_2$-receptor blockade in the mesenteric circulation allows unopposed action of $β_1$-adrenergic receptors, which results in vasoconstriction. The combination of decreased cardiac output and decreased splanchnic flow results in decreased portal bloodflow.

Propranolol is usually started at a dose of 20 mg twice a day. Nadolol is usually started at a dose of 40 mg once a day. Long-acting and evening dosing of β-blockers has been advocated, as the risk of bleeding is highest at nighttime [6]. Carvedilol, a non-selective β-blocker and alpha-1-adrenergic blocker is preferred in patients with hypertension or cardiovascular disease (CVD). Discontinuation of β-blockers may be necessary when patients develop refractory ascites.

Primary Prophylaxis

In patients with compensated cirrhosis who do not have varices on initial EGD, non-selective β-blockers are not indicated for prevention of bleeding. A repeat endoscopy should be performed in 3 years. If hepatic decompensation occurs, EGD should be done earlier, and annually thereafter [5].

In patients with cirrhosis and small varices that have never bled, increased risk criteria for hemorrhage (child B/C or presence of red wale marks on varices) will determine the need for intervention. In the presence of high-risk criteria, non-selective β-blockers are recommended to prevent the first variceal hemorrhage. In patients with small esophageal varices and child B'C cirrhosis, non-selective β-blockers can be initiated, though their long term benefit has not been established. Alternatively, repeat EGD can be accomplished in 1–2 years if cirrhosis remains compensated, or shortly after hepatic decompensation and yearly thereafter [5].

In patients with medium/large varices that have never bled and which have high-risk features for hemorrhage, non-selective β-blockers or EVL is recommended for the prevention of first variceal hemorrhage. EVL can be used if there are contraindications, intolerances, or difficulties with adherence to β-blockers [5].

Management of Acute Variceal Bleeding

Acute variceal bleeding is associated with a 6-week mortality rate of 20%. Treatment includes resuscitation of the patient, control of the bleed, and prevention of complications.

Two large-bore intravenous access lines should be established, and the airway should be protected with a low threshold for endotracheal intubation. Packed red blood cell (RBC) transfusions are indicated when the hemoglobin drops below 7 G/dL; overtransfusion may worsen the portal hypertension and be associated with worse outcomes.

A 7-day course of norfloxacin 400 mg orally, ciprofloxacin 400 mg intravenously, or levofloxacin 500 mg intravenously, all administered every 12 hours, may be used to prevent SBP and bacteremia [8]. In patients with advanced cirrhosis (child B/C) and GI hemorrhage, intravenous (IV) ceftriaxone (1 g/day) is more effective than oral norfloxacin in preventing bacterial infections – mostly those caused by Gram-positive organisms [9].

Pharmacotherapy

Vasopressin is the most potent splanchnic vasoconstrictor, but is seldom used nowadays because of its side effects (including bowel necrosis, bradycardia, hyponatremia, and myocardial infarction) [10].

Terlipressin, a vasopressin analogue with lower risk of side effects, is widely used in Europe but is not available in the United States.

Somatostatin and its analogues decrease portal pressure by inhibiting release of glucagon [11]. They constrict the splanchnic arterioles and decrease postprandial portal bloodflow. Octreotide is given as an initial IV bolus (50 µg), followed by a continuous infusion of 50 µg/hour. Somatostatin and its analogues are safe and are used continuously for up to 5 days [5].

Endoscopic Therapy

1 Band ligation, the preferred method of control of bleeding from esophageal varices, should be performed as soon as the patient is hemodynamically stable, and after the vasoactive agent has been infused for at least 30 minutes. Variceal ligation involves suctioning of a varix into the channel of the endoscope and then firing a band around the base of the varix. The optimal site of ligation is at, or immediately distal to, the point of bleeding. If evidence of a recent bleed is seen, such as a white fibrin plug or thrombus over a varix, or any red signs, the site should be banded. If active bleeding is not seen but large varices are present, the varices should be banded, starting at the gastroesophageal junction and moving proximally in a spiral fashion at intervals of 2 cm. Complications of banding include esophageal ulcers, strictures, dysmotility, and rebleeding after the band sloughs off.

2 Sclerotherapy is seldom used as first-line treatment of variceal bleeding [12]. It involves injection of a sclerosant (e.g., sodium tetradecylsulfate) either into (intravariceal) or adjacent to (paravariceal) a varix. Sclerotherapy should be used when EVL is not available. Complications include retrosternal discomfort, ulcers, strictures, and perforation.

Transjugular Intrahepatic Portosystemic Shunts

If bleeding from varices cannot be controlled after two sessions of endoscopic therapy within a 24-hour period, TIPS placement is recommended. TIPS are also used to prevent rebleeding. Once variceal bleeding has been controlled in patients at high risk of rebleeding, TIPS should be inserted within 72 hours – preferably as early as possible. Patients at high risk of bleeding include those with Child–Turcotte–Pugh (CTP) class C, those with CTP class B with active bleeding, and those with Model for End-Stage Liver Disease (MELD) score >18. Patients with early treatment have better survival (86 vs. 61%) and lower rebleeding rates (3 vs. 50%) at 1 year.

TIPS create a communication between the hepatic vein and an intrahepatic branch of the portal vein using an expandable metallic stent, and so decompress the high portal pressures. The shunt is placed by an interventional radiologist via a transjugular approach, and dilated as needed to reduce the portacaval pressure gradient to below 12 mmHg. Nowadays, coated stents are used to reduce the frequency of shunt stenosis.

Immediate complications of TIPS placement include intraperitoneal hemorrhage, sepsis, and cardiopulmonary failure due to excessive right heart volume. Early complications include shunt thrombosis or migration, hepatic encephalopathy, progressive hepatic failure, and pulmonary artery hypertension. Late complications include shunt stenosis, progressive hepatic encephalopathy, portal vein thrombosis, and heart failure.

The best indicator of failure of a TIPS is recurrence of GI bleeding. TIPS should be avoided in patients with a MELD score >24, as they have a reduced survival [13]. In patients with a MELD score ≤14, survival is excellent. Severe hepatic encephalopathy is a relative contraindication for TIPS. The best method of evaluating the patency of TIPS is through hepatic venogram and measurement of the portacaval pressure gradient.

Secondary Prophylaxis

Following the first variceal bleed, up to 80% of patients rebleed at 2 years. Therefore, secondary prophylaxis with β-blockers, or variceal ligation, or the combination, should be initiated. Isosorbide mononitrate can be added to β-blockers to decrease the portal pressure further, but nitrates are not usually well tolerated, due to headaches and hypotension.

Patients who have a variceal bleed despite β-blockers and band ligation should be considered for a portosystemic shunt placement. If a patient has Child–Pugh class A cirrhosis, a distal splenorenal surgical shunt can be considered; in all others, TIPS should be considered.

Varices at Other Sites

Gastric Varices

- Type 1 gastroesophageal varices (GOV1) extend 2–5 cm below the gastroesophageal junction and in continuity with esophageal varices.
- Type 2 gastroesophageal varices (GOV2) occur in the fundus of the stomach and in continuity with esophageal varices.
- Isolated gastric varices occur in the fundus (IGV1) or distal stomach (IGV2) in the absence of esophageal varices [14].

GOV1 make up 70% of all gastric varices. IGV1 can result from splenic vein thrombosis, but the most common cause is cirrhosis. Bleeding is most common from large gastric fundal varices (≥10 mm in diameter). β-blockers may be used for primary prophylaxis, but endoscopic treatment is not currently recommended. Treatment of acute bleeding from gastric varices is similar to that of esophageal variceal bleeding, except that the preferred endoscopic therapy is injection of polymers of cyanoacrylate into the varices [15]. Complications of cyanoacrylate injection include bacteremia, ulceration, and cerebral and pulmonary emboli. Ligation is safe if the varices are in the cardia of the stomach (GOV1) and <10 mm in diameter. Most patients with refractory bleeding from gastric varices require a TIPS that controls 90% of bleeding [16,17].

Ectopic Varices

Ectopic varices are varices that occur elsewhere than in the esophagus and stomach. They account for <5% of all variceal bleeds. Ectopic varices usually present with melena. Cirrhosis is a cause of duodenal varices, but typically duodenal varices are associated with portal vein thrombosis [18]. Peristomal varices are seen especially often in patients with primary sclerosing cholangitis and ulcerative colitis after a proctocolectomy [19]. They appear as a bluish halo around the stoma, with the stoma appearing dusky and friable. Anorectal varices are formed by dilated superior and middle hemorrhoidal veins. They collapse with digital pressure, unlike hemorrhoids, which do not.

Clinical evidence of bleeding from ectopic intra-abdominal varices includes a sudden increase in baseline ascites with abdominal pain, hypotension, and a fall in the hematocrit. A CT of the abdomen can help make the diagnosis, but confirmation is by paracentesis of bloody fluid.

There is no evidence to support primary prophylaxis against bleeding from ectopic varices. Control of bleeding and secondary prophylaxis is essentially the same as with gastroesophageal varices. To prevent rebleeding, β-blockers, surgery, or TIPS can be considered.

Portal Hypertensive Gastropathy and Gastric Antral Vascular Ectasia

Mild PHG is diagnosed by the endoscopic appearance of a mosaic-like pattern of the gastric mucosa; severe PHG has a mosaic-like pattern with superimposed red spots [20].

The usual presentation of PHG bleeding is with anemia, but primary prophylaxis is not recommended. β-blockers are recommended only in patients with anemia [21, 22]. TIPS are effective in decreasing transfusion dependence in patients who bleed despite β-blocker therapy [23].

GAVE is diagnosed by the endoscopic appearance of red spots without a background mosaic pattern of the mucosa, usually confined to the antrum [24]. In "watermelon stomach," the lesions are linear in arrangement. Red spots distributed throughout the stomach are termed "diffuse gastric vascular ectasia." Mucosal biopsies show dilated mucosal capillaries with ectasia and foci of fibrin thrombi.

GAVE also presents with chronic bleeding. Treatment involves iron replacement and RBC transfusions. Argon plasma coagulation (APC) is normally used. Cryotherapy is another treatment modality. Oral estrogen 35 μg with norethindrone 1 mg daily can be employed, but side effects of gynecomastia may limit its use. TIPS are not recommended for GAVE, because they do not reduce the bleeding risk [23]. GAVE resolves with liver transplantation, but few patients are actually candidates for the procedure because the lesions typically occur in older people.

Ascites

Ascites is an increase in fluid in the abdominal cavity beyond the normal 50–100 mL.

Case 2

A 59-year-old woman presents to the clinic complaining that her clothes are steadily getting tighter, especially around the waist. She also complains of worsening swelling in her feet. She has a history of primary biliary cirrhosis diagnosed 10 years ago, for which she has been on ursodiol. She has had no other complications of her disease, and has no other medical problems.

On examination, she is afebrile, pulse 68, blood pressure 106/78. Abdominal examination reveals mild distension, positive for shifting dullness on percussion. Abdominal ultrasonography confirms the presence of ascites.

Pathophysiology

The most common cause of ascites in the United States is cirrhosis (about 85% of patients) [25]. Ascites in cirrhosis results from increased renal retention of sodium and water and elevated hepatic sinusoidal pressure, which leads to localization of fluid to the peritoneal space.

Vasodilation in the splanchnic and systemic vascular beds leads to effective hypovolemia [26]. This decrease in effective arterial blood volume activates vasoconstrictive pathways, including the renin–angiotensin–aldosterone pathway, the sympathetic nervous system, and antidiuretic hormone (ADH). The result is sodium and water retention and an increase in the intra-arterial blood volume. ADH hypersecretion leads to water retention and hyponatremia, a marker for advanced disease [27]. The increased sinusoidal hydrostatic pressure causes movement of fluid out of the sinusoids into the space of Disse. As portal hypertension worsens, the lymphatics become overwhelmed and excess lymph spills into the peritoneal cavity. Over time, the leaky sinusoidal basement membranes become less permeable to albumin, with less loss of albumin into the peritoneal cavity. This results in a low ascitic fluid albumin and high serum ascites–albumin gradient (SAAG) [28].

Clinical Features

History

Ascites presents as increasing abdominal girth, and may be associated with other clinical features of chronic liver disease. In patients with ascites, a history of risk factors for liver disease should be obtained. Other important questions are country of origin, family history of liver disease, autoimmune disease, exposure to herbal teas or supplements, and history of obesity.

If a patient with compensated cirrhosis has sudden development of ascites, then hepatocellular carcinoma (HCC), portal vein thrombosis, hepatic venous outflow obstruction, and worsening renal function should be considered. In a patient with a history of malignancy, peritoneal carcinomatosis is suspected. Tuberculous peritonitis is suspected in patients from endemic countries, or those with acquired immunodeficiency syndrome (AIDS). Myxedema may present with ascites, and therefore thyroid function must be evaluated.

Physical Examination

Ascites is demonstrated by shifting dullness. Approximately 1500 mL of fluid is needed in the abdomen for flank dullness to be present [29]. Demonstration of ascites is more difficult in patients with obesity or gaseous bowel distension. Abdominal ultrasonography is necessary to diagnose small-volume ascites. During the physical exam, other features of chronic liver disease, congestive heart failure, nephrotic syndrome, or malignancy should be noted.

Diagnosis

Ultrasonography, CT, or MRI is used to determine the cause of ascites. However, ascitic fluid analysis is imperative for confirmation of the diagnosis. Paracentesis must be performed when ascites is diagnosed for the first time and whenever a patient with ascites is hospitalized. Paracentesis can be repeated if signs or symptoms of an infection, including SBP, develop.

Complications of paracentesis are rare; they include abdominal wall and retroperitoneal hematomas and bowel perforations [30]. Measurement of platelet counts and prothrombin time and prophylactic transfusions of blood products are not recommended routinely before paracentesis [31]. Coagulopathy should preclude paracentesis only when there is clinically evident hyperfibrinolysis or disseminated intravascular coagulation [32].

The site for paracentesis may be guided by ultrasonography; if ultrasonography is not available, the left lower quadrant can be used (the right lower quadrant may contain distended cecum or scar tissue from a previous appendectomy). A point lateral to the midpoint between the umbilicus and left anterosuperior iliac spine is usually a safe location. The midline below the umbilicus may also be used, provided that the bladder is not distended. Paracenteses must be performed using sterile precautions and a local anesthetic; fluid is sent for a total and a differential cell count and for albumin. If there is suspicion of SBP, ascitic fluid is cultured.

SAAG is used to differentiate between causes of ascites (Table 87.1). It is calculated by subtracting the ascitic fluid albumin concentration from the serum albumin concentration. A SAAG ≥1.1 indicates portal hypertension as the cause of ascites [33]. The characteristics of other causes of ascites are shown in Table 87.2.

Table 87.1 Differentiation of causes of ascites using the serum ascites–albumin gradient (SAAG).

High SAAG (≥1.1)	Low SAAG (<1.1)
Cirrhosis	Tuberculous peritonitis
Alcoholic hepatitis	Peritoneal carcinomatosis
Fulminant hepatic failure	Pancreatic ascites
Cardiac failure	Biliary ascites
Budd–Chiari syndrome	Nephrotic syndrome
Sinusoidal obstruction	Bowel infarction
Portal vein thrombosis	Serositis in connective-tissue disease

Treatment

New-Onset Ascites

Management of non-cirrhotic ascites involves treatment of the underlying disease, and is not discussed here.

Ascites secondary to alcoholic hepatitis is unique in that it occurs secondary to portal hypertension, but may be reversed by abstinence from alcohol [34]. Patients are otherwise treated as for other forms of ascites.

Sodium restriction (90 mmol/day) is a very important part of the treatment, and requires rigorous dietary education.

Oral diuretics are the other component of management. The recommended initial doses of diuretics are furosemide 40 mg/day and spironolactone 100 mg/day; the maximum recommended doses are furosemide 160 mg/day and spironolactone 400 mg/day. When adjusting diuretic dose, a ratio of 40 : 100 should be maintained. Furosemide can produce side effects of hypokalemia, hyponatremia, and dehydration [32], so bumetanide (0.5–2.0 mg once a day) can be used as an alternative. To convert furosemide to bumetanide, divide the furosemide dose by 40. Spironolactone, used alone, can cause hyperkalemia. The most common reason for discontinuation of spironolactone is painful gynecomastia, however. If this occurs, spironolactone can be replaced with amiloride at a starting dose of 10 mg/day. Diuretic doses may be increased every 5–6 days, as long as serum creatinine and electrolytes are stable.

The maximum recommended weight loss during diuretic therapy is 0.5 kg/day in patients without lower limb edema and 1 kg/day in patients with edema [35].

To evaluate compliance with salt restriction and response to diuretics, either a random or a 24-hour urine sodium is measured; the latter is more accurate.

All diuretics should be discontinued if there is severe hyponatremia (serum sodium <120 mmol/L), progressive renal failure, worsening hepatic encephalopathy, or incapacitating muscle cramps. Diuretics are generally contraindicated in patients with overt hepatic encephalopathy [35].

The goal of long-term diuretic therapy is to maintain patients free of ascites with the minimum dose of diuretics. Once ascites has largely resolved, the dose of diuretics should be reduced and an attempt to discontinue them should be made whenever possible. Caution should be used when starting treatment with diuretics in patients with renal impairment, but there is no good evidence for what level of impairment is too severe for their use. Frequent monitoring of kidney function, sodium, potassium and other electrolytes should be carried out in this setting [35].

Non-steroidal anti-inflammatory drugs (NSAIDs) are contraindicated in patients with ascites because of the high risk of developing further sodium retention, hyponatremia, and renal failure. Angiotensin-converting enzyme (ACE) inhibitors, angiotensin II antagonists, and alpha-1-adrenergic receptor blockers decrease arterial pressure and renal bloodflow and so should not be used in the setting of ascites. Aminoglycosides are associated with an increased risk of renal failure, so their use should be reserved for patients with bacterial infections

If ascites is tense, a large-volume paracentesis (LVP) may be performed. Whenever more than 5 L of ascitic fluid is removed, or in a patient without lower limb edema, albumin replacement should be provided intravenously during or immediately after the procedure, at a dose of 6–8 g of albumin per liter of fluid removed. Albumin administration prevents postparacentesis circulatory dysfunction, which is associated with worsening renal function, rapid reaccumulation of ascites, and reduced survival [36, 37].

Refractory Ascites

Refractory ascites is defined as ascites that is unresponsive to maximal doses of diuretics or that recurs rapidly after paracenteses [38]. Refractory ascites may be diuretic-resistant or diuretic-intractable.

Repeated LVP can be used to treat diuretic-resistant ascites with albumin replacement after each tap. However, survival is not improved [39].

TIPS are used if patients require frequent LVP [40, 41]. TIPS are associated with an increased risk of hepatic encephalopathy. Sodium restriction and diuretics may need to be continued after TIPS placement, albeit at lower doses. Since the advent of TIPS, peritoneovenous shunts are seldom used.

The prognosis of patients with refractory ascites is poor, so they should be considered for liver transplantation [32].

Complications

Dilutional hyponatremia, associated with worsening of the underlying cirrhosis, results from excess free water retention. Hyponatremia is best treated with fluid restriction to 1000 mL/day. Hypertonic saline administration is required only if hyponatremia is secondary to overdiuresis.

Hepatic hydrothorax is a transudative pleural effusion, usually >500 mL, that occurs in patients with portal hypertension without any other underlying primary cardiopulmonary cause. Such effusions are found in approximately 5% of patients with cirrhosis and ascites. Hydrothorax results from movement of ascites across the diaphragmatic apertures into the pleural cavity, most often on the right side [42].

First-line treatment includes sodium restriction and diuretics. Thoracocentesis should be performed to relieve dyspnea. A chest

Table 87.2 Causes of ascites.

Ascitic fluid test	Abnormality	Disease condition
Bilirubin (mg/dL)	>6	Bile duct or upper small-intestinal perforation
Glucose (mg/dL)	<50	Secondary peritonitis
LDH (mU/mL)	≥225	Secondary peritonitis
Amylase	Highly increased	Acute pancreatitis or small intestinal perforation
Triglyceride (mg/dL)	>200	Chylous ascites
Absolute PMN count (cells/mm³)	>250	SBP
Absolute lymphocyte count	Highly increased	Tuberculous peritonitis

LDH, lactate dehydrogenase; PMN, polymorphonuclear leukocytes; SBP, spontaneous bacterial peritonitis.

tube should not be placed, because persistent leakage of fluid worsens survival. Use of TIPS is a second-line treatment and should be considered in refractory hepatic hydrothorax. Other, less well studied treatments include surgical repair of diaphragmatic defects and pleurodesis [42].

Analysis of the pleural fluid and the ascitic fluid demonstrates similar, but not identical, chemistry. Spontaneous bacterial empyema (SBE) is an infection of the hydrothorax in the absence of pneumonia. There is typically no pus or abscess in the thoracic cavity. Diagnostic criteria include a positive pleural culture and a polymorphonuclear >250 cells/mm^3 or a negative pleural culture with a polymorphonuclear count >500 cells/mm^3. SBE has been reported in up to 13% of hospitalized cirrhotic patients. It can occur without SBP in up to 40% of patients. Treatment is similar to that for SBP [42]. The use of albumin to prevent HRS has not been well studied. Long-term prophylaxis should be recommended.

Prognosis

The mortality rate after onset of ascites is approximately 15% in 1 year and 44% in 5 years [43]. Hyponatremia is an independent predictor of poor outcome [27,45]. Patients with ascites should be referred for consideration of liver transplantation.

Spontaneous Bacterial Peritonitis

SBP is diagnosed when the absolute polymorphonuclear leukocyte (PMN) count is >250 cells/mm^3 (neutrocytic ascites) with positive bacterial culture (usually a single organism) in the absence of an intra-abdominal source of infection [25]. Culture-negative neutrocytic ascites (CNNA) occurs when ascitic cultures are negative in the presence of neutrocytic ascites. "Bacterascites" describes positive ascitic cultures in the absence of neutrocytic ascites.

Case 3

A 48-year-old man with a history of cirrhosis secondary to hemochromatosis presents with his wife. She complains that he has been confused for the past 2 days. He has a history of ascites, which is treated with furosemide 40 mg/day and spironolactone 100 mg/day. However, he is not very compliant with his salt restriction, and hence his ascites has been hard to control completely.

On examination, he is febrile, pulse 82, blood pressure 94/70. Abdominal examination reveals a positive fluid wave, and the abdomen is diffusely tender to deep palpation. Asterixis is also present.

A paracentesis is performed and the cell count shows 800 white blood cells (WBCs) with 98% neutrophils. Cultures are pending.

Pathophysiology

Increased translocation of bowel bacteria into the circulation through the mesenteric lymph nodes results in transient bacteremia; subsequently, colonization of ascitic fluid takes place. When immune defenses are compromised, as in low protein ascites [46], intercurrent infections, and advanced liver disease, the patient develops SBP.

SBP may be associated with bacteremia from pneumonia or urinary tract infections (UTIs).

Secondary bacterial peritonitis, occurring secondary to intra-abdominal infection, is usually polymicrobial, including anaerobes.

Organisms

The most common organisms causing SBP are *Escherichia coli*, *Klebsiella pneumoniae*, and pneumococci. Other enteric Gram-negative and Gram-positive organisms may be cultured.

Oral selective bowel decontamination can alter the enteric flora, and patients may get SBP secondary to Gram-positive organisms, including enterococci [47].

Clinical Features

Patients with SBP may be symptomatic, but SBP should be ruled out in any hospitalized patient with ascites, especially with variceal bleeding [48]. Fever is the most common symptom associated with SBP [29]. Also noted are abdominal pain or tenderness, altered mental status, and HRS.

Diagnosis

The diagnosis of SBP requires demonstration of an absolute neutrophil count >250/mm^3 in ascitic fluid. The optimal method of ascitic fluid culture is inoculation of at least 10 mL of ascitic fluid in blood culture bottles at the bedside immediately after paracentesis.

Rare causes of neutrocytic ascitic fluid include tuberculosis, peritoneal carcinomatosis, and pancreatitis, though these conditions are more likely to have a lymphocytic predominance.

Treatment

Empirical antibiotic therapy for suspected SBP is warranted if a patient has convincing symptoms or signs of an infection (ascitic fluid neutrophil count >250 cells/mm^3) but culture results are pending [49].

Initially, cefotaxime 2 g IV every 8 hours or a similar third-generation cephalosporin is used [49], with dose adjusted in renal impairment. Alternative options include amoxicillin/clavulanic acid and quinolones such as ciprofloxacin or ofloxacin. However, the use of quinolones should not be considered in patients who are taking these drugs for prophylaxis against SBP, in areas of high prevalence of quinolone-resistant bacteria, or in nosocomial SBP [35].

Antibiotic coverage for anaerobes, *Pseudomonas*, and *Staphylococcus* spp. is not usually needed. If secondary peritonitis is suspected, metronidazole 400 mg IV every 8 hours or piperacillin–tazobactam 3.375 g IV every 6 hours is recommended. Antibiotics are tailored according to susceptibility results.

Intravenous albumin at a dose of 1.5 g/kg body weight on day 1 and 1.0 g/kg body weight on day 3 decreases the risk of renal failure and improves survival [50, 51].

Duration of treatment is usually 5 days. The ascitic fluid culture can become sterile after a single dose of cefotaxime in 86% of patients. Repeat paracentesis can be performed to document the decrease in PMN count. A decrease in ascitic neutrophil count >25% after 48 hours demonstrates response to treatment. If the neutrophil count does not decrease, secondary peritonitis is suspected [32].

Prognosis

SBP resolves with antibiotic therapy in approximately 90% of patients. Prognosis for patients with SBP may be improved with early detection and antibiotic therapy after an episode of SBP.

Secondary prophylaxis with norfloxacin 400 mg once daily is recommended. Alternative regimens include ciprofloxacin (750 mg once weekly, orally) and co-trimoxazole (800 mg sulfamethoxazole and 160 mg trimethoprim daily, orally), but evidence is not as strong as that with norfloxacin [35]. Primary prophylaxis is also used in patients without a history of SBP but with low protein ascites (<1.0 g/dL) [32].

Hepatorenal Syndrome

HRS is a functional renal failure occurring in patients with advanced liver disease [52]. Type 1 HRS, with median survival <30 days, is rapidly progressive; type 2 HRS is more indolent, with a median survival <6 months.

Case 4

A 75-year-old woman with a history of cirrhosis secondary to alcohol is admitted with SBP. She has had ascites for 2 years, controlled with diet and diuretics. On admission, her serum creatinine is 1.3 mg/dL. She is treated with intravenous cefuroxime for her SBP. On day 3, her serum creatinine rises to 2.8 mg/dL.

Pathophysiology

The pathophysiology of HRS represents the extreme end of renal vasoconstriction and renal sodium retention. A precipitating event such as SBP results in further systemic and renal vasoconstriction, and type 1 HRS can develop. Type 2 HRS develops when this circulatory imbalance continues for a prolonged period, but to a lesser degree.

Clinical Features

- Type 1 HRS is a severe and rapidly progressive renal failure, with doubling of serum creatinine to >2.5 mg/dL in <2 weeks [53].
- It almost always follows a precipitating event, such as SBP and variceal bleed [54]. About 25% of patients with SBP can develop type 1 HRS.
- Type 2 HRS is a more slowly progressive renal failure; the serum creatinine levels are usually between 1.5 and 2.5 g/dL.
- Type 2 HRS is usually associated with refractory ascites.
- Patients with type 2 HRS can develop type 1 HRS as well if there is a precipitating event.

Diagnosis

The current diagnostic criteria for HRS are:
- Cirrhosis with ascites.
- Serum creatinine >1.5 mg/dL.
- No improvement in serum creatinine (to <1.5 mg/dL) after at least 2 days of diuretic withdrawal and volume expansion with albumin (1 g/kg of body weight per day daily).
- Absence of shock.
- No current or recent treatment with nephrotoxic drugs.
- Absence of parenchymal kidney disease, as indicated by proteinuria >500 mg/day, microhematuria (>50 RBCs/high-power field), and/or abnormal renal ultrasonography.

HRS always needs to be differentiated from other etiologies of renal failure, including pre-renal causes such as overdiuresis, acute tubular necrosis, and, rarely, obstructive uropathy. Drugs such as aminoglycosides [55], NSAIDs [56], and vasodilators (e.g., prazosin, nitrates) can cause renal failure and must be avoided. Intrinsic renal diseases such as glomerulonephritis in patients with hepatitis B or C must be ruled out.

Treatment

The aim of treatment in HRS is correction of the circulatory dysfunction, including expansion of the intra-arterial volume with albumin and splanchnic vasoconstrictors, and correction of the portal hypertension.

Albumin

Albumin expands the central blood volume and increases cardiac output. It is most effective in type 1 HRS, but must also be used in type 2 HRS when therapeutic paracentesis is carried out. It is usually given intravenously as 1 g/kg body weight/day, up to 100 g/day.

Vasoconstrictor Agents

Terlipressin (initial dose 0.5–1.0 mg IV every 4–6 hours or continuous IV infusion starting at 2 mg/day) is the most widely used splanchnic vasoconstrictor worldwide [56]; however, it is not available in the United States. Oral midodrine (an α-agonist) at a dose of 7.5–15.0 mg three times a day plus subcutaneous octreotide at a dose of 100 μg/day is the combination most often used in the United States [57]. Norepinephrine has also been shown to be an effective and safe vasoconstrictor [58], but it is not often used.

With vasoconstrictors and albumin, about 60% of type 1 HRS will resolve. If a relapse occurs, the same agents are used.

TIPS

TIPS work by improving renal perfusion and the glomerular filtration rate (GFR), increasing urine sodium and water excretion, and correcting hyponatremia [59]. They thus help to eliminate the refractory ascites in patients with type 2 HRS. However, they can worsen hepatic encephalopathy. The role of TIPS in type I HRS is less clear.

Liver Transplantation

The ideal treatment for both types of HRS is liver transplantation.

After receipt of a liver transplant in patients with HRS, GFR may continue to decline for a brief period before it starts to recover. These patients have more complications and higher mortality rates than those without HRS [52, 53].

Hepatic Encephalopathy

Hepatic encephalopathy is the neuropsychiatric manifestation of acute and chronic liver disease. It results from a combination of portosystemic shunting and liver dysfunction.

Case 5

A 68-year-old man with cirrhosis secondary to hepatitis C presents for a routine visit. He feels well and his ascites is well controlled with diuretics. However, he says that he has been feeling very tired recently and is unable to get a good night's rest. He is sleeping a lot during the day. Also, he has noticed that his wife is always upset at him for forgetting about routine chores that she has asked him to perform.

On exam, he is afebrile, pulse 59, blood pressure 98/64. Abdomen is soft, non-tender. Asterixis not present.

Pathophysiology

In cirrhosis, hepatocellular dysfunction and portosystemic collaterals allow a rise in ammonia concentration in the bloodstream that crosses the blood–brain barrier (BBB). Gamma-aminobutyric acid (GABA), the major inhibitory transmitter in the brain, may be responsible for the neuroinhibition. The initial step is ammonia accumulation, due to impaired clearance by the liver. Ammonia exposure to cerebral structures leads to astrocyte swelling, through a number of different mechanisms. Once ammonia is present in the astrocyte, glutamate synthetase forms glutamine from glutamate. Glutamine then enters the mitochondria, producing glutaminase and ammonia, which results in a further increase in intracellular ammonia and consequent production of reactive nitrogen and oxygen species, perpetuating the edema. Benzodiazepine-like compounds (arising from intestinal flora, diet, and medications) may accumulate in the brain of cirrhotic patients due to impaired clearance. Benzodiazepine-like compounds bind to GABA receptors, inducing GABA release, neuroinhibition, and upregulation of peripheral-type benzodiazepine receptors (PBRs). The PBRs trigger the synthesis of neurosteroids, strong GABA agonists that, which induce cortical depression and thus hepatic encephalopathy [60]. A microsatellite in the promoter region of the glutaminase gene (TACC and CACC) has been linked to the development of overt hepatic encephalopathy in patients with cirrhosis. This might help identify patients at risk of overt hepatic encephalopathy [61].

The use of TIPS for treatment of variceal hemorrhage or ascites can result in post-TIPS-induced hepatic encephalopathy. Episodes are usually mild, present early, and respond to conventional medical therapy. Severe or refractory cases may require closure of the shunt. Post-TIPS hepatic encephalopathy occurs in 30–35% of patients; the main risk factors are prior history of hepatic encephalopathy, advanced age, and a high Child–Pugh score pre-TIPS [60].

Clinical Features

Hepatic encephalopathy usually presents as altered mental status or consciousness, and is classified as follows:
- Type A, associated with **a**cute liver disease.
- Type B, secondary to portosystemic shunts (**b**ypass), without chronic liver disease.
- Type C, due to **c**irrhosis [62].

The classification is based on clinical presentation, as shown in Table 87.3. Alternatively, the West Haven classification scores level of consciousness, intellect, behavior, and other neurologic abnormalities (Table 87.4).

Severe symptoms, such as drowsiness, can easily be identified in order to diagnose overt hepatic encephalopathy. Mild symptoms, on the other hand, require specialized testing, as they comprise cognitive and attention deficits. This stage is called "hepatic encephalopathy." Patients experience no disorientation, but abnormalities can be detected by neuropsychiatric testing. They are at risk of developing overt hepatic encephalopathy. Attention, vigilance, response inhibition, executive function, safety, and quality of life are impaired. Driving is not advised.

It has recently been proposed that minimal and stage 1 hepatic encephalopathy be combined under the heading "covert hepatic encephalopathy" and differentiated from "overt hepatic encephalopathy," which includes stages 2–4, where disorientation is a hallmark [63].

Table 87.3 Classification of hepatic encephalopathy.

Type	Characteristics
Episodic	Occurs intermittently
Precipitated	Occurs in the presence of a specific precipitant
Spontaneous	Occurs without a precipitant
Persistent	Affects the patient's daily living and activities

Table 87.4 Modified West Haven classification of hepatic encephalopathy.

Grade	Description
0	No abnormality detected
Minimal	No neurological symptoms
	Normal clinical examination
	Abnormal psychometric test performance
1	Trivial lack of awareness
	Euphoria or anxiety
	Shortened attention span
	Impairment of addition or substraction
2	Lethargy or apathy
	Disorientation to time
	Obvious personality change
	Inappropriate behaviors
3	Somnolence to semi-stupor
	Responsiveness to stimuli
	Confusion
	Gross disorientation
	Bizarre behavior
4	Coma – unable to test mental status

Diagnosis

The diagnosis of hepatic encephalopathy can be made on history and physical examination alone, but may require formal neuropsychiatric testing when mild. Altered sleep patterns and collateral history from the patient's family may provide clues to the diagnosis. The cranial nerves are usually spared, and sensory functions are intact. However, increased tone, motor slowing, impaired posture, and increased deep-tendon reflexes may be seen.

As there is no pathognomonic feature, other causes of altered sensorium, such as neurologic disorders, encephalopathies, and toxin or drug ingestions, must be excluded.

The most common precipitants are excess dietary protein, constipation, GI bleeding, infection (especially SBP), renal failure, overdiuresis and dehydration, hypokalemia, spontaneous or iatrogenic portosystemic shunts, decompensation of liver disease, HCC, and use of benzodiazepines and narcotics.

Hepatic encephalopathy after a TIPS procedure is more common in patients over the age of 60 and in those with a prior history of hepatic encephalopathy [64].

Asterixis, also called "flapping tremor," is present in stage 2 and 3 hepatic encephalopathy. It is elicited by having the patient fully extend the elbows and dorsiflex the wrists with the fingers spread apart. Asterixis appears as a rapid flexion–extension movement at the wrist and the metacarpophalangeal joints, with flexion being the more rapid component. Other causes of asterixis include uremia, hypercapnia, and drugs such as phenytoin, carbamazepine, and lithium.

Treatment

Chronic Hepatic Encephalopathy

Treatment of the precipitant factor depends on its correct identification. Hydration and management of renal insufficiency are key. The overall goal of pharmacological treatment is to target the reduction in production and/or absorption of ammonia.

Dietary protein must be limited to 1.0–1.5 g protein/kg/day. A low-protein diet is not recommended. Dairy and vegetable proteins are preferred to animal protein. Branched-chain amino acids prolong time to decompensation with hepatic encephalopathy [65, 66] but are not routinely recommended.

Non-absorbable disaccharides, including lactulose and lactitol (not approved for use in the United States), act by acidifying the colonic contents, which causes ionic trapping of ammonia, and reduces ammonia-producing bacteria through a cathartic effect [67]. Lactulose dosage must be titrated to achieve two to four semi-formed bowel movements a day. Lactulose is the first-line agent. Side effects include abdominal distention, cramping, diarrhea, and electrolyte abnormalities. The latter two can precipitate hepatic encephalopathy.

The antibiotics neomycin (4–6 g/day), metronidazole (250 mg three times daily), and rifaximin (550 two times daily) are believed to reduce the burden of ammonia-producing organisms in the gut. However, systemic absorption may occur and produce side effects: neomycin can cause ototoxicity and nephrotoxicity (long-term use requires annual auditory testing and continuos renal function monitoring), and metronidazole can cause peripheral neuropathy. Rifaximin is the antibiotic of choice, as it is minimally absorbed, has a broad spectrum for gut bacteria, and has a low risk of inducing bacterial resistance. Rifaximin has been shown to maintain remission and prevent hospitalizations from hepatic encephalopathy [68]. It is a second-line agent but is being used with increased frequency, in combination with lactulose or as monotherapy (where there are side effects to lactulose). The main limitation is its high cost.

L-ornithine-L-aspartate (LOLA), given orally or parenterally, increases ammonia fixation by the liver. It provides ornithine as a substrate in the urea cycle, which is defective in patients with cirrhosis, and improves hepatic ammonia clearance [69]. LOLA is not available for use in the United States.

Zinc is a trace element that is a critical cofactor of ammonia metabolism. Ammonia is converted to urea via ornithine transcarbamylase in the liver and to glutamic acid via glutamine synthetase in the skeletal muscle. Zinc deficiency is observed frequently in patients with cirrhosis and hepatic encephalopathy. Though still controversial, some studies have shown that zinc supplementation decreases the grade of hepatic encephalopathy and improves neuropsychiatric testing. Zinc sulfate is administered orally at 600 mg/day. It takes approximately 3 months to show results. Patients with zinc deficiency should be treated [70,71].

Flumazenil, a benzodiazepine receptor antagonist administered intravenously, is short-acting and not practical to use.

Large spontaneous portosystemic shunts (SPSS) are recognized as a cause of chronic protracted or recurrent hepatic encephalopathy. Embolization of large SPSS is safe and effective in most patients. Spontaneous portosystemic shunts must be considered as a cause in patients with refractory hepatic encephalopathy and MELD scores <15. [72].

Data on other therapies are very limited. Sodium benzoate (5 g orally twice daily) interacts with glycine to form hippurate, which is excreted renally, leading to loss of ammonia ions. Its use is limited by unpleasant taste and potential salt overload. Acarbose (150–300 mg/day) inhibits the conversion of carbohydrates into monosaccharides and facilitates the reduction of proteolytic bacteria, which produce benzodiazepine-like substances, mercaptans, and ammonia. Benefit has been reported in patients with diabetes and cirrhosis with mild to moderate hepatic encephalopathy. Side effects (abdominal bloating and pain, diarrhea, and flatulence) limit its use. Probiotics appears to reduce the serum ammonia concentrations by modulating intestinal bacteria and colonization of non-urease-producing bacteria. Improvement has been reported in patients with minimal hepatic encephalopathy [73].

Extracorporeal albumin dialysis using the molecular adsorbent recirculating system (MARS) has been used in the treatment of hepatic encephalopathy. In a short-term randomized controlled multicenter study, MARS was found to improve quicker and more frequently severe hepatic encephalopathy (stage 3 and 4) than standard medical therapy. MARS removes both protein-bound and water-soluble toxins from the blood using a recirculating albumin solution regenerated by charcoal and resin absorbers [74]. A session of treatment lasts 6–8 hours. MARS is currently approved by the US Food and Drug Administration (FDA) for treatment of chronic hepatic encephalopathy. Cost, invasiveness, and availability may limit its use.

Liver transplantation is the definitive treatment for hepatic encephalopathy.

Hepatic Encephalopathy Associated with Fulminant Hepatic Failure

Patients with grade 3 or 4 hepatic encephalopathy should be kept in an intensive care unit (ICU), sedated, paralyzed, and electively ventilated.

Intracranial pressure (ICP) catheters are used to monitor ICP. However, epidural catheters or subdural bolts carry a risk of hemorrhage as high as 20%.

Blood pressure should be tightly controlled, using phenylephrine if low or sodium nitroprusside or hydralazine if high, to maintain a cerebral perfusion pressure >60 mmHg.

Hyperventilation, mannitol boluses (100 mL 20% mannitol at 10-minutes intervals), or intravenous furosemide is used to decrease ICP. Mannitol is contraindicated if serum osmolality is greater than 320 mosmol/L or if there is oliguric renal failure. Hypothermia to 32–33 °C can also reduce ICP.

Specific therapy for the underlying disease should be started simultaneously: N-acetylcysteine for acetaminophen toxicity, penicillamine for Wilson's disease, or corticosteroid therapy for autoimmune hepatitis. A placebo-controlled trial involving patients with acute liver failure (ALF) due to causes other than acetaminophen found significantly higher transplant-free survival (40 vs. 27%) in patients randomized to N-acetylcysteine. The benefit was limited to patients with early-stage hepatic encephalopathy [75]. Additional studies are needed before this therapy can be routinely recommended, but its low side effect profile and potential benefits make it attractive, especially for patients who are not candidates for liver transplantation.

Liver transplantation must also be considered urgently in these patients.

Prognosis

Hepatic encephalopathy is a manifestation of both decompensation of chronic liver disease and acute hepatic failure, and is associated with decreased survival [76].

Hepatopulmonary Syndrome and Portopulmonary Hypertension

The pulmonary vascular complications of portal hypertension – HPS and portopulmonary hypertension (PPH) – significantly impact both survival and quality of life.

Case 6

A 55-year-old woman with cirrhosis secondary to hepatitis B complains of worsening dyspnea with exercise. Her cirrhosis has been well compensated so far, and in fact she has continued to work full time. Now, she is unable to walk up a single flight of stairs without needing to stop for air.

On exam, she is afebrile, pulse is 76 bpm, blood pressure 108/80 mmHg. Heart exam is normal, including jugular venous pressure. Lungs are clear. Abdomen is soft, non-tender. No pedal edema is seen.

Pulse oximetry on room air shows oxygen saturation of 88% at rest.

Hepatopulmonary Syndrome

Pathophysiology

HPS is primarily an arterial oxygenation defect, induced by dilation of the pulmonary precapillary and capillary vessels (15 μm diameter). Pleural and portopulmonary venous anastomoses may rarely be present. Intrapulmonary vascular dilation (IPVD) results in rapid shunting of mixed venous blood into the pulmonary veins, producing a ventilation–perfusion defect and causing hypoxemia. As a result of attenuation in the hypoxic vasoconstriction response in patients with cirrhosis, vasodilation is unopposed.

In advanced stages of the disease, an alveolar–capillary diffusion limitation to oxygen develops. This, along with the increased cardiac output seen in advanced cirrhosis, leads to further worsening of the total oxygenation of blood in the lungs.

Enhanced pulmonary production of NO through increased pulmonary vascular endothelial NO synthase (eNOS) and inducible NO synthase (iNOS in macrophages) causes vasodilation.

Clinical Features

HPS occurs in association with portal hypertension of all causes, as well as in patients with acute [77] and chronic hepatitis [78].

Dyspnea with exertion, or at rest, is the most common symptom. However, dyspnea is fairly common in patients with liver disease because of anemia, ascites, and muscle wasting. The diagnosis of HPS is made by measuring arterial blood gases, echocardiography, and brain–lung perfusion scanning.

Platypnea (worsened dyspnea from the supine to the upright position) is the pathognomonic symptom of HPS. Platypnea results from worsening of the ventilation–perfusion mismatch on standing due to orthodeoxia (decrease in arterial partial pressure of oxygen $\geq$5% or $\geq$4 mmHg).

In advanced HPS, digital clubbing and cyanosis of the lips and nail beds occur. Rarely, complications of right-to-left pulmonary communications may be seen, such as brain abscesses or polycythemia [79].

Diagnosis

The criteria for diagnosis include:
- Oxygenation defect: a PaO_2 <70 mmHg and/or PA–aO_2 $\geq$15 mmHg in the presence of portal hypertension and in the absence of other factors.
- Pulmonary vascular dilation:
  - Contrast-enhanced transthoracic echocardiography is a qualitative screening method used to demonstrate pulmonary vascular dilation. Agitated saline microbubbles, when injected into a peripheral vein, normally do not appear in the left heart. Appearance of bubbles in the left heart in fewer than three cardiac cycles suggests an intracardiac right-to-left communication. Appearance of microbubbles after three to six cardiac cycles confirms IPVD. Transesophageal echocardiography is more sensitive but is not used routinely.
  - ^{99m}Tc-labeled macroaggregated albumin injected into a peripheral vein is normally trapped in the lung, because the particle size is >20 μm. In HPS, particles pass through the dilated vasculature and are retained in the brain. Measurement of the uptake in the lungs and brain allows quantification of the pulmonary shunting. A brain shunt fraction >6% suggests HPS.
  - Pulmonary angiography is used only when embolization of macroscopic shunts is planned.

Treatment

There are currently no curative medical or pharmacological therapies for HPS. Liver transplantation is the only curative treatment.

Long-term oxygen therapy is used. Coil embolization of the IPVD is attempted only when a macroscopic IPVD is demonstrated on a chest CT scan.

Prognosis

Median survival after diagnosis of HPS for patients not undergoing liver transplantation is about 41 months [80]. Mortality usually results from complications of the liver disease. After transplantation, most patients experience complete resolution of HPS.

Portopulmonary Hypertension

Pathophysiology

Pulmonary arterial hypertension associated with portal hypertension results from pulmonary vasoconstriction. Endothelial and smooth-muscle proliferation, *in situ* thrombosis, and plexogenic arteriopathy ultimately result in increased resistance to pulmonary arterial bloodflow and pulmonary hypertension. Eventually, right ventricular hypertrophy, tricuspid regurgitation, right atrial dilation, and right heart failure develop. The resulting decrease in cardiac output worsens symptoms. TIPS in PPH may worsen the pulmonary hypertension by increasing right ventricular preload.

A variety of mechanisms have been proposed for the vasoconstriction. Vasoactive substances that escape the liver metabolism due to portosystemic shunting reach the lungs. Neurohormones such as serotonin and endothelin are implicated in vasoconstriction and mitogenesis. Release of cytokines such as tumor necrosis factor (TNF)-β and growth factors promotes vascular proliferation.

Clinical Features

Dyspnea and fatigue are the most common presenting manifestations. As PPH worsens, symptoms of right heart failure develop, including lower-extremity edema. In advanced PPH, chest discomfort and syncope may be seen.

Diagnosis

Transthoracic Doppler echocardiography is used to screen for PPH. Echocardiography can estimate only right ventricular systolic pressure (RVSP). However, right heart catheterization (RHC) is necessary to measure mean pulmonary arterial pressure (MPAP). RHC is indicated to evaluate RVSP >40 mmHg.

RHC is used to measure MPAP, pulmonary vascular resistance, and cardiac output. The hemodynamic response to vasodilators can also be measured to guide treatment. PPH is confirmed in a patient with portal hypertension with an MPAP $\geq$25 mmHg, pulmonary capillary wedge pressure <15 mmHg, and pulmonary vascular resistance >240 dyn s/cm^5.

Treatment

Diuretics may be used when pulmonary hypertension is secondary to volume overload. Hypovolemia can worsen cardiac output and precipitate HRS, however.

Oral anticoagulants are not usually recommended in PPH because of the risk of variceal bleeding.

Vasodilators are the mainstay of medical therapy. They can reverse vasoconstriction, but have no effect on the fibrotic and proliferative vascular changes. They should be used only after the diagnosis has been hemodynamically confirmed by RHC.

Prostacyclin (epoprostenol), a systemic and pulmonary vasodilator and platelet inhibitor, is derived from the metabolism of arachidonic acid. It is administered by continuous intravenous infusion and has a short half-life (3–5 minutes). It decreases the MPAP, PVR, and SVR by 11.8, 24.0, and 28.0%, respectively. Adverse effects include jaw pain, headaches, nausea, diarrhea, flushing, and catheter-related infections and thromboses. Interruption of the infusion can be life–threatening, due to the sudden loss of vasodilation. The inhaled form of treprostinil (Tyvaso) is approved in the United States.

PDE5 inhibitors (sildenafil, tadalafil, and vardenafil) prevent the breakdown of cyclic guanosine monophosphate, which mediates NO-induced vasodilation and reduces pulmonary artery pressure. They are administered orally. Sildenafil decreases MPAP and PVR, and is the most widely used PDE5 inhibitor.

Oral endothelin receptor antagonists (bosentan and ambrisentan) are used with increased frequency, alone or as combination therapy. Bosentan is a non-specific endothelin antagonist, while ambrisentan is a specific endothelin A antagonist [81, 82].

Unlike HPS, PPH is not considered an indication for liver transplantation. In fact, moderate-to-severe pulmonary hypertension has been shown to increase perioperative mortality and morbidity [83, 84], and is hence a contraindication to liver transplantation. Liver transplantation should not be attempted unless significant hemodynamic improvement and improved right heart function can be documented. Current United Network for Organ Sharing (UNOS) policy provides for MELD exceptions to facilitate timely liver transplant if significant hemodynamic improvement (mean pulmonary artery pressure <35 mm Hg) can be attained with pulmonary vasodilators. Within a couple of months after liver transplant, 40–50% of patients are able to be weaned off all forms of vasodilator therapy. Most patients on intravenous prostacyclin can be weaned off the infusion therapy, but some require oral vasodilators [81].

Prognosis

PPH implies a poor prognosis. The 5-year survival among untreated PPH patients is 14%; vasodilatory therapy improves this to 68% [81].

Take Home Points

Varices:
- Varices are dilated veins that develop as a result portal hypertension. They can be seen in the esophagus, stomach, rectum, umbilicus, and retroperitoneum. Those in the lower third of the esophagus are most likely to bleed.
- Screening for varices should be done when cirrhosis is diagnosed. Varices are most accurately diagnosed by EGD. If no varices are seen on the initial EGD, it should be repeated in 3 years. If small varices are present, repeat in 2 years. If hepatic decompensation occurs, perform EGD immediately and then annually.

- Primary prophylaxis for large varices is with non-selective β-blockers or endoscopic variceal ligation. Small varices with high-risk bleeding features can be managed with β-blockers.
- Acute variceal bleeding is treated with supportive measures, octreotide, and vasopressin analogues, and endoscopic therapy in the form of variceal banding. Antibiotic prophylaxis to prevent development of spontaneous bacterial peritonitis (SBP) is also needed. If bleeding is recurrent or intractable, TIPS may be beneficial, but hepatic encephalopathy is a limiting factor.
- Portal hypertension is diagnosed by measurement of the hepatic vein pressure gradient (HVPG) at ≥ 6 mmHg.
- Portal hypertensive gastropathy (PHG) may be mild (mosaic pattern of mucosa) or severe (with superimposed red spots). β-blockers are recommended when significant blood loss occurs. TIPS are reserved for selected cases that are refractory to medical therapy.
- Gastric antral vascular ectasia (GAVE) appears as red spots, without the mosaic background. It most commonly involves the antrum. It resolves with liver transplantation. Thermoablative therapies may be helpful.

Ascites:
- The most common cause of ascites is cirrhosis. Other causes include congestive heart failure, nephrotic syndrome, peritoneal carcinomatosis, and infections, including tuberculosis.
- A diagnostic paracentesis must be performed when ascites is diagnosed and whenever a patient with ascites is admitted to the hospital for any reason. Ascitic fluid should be evaluated for albumin and protein concentrations, cell count with differential, and culture.
- Management of ascites involves dietary restriction of sodium to 90 mmol/day and diuretics (furosemide and spironolactone). If ascites becomes refractory to diuretics, repeated paracenteses and TIPS are treatment options.
- Hepatic hydrothorax should be treated similarly. Avoid placement of chest tubes.
- Hyponatremia is an independent predictor of mortality and is treated with restriction of free water.

Spontaneous bacterial peritonitis:
- SBP is defined as ascitic fluid with a neutrophil count >250 cells/mm³ and a positive bacterial culture. The most common causative organisms are Gram-negative enteric flora (*E. coli*, *Klebsiella* sp., and pneumococci). In patients on chronic suppressive antibiotics or oral selective bowel decontamination, Gram-positive organisms are more common.
- SBP may present with fever or abdominal pain. It must be ruled out in patients who present with hepatorenal syndrome (HRS), variceal bleeding, or encephalopathy. SBP can also be asymptomatic.
- Treatment is with antibiotics, initially cefotaxime 2 g IV every 8 hours or equivalent. Duration of treatment is 5 days in uncomplicated cases.
- Intravenous albumin should be given on days 1 and 3 to prevent HRS.

Hepatorenal syndrome:
- Type 1 HRS is rapidly progressive, is usually associated with a precipitating event, and has a very poor prognosis.
- Type 2 HRS is more slowly progressive, is usually associated with refractory ascites, and has a longer survival, but still has a 100% mortality rate without treatment.
- Precipitating events include SBP, variceal bleeds, and other bacterial infections.
- All diuretics must be discontinued. Volume resuscitation with intravenous albumin must be started, followed by vasoconstrictor agents such as midodrine and octreotide. TIPS can be performed, but liver transplantation is the only cure.

Hepatic encephalopathy:
- Hyperammonemia is implicated in the pathogenesis of hepatic encephalopathy.
- Diagnosis is by history, clinical exam, and neuropsychiatric testing.

- Management includes dietary protein restriction, use of lactulose, antibiotics such as neomycin and rifaximin, and, ultimately, liver transplantation.
- Fulminant hepatic failure occurs when hepatic encephalopathy develops within 8 weeks of the onset of symptoms or within 2 weeks of the onset of jaundice.
- Hepatic encephalopathy associated with acute hepatic failure can cause cerebral edema, herniation, and death. It is treated more aggressively with intubation, intracranial pressure (ICP) monitoring, and mannitol.

Hepatopulmonary syndrome and portopulmonary hypertension:

- Hepatopulmonary syndrome (HPS) is caused by dilatation of the pulmonary capillary and precapillary vessels. Thus, there is rapid shunting of blood throughout the lungs, which results in an oxygenation defect. HPS is a problem of gas exchange.
- Pulmonary arterial hypertension (PPH) is caused by pulmonary vasoconstriction with endothelial and smooth-muscle proliferation. It eventually causes right-sided heart failure and decreased cardiac output. PPH is a hemodynamic problem.
- Both HPS and PPH may present with dyspnea on exercise and at rest. Platypnea is characteristic of HPS.
- In HPS, the dilated arterial bed is diagnosed by contrast-enhanced transthoracic echocardiography with agitated saline and a perfusion lung scan. In PPH, transthoracic echocardiography suggests the diagnosis, but right heart catheterization (RHC) is needed to confirm and monitor effectiveness of therapy.
- HPS is treated only by liver transplantation. It is a criterion for receiving a higher model for end-stage liver disease (MELD) exception score for liver transplantation. Supplemental oxygen is usually needed till transplantation.
- PPH can be treated medically with diuretics, vasodilators, and supplemental oxygen. TIPS are contraindicated, because they may worsen right heart failure.

References

1 Shah VH, Kamath PS. Portal hypertension and gastrointestinal bleeding. In: Marvin H, Sleisenger M, eds. *Sleisenger & Fordtran's Gastrointestinal and Liver Disease.* Philadelphia, PA: Saunders Elsevier, 2006.

2 Perri RE, Chiorean MV, Fidler JL, *et al.* A prospective evaluation of computerized tomographic (CT) scanning as a screening modality for esophageal varices. *Hepatology* 2008; **47**: 1587–94.

3 Vianna A, Hayes PC, Moscoso G, *et al.* Normal venous circulation of the gastroesophageal junction. A route to understanding varices. *Gastroenterology* 1987; **93**: 876–89.

4 Escorsell A, Gines A, Llach J, *et al.* Increasing intra-abdominal pressure increases pressure, volume, and wall tension in esophageal varices. *Hepatology* 2002; **36**(4 Pt. 1): 936–40.

5 Garcia-Tsao G, Sanyal A, Grace ND, Carey W. Prevention and management of gastroesophageal varices and variceal hemorrhage in cirrhosis. *Hepatology* 2007; **46**: 923–38.

6 Sugano S, Yamamoto K, Sasao K, *et al.* Daily variation of azygos and portal blood flow and the effect of propranolol administration once an evening in cirrhotics. *J Hepatol* 2001; **34**: 26–31.

7 Tripathi D, Ferguson JW, Kochar N, *et al.* Randomized controlled trial of carvedilol versus variceal band ligation for the prevention of the first variceal bleed. *Hepatology* 2009; **50**: 825–33.

8 Bernard B, Grange JD, Khac EN, *et al.* Antibiotic prophylaxis for the prevention of bacterial infections in cirrhotic patients with gastrointestinal bleeding: a meta-analysis. *Hepatology* 1999; **29**: 1655–61.

9 Fernandez J, Ruiz del Arbol L, Gomez C, *et al.* Norfloxacin vs ceftriaxone in the prophylaxis of infections in patients with advanced cirrhosis and hemorrhage. *Gastroenterology* 2006; **131**: 1049–56.

10 Bolognesi M, Balducci G, Garcia-Tsao G, *et al.* Complications in the medical treatment of portal hypertension. In: de Franchis R, ed. *Portal Hypertension III. Proceedings of the Third Baveno International Consensus Workshop on Definitions, Methodology and Therapeutic Strategies.* Oxford: Blackwell Science, 2001: 180–203.

11 Bosch J, Kravetz D, Rodes J. Effects of somatostatin on hepatic and systemic hemodynamics in patients with cirrhosis of the liver: comparison with vasopressin. *Gastroenterology* 1981; **80**: 518–25.

12 D'Amico G, Pietrosi G, Tarantino I, Pagliaro L. Emergency sclerotherapy versus vasoactive drugs for variceal bleeding in cirrhosis: a Cochrane meta-analysis. *Gastroenterology* 2003; **124**: 1277–91.

13 Malinchoc M, Kamath PS, Gordon FD, *et al.* A model to predict poor survival in patients undergoing transjugular intrahepatic portosystemic shunts. *Hepatology* 2000; **31**: 864–71.

14 Sarin SK, Lahoti D, Saxena SP, *et al.* Prevalence, classification and natural history of gastric varices: a long-term follow-up study in 568 portal hypertension patients. *Hepatology* 1992; **16**: 1343–9.

15 Sarin SK, Jain AK, Jain M, Gupta R. A randomized controlled trial of cyanoacrylate versus alcohol injection in patients with isolated fundic varices. *Am J Gastroenterol* 2002; **97**: 1010–15.

16 Barange K, Peron JM, Imani K, *et al.* Transjugular intrahepatic portosystemic shunt in the treatment of refractory bleeding from ruptured gastric varices. *Hepatology* 1999; **30**: 1139–43.

17 Chau TN, Patch D, Chan YW, *et al.* "Salvage" transjugular intrahepatic portosystemic shunts: gastric fundal compared with esophageal variceal bleeding. *Gastroenterology* 1998; **114**: 981–7.

18 Itzchak Y, Glickman MG. Duodenal varices in extrahepatic portal obstruction. *Radiology* 1977; **124**: 619–24.

19 Wiesner RH, LaRusso NF, Dozois RR, Beaver SJ. Peristomal varices after proctocolectomy in patients with primary sclerosing cholangitis. *Gastroenterology* 1986; **90**: 316–22.

20 Primignani M, Carpinelli L, Preatoni P, *et al.* Natural history of portal hypertensive gastropathy in patients with liver cirrhosis. The New Italian Endoscopic Club for the study and treatment of esophageal varices (NIEC). *Gastroenterology* 2000; **119**: 181–7.

21 Panes J, Bordas JM, Pique JM, *et al.* Effects of propranolol on gastric mucosal perfusion in cirrhotic patients with portal hypertensive gastropathy. *Hepatology* 1993; **17**: 213–18.

22 Perez-Ayuso RM, Pique JM, Bosch J, *et al.* Propranolol in prevention of recurrent bleeding from severe portal hypertensive gastropathy in cirrhosis. *Lancet* 1991; **337**: 1431–4.

23 Kamath PS, Lacerda M, Ahlquist DA, *et al.* Gastric mucosal responses to intrahepatic portosystemic shunting in patients with cirrhosis. *Gastroenterology* 2000; **118**: 905–11.

24 Jabbari M, Cherry R, Lough JO, *et al.* Gastric antral vascular ectasia: the watermelon stomach. *Gastroenterology* 1984; **87**: 1165–70.

25 Runyon BA. Management of adult patients with ascites due to cirrhosis. *Hepatology* 2004; **39**: 841–56.

26 Ruiz-del-Arbol L, Monescillo A, Arocena C, *et al.* Circulatory function and hepatorenal syndrome in cirrhosis. *Hepatology* 2005; **42**: 439–47.

27 Kim WR, Biggins SW, Kremers WK, *et al.* Hyponatremia and mortality among patients on the liver-transplant waiting list. *N Engl J Med* 2008; **359**: 1018–26.

28 Hoefs JC. Serum protein concentration and portal pressure determine the ascitic fluid protein concentration in patients with chronic liver disease. *J Lab Clin Med* 1983; **102**: 260–73.

29 Cattau EL Jr., Benjamin SB, Knuff TE, Castell DO. The accuracy of the physical examination in the diagnosis of suspected ascites. *JAMA* 1982; **247**: 1164–6.

30 Runyon BA. Paracentesis of ascitic fluid. A safe procedure. *Arch Intern Med* 1986; **146**: 2259–61.

31 Grabau CM, Crago SF, Hoff LK, *et al.* Performance standards for therapeutic abdominal paracentesis. *Hepatology* 2004; **40**: 484–8.

32 Runyon B. Management of adult patients with ascites due to cirrhosis: update 2012. Available from: https://www.aasld.org/sites/default/files/guideline_documents/adultascitesenhanced.pdf (last accessed February 15, 2016).

33 Runyon BA, Montano AA, Akriviadis EA, *et al.* The serum-ascites albumin gradient is superior to the exudate-transudate concept in the differential diagnosis of ascites. *Ann Intern Med* 1992; **117**: 215–20.

34 Runyon BA. *Ascites and Spontaneous Bacterial Peritonitis*, 7th edn. Philadelphia, PA: Saunders, 2002.

35 European Association for the Study of the Liver. EASL clinical practice guidelines on the management of ascites, spontaneous bacterial peritonitis, and hepatorenal syndrome in cirrhosis. *J Hepatology* 2010; **53**: 397–417.

36 Gines A, Fernandez-Esparrach G, Monescillo A, *et al.* Randomized trial comparing albumin, Dextran 70, and polygeline in cirrhotic patients with ascites treated by paracentesis. *Gastroenterology* 1996; **111**: 1002–10.

37 Gines P, Tito L, Arroyo V, *et al.* Randomized comparative study of therapeutic paracentesis with and without intravenous albumin in cirrhosis. *Gastroenterology* 1988; **94**: 1493–502.

CHAPTER 87

38 Blendis L, Wong F. The natural history and management of hepatorenal disorders: from pre-ascites to hepatorenal syndrome. *Clin Med* 2003; **3**: 154–9.

39 Gines P, Arroyo V, Vargas V, *et al*. Paracentesis with intravenous infusion of albumin as compared with peritoneovenous shunting in cirrhosis with refractory ascites. *N Engl J Med* 1991; **325**: 829–35.

40 Albillos A, Banares R, Gonzalez M, *et al*. A meta-analysis of transjugular intrahepatic portosystemic shunt versus paracentesis for refractory ascites. *J Hepatol* 2005; **43**: 990–6.

41 Saab S, Nieto JM, Ly D, Runyon BA. TIPS versus paracentesis for cirrhotic patients with refractory ascites. *Cochrane Database Syst Rev* 2004(3):CD004889.

42 Krok KL, Cardenas A. Hepatic hydrothorax. *Semin Respir Crit Care Med* 2012; **33**: 3–10.

43 Planas R, Montoliu S, Balleste B, *et al*. Natural history of patients hospitalized for management of cirrhotic ascites. *Clin Gastroenterol Hepatol* 2006; **4**: 1385–94.

44 D'Amico G, Morabito A, Pagliaro L, Marubini E. Survival and prognostic indicators in compensated and decompensated cirrhosis. *Digest Dis Sci* 1986; **31**: 468–75.

45 Heuman DM, Abou-Assi SG, Habib A, *et al*. Persistent ascites and low serum sodium identify patients with cirrhosis and low MELD scores who are at high risk for early death. *Hepatology* 2004; **40**: 802–10.

46 Runyon BA. Low-protein-concentration ascitic fluid is predisposed to spontaneous bacterial peritonitis. *Gastroenterology* 1986; **91**: 1343–6.

47 Llovet JM, Rodriguez-Iglesias P, Moitinho E, *et al*. Spontaneous bacterial peritonitis in patients with cirrhosis undergoing selective intestinal decontamination. A retrospective study of 229 spontaneous bacterial peritonitis episodes. *J Hepatol* 1997; **26**: 88–95.

48 Bernard B, Cadranel JF, Valla D, *et al*. Prognostic significance of bacterial infection in bleeding cirrhotic patients: a prospective study. *Gastroenterology* 1995; **108**: 1828–34.

49 Rimola A, Garcia-Tsao G, Navasa M, *et al*. Diagnosis, treatment and prophylaxis of spontaneous bacterial peritonitis: a consensus document. International Ascites Club. *J Hepatol* 2000; **32**: 142–53.

50 Ruiz-del-Arbol L, Urman J, Fernandez J, *et al*. Systemic, renal, and hepatic hemodynamic derangement in cirrhotic patients with spontaneous bacterial peritonitis. *Hepatology* 2003; **38**: 1210–18.

51 Sort P, Navasa M, Arroyo V, *et al*. Effect of intravenous albumin on renal impairment and mortality in patients with cirrhosis and spontaneous bacterial peritonitis. *N Engl J Med* 1999; **341**: 403–9.

52 Salerno F, Gerbes A, Gines P, *et al*. Diagnosis, prevention and treatment of hepatorenal syndrome in cirrhosis. *Gut* 2007; **56**: 1310–18.

53 Arroyo V, Fernandez J, Gines P. Pathogenesis and treatment of hepatorenal syndrome. *Semin Liver Dis* 2008; **28**: 81–95.

54 Fasolato S, Angeli P, Dallagnese L, *et al*. Renal failure and bacterial infections in patients with cirrhosis: epidemiology and clinical features. *Hepatology* 2007; **45**: 223–9.

55 Hampel H, Bynum GD, Zamora E, El-Serag HB. Risk factors for the development of renal dysfunction in hospitalized patients with cirrhosis. *Am J Gastroenterol* 2001; **96**: 2206–10.

56 Brater DC, Anderson SA, Brown-Cartwright D, Toto RD. Effects of nonsteroidal antiinflammatory drugs on renal function in patients with renal insufficiency and in cirrhotics. *Am J Kidney Dis* 1986; **8**: 351–5.

57 Wong F, Pantea L, Sniderman K. Midodrine, octreotide, albumin, and TIPS in selected patients with cirrhosis and type 1 hepatorenal syndrome. *Hepatology* 2004; **40**: 55–64.

58 Alessandria C, Ottobrelli A, Debernardi-Venon W, *et al*. Noradrenaline vs terlipressin in patients with hepatorenal syndrome: a prospective, randomized, unblinded, pilot study. *J Hepatol* 2007; **47**: 499–505.

59 Schwartz JM, Beymer C, Althaus SJ, *et al*. Cardiopulmonary consequences of transjugular intrahepatic portosystemic shunts: role of increased pulmonary artery pressure. *J Clin Gastroenterol* 2004; **38**: 590–4.

60 Sundaram V, Shaikh O. Hepatic encephalopathy: pathophysiology and emerging therapies. *Med Clin N Am* 2009; **93**: 819–36.

61 Romero-Gómez M, Jover M, Del Campo JA, *et al*. Variations in the promoter region of the glutaminase gene and the development of hepatic encephalopathy in patients with cirrhosis. *Ann Int Med* 2010; **153**: 281–8.

62 Ferenci P, Lockwood A, Mullen K, *et al*. Hepatic encephalopathy – definition, nomenclature, diagnosis, and quantification: final report of the working party at the 11th World Congresses of Gastroenterology, Vienna, 1998. *Hepatology* 2002; **35**: 716–21.

63 Kappus M, Bajaj JS. Covert hepatic encephalopathy: not as minimal as you might think. *Clin Gastroenterol Hepatol* 2012; **10**: 1208–19.

64 Sanyal AJ, Freedman AM, Luketic VA, *et al*. Transjugular intrahepatic portosystemic shunts compared with endoscopic sclerotherapy for the prevention of recurrent variceal hemorrhage. A randomized, controlled trial. *Ann Intern Med* 1997; **126**: 849–57.

65 Ghanta RK, Salvino RM, Mullen KD. Branched chain amino acid supplements in liver disease. *Clin Gastroenterol Hepatol* 2005; **3**: 631–2.

66 Marchesini G, Bianchi G, Merli M, *et al*. Nutritional supplementation with branched-chain amino acids in advanced cirrhosis: a double-blind, randomized trial. *Gastroenterology* 2003; **124**: 1792–801.

67 Shawcross D, Jalan R. Dispelling myths in the treatment of hepatic encephalopathy. *Lancet* 2005; **365**: 431–3.

68 Bass NM, Mullen KD, Sanyal A, *et al*. Rifaximin treatment in hepatic encephalopathy. *N Engl J Med* 2010; **362**: 1071–81.

69 Kircheis G, Wettstein M, Dahl S, Haussinger D. Clinical efficacy of L-ornithine-L-aspartate in the management of hepatic encephalopathy. *Metab Brain Dis* 2002; **17**: 453–62.

70 Chavez-Tapia N, Cesar-Arce A, Barrientos-Gutiérrez T, *et al*. Systematic review and meta-analysis of the use of oral zinc in the treatment of hepatic encephalopathy. *Nutr J* 2013; **12**: 74.

71 Takuma Y, Nouso K, Makino Y, *et al*. Clinical trial: oral zinc in hepatic encephalopathy. *Aliment Pharmacol Ther* 2010; **32**: 1080–90.

72 Laleman, W, Simon-Talero M, Maleux G, *et al*. Embolization of large spontaneous portosystemic shunts for refractory hepatic encephalopathy: a multicenter survey on safety and efficacy. *Hepatology* 2013; **57**: 2448–57.

73 Phongsamran P, Kim JW, Abbott JC, Rosenblatt A. Pharmacotherapy for hepatic encephalopathy. *Drugs* 2010; **70**: 1131–48.

74 Hassanein T, Tofteng F, Brown RS, *et al*. Randomized controlled study of extracorporeal albumin dialysis for hepatic encephalopathy in advanced cirrhosis. *Hepatology* 2007; **46**: 1853–62.

75 Lee WM, Hynan LS, Rossaro L, *et al*. Intravenous N-acetylcysteine improves transplant-free survival in early stage non-acetaminophen acute liver failure. *Gastroenterology*. 2009; **137**: 856–64.

76 Stewart CA, Malinchoc M, Kim WR, Kamath PS. Hepatic encephalopathy as a predictor of survival in patients with end-stage liver disease. *Liver Transpl* 2007; **13**: 1366–71.

77 Regev A, Yeshurun M, Rodriguez M, *et al*. Transient hepatopulmonary syndrome in a patient with acute hepatitis A. *J Viral Hepatitis* 2001; **8**: 83–6.

78 Teuber G, Teupe C, Dietrich CF, *et al*. Pulmonary dysfunction in non-cirrhotic patients with chronic viral hepatitis. *Eur J Intern Med* 2002; **13**: 311–18.

79 Rodriguez-Roisin R, Krowka MJ. Hepatopulmonary syndrome – a liver-induced lung vascular disorder. *N Engl J Med* 2008; **358**: 2378–87.

80 Swanson KLWR, Krowka MJ. Long-term survival in hepatopulmonary syndrome. *Chest* 2002; **122**: 210S–11S.

81 Krowka M. Portopulmonary hypertension. *Semin Respir Crit Care Med* 2012; **33**: 17–25.

82 Safdar Z, Bartolome S, Sussman N. Portopulmonary hypertension: an update. *Liver Transplantation* 2012; **18**: 881–91.

83 Krowka MJ, Swanson KL, Frantz RP, *et al*. Portopulmonary hypertension: results from a 10-year screening algorithm. *Hepatology* 2006; **44**: 1502–10.

84 Fallon MB, Krowka MJ, Brown RS, *et al*. Impact of hepatopulmonary syndrome on quality of life and survival in liver transplant candidates. *Gastroenterology* 2008; **135**: 1168–75.

CHAPTER 88

TIPS

Santiago Cornejo and Sailendra Naidu

Department of Radiology, Mayo Clinic, Scottsdale AZ, USA

Summary

Transjugular intrahepatic portosystemic shunts (TIPS) are percutaneously created shunts for the treatment of complications related to portal hypertension, most commonly variceal bleeding and refractory ascites. Techniques and technology have improved significantly since the first live human experience in 1982 [1, 2], yielding more durable results and reduced complication rates. New indications are being explored, but morbidity limits the role of TIPS as a first-line therapy. Appropriate patient selection and an experienced operator can maximize benefit and maintain risks at an acceptable level. The decision to perform a TIPS requires multidisciplinary input from gastroenterology/hepatology, interventional radiology, and, when appropriate, transplant surgery.

Equipment and Review of Technology

Several TIPS access sets are available for use, each with their own advantages and disadvantages. In general, a TIPS set consists of a long access sheath, an angled catheter for selection of the hepatic veins, a puncture needle (which is loaded through a straight catheter also provided in the set), and a wire. A pressure transducer is frequently used to measure right atrial and portal venous pressures. Carbon dioxide portography can be performed via a balloon occlusion catheter, wedged selection catheter, or skinny needle placed in the liver parenchyma. A pigtail marking catheter is used for direct portography and to determine appropriate stent length. The Viatorr stent graft (GORE, Flagstaff, AZ) is now the preferred conduit for TIPS. It is specially designed for TIPS, consisting of a 2 cm uncovered distal end and a variable-length ePTFE-covered portion, depending on the tract length. Bare metal stents were initially used but were plagued by dysfunction rates of 55–80% [3, 4], requiring frequent reintervention. In general, 1-year patency rates for Viatorr hover around 80%. All studies comparing Viatorr against bare metal stents have shown improved patency rates and decreased dysfunction rates in the statistically significant range.

Application

We prefer the use of general anesthesia for our TIPS procedure. A TIPS is generally performed from the right internal jugular vein, but can be performed from the left. Once the sheath is in place, the selection catheter is used to select an appropriate hepatic vein (usually the right hepatic vein). The most challenging step in TIPS creation is accessing the portal vein. This can be accomplished using fluoroscopic landmarks, ultrasound guidance, or other advanced techniques. Carbon dioxide portography is performed as already discussed (Figure 88.1a); the high diffusion capacity of CO_2 results in retrograde filling of the portal vein. The selection catheter is then exchanged for the puncture needle or a metal cannula with a skinny puncture needle. Based on the CO_2 portogram, the needle is advanced toward the portal vein target. This is usually the right portal vein when puncture from the right hepatic vein is being attempted. The needle is slowly withdrawn, while maintaining negative pressure with a syringe. Return of blood indicates the intravascular needle tip location. If a contrast injection confirms portal vein entry, the access is secured with wire. A marking pigtail catheter is placed into the portal vein and pressure measurements are obtained. Simultaneous pressure measurement of the right atrium is obtained to calculate the baseline portosystemic (PS) gradient. A contrast portogram is then performed to define the portal venous anatomy, assess the extent of variceal filling, and measure the tract length for appropriate stent graft selection (Figure 88.1b). It is critical that the uncovered portion of the stent graft be within the portal vein and that the covered portion extends to within 1 cm of the hepatic vein/inferior vena cava (IVC) confluence, to prevent the development of a stenosis at the hepatic venous end. Balloon dilation of the stent graft is performed to obtain good stent apposition, and subsequently a portal systemic gradient is measured. Reducing the gradient to <12 mmHg is considered technical success. Further dilatation to maximal stent diameter can be performed to achieve the needed reduction. Many advocate not bringing the PS gradient below 5 mmHg in order to help prevent encephalopathy [5]. Formal portogram is then performed to assess the caliber of the TIPS, ensure accurate deployment and stent length, and evaluate for residual variceal filling (Figure 88.1c). The sheath is removed and hemostasis is achieved by holding manual pressure at the internal jugular vein access site.

Diagnostic Methods

Portal hypertension is defined as portal pressure >10 mmHg. In cirrhotics, corrected sinusoidal pressure (CSP) reflects the portal pressure. CSP can be measured via transjugular hepatic vein access with a catheter in order to obtain free and wedged hepatic venous pressures. The free hepatic venous pressure is subtracted from the wedged hepatic venous pressure to obtain the CSP. A gradient of

Practical Gastroenterology and Hepatology Board Review Toolkit, Second Edition. Edited by Nicholas J. Talley, Kenneth R. DeVault, Michael B. Wallace, Bashar A. Aqel and Keith D. Lindor.
© 2016 John Wiley & Sons, Ltd. Published 2016 by John Wiley & Sons, Ltd. Companion website: www.practicalgastrohep.com

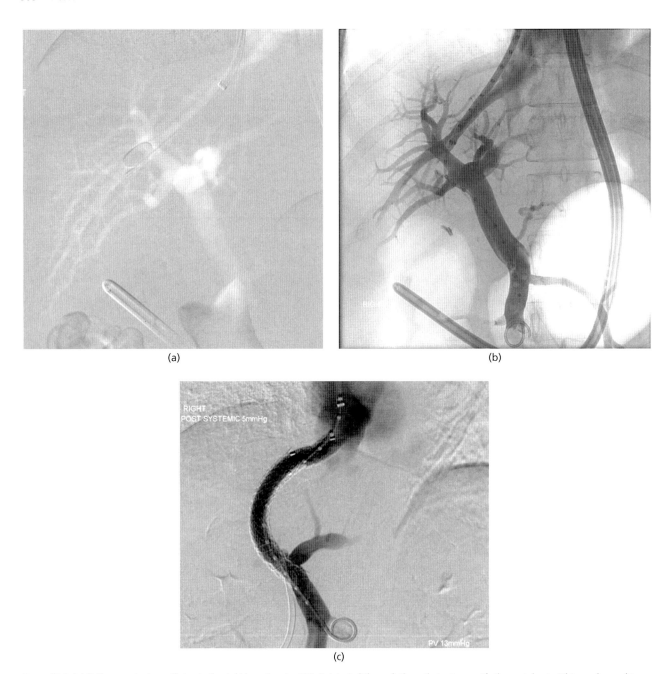

(a)

(b)

(c)

Figure 88.1 (a) Balloon occlusion catheter in the right hepatic vein. CO_2 is injected through the catheter to opacify the portal vein. This can be used to help target the portal vein for needle puncture. (b) After successful puncture of the portal vein from the hepatic vein, contrast is injected to assess varices and to allow stent graft deployment planning. Portal pressures are also measured. (c) Following placement of the stent graft, blood is shunted through the covered stent, with decreased filling of the intrahepatic portal vein branches. In this example, an extra stent was placed to extend the shunt near the hepatic vein/inferior vena cava confluence.

<5 mmHg is normal. CSP >5 and <10 mmHg in the absence of clinical manifestations is considered subclinical portal hypertension. CSP ≥10 mmHg is clinically significant portal hypertension and CSP >12 mmHg is the threshold for variceal rupture [6].

The use of preprocedural imaging varies between institutions, though it is generally recommended that some form of imaging be obtained. Spectral Doppler of the liver, computed tomography (CT), or magnetic resonance imaging (MRI) can be used to confirm patency of the hepatic and portal veins, detect liver masses, and provide information regarding the hepatic vein relationship to the portal vein. In patients with a cardiac history, pre-procedure

evaluation of their condition is warranted. In the absence of a cardiac history, pre-procedure echocardiogram is unnecessary [7].

In the days when bare metal stents were deployed for TIPS, ultrasound surveillance of the TIPS stent was necessary. Velocity in the TIPS ranges between 90 and 190 cm/s. When there is an increase or decrease in velocities, a stenosis should be considered. Elevated velocities at the level of a narrowing may indicate a physiologically significant stenosis. Conversely, downstream from the stenosis, the velocities may decrease. Main portal vein velocity <30 cm/s has also been described as a sign of TIPS stent stenosis [8]. Hepatopetal (antegrade) flow within intrahepatic portal vein branches may be a sign of TIPS dysfunction, particularly if it represents a new finding compared to previous studies. Some authors have suggested a temporal change in shunt or hepatic vein velocity >50 cm/s to be a sign of stenosis [9]. Lack of flow within the stent suggests thrombosis. Any of these findings warrants referral to interventional radiology for venography assessment of the TIPS. Recurrent symptoms (ascites, variceal bleeding) despite negative ultrasound also warrants venographic assessment of the TIPS. An accepted surveillance protocol for bare metallic stents consists of baseline color Doppler ultrasound within 24–72 hours of implantation and follow-up ultrasound at 1, 3, and 6 months after stent placement and every 6 months thereafter [10]. Given the improved patency rate with stent grafts, the current role of ultrasound surveillance is less clear, and some authors have argued that routine ultrasound surveillance may not be warranted in the absence of clinical signs/symptoms of complications [11]. A recent retrospective study [10] suggested that a single Doppler ultrasound after stent graft implantation serves as an effective means of assessing TIPS patency in the short term and can act as a baseline reference should clinical symptoms warrant ultrasound evaluation. For the TIPS made with a stent graft, it is recommended to wait at least 5 days after implantation before obtaining an ultrasound of the TIPS, as air within the stent graft fabric does not allow ultrasound penetration, rendering the study non-diagnostic.

Evidence-Based Therapeutics

A list of generally accepted indications for TIPS and the strength of evidence for each is given in Table 88.1.

Patients presenting with acute variceal bleeding are initially managed with pharmacological and endoscopic methods as first-line therapy. Child–Pugh score, active bleeding at index endoscopy, refractory bleeding after endoscopy, and hepatic vein-to-portal vein gradient (HVPG) >20 [13–15] are predictors of endoscopic treatment failure and early rebleeding. A recent European study [16] found lower rates of rebleeding or failure to control bleeding and improved 1-year survival in patients at high risk of treatment failure (Child–Pugh C or Child–Pugh B with active bleeding at index endoscopy) who received early TIPS versus continued endoscopic and pharmacologic treatment. In this situation, and due to lack of better alternatives, TIPS should be considered. The 2009 American Association for the Study of Liver Diseases (AASLD) Practice Guidelines [7] endorse TIPS in controlling acute bleeding from varices refractory to medical therapy.

One of the most studied indications for TIPS is in the secondary prevention of variceal bleeding. This is not uncommon, as

bleeding varices have at least a 50% chance of rebleeding [7,17,18]. Meta-analyses [12,19,20] have shown recurrent bleeding rates after TIPS of 9.0–40.6%, compared with 20.5–60.6% with continued endoscopic therapy in this patient population. Despite this, there is no significant difference in survival, though, as expected, patients who have undergone TIPS have a higher rate of morbidity in the form of encephalopathy.

It is worth special mention that gastric varices should be considered a distinct entity from esophageal varices. Bleeding tends to be more severe and can occur at a lower PS gradient. Gastric varices also are not as amenable to endoscopic intervention, such as banding, as are esophageal varices. TIPS has been used to control active gastric variceal bleeding and prevent rebleeding, It has been reported to control active bleeding in 90–96% of cases [21,22], which is comparable with the higher end of reported success by endoscopy. Rebleeding rates have been reported as 26–29% at 6–7 months and 31% at 12 months, whcih is lower than the best reported rates by endoscopy. In more recent studies, the rebleed rate has been reported as 11–20% at 12–24 months post-TIPS [23–26]. The current data reflect the use of bare stents, and the rebleed rate in the era of ePTFE-covered stents is likely lower. In some cases of bleeding gastric varices, the patient may benefit more from balloon-occluded retrograde transvenous obliteration of gastric varices (BRTO) than from TIPS. The primary advantage of BRTO is the lack of an increased risk of encephalopathy. TIPS is the preferred approach for prevention of rebleeding from gastric and ectopic (intestinal, stomal, anorectal) varices [7].

Diagnostic criteria for refractory ascites generally include failure of maximal diuretic therapy, intolerance of diuretic therapy, and rapid reaccumulation of drained ascites. The presence of refractory ascites is a poor prognostic indicator [27]. Large-volume paracentesis (LVP) with volume replacement and TIPS are the mainstays of treatment. The available randomized controlled trials (RCTs) comparing TIPS with LVP (± albumin replacement) show some variability in numbers, but some conclusions can be made on the basis of two quality meta-analysis [28,29]. First, TIPS outperforms LVP in the treatment of refractory ascites, with recurrence of tense ascites in 42–44% of patients treated with TIPS versus 87–89% of patients treated with LVP. However, this is counterbalanced by a nearly 2.3-fold increase in the risk of encephalopathy associated with TIPS [28]. The survival data on this subset of patients are inconsistent, but two of the more recent RCTs have suggested some survival benefit [30, 31]. The current data are derived from TIPS created with bare stents; it is reasonable to expect that the use of ePTFE-covered stents will impact treatment outcomes.

Patients may present with hepatic hydrothorax where the ascites flows from the peritoneum into the pleural space via small diaphragmatic communications. Analogous to ascites, patients can first be managed with medical therapy and thoracentesis. When symptoms are refractory to medical management, TIPS can be considered. Fewer studies are available to demonstrate the efficacy of TIPS in this setting, however; those that do exist have shown favorable results. Chest tube placement in these patients carries high morbidity and mortality and should be avoided [32]. AASLD guidelines [7] recommend TIPS for refractory ascites in patients intolerant of LVP and in those with hepatic hydrothorax whose effusion cannot be controlled by diuretics and sodium restriction.

Hepatorenal syndrome can present as rapidly deteriorating renal function (type 1) or as a slower, progressive rise in creatinine (type 2). Type 1 hepatorenal syndrome carries a poor prognosis: less than 10% survival rate by 6 months [27]. Survival rates of 20 and 70%

Table 88.1 Typical indications for TIPS.

Indication	Best available level of evidence	References
Secondary prevention of variceal bleeding	1A	[10,19]
Refractory ascites	1A	[28]
Budd–Chiari syndrome	4	[38,50]
Hepatic hydrothorax	4	[51–54]
Hepatic venoocclusive disease	4	[55]
Hepatorenal syndromes (types 1 and 2)	2B	[33]
Hepatopulmonary syndrome	4	[56]
Portal hypertensive gastropathy	2B	[57]
Refractory acute variceal bleeding	1B	[16]

Source: Fidelman 2012 [12]. Reproduced with permission of AJR.

have been reported at 1 year in type 1 and type 2 patients receiving TIPS, respectively [33]. These numbers are favorable compared to less than 20% survival by 13 weeks in the non-TIPS group. Standard treatment consists of medical management, but TIPS may prolong renal function in patients who initially respond to medical management [34]. Several studies [33–35] have shown improvement in renal function parameters and even vasoactive systems following TIPS placement. Liver transplant remains the definitive treatment. Despite the promising data, to date a clear position has not been found for TIPS in the treatment algorithm.

Budd–Chiari syndrome is a disorder of hepatic venous obstruction occurring at any level between the small hepatic veins and the right atrium [36]. Its relatively low incidence is evident from the limited data available. Patients may be asymptomatic or may present with fulminant liver failure. An expert panel [36] has outlined a step-by-step approach to treatment of Budd–Chiari syndrome, which ranges from conservative measures such as anticoagulation and medical therapy to liver transplant, surgical shunts, and TIPS creation. A classification scheme, the Rotterdam BCS index, stratifies patients into high-, intermediate-, and low-risk groups [37]. A recent study [38] found that patients at intermediate and high risk according to the Rotterdam BCS index treated with TIPS had 1- and 5-year transplant-free survival of 88 and 78%, respectively, which is quite favorable compared with the 74 and 42% survival predicted by the Rotterdam BCS index. Encouraging results have also been seen in a more recent, smaller study [39]. The extent and location of venous occlusion can complicate TIPS placement. Not all centers have the experience or capacity to undertake these cases.

There has been some interest in the use of TIPS to maintain the patency of partially thrombosed portal veins in liver transplant candidates. The data are limited, and this is still not a widely accepted indication for TIPS.

There are numerous contraindications to TIPS (Table 88.2). These should be weighed against the potential benefits.

Numerous scoring systems and laboratory values have been used to predict post-TIPS mortality. A recent study [40] compared the performance of different liver disease scoring systems in predicting early (30- and 90-day) mortality after TIPS creation. When all TIPS placements were considered, regardless of indication or stent type (bare stent vs. covered stent), the Model for End-Stage Liver Disease (MELD) and serum sodium (MELD-Na) scores showed the best performance, achieving area under the curve (AUC) operator characteristics of 0.878 and 0.816 for MELD and 0.863 and 0.823 for MELD-Na at 30 and 90 days, respectively (with no statistically significant difference between MELD and MELD-Na).

Table 88.2 Contraindications to TIPS placement.

Absolute	Relative
Primary prevention of variceal bleeding	Hepatocellular carcinoma, especially central
Congestive heart failure	Obstruction of all hepatic veins
Severe tricuspid regurgitation	Portal vein thrombosis
Severe pulmonary hypertension	Moderate pulmonary hypertension
Mulitple hepatic cysts	Severe coagulopathy (INR >5)
Uncontrolled systemic infection or sepsis	Thrombocytopenia <20 000 cells/cm³
Unrelieved biliary obstruction	Hepatic encephalopathy

INR, International Normalized Ratio.
Source: Fidelman 2012 [12]. Reproduced with permission of AJR.

Table 88.3 Risk stratification based on MELD score.

MELD score	Risk category	30-day mortality	90-day mortality
<10	Minimal	0%	4%
10–18	Low	8%	16%
19–25	Intermediate	18%	33%
>25	High	72%	80%

Source: Gaba 2013 [40]. Reproduced with permission of Elsevier.

The MELD score showed statistical superiority over bilirubin level, Emory score, and Bonn TIPS early mortality (BOTEM) score at 30 and 90 days. The authors of the study suggest risk stratification based on MELD score (Table 88.3).

The present authors recommend using a MELD-based scoring system to optimize patient selection for TIPS and providing more accurate counseling of patients on expected outcome. Other scoring systems, including bilirubin level, Childs–Pugh class, Emory score, Prognostic Index, Acute Physiology and Chronic Health Evaluation (APACHE 2) score, and BOTEM score, should be used as secondary options. That being said, there are data showing improved renal function following TIPS placement [24,33–35], and patients with high MELD scores driven primarily by high creatinine levels deserve some special consideration.

Complications

Intraprocedural complications range from quite minor to catastrophic. Inadvertent puncture of the carotid artery has been described. Life-threatening bleeding can result from liver capsular perforation during wedged or balloon occlusion portography or extrahepatic portal vein access (Figure 88.2). Puncture of the hepatic arteries and intrahepatic bile ducts is not uncommon while trying

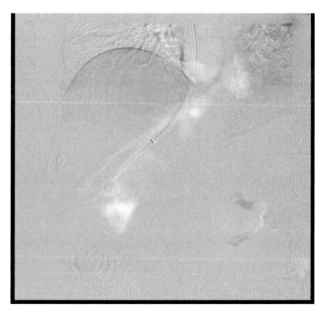

Figure 88.2 Balloon occlusion retrograde CO_2 portogram from a peripheral location, resulting in capsular liver perforation and intraperitoneal extravasation of CO_2. Note the short tract defining the hepatic injury. Though capsular perforation can be life-threatening, this patient exhibited no hemodynamic changes.

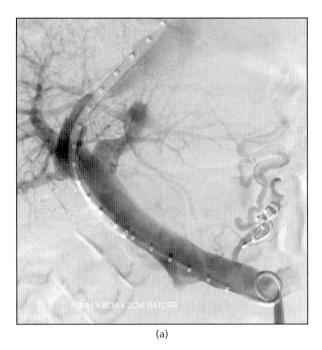
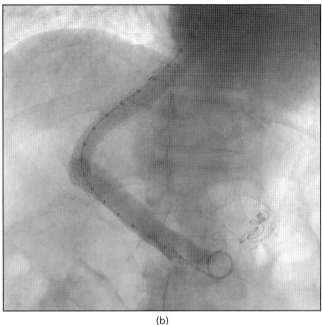

(a)   (b)

Figure 88.3 (a) TIPS venogram from a patient with bare metal stent TIPS, showing narrowing near the mid portion of the shunt. Hemodynamic significance is suggested by prominent filling of the intrahepatic portal vein branches and the coronary vein. (b) The bare stent after re-lining with a Viatorr stent. The stenosis resolved with reduction in the portal pressure and resolution of the varices.

to establish portal vein access, and such injuries are generally of no clinical consequence. Arrhythmias caused by right atrial irritation may occur but are generally self-limited, rarely requiring treatment. Stent migration or dislodgement may be seen during the procedure.

In the post-procedural period, complications may arise despite successful and uncomplicated placement of a TIPS. Patients with poor cardiac reserve or pulmonary hypertension can exhibit decompensation after TIPS due to significant elevation of pulmonary artery pressure, right atrial pressure, cardiac index, and pulmonary vascular resistance following the procedure. Patients should be managed medically, but adequate pre-TIPS screening can reduce the possibility of cardiopulmonary complications. Review of the recent literature indicates new or worsened encephalopathy complicating TIPS in 30–46% of cases [12]. A recent meta-analysis [41] found increased age, higher Child–Pugh score, and prior hepatic encephalopathy to be the most robust predictors of post-TIPS hepatic encephalopathy. In most cases, this can be controlled medically with protein-restricted diet, branched-chain amino acids, and oral lactulose. In the minority of patients with encephalopathy refractory to medical management after TIPS, shunt reduction and even occlusion may need to be performed. Over-shunting of blood away from the intrahepatic portal branches, resulting in deteriorating liver function, occurs in approximately 10% of patients [20]. Progression to fulminant liver failure may occur, especially in patients with poor hepatic artery buffer response. Sudden elevation of bilirubin and moderate elevation of liver enzymes can be seen. Shunt reduction or occlusion may be necessary.

Delayed complications (rebleeding, recurrent ascites) are almost exclusively related to shunt dysfunction. Bare stents were plagued with dysfunction rates of 50% at 1 year and 80% at 2 years [42,43]. In a large number of cases, dysfunction is the result of in-stent stenosis (Figure 88.3). Bile leakage across the stent interstices is implicated in acute thrombogenic occlusion and non-thrombogenic stenosis due to pseudointimal hyperplasia [44, 45]. Great advances were made

with the introduction of the Viatorr stent graft. In 2004, the first randomized trial comparing the patency rates of bare stents versus Viatorr was published [46]. The results demonstrated a 13% shunt dysfunction rate at median follow-up of 300 days for Viatorr, compared with 44% for bare stents. This was validated in the follow-up study, showing 2-year actuarial primary patency rates of 76 and 36% for Viatorr and bare stents, respectively [47]. Subsequent studies have shown similar benefit from Viatorr. Importantly, encephalopathy rates are not statistically significantly increased with Viatorr. A study comparing Viatorr with a generic stent graft/bare metal stent combination showed a statistically significant difference between primary unassisted patency rates at 1 year: 89% for Viatorr versus 81% for generic stent graft/bare metal stent combination [48]. Covered stents, whether a Viatorr or a bare stent/covered stent combination, result in lower TIPS dysfunction rates compared with bare stents alone [49]. Pseudointimal hyperplasia may still occur if the entire transhepatic tract is not covered by the ePTFE portion of the Viatorr.

> ### Take Home Points
>
> - Use of covered stent grafts for transjugular intrahepatic portosystemic shunts (TIPS) has resulted in improved patency rates compared to bare metal stents.
> - Preoperative imaging in the form of ultrasound, computed tomography (CT), or magnetic resonance imaging (MRI) is useful in documenting patency of the portal vein, identifying the relationship of the hepatic vein to the portal vein, and evaluating for liver masses.
> - The portosystemic (PS) gradient should be brought under 12 mmHg following TIPS.
> - While surveillance ultrasound is recommended for TIPS made with bare metal stents, it is not necessary in a TIPS constructed with a covered stent graft, due to the improved patency rates. Most

authorities recommend a baseline Doppler ultrasound shortly after TIPS creation.

- TIPS is used for the secondary prevention of esophageal variceal bleeding. First-line therapy is medical management with endoscopic intervention.
- Refractory ascites may be better controlled with TIPS than with large-volume paracentesis (LVP) and volume replacement, but the rate of encephalopathy is higher in patients who have undergone TIPS.
- Procedural complications include bleeding, arrhythmias, and stent migration.
- Post-procedural complications include congestive heart failure due to increased right heart flow, liver decompensation, and encephalopathy.

References

1 Colapinto RF, Stronell RD, Birch SJ, *et al.* Creation of an intrahepatic portosystemic shunt with a Grüntzig balloon catheter. *Can Med Assoc J* 1982; **126**: 267–8.

2 Gordon JD, Colapinto RF, Abecassis M, *et al.* Transjugular intrahepatic portosystemic shunt: a nonoperative approach to life-threatening variceal bleeding. *Can J Surg* 1987; **30**: 45–9.

3 Luca A, D'Amico G, La Galla R, *et al.* TIPS for prevention of recurrent bleeding in patients with cirrhosis: meta-analysis of randomized trials. *Radiology* 1999; **212**: 411–21.

4 Hausegger KA, Sternthal HM, Klein GE, *et al.* Transjugular intrahepatic portosystemic shunt: angiographic follow-up and secondary interventions. *Radiology* 1994; **191**: 177–81.

5 Chung HH, Razavi MK, Sze DY, *et al.* Portosystemic pressure gradient during transjugular intrahepatic portosystemic shunt with Viatorr stent graft: what is the critical low threshold to avoid medically uncontrolled low pressure gradient related complications? *J Gastroenterol Hepatol* 2008; **23**: 95–101.

6 Kumar A, Sharma P, Sarin SK. Hepatic venous pressure gradient measurement: time to learn! *Indian J Gastroenterol* 2008; **27**: 74–80.

7 Boyer TD, Haskal ZJ. The role of transjugular intrahepatic portosystemic shunt (TIPS) in the management of portal hypertension: update 2009. *Hepatology* 2010; **51**(1): 306.

8 Darcy M. Evaluation and management of transjugular intrahepatic portosystemic shunts. *Am J Roentgenol* 2012; **199**: 7306.

9 Dodd GD 3rd, Zajko AB, Orons PD, *et al.* Detection of transjugular intrahepatic portosystemic shunt dysfunction: value of duplex Doppler sonography. *Am J Roentgenol* 1995; **164**: 1119–24.

10 Carr CE, Tuite CM, Soulen MC, *et al.* Role of ultrasound surveillance of transjugular intrahepatic portosystemic shunts in the covered stent era. *J Vasc Interv Radiol* 2006; **17**: 1297–305.

11 Huang Q, Wu X, Fan X, *et al.* Comparison study of Doppler ultrasound surveillance of expanded polytetrafluoroethylene-covered stent versus bare stent in transjugular intrahepatic portosystemic shunt. *J Clin Ultrasound* 2010; **38**: 353–60.

12 Fidelman N, Kwan SW, LaBerge JM, *et al.* The transjugular intrahepatic portosystemic shunt: an update. *Am J Roentgenol* 2012; **199**: 746–55.

13 Monescillo A, Martinez-Lagarez F, Ruiz-del-Arbol L, *et al.* Influence of portal hypertension and its early decompression by TIPS placement on the outcome of variceal bleeding. *Hepatology* 2004; **40**: 793–801.

14 Moitinho E, Escorsell A, Bandi JC, *et al.* Prognostic value of early measurements of portal pressure in acute variceal bleeding. *Gastroenterology* 1999; **117**: 626–31.

15 D'Amico G, de Franchis R. Upper digestive bleeding in cirrhosis. Post-therapeutic outcome and prognostic indicators. *Hepatology* 2003; **38**: 599–612.

16 Garcia-Pagan JC, Caca K, Bureau C, *et al.* Early use of TIPS in patients with cirrhosis and variceal bleeding. *N Engl J Med* 2010; **362**: 2370–9.

17 Sharara AI, Rockey DC. Gastroesophageal variceal hemorrhage. *N Engl J Med* 2001; **345**: 669–81.

18 Chalasani N, Kahi C, Francois F, *et al.* Improved patient survival after acute variceal bleeding: a multicenter, cohort study. *Am J Gastroenterol* 2003; **98**: 653–9.

19 Burroughs AK, Vangeli M. Transjugular intrahepatic portosystemic shunt versus endoscopic therapy: randomized trials for secondary prophylaxis of variceal bleeding: an updated meta-analysis. *Scand J Gastroenterol* 2002; **37**: 249–52.

20 Zheng M, Chen Y, Bai J, *et al.* Transjugular intrahepatic portosystemic shunt versus endoscopic therapy in the secondary prophylaxis of variceal rebleeding in cirrhotic patients: meat-analysis update. *J Clin Gastroenterol* 2008; **42**: 507–16.

21 Choi YH, Yoon CJ, Park JH, *et al.* Balloon-occluded retrograde transvenous obliteration for gastric variceal bleeding: its feasibility compared with transjugular intrahepatic portosystemic shunt. *Korean J Radiol* 2003; **4**: 109–16.

22 Chau TN, Patch D, Chan YW, *et al.* "Salvage" transjugular intrahepatic portosystemic shunts: gastric fundal compared with esophageal variceal bleeding. *Gastroenterology* 1998; **114**: 981–7.

23 Kitamoto M, Imamura M, Kamada K, *et al.* Balloon occluded retrograde transvenous obliteration of gastric fundal varices with hemorrhage. *Am J Roentgenol* 2002; **178**: 1167–74.

24 Anderson CL, Saad WE, Kalagher SD, *et al.* Effect of transjugular intrahepatic portosystemic shunt placement on renal function: a 7-year, single-center experience. *J Vasc Interv Radiol* 2010; **2**: 1370–6.

25 Barange K, Péron J-M, Imani K, *et al.* Transjugular intrahepatic portosystemic shunt in the treatment of refractory bleeding from ruptured gastric varices. *Hepatology* 1999; **30**: 1139–43.

26 Lo G-H, Liang H-L, Chen W-C, *et al.* A prospective, randomized controlled trial of transjugular intrahepatic portosystemic shunt versus cyanoacrylate injection in the prevention of gastric variceal rebleeding. *Endoscopy* 2007; **39**: 679–85.

27 Gines P, Cardenas A, Arroyo V, Rodes J. Management of cirrhosis and ascites. *N Engl J Med* 2004; **350**: 1646–54.

28 D'Amico G, Luca A, Morabito A, *et al.* Uncovered transjugular intrahepatic portosystemic shunt for refractory ascites: a meta-analysis. *Gastroenterology* 2005; **129**: 1282–93.

29 Salerno F, Camma C, Enea A, *et al.* Transjugular intrahepatic portosystemic shunt for refractory ascites: a meta-analysis of individual patient data. *Gastroenterology* 2007; **133**: 825–34.

30 Salerno F, Merli M, Riggio O, *et al.* Randomized controlled study of TIPS versus paracentesis plus albumin in cirrhosis with severe ascites. *Hepatology* 2004; **40**: 629–35.

31 Narahara Y, Kanazawa H, Fukuda T, *et al.* Transjugular intrahepatic portosystemic shunt versus paracentesis plus albumin in patients with refractory ascites who have good hepatic and renal function: a prospective randomized trial. *J Gastroenterol* 2011; **46**: 78–85.

32 Orman ES, Lok AS. Outcomes of patients with chest insertion for hepatic hydrothorax. *Hepatol Int* 2009; **3**: 582–6.

33 Brensing KA, Textor J, Perz J, *et al.* Long term outcome after transjugular intrahepatic portosystemic stent-shunt in non-transplant cirrhotics with hepatorenal syndrome: a phase II study. *Gut* 2000; **47**: 288–95.

34 Wong F, Pantea L, Sniderman K. Midodrine, octreotide, albumin, and TIPS in selected patients with cirrhosis and type 1 hepatorenal syndrome. *Hepatology* 2004; **40**: 55–64.

35 Guevara M, Gines P, Bandi JC, *et al.* Transjugular intrahepatic portosystemic shunt in hepatorenal syndrome: effects on renal function and vasoactive systems. *Hepatology* 1998; **28**: 416–22.

36 Janssen HL, Garcia-Pagan JC, Elias E, *et al.* Budd-Chiari syndrome: a review by an expert panel. *J Hepatol* 2003; **38**: 364–71.

37 Murad SD, Valla DC, de Groen PC, *et al.* Determinants or survival and the effect of portosystemic shunting in patients with Budd-Chiari syndrome. *Hepatology* 2004; **39**: 500–8.

38 García-Pagán JC, Heydtmann M, Raffa S, *et al.* TIPS for Budd-Chiari syndrome: long-term results and prognostics factors in 124 patients. *Gastroenterology* 2008; **135**: 808–15.

39 Fitsiori K, Tsitskair M, Kelekis A, *et al.* Transjugular intrahepatic portosystemic shunt for the treatment of Budd-Chiari syndrome patients: results from a single center. *Cardiovasc Intervent Radiol* 2014; **37**(3): 691–7.

40 Gaba RC, Couture PM, Bui JT, *et al.* Prognostic capability of different liver disease scoring systems for prediction of early mortality after transjugular intrahepatic portosystemic shunt creation. *J Vasc Interv Radiol* 2013; **24**: 411–20.

41 Bai M, Qi X, Yang Z, *et al.* Predictors of hepatic encephalopathy after transjugular intrahepatic portosystemic shunt in cirrhotic patients: a systematic review. *J Gastroenterol Hepatol* 2011; **26**: 943–51.

42 Sanyal AJ, Freedman AM, Luketic VA, *et al.* The natural history of portal hypertension after transjugular intrahepatic portosystemic shunts. *Gastroenterology* 1997; **112**: 889–98.

43 Casado M, Bosch J, Garcia-Pagan JC, *et al.* Clinical events after transjugular intrahepatic portosystemic shunt: correlation with hemodynamic findings. *Gastroenterology* 1998; **114**: 1296–303.

44 Saxon RR, Mendel-Hartvig J, Corless CL, *et al.* Bile duct injury as a major cause of stenosis and occlusion in the transjugular intrahepatic portosystemic shunts: comparative histopathologic analysis in humans and swine. *J Vasc Interv Radiol* 1996; **7**: 487–97.

45 Ducoin H, El-Khoury J, Rousseau H, *et al.* Histopathologic analysis of transjugular intrahepatic portosystemic shunts. *Hepatology* 1997; **25**: 1064–9.

46 Bureau C, Garcia-Pagan JC, Otal P, *et al.* Improved clinical outcome using polytetrafluoroethylene-coated stents for TIPS: results of a randomized study. *Gastroenterology* 2004; **126**: 469–75.

47 Bureau C, Garcia Pagan JC, Layrargues GP, *et al.* Patency of stents covered with polytetrafluoroethylene in patients treated by transjugular intrahepatic portosystemic shunts: long-term results of a randomized multicentre study. *Liver Int* 2007; **27**: 742–7.

48 Saad WE, Darwish WM, Davies MG, Waldman DL. Stent-grafts for transjugular intrahepatic portosystemic shunt creation: specialized TIPS stent-graft versus generic stent-graft/bare stent combination. *J Vasc Interv Radiol* 2010; **21**: 1512–20.

49 Perarnau JM, Le Gouge A, Nicolas C, *et al.* Covered versus uncovered stents for transjugular intrahepatic portosystemic shunt: a randomized controlled trial. *J Hepatol* 2014; **60**(5): 962–8.

50 Hernández-Guerra M, Turnes J, Rubinstein P, *et al.* PTFE-covered stents improve TIPS patency in Budd-Chiari syndrome. *Hepatology* 2004; **40**: 1197–202.

51 Dhanasekaran R, West JK, Gonzales PC, *et al.* Transjugular intrahepatic portosystemic shunt for symptomatic refractory hepatic hydrothorax in patients with cirrhosis. *Am J Gastroenterol* 2010; **105**: 635–41.

52 Siegerstetter V, Deibert P, Ochs A, *et al.* Treatment of refractory hepatic hydrothorax with transjugular intrahepatic portosystemic shunt: long-term results in 40 patients. *Eur J Gastroenterol Hepatol* 2001; **13**: 529–34.

53 Wilputte JY, Goffette P, Zech F, *et al.* The outcome after transjugular intrahepatic portosystemic shunt (TIPS) for hepatic hydrothorax is closely related to liver dysfunction: a long-term study in 28 patients. *Acta Gastroenterol Belg* 2007; **70**: 6–10.

54 Spencer EB, Cohen DT, Darcy MD. Safety and efficacy of transjugular intrahepatic portosystemic shunt creation for the treatment of hepatic hydrothorax. *J Vasc Interv Radiol* 2002; **13**: 385–90.

55 Azoulay D, Castaing D, Lemoine A, *et al.* Transjugular intrahepatic portosystemic shunt (TIPS) for severe veno-occlusive disease of the liver following bone marrow transplantation. *Bone Marrow Transplant* 2000; **25**: 987–92.

56 Martinez-Palli G, Drake BB, García-Pagán JC, *et al.* Effect of transjugular intrahepatic portosystemic shunt on pulmonary gas exchange in patients with portal hypertension and hepatopulmonary syndrome. *World J Gastroenterol* 2005; **11**: 6858–62.

57 Urata J, Yamashita Y, Tsuchigame T, *et al.* The effects of transjugular intrahepatic portosystemic shunt on portal hypertensive gastropathy. *J Gastroenterol Hepatol* 1998; **13**: 1061–7.

CHAPTER 88

CHAPTER 89

Primary Carcinoma of the Liver

Renumathy Dhanasekaran,[1] Julie K. Heimbach,[2] and Lewis R. Roberts[1]

[1] Division of Gastroenterology and Hepatology, Mayo Clinic, Rochester, MN, USA
[2] Division of Transplantation Surgery, Mayo Clinic, Rochester, MN, USA

Summary

Hepatocellular carcinoma (HCC) and cholangiocarcinoma (CCA) are the two most common primary liver malignancies, HCC accounting for almost 90% of all such malignancies and CCA for less than 10%. HCC and CCA differ in terms of epidemiology, risk factors, clinical presentation, and prognosis. Both are relatively rare in Western countries compared to other regions of the world, but their incidence has been reported to be rising. Substantial advances have been made in liver transplantation for HCC, and patients with early-stage disease can achieve a 5-year survival rate of over 70%. These results, along with advances in surgical resection, local ablation, and transarterial therapies, have led to an increased emphasis on identification and surveillance of individuals at risk for HCC, to allow for early diagnosis, more effective treatment, and improved long-term outcomes. For patients with advanced, unresectable HCC, the multikinase inhibitor sorafenib, which has been shown to moderately extend patient survival, is the current standard of care. Meanwhile, CCA remains an aggressive tumor associated with poor prognosis; early diagnosis to identify patients eligible for curative surgical resection or liver transplantation is crucial.

Hepatocellular Carcinoma

Epidemiology

HCC is the fifth most common cancer in men worldwide and the second most frequent cause of cancer-related mortality; it was estimated to be responsible for nearly 746 000 deaths in 2012 [1]. The prognosis for liver cancer is very poor, with an overall ratio of mortality to incidence of 0.95 in both developed and developing countries. More than 80% of HCC is diagnosed in less developed regions of the world, such as Asia and sub-Saharan Africa, with the age-standardized rate of HCC being four times higher in less developed regions (8.8 per 100 000) than in more developed ones (2.2 per 100 000). In the United States, the incidence of liver and intrahepatic bile duct cancer has been rising at an average of 4.1% per year over the last 10 years [2]. The risk of HCC increases with age, and the age-specific incidence for HCC in the United States is highest among those older than 65 years [2]. In all regions of the world, men have a higher risk of developing HCC than women, with a worldwide male/female incidence ratio of 2.4 : 1 [1].

Risk Factors

The major risk factor for HCC is cirrhosis secondary to chronic hepatitis B or C, which accounts for about 80% of the global HCC burden. Individuals with chronic hepatitis B in the absence of cirrhosis are also at risk for HCC, particularly Africans over the age of 20, Asian males over the age of 40, Asian females over the age of 50, those with active inflammation, those with a family history of HCC, and those with high hepatitis B virus (HBV) DNA levels. Other important risk factors are dietary aflatoxin exposure, alcoholic cirrhosis, and other causes of cirrhosis such as hemochromatosis and non-alcoholic steatohepatitis (NASH).

Chronic Hepatitis B

There are 240 million individuals with chronic HBV infection worldwide, and around 600 000 people die every year as a consequence of hepatitis B infection. The majority of patients infected with hepatitis B who develop HCC have underlying cirrhosis, but hepatitis B can cause cancer even without cirrhosis. High HBV DNA levels are the strongest predictor of progression to cancer; in addition, hepatitis B "e" antigen (HBeAg) positivity, abnormal alanine transaminase (ALT) levels, male sex, and older age are associated with an increased risk of HCC [3]. Nomograms into which these variables can be input to predict an individual's risk for HCC have been developed and validated in Asian populations [4]. Treatment of hepatitis B has been shown to decrease the risk for HCC development, but does not completely protect against it; individuals on treatment therefore need to remain on surveillance for HCC [5]. Reassuringly, immunization of infants and at-risk individuals decreases the prevalence of chronic hepatitis B infection and the incidence of HCC [6].

Chronic Hepatitis C

About 150 million people worldwide are infected with hepatitis C virus (HCV), and 350 000 people die every year due to hepatitis C-related liver disease. Major risk factors for acquiring HCV include contaminated blood transfusions, use of contaminated needles, and other unhygienic practices among intravenous drug users and in substandard health care facilities. Chronic hepatitis C is a slowly progressive disease, and HCC usually develops only in those with HCV-induced cirrhosis. Older age, male gender, concurrent tobacco or alcohol use, persistently high ALT levels, increased stage of liver

Practical Gastroenterology and Hepatology Board Review Toolkit, Second Edition. Edited by Nicholas J. Talley, Kenneth R. DeVault, Michael B. Wallace, Bashar A. Aqel and Keith D. Lindor.

fibrosis, co-infection with hepatitis B or human immunodeficiency virus (HIV), diabetes, and obesity have all been reported to increase risk for HCC in patients with chronic HCV. Treatment of hepatitis C with a sustained virological response (SVR) is protective against the initial development of HCC or recurrence after surgical resection. However, patients with HCV and cirrhosis remain at risk for HCC even after achieving SVR and should remain in a surveillance program indefinitely [7].

Dietary Aflatoxin Exposure

Aflatoxins are mycotoxins produced by the ubiquitous fungi *Aspergillus flavus* and *A. parasiticus*. They are known liver carcinogens; of the related compounds, aflatoxin B1 is the most carcinogenic. Aflatoxins contribute substantially to the incidence of HCC in areas where the food supply is contaminated with Aspergillus fungi, including sub-Saharan Africa, South East Asia, and China [8]. Aflatoxin B1 is a procarcinogen that is converted by the cytochrome P-450 system in the liver to a mutagenic metabolite, which induces mutations in the *p53* gene, normally an important suppressor of liver tumorigenesis. Aflatoxin exposure is synergistic with chronic HBV and HCV infection in inducing liver tumorigenesis [3].

Other Causes

A possible link between diabetes, obesity, metabolic syndrome, and development of HCC is increasingly being recognized based on epidemiologic studies [9, 10]. Non-alcoholic fatty liver disease (NAFLD), which is a rising epidemic, is associated with a smaller but substantial risk for HCC, especially in cirrhotics. Hemochromatosis, alpha-1-antitrypsin (A1AT) deficiency, and other causes of chronic hepatitis also increase risk for HCC.

Pathogenesis

HCC occurs in multiple genetic and environmental contexts, and oncogene activation and tumor-suppressor inactivation play key roles in the carcinogenesis of HCC (Figure 89.1). In cirrhotic livers, macroregenerative nodules with foci of hepatocyte dysplasia have been identified as precancerous lesions. The sequence of persistent hepatitis with regenerative hepatocellular turnover, premature senescence of the liver, abrogation of the ability of the liver to regenerate its normal architecture, and eventual development of cirrhosis is presumed to play a major role in carcinogenesis.

Clinical Features

Most patients with HCC are asymptomatic early in the disease, except for symptoms associated with the underlying chronic liver

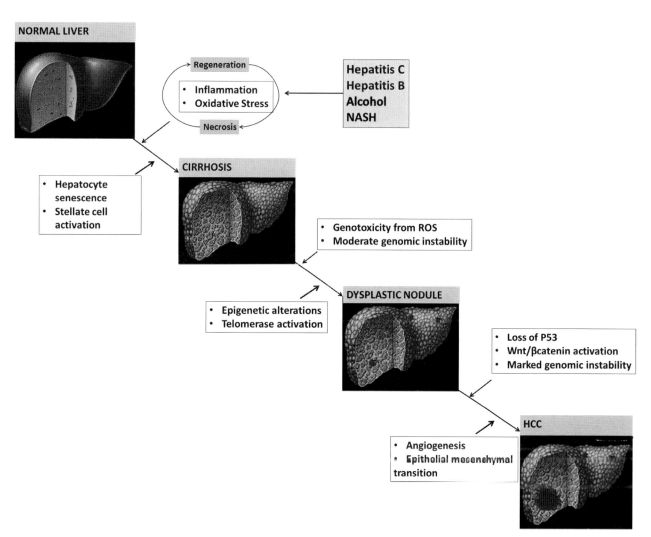

Figure 89.1 Simplified schematic representation of HCC pathogenesis. NASH, non-alcoholic steatohepatitis; ROS, reactive oxygen species; HCC, hepatocellular carcinoma.

CHAPTER 89

disease. Early-stage HCC is usually identified during surveillance of patients at risk for HCC. Rapid decompensation of cirrhosis, worsening portal hypertension, and ascites should raise suspicion for development of HCC with associated vascular invasion. Tumor infiltration of the hepatic sinusoids also worsens hepatic function, resulting in hyperbilirubinemia, coagulopathy, and encephalopathy. The development of spontaneous bacterial peritonitis (SBP) may be the first sign of HCC; therefore, patients diagnosed with SBP should be screened for HCC. Patients with advanced HCC may present with an abdominal mass, obstructive jaundice due to pressure effects on the central bile ducts, an acute abdomen due to intratumoral hemorrhage or intraperitoneal rupture, fever of unknown origin, metastatic disease, or constitutional symptoms. Paraneoplastic phenomena associated with HCC include hypercalcemia, hypoglycemia, thrombophlebitis migrans, erythrocytosis, and diarrhea. Laboratory features associated with HCC include changes of advanced liver disease, such as elevated bilirubin, alkaline phosphatase, and transaminases, with low albumin levels and prolongation of the prothrombin time.

Diagnosis

Surveillance and Screening Tests

Table 89.1 identifies the high-risk populations that should be enrolled in a surveillance program for HCC, based on American Association for the Study of Liver Diseases (AASLD) guidelines [11]. At-risk individuals should be screened at 6-month intervals with abdominal ultrasonography, which has a reported sensitivity of 94% [12]. The serum tumor marker alpha-fetoprotein (AFP) should not be used as a standalone diagnostic test, as it has a relatively low sensitivity (41–65%). Though the combined use of AFP and ultrasonography increases detection rates [13], the 2010 AASLD guidelines do not recommend the use of AFP due to concern that it increases costs through high false-positive rates. Other serum tumor markers include des-gamma-carboxyprothrombin (DCP) and the AFP-L3 isoform of AFP. These latter markers have not shown superior performance over the serum AFP, but may be helpful when used in combination with ultrasonography and AFP [14, 15].

Diagnosis and Staging

Once a new nodule has been found by screening ultrasonography in a cirrhotic liver, further cross-sectional liver imaging with computed tomography (CT) or magnetic resonance imaging (MRI) should be pursued. Figure 89.2 provides an algorithm for the evaluation of nodules found on ultrasound surveillance. For the most part, HCC

Table 89.1 High-risk pool to enroll in an HCC surveillance program. Based on AASLD 2010 guidelines [11].

Recommended surveillance for **cirrhotics**	Hepatitis B cirrhosis
	Hepatitis C cirrhosis (fibrosis ≥3)
	Alcoholic cirrhosis
	Genetic hemochromatosis
	NASH
	A1AT deficiency
	Autoimmune hepatitis
Recommended surveillance for **non-cirrhotics**	Hepatitis B:
	• Asian males >40 years
	• Asian females >50 years
	• Africans >20 years
	• Family history of HCC
	• High HBV DNA, high ALT

NASH, non-alcoholic steatohepatitis; A1AT, alpha-1-antitrypsin; HCC, hepatocellular carcinoma; HBV, hepatitis B virus; ALT, alanine aminotransferase.

can be diagnosed based on imaging alone, and biopsies are seldom required. The risks of biopsy include bleeding, a small but significant risk of tumor seeding (in perhaps 0.5% of cases), and a more substantial risk of a false-negative result (up to 10% for attempted biopsies of small lesions) [16]. The current United Network for Organ Sharing (UNOS) guidelines grant standard Model for End-Stage Liver Disease (MELD) exception scores only to individuals who meet the Milan criteria (one lesion between 2 and 5 cm in maximal diameter or up to three lesions, none of which is >3 cm in maximal diameter), though patients successfully treated with downsizing protocols and those with tumors that exceed the Milan criteria may be considered on an individual basis at the level of the regional review boards. Patients who are granted MELD exception points must meet the recently revised, more rigorous radiographic criteria for the diagnosis of HCC.

The Barcelona Clinic Liver Cancer (BCLC) staging system is endorsed by the AASLD and the European Association for the Study of the Liver (EASL). HCCs are classified into five stages based on the extent of the primary lesion, performance status, underlying liver synthetic function, presence of constitutional symptoms, vascular invasion, and extrahepatic spread [17] (Figure 89.3).

Treatment

The stage of the tumor at presentation determines the treatment options. Figure 89.3 outlines treatment options for patients with HCC based on BCLC staging.

Early Stage (BCLC Stages 0 and A)

Surgical Resection

Resection is a potentially curative option for patients with early-stage HCC with well-compensated liver disease. Unfortunately, only a very small proportion of patients with chronic liver disease are eligible for resection. The ideal candidate for resection is a patient with BCLC stage 0 or A with Child–Pugh class A cirrhosis (characterized by normal portal pressures (hepatic venous pressure gradient <10 mmHg), normal bilirubin (total bilirubin <1 mg/dL), and absence of clinically significant portal hypertension (lack of esophageal varices and splenomegaly, with platelet count >100 000)) [10]. In carefully selected patients who achieve negative margins after resection and do not have microvascular invasion, 5-year survival rates up to 80% have been reported. As the neoplastic potential of the non-resected cirrhotic liver remains unchanged, intrahepatic recurrence of HCC frequently occurs after an apparently curative resection; recurrence rates are up to 50% at 3 years and 75% at 5 years after resection.

Liver Transplantation

Liver transplantation is the optimal therapy for patients with early-stage HCC with moderate to severe liver dysfunction, who are thus not eligible for surgical resection. Liver transplantation offers a couple of advantages over partial hepatectomy: it can be employed for patients with all stages of liver disease and it addresses the cancer, the neoplastic potential of the surrounding liver, and the chronic liver disease itself. The best outcomes are achieved in patients without extrahepatic metastases who have a single tumor 2–5 cm in maximal diameter or up to three lesions, the largest of which is not more than 3 cm in maximal diameter (the Milan criteria) [19]. The most important limitation of liver transplantation is an increasing donor organ shortage. Current UNOS policy assigns additional MELD points to patients with HCC listed for liver transplantation,

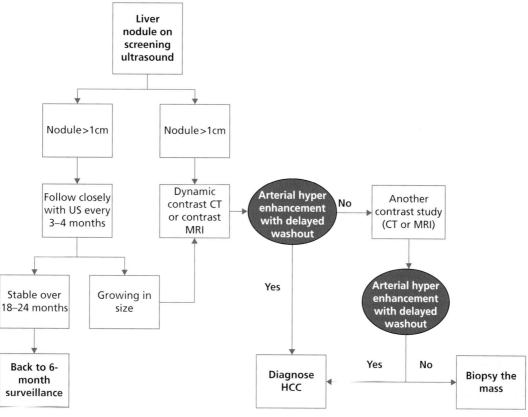

Figure 89.2 Algorithm for the evaluation of nodules found on ultrasound surveillance in patients with cirrhosis. US, ultrasound; CT, computed tomography; MRI, magnetic resonance imaging; HCC, hepatocellular carcinoma.

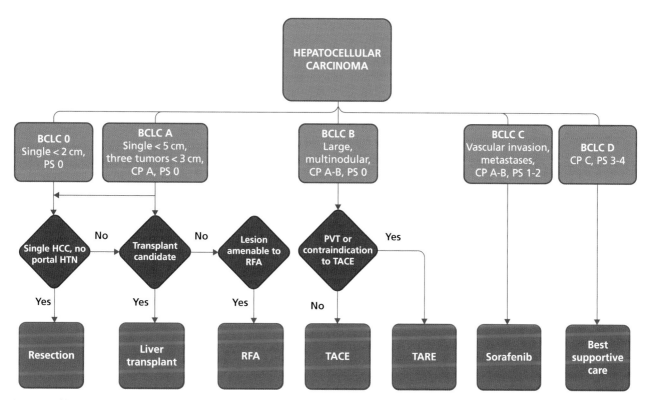

Figure 89.3 Treatment options for patients with HCC, based on BCLC staging. BCLC, Barcelona Clinic Liver Cancer; PS, performance status; CP, Child–Pugh class; HCC, hepatocellular carcinoma; HTN, hypertension; RFA, radiofrequency ablation; PVT, portal vein thrombosis; TACE, transarterial chemoembolization; TARE, transarterial radioembolization.

with the goal of achieving the same rate of transplantation as found in patients with non-malignant liver diseases. The data currently demonstrate that patients with HCC are overprioritized, with higher transplant rates and lower waitlist drop-out rates compared to non-HCC patients [20]. To prevent tumor growth and metastasis while patients await liver transplantation, many transplant centers treat these lesions using bridging locoregional therapy prior to transplantation. Liver transplantation for HCC is associated with excellent survival rates (5-year survival: 60–70%), similar to those for non-malignant diseases.

Intermediate Stage (BCLC Stage B)

In patients who do not meet the criteria for surgical resection or liver transplantation, local ablation techniques such as radiofrequency ablation (RFA), microwave ablation, laser ablation, and percutaneous ethanol injection (PEI) are used to treat early-stage HCC with two to four lesions of up to 4 cm diameter. Patients with intermediate-stage disease with bilateral multinodular disease are treated with transarterial chemoembolization (TACE) or transarterial radioembolization (TARE), if feasible.

Ablation Therapies

RFA destroys cancer tissues using thermal energy generated by an alternating electric current generator operating in the radiofrequency range 200–1200 kHz. In PEI, the injection of absolute alcohol destroys tumor cells through cellular dehydration, coagulation necrosis, and vascular thrombosis, followed by ischemia. The decision regarding which technique to employ is usually based on tumor size, tumor location, presence of portal vein thrombus, and local expertise. RFA has been shown to be more efficacious than PEI for small tumors, both in a meta-analysis and in a randomized controlled trial (RCT) [21, 22]. However, RFA is contraindicated for lesions adjacent to the diaphragm or large vessels, due to potential damage to adjacent tissues and potential loss of efficacy through the heatsink effect of large blood vessels. In those small tumors not eligible for RFA, PEI can be considered.

Transarterial Chemoembolization

TACE uses angiography to selectively deliver chemotherapeutic drugs and embolizing agents directly into the arterial supply of the HCC. It causes selective ischemia and traps the chemotherapy agent(s) within the tumor, allowing high-dose chemotherapeutic effects on the HCC. Two RCTs have demonstrated a survival benefit of TACE over best supportive care in patients with intermediate-stage multifocal HCC with Child–Pugh class A [23, 24]. Most patients receiving TACE should be hospitalized for observation, because of the high frequency of post-embolization syndrome, characterized by fever, nausea, abdominal pain, and elevated transaminases. Fortunately, this syndrome is usually self-limited, and resolves in 24–48 hours. Other potential complications of TACE include contrast allergy, contrast nephropathy, bleeding, pseudoaneurysm formation, and hepatic abscess. Advanced Child class C cirrhosis is a relative contraindication for TACE, because of the high risk of fatal complications such as liver failure. Portal vein thrombosis (PVT) is also a contraindication, because additional occlusion of the hepatic artery branches with TACE results in complete ischemia of the treated liver segments. Other contraindications include hepatic encephalopathy, biliary obstruction, and the presence of a transjugular intrahepatic portosystemic shunt (TIPS).

Transarterial Radioembolization

TARE employs yttrium-90-labeled (Y90) microspheres and is similar to TACE in that radiolabeled particles are infused into the hepatic artery and flow into the vascular bed of the HCC, sparing normal liver tissue, which is primarily perfused by the portal vein. Staging hepatic angiography is performed before radioembolization, and if hepatic arterial branches that might result in extrahepatic deposition of the microspheres are identified, they are occluded using standard angiographic techniques. A technetium-99m (^{99m}Tc)-macro aggregated albumin study is then performed to calculate the proportion of infused radiation that will be shunted to the lungs. The two subgroups in which TARE appears to have an advantage over TACE include patients on the transplant waiting list and patients with PVT. TARE has been shown to be safe and effective in downstaging HCC prior to transplantation [25]. In addition, because the Y90 microspheres do not completely occlude the arterial vascular bed, patients with PVT remain candidates for TARE [26]. Complications of radioembolization include worsening hepatic dysfunction, cholecystitis, gastric or duodenal ulcers, allergic reactions, fatigue, and abdominal pain.

Advanced Stage (BCLC Stages C and D)

HCC has traditionally been considered relatively resistant to systemic chemotherapy, and patients with cirrhosis and resultant cytopenias usually do not tolerate the side effects associated with conventional cytotoxic chemotherapy. Sorafenib, an oral multikinase/tyrosine kinase inhibitor, has been shown to provide a survival benefit over best supportive care in two pivotal studies: the SHARP trial (a phase III study of sorafenib in patients with advanced HCC) and the Asia-Pacific sorafenib trial. These studies predominantly included patients with Child–Pugh class A cirrhosis and advanced BCLC stage C HCC [27,28]. The primary end point, overall survival, was improved by 3 months in the sorafenib group when compared with placebo (7.9 versus 10.7 months). Treatment with sorafenib is relatively well tolerated: the most significant side effects are fatigue, diarrhea, hypertension, and hand–foot skin reaction. Multiple other molecular targeted therapies for management of HCC are currently in clinical trials. Patients with Child–Pugh class C and poor performance status are usually not candidates for any of the therapies mentioned in this section and should be provided best supportive care.

Cholangiocarcinoma

Epidemiology and Risk Factors

CCAs are malignant tumors that arise from the bile duct epithelium and are the second most common form of primary liver cancer. They are usually aggressive tumors with a dismal prognosis, with a 5-year survival of less than 10% [29]. CCAs are classified into three subtypes based on location (Figure 89.4): intrahepatic cholangiocarcinomas (iCCAs) are located within the hepatic parenchyma; perihilar cholangiocarcinomas (pCCAs) arise between the second-order bile ducts and the origin of the cystic duct; and distal cholangiocarcinomas (dCCAs) arise between the origin of the cystic duct and the ampulla of Vater. Of the three, pCCA is the most common subtype, but the incidence of iCCA has been reported to be on the rise. Most CCAs are sporadic in nature and are not associated with any underlying liver disease or risk factors. A minority of patients have established predisposing risk factors for CCA, including primary sclerosing cholangitis (PSC), Caroli's disease, choledochal cysts, inflammatory bowel disease (IBD), and hepatobiliary flukes.

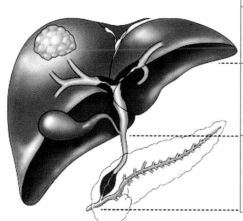

CHOLANGIOCARCINOMA CLASSIFICATION

Intrahepatic CCA (iCCA)
Arise from the intrahepatic biliary tract proximal to the second-order biliary ducts

Perihilar CCA (pCCA)
Arise between the second-order biliary ducts and the site of cystic duct origin

Distal CCA (dCCA)
Arise between the cystic duct origin and the ampulla of Vater

Figure 89.4 The anatomic landmarks that help classify CCA.

Patients with PSC carry a high risk for CCA, with a lifetime cumulative risk of 7–13%, which is substantially higher than that in the general population [30]. Other, less well established risk factors reported in the literature include biliary cirrhosis, cholelithiasis, diabetes, obesity, chronic liver disease, chronic HCV infection, and smoking.

Clinical Features and Diagnosis
Patients with perihilar and distal CCA usually present with painless obstructive jaundice and laboratory features of direct hyperbilirubinemia and elevated alkaline phosphatase. Patients with intrahepatic CCA are less likely to be jaundiced and usually present with abdominal pain or other constitutional symptoms, such as weight loss. Patients with PSC may present with rapid decompensation or recurrent cholangitis. Perihilar CCA frequently arises unilaterally, causing ipsilateral ductal obstruction and vascular encasement for a period of time before extension into the confluence and development of bilateral biliary obstruction. During the initial period of unilateral obstruction, an atrophy–hypertrophy complex develops; this is characterized by ipsilateral liver lobe atrophy, with associated marked biliary dilatation, and simultaneous contralateral lobe compensatory hypertrophy (Figure 89.5).

The diagnosis of CCA can be challenging, especially when the tumor is intraductal in location. The tumor marker CA19-9 has low sensitivity and specificity, but can be useful as a confirmatory test, though results need to be interpreted cautiously as biliary obstruction and cholangitis can also raise CA19-9. Non-invasive modalities like contrast CT and MRI/magnetic resonance cholangiopancreatography (MRCP) are the initial tests of choice, and CCA is usually characterized by delayed venous phase enhancement. If intrahepatic masses are found, biopsy can be considered for diagnosis of iCCA. For pCCA or dCCA, initial imaging studies are usually followed by endoscopic retrograde cholangiopancreatography (ERCP) and, less commonly, PTC to look for dominant strictures, which are then brushed for cytology and fluorescent in situ hybridization (FISH) and biopsied, if feasible. The yield of cytology from brushings is low, at around 20%, due to the intense desmoplastic reaction associated with this tumor, which results in sampling of a limited number of tumor cells. In patients with pCCA who are potential surgical candidates, a percutaneous or endoscopic ultrasonography (EUS)-guided biopsy should be avoided as it increases the risk of metastatic spread and renders the patient ineligible for transplant. Chromosomal analysis using FISH increases the diagnostic yield of the brushings if polysomy of chromosomes 3, 7, and 17 or loss at the 9p21 locus is found. Though none of these tests can be used in isolation to diagnose CCA, a combination of clinical features, radiologic findings, cytology, and FISH aids physicians in arriving at the diagnosis.

Treatment
CCA generally has a poor prognosis and limited therapeutic options. The mainstay of potentially curative therapy remains surgical resection or liver transplantation in selected patients. Once the diagnosis of CCA is made and local or distant metastatic disease is ruled out, the patient needs to be referred to an experienced hepatobiliary surgeon for consideration for resection. Distal CCAs have the highest possibility of resection, and pCCAs the lowest. Resectability is generally determined during surgery, as the presence of vascular invasion is not always evident on preoperative imaging. Postoperative adjuvant chemotherapy is usually used in patients

CHAPTER 89

Figure 89.5 (a) MRI of liver with arterial enhancement. (b) Venous washout of the same lesion. (c) MRI liver demonstrating atrophy–hypertrophy with biliary ductal dilation of the left hepatic lobe.

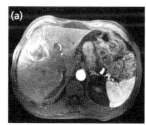
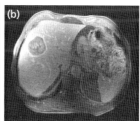
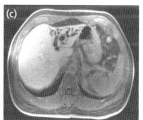

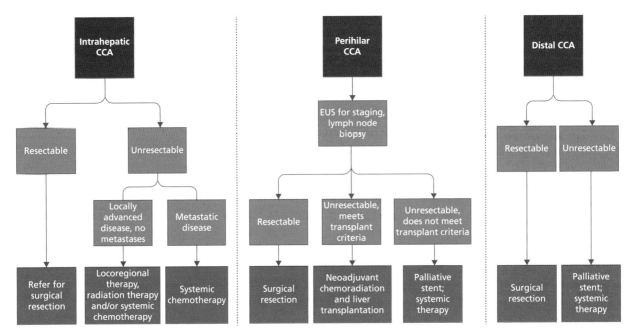

Figure 89.6 Treatment algorithm for patients with cholangiocarcinoma. CCA, cholangiocarcinoma; EUS, endoscopic ultrasound.

with high-risk features such as lymph node positivity and positive surgical margins after surgery with curative intent, but its benefit has not been clearly established. Another potentially curative treatment option is combined neoadjuvant chemoradiotherapy followed by liver transplantation, which is available only for a highly select group of patients with early-stage pCCA. The diagnosis and staging criteria are stringent, and patients receive neoadjuvant chemoradiotherapy prior to liver transplantation. In our single-center experience, we have reported excellent 1- and 5-year patient survival rates of 90 and 71%, respectively [31]. Similar results (5-year disease-free survival of 65%) have recently been demonstrated in a multicenter report incorporating data from 12 US centers [32]. These results are exceptional for this aggressive tumor.

For patients with advanced CCA, systemic chemotherapy is offered, but no single chemotherapeutic agent or combination regimen has been shown to be reliably associated with better local tumor control or survival benefit. The most commonly used combination therapy consists of gemcitabine plus cisplatin or oxaliplatin. A randomized controlled study has demonstrated that combination gemcitabine/cisplatin is associated with improved median survival when compared to gemcitabine alone (11.7 versus 8.1 months) [33]. Combinations of existing chemotherapeutic regimens with newer molecular targeted therapies for advanced CCA are in clinical trials. In patients with unresectable iCCAs, locoregional therapies such as TACE or TARE can also be employed to achieve local tumor control. Figure 89.6 outlines a treatment algorithm for patients with CCA.

- Individuals with early-stage HCC should be considered for surgical resection if they do not have cirrhosis or have cirrhosis with a normal bilirubin and without clinically significant portal hypertension.
- Liver transplantation is the most effective therapy for HCC, and is offered for eligible candidates with tumor burden within the Milan criteria (one lesion between 2 and 5 cm in maximal diameter or up to three lesions, none of which is >3 cm in maximal diameter).
- HCC patients who are not surgical candidates should be considered for local ablation with radiofrequency ablation (RFA) or percutaneous ethanol injection (PEI) if they have early-stage disease. Individuals with intermediate-stage disease are candidates for transarterial chemoembolization (TACE) or transarterial radioembolization (TARE).
- Patients with advanced HCC are candidates for treatment with the multikinase inhibitor sorafenib. Major side effects of sorafenib include fatigue, diarrhea, hypertension, and hand–foot reaction.
- Cholangiocarcinomas (CCAs) are classified as intrahepatic (iCCA), perihilar (pCCA), or distal (dCCA) based on anatomic location.
- The diagnosis of CCA is challenging and requires a combination of clinical features, radiologic findings, and retrograde cholangiopancreatography (ERCP) or percutaneous transhepatic cholangiography (PTC) with brushings for cytology and fluorescent in situ hybridization (FISH).
- Resection is the best curative option for early-stage patients with de novo disease. Those with early-stage pCCA and underlying primary sclerosing cholangitis (PSC) are best served by neoadjuvant therapy and transplantation protocol. Neoadjuvant chemoradiotherapy followed by liver transplantation is offered for a highly select group of individuals with early-stage pCCA. Transperitoneal biopsy of the primary tumor should be avoided due to the high risk of peritoneal seed.

Take Home Points

- Individuals with cirrhosis of any cause or with chronic hepatitis B virus (HBV) infection without cirrhosis (in Africans >20 years, Asian males >40 years, and Asian females >50 years) should be enrolled in a surveillance program for hepatocellular carcinoma (HCC).
- Current surveillance recommendations are for patients to have liver ultrasonography every 6 months.

References

1 International Agency for Reaserch on Cancer; World Health Organization. GLOBOCAN 2012: estimated cancer incidence, mortality and prevalance worldwide in 2012. Available from: http://globocan.iarc.fr (last accessed February 15, 2016).
2 National Cancer Institute. SEER Stat Fact Sheets: liver and intrahepatic bile duct cancer. Available from: http://seer.cancer.gov/statfacts/html/livibd.html (last accessed February 15, 2016).

3 Iloeje UH, Yang HI, Su J, *et al.* Predicting cirrhosis risk based on the level of circulating hepatitis B viral load. *Gastroenterology* 2006; **130**(3): 678–86.

4 Yang H-I, Sherman M, Su J, *et al.* Nomograms for risk of hepatocellular carcinoma in patients with chronic hepatitis B virus infection. *J Clin Oncol* 2010; **28**(14): 2437–44.

5 Papatheodoridis GV, Lampertico P, Manolakopoulos S, Lok A. Incidence of hepatocellular carcinoma in chronic hepatitis B patients receiving nucleos(t)ide therapy: a systematic review. *J Hepatol* 2010; **53**(2): 348–56.

6 Chang MH, Chen TH, Hsu HM, *et al.* Prevention of hepatocellular carcinoma by universal vaccination against hepatitis B virus: the effect and problems. *Clin Cancer Res* 2005; **11**(21): 7953–7.

7 George SL, Bacon BR, Brunt EM, *et al.* Clinical, virologic, histologic, and biochemical outcomes after successful HCV therapy: a 5-year follow-up of 150 patients. *Hepatology* 2009; **49**(3): 729–38.

8 Liu Y, Wu F. Global burden of aflatoxin-induced hepatocellular carcinoma: a risk assessment. *Environ Health Perspect* 2010; **118**(6): 818–24.

9 El-Serag HB, Tran T, Everhart JE. Diabetes increases the risk of chronic liver disease and hepatocellular carcinoma. *Gastroenterology* 2004; **126**(2): 460–8.

10 Wang C, Wang X, Gong G, *et al.* Increased risk of hepatocellular carcinoma in patients with diabetes mellitus: a systematic review and meta-analysis of cohort studies. *Int J Cancer* 2012; **130**(7): 1639–48.

11 Bruix J, Sherman M, Practice Guidelines Committee, American Association for the Study of Liver Diseases. Management of hepatocellular carcinoma. *Hepatology* 2005; **42**(5): 1208–36.

12 Singal A, Volk ML, Waljee A, *et al.* Meta-analysis: surveillance with ultrasound for early-stage hepatocellular carcinoma in patients with cirrhosis. *Aliment Pharmacol Ther* 2009; **30**(1): 37–47.

13 Gupta S, Bent S, Kohlwes J. Test characteristics of alpha-fetoprotein for detecting hepatocellular carcinoma in patients with hepatitis C. A systematic review and critical analysis. *Ann Intern Med* 2003; **139**(1): 46–50.

14 Morimoto M, Numata K, Nozaki A, *et al.* Novel Lens culinaris agglutinin-reactive fraction of alpha-fetoprotein: a biomarker of hepatocellular carcinoma recurrence in patients with low alpha-fetoprotein concentrations. *Int J Clin Oncol* 2012; **17**(4): 373–9.

15 Marrero JA, Su GL, Wei W, *et al.* Des-gamma carboxyprothrombin can differentiate hepatocellular carcinoma from nonmalignant chronic liver disease in american patients. *Hepatology* 2003; **37**(5): 1114–21.

16 Perkins JD. Seeding risk following percutaneous approach to hepatocellular carcinoma. *Liver Transpl* 2007; **13**(11): 1603.

17 Llovet JM, Bru C, Bruix J. Prognosis of hepatocellular carcinoma: the BCLC staging classification. *Semin Liver Dis* 1999; **19**(3): 329–38.

18 Llovet JM, Fuster J, Bruix J. Intention-to-treat analysis of surgical treatment for early hepatocellular carcinoma: resection versus transplantation. *Hepatology* 1999; **30**(6): 1434–40.

19 Mazzaferro V, Regalia E, Doci R, *et al.* Liver transplantation for the treatment of small hepatocellular carcinomas in patients with cirrhosis. *N Engl J Med* 1996; **334**(11): 693–9.

20 Goldberg D, French B, Abt P, *et al.* Increasing disparity in waitlist mortality rates with increased model for end-stage liver disease scores for candidates with hepatocellular carcinoma versus candidates without hepatocellular carcinoma. *Liver Transpl* 2012; **18**(4): 434–43.

21 Bouza C, Lopez-Cuadrado T, Alcazar R, *et al.* Meta-analysis of percutaneous radiofrequency ablation versus ethanol injection in hepatocellular carcinoma. *BMC Gastroenterol* 2009; **9**: 31.

22 Lencioni RA, Allgaier HP, Cioni D, *et al.* Small hepatocellular carcinoma in cirrhosis: randomized comparison of radio-frequency thermal ablation versus percutaneous ethanol injection. *Radiology* 2003; **228**(1): 235–40.

23 Llovet JM, Real MI, Montana X, *et al.* Arterial embolisation or chemoembolisation versus symptomatic treatment in patients with unresectable hepatocellular carcinoma: a randomised controlled trial. *Lancet* 2002; **359**(9319): 1734–9.

24 Lo CM, Ngan H, Tso WK, *et al.* Randomized controlled trial of transarterial lipiodol chemoembolization for unresectable hepatocellular carcinoma. *Hepatology* 2002; **35**(5): 1164–71.

25 Lewandowski RJ, Kulik LM, Riaz A, *et al.* A comparative analysis of transarterial downstaging for hepatocellular carcinoma: chemoembolization versus radioembolization. *Am J Transplant* 2009; **9**(8): 1920–8.

26 Kulik LM, Carr BI, Mulcahy MF, *et al.* Safety and efficacy of 90Y radiotherapy for hepatocellular carcinoma with and without portal vein thrombosis. *Hepatology* 2008; **47**(1): 71–81.

27 Llovet JM, Ricci S, Mazzaferro V, *et al.* Sorafenib in advanced hepatocellular carcinoma. *N Engl J Med* 2008; **359**(4): 378–90.

28 Cheng AL, Kang YK, Chen Z, *et al.* Efficacy and safety of sorafenib in patients in the Asia-Pacific region with advanced hepatocellular carcinoma: a phase III randomised, double-blind, placebo-controlled trial. *Lancet Oncol* 2009; **10**(1): 25–34.

29 Everhart JE, Ruhl CE. Burden of digestive diseases in the United States Part III: Liver, biliary tract, and pancreas. *Gastroenterology* 2009; **136**(4): 1134–44.

30 Burak K, Angulo P, Pasha TM, *et al.* Incidence and risk factors for cholangiocarcinoma in primary sclerosing cholangitis. *Am J Gastroenterol* 2004; **99**(3): 523–6.

31 Rosen CB, Heimbach JK, Gores GJ. Surgery for cholangiocarcinoma: the role of liver transplantation. *HPB (Oxford)* 2008; **10**(3): 186–9.

32 Darwish Murad S, Kim WR, Harnois DM, *et al.* Efficacy of neoadjuvant chemoradiation, followed by liver transplantation, for perihilar cholangiocarcinoma at 12 US centers. *Gastroenterology* 2012; **143**(1): 88–98.e3, quiz e14.

33 Valle JW, Wasan H, Johnson P, *et al.* Gemcitabine alone or in combination with cisplatin in patients with advanced or metastatic cholangiocarcinomas or other biliary tract tumours: a multicentre randomised phase II study – The UK ABC-01 Study. *Br J Cancer* 2009; **101**(4): 621–7.

CHAPTER 89

Pregnancy and Liver Disease

J. Eileen Hay

Division of Gastroenterology and Hepatology, Mayo Clinic, Rochester, MN, USA

Summary

Liver dysfunction occurs in 3% of pregnancies and is usually pregnancy-related. Hyperemesis gravidarum occurs in the first trimester, with intractable nausea, vomiting, and dehydration. Intrahepatic cholestasis of pregnancy (ICP) occurs in the second half of pregnancy and causes intense pruritus associated with elevated serum bile acid levels; maternal outcomes are excellent, but the fetus requires intense fetal monitoring and early delivery to prevent intrauterine death. Ursodeoxycholic acid (UDCA) is the treatment of choice. The third-trimester diseases are pre-eclampsia-associated liver diseases. Pre-eclampsia/eclampsia itself is the commonest cause of liver tenderness and abnormal liver tests in pregnancy. The HELLP syndrome (hemolysis, elevated liver tests, and low platelet count) is a life-threatening condition for which immediate delivery is the only definitive therapy. Acute fatty liver of pregnancy (AFLP) causes acute liver failure via microvesicular fat accumulation in hepatocytes; rapid clinical diagnosis and delivery of the fetus are life-saving.

Case

A 32-year-old G2P1 woman at 24 weeks' gestation presents with 2 weeks of severe pruritus, which is generalized, but occurs especially in the palms and soles; this is present constantly, but has nocturnal exacerbation, preventing sleep. Her last pregnancy was notable for mild pruritus with abnormal liver chemistries. She denies fever, nausea, jaundice, or abdominal pain. Examination shows a gravid uterus and a few skin excoriations.

Aspartate aminotransferase (AST) is 177 IU/L, alanine aminotransferase (ALT) 355 IU/L, total bilirubin 2.1 mg/dL; complete blood count (CBC), electrolyte panel, and renal function are normal.

Definition and Epidemiology

Liver dysfunction in pregnancy occurs due to (i) coincidental liver disease, (ii) underlying chronic liver disease, or (iii) one of the five liver diseases unique to pregnancy (Table 90.1). Most liver dysfunction in pregnancy is pregnancy-related [1], but other causes must be excluded. In a normal pregnancy, elevation of alkaline phosphatase and falls in albumin and hemoglobin levels occur, but no changes in AST, ALT, bilirubin, serum bile acids, prothrombin time, or liver-spleen size are seen.

This chapter focuses on the five liver diseases unique to pregnancy. Hyperemesis gravidarum occurs in 0.3% of pregnancies. It consists of intractable nausea and vomiting leading to severe dehydration in the first trimester. ICP is reversible cholestasis with severe pruritus in the second and third trimesters and elevated serum bile acid levels [2]. In the United States, it occurs in 0.1–0.3% of pregnancies, but its incidence has a striking geographic, ethnic, and seasonal variability worldwide.

The other three pregnancy-related liver diseases are all third-trimester diseases and are associated with pre-eclampsia. Pre-eclampsia itself is the commonest cause of hepatic tenderness and liver dysfunction in pregnancy, with abnormal liver tests in 10% of cases [1]. Severe pre-eclampsia is complicated in 2–12% patients by HELLP syndrome. AFLP is the most severe and rarest of the pregnancy-related liver diseases. It involves microvesicular fatty infiltration of hepatocytes, causing acute liver failure. It occurs in 0.005–0.100% pregnancies [3].

Pathophysiology

Hyperemesis Gravidarum

The etiology of hyperemesis gravidarum remains unknown, with potential effects from immunologic, hormonal, and psychologic factors associated with pregnancy. Risk factors include hyperthyroidism, psychiatric illness, molar pregnancy, pre-existing diabetes, multiple gestations, and gastrointestinal (GI) disorders [4].

Intrahepatic Cholestasis of Pregnancy

ICP is cholestasis due to abnormal biliary transport across the canalicular membrane, resulting in high levels of bile acids (>10 umol/L) in maternal serum. Genetic and exogenous factors are etiologically involved. The temporal relationship to hormone levels in late pregnancy, the increased incidence in twin pregnancies, the precipitation by exogenous progesterone, and the resolution after pregnancy all suggest that ICP is strongly influenced by estrogen and/or progesterone. Sex hormones have known cholestatic effects. Impaired sulfation and abnormalities in progesterone metabolism have been found in ICP.

Familial cases and ethnic variability have long suggested a genetic predisposition. Studies of genetic polymorphisms in bile acid-associated genes have identified at least 10 mutations in the *MDR3* (*ABCB4*) gene that have an association with ICP in about 15% cases

Practical Gastroenterology and Hepatology Board Review Toolkit, Second Edition. Edited by Nicholas J. Talley, Kenneth R. DeVault, Michael B. Wallace, Bashar A. Aqel and Keith D. Lindor.
© 2016 John Wiley & Sons, Ltd. Published 2016 by John Wiley & Sons, Ltd. Companion website: www.practicalgastrohep.com

Table 90.1 Causes of liver dysfunction in pregnancy.

Coincidental liver diseases	Acute viral hepatitis
	Gallstones
	Drugs or toxins
	Sepsis
	Budd–Chiari syndrome
Chronic liver diseases	Autoimmune hepatitis
	PSC (rarely, PBC)
	Hepatitis C or chronic B
	Wilson's, A1AT deficiency
	Cirrhosis of any cause
Liver diseases unique to pregnancy	Hyperemesis gravidarum
	ICP
	Pre-eclampsia
	HELLP syndrome
	AFLP

PSC, primary sclerosing cholangitis; PBC, primary biliary cirrhosis; A1AT, alpha-1-antitrypsin; ICP, intrahepatic cholestasis of pregnancy; HELLP, hemolysis, elevated liver tests, low platelets; AFLP, acute fatty liver of pregnancy.

[5,6]. *MDR3* is the transporter for phospholipids across the canalicular membrane; mutations may result in loss of function, causing elevated bile acid levels. Similarly, risk alleles for ICP have been shown for *ABCB11* (the gene associated with bile salt export) [7]. The fact that recurrence is seen in only 45–70% of pregnancies and the clear seasonal variability in areas of high prevalence suggest the influence of exogenous factors, such as selenium or vitamin D deficiency [8,9].

High maternal levels of bile acid in ICP correlate with fetal morbidity and mortality [10]. Abnormal placental bile acid transport from fetal to maternal circulation, increased maternal bile acid levels, and immature fetal transport systems may all contribute to elevated fetal bile acid levels in ICP.

HELLP Syndrome

HELLP syndrome is a microangiopathic hemolytic anemia associated with vascular endothelial injury and platelet activation. Small to diffuse areas of hemorrhage and necrosis occur in the liver, with large hematomas, capsular tears, and risk of hepatic rupture. No precipitating injury or single genetic predisposition is known [11], though some cases are associated with maternal heterozygosity for factor V Leiden [12]. It is considered a complication of pre-eclampsia and has some overlap with AFLP.

Acute Fatty Liver of Pregnancy

AFLP causes acute liver failure from microvesicular fatty infiltration of hepatocytes. Autosomal recessive genetic mutations of the enzymes necessary for the beta-oxidation of fatty acids in hepatic mitochondria are implicated in the pathogenesis of AFLP [13], especially deficiency of the enzyme long-chain 3-hydroxyacyl CoA dehydrogenase (LCHAD) – particularly its *G1548C* mutation. Mothers of babies with defects in fatty acid oxidation (FAO) have a very high incidence of AFLP, and 20% of babies of mothers with AFLP have LCHAD deficiency. It is hypothesized that maternal heterozygosity for LCHAD deficiency reduces the maternal capacity to oxidize long-chain fatty acids in both liver and placenta. This, together with the metabolic stress of pregnancy and fetal homozygosity for LCHAD deficiency, causes accumulation in the maternal circulation of hepatotoxic LCHAD metabolites. External factors, such as carnitine deficiency or other dietary factors, may exacerbate this situation.

Clinical Features

Hyperemesis Gravidarum

Hyperemesis gravidarum is intractable, dehydrating vomiting, typically starting at 4–10 weeks' gestation, most often in young primigravidae. Liver dysfunction is present in half of hospitalized patients and parallels the severity of vomiting. Transaminases may rise 20-fold, and mild jaundice (bilirubin <5 mg/dL) may occasionally occur.

Intrahepatic Cholestasis of Pregnancy

Pruritus occurring at around 25–32 weeks' gestation in a patient with no other signs of liver disease is strongly suggestive of ICP. It may occasionally occur earlier than 25 weeks, but 80% of cases have pruritus after 30 weeks. The pruritus affects all parts of the body (especially the palms and soles), is worse at night, and may lead to suicidal ideation. Excoriations are obvious, with jaundice in 10–25% of patients, usually following the pruritus by 2–4 weeks. Transaminase elevations are mild to >1000 IU/L; bilirubin is usually <5 mg/dL. The most specific marker is serum bile acid levels, which are always >10 umol/L and may be 100 times elevated. The main risk of ICP is for the fetus, with placental insufficiency, premature labor, and sudden fetal death. The risk correlates with severe elevations of bile acids [10].

Pre-eclampsia

Severe pre-eclampsia may present with right upper abdominal pain, jaundice, and a tender, normal-sized liver. Transaminases are variably elevated, from mild to 10–20 times elevation; bilirubin is usually <5 mg/dL.

HELLP Syndrome

Most patients present at between 27 and 36 weeks' gestation, occasionally earlier, and in 20–30% cases, after delivery. HELLP is more common in white, multiparous, older women. The most common presentations are epigastric/right upper quadrant pain and tenderness, nausea and vomiting, and features of pre-eclampsia (edema, hypertension, and proteinuria) [14]. Jaundice is uncommon (5%). Transaminase elevation is variable, from mild to 10–20-fold, and bilirubin is usually <5 mg/dL.

HELLP syndrome is a progressive condition, with significant maternal morbidity from complications, including disseminated intravascular coagulation (DIC), abruptio placentae, eclampsia, acute renal failure, subcapsular hematoma, and, rarely, hepatic failure (1–2%). Hepatic rupture of a subcapsular hematoma is a life-threatening complication [15].

Acute Fatty Liver of Pregnancy

AFLP occurs almost exclusively in the third trimester, from 28 to 40 weeks, and only rarely earlier. Some 40–50% patients with AFLP are nulliparous, with an increased incidence in twin pregnancies. The typical presentation is the patient with 1–2 weeks of anorexia, nausea and vomiting, upper abdominal discomfort, and jaundice, leading to acute liver failure with coagulopathy, jaundice, and hepatic encephalopathy [2,16]. Intrauterine fetal death may occur. Pre-eclampsia occurs in 50%, with overlap with HELLP syndrome.

Transaminases and bilirubin are always elevated. AST is usually 300–500 IU/L, and occasionally higher. Typical abnormalities are anemia, leukocytosis, normal–low platelets, coagulopathy with or without DIC, metabolic acidosis, renal dysfunction (often

Table 90.2 Diagnostic algorithm for liver dysfunction in pregnancy.

1. Any clinical evidence of chronic liver disease?
2. Is this viral hepatitis?
3. Is this biliary disease? (symptomatic gallstones?)
4. Any drugs or toxins?
5. Any infection?
6. Any features of Budd–Chiari syndrome?
7. If "no" to all the preceding, is this pregnancy-related disease?
   THEN
8. Intractable vomiting in first trimester → hyperemesis gravidarum
9. Severe pruritus in second half of pregnancy → ICP (can confirm with bile acid levels)
10. Severe disease in third trimester, with (usually) or without pre-eclampsia:
    • Hemolysis + low platelets → HELLP syndrome
    • Acute liver failure → AFLP
    • No HELLP syndrome or AFLP → severe pre-eclampsia

progressing to oliguric renal failure), hypoglycemia, high ammonia, and biochemical pancreatitis.

Case Continued

Hepatic ultrasound shows mobile gallstones without ductal dilation or signs of cholecystitis. This characteristic clinical picture with benign ultrasound findings suggests ICP. Treatment is started while awaiting the results of serum bile acids, which are >40 mol/L, confirming the diagnosis.

Diagnosis

A diagnostic algorithm is presented in Table 90.2.

Hyperemesis Gravidarum

The diagnosis of hyperemesis gravidarum is clinical, with severe intractable vomiting necessitating intravenous hydration. Viral hepatitis should be excluded if transaminases are high.

Intrahepatic Cholestasis of Pregnancy

Intense pruritus with elevated serum bile acids in the second half of pregnancy in an otherwise healthy patient characterizes ICP. The diagnosis is confirmed by rapid postpartum resolution. During the first pregnancy, the diagnosis is presumptive, and usually made on clinical grounds alone. Elevated serum total bile acid level will confirm it. Hepatic synthetic function and bile ducts by ultrasonography are normal. Liver biopsy is needed only to exclude more serious liver disease.

HELLP Syndrome

No clinical criteria differentiate HELLP syndrome from pre-eclampsia, but a rapid diagnosis on routine blood tests is essential for early therapy. Criteria for diagnosis are the triad of hemolysis (abnormal blood smear, elevated lactate dehydrogenase of >600 IU/L, and increase in indirect bilirubin), AST >70 IU/L, and platelet count <100 000. The nadir of platelet count further stratifies into severe (class I), moderate (class II), and mild (class III) disease (Table 90.3). Most maternal and fetal mortality and morbidity occurs in class I disease. Hepatic computed tomography (CT) is done to show subcapsular hematomas, intraparenchymal hemorrhage, infarction, or hepatic rupture.

Acute Fatty Liver of Pregnancy

A presumptive clinical diagnosis of AFLP is made based on typical clinical presentation, laboratory abnormalities, and complications

Table 90.3 Diagnostic criteria (Mississippi classification) for the HELLP (hemolysis, elevated liver tests, and low platelet count) syndrome.

Class	Platelet count	AST (IU/L)	LDH[a]
I	≤50 000	≥70	≥600
II	50–100 000	≥70	≥600
III	100–150 000	≥70	≥600

[a]Requires hemolysis on blood smear and elevated indirect bilirubin.
AST, aspartate transaminase; LDH, lactate dehydrogenase.

[2]. Swansea criteria can be used for a more specific diagnosis [16]. The definitive diagnosis is histologic, but biopsy is rarely indicated, given the need for expeditious therapy and the presence of coagulopathy. Histology shows microvesicular fatty infiltration occurring predominantly in zone 3.

Case Continued

The patient is started on UDCA 900 mg/day. Pruritus and liver tests improve significantly. Careful fetal monitoring is continued throughout the pregnancy and shows normal fetal growth; delivery of a healthy baby is effected at 37 weeks. Pruritus resolves immediately after delivery and liver tests normalize.

Therapeutics

Hyperemesis Gravidarum

Hospitalization is necessary for hydration and parenteral nutrition; otherwise, therapy is symptomatic, with pyridoxine, powdered ginger, antiemetics, and avoidance of environmental triggers. Controlled trials of corticosteroids have yielded conflicting results.

Intrahepatic Cholestasis of Pregnancy

Management of ICP is twofold: fetal and maternal. Maternal therapy is symptomatic. UDCA 10–20 mg/kg is the treatment of choice, with relief of pruritus and liver dysfunction and probable improved fetal outcome [17]. High-dose UDCA (1.5–2.0 g/day) reduces abnormal maternal and fetal bile acid levels. UDCA is more effective than cholestyramine [18] and dexamethasone (12 mg/day for 7 days), though the latter has the advantage of promoting fetal lung maturity [19]. S-adenosyl-l-methionine may have an additive effect to UDCA.

The main risk in ICP is to the fetus, necessitating referral to a high-risk obstetrician. Monitoring for chronic placental insufficiency is essential, but will not prevent all fetal deaths from acute anoxia; these occur mostly in the last month of pregnancy and can be prevented only by early delivery – 60% of babies are delivered before term. Fetal complications correlate with maternal bile acid levels of >40 umol/L [10].

Pre-eclampsia

No specific therapy is needed for the hepatic involvement of pre-eclampsia, but it indicates severe disease, necessitating immediate delivery to avoid significant fetal and maternal morbidity.

HELLP Syndrome

Delivery is the only definitive therapy. The condition is progressive and may suddenly deteriorate. Hypertension and intravenous magnesium sulfate [15] should be given, limited hepatic CT performed, and the patient transferred to a center with high-risk obstetric care.

Immediate delivery is indicated if the patient is beyond 34 weeks or has multiorgan dysfunction, DIC, renal failure, or abruptio placentae. Cesarean section is often used, but well-established uncomplicated labor should be allowed to proceed. Blood, blood products, and prophylactic antibiotics are given.

The optimal management of the patient remote from term is unknown. Corticosteroids are commonly used, but their benefit is controversial, and a recent Cochrane analysis of 11 randomized trials showed no clear evidence of benefit [20]. For patients at less than 34 weeks' gestation and with stable, mild disease, stabilization of the maternal condition and corticosteroid therapy for 24–48 hours may be an option, but delivery must be effected with any maternal deterioration. With conservative therapy for 24–72 hours, prognosis is poor, with a high risk of fetal loss.

Most patients have rapid resolution of HELLP syndrome after delivery, with normalization of platelets by 5 days. Some experts recommend the routine use of intravenous corticosteroids from diagnosis, through delivery, and into the early postpartum period. Persistent thrombocytopenia, hemolysis, and progressive elevation of bilirubin and creatinine for >72 hours with no improvement is usually taken as an indication for specific therapy (plasma exchange with fresh frozen plasma (FFP) and plasmapheresis are most commonly used, after steroids), but there are no supporting data from clinical trials. Indications to proceed with liver transplantation are very limited: hepatic rupture, persistent bleeding from a hematoma, liver failure from extensive necrosis.

Subcapsular hematomas are managed conservatively, with close hemodynamic monitoring, immediate provision of blood products and imaging, and avoidance of exogenous trauma. Liver rupture is a rare, life-threatening complication, usually preceded by a right lobe subcapsular hematoma in patients with severe thrombocytopenia. Management requires rapid, aggressive, supportive care; immediate laparotomy with pressure packing and drainage is probably optimal, followed by consideration of hepatic artery embolization or ligation, partial hepatectomy, or oversewing of the laceration.

Acute Fatty Liver of Pregnancy

Early diagnosis of AFLP and immediate delivery of the fetus are essential for maternal and fetal survival. Delivery is usually by Caesarian section, but rapid controlled vaginal delivery with fetal monitoring is probably safer in later pregnancy, with less bleeding and infection. Normalization of coagulopathy (International Normalized Ratio (INR) <1.5; platelets >50,000) during and after delivery and the use of prophylactic antibiotics are recommended. Epidural anesthesia allows better ongoing assessment of maternal level of consciousness but is contraindicated with coagulopathy.

Clinical improvement occurs within 48–72 hours of delivery, but intensive supportive care is needed until recovery is established and usually for 1–4 weeks postpartum, though there may be prolonged cholestasis for months, with infectious and bleeding complications. Patients who are critically ill at presentation or who continue to deteriorate despite emergency delivery should be transferred to a liver transplant center. Liver transplantation is necessary only for patients who continue to deteriorate with liver failure after delivery.

Prognosis and Recurrence of Disease in Future Pregnancies

Hyperemesis Gravidarum

Maternal and infant outcomes in hyperemesis gravidarum are usually excellent, but poor maternal weight gain is associated with adverse infant outcome. Hyperemesis gravidarum resolves with delivery, but psychologic sequelae are common. The recurrence rate in subsequent pregnancies is 15–20%.

Intrahepatic Cholestasis of Pregnancy

ICP resolves with fetal delivery but recurs in 45–70% of subsequent pregnancies. Pruritus may occur with use of oral contraceptives. Rare familial cases of apparent ICP have persisted postpartum, with progression to subsequent fibrosis and cirrhosis. Two large population studies have now confirmed that ICP patients have an increased risk of subsequent hepatobiliary disease: more symptomatic gallstones, perhaps through shared genetic risk factors; more hepatitis C; and more non-alcoholic cirrhosis [21, 22]. Patients with ICP should be tested for hepatitis C. Fetal outcome is poorer than maternal outcome and correlates with maternal serum bile acid levels [10]. Premature delivery occurs in 40–100% of cases, with fetal demise in 1–5%, usually in the last month of pregnancy. Early delivery improves fetal outcome.

HELLP Syndrome and Acute Fatty Liver of Pregnancy

Adverse maternal outcome in pre-eclampsia is higher in patients with liver dysfunction [23] and in HELLP syndrome, with mortality correlating with MELD score [24]. The maternal mortality rate from hepatic rupture remains very high at 50%, with significant fetal loss (10–60%). Among the selected women who undergo liver transplantation for HELLP syndrome, the 1-year survival rate is about 80%. Fetal mortality in HELLP ranges from 7 to 20% and is usually related to prematurity (70%), intrauterine growth restriction, or abruptio placentae. Neonatal thrombocytopenia may occur, with intraventricular hemorrhage and long-term neurologic complications. Recurrence of HELLP syndrome is low (2–6%), but subsequent pregnancies carry a high risk of pre-eclampsia, prematurity, intrauterine growth retardation, abruptio placentae, and perinatal mortality.

The maternal and fetal mortality rates in AFLP are now 10–18 and 9–23%, respectively. Many women do not become pregnant again after AFLP, either by choice or due to hysterectomy to control postpartum bleeding. All babies of mothers with AFLP are tested for LCHAD deficiency. In mothers without identifiable genetic abnormalities, AFLP does not tend to recur in subsequent pregnancies, though rare cases have been reported.

Take Home Points

- Liver dysfunction in pregnancy is usually pregnancy-related.
- The liver diseases unique to pregnancy are hyperemesis gravidarum, intrahepatic cholestasis of pregnancy (ICP), and the three pre-eclampsia-related diseases: pre-eclampsia itself, HELLP syndrome, and acute fatty liver of pregnancy (AFLP).
- Liver abnormalities exist in 50% of patients hospitalized for hyperemesis gravidarum; care is supportive, with excellent maternal and fetal outcomes.
- ICP is a condition of reversible cholestasis, with severe pruritus and elevated serum bile acids; ursodeoxycholic acid (UDCA) is the treatment of choice. Maternal prognosis is excellent, but the fetus requires close monitoring and early delivery.
- HELLP syndrome is a life-threatening condition, for which immediate delivery is the only definitive therapy; corticosteroids may be given to promote fetal lung maturity and perhaps aid maternal stabilization.

- AFLP causes acute liver failure, with coagulopathy and encephalopathy. It requires rapid clinical diagnosis and prompt delivery of the fetus.

References

1 Ch'ng CL, Morgan M, Hainsworth I, Kingham JG. Prospective study of liver dysfunction in pregnancy in Southwest Wales. *Gut* 2002; **51**(6): 876–80.

2 Beuers U. EASL Recognition Awardee 2009: Prof. Raoul Poupon. *J Hepatol* 2009; **51**(4): 617–19.

3 Nelson DB, Yost NP, Cunningham FG. Acute fatty liver of pregnancy: clinical outcomes and expected duration of recovery. *Am J Obstet Gynecol* 2013; **209**(5): 456.e1–7.

4 Fell DB, Dodds L, Joseph KS, *et al.* Risk factors for hyperemesis gravidarum requiring hospital admission during pregnancy. *Obstet Gynecol* 2006; **107**(2 Pt. 1): 277–84.

5 Keitel V, Vogt C, Häussinger D, Kubitz R. Combined mutations of canalicular transporter proteins cause severe intrahepatic cholestasis of pregnancy. *Gastroenterology* 2006; **131**(2): 624–9.

6 Schneider G, Paus TC, Kullak-Ublick GA, *et al.* Linkage between a new splicing site mutation in the MDR3 alias ABCB4 gene and intrahepatic cholestasis of pregnancy. *Hepatology* 2007; **45**(1): 150–8.

7 Dixon PH, Wadsworth CA, Chambers J, *et al.* A comprehensive analysis of common genetic variation around six candidate Loci for intrahepatic cholestasis of pregnancy. *Am J Gastroenterol* 2014; **109**(1): 76–84.

8 Reyes H, Báez ME, González MC, *et al.* Selenium, zinc and copper plasma levels in intrahepatic cholestasis of pregnancy, in normal pregnancies and in healthy individuals, in Chile. *J Hepatol* 2000; **32**(4): 542–9.

9 Wikström Shemer E, Marschall HU. Decreased 1,25-dihydroxy vitamin D levels in women with intrahepatic cholestasis of pregnancy. *Acta Obstet Gynecol Scand* 2010; **89**(11): 1420–3.

10 Glantz A, Marschall HU, Mattsson LA. Intrahepatic cholestasis of pregnancy: relationships between bile acid levels and fetal complication rates. *Hepatology* 2004; **40**(2): 467–74.

11 Abildgaard U, Heimdal K. Pathogenesis of the syndrome of hemolysis, elevated liver enzymes, and low platelet count (HELLP): a review. *Eur J Obstet Gynecol Reprod Biol* 2013; **166**(2): 117–23.

12 Muetze S, Leeners B, Ortlepp JR, *et al.* Maternal factor V Leiden mutation is associated with HELLP syndrome in Caucasian women. *Acta Obstet Gynecol Scand* 2008; **87**(6): 635–42.

13 Ibdah JA. Acute fatty liver of pregnancy: an update on pathogenesis and clinical implications. *World J Gastroenterol* 2006; **12**(46): 7397–404.

14 Haram K, Svendsen E, Abildgaard U. The HELLP syndrome: clinical issues and management. A review. *BMC Pregnancy Childbirth* 2009; **9**: 8.

15 Martin JN Jr. Milestones in the quest for best management of patients with HELLP syndrome (microangiopathic hemolytic anemia, hepatic dysfunction, thrombocytopenia). *Int J Gynaecol Obstet* 2013; **121**(3): 202–7.

16 Knight M, Nelson-Piercy C, Kurinczuk JJ, *et al.* A prospective national study of acute fatty liver of pregnancy in the UK. *Gut* 2008; **57**(7): 951–6.

17 Bacq Y, Sentilhes L, Reyes HB, *et al.* Efficacy of ursodeoxycholic acid in treating intrahepatic cholestasis of pregnancy: a meta-analysis. *Gastroenterology* 2012; **143**(6): 1492–501.

18 Kondrackiene J, Beuers U, Kupcinskas L. Efficacy and safety of ursodeoxycholic acid versus cholestyramine in intrahepatic cholestasis of pregnancy. *Gastroenterology* 2005; **129**(3): 894–901.

19 Glantz A, Marschall HU, Lammert F, Mattsson LA. Intrahepatic cholestasis of pregnancy: a randomized controlled trial comparing dexamethasone and ursodeoxycholic acid. *Hepatology* 2005; **42**(6): 1399–405.

20 Woudstra DM, Chandra S, Hofmeyr GJ, Dowswell T. Corticosteroids for HELLP (hemolysis, elevated liver enzymes, low platelets) syndrome in pregnancy. *Cochrane Database Syst Rev* 2010(9):CD008148.

21 Ropponen A, Sund R, Riikonen S, *et al.* Intrahepatic cholestasis of pregnancy as an indicator of liver and biliary diseases: a population-based study. *Hepatology* 2006; **43**(4): 723–8.

22 Marschall HU, Wikström Shemer E, Ludvigsson JF, Stephansson O. Intrahepatic cholestasis of pregnancy and associated hepatobiliary disease: a population-based cohort study. *Hepatology* 2013; **58**(4): 1385–91.

23 Kozic JR, Benton SJ, Hutcheon JA, *et al.* Abnormal liver function tests as predictors of adverse maternal outcomes in women with preeclampsia. *J Obstet Gynaecol Can* 2011; **33**(10): 995–1004.

24 Murali AR, Devarbhavi H, Venkatachala PR, *et al.* Factors that predict 1-month mortality in patients with pregnancy-specific liver disease. *Clin Gastroenterol Hepatol* 2014; **12**(1): 109–13.

CHAPTER 91

Pediatric Liver Disease

Tamir Miloh

Phoenix Children's Hospital, Phoenix, AZ, USA

Summary

Pediatric liver disease is a unique field, as children are not little adults. The etiology, presentation, and natural progression are different in children. Special consideration needs to be given to growth, nutrition, development, psychosocial aspects, parents, school performance, medication choice, and dosing, among many other factors. Children are usually cared for by a pediatric subspecialist and are transitioned to the care of an adult specialist. The transfer of care is a very delicate and complex process. The aim of this chapter is to educate adult providers in the management of certain liver diseases that more commonly present in children, including biliary atresia, cystic fibrosis, alpha 1 antitrypsin (A1AT) deficiency, progressive familial intrahepatic cholestasis (PFIC), benign recurrent intrahepatic cholestasis (BRIC), alagille syndrome (AGS), disorders of bilirubin (Dubin–Johnson and Crigler–Najjar syndrome), and a few of the more common metabolic conditions. Annually, approximately 600 children receive a liver transplant, and as they become adults, these transplant recipients will need to transition care. There are distinctive surgical and medical aspects in managing pediatric liver transplant recipients, and an effective transition is essential for good long-term outcome.

Biliary Atresia

Biliary atresia is a progressive fibroinflammatory disease of the biliary system and is the leading cause of liver transplantation in pediatrics [1]. The incidence is 1 : 10 000 newborns, and it is fatal if not corrected surgically by 2 years of age [2]. The classical presentation is in infancy, with jaundice, pale stools, hepatosplenomegaly, and conjugated hyperbilirubinemia. Ultrasonography may show an absent gallbladder or the triangular cord sign [3, 4]. Radionuclide hepatobiliary scintigraphy after priming with phenobarbitone is often used in the workup of cholestatic jaundice. Typically, there is no excretion of dye in biliary atresia. Endoscopic retrograde cholangiopancreatography (ERCP) and magnetic resonance cholangiopancreatography (MRCP) have been used in the diagnosis. Liver biopsy characteristically shows expanded portal tracts with biliary ductular proliferation, consistent with biliary obstruction. Choledochal cyst and A1AT deficiency should be ruled out by appropriate testing, as they have a similar histological picture. Paucity of bile ducts is rare and is more commonly associated with AGS.

Case

A 24-year-old woman with biliary atresia is contemplating pregnancy and would like to discuss her clinical status. She had a Kasai portoenterostomy in infancy and was previously managed in a pediatric facility. She has been stable, with no history of cholangitis or gastrointestinal (GI) bleeding. Her examination is normal apart from mild splenomegaly. Laboratory tests reveal a platelet count of $94 \times 10^3/mm^3$ and a white blood cell (WBC) count of $4.6 \times 10^3/mm^3$. Her gamma-glutamyltransferase (GGT) is elevated at 120 IU/L, alanine transaminase (ALT) 55 IU/L, total bilirubin 1.3 mg/dL with a direct fraction of 0.6 mg/dL, total protein 5.8g/dL, albumin 3.8 g/dL, and International Normalized Ratio (INR) 1.1. Abdominal ultrasound reveals splenomegaly but no ascites. Her pulse oximetry is 98% in an upright position in room air.

Pathophysiology and Types

The etiology of biliary atresia is not known, though viral, autoimmune, embryological, vascular, and other mechanisms have been proposed [5]. The Childhood Liver Disease Research Network (ChiLDReN), an NIDDK/NIH funded consortium, has developed a database of children with cholestatic disease, including biliary atresia, and initiated studies of etiology with the aim of improving outcomes in the disease. Biliary atresia may present at birth (the so-called "fetal/embryonic" type) or develop later (the peri/postnatal type) [6]. The less common (10–35%) fetal form has a high frequency of associated malformations, including biliary atresia splenic malformation (BASM), which includes polysplenia/asplenia, abdominal situs, intestinal anomalies, preduodenal portal vein, and cardiovascular defects [7, 8]. Recently, a group of biliary atresia distinct from syndromic BASM has been identified, which is defined by multiple malformations without laterality defects [9].

Biliary atresia has also been divided into three types based on anatomic variants: type 1, atresia of the common bile duct; type 2, atresia of the common hepatic duct; and type 3, atresia of the right and left hepatic ducts. In terms of biliary drainage after Kasai, type 1 has the best prognosis and type 3 (the most common) the worst. Type 2 is rare.

Practical Gastroenterology and Hepatology Board Review Toolkit, Second Edition. Edited by Nicholas J. Talley, Kenneth R. DeVault, Michael B. Wallace, Bashar A. Aqel and Keith D. Lindor.

Diagnosis and Management

The gold standard for diagnosis of biliary atresia is intraoperative cholangiography, and current management is Kasai portoenterostomy [10]. Ideally, the procedure should be performed before 8 weeks of age. Children need intensive nutritional rehabilitation with a high medium-chain triglyceride (MCT) formula and supplementation of fat-soluble vitamins (shneider) and ursodeoxycholic acid (UDCA) until they achieve biliary drainage or receive a liver transplant. The classic Kasai procedure involves excision of the atretic portion of the bile ducts, including the fibrotic portal plate, and anastomosis of a Roux limb of the jejunum to the cut edge of the liver parenchyma [11]. Though the Japanese surgeon Dr. Morio Kasai introduced portoenterostomy in 1959, it took almost 2 decades for the technique to gain acceptance. A worldwide review of cases in 1977 showed only 1.1% survival [12], but as reports of better results became available, the procedure became standard of care for biliary atresia. Currently, biliary drainage is achieved in 50–80% of cases, and the Kasai portoenterostomy is regarded as treatment but not cure for biliary atresia – largely because biliary atresia is not restricted to the extrahepatic bile duct and there is a varying degree of ongoing intrahepatic biliary inflammation and fibrosis. Cholangiograms in adults with biliary atresia look similar to those seen in adults with sclerosing cholangitis, and the complications are similar, with ongoing cholestasis and bacterial cholangitis in the majority of adults surviving with their native liver.

Survival with Native Liver

Earlier diagnosis and standardized operative interventions have increased survival with native liver, but biliary atresia remains the most common indication for liver transplantation in children worldwide. An interesting study from King's College Hospital in 2001 comparing Japanese patients to an age-matched English cohort reported that median survival time in the Japanese patients was less than 1 year before 1975 but increased to 18 years after 1975 [13]. Survival with native liver in the first decade of life was reported in the United States and Europe to be between 28 and 43% [13–15]. The calculated survival rate (with failure defined as death or transplantation) at 5 years was 49% in the United States, and median survival was 15 years when bile drainage was established; however, long-term outcome and complications were not described in this series [14]. With improving outcomes after Kasai portoenterostomy, long-term survivors with native liver are becoming more common, and 20-year native liver survival of between 23 and 44% has been reported [16–19]. The two largest clinical reports of long-term survivors with biliary atresia with a native liver come from Sendai, Japan and Paris, France. The French series reported a 20-year transplant-free survival in 63 of 271 (23%) cases of biliary atresia in infants operated on during the years 1968–83 [19]. After age 20, 2 patients died of liver failure and 14 underwent or were waiting for liver transplantation. The authors attributed better outcomes to those who were operated on earlier and to those who had type 1 biliary atresia and not BASM. Long-term survival was significantly greater in those whose biliary atresia affected only the common bile duct (type 1 or so-called correctable biliary atresia) [20].

Clinical Features

Given a prevalence of 1 : 15 000 for biliary atresia, it is estimated that there may be as many as 4000 adults with biliary atresia in the United States. Up to two-thirds of patients have evidence of chronic biliary disease with transient or persistent cholestasis and variable elevations in GGT and portal hypertension, 33% of whom have bacterial cholangitis and around 10% gallstones [19, 21, 22].

Intrapulmonic shunting has been observed in adult patients with biliary atresia and portal hypertension [19, 23]. Hepatopulmonary syndrome (HPS) and portopulmonary hypertension (PPHTN) have also been described in patients with biliary atresia and portal hypertension. Patients with new-onset dyspnea, syncope, and murmur, and those undergoing evaluation for liver transplantation, should be screened for PPHTN with echocardiography. Confirmation of the diagnosis is made with cardiac catheterization. Diagnosis of and differentiation between HPS and PPHTN, along with appropriate grading of severity of pulmonary disease, are critical to determining whether medical management or transplantation is a treatment option [24, 25].

Recurrent cholangitis is a complication in children who achieve biliary drainage after Kasai portoenterostomy and is an indication for liver transplantation. Multiple theories as to the pathogenesis of cholangitis after hepatoportoenterostomy (HPE) have been presented, including direct infection via colonization in the Roux limb, bacterial translocation via the lymphatics, and hematogenous infection via the portal vein [26]. Widely accepted diagnostic criteria for cholangitis include fever, abdominal pain, acholic stools, and rise in conjugated bilirubin. If a child who is post Kasai portoenterostomy has fever of unknown etiology, it is standard of care to treat with intravenous (IV) antibiotics for presumed cholangitis. Cholangitis episodes clearly occur during adulthood as well: in one study, 35 of 131 (27%) long-term survivors had at least one episode after the age of 20 [19, 27]. Antibiotic treatment of cholangitis should be chosen for broad-spectrum coverage of enteric organisms. Diagnostic imaging (computed tomography (CT), magnetic resonance imaging (MRI), and hepatobiliary scintigraphy) used to determine underlying risk factors for infection in one series showed the presence of fibrosis, dilated intrahepatic ducts, and intrahepatic stones in 70% of patients who developed cholangitis. Surgical intervention for mechanical obstruction of the Roux loop has been described with mixed short-term results [26, 27].

Overall, intrahepatic bile duct abnormalities (dilation, cyst formation) and lithiasis develop in about 10–15% of patients and present with jaundice or cholangitis or as an incidental finding. Yearly screening with ultrasonography or CT has been proposed for long-term survivors following HPE, particularly in order to detect and treat intrahepatic stones [21]. Antibiotic prophylaxis may be considered in adults who have undergone HPE and have recurrent cholangitis with ductal abnormalities. Interestingly, there are no reports of cholangiocarcinoma in these adult patients. Hepatocellular carcinoma (HCC) has been reported in younger patients with biliary atresia, but not in the cohort of long-term survivors.

Adolescents and Adults without Chronic Liver Disease

In one series, chronic liver disease was described as normal bilirubin, AST, albumin, INR, and platelet count in the absence of surgical complications [28]. Of 244 children who had a Kasai HPE in a single center between 1979 and 1991, 28 (11%, all adolescents) were deemed to have no chronic liver disease. However, 12 (43%) had a history of cholangitis at a median age of 3.4 years. Liver biopsy showed fibrosis in the majority who underwent biopsy, but no child had GI bleeding during follow-up. Surveillance endoscopy was normal in all 13 (46%) who underwent the procedure. Eventually, 26 (93%) went on to mainstream education, and 2 attended special school secondary to reasons unrelated to liver disease. The authors concluded that the good outcome in these children was not impaired by isolated episodes of cholangitis and that the impact of fibrosis on outcomes in their lifetime was unclear.

Among the 20-year survivors post HPE, 6 of 28 (21%) had normal liver biochemistry and no clinical or ultrasonographic signs of cirrhosis or portal hypertension [18]. In the French series, 12 of 63 had completely normal bilirubin and aminotransferases [19]. However, biopsies in patients without evidence of portal hypertension or hypersplenism and/or who have normal biochemical parameters may still show evidence of fibrosis and cirrhosis. The long-term implications of these histologic changes have not been examined, as most reported biopsy results were obtained within 8 years of HPE [28].

Quality of Life

A cross-sectional survey of health-related quality of life (HRQOL) in patients with biliary atresia with their native livers (ages 2–25) was conducted by the ChiLDReN group and compared with healthy and post-liver transplantation biliary atresia [36]. In total, 221 children (54% female, 67% white) were studied. Patient self and parent proxy reports showed significantly poorer HRQOL compared to healthy children in all domains (p <0.001), particularly in emotional and psychosocial settings. The HRQOL in the children with native liver was similar to that of children post liver transplantation with biliary atresia.

Quality-of-life data were available in 52 of 63 patients who had survived for over 20 years post HPE [19]: 38 were considered to lead a normal life, 21 were regularly employed, and 17 were university students; 20 were married or in a stable relationship, 7 female patients gave birth to 9 children, and 3 male patients fathered 6 children. In the Dutch study, general health perception (RAND-36) data were collected for 28 adults with a 20-year transplant-free survival, and it was noted that women with biliary atresia had a reduced perception of their health compared to controls, but not men [18]. The British study compared quality of life in Japanese survivors with native liver with the matched English cohort and found that it was comparable [13].

Transplantation

Biliary atresia remains the primary indication for liver transplantation in children both in the United States and in many countries around the world. Public insurance coverage is an independent risk factor for significantly increased waitlist and post-transplant mortality in children with biliary atresia [37]. In pediatric series, the 10-year survival rate in patients with biliary atresia undergoing liver transplantation after HPE is 80–90%. The largest adult series of patients undergoing living-related donor transplant reveals a 5-year survival rate of 90% [38]. Looking at the United Network for Organ Sharing (UNOS) database, only 56 adults with biliary atresia received their first liver transplant, out of 79 400 adults transplanted between October 1987 and May 2008 [39]. The 1- and 5-year patient (89.3 and 87.5%) and graft (82.1 and 78.6%) survivals in adults with biliary atresia who had their first transplant were comparable to those in transplants performed for other indications.

Cystic Fibrosis

Pathophysiology/Definition

Cystic fibrosis is an autosomal recessive disorder. It is more common in Caucasians, with a frequency of 1 in 2000–3000 live births.

It is characterized by abnormal transport of electrolytes by the cystic fibrosis transmembrane conductance regulator (CFTR) [40]. The ubiquitous nature of the transporter leads to multisystem involvement, including chronic lung disease, chronic sinusitis, distal intestinal obstruction, pancreatic insufficiency, reproductive system disorders, musculoskeletal disorders, recurrent venous thrombosis, renal stones, and hepatobiliary manifestations. The CFTR is located on the apical membrane of cholangiocytes. An abnormal CFTR is hypothesized to impair bile flow, leading to obstruction and subsequent injury. Cystic fibrosis may present in classic form, with elevated sweat chloride ($\geq$60 mmol/L), or in non-classic form, with phenotypic spectrum and normal or intermediate sweat chloride (diagnosed based on genetics or on measurement of nasal potential difference) [41, 42].

Epidemiology

The pathognomonic hepatobiliary manifestation of cystic fibrosis, referred to as cystic fibrosis liver disease (CFLD), is focal biliary cirrhosis caused by inspissated bile [43]. Among patients with focal biliary cirrhosis, 10% will progress to multilobular cirrhosis [44]. Most patients with severe CFLD are diagnosed before age 20. Improvements in medical management and survival in the last 30 years have led to a dramatic increase in the number of adult patients with cystic fibrosis. Adults with cystic fibrosis represent more than 40% of patients in the Cystic Fibrosis Foundation Patient Registry. Increasing patient survival and an increased awareness of hepatobiliary involvement have led to greater recognition of CFLD. However, its clinically silent course requires active screening [45].

The hepatobiliary manifestations of cystic fibrosis are [46, 47]:
- elevated liver enzymes (30%), with unclear clinical significance;
- micro gallbladder;
- cholelithiasis (12%);
- bile duct stricture;
- cholestasis;
- cholecystitis;
- portal hypertension ($\leq$5%);
- hepatolithiasis;
- focal biliary cirrhosis;
- multilobular cirrhosis;
- steatosis, mostly due to malnutrition;
- hepatomegaly and congestive hepatopathy;
- end-stage liver disease;
- cholangiocarcinoma.

CFLD most commonly presents in the first decade of life, in boys, in patients with a history of meconium ileus in infancy or failure to thrive, and in those with a pancreatic insufficiency phenotype. Just 7% are diagnosed at age $\geq$18 years. Most adults with CFLD have a benign course, with slowly progressive disease. Patients diagnosed with cystic fibrosis as adults are more likely to have a milder pulmonary disease and to have GI symptoms, diabetes mellitus, and infertility with normal or intermediate sweat chloride results. There is a higher frequency of non-delta F508 mutations [46]. It is not clear that improved survival into adulthood translates into an increased incidence of CFLD. However, complications of end-stage liver disease and portal hypertension will impact clinical course. CFLD at baseline appears as an independent factor associated with death or lung transplantation.

Diagnosis

The diagnosis of cystic fibrosis is based upon compatible clinical findings with biochemical (abnormal sweat chloride >60 mmol/L twice or abnormal nasal potential difference) or genetic confirmation. Most cases are diagnosed through newborn screening testing of serum immunoreactive trypsin, followed by DNA testing. Newborn screening has shown improved cystic fibrosis-related morbidity and mortality [48].

Current consensus recommendations suggest examination of liver and spleen size at every clinic visit and yearly biochemical screening with a hepatic panel including ALP, GGT, and bilirubin. Abnormal values (>1.5 times the upper limit of normal (ULN)) should prompt repeat laboratory testing in 3–6 months. Persistent elevation for >6 months or high elevation (>5 times ULN) should prompt further evaluation. Significant liver disease can be seen in patients with relatively normal liver biochemistries, highlighting the importance of a careful physical examination in patients with cystic fibrosis. Other manifestations of chronic liver disease (such as jaundice, spider angiomata, palmar erythema, and ascites) are uncommon, and nutrition should be assessed.

Ultrasonography of the liver and gallbladder is the imaging modality of highest yield in the diagnosis of the hepatobiliary manifestations of cystic fibrosis. Commonly seen findings on ultrasonography include parenchymal heterogeneity, nodularity, and evidence of portal hypertension, sometimes preceding biochemical abnormality Transient elastography is an evolving non-invasive tool for the assessment liver fibrosis. Esophagogastroduodenoscopy (EGD) to screen for varices should be considered in patients with evidence of portal hypertension [49]. Liver biopsy is not routinely recommended in the diagnosis of CFLD, because of the patchy distribution of the disease.

Differential Diagnosis

Biochemical evidence of hepatitis and/or hepatomegaly in cystic fibrosis patients may also reflect steatosis associated with malnutrition [50], hyperexpansion of lung volumes, or cor pulmonale with hepatic congestion. Cholestasis is a worrisome and late finding in CFLD. Cholestasis may alternatively represent cholelithiasis and, rarely, bile duct stricture hepatolithiasis and cholangiocarcinoma [51]. Patients with CFLD are not considered high-risk for HCC. Screening in this population is not currently recommended. Evaluation should include a review of medication and toxin effect, as well as screening for common viral hepatitis.

Alpha-1-Antitrypsin Deficiency

A1AT deficiency is the most common metabolic liver disease requiring liver transplantation in children (perlmutter, suchy). The incidence is estimated to be 1 in 2000 live births, and is highest in Northern Europeans. A1AT is a glycoprotein synthesized in the liver that inhibits neutrophil elastase-induced host pulmonary injury. Early studies using acid starch electrophoresis show that A1AT exists in a number of biochemical forms, known collectively as the protease inhibitor (Pi) system [52]. Each variant is labeled according to its mobility on the gel: Z is very slow, S is slow, M is medium, and F is fast. A1AT deficiency is an autosomal codominant disorder, with equal contribution to the phenotype from both alleles. The A1AT gene (SERPINA 1) is located on chromosome 14 [53]. The most common deficiency allele is PiZ: 95% of individuals with A1AT deficiency have PiZZ phenotype.

Case

A 29-year-old woman who is completely asymptomatic has been told that she has the PiZZ phenotype. She underwent screening after her baby with neonatal jaundice was diagnosed as having A1AT deficiency. She would like to know her chances of developing liver and/or lung disease and wants to obtain genetic counseling.

Pathophysiology

Homozygotes (PiZZ phenotype) are more likely to develop emphysema through a "loss of function" mechanism, where absence of A1AT causes unopposed proteolytic damage to the pulmonary connective tissue matrix. Around 10% of of PiZZ patients experience liver disease [54]. Liver injury is thought to result from a "gain of toxic function" mechanism, where the mutant A1AT is retained in the endoplasmic reticulum [55]. It has been hypothesized that the accumulation of A1AT (i) causes mitochondrial dysfunction, (ii) activates autophagic response, and (iii) activates transcription factor NF-κB. The latter has been shown to play a key role in inflammation-associated carcinogenesis and has been postulated to play a role in the development of HCC in A1AT deficiency.

Clinical Features and Diagnosis

Infants usually present with prolonged jaundice and hepatosplenomegaly with or without ascites. Biochemical tests typically show a conjugated hyperbilurubinemia, elevated aminotransferases, and GGT. The cholestatic jaundice may resolve spontaneously in childhood or may progress to cirrhosis requiring liver transplantation at any time from infancy to adulthood. Some patients may show evidence of synthetic dysfunction, with prolonged INR and low serum albumin levels. The histological picture can be similar to that in biliary atresia, and it is important to rule out A1AT deficiency before subjecting an infant to intraoperative cholangiography. The hallmark of A1AT deficiency is periodic acid–Schiff (PAS)-positive, diastase-resistant red glycoprotein granules. A1AT phenotyping by isoelectric focusing is the gold standard for establishing diagnosis. The normal variant is PiMM, but those with A1AT deficiency have PiZZ. A1AT is an acute-phase reactant, and A1AT levels may be elevated during infection or inflammation, making them unreliable in making a diagnosis. Liver disease can present for the first time in late childhood or adolescence. The frequency with which adults develop liver disease is not clear, but it is estimated that 10% of adults with homozygous deficiency will develop cirrhosis and end-stage liver disease. This is similar to the frequency with which homozygotes develop emphysema. The major pulmonary manifestation is development of panacinar emphysema, predominantly affecting the lower lobes before the age of 50. Cigarette smoking is strongly associated with more rapid disease progression. Smoking should be strictly avoided in subjects with A1AT deficiency and in the households of children diagnosed with A1AT deficiency. Approximately two-thirds of adults with homozygous deficiency (PiZZ) will be recognized medically at some point in their lifetime; the remaining third will be completely asymptomatic. There is a very high incidence of HCC in A1AT deficiency.

During the period 1989–2002, at one tertiary center in England, 11 families with an affected child with A1AT deficiency and liver disease obtained antenatal diagnosis for subsequent pregnancies, and 8 pregnancies with PiZZ phenotype were terminated [56]. The same center investigated the clinical course of siblings with PiZZ phenotype, identifying 58 PiZZ children (32 boys) from 29 families. These 29 probands and 29 siblings with PiZZ phenotype were followed for a median of 80 months: 21 (72%) PiZZ siblings had liver involvement, 6 (29%) with the same severity as the proband.

The authors concluded that while there was concordance for liver involvement in PIZZ siblings, the severity of liver disease was variable.

The prevalences of the PiZ and PiS alleles in the European population are estimated to be 0.5–2.0% and 1–9%, respectively. In one study, around 10% of 162 children with A1AT deficiency had PiSS or PiSZ phenotype, 14 of whom were male. Additionally, 12 asymptomatic siblings were also found to be PiSS/PiSZ on family screening [57]. The authors reported that PAS-positive, diastase-negative granules were not detected in any of the five biopsies of children with PiSS phenotype, but were present in two of eight liver biopsies in PiSZ patients. The disease was not in any way different than the underlying diagnosis.

Progressive Familial Intrahepatic Cholestasis

PFIC is an autosomal recessive disease. It is the cause of cholestasis in approximately 10–15% of children, with an estimated incidence of 1 : 50 000–100 000 births. There are three types of PFIC: patients with PFIC-1 and PFIC-2 present with low-serum GGT, while patients with PFIC-3 have high-serum GGT [58].

PFIC-1, also known as Byler's disease, is caused by a mutation of the FIC1 gene on chromosome 18q21-22, which encodes a P-type ATPase (ATP8Bl) involved in aminophospholipid flippase. FIC1 is expressed in the intestine (highly expressed), liver, biliary tract, pancreas, and kidney [59]. Patients with PFIC-1 usually present in the first weeks of life with severe pruritus disproportionate to the degree of jaundice. Progression to cirrhosis and end-stage liver disease occurs at a variable rate. Extrahepatic manifestations include chronic diarrhea, short stature, failure to thrive, deafness, pancreatitis, biliary stones, and respiratory symptoms. PFIC-1 is characterized by low-serum GGT, high bilirubin and serum bile salts, moderately elevated liver enzymes, and normal serum cholesterol. Liver imaging is normal [60,61]. Liver histology reveals "bland" cholestasis, and electron microscopy may show coarse granular bile [62]. Diagnosis is supported by genetic analysis of the ATP8B1 gene, but many patients are compound-heterozygous [63].

Medical management is mostly supportive: nutrition, prevention of fat-soluble vitamins deficiency, UDCA in some patients [61]. Treating pruritus may require partial external biliary diversion (PEBD: a gallbladder cutaneous stoma alongside a loop of small bowel) or internal biliary diversions (intestinal conduits between the gallbladder and cecum, bypassing the terminal ileum). Recurrence of cholestasis or ileal bypass (ileocolonic anastomosis bypassing the terminal ileum) has been reported in a few cases [64]. Nasobiliary drainage may help select potential responders to biliary diversion.

Liver transplantation is performed in cirrhosis, portal hypertension, and refractory pruritus, but may lead to worsening watery diarrhea (responsive to bile salt sequestrants) and steatohepatitis of the graft [65].

PFIC-2 is caused by a mutation in the ABCB11 gene on chromosome 2q24, which encodes the bile salt export pump (BSEP). Patients with PFIC-2 usually have a more severe presentation that those with PFIC-1, with jaundice, pruritus, failure to thrive, hepatosplenomegaly, coagulopathy, and hypocalcemia due to vitamin D deficiency [66]. They have an increased risk of HCC at a young age and require surveillance. There are no extrahepatic manifestations [66]. PFIC-2 is characterized by direct hyperbilirubinemia, elevated aminotransferase and alpha fetoprotein (higher than in PFIC-1), normal GGT, elevated serum bile acids, and decreased biliary bile salts [61]. Liver imaging is normal. Liver biopsy reveals giant cell transformation with canalicular cholestasis. Immunostaining for BSEP protein is negative. Electron microscopy reveals amorphous or finely filamentous bile [62].

Medical management is mostly supportive (like PFIC-1) and often unsatisfactory. Surgical diversions may be effective. Liver transplantation is indicated in cirrhosis, failed medical and surgical approaches, intractable pruritus, or HCC. Allo-immune-mediated BSEP dysfunction may occur after liver transplantation in PFIC-2 patients, leading to a PFIC-2-like phenotype after transplantation [67].

PFIC-3 is caused by a mutation of the multidrug resistance 3 (MDR3) glycoprotein, which is coded by the ABCB4 gene on chromosome 7q21. MDR3 protein is an adenosine triphosphate (ATP)-dependent phosphatidylcholine flippase that is responsible for biliary phospholipid and has a wide genotype–phenotype expression spectrum. MDR3 deficiency has been documented in several disease phenotypes, including intrahepatic and gallbladder cholesterol lithiasis, intrahepatic cholestasis of pregnancy, and PFIC3 [68].

PFIC-3 is characterized by neonatal presentation in 50% of cases, leading to jaundice, pale stools, pruritus, hepatosplenomegaly, high risk of intrahepatic and gallbladder cholesterol cholelithiasis, and drug-induced cholestasis. Laboratory testing reveals elevated aminotransferases, ALP, GGT, total serum bile acid, and direct hyperbilirubinemia, and absent serum lipoprotein X. Bile analysis reveals low concentrations of phospholipids. Liver imaging is typically normal, but may show a huge gallbladder or biliary stones [61]. Liver biopsy reveals ductular proliferation, and biliary fibrosis and immunohistochemical staining for MDR3 show a complete absence of canalicular staining. Treatment with UDCA has variable results depending on the severity of the mutation, with complete normalization of liver function test (LFT) in 41% of cases, negative response in 37%, and partial improvement in 20%. Refractory progressive cases may require liver transplantation [69].

Benign Recurrent Intrahepatic Cholestasis

BRIC is characterized by intermittent attacks of jaundice and pruritus, separated by symptom-free intervals. It usually manifests at adolescence. BRIC-1 affects the ATP8B1 gene and BRIC-2 ABCB11. The BRIC protein is only partially impaired in comparison to PFIC, and there is no progression to cirrhosis. Clinical flares consist of malaise, anorexia, and pruritus, with an icteric phase usually lasting from 2 to 3 months. Over time, the cholestatic episodes become less frequent, ranging from several times a year to once a decade. Flares may exacerbate with seasons, infection, pregnancy, or contraception [61]. Patients with BRIC-1 may have significant weight loss, pancreatitis, and steatorrhea. Patients with BRIC-2 have a higher incidence of cholelithiasis [70]. During a flare, there is a characteristic cholestatic liver enzyme panel, except that serum GGT remains low, normalizing between flares. Liver biopsy is normal.

Medical therapies during the BRIC pruritic flare include UDCA and bile salt sequestrates, with conflicting results. Nasobiliary drain, extracorporeal albumin dialysis (with the Molecular Adsorbent Recirculating System (MARS)), and the extracorporeal artificial liver support have been shown to alleviate pruritus in refractory cases [71,72]. No therapy has proven effective in avoiding or shortening the cholestatic episodes.

Alagille Syndrome

AGS is an autosomal dominant condition that affects approximately 1 in 70 000 live births [73]. The majority of cases are caused by a JAG 1 mutation. There is a wide phenotypic expression, even within the same family. The main clinical and pathological features are intrahepatic bile duct paucity (resulting in chronic cholestasis), peripheral pulmonary artery stenosis (or other cardiac defects), vertebral anomalies, characteristic facies, posterior embryotoxon, pigmentary retinopathy, dysplastic kidneys, and vascular abnormalities (which may lead to cerebrovascular accident (CVA) or intracranial bleeding) [74]. Patients may present with progressive cholestasis, pruritus, cirrhosis, or liver failure. There are currently no effective medical therapies for AGS. Supportive measures include management of pruritus and end-stage liver disease and monitoring of nutrition and fat-soluble vitamin levels [75].

Liver transplantation is required in approximately 15% of cases. Patient survival at 1 year post liver transplantation for AGS patients is 87%, compared to 96% for biliary atresia patients. Deaths in AGS patients mostly occur within the first month post transplantation. Biliary, vascular, central nervous system (CNS), and renal complications following liver transplantation are associated with death in AGS patients. Renal insufficiency usually worsens after liver transplantation [76].

Dubin–Johnson Syndrome

Dubin–Johnson syndrome is a rare, autosomal recessive liver disorder linked to deficient hepatic excretion of non-bile salt organic anions by the ATP-binding cassette (ABC) transport system, encoded by MRP2 (ABCC2) on chromosome 10q24. It is characterized by elevation of both conjugated and unconjugated bilirubin, with more than 50% of the total bilirubin being conjugated. Liver enzymes, GGT, and bile acids are within normal limits. Total urine excretion of coproporphyrin isomer I is >80% (normal 25%). Jaundice can worsen with use of oral contraceptives and pregnancy. Liver biopsy shows characteristic brown to black discoloration of the liver, with otherwise normal histology. Jaundice is lifelong, and no specific therapy is required [77,78].

Crigler–Najjar Syndrome

Crigler–Najjar syndrome is caused by an autosomal recessive defect in the UGTJA1 gene complex responsible for bilirubin conjugation. In Crigler–Najjar type I, complete absence of activity leads to substantial unconjugated hyperbilirubinemia, which can lead in turn to significant neurologic impairment due to bilirubin encephalopathy and permanent sequelae (kernicterus). Liver enzymes, serum bile acids, and liver histology are normal. Crigler–Najjar type 2 (also known as Arias syndrome) is a milder version that is responsive to phenobarbital. Treatment includes phototherapy, plasmapheresis (removes albumin-bound bilirubin), liver transplantation, and hepatocyte transplantation [79].

Urea Cycle Defects

Urea cycle disorders result from defects in the metabolism of the extra nitrogen produced by the breakdown of protein and other nitrogen-containing molecules. The majority of the nitrogen is produced by metabolism of amino acids. About 75% of the urea produced by the Kreb's cycle is excreted by the kidneys, and the remaining 25% is excreted in the gut, where bacteria convert it to ammonia or bacterial protein.

The incidence of urea cycle defects is 1 in 25 000 births. Severe deficiency or complete absence of activity of the first four enzymes of the urea cycle (carbamyl phosphate synthetase 1, ornithine transcarbamylase, argininosuccinate synthetase, argininosuccinate lyase) or of the cofactor n-acetyl glutamate synthetase results in profound hyperammonemia in the newborn period. This hyperammonemia can cause alterations in sensorium, with rapid progress to coma, seizures, hypothermia, hyperventilation (to compensate for acidosis), and eventually death, unless therapy is instituted. In partial deficiency of enzymes, presentation is usually later and may be triggered by illness or stress at any point in the person's lifetime.

Laboratory data useful in making a diagnosis include plasma ammonia, pH, plasma amino acids, and urine organic acids. Definitive enzymatic and genetic diagnosis is possible. Management is based on (i) removal of the ammonia by dialysis or continuous venovenous hemofiltration (CVVH), (ii) removal of excess nitrogen by scavengers such as phenyl acetate or benzoate, and (iii) reversing the catabolic state with fluid and calorie supplementation (dextrose and intralipid). Liver transplantation is an option in suitable candidates.

Glycogen Storage Diseases

Glycogen is the main storage form of carbohydrate and is found mainly in the liver and muscle. Glycogen storage diseases (GSDs) result from abnormal glycogen synthesis or breakdown secondary to specific enzyme defects. The incidence is 1 in 25,000 live births. Other disorders of carbohydrate metabolism include galactosemia and hereditary fructose intolerance (Table 91.1).

The GSDs are denoted by a number relating to the historical sequence in which they were first described. Types I, III, IV, VI, IX, and XI characteristically involve the liver. Von Gierke's disease, GSD I, is the most common. It involves deficiency of glucose-6-phosphatase activity. The gene has been mapped to chromosome 17. Presentation is in the neonatal period, with hepatomegaly, hypoglycemia, metabolic acidosis with increased lactate, hypophosphatemia, hyperlipidemia, and hyperuricemia. The main management strategy is to control the metabolic derangements, particularly the hypoglycemia, with regular feeding and cornstarch around the clock. Raw cornstarch is hydrolyzed in the gut and enables slow release of glucose, allowing subjects to stop continuous enteral or parenteral feeding. Liver transplantation is an option when there is development of adenomas or when medical treatment fails.

Inborn Errors of Mitochondrial Fatty Acid Oxidation

During fasting and hypoglycemia, mitochondrial fatty acid β-oxidation (FAO) in the liver provides ketone bodies as an alternative source of energy for the brain and extrahepatic tissues, such as muscle and heart. After a 24 hour period of fasting, adults obtain 80% of their calories via FAO. Infants rely on FAO within 12 hours of a fast, so they are more susceptible to FAO defects. The hallmark of FAO defects is hypoketotic hypoglycemia resulting from glucose depletion and impaired gluconeogenesis. The most common FAO is medium-chain fatty acid disorder (MCAD). The clinical presentation in FAO may be severe, with fulminant liver failure, cardiomyopathy, and sudden death if not diagnosed and treated in a timely manner. Liver histology reveals a microvesicular steatosis. Analysis of the acyl carnitine profile and urine organic acids during a metabolic crisis is helpful. Diagnosis can be confirmed by fibroblastic enzymatic assays and/or molecular genetic testing.

Maternal liver disease has been associated with FAO, including acute fatty liver of pregnancy (AFLP) and HELLP (hemolysis, elevated liver enzymes, and low platelets). In AFLP, women

Table 91.1 Disorders of carbohydrate metabolism.

Disease	Clinical presentation	Diagnostic approach
Galactosemia	Vomiting and hypoglycemia after ingesting lactose (breast milk) Fulminant liver failure *Escherichia coli* sepsis Cataracts	Results of newborn screening Positive non-glucose urine-reducing substances Low activity of galactose-1-phosphate uridyl transferase in RBCs
Hereditary fructosemia	Vomiting Hypoglycemia Tremor after exposure to fructose (fruit) Fulminant liver failure Renal dysfunction	Low fructose-1-phosphate aldolase B activity in liver tissue Liver biopsy with electron miscroscopy Genetic analysis
Tyrosinemia	Fulminant liver failure Cirrhosis Early HCC Neurologic crisis Renal dysfunction	Results of newborn screening High serum tyrosine and methionine levels High serum α-fetoprotein level Succinylacetone detection in urine
Neonatal hemochromatosis	Fulminant liver failure Coagulopathy in the presence of near-normal transaminase levels	High ferritin level (>1000 µg/L) Low total iron-binding capacity Liver biopsy with iron stain or buccal mucosal biopsy MRI (of the abdomen for typical pattern of iron deposition)
Inborn errors of bile acid metabolism	Jaundice without pruritus	Low serum GGT and bile acid levels Urinalysis for bile acids
Propionic academia Methylmalonic acidemia	Metabolic crisis Fulminant liver failure	Acidosis Hyperammonemia Fatty infiltration on liver biopsy Genetic analysis
Wolman's disease Cholesterol ester storage disease	FTT, vomiting, diarrhea Hepatosplenomegaly Wolman's: fatal in infancy Jaundice, anemia, leukopenia CESD: later presentation and less severe	Adrenal calcification Hyperlipidemia Vacuolated lymphocytes on peripheral blood film Sea-blue histiocytes in bone marrow aspirate Genetic analysis
Respiratory chain defects Complex I, IV, III deficiencies	Jaundice, hypotonia, seizures, FTT Neonatal liver failure Hypertrophic obstructive cardiomyopathy	Lactic acidosis Hyperammonemia Ketotic hypoglycemia High lactate pyruvate ratio Steatosis: microvesicular and macrovesicular e/m abnormal mitochondria Genetic and enzymatic analysis
Alpers' syndrome POLG mutation	Dysmorphic features Lethargy, hypotonia Intractable seizures Developmental delay Hepatomegaly, delayed liver failure Hypertrophic cardiomyopathy	High blood lactate High CSF/blood lactate ratio Microvesicular steatosis on liver histology, e/m abnormal mitochondria Abnormal MRI, EEG, and visual evoked response Genetic analysiss
Pearson's syndrome	Exocrine pancreatic insufficiency Sideroblastic anemia Progressive liver disease Renal Fanconi's syndrome	High blood lactate Ragged red fibers on muscle biopsy Respiratory chain enzyme analysis e/m abnormal mitochondria, histology steatosis, cholestasis, fibrosis, necrosis Genetic analysis

RBC, red blood cell; MRI, magnetic resonance imaging; GGT, gamma-glutamyltransferase; FTT, failure to thrive; CESD, cholesterol ester storage disease; CSF, cerebrospinal fluid; EEG, electroencephologram.

present in the third trimester with abdominal pain, nausea, and vomiting, and rapidly develop fulminant liver failure. Liver biopsy shows microvesicular steatosis and abnormal mitochondria on electron microscopy. HELLP is thought to be a complication of severe ecclampsia, but liver biopsy here may show micro- and macrovesicular steatosis. In both cases, early diagnosis and prompt delivery is lifesaving.

Liver Transplantation in Children

Liver transplantation is now considered standard of care in children with end-stage liver disease and fulminant liver failure. Thomas Starzl attempted the first liver transplant in a child with biliary atresia in 1963 in Denver, CO [80]. This was unsuccessful, but 7 years later he transplanted another child with biliary atresia, who is currently the oldest living survivor of a liver transplant in the world. Over 12 000 liver transplants have been performed in children in

the United States, with around 600 pediatric liver transplantations performed annually.

Indications and Contraindications

The most common indication for liver transplantation in children is biliary atresia (versus hepatitis C in adults). Hepatoblastoma is the most common tumor requiring liver transplantation in children (versus HCC in adults). Drug overdose requiring liver transplantation in children is relatively rare compared to adults. Common indications for liver transplantation include (i) cholestatic liver disease (biliary atresia, sclerosing cholangitis), (ii) fulminant liver failure, (iii) metabolic liver disease (Wilson's disease, A1AT deficiency, GSDs, urea cycle defects), (iv) autoimmune hepatitis, (v) hepatoblastoma, (vi) cryptogenic cirrhosis, (vii) and retransplantation secondary to complications of first transplant [81]. Contraindications are similar to those in adults, and include (i) coma with irreversible brain injury, (ii) uncontrolled systemic infection, (iii) inoperable extrahepatic metastasis, (iv) terminal or progressive systemic disease, and (v) insufficient cardiac or pulmonary reserve.

After establishing that liver transplantation is indicated, the child undergoes transplant evaluation by a multidisciplinary team and gets placed on the waitlist, and preoperative intervention is initiated (including intensive nutritional rehabilitation, immunizations (particularly the live vaccines), and education).

Position on Waitlist

The Organ Procurement and Transplantation Network (OPTN) was established in the early 1980s in the United States to distribute organs in an equitable fashion. Traditionally, position on the waitlist was determined by waiting time and severity of disease, as determined by patient location (home/hospital or intensive care unit (ICU)), but this did not accurately stratify patients. In 2002, a new system was developed: Pediatric End-Stage Liver Disease (PELD) for children and the Model for End-Stage Liver Disease (MELD) for adults [82]. The PELD was developed as a means of stratifying children awaiting liver transplantation based upon a continuous objective score that reflects risk of death and/or movement to ICU in the ensuing 3 months. The formula for calculating PELD is 0.436 (Age (<1 year)) − 0.687 × Loge (albumin g/dL) + 0.480 × Loge (total bilirubin mg/dL) + 1.87 × Loge (INR) + 0.667 (growth failure (< −2SD present). The MELD score is based on bilirubin, INR, and serum creatinine. It is used in adults and children over 12 years of age, as it has been recognized that MELD and not PELD is more accurate in older children. When the PELD/MELD score is not believed to be reflective of a child's true mortality risk, there is a system for appealing to the Regional Review Board (RRB) for more points.

The highest priority for liver transplant in the UNOS waitlist is designated as status 1a, which is for (i) fulminant liver failure, (ii) primary non-function, (iii) hepatic artery thrombosis, and (iv) acute decompensated Wilson's disease. Status 1b is allocated to children who do not typically have abnormalities of liver function, including (i) metabolic disease and (ii) liver tumors (e.g., hepatoblastoma). Status 1b designation is also allocated to children with chronic liver disease with calculated MELD/PELD >25 and one of the following: (i) ventilated; (ii) Glasgow coma scale <10, within 48 hours of listing; (iii) GI bleed requiring at least 30 mL/kg of packed red blood cell (RBC) replacement in the previous 24 hours; or (iv) renal failure/insufficiency requiring dialysis/continuous venovenous filtration.

Technical Aspects of Liver Transplantation in Children

The organ used may be from a deceased or a living donor. The graft may be whole from a size-matched pediatric donor or, in the current climate of organ shortage, reduced [83, 84] or split between a pediatric and an adult recipient or two pediatric recipients [85]. The liver constitutes about 2% of body weight. As a rule of thumb, infants get the left lateral segment (25% of the liver), children below the age of 12 get the left lobe (40% of the liver), and children over 12 and adults get the right lobe (60% of the liver) [81]. Neonates may get monosegment grafts, where the transplant is technically challenging and requires great surgical expertise. Small-for-size, where the graft/recipient ratio (expressed as percentage of body weight) is below the recommended 0.8–4.0% range, is not common in children.

In adults, conventional liver transplantation involves removal of the recipient native liver along with the retrohepatic vena cava, followed by implantation of the donor liver. Venovenous bypass is used to avoid cardiovascular instability. The venous anastomosis is done first; the liver is then reperfused with recipient's blood, and then the arterial anastomosis is performed. The biliary anastomosis is performed last [86]. In children, the "piggyback technique" is often used, where the native retrohepatic vena cava is preserved and the new liver is anastomosed to a cuff from one or more of the main suprahepatic veins in order to avoid venovenous bypass. The diameter of the vessels is very small, and vascular grafts may be used in arterial and venous anastomoses. Use of an operating microscope has reduced the incidence of hepatic artery thrombosis. The bile ducts are also very small, and are absent if the child has biliary atresia. The biliary anastomosis in infants and small children is often a choledochojejunostomy (to a Roux-en-Y defunctioning intestinal loop) rather than a "duct-to-duct," as seen in adults. Other advances in liver transplantation include transfusion-free liver transplantation, which is important to Jehova's Witness patients who require transplant [87].

Living Donor Transplantation in Children

Living donor liver transplantation was started in children in response to the organ shortage and a childhood waitlist mortality of >25%. The first living donor liver transplantation was performed in Chicago in 1991 [84]. For the doctor, the advantages are mainly psychological. For the recipient, there are several advantages: the operation is elective instead of emergent, the organ does not undergo ischemic liver injury as the donor is usually healthy, and the total ischemia time (the interval between hepatectomy and reperfusion in the donor) is considerably reduced [88]. There may also be an immunological advantage, but this remains to be established. One must always keep in mind the risk to the healthy living donor.

Complications of Liver Transplantation

Many pediatric post-liver transplant complications are similar to those in adults, including primary graft non-function, hepatic artery thrombosis, portal vein thrombosis, hemorrhage, sepsis, biliary complications, and rejection. Additionally, children are usually seronegative for Epstein–Barr virus (EBV) and cytomegalovirus (CMV), and first exposure to such viruses from the donor graft while on immunosuppressive anti-rejection therapy makes them susceptible to viral infections and EBV-related post-transplant proliferative disease. Regular surveillance of EBV and CMV polymerase chain reactions (PCRs) and various prophylactic protocols are used by pediatric programs to reduce the incidence of this virus-related complication [89]. Recurrence of disease is not common in pediatric liver transplantation, but "*de novo* autoimmune hepatitis" has been described more often in pediatric than in adult recipients [90]. Another issue unique to children is intensive nutritional rehabilitation, particularly in the first few months post transplant, as a lot of catch-up growth needs to be achieved once the child has a normally functioning liver.

Quality of Life

The parameters for measuring success in liver transplantation include not only improved patient and graft survival but also optimal quality of life. Longitudinal growth is an important component of quality of life [91]. Post-transplant obesity [92], diabetes [93], hypertension, and hyperlipidemia can all affect quality of life, as can other medical issues, such as renal dysfunction, infections, and malignancy. Sexual and reproductive health is important, as many adolescent recipients have amenorrhea or menstrual irregularities pre-transplant. In general, solid organ recipients report good psychosocial outcomes compared to pre-transplant. However, liver transplant recipients have reported lower quality of life compared with healthy peers [94, 95].

Adherence

Non-adherence to medical recommendations is a leading cause of rejection in children and adolescent transplant recipients. There is significant morbidity and risk of graft loss related to non-adherence in pediatric liver transplantation [96].

Parents take responsibility for administering medications in children, but it is adolescents who are most likely to have problems with non-adherence. The responsibility for taking medications is usually shifted to the child at around the age of 12, but it can occur as late as 16. In order to improve outcomes by improving adherence, the non-adherent liver transplant recipient must first be identified. Subjective measures such as direct questioning of the child/parent and physician/nursing impression have not been successful in assessing the status of adherence. Objective measures like pill counting, prescription refills, clinic attendance, electronic monitoring devices, and medication levels yield a more realistic assessment. These indirect markers can allow intervention before the recipient presents with graft dysfunction or rejection.

Underlying risk factors for non-adherence include low socioeconomic status, problems with medical insurance, post-traumatic stress syndrome, and complicated medical status. Surprisingly, medication side effects are not a common cause. Once the non-adherent recipient is identified, it is helpful to have a consult with them in-clinic to look into the underlying cause and provide appropriate help, by linking them with a socialworker or psychologist. These patients require more frequent blood draws and regular office visits, where the importance of adherence is reinforced by multiple transplant team members. Simplifying the medication regimen may also help: forgetfulness is a common reason cited by many for non-adherence. Sending reminder text messages or putting an alarm on their phones may be a simple means of improving adherence, particularly in adolescents and young adults. In a prospective study of 41 pediatric liver transplant recipients, text messaging reduced the incidence of acute cellular ejection episodes from 12 to 2. Risk factors for rejection were older age and administration of more than one immunosuppressant [97].

Transition to Adult Service

For long-term patient and graft survival, successful transition to adult services is essential. Unfortunately, all too often transplant recipients transfer from pediatric to adult care services without adequate preparation. A study examining adherence and outcomes in patients who were recently transferred to adult facilities showed that adherence declined significantly, and there were four deaths after transfer [98, 99]. Teaching the recipient health care management skills while still at the pediatric facility and implementing standarsized communication with the adult facility may be necessary to achieve successful transition [100]. While multidisciplinary input is essential, having one point person (e.g., a transition coordinator) take responsibility and oversee the transition process can improve outcomes [101]. Funding is sometimes the main hurdle, but perhaps providing salary support to have a person focus on transition would save a lot of hospitalizations and rejection-related morbidities and mortalities, which could turn out to be so much more expensive in

the long term. Ongoing research and dedicated funding is needed to ensure successful transition.

Take Home Points

Biliary atresia:
* Biliary atresia is a progressive fibroinflammatory disorder of the biliary tree of unknown etiology and is fatal if not corrected surgically by 2 years of age.
* Presentation is in infancy, with jaundice, pale stools, hepatosplenomegaly, and conjugated hyperbiliurubinemia.
* The gold standard for diagnosis in intraoperative cholangiography.
* Kasai portoenterostomy is currently the standard of care, but biliary drainage can be established successfully in only 50–80% of cases.

Cystic fibrosis:
* Cystic fibrosis is a multisystem disease with pulmonary, sinus, pancreatic, intestinal, reproductive, and renal and hepatobiliary manifestations.
* Diagnosis is made by annual screening with physical exam, biochemical tests, and ultrasonography. Nutrition, fat-soluble vitamins levels, bone health, pancreatic function, and portal hypertension should be monitored.
* Liver transplantation should be considered in the context of evidence of true synthetic liver failure (i.e., coagulopathy unresponsive to parenteral vitamin K), intractable ascites, or severe mechanical pulmonary compromise secondary to organomegaly and/or ascites, and should take into account the multiorgan involvement in cystic fibrosis.
* Multivisceral transplant with combined liver–lung or pancreas should be considered in selective cases.

Alpha-1-antitrypsin deficiency:
* Alpha-1-antitrypsin (A1AT) deficiency presents with liver disease in pediatrics and lung disease in adults.
* Diagnosis is made by obtaining a phenotype through isoelectric focusing; the disease phenotype is PiZZ. Histologically, periodic acid–Schiff (PAS)-positive diastase-resistant granules are the hallmark of A1AT deficiency liver disease. 10% of homozygotes with PiZZ deficiency will develop liver disease.
* Heterozygosity for A1AT deficiency (PiMZ) has been found to be a risk factor for developing chronic liver disease in adults and a marker for disease severity in children with biliary atresia.
* Transplantation considerably improves prognosis in those affected with A1AT deficiency.

Liver transplantation in children:
* Biliary atresia is the most common indication for liver transplantation in children.
* Pediatric End-Stage Liver Disease (PELD) is used to allocate waitlist positions for children below 12 years of age; the Model for End-Stage Liver Disease (MELD) is used for those over 12, as for adults.
* Living donor and split liver transplants are increasingly being performed in pediatric recipients due to organ shortage.
* Adherence to medications requires special attention.
* Successfully transitioning pediatric recipients to adult services requires dedicated effort and resources.
* Good outcomes in liver transplantation requires good quality of life post transplant, in addition to improvement in patient and graft survival.

References

1 Balistreri WF, Bezerra J, Ryckman FC. Biliary atresia and other disorders of the extrahepatic bile duct. In: Suchy FJ, Sokol RJ, Balistreri WF, eds. *Liver Disease in Children.* Cambridge: Cambridge University Press, 2014; 155–76.
2 Hays DM, Snyder WH Jr. Life-span in untreated biliary atresia. *Surgery* 1963; **54**: 373–5.

3 Farrant P, Meire HB, Mieli-Vergani G. Ultrasound features of the gall bladder in infants presenting with conjugated hyperbilirubinaemia. *Br J Radiol* 2000; **73**(875): 1154–8.

4 Choi SO, Park WH, Lee HJ, Woo SK. "Triangular cord": a sonographic finding applicable in the diagnosis of biliary atresia. *J Pediatr Surg* 1996; **31**(3): 363–6.

5 Mack CL, Sokol RJ. Unraveling the pathogenesis and etiology of biliary atresia. *Pediatr Res* 2005; **57**(5 Pt. 2):87R–94R.

6 Schweizer P. [Long-term results in the treatment of extrahepatic bile duct atresia]. *Z Kinderchir* 1985; **40**(5): 263–7.

7 Davenport M, Savage M, Mowat AP, Howard ER. Biliary atresia splenic malformation syndrome: an etiologic and prognostic subgroup. *Surgery* 1993; **113**(6): 662–8.

8 Davenport M, Tizzard SA, Underhill J, et al. The biliary atresia splenic malformation syndrome: a 28-year single-center retrospective study. *J Pediatr* 2006; **149**(3): 393–400.

9 Schwarz KB, Haber BH, Rosenthal P, et al. Extrahepatic anomalies in infants with biliary atresia: results of a large prospective North American multicenter study. *Hepatology* 2013; **58**(5): 1724–31.

10 Sokol RJ, Shepherd RW, Superina R, et al. Screening and outcomes in biliary atresia: summary of a National Institutes of Health workshop. *Hepatology* 2007; **46**(2): 566–81.

11 Kasai M, Asakura Y. [Surgery of congenital obstruction of the bile ducts in our clinics]. *Shujutsu* 1968; **22**(12): 1228–35.

12 Carcassonne M, Bensoussan A. Long term results in treatment of biliary atresia. *Prog Pediatr Surg* 1977; **10**: 151–60.

13 Howard ER, MacLean G, Nio M, et al. Survival patterns in biliary atresia and comparison of quality of life of long-term survivors in Japan and England. *J Pediatr Surg* 2001; **36**(6): 892–7.

14 Altman RP, Lilly JR, Greenfeld J, et al. A multivariable risk factor analysis of the portoenterostomy (Kasai) procedure for biliary atresia: twenty-five years of experience from two centers. *Ann Surg* 1997; **226**(3): 348–53, disc. 53–5.

15 Laurent J, Gauthier F, Bernard O, et al. Long-term outcome after surgery for biliary atresia. Study of 40 patients surviving for more than 10 years. *Gastroenterology* 1990; **99**(6): 1793–7.

16 Nio M, Ohi R, Hayashi Y, et al. Current status of 21 patients who have survived more than 20 years since undergoing surgery for biliary atresia. *J Pediatr Surg* 1996; **31**(3): 381–4.

17 Shinkai M, Ohhama Y, Take H, et al. Long-term outcome of children with biliary atresia who were not transplanted after the Kasai operation: >20-year experience at a children's hospital. *J Pediatr Gastroenterol Nutr* 2009; **48**(4): 443–50.

18 de Vries W, Homan-Van der Veen J, Hulscher JB, et al. Twenty-year transplant-free survival rate among patients with biliary atresia. *Clin Gastroenterol Hepatol* 2011; **9**(12): 1086–91.

19 Lykavieris P, Chardot C, Sokhn M, et al. Outcome in adulthood of biliary atresia: a study of 63 patients who survived for over 20 years with their native liver. *Hepatology* 2005; **41**(2): 366–71.

20 Nio M, Sano N, Ishii T, et al. Long-term outcome in type I biliary atresia. *J Pediatr Surg* 2006; **41**(12): 1973–5.

21 Nio M, Ohi R, Shimaoka S, et al. The outcome of surgery for biliary atresia and the current status of long-term survivors. *Tohoku J Exp Med* 1997; **181**(1): 235–44.

22 Okazaki T, Kobayashi H, Yamataka A, et al. Long-term postsurgical outcome of biliary atresia. *J Pediatr Surg* 1999; **34**(2): 312–15.

23 Ohi R, Hanamatsu M, Mochizuki I, et al. Progress in the treatment of biliary atresia. *World J Surg* 1985; **9**(2): 285–93.

24 Arguedas MR, Abrams GA, Krowka MJ, Fallon MB. Prospective evaluation of outcomes and predictors of mortality in patients with hepatopulmonary syndrome undergoing liver transplantation. *Hepatology* 2003; **37**(1): 192–7.

25 Rodriguez-Roisin R, Krowka MJ, Herve P, Fallon MB. Pulmonary-hepatic vascular disorders (PHD). *Eur Respir J* 2004; **24**(5): 861–80.

26 Houben C, Phelan S, Davenport M. Late-presenting cholangitis and Roux loop obstruction after Kasai portoenterostomy for biliary atresia. *J Pediatr Surg* 2006; **41**(6): 1159–64.

27 Nio M, Sano N, Ishii T, et al. Cholangitis as a late complication in long-term survivors after surgery for biliary atresia. *J Pediatr Surg* 2004; **39**(12): 1797–9.

28 Hadzic N, Davenport M, Tizzard S, et al. Long-term survival following Kasai portoenterostomy: is chronic liver disease inevitable? *J Pediatr Gastroenterol Nutr* 2003; **37**(4): 430–3.

29 Nio M, Wada M, Sasaki H, et al. Risk factors affecting late-presenting liver failure in adult patients with biliary atresia. *J Pediatr Surg* 2012; **47**(12): 2179–83.

30 Davenport M, Kerkar N, Mieli-Vergani G, et al. Biliary atresia: the King's College Hospital experience (1974–1995). *J Pediatr Surg* 1997; **32**(3): 479–85.

31 Kuroda T, Saeki M, Morikawa N, Fuchimoto Y. Biliary atresia and pregnancy: puberty may be an important point for predicting the outcome. *J Pediatr Surg* 2005; **40**(12): 1852–5.

32 Sasaki H, Nio M, Hayashi Y, et al. Problems during and after pregnancy in female patients with biliary atresia. *J Pediatr Surg* 2007; **42**(8): 1329–32.

33 Kuroda T, Saeki M, Morikawa N, Watanabe K. Management of adult biliary atresia patients: should hard work and pregnancy be discouraged? *J Pediatr Surg* 2007; **42**(12): 2106–9.

34 Kuroda T, Saeki M, Nakano M, Morikawa N. Biliary atresia, the next generation: a review of liver function, social activity, and sexual development in the late postoperative period. *J Pediatr Surg* 2002; **37**(12): 1709–12.

35 Russell MA, Craigo SD. Cirrhosis and portal hypertension in pregnancy. *Semin Perinatol* 1998; **22**(2). 156–65.

36 Sundaram SS, Alonso EM, Haber B, et al. Health related quality of life in patients with biliary atresia surviving with their native liver. *J Pediatr* 2013; **163**(4): 1052–7.e2.

37 Arnon R, Annunziato RA, Willis A, et al. Liver transplantation for children with biliary atresia in the pediatric end-stage liver disease era: the role of insurance status. *Liver Transpl* 2013; **19**(5): 543–50.

38 Kyoden Y, Tamura S, Sugawara Y, et al. Outcome of living donor liver transplantation for post-Kasai biliary atresia in adults. *Liver Transpl* 2008; **14**(2): 186–92.

39 Arnon R, Annunziato R, Schiano T, et al. Orthotopic liver transplantation for adults with Alagille syndrome. *Clin Transplant* 2011; **26**(2): E94–100.

40 Salvatore D, Buzzetti R, Baldo E, et al. An overview of international literature from cystic fibrosis registries. Part 4: update 2011. *J Cyst Fibros* 2012; **11**(6): 480–93.

41 Boyle MP. Nonclassic cystic fibrosis and CFTR-related diseases. *Curr Opin Pulm Med* 2003; **9**(6): 498–503.

42 De Boeck K, Wilschanski M, Castellani C, et al. Cystic fibrosis: terminology and diagnostic algorithms. *Thorax* 2006; **61**(7): 627–35.

43 Colombo C, Battezzati PM. Hepatobiliary manifestations of cystic fibrosis. *Eur J Gastroenterol Hepatol* 1996; **8**(5): 748–54.

44 Scott-Jupp R, Lama M, Tanner MS. Prevalence of liver disease in cystic fibrosis. *Arch Dis Child* 1991; **66**(6): 698–701.

45 Nazareth D, Walshaw M. Coming of age in cystic fibrosis - transition from paediatric to adult care. *Clin Med* 2013; **13**(5): 482–6.

46 Parisi GF, Di Dio G, Franzonello C, et al. Liver disease in cystic fibrosis: an update. *Hepat Mon* 2013; **13**(8): e11215.

47 Sokol RJ, Durie PR. Recommendations for management of liver and biliary tract disease in cystic fibrosis. Cystic Fibrosis Foundation Hepatobiliary Disease Consensus Group. *J Pediatr Gastroenterol Nutr* 1999; **28**(Suppl. 1): S1–13.

48 Farrell PM, Rosenstein BJ, White TB, et al. Guidelines for diagnosis of cystic fibrosis in newborns through older adults: Cystic Fibrosis Foundation consensus report. *J Pediatr* 2008; **153**(2): S4–14.

49 Kitson MT, Kemp WW, Iser DM, et al. Utility of transient elastography in the non-invasive evaluation of cystic fibrosis liver disease. *Liver Int* 2013; **33**(5): 698–705.

50 Dodge JA, Turck D. Cystic fibrosis: nutritional consequences and management. *Best Pract Res Clin Gastroenterol* 2006; **20**(3): 531–46.

51 Perdue DG, Cass OW, Milla C, et al. Hepatolithiasis and cholangiocarcinoma in cystic fibrosis: a case series and review of the literature. *Dig Dis Sci* 2007; **52**(10): 2638–42.

52 Laurell CB, Eriksson S. The serum alpha-L-antitrypsin in families with hypo-alpha-L-antitrypsinemia. *Clin Chim Acta* 1965; **11**: 395–8.

53 Lai EC, Kao FT, Law ML, Woo SL. Assignment of the alpha 1-antitrypsin gene and a sequence-related gene to human chromosome 14 by molecular hybridization. *Am J Hum Genet* 1983; **35**(3): 385–92.

54 Sveger T. Liver disease in alpha1-antitrypsin deficiency detected by screening of 200 000 infants. *N Engl J Med* 1976; **294**(24): 1316–21.

55 Perlmutter DH. Pathogenesis of chronic liver injury and hepatocellular carcinoma in alpha-1-antitrypsin deficiency. *Pediatr Res* 2006; **60**(2): 233–8.

56 Hinds R, Hadchouel A, Shanmugam NP, et al. Variable degree of liver involvement in siblings with PiZZ alpha-1-antitrypsin deficiency-related liver disease. *J Ped Gastroenterol Nutr* 2006; **43**(1): 136–8.

57 Hadzic N, Francavilla R, Chambers SM, et al. Outcome of PiSS and PiSZ alpha-1-antitrypsin deficiency presenting with liver involvement. *Eur J Pediatr* 2005; **164**(4): 250–2.

58 Jacquemin E. Progressive familial intrahepatic cholestasis. *J Gastroenterol Hepatol* 1999; **14**(6): 594–9.

59 Klomp LW, Bull LN, Knisely AS, et al. A missense mutation in FIC1 is associated with greenland familial cholestasis. *Hepatology* 2000; **32**(6): 1337–41.

60 Whitington PF, Freese DK, Alonso EM, et al. Clinical and biochemical findings in progressive familial intrahepatic cholestasis. *J Pediatr Gastroenterol Nutr* 1994; **18**(2): 134–41.

61 Alissa FT, Jaffe R, Shneider BL. Update on progressive familial intrahepatic cholestasis. *J Pediatr Gastroenterol Nutr* 2008; **46**(3): 241–52.

62 Morotti RA, Suchy FJ, Magid MS. Progressive familial intrahepatic cholestasis (PFIC) type 1, 2, and 3: a review of the liver pathology findings. *Semin Liv Dis* 2011; **31**(1): 3–10.

63 Gonzales E, Spraul A, Jacquemin E. Clinical utility gene card for: progressive familial intrahepatic cholestasis type 1. *Eur J Hum Genet* 2014; **22**(4).

64 Davis AR, Rosenthal P, Newman TB. Nontransplant surgical interventions in progressive familial intrahepatic cholestasis. *J Pediatr Surg* 2009; **44**(4): 821–7.

65 Egawa H, Yorifuji T, Sumazaki R, *et al.* Intractable diarrhea after liver transplantation for Byler's disease: successful treatment with bile adsorptive resin. *Liver Transpl* 2002; **8**(8): 714–16.

66 Pawlikowska L, Strautnieks S, Jankowska I, *et al.* Differences in presentation and progression between severe FIC1 and BSEP deficiencies. *J Hepatol* 2010; **53**(1): 170–8.

67 Maggiore G, Gonzales E, Sciveres M, *et al.* Relapsing features of bile salt export pump deficiency after liver transplantation in two patients with progressive familial intrahepatic cholestasis type 2. *J Hepatol* 2010; **53**(5): 981–6.

68 Jacquemin E, De Vree JM, Cresteil D, *et al.* The wide spectrum of multidrug resistance 3 deficiency: from neonatal cholestasis to cirrhosis of adulthood. *Gastroenterology* 2001; **120**(6): 1448–58.

69 Davit-Spraul A, Gonzales E, Baussan C, Jacquemin E. The spectrum of liver diseases related to ABCB4 gene mutations: pathophysiology and clinical aspects. *Semin Liv Dis* 2010; **30**(2): 134–46.

70 van Mil SW, van der Woerd WL, van der Brugge G, *et al.* Benign recurrent intrahepatic cholestasis type 2 is caused by mutations in ABCB11. *Gastroenterology* 2004; **127**(2): 379–84.

71 Stapelbroek JM, van Erpecum KJ, Klomp LW, *et al.* Nasobiliary drainage induces long-lasting remission in benign recurrent intrahepatic cholestasis. *Hepatology* 2006; **43**(1): 51–3.

72 Sturm E, Franssen CF, Gouw A, *et al.* Extracorporal albumin dialysis (MARS) improves cholestasis and normalizes low apo A-I levels in a patient with benign recurrent intrahepatic cholestasis (BRIC). *Liver* 2002; **22**(Suppl. 2): 72–5.

73 Danks DM, Campbell PE, Jack I, *et al.* Studies of the aetiology of neonatal hepatitis and biliary atresia. *Arch Dis Child* 1977; **52**(5): 360–7.

74 Piccoli DA, Spinner NB. Alagille syndrome and the Jagged1 gene. *Semin Liv Dis* 2001; **21**(4): 525–34.

75 Kronsten V, Fitzpatrick E, Baker A. Management of cholestatic pruritus in paediatric patients with alagille syndrome: the King's College Hospital experience. *J Pediatr Gastroenterol Nutr* 2013; **57**(2): 149–54.

76 Kamath BM, Yin W, Miller H, *et al.* Outcomes of liver transplantation for patients with Alagille syndrome: the studies of pediatric liver transplantation experience. *Liver Transpl* 2012; **18**(8): 940–8.

77 Paulusma CC, Kool M, Bosma PJ, *et al.* A mutation in the human canalicular multispecific organic anion transporter gene causes the Dubin-Johnson syndrome. *Hepatology* 1997; **25**(6): 1539–42.

78 Kondo T, Kuchiba K, Shimizu Y. Coproporphyrin isomers in Dubin-Johnson syndrome. *Gastroenterology* 1976; **70**(6): 1117–20.

79 van der Veere CN, Sinaasappel M, McDonagh AF, *et al.* Current therapy for Crigler-Najjar syndrome type 1: report of a world registry. *Hepatology* 1996; **24**(2): 311–15.

80 Starzl TE, Kaulla KN, Hermann G, *et al.* Homotransplantation of the liver in humans. *Surg Gynnecol Obstet* 1963; **117**: 659–76.

81 Kerkar N, Emre S. Issues unique to pediatric liver transplantation. *Clin Liver Dis* 2007; **11**: 323–37.

82 McDiarmid SV, Anand R, Lindblad AS. Development of a pediatric end-stage liver disease score to predict poor outcome in children awaiting liver transplantation. *Transplantation* 2002; **74**(2): 173–81.

83 Bismuth H, Houssin D. Reduced-sized orthotopic liver graft in hepatic transplantation in children. *Surgery* 1984; **95**(3): 367–70.

84 Broelsch CE, Emond JC, Thistlethwaite JR, *et al.* Liver transplantation with reduced-size donor organs. *Transplantation* 1988; **45**(3): 519–24.

85 Rogiers X, Malago M, Gawad K, *et al.* In situ splitting of cadaveric livers. The ultimate expansion of a limited donor pool. *Ann Surg* 1996; **224**(3): 331–9, disc. 9–41.

86 Eghtesad B, Kadry Z, Fung J. Technical considerations in liver transplantation: what a hepatologist needs to know (and every surgeon should practice). *Liver Transpl* 2005; **11**(8): 861–71.

87 Jabbour N, Gagandeep S, Thomas D, *et al.* Transfusion-free techniques in pediatric live donor liver transplantation. *J Pediatr Gastroenterol Nutr* 2005; **40**(4): 521–3.

88 Emre S. Living-donor liver transplantation in children. *Pediatr Transplant* 2002; **6**(1): 43–6.

89 Kerkar N, Morotti RA, Madan RP, *et al.* The changing face of post-transplant lymphoproliferative disease in the era of molecular EBV monitoring. *Pediatr Transplant* 2010; **14**(4): 504–11.

90 Kerkar N, Hadzic N, Davies ET, *et al.* De-novo autoimmune hepatitis after liver transplantation. *Lancet* 1998; **351**(9100): 409–13.

91 LaRosa C, Baluarte HJ, Meyers KE. Outcomes in pediatric solid-organ transplantation. *Pediatr Transplant* 2011; **15**(2): 128–41.

92 Sundaram SS, Alonso EM, Zeitler P, *et al.* Obesity after pediatric liver transplantation: prevalence and risk factors. *J Pediatr Gastroenterol Nutr* 2012; **55**(6): 657–62.

93 Greig F, Rapaport R, Klein G, *et al.* Characteristics of diabetes after pediatric liver transplant. *Pediatr Transplant* 2013; **17**(1): 27–33.

94 Shemesh E, Shneider BL, Emre S. Adherence to medical recommendations in pediatric transplant recipients: time for action. *Pediatr Transplant* 2008; **12**(3): 281–3.

95 Taylor R, Franck LS, Gibson F, Dhawan A. A critical review of the health-related quality of life of children and adolescents after liver transplantation. *Liver Transpl* 2005; **11**(1): 51–60, disc. 7–9.

96 Lurie S, Shemesh E, Sheiner PA, *et al.* Non-adherence in pediatric liver transplant recipients – an assessment of risk factors and natural history. *Pediatr Transplant* 2000; **4**(3): 200–6.

97 Miloh T, Annunziato R, Arnon R, *et al.* Improved adherence and outcomes for pediatric liver transplant recipients by using text messaging. *Pediatrics* 2009; **124**(5): e844–50.

98 Annunziato RA, Emre S, Shneider B, *et al.* Adherence and medical outcomes in pediatric liver transplant recipients who transition to adult services. *Pediatr Transplant* 2007; **11**(6): 608–14.

99 Shemesh E, Annunziato RA, Yehuda R, *et al.* Childhood abuse, nonadherence, and medical outcome in pediatric liver transplant recipients. *J Am Acad Child Adolesc Psychiatry* 2007; **46**(10): 1280–9.

100 Fredericks EM, Dore-Stites D, Lopez MJ, *et al.* Transition of pediatric liver transplant recipients to adult care: patient and parent perspectives. *Pediatr Transplant* 2011; **15**(4): 414–24.

101 Annunziato RA, Baisley MC, Arrato N, *et al.* Strangers headed to a strange land? A pilot study of using a transition coordinator to improve transfer from pediatric to adult services. *J Pediatr* 2013; **163**(6): 1628–33.

CHAPTER 91

PART 3

Liver Transplantation

92 Indications and Selection of Patients for Liver Transplantation, 601
Michael D. Leise and Marie A. Laryea

93 What Every Hepatologist Should Know about Liver Transplantation, 608
Peter S. Yoo and David C. Mulligan

94 Immunosuppression Used in Liver Transplantation, 617
Rebecca L. Corey and David D. Douglas

95 Medical Management of the Liver Transplant Patient, 626
William C. Palmer and Denise M. Harnois

96 Organ Allocation Policy: Practical Issues and Challenges to the Gastroenterologist, 632
Jessica Yu and Pratima Sharma

97 Endoscopic Ultrasound, 637
Thomas J. Savides

CHAPTER 92

Indications and Selection of Patients for Liver Transplantation

Michael D. Leise[1] and Marie A. Laryea[2]

[1]William J. von Liebig Center for Transplantation and Clinical Regeneration, Rochester, MN, USA
[2]Division of Gastroenterology and Hepatology, Dalhousie University, Halifax, NS, Canada

Summary

Liver transplantation is an effective treatment for patients with end-stage liver disease, acute liver failure (ALF), specific hepatobiliary malignancies, and certain metabolic diseases. Patient and graft survival are excellent (Figure 92.1). The field of liver transplantation has evolved significantly since the first liver transplant performed by Dr. Thomas E. Starzl in 1967. Recipients now enjoy 1- and 5-year survivals of approximately 89 and 71%, respectively. Advances in surgical technique, anesthesia, immunosuppression, care of patients with end-stage liver disease, and survival prediction models have contributed to this. In 2012, 6256 liver transplants were performed in the United States, while 2187 died on the waiting list and 815 were removed because they were too sick [2]. Currently, the demand for liver transplantation outstrips the supply of donor organs. This chapter will focus on the indications for liver transplantation according to disease and the selection of appropriate candidates, which are crucial issues given donor organ shortages.

Case

A 66-year-old male with alcohol-related liver disease is seen for increased abdominal girth and is noted to have ascites on clinical exam. He is known to have had cirrhosis for approximately 4 years, and has had no previous decompensation. He quit drinking alcohol 2 years ago and attends Alcoholics Anonymous. An abdominal ultrasound reveals a 2.8 cm lesion in the left lobe, with arterial enhancement and portal venous phase washout. Laboratory studies reveal a bilirubin of 1.5 mg/dL, albumin of 3.4 g/dL, International Normalized Ratio (INR) 1.4, and creatinine 1.1 mg/dL. Other medical problems include benign prostatic hypertrophy and gout. His Model for End-Stage Liver Disease (MELD) score is 13 and his Child–Turcotte–Pugh score is 6. Subsequent computed tomography (CT) scan confirms the 2.8 cm lesion in the left lobe, which is suspicious for hepatocellular carcinoma (HCC), as well as a small 0.9 cm indeterminate lesion in the right lobe. The patient asks if liver transplantation is an option for him.

Prognosis and Allocation

Prognosis and organ allocation are intimately linked. In the past, liver allocation in the United States was based on both waiting time and severity of liver disease. Prior to 2002, The Child–Turcotte–Pugh criteria (Table 92.1) were utilized to define liver disease severity. However, these criteria have multiple flaws, including using subjective parameters of ascites and hepatic encephalopathy and providing a limited range of scores. The US Department of Health and Human Services (HHS) issued a Final Rule in 1998, which recommends elimination of waiting time and subjective variables as a foundation for allocation.

Currently, allocation of donor livers is based on the MELD score: an urgency or "sickest-first" system in which waitlisted candidates are prioritized based on objective laboratory values, specifically bilirubin, INR, and creatinine.

The MELD score (range 6–40) is calculated as follows:

$$\text{MELD score} = (0.957 \times \ln(\text{serum creatinine}) + 0.378$$
$$\times \ln(\text{serum bilirubin}) + 1.120 \times \ln(\text{INR}) + 0.643)$$
$$\times 10 \text{ (if on hemodialysis, the value for creatinine is}$$
$$\text{automatically set to 4.0)}$$

This predictive model was derived from patients undergoing placement of a transjugular portosystemic shunt and is an accurate predictor of 3-month mortality in patients with cirrhosis waiting for liver transplantation [3]. After it was adopted in the United States in 2002, waitlist mortality decreased by 15%, liver transplantation increased by 6%, and median time to transplantation decreased from 656 to 300 days [4].

Since the inception of the MELD-based allocation system, there have been numerous attempts to improve its predictive potential, by adding different variables or reweighting the coefficients. When sodium is included (MELD-Na), it improves the ability to predict 3-month mortality (patients with lower sodium values have a higher likelihood of 3-month mortality) [5,6]. Hyponatremia is thought to be a marker for poor renal function, which is complementary to the creatinine. The MELD-Na has recently replaced the MELD score as the organ allocation model in the U.S.

The MELD system does have some disadvantages. It was developed and implemented to avoid the subjective parameters (ascites, hepatic encephalopathy) and waitlist time used by the Child–Turcotte–Pugh system, but as a result it does not capture patients with conditions which significantly affect quality of life, such as refractory pruritus, ascites, hepatic encephalopathy, and recurrent

Practical Gastroenterology and Hepatology Board Review Toolkit, Second Edition. Edited by Nicholas J. Talley, Kenneth R. DeVault, Michael B. Wallace, Bashar A. Aqel and Keith D. Lindor.

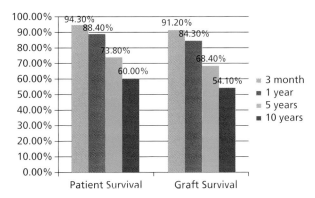

Figure 92.1 Patient and graft survival after liver transplantation in the United States between 1999 and 2008. Source: Thuluvath 2010 [1]. Reproduced with permission of *American Journal of Transplantation*.

cholangitis. Also, the MELD score does not represent poor prognosis in some conditions. Certain conditions can thus receive exception MELD scores, as listed in Table 92.2. HCC is the most common indication for an exception score, accounting for 21% of all liver transplants in 2011.

Indication and Timing of Liver Transplantation Evaluation

The indications for liver transplantation are diverse, but they may be broadly categorized as end-stage liver disease, malignancy, metabolic disorders, and ALF (Table 92.3).

Evaluation for liver transplantation is indicated for patients with decompensated end-stage liver disease, a Child–Turcotte–Pugh Score ≥7, or a MELD > or = to 15. Decompensated end-stage liver disease is defined by cirrhosis with one or more complications of portal hypertension, including hepatic encephalopathy, variceal hemorrhage, ascites, hepatorenal syndrome, hepatopulmonary syndrome (HPS), or HCC. The 2-year survival of patients with decompensated cirrhosis is approximately 50%, as compared to ≥80% in their compensated counterparts. Patients with ALF should be referred to a liver transplant center immediately.

Table 92.1 Child–Turcotte–Pugh scoring system.

Parameter	Points assigned		
	1	2	3
Ascites	Absent	Slight	Moderate
Bilirubin (mg/dL)	<2	2–3	>3
Albumin (g/dL)	>3.5	2.8–3.5	<2.8
INR	<1.7	1.7–2.3	>2.3
Encephalopathy	None	Grade 1–2	Grade 3–4

Scores of 5–6 = Child A; 7–9 = Child B; 10–15 = Child C.
1-year patient survival: A = 100%; B = 80%; C = 45%.
INR, International Normalized Ratio.

Table 92.2 Conditions granted exception MELD points.

Hepatocellular carcinoma (HCC) with Milan criteria
Hilar cholangiocarcinoma (CCA) within United Network for Organ Sharing (UNOS) criteria
Familial amyloidotic polyneuropathy
Portopulmonary hypertension
Hepatopulmonary syndrome (HPS)
Primary hyperoxaluria
Cystic fibrosis

Table 92.3 Indications for liver transplantation

Complications of end-stage liver disease of any etiology:
* Refractory ascites
* Hepatorenal syndrome
* Encephalopathy
* Gastrointestinal (GI) bleed due to portal hypertension
* Portopulmonary hypertension
* Hepatopulmonary syndrome (HPS)
* Hepatocellular carcinoma (HCC)
* Cholangiocarcinoma (CCA)
Fulminant hepatic failure

Metabolic or genetic diseases:
* Hyperoxaluria
* Familial amyloidosis
* Polycystic liver disease
* Caroli's disease
* Glycogen storage disease I, IV
* Hemophilia A, B
* Byler disease
* Crigler–Najjar syndrome
* Alagille syndrome

Miscellaneous diseases:
* Budd–Chiari syndrome
* Sinusoidal obstruction syndrome (veno-occlusive disease)
* Graft-versus-host disease (GVHD)
* Nodular regenerative hyperplasia
* Hepatic tumors (adenoma, carcinoid, pancreatic islet cell tumors, epithelioid hemangioendothelioma, fibrolamellar carcinoma, hepatoblastoma)
* Hepatic trauma

General Assessment of the Potential Liver Transplant Candidate

A thorough multidisciplinary evaluation should be tailored to each potential candidate's liver disease and medical comorbidities. Most transplant centers have specific protocols that are utilized to evaluate patients in a systematic fashion. At a minimum, each patient should undergo a history and physical examination, an in-depth psychiatric, substance, and tobacco use history, routine blood work (including complete blood count (CBC), chemistry panel, liver biochemistries, and arterial blood gas), evaluation for coexisting or previous infections (including hepatitis B and C, Epstein–Barr virus (EBV), cytomegalovirus (CMV), and human immunodeficiency virus (HIV)), transthoracic echocardiogram with agitated saline injection (to evaluate for possible portopulmonary hypertension and HPS) and dobutamine stress echocardiogram (for patients >50 years, smokers, or those with diabetes or a strong family history of cardiovascular disease (CVD)), contrast-enhanced CT or ultrasound with Doppler of the abdomen (to determine presurgical anatomy and screen for HCC), chest radiograph, and age-appropriate cancer screening. The psychosocial evaluation is crucial to identifying patients who have adequate social support, strong probability of medical compliance, and low risk of chemical dependency relapse. In the context of ALF, these steps may need to be truncated in order to avoid a delay in providing liver transplantation for those patients at the highest risk of death.

Absolute contraindications to transplantation include brainstem herniation (ALF), severe intracranial hypertension (ICH; >50 mmHg) (ALF), severe/progressive primary neurologic disease, advanced cardiopulmonary disease, hemodynamic instability requiring high-dose or multiple pressors, severe portopulmonary hypertension despite treatment, uncontrolled infection, multiorgan failure, current/recent extrahepatic malignancy (excluding superficial non-melanoma skin cancer; unless tumor-free ≥2 years and with a low risk of recurrence), hilar cholangiocarcinoma (CCA) that has been percutaneously sampled, untreated alcoholism/drug use, and severe, uncontrolled mood disorder [7].

Relative contraindications are a moving target. Advanced age is one. The rate of liver transplantation for patients >65 years increased from 7.6% (363) to 14.6% (835) between 2002 and 2012 [2]. In general, patients >65 years usually are good candidates for liver transplantation in the absence of any other serious comorbidity. Obesity is an increasingly common challenge. Class III obesity was once viewed as a contraindication to liver transplantation, but recent studies have demonstrated that it is not independently associated with diminished survival. The Mayo Clinic is currently performing a sleeve gastrectomy weight-loss surgery at the time of liver transplantation for highly selected candidates. Other centers are performing Roux-en-Y bariatric gastric bypass after recovery from liver transplantation. HIV was previously an absolute contraindication, due to poor outcomes, but with the availability of highly active antiretroviral therapy (HAART), specialized centers have now demonstrated acceptable outcomes in this population when the HIV is well controlled. Other relative contraindications include severe muscle wasting/deconditioning, extensive previous abdominal surgeries or radiation treatment, extensive portomesenteric thromboses, and lack of social support.

Deceased versus Living Donor Liver Transplantation

In the year 2012, 6256 adult liver transplants were performed: 6010 were deceased donor transplants and 246 were living donor transplants. Meanwhile, 2187 patients died while awaiting transplantation and 815 were removed from the waitlist because they were too sick. About 12,427 patients remained active on the liver transplantation waitlist at the end of 2012 [2]. These numbers reflect general organ scarcity. Organ donation has been relatively stable at about 10 donations per 1000 deaths. Options to help narrow the gap between the supply of deceased donor livers and demand by waitlisted patients include the use of extended-criteria deceased donor livers and living donor liver transplantation.

Extended-criteria donors (ECDs) include those who died in old age, those with allograft steatosis, those with prolonged cold ischemia time, those with previous malignancy, those with ABO incompatibility, and those with donor infection. Donation after cardiac death (DCD) is a form of ECD that is different from the typical deceased-after-brain-death (DBD) donor and is at higher risk for primary non-function of the allograft following transplant and ischemic cholangiopathy. Split-liver grafts, which are donated to two individuals, and domino transplantation, using a familial amyloidotic polyneuropathy donor, are also examples of ECD.

Living donor liver transplantation reached its peak in 2001 with 519 live donations. Since that time, it has been performed less frequently, due to donor deaths and increased use of ECD grafts. Living donor liver transplantation and deceased donor liver transplantation have similar rates of graft and patient survival. The benefits of living donor liver transplantation are the availability of a presumed high-quality graft, control over timing of the operation, decreased cold ischemia, and expansion of the donor pool. The disadvantage is the risk to the donor, including a 0.5–1.0% risk of mortality and an up to 38% risk of complication, with biliary complications in 10% and incisional hernia in 5%. In the recipient, vascular complications are more common than in DBD, and biliary leaks can occur in 20–30% [8]. Overall, the decision to pursue living donor liver transplantation by a patient and physician is a complex one,

taking into account the patient's age, the indication for liver transplantation, blood group, MELD score, predicted waiting time, and the availability of live donors.

Listing for Simultaneous Liver–Kidney Transplantation

The MELD score emphasizes creatinine in the allocation of donor organs. Since it went into effect in 2002, there has been a significant increase in the frequency of simultaneous liver–kidney transplantation (SLKT), which accounts for about 5% of all liver transplants in the United States today. It is challenging to determine which patients may regain renal function after liver transplantation and which will remain in stage V chronic kidney disease requiring dialysis. A consensus guideline formulated in 2008 recommends SLKT when one of the following three criteria is met: (i) patients with end-stage liver disease and chronic kidney disease with glomerular filtration rate (GFR) ≤30 mL/min; (ii) patients with acute kidney injury (AKI), including hepatorenal syndrome, with creatinine ≥2.0 mg/dL and dialysis ≥8 weeks; or (iii) patients with end-stage liver disease, evidence of chronic kidney disease, and kidney biopsy demonstrating >30% glomerulosclerosis or 30% fibrosis [9]. Even with these guidelines, there continues to be much debate about the most appropriate candidates for SLKT, especially given the severe shortage of kidney allografts for primary kidney transplantation. It is highly likely that the United Network for Organ Sharing (UNOS) will introduce new policies in this area in the coming years.

Disease-Specific Considerations

Acute Liver Failure

Diagnostic criteria for ALF include an absence of pre-existing liver disease, INR ≥1.5, and hepatic encephalopathy with total illness duration <26 weeks. Patients meeting the criteria for ALF who also require mechanical ventilation or dialysis or who have an INR >2.0 receive the highest priority for liver transplantation, called status 1. Patients with hepatitis B, Wilson's disease, and autoimmune hepatitis (AIH) may have evidence of cirrhosis at the initial presentation and are exceptions to the "no pre-existing liver disease" rule. The most common causes of ALF in the United States are acetaminophen and indeterminate, idiosyncratic drug-induced liver injury (DILI), followed by hepatitis B. ALF is a medical emergency that merits immediate consideration of transfer to a transplant center for appropriate candidates. Transfer is preferable when the patient has early-grade hepatic encephalopathy. A detailed discussion of the management of ALF is beyond the scope of this chapter. An excellent treatment guideline has been published by the American Association for the Study of Liver Diseases (AASLD) [10,11]. Transplant-free survival is highest (>50%) for patients with acetaminophen, hepatitis A, and pregnancy-related ALF. The King's College criteria (Table 92.4) can help determine which patients are at highest risk of death and should proceed to liver transplantation, but are unfortunately imperfect in predicting mortality.

Alcoholic Liver Disease

Alcoholic cirrhosis is the second most common indication for liver transplantation in the United States, accounting for approximately 24% of all liver transplants. Evaluation of the patient with alcoholism requires extra measures, including examination by a psychiatrist and a chemical dependency counselor to assess the severity of

Table 92.4 King's College criteria. Source: Lee *et al.* 2011 [11]. Reproduced with permission of Wiley.

Acetaminophen-induced ALF

Strongly consider OLT listing if:
- arterial lactate >3.5 mmol/L after early fluid resuscitation

List for OLT if:
- pH <7.3; or
- arterial lactate >3.0 mmol/L after adequate fluid resuscitation

List for OLT if all three of the following occur within a 24-hour period:
- grade 3 or 4 hepatic encephalopathy
- INR >6.5
- creatinine >3.4 mg/dL

Non-acetaminophen-induced ALF

List for OLT if:
- INR >6.5 and encephalopathy present (irrespective of grade)

List for OLT if any three of the following are true (encephalopathy present; irrespective of grade):
- age <10 or >40 years
- jaundice for >7 days before development of encephalopathy
- INR ≥3.5
- serum bilirubin ≥17 mg/dL
- unfavorable etiology, such as Wilson's disease
- idiosyncratic drug reaction
- seronegative hepatitis

ALF, acute liver failure; OLT, orthotopic liver transplantation; INR, International Normalized Ratio.

alcohol abuse and/or dependence, abuse of or dependence on other substances, the need for chemical dependency treatment, and the risk of relapse. Most programs require 6 months of sobriety before listing for liver transplantation. A substantial proportion of patients may have improvement in liver function and portal hypertension with sustained abstinence, such that liver transplantation is no longer necessary.

A French multicenter study prospectively examined the outcomes of early liver transplantation for severe alcoholic hepatitis (n = 26) and found a dramatic improvement in 6-month survival as compared to standard medical care (77 ± 8% vs. 23 ± 8%, p <0.001), which was sustained at 2 years (71 ± 9% vs. 23 ± 8%, p <0.001) [12]. However, liver transplantation for alcoholic hepatitis is a controversial issue, and this practice has not been adopted for widespread use in the United States. In general, patients with alcoholic cirrhosis have excellent post-transplant survival, with >90% 1-year survival. These patients are 1.5–2.0 times more likely to experience *de novo* malignancy and 10 times more likely to develop upper aerodigestive cancers after liver transplantation compared to non-alcoholic counterparts. Alcohol relapse (any use) occurs in approximately 40% in the first 4.5 years, while more serious binge and frequent use occur in about 25% over 5 years.

Non-Alcoholic Steatohepatitis

Current estimates suggest that the prevalence of obesity in the United States is 29% for males and 34% for females. The prevalence of non-alcoholic fatty liver disease (NAFLD) is approximately 30%. The proportion of individuals who will go on to develop cirrhosis and decompensated cirrhosis is not entirely known. However, it has been shown that the rate of liver transplantation for non-alcoholic steatohepatitis (NASH)-related cirrhosis in the United States has increased from 1% in 2001 to 8.5% in 2009, suggesting a significant burden of illness [13]. If patients with cryptogenic cirrhosis and body mass index (BMI) >30 are classified as having NASH, the 2009 liver transplantation frequency increases to 12.5%. NASH is

projected to become the most common indication for liver transplantation between 2020 and 2025, and is currently third most common.

While initial reports suggested increased morbidity and mortality after liver transplantation in patients with obesity, recent data in the NASH population support similar short-term survival (up to 3 years) for both obese and non-obese populations.

The most important aspect of liver transplantation for patients with NASH is careful selection. The majority of patients have concomitant conditions, including hypertension, dyslipidemia, and diabetes, which are shared risk factors for coronary artery disease. The most common cause of death in patients with NAFLD is CVD, rather than liver disease. Thus, intensified screening for coronary artery disease is important. Individual transplant programs may take different approaches to this screening.

Post transplantation, calcineurin inhibitors contribute to worsening hypertension, hyperlipidemia, and diabetes. Patients need close medical follow-up for optimal management of these problems, especially given the risks of drug–drug interactions. Many patients will also gain weight as they begin to feel well following liver transplantation, further compounding these metabolic conditions.

Hepatitis C

Hepatitis C continues to be the most common indication for liver transplantation (30%). However, it is currently undergoing a major paradigm shift with respect to liver transplantation, with the emergence of many new direct-acting viral agents that have displaced the need for pegylated inteferon. The need for pegylated interferon. It is anticipated that screening strategies for all individuals born between 1945 and 1965 and more effective and better tolerated therapies will reduce the need for liver transplantation for this indication in future years.

An arsenal of new direct acting antivirals have been approved in North America and Europe including Elbasvir/Grazoprevir, Ritonavir boosted Paritaprevir with Dasabuvir and Ombitasvir, Sofosbuvir, Sofosbuivr/Ledipasvir, Sofosbuvir/Daclatasvir, and Sofosbuvir/Simeprevir. The intricacies of managing hepatitis C in individual patients is beyond the scope of this chapter and the authors recommend the HCV guidance document (www.hcvguidance.org) sponsored by the AASLD and Infectious Diseases Society of America (IDSA) for further reference. A particularly exciting issue pertaining to hepatis C and LT is the decision to treat HCV before or after liver transplantation. In the era of pegylated interferon and ribavirin, decompensated cirrhotics and even compensated cirrhotics had difficulty tolerating this regimen and achieved low sustained virologic response (cure) rates. Post liver transplantation, SVR rates were also <50% and the risk of interferon mediated graft dysfunction was approximately 7% [14]. Recent trials including SOLAR-1, SOLAR-2, and ASTRAL-4 [15] have demonstrated high cure rates with direct acting antivirals (without pegylated interferon) approximating 85–95% in Child B cirrhotics, approximately 70–90% response rates in Child C cirrhotics, and >90% cure rates in patients treated post liver transplantation with compensated graft function. Most of the decompensated patients in these trials had MELD scores ≤ 20. Many programs will treat patients awaiting LT who have MELD scores < 20 and long enough expected wait times to complete treatment. A small percentage of patients will have 're-compensation' of their cirrhosis though this cannot be predicted and occurs in a small fraction of patients. It is important to note that the MELD-Na score may improve while symptoms might not (ie ascites), leaving patients in a wait list "purgatory". For example, the ASTRAL-4 study, 81% of patients with baseline MELD ≥ 15 experienced improvement in their MELD score after treatment.Additionally, patients who have their HCV treated while awaiting LT would not be able to receive a hepatitis C positive donor (extended criteria donor). Antiviral resistance can be a significant problem, particularly with NS5A inhibitors where the resistant viruses persist post treatment for years. Thus, a patient failing a regimen with an NS5A inhibitor (daclatasvir, elbasvir, ledipasvir, or ombitasvir) before LT would have difficulty receiving effective HCV post LT. Therefore, one can also make a compelling argument to treat post LT where the SVR rates are more consistently >90%. This decision requires careful thought and collaboration with the patient with reflection on their values.

With respect to post-liver transplantation immunosuppression, there continues to be some debate about whether or not tacrolimus is better than cyclosporine for patients with hepatitis C. Recurrence of hepatitis C is more severe in patients with acute cellular rejection treated with bolus corticosteroids or thymoglobulin. Since tacrolimus is more effective at preventing acute cellular rejection, many opt to use it in this population. Elimination of maintenance corticosteroids has not been shown to improve the severity of HCV recurrence.

Hepatitis B

Prior to the advent of hepatitis B immune globulin (HBIG) in the early 1990s, outcomes after liver transplantation for hepatitis B were poor due to recurrence of the disease. In fact, hepatitis B was considered a contraindication to liver transplantation. With HBIG and the availability of effective oral antiviral therapy, patients with hepatitis B now have equivalent, if not better, post-transplant outcomes to other liver diseases [16].

Before liver transplantation, all candidates with hepatitis B and detectable hepatitis B virus (HBV) should be started on oral antiviral therapy. The most important predictor of HBV recurrence risk is the HBV viral load at the time of liver transplantation. Patients with a low or undetectable load can be treated with short-term (1–6 months) HBIG after transplantation, combined with indefinite oral antiviral therapy. Those with high levels of HBV DNA (>10 000 U/mL) at transplantation should remain on long-term HBIG with oral antiviral therapy.

Autoimmune Hepatitis

AIH can require liver transplantation for those who develop ALF or decompensated cirrhosis. This is a relatively infrequent indication for liver transplantation, representing about 4–6% of cases in the United States and Europe. Those who present with acute hepatitis require immediate treatment with corticosteroids. Patients with ALF secondary to AIH can be treated with corticosteroids if they do not have an infection and have a MELD score <28 [17]. Higher MELD scores predict non-response and put the patient at risk for serious infections. Liver transplant outcomes are generally excellent for this population, though a recent report from Europe suggested a higher risk of death after the first year post transplantation. Recurrent AIH can occur in approximately 22% of recipients, and usually responds to the addition of prednisone to the usual calcineurin inhibitor immunosuppressive regimen.

Cholestatic Liver Diseases

Cholestatic liver diseases account for 8.5% of liver transplantation in the United States.

Patients with cirrhotic-stage primary sclerosing cholangitis (PSC) and complications of portal hypertension or unresectable CCA should be considered for liver transplantation and should receive prioritization based on their MELD score. This is the fifth most common indication for liver transplantation in the United States. Many patients with PSC do not develop high MELD scores, and it has been argued that they are disadvantaged by the MELD system. In particular, patients may develop recurrent episodes of bacterial cholangitis or intractable pruritus without sufficiently increasing their MELD score to be prioritized for deceased donor liver transplantation. Quality of life can be severely diminished in these scenarios. Petitions for exception (higher) MELD scores can be made for these individuals, or they can be considered for living donor liver transplantation. MELD score exceptions were granted in 12% of cases between 2002 and 2011. Recently, however, an analysis at two transplant centers demonstrated that bacterial cholangitis was not a risk factor for death or removal from the waitlist, calling into question the need to grant MELD exception points [18]. Another large database analysis demonstrated that PSC patients have superior waitlist survival to non-PSC patients [19]. Patients with PSC have among the best post-liver transplantation survivals relative to other conditions, but recurrent PSC can occur in 20–37%, resulting in the need for retransplantation in a minority.

Primary biliary cirrhosis (PBC) is the sixth most common indication for liver transplantation in the United States. Patients receive prioritization through a calculated MELD score. A Mayo PBC risk score >7.8 is associated with decreased survival without liver transplantation, but this scoring system is not used for organ allocation [20]. Intractable pruritus may occur in this population, which also merits consideration for living donor liver transplantation or petition for MELD exception points on the basis of quality of life. All medical options for control of pruritus should be explored, including cholestyramine, sertraline, rifampin, naloxone, and Molecular Adsorbent Recirculating System (MARS), as pruritus does not impact pretransplant survival. PBC may recur in 21–37% of patients at a median 3–5 years but does not affect graft or patient survival [21].

Metabolic Diseases

Liver transplantation is curative for patients with hemochromatosis, Wilson's disease, alpha-1-antitrypsin (A1AT) deficiency (liver disease), and hyperoxaluria, as well as a number of other, less common metabolic diseases. The acute Wilsonian crisis, or ALF secondary to Wilson's disease, accounts for only 2–3% of ALF cases in the United States. Classic features include a high bilirubin (>20 mg/dL) with elevated indirect fraction, low alkaline phosphatase and uric acid, and Coombs-negative hemolytic anemia in a young person. These patients receive top priority (status 1) for liver transplantation, and rarely survive without it. Liver transplantation is indicated for patients with hereditary hemochromatosis and decompensated cirrhosis or HCC. Iron-depletion therapy will not reverse the consequences of end-stage liver disease, so it is ideal to make the diagnosis of hereditary hemochromatosis and begin phlebotomy early. Patients with adequate iron depletion prior to liver transplantation probably have similar post-liver transplantation survival when compared to other indications for liver transplantation. End-stage liver disease secondary to A1AT deficiency is cured by liver transplantation, and pulmonary disease does not seem to be a major problem in this population. In type 1 hyperoxaluria, there is a deficiency of hepatic alanine glyoxylate aminotransferase, with increased conversion of glyoxylate to oxalate and resultant renal failure. SLKT is the best treatment for the majority of patients. Type 1 primary hyperoxaluria receives exception MELD points, starting at a MELD of 28 and increasing every 3 months thereafter. Familial amyloidotic polyneuropathy is another metabolic condition in which abnormal amyloid is produced by an otherwise normally functioning liver. Patients without significant cardiac involvement, advanced neuropathies, or malnutrition benefit from liver transplantation and receive exception MELD points [22].

Hepatocellular Carcinoma

Most HCCs arise in the setting of cirrhosis. Liver transplantation for HCC in patients with end-stage liver disease has increased significantly since the introduction of the MELD system. Currently, patients with HCC within Milan criteria receive exception MELD points starting at MELD 22 and increasing by 10% every 3 months. The Milan criteria are one tumor $\leq$5 cm or two or three tumors no larger than 3cm [23]. A chest CT must be obtained at baseline to exclude pulmonary metastases. Some programs also perform a bone scan to exclude skeletal metastases. A targeted biopsy of the liver lesion(s) is not necessary, as the majority of HCCs have characteristic radiologic features, including arterial enhancement, portal venous washout of contrast, and occasionally a pseudocapsule. For lesions that do not possess these radiologic features, but are growing, a high degree of suspicion must be maintained, and a targeted biopsy is usually required. The risk of needle-track seeding with percutaneous liver biopsy is about 1–2%.

Patients who are listed for liver transplantation with HCC within Milan criteria should undergo locoregional therapy if the waiting period is expected to be >6 months, which is the case for the vast majority who are awaiting a deceased donor liver transplant [24]. The locoregional therapy of choice depends on tumor size, number, location, proximity to vasculature, and portal vein patency, as well as local expertise. For patients undergoing living donor liver transplant, a waiting period of 6 months after locoregional therapy has been advised to allow for observation of tumor behavior. If there is concerning progression with large tumors or multiple tumors during the period of observation, liver transplantation is not likely to provide long-term survival, due to the high risk of HCC post transplant.

Cholangiocarcinoma

CCA is the second most primary hepatic malignancy. It is classified according to location as intrahepatic, hilar, or distal. Intrahepatic CCA (above the biliary secondary radicles), when found incidentally on explants, portends a very poor post-transplantation survival due to recurrence. Distal CCA is best treated with a Whipple's resection, if staging allows. Hilar CCA arises between the secondary biliary radicles and the cystic duct insertion. Resection is the treatment of choice, if possible. Non-resectable CCA, either *de novo* or arising in the setting of PSC, may be a candidate for liver transplantation. It is important to note that transperitoneal biopsy should not be used to diagnose a presumed unresectable hilar CCA, as this is an exclusion criterion for liver transplantation due to its high risk of seeding.

Diagnosis of hilar CCA can be made based on the presence of a dominant stricture or hilar mass and a positive biopsy or cytology, CA19-9 >100 U/mL, or positive fluorescent *in situ* hybridization (FISH). The mass must be <3 cm in radial diameter, without intrahepatic or extrahepatic metastases, to be eligible for liver transplantation. An endoscopic ultrasonography (EUS) is performed before

enrollment into a transplant protocol in order to exclude malignant perihepatic lymphadenopathy.

Pretransplant protocols include external beam radiation, brachytherapy applied via a nasobiliary tube, chemotherapy, and laparoscopic operative staging [25]. Patients meeting all of the aforementioned criteria and enrolled in a pretransplant chemoradiation protocol start with 22 MELD exception points, which increase by 10% every 3 months. Survival at 5 years post liver transplantation is approximately 70%. Of the patients enrolled in a pre-liver transplantation protocol at the Mayo Clinic, approximately two-thirds went on to complete chemoradiation and received a liver transplant. Risk factors for recurrence of CCA after liver transplantation include residual viable tumor at explant, lymph node, perineural, or vascular invasion on explant, and tumor grade [25].

Hepatopulmonary and Portopulmonary Syndromes

HPS is defined by evidence of portal hypertension, intrapulmonary shunting seen on transthoracic echocardiogram with agitated saline or a technetium 99m macroaggregated albumin scan, and hypoxemia evidenced by low PaO_2 or elevated A–a gradient. Classic features of this condition include platypnea and orthodeoxia. Patients with a PaO_2 <60 mmHg qualify for exception MELD points, starting with a MELD of 22 and increasing by 10% every 3 months, provided the PaO_2 remains below 60 mmHg. Patients with HPS have improved 5-year survival with liver transplantation (76%) as compared to without (23%). The more severe the hypoxemia prior to liver transplantation, the longer it generally takes for patients to be weaned from supplemental oxygen after transplant, but liberation from supplemental oxygen is expected [26].

Portopulmonary syndrome should be suspected in patients with a high right ventricular systolic pressure >50 mmHg on transthoracic echocardiogram in the presence of portal hypertension. The typical accompanying symptom is dyspnea on exertion. A right heart catheterization is required to make the diagnosis. Diagnostic criteria include a mean pulmonary artery pressure (MPAP) >25 mmHg, a pulmonary capillary wedge pressure <15 mmHg, and a pulmonary vascular resistance (PVR) >240 dyne/s/cm^5 (or 3 woods units). Those with an MPAP <35 mmHg and PVR <400 dyne/s/cm^5 after medical treatment qualify for MELD exception points, starting at 22 and increasing every by 10% every 3 months, provided that the pulmonary circulation hemodynamics remain within the aforementioned criteria. Patients can be treated with endothelin antagonists (i.e., bosentan, ambrisentan), prostacyclin analogues (i.e., epoprostenol, iloprost), and/or phosphodiesterase inhibitors (i.e., sildenafil). Resolution of portopulmonary hypertension post liver transplantation is less reliable, and about 50% of patients continue to need vasoactive therapy after transplant [26].

Case Continued

The patient is in otherwise good health, is abstinent, and is attending Alcoholics Anonymous. His tumor size and number are within the Milan criteria for transplantation for HCC. He will be a transplant candidate if the remainder of his pre-liver transplantation evaluation is satisfactory.

Conclusion

Liver transplantation evaluation is warranted in any patient with ALF or decompensated cirrhosis with MELD ≥15 or Child–Turcotte–Pugh ≥7, as well as in some patients with hepatic malignancies or metabolic disorders. Early referral of patients to a transplant center is preferable, to allow adequate time for evaluation and stabilization and so maximize the likelihood of a good outcome. If in doubt, always call the local transplant center before deeming a patient a poor candidate.

Take Home Points

- Successful liver transplantation requires optimal patient selection and transplantation timing.
- Indications and patient selection for transplantation are similar across most transplant centers, and have changed only slightly in recent years.
- Contraindications to transplantation are dynamic and may differ between centers, reflecting local expertise.
- Model for End-Stage Liver Disease (MELD) scores are a more accurate and less easily manipulated method of predicting mortality in patients with liver disease than are Child–Turcotte–Pugh scores, and are currently used to prioritize organ allocation.

References

1 Thuluvath PJ, Guidinger MK, Fung JJ, *et al.* Liver transplantation in the United States, 1999–2008. *Am J Transpl* 2010; **10**(4): 1003–19.

2 Kim WR, Smith JM, Skeans MA, *et al.* OPTN/SRTR 2012 annual data report: liver. *Am J Transplant* 2014; **14**(Suppl. 1): 69–96.

3 Wiesner R, Edwards E, Freeman R, *et al.* Model for End-Stage Liver Disease (MELD) and allocation of donor livers. *Gastroenterology* 2003; **124**(1): 91–6.

4 Freeman RB Jr., Wiesner RH, Roberts JP, *et al.* Improving liver allocation: MELD and PELD. *Am J Transplant* 2004; **4**(Suppl. 9): 114–31.

5 Kim WR, Biggins SW, Kremers WK, *et al.* Hyponatremia and mortality among patients on the liver-transplant waiting list. *N Engl J Med* 2008; **359**(10): 1018–26.

6 Leise MD, Kim WR, Kremers WK, *et al.* A revised Model for End-Stage Liver Disease optimizes prediction of mortality among patients awaiting liver transplantation. *Gastroenterology* 2011; **140**(7): 1952–60.

7 Murray KF, Carithers RL Jr. AASLD practice guidelines: evaluation of the patient for liver transplantation. *Hepatology* 2005; **41**(6): 1407–32.

8 Abecassis MM, Fisher RA, Olthoff KM, *et al.* Complications of living donor hepatic lobectomy – a comprehensive report. *Am J Transplant* 2012; **12**(5): 1208–17.

9 Eason JD, Gonwa TA, Davis CL, *et al.* Proceedings of consensus conference on simultaneous liver kidney transplantation (SLK). *Am J Transplant* 2008; **8**(11): 2243–51.

10 Lee WM, Larson AM, Stravitz RT. AASLD Position Papter: The Management of Acute Liver Failure: Update 2011. Available from: http://www.aasld.org/practiceguidelines/Documents/AcuteLiverFailureUpdate2011.pdf (last accessed February 15, 2016).

11 Lee WM, Stravitz RT, Larson AM. Introduction to the revised American Association for the Study of Liver Diseases position paper on acute liver failure 2011. *Hepatology* 2012; **55**(3): 965–7.

12 Mathurin P, Moreno C, Samuel D, *et al.* Early liver transplantation for severe alcoholic hepatitis. *N Engl J Med* 2011; **365**(19): 1790–800.

13 Charlton MR, Burns JM, Pedersen RA, *et al.* Frequency and outcomes of liver transplantation for nonalcoholic steatohepatitis in the United States. *Gastroenterology* 2011; **141**(4): 1249–53.

14 Curry MP, Forns X, Chung RT, *et al.* Pretransplant sofosbuvir and ribavirin to prevent recurrence of hCV infection after liver transplantation. Program and Abstracts of the 64th Annual Meeting of the American Association for the Study of Liver Diseases. Washington, DC, 2013.

15 Jacobson IM, Ghalib R, Rodriguez-Torres M, *et al.* SVR results of a once-daily regimen of simeprevir (TMC435) plus sofosbuvir (GS7977) with or without ribavirin in cirrhotic and non-cirrhotic hcv genotype 1 treatment-naive and prior null responder patients: the COSMOS study. Program and Abstracts of the 64th Annual Meeting of the American Association for the Study of Liver Diseases. Washington, DC, 2013.

16 Crespo G, Marino Z, Navasa M, Forns X. Viral hepatitis in liver transplantation. *Gastroenterology* 2012; **142**(6): 1373–83.e1.

17 Verma S, Maheshwari A, Thuluvath P. Liver failure as initial presentation of autoimmune hepatitis: clinical characteristics, predictors of response to steroid therapy, and outcomes. *Hepatology* 2009; **49**(4): 1396–7.

18 Goldberg DS, Camp A, Martinez-Camacho A, *et al.* Risk of waitlist mortality in patients with primary sclerosing cholangitis and bacterial cholangitis. *Liver Transpl* 2013; **19**(3): 250–8.

19 Goldberg D, French B, Thomasson A, *et al.* Waitlist survival of patients with primary sclerosing cholangitis in the Model for End-Stage Liver Disease era. *Liver Transpl* 2011; **17**(11): 1355–63.

20 Kim WR, Wiesner RH, Therneau TM, *et al.* Optimal timing of liver transplantation for primary biliary cirrhosis. *Hepatology* 1998; **28**(1): 33–8.

21 Ilyas JA, O'Mahony CA, Vierling JM. Liver transplantation in autoimmune liver diseases. *Best Pract Res Clin Gastroenterol* 2011; **25**(6): 765–82.

22 Freeman RB Jr., Gish RG, Harper A, *et al.* Model for End-Stage Liver Disease (MELD) exception guidelines: results and recommendations from the meld exception study group and conference (message) for the approval of patients who need liver transplantation with diseases not considered by the standard meld formula. *Liver Transpl* 2006; **12**(Suppl. 3): S128–36.

23 Mazzaferro V, Regalia E, Doci R, *et al.* Liver transplantation for the treatment of small hepatocellular carcinomas in patients with cirrhosis. *N Engl J Med* 1996; **334**(11): 693–9.

24 Bruix J, Sherman M. Management of hepatocellular carcinoma: an update. *Hepatology* 2011; **53**(3): 1020–2.

25 Darwish Murad S, Kim WR, Harnois DM, *et al.* Efficacy of neoadjuvant chemoradiation, followed by liver transplantation, for perihilar cholangiocarcinoma at 12 US centers. *Gastroenterology* 2012; **143**(1): 88–98.e3, quiz e14.

26 Krowka MJ, Wiesner RH, Heimbach JK. Pulmonary contraindications, indications and meld exceptions for liver transplantation: a contemporary view and look forward. *J Hepatol* 2013; **59**(2): 367–74.

CHAPTER 92

What Every Hepatologist Should Know about Liver Transplantation

Peter S. Yoo and David C. Mulligan

Section of Transplantation and Immunology, Department of Surgery, Yale University School of Medicine, New Haven, CT, USA

Summary

The techniques of liver transplantation have evolved significantly over the last few decades, and the development of collaborative, multidisciplinary care has become a key component of successful outcomes in transplant recipients. Fundamentals of organ allocation, hepatic anatomy, surgical technique, and risks of complications must be understood by all clinicians caring for liver transplant patients. Each phase of the transplant operation has unique physiologic circumstances, each with its own potential for success or failure. Biliary complications are most common, followed by hepatic arterial, portal venous, and hepatic venous complications. Finally, new techniques – especially the introduction of living donor liver transplantation (LDLT) – have been used to further expand the donor pool and provide excellent long-term patient outcomes.

Introduction

Orthotopic liver transplantation remains the only definitive treatment for end-stage liver disease. The first liver transplant was performed in 1963 by Dr. Thomas Starzl, and the first time a recipient survived beyond 1 year was in 1967. Though techniques have been refined and patient and graft survival have improved since 1963, liver transplantation remains a formidable surgical challenge. The technical complexities of the procedure can result in a variety of postoperative complications. Transplant hepatologists should be familiar with organ allocation, hepatic anatomy, and technical aspects of liver transplantation and its potential complications, in order to provide excellent care for these patients.

Liver Allocation

In the United States, organ allocation is governed by the United Network for Organ Sharing (UNOS), which divides the country into 11 geographic regions (Figure 93.1). Each region is further subdivided into Donor Service Areas (DSAs), managed by a local organ procurement organization. Using this geographic framework, an individual recipient's priority on the waiting list for a given organ depends on the location of the recipient center (in or out of region), ABO blood group, degree of medical urgency (based upon their Model for End-Stage Liver Disease (MELD) score), and size match. The highest level of priority (status 1a) is given to patients with fulminant liver failure with an expected survival without transplant of less than 7 days. This includes patients with advanced acute liver failure (ALF), primary non-function (PNF) or hepatic artery thrombosis (HAT) of a transplanted liver within 7 days of transplantation, or acute decompensated Wilson's disease. Additional priority is also given to children, to neutralize the difficulty of identifying size-matched organs.

The majority of the remaining waitlisted patients will be transplanted according to a point system based on their MELD score [1]. This score is derived from three blood tests: serum creatinine, total bilirubin, and protime reported as International Normalized Ratio (INR). The MELD score predicts 90-day survival without transplantation, and has a range of 6–40 points. Several conditions are associated with a high degree of mortality not expressed in the MELD score, and for these conditions, so-called "exception points" may be awarded to allow patients access to life-saving transplantation. These conditions include hepatocellular carcinoma (HCC), hepatopulmonary syndrome, familial amyloidosis, and primary oxaluria.

The federal government's regulation governing organ allocation, the Organ Procurement and Transplantation Network (OPTN) "Final Rule," stipulates that allocation of organs "Shall not be based on the candidate's place of residence or place of listing," except to the extent necessary to maximize the quality and utility of the organ. In June 2013, UNOS enacted a policy called "Share 35R," which allows for patients with MELD scores >35 to have priority region wide, rather than confined to their own local DSA. It is expected that this new policy change will allow timely transplant and decrease waitlist mortality for some gravely ill patients. The impact of broader sharing at MELD 35 will be to provide a greater organ availability to patients with the same waitlist mortality as those who are status 1a, but it does not address the need for a reduction in the large variability in access to donor livers across the regions. Plans are underway to utilize novel mathematical modeling to address these disparities and reduce variations in MELD at transplant throughout the country. Similarly, a national Share 15 algorithm ensures donor livers go to patients with MELD 15 and above who have a transplant survival benefit at 1 year, regardless of geography.

Future Trends in Organ Allocation

Several new directions in organ allocation can be anticipated in the coming years. First, it is thought there will be a significant

Practical Gastroenterology and Hepatology Board Review Toolkit, Second Edition. Edited by Nicholas J. Talley, Kenneth R. DeVault, Michael B. Wallace, Bashar A. Aqel and Keith D. Lindor.

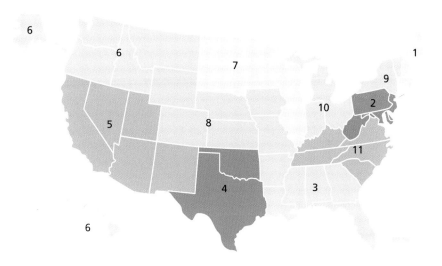

Figure 93.1 UNOS regions. Region 1: Connecticut, Maine, Massachusetts, New Hampshire, Rhode Island, Eastern Vermont. Region 2: Delaware, District of Columbia, Maryland, New Jersey, Pennsylvania, West Virginia, Northern Virginia. Region 3: Alabama, Arkansas, Florida, Georgia, Louisiana, Mississippi, Puerto Rico. Region 4: Oklahoma, Texas. Region 5: Arizona, California, Nevada, New Mexico, Utah. Region 6: Alaska, Hawaii, Idaho, Montana, Oregon, Washington. Region 7: Illinois, Minnesota, North Dakota, South Dakota, Wisconsin. Region 8: Colorado, Iowa, Kansas, Missouri, Nebraska, Wyoming. Region 9: New York, Western Vermont. Region 10: Indiana, Michigan, Ohio. Region 11: Kentucky, North Carolina, South Carolina, Tennessee, Virginia. Source: http://optn.transplant. hrsa.gov/converge/members/regions.asp.

redistricting of the UNOS regions, to enhance compliance with the spirit of the "Final Rule." Changing the geographic boundaries of the current 11 UNOS regions will dramatically change the distribution of organs between centers. Second, the MELD score is expected to be modified in order to take into account a patient's serum sodium level and so better reflect the degree of illness and medical urgency of liver transplantation. Third, the HIV Organ Policy Equity (HOPE) act was recently signed into law. This statute reverses the previous ban on the transplantation of organs from donors who are known to be human immunodeficiency virus (HIV) positive. The HOPE act opens the door for research to begin on how best to transplant organs from HIV-positive donors to HIV-positive recipients.

Donor Selection

As with all organ transplantation, the availability and selection of donor organs are the foundations of successful liver transplantation. Considerations known to affect the quality of the organ include: cause of death (brain or cardiac death), donor age, whole or partial graft, donor race/ethnicity, size, steatosis, cold ischemia time, hypernatremia, and hemodynamic instability [2].

Organ donors fall into two broad classifications: living and deceased. Living donor selection is covered in Chapter 92. Deceased donors can be further subdivided into donors after brain death (DBDs) and donors after cardiac death (DCDs). In the early days of liver transplantation, Starzl and colleagues routinely recovered livers from donors after the cessation of cardiac activity, and prior to 1968, deceased donor organs were almost exclusively recovered from DCDs. That year, however, criteria for determining brain death were described by an *ad hoc* committee at Harvard Medical School and reported in the *Journal of the American Medical Association* [3]. This report defined brain death, providing the foundation for the recognition of brain death in all 50 states. Organ donation after brain death allowed procurement of organs with minimal warm ischemic time and ushered in a new era in organ transplantation, which lasted a generation.

By the 1990s, however, a mounting crisis of organ shortage led to a renewed interest in DCD organs. Furthermore, there was a growing recognition that for a patient and family with a hopeless prognosis, DCD offers the option to donate when brain death criteria will not be met. The Pittsburgh group released a set of guidelines for recovering organs after the palliative withdrawal of life-prolonging measures leading to cardiac death [4, 5]. This led to a resurgence in the use of DCD livers for transplantation, and unmasked some of the intrinsic differences in quality between DCD and DBD livers. DCD livers are associated with ischemic cholangiopathy and poorer overall survival when compared to otherwise equivalent DBD liver grafts [6–9]. However, recent analysis has revealed that the risks associated with DCD liver transplantation may be outweighed by the benefits in patients with MELD scores >20 points, or in those with HCC but without augmentation by exception points. The appropriate use of DCD livers is an area of continued controversy, especially in UNOS regions where organ shortage is dire and waitlist mortality is grave.

Surgical Anatomy of the Liver

A thorough knowledge of hepatic anatomy, in particular the blood vessels and their relationship to the liver parenchyma, is important to understanding the nuances of liver transplantation. The liver lies in the right upper quadrant of the abdomen, suspended from the diaphragm by the triangular and coronary ligaments. The liver can be divided into eight segments, based upon the portal venous vascular supply and hepatic venous drainage. Each of these segments has its own arterial and portal blood supply and venous and biliary drainage, rendering each capable of functioning independently of the others. A central vertical division plane called Cantlie's line extends from the suprahepatic vena cava to the gallbladder fossa and divides the liver into left and right lobes (Figure 93.2). The caudate lobe encircles the inferior vena cava (IVC). It is often disproportionally large in patients with cirrhosis, especially in conditions like Budd–Chiari syndrome, as the outflow from the caudate lobe is separate from the right, middle, and left hepatic venous drainage utilized by the rest of the liver.

The liver is the only organ in the body that has dual inflow, through the portal vein and hepatic artery. The portal vein is formed posterior to the neck of the pancreas, at the confluence of the superior mesenteric vein (SMV) and splenic vein, and tracks in the substance of the hepatoduodenal ligament *en route* to the liver. Unlike the hepatic artery, the portal vein has few anatomic anomalies, the most common being trifurcation rather than classical bifurcation. Pediatric patients can have congenital malformation or agenesis of the portal vein, or direct drainage of the portal vein into the IVC. Adult patients with cirrhosis are prone to developing thrombus in the portal vein due to stagnant venous flow. Patients with chronic thrombus may develop cavernous transformation as well.

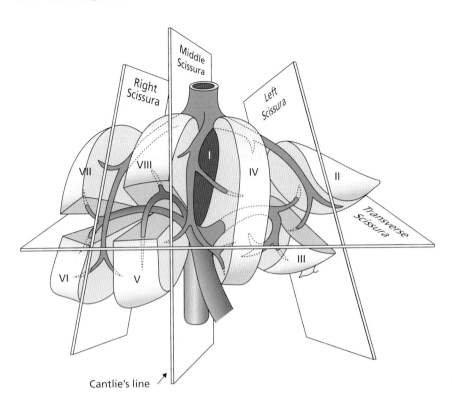

Right
Scissura

Middle
Scissura

Left
Scissura

VII

VIII

I

IV

II

Transverse
Scissura

VI

V

III

Cantlie's line

Figure 93.2 Hepatic segmental anatomy.

At the time of transplantation, portal venous thrombus can be carefully extracted from the portal vein in most cases. However, if the thrombus cannot be extracted, then an interposition graft (donor iliac vein harvested at the time of organ recovery) is usually interposed between the recipient SMV and the donor graft portal vein. It is imperative that potential recipients with portal vein thrombosis (PVT) have a patent SMV in case a graft is necessary. The surgical techniques used to deal with this condition are quite harrowing and may lead to a greater risk of post-transplant complications and intraoperative blood loss. In patients undergoing LDLT, PVT may prevent successful transplantation, and thrombosis rates of SMV–portal vein conduits can be as high as 20%. Patients with thrombosis of the portal–superior mesenteric–splenic confluence into the SMV are not candidates for transplantation. Portal venous thrombosis in the setting of HCC is also a contraindication to transplant.

The hepatic artery can have multiple variations. Hiatt and colleagues described five classes of hepatic arterial anatomy in 1000 cases [10]. In three-quarters of all cases, the common hepatic artery arises as a branch of the celiac artery. The common hepatic artery usually gives rise to two branches – the right gastric artery and the gastroduodenal artery (GDA) – and then proceeds as the proper hepatic artery. The proper hepatic artery divides to form the right and left hepatic arteries in the porta hepatis. The major hepatic arterial anomalies are a replaced or accessory right hepatic artery, which arises from the superior mesenteric artery (SMA), and a replaced or accessory left hepatic artery, which arises from the left gastric artery. Each anomaly is present in about 10% of cases. Other anomalies include a completely replaced hepatic arterial system arising from the SMA, a right hepatic artery arising from the GDA, and an independent common hepatic artery arising from the aorta. In less than 1% of people, a triple artery configuration exists, namely a simultaneous replaced or accessory right, left, and main hepatic arterial system. These anomalies are more important to recognize in the donor than in the recipient, as failure to notice and properly reconstruct the arterial inflow during a liver transplant can result in significant ischemia, especially to the biliary tree.

Techniques of Liver Transplantation

The principal distinction in the technical aspects of liver transplantation has to do with the management of the vena cava. As previously noted, the segment of vena cava between the renal veins and the right atrium of the heart is intimately invested by hepatic parenchyma of the caudate lobe. The three main hepatic veins and numerous short hepatic veins drain directly from the liver into the vena cava. Orthotopic deceased donor liver transplantation can be performed either by completely replacing the retrohepatic IVC (conventional) or by sparing the vena cava using the Barcelona or "piggyback" technique (Figure 93.3). Until the late 1990s, liver transplantation was almost always completed by completely replacing the IVC. This maneuver requires clamping the vena cava above and below the liver. In order to maintain preload to the right heart, veno-venous bypass can be employed. Inflow to the circuit is supplied by the portal and femoral veins. An extracorporeal pump is used to propagate the blood to the outflow, which terminates in the superior vena cava (SVC), accessed by a jugular, subclavian or axillary approach. Compared to caval clamp without bypass, veno-venous bypass enables decompression of the portal system, allowing for completion of the hepatectomy without bowel congestion, protecting renal function by decreasing renal venous hypertension and preventing the hemodynamic instability associated with clamping of the IVC (decreased venous return to the right heart can cause severe hypotension). The complications of veno-venous bypass include hemorrhage, coagulopathy, platelet consumption, air embolus, thrombotic events, and venous injury in 30% of patients [11, 12]. The bypass is also time-consuming and increases the cost of the liver transplant procedure.

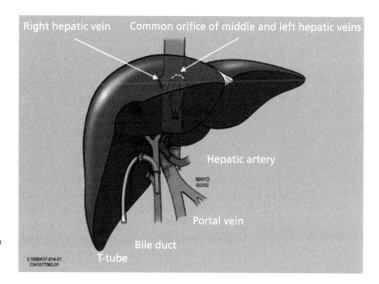

Figure 93.3 Classic "piggyback" technique. The Barcelona modification includes the right hepatic vein to the outflow anastomosis, to reduce hepatic congestion. Source: By permission of Mayo Foundation for Medical Education and Research. All rights reserved.

In 1968, Sir Roy Calne described the caval sparing technique, where the retrohepatic IVC is not resected. Instead, the hepatic vein orifices are clamped and made into a common orifice to which the graft suprahepatic vena cava orifice is anastomosed. However, this took several decades to become a routine practice [13]. The most significant benefit of the so-called *piggyback* technique was that veno-venous bypass was no longer needed, though technically it can be more challenging to dissect the liver from the vena cava, and there is an increased risk of stenosis and subsequent outflow obstruction at the level of the suprahepatic vena cava anastomosis. Originally, the technique utilized the middle and left hepatic vein orifices as a common cloaca or orifice, but the team from Barcelona demonstrated that frequently this created an outflow gradient for the liver allograft, and that adding the right hepatic vein to the middle/left combined orifice would ensure widely patent outflow with no gradient. This technique has been further modified by Belghiti *et al.* [14], who advocate a side-to-side vena cava anastomosis to prevent outflow obstruction. As the anesthetic techniques and comfort with liver transplantation have improved over time, even caval replacement can now be safely accomplished without veno-venous bypass. However, a few prominent centers still employ bypass, as they consider it a safer procedure, especially as teaching the surgical techniques to new trainees may require longer anastomotic times. Occasionally, veno-venous bypass may be indicated in patients with significant cardiac disease, large graft size, or reduced space, in retransplants requiring IVC replacement, and in hemodynamic instability [15].

The development of piggyback techniques also facilitated the capability of split liver and LDLT. As the retrohepatic vena cava must stay with the donor, all living donor transplants (both right- and left-lobe grafts) are completed using piggyback techniques.

Phases of Liver Transplantation

Total Hepatectomy

The first phase of liver transplantation is the complete resection of the native diseased liver. Historically, heterotopic auxiliary liver transplantation has been attempted in animal models and human subjects, with limited success [16]. Many functions of the liver are dependent on its location in the abdomen, particularly biochemical functions related to the portal venous drainage and the drainage of the biliary system. In addition, the increased risk for HCC in any patient with cirrhosis mandates that the entire liver is resected. This is often the most difficult phase of a liver transplant, due to coagulopathy and portal hypertension. In patients with cirrhosis, the ligaments that suspend the liver (triangular and coronary) often become thickened and lined with dilated venous collaterals. The venous collaterals are often present throughout the porta hepatis, falciform ligament, and even the abdominal wall, and can bleed excessively, especially in a coagulopathic patient. The liver is resected from its attachments and the portal triad is dissected free to isolate its constituents. Both the common bile duct and the hepatic artery are ligated at this time: the bile duct is legated at the junction of the cystic duct, while in the case of the proper hepatic artery, either the junction of the right and left hepatic arteries is ligated, or the right and left hepatic arteries are ligated separately. The portal vein is left intact until the hepatectomy is almost complete, in order to reduce venous congestion and edema of the bowel, especially when veno-venous bypass is avoided.

The retrohepatic vena cava can present a major challenge during hepatectomy. The retrohepatic vena cava is surrounded by the caudate lobe and the posterior segments of the right lobe of the liver. The caudate lobe often has a small band of tissue that runs posterior to the vena cava. In patients with cirrhosis, the caudate lobe hypertrophies, and this band of tissue can become a circumferential ring of liver parenchyma. In a piggyback operation, there are multiple small hepatic veins that run from the retrohepatic vein cava to the caudate and right lobe of the liver, which need to be carefully ligated for a caval sparing (piggyback) hepatectomy.

Hemodynamic instability is the hallmark of this stage of a liver transplant, and careful volume regulation by the anesthesia team is mandatory. Excessive bleeding can lead to incredible management issues during the following phase of the operation, the anhepatic phase, which can in turn set the stage for significant patient compromise.

Anhepatic Phase

For a caval-sparing liver transplant, a single vascular clamp is placed across a common cloaca or orifice, created by joining the openings of the right, middle, and left hepatic veins above their junction with the IVC, allowing the continuation of caval flow to the heart. For a conventional liver transplant, vascular clamps are placed on the supra- and infrahepatic vena cava, and the retrohepatic vena cava is removed with the liver. If the patient becomes hemodynamically unstable at the time of caval clamping, veno-venous bypass must be considered. Even in a caval-sparing procedure, the vena cava may be partially occluded by the hepatic vein clamp, and hemodynamic instability may be seen [17].

A second clamp is placed on the portal vein prior to completion of the hepatectomy. Prolonged clamping of the portal vein can result in significant venous congestion of the bowel, especially in patients who have not had time to develop venous collaterals (fulminant hepatic failure). The liver is then removed from the field. For a piggyback procedure, the common orifices of the hepatic veins of the recipient are anastomosed in an end-to-end fashion to the suprahepatic vena cava of the donor, and the infrahepatic vena cava is then ligated, either with a tie or with a vascular stapler. This leaves a redundant segment of donor retrohepatic vena cava, which thromboses over time in most patients. In conventional liver transplant, two separate end-to-end caval anastomoses are completed between the supra- and infrahepatic vena cavae of the donor and recipient.

After the caval anastomoses are complete, most surgeons then complete the portal vein anastomosis, also in an end-to-end fashion. Care must be taken to trim the portal vein to an appropriate length and prevent kinking, which could compromise portal flow to the liver graft. Between 2 and 26% of patients with cirrhosis have PVT at the time of transplantation, which carries an increased risk of perioperative complications and decreased long-term survival. In most cases, the thrombus can be carefully separated from the intima of the portal vein and removed prior to anastomosis. However, in cases where it has become so organized or extensive that portal venous flow cannot be restored, an alternative inflow must be created. A segment of donor iliac vein or autologous vein (renal, saphenous, or jugular) can be used as a jump graft from the SMV to the donor portal vein. In cases where this cannot be done due to thrombosis or fragility of the SMV, the only choice is to anastomose the portal vein to the IVC or renal vein (cavoportal or renoportal transposition), which usually results in a poor outcome [18].

If the team is able to make the appropriate vascular anastomoses in a reasonably short period of time and the hepatectomy is associated with a minimal blood loss, the hepatectomy phase can be relatively uneventful. However, there can be significant metabolic and electrolyte derangements during this phase, which can alter cardiac physiology and, coupled with the blunted response of vasopressors in an acidic environment, make management of the patient challenging.

Reperfusion

Standard practice is to reperfuse the liver after completion of the portal vein anastomosis in order to minimize ischemia. The hepatic artery anastomosis is then completed after portal reperfusion. Some surgical teams will not reperfuse until they complete the hepatic arterial anastomosis, in theory to decrease the risk of biliary ischemia. Similarly, there has been some evidence that initial arterial reperfusion may decrease hemodynamic instability at the time of reperfusion and may be indicated in patients with poor cardiac reserve, though this benefit may only be temporary until the portal vein is reperfused. The order of vascular reperfusion in adult liver transplantation has not been proven to impart any significant clinical benefit.

At the time of procurement, most livers are preserved with University of Wisconsin (UW, SPS, or Viaspan) solution, though histidine–ketogluturate–tryptophan (HTK or Custodial) solution is becoming more widely used. UW solution has a high concentration of potassium (125 mEq/L). To prevent severe life-threatening hyperkalemia upon reperfusion, the liver needs to be flushed with blood or a low-potassium solution before continuity is restored from the hepatic venous outflow to the right heart. HTK solution does not need to be flushed out prior to reperfusion unless cold ischemia has been prolonged.

First the vena cava clamp or clamps are removed, and then the portal clamps, allowing blood to slowly flow through the liver, which is visible as the liver parenchyma changes color from grey and tan to its usual deep pink. Even with flushing prior to reperfusion, severe metabolic derangements, cardiac arrhythmias, and hemodynamic instability can occur. Hyperkalemia is common, usually from the accumulation of potassium and acid species in the bowel secondary to portal vein occlusion. Arrhythmias can also occur from the cold preservation solution, creating hypothermia in the myocardium. Experienced, specialty-trained liver transplant anesthesiologists are essential in anticipating and correcting these derangements, and getting the patient safely through the reperfusion stage [19].

As soon as the patient is stable, the hepatic arterial anastomosis is completed. Most surgeons use a bifurcation of either the right and left or the common hepatic artery and GDA as an end-to-end anastomosis to the common hepatic artery of the donor. If the donor has aberrant hepatic arterial anatomy, reconstruction is completed at the back table prior to transplantation. If the recipient has variant arterial anatomy, the most substantial artery is used for the anastomosis. If the hepatic artery is damaged (not uncommon currently, due to the increasing frequency of preoperative chemoembolization), it may be necessary to use a graft of iliac artery from the donor to connect between the donor hepatic artery and either the supraceliac or the infrarenal abdominal aorta [20, 21]. These grafts have a slightly decreased long-term patency rate compared to the native hepatic artery, but long-term outcomes are similar [22, 23]. In select cases, the recipient splenic artery, left gastric artery, or GDA may be used as a conduit.

Biliary Anastomosis

After bloodflow is restored to the liver and adequate hemostasis is achieved, biliary anastomosis is the last step. First, the donor gallbladder is removed and the donor cystic artery and duct are ligated. During both the donor and the recipient hepatectomies, care must be taken not to strip the vascular complex from the bile duct, which can compromise bloodflow and lead to ischemic strictures. In most cases, a choledochocholedochostomy (duct-to-duct anastomosis) is performed, in which the donor and recipient bile ducts are anastomosed together in an end-to-end fashion using absorbable suture. Historically, T-tubes were used in all biliary reconstructions, but this has fallen out of practice for most transplant programs, because of a risk of biliary complications of between 10 and 60%, especially at the time of removal [24, 25] (Figure 93.4). Multiple studies have examined the use of perioperative biliary stents and compared running suture to interrupted sutures, without conclusive evidence that the risk of strictures and/or bile leaks is different [26, 27]. Most surgeons complete this anastomosis in an end-to-end manner, but there is some evidence that a side-to-side anastomosis may decrease the risk of postoperative stenosis [28]. In patients with primary sclerosing cholangitis or an otherwise abnormal native biliary system, a Roux-en-Y choledochojejunostomy is used to prevent further strictures resulting from native disease. Whenever a recipient common bile duct appears unfavorable, a hepaticojejunostomy is performed.

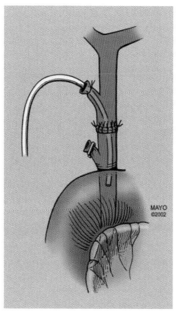 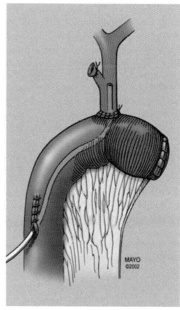

Duct-to-duct   Roux-en-Y

Figure 93.4 Biliary reconstruction with T-tubes. Source: By permission of Mayo Foundation for Medical Education and Research. All rights reserved.

After completion of the transplant, closed suction drains are placed to detect bleeding and bile leakage, usually under the right lobe, under the left lobe, and behind the porta hepatis.

Surgical Complications of Liver Transplantation

Surgical complications affect over 25% of liver transplants and can have a significant impact on their long-term outcome and cost [29, 30]. The risk of complication depends on a variety of donor and recipient factors, as well as the ischemic time and technical aspects of the operation. Timely diagnosis is critical to long-term graft and patient survival.

Hemorrhage

Postoperative hemorrhage is the most common complication after liver transplantation, occurring in 10–15% of liver transplant recipients and requiring reoperation and hemorrhage control in 50% of cases [31]. At the time of re-exploration, few will have an identifiable cause of bleeding. Hemorrhage is the result of ongoing coagulopathy, which can be worsened by poor or delayed graft function and insufficient resuscitation of the recipient in the operating room. However, vascular anastomoses, injuries to the right adrenal gland, and liver lacerations can also result in postoperative bleeding. Patients who need re-exploration have an increased risk of intra-abdominal infection, and there is a significantly increased cost.

Hepatic Arterial Complications

Both hepatic artery stenosis (HAS) and HAT are diagnosed initially by Doppler ultrasonography of the liver graft, which is readily available and cost-effective. The ultrasound may show an absence of arterial flow, or resistive indices of less than 0.5 with delayed upstroke of the arterial waveform. To confirm the ultrasound results, computed tomography angiography (CTA) is the best option. However, for patients with renal insufficiency, magnetic resonance angiography without gadolinium can also be used. Conventional

angiography may be used, particularly in cases where stenosis is suspected with a therapeutic intent. Most interventional radiologists prefer not to intervene with angioplasty and/or stenting until at least 21 days post liver transplant.

If there is decreased inflow arising from the recipient's native arterial system, whether due to vascular disease, arcuate ligament tethering of the celiac artery, or small native vasculature, alternative inflow must be identified. In these cases, a graft (usually the iliac artery from a deceased donor) can be anastomosed from the aorta to the donor hepatic artery. As transplant specialists become more aggressive with preoperative chemoembolization of hepatic lesions, the hepatic artery can be injured, especially with repeat treatments [20]. In such cases, or when an artery is injured intraoperatively, an arterial interposition graft may be necessary.

Thrombosis

HAT is a vexing clinical problem, and a high degree of suspicion of this entity must be present at all times following liver transplantation. The presentation can be dramatic, as in florid graft failure, or it can be subtle and clinically irrelevant. Most cases are somewhere in between. HAT can be divided into early (within 14 days) and late (after 14 days) occurrence. The risk of early HAT in adult cadaveric liver transplant is 3–10% [32, 33], increasing to 6.5% in adult-to-adult LDLT [34] and to over 20% in pediatric liver transplantation, secondary to smaller-diameter arterial blood vessels. Other risk factors include arteriosclerosis, stenosis, aneurysm, splenic artery steal syndrome, and celiac stenosis or occlusion. Intraoperative arterial damage, including mural thrombus, intimal flap injury, and clamp injury, can lead to HAT. Acute HAT can lead to massive liver necrosis, with a mortality >80% without emergent revascularization or transplantation. With early recognition (within 24–48 hours of thrombosis), revascularization, either by revising the initial anastomosis or by using an iliac artery conduit from the aorta, can salvage over 80% of asymptomatic patients, but only 40% of symptomatic patients. Since the hepatic artery provides arterial supply to the biliary tree, late HAT often presents as bile leaks, bilomas, bile duct necrosis, and ischemic intrahepatic biliary strictures, which require retransplantation. However, some patients (especially children) with late HAT may develop collateralization, and graft function will remain stable without retransplantation.

Stenosis

HAS is defined as angiographic evidence of >50% reduction in the caliber of the arterial lumen, and has an incidence of 5–11%. The majority of HAS occurs at the anastomosis and is related to technical factors. Therapeutic angiography with balloon angioplasty and stenting is successful in >90% of cases. If stenosis occurs within the first 3 weeks after transplantation, it is best revised surgically, using donor iliac artery conduit if necessary.

Portal Vein Complications

Thrombosis

PVT is a rare but life-threatening complication after liver transplantation. It is manifested by significant and rapid graft dysfunction, variceal bleeding, and massive ascites. It can be the result of technical factors (portal vein kinking or stenosis), recurrence or propagation of prior portal, splenic, or mesenteric vein thrombus, or poor mesenteric flow, often because large venous collaterals are stealing flow away from the liver. It requires immediate surgical thrombectomy and revascularization. Inspection and ligation of large collaterals must be performed. A bypass graft may be necessary for rethrombosis. Retransplantation is necessary for cases that are recalcitrant to revascularization, though the outcomes are poor.

Stenosis

Portal vein stenosis (PVS) is a rare complication of liver transplantation, occurring in less than 3% of adults and 7% of pediatric recipients. Patients present with symptoms of portal hypertension. As with HAS, it is usually seen at the anastomosis. Intraoperatively, it can be prevented by allowing a "growth factor" or "air knot" in the suture, which enables vein expansion with flow, preventing the anastomotic waist from occurring as a result of a too tight suturing technique. As with HAS, ultrasound and CTA are diagnostic. Early PVS should be revised surgically, and late PVS can undergo transluminal angioplasty and stenting.

Hepatic Vein and IVC Complications

With conventional liver transplants, stenosis at the suprahepatic vena cava occurs in 1.0–2.5% of patients. The risk is increased to 6% with the caval sparing technique [35], and can be prevented intraoperatively by including all three hepatic veins in a broad orifice or a side-to-side cavoplasty. The risk of complete outflow obstruction is very low, but has a mortality >50% and requires immediate operative intervention. Vena cava obstruction can be caused by too long a donor vena cava, resulting in kinking, anastomotic narrowing, recurrence of Budd–Chiari syndrome, or anatomical anomalies of donor or recipient vena cava. Clinically, the patients present like Budd–Chiari syndrome, with liver dysfunction, ascites, and impaired renal function. Stenosis of the infrahepatic vena cava from a conventional liver transplant presents with lower-body and extremity edema and impaired renal function. The first-line therapy is endovascular balloon angioplasty and stenting. If that is not successful, the surgical options are limited. If the patient had a caval-sparing approach, the retrohepatic donor vena cava can be anastomosed to the recipient vena cava to improve outflow. Other surgical options for venoplasty or conventional revision are treacherous, and retransplantation may be the only option.

Biliary Complications

The overall incidence of postoperative biliary complications is 15–20%, increasing to up to 50% in split and reduced liver transplantation, making them the most frequent complication following liver transplant. Mortality related to persistent biliary complications is 10%. The diagnosis of both bile leak and stricture is non-specific, though elevated bilirubin and alkaline phosphatase are suggestive of problems. Biliary ductal dilation is often not seen in transplant recipients, and significant strictures can be present in the face of normal bile ducts. Diagnosis can be made with magnetic resonance or CT cholangiopancreatography. Endoscopic retrograde pancreatography (ERCP) or percutaneous transhepatic cholangiography (PTC) can be both diagnostic and therapeutic. Postoperative leakage is more common after choledochojejunostomy, and stenosis after choledochocholedochostomy [36].

Leak

Bile leaks occur in 10–15% of patients following liver transplantation and can cause significant morbidity. Risk factors for leaks include hepatic arterial insufficiency and technical factors that compromise the blood supply to the bile duct, including excessive bile duct dissection, excessive suturing, and increased bile duct length. T-tube placement at the time of transplantation may increase the risk of postoperative biliary leak. Leaks can easily become infected and inflame the surrounding structures, putting the vascular anastomoses at risk for the development of mycotic aneurysms and rupture. Initial treatment with antibiotics (including antifungal treatment) is mandatory, as are drainage and biliary stenting. If the leaks continue or are unable to be fixed with stenting, re-exploration and conversion to a Roux-en-Y hepaticojejunostomy is necessary. At the time of diagnosis, it is imperative to rule out an HAT/HAS, which can lead to biliary ischemia and leak.

Stenosis

Biliary strictures and stenosis are the most common biliary complications following liver transplantation, occurring in 2.5–20.0% of deceased donor transplantations and 18–32% of LDLTs [34, 37]. They can result from a technical complication from the anastomosis, particularly a duct size mismatch or bile duct ischemia. They are usually at or proximal to the biliary anastomosis. ERCP and PTC can be used to both balloon dilate and stent the anastomosis, and in almost all cases the strictures resolve over time, though it may take several treatments [38]. For recalcitrant strictures, revision to a Roux-en-Y hepaticojejunostomy is recommended. Prolonged stenosis can result in secondary intrahepatic biliary stricturing and graft dysfunction, which may need retransplantation to resolve.

Donor-Related Complications

PNF occurs in up to 6% of liver transplants and is associated with a high risk of mortality [39]. The etiology of PNF remains unclear, and it is difficult to predict. Donation after cardiac death, older donors, high donor sodium, graft steatosis, and prolonged ischemic time have all been identified as risk factors. PNF is often detected in the operating room or immediately postoperatively, presenting as significant coagulopathy, refractory acidosis, hemodynamic instability, and liver dysfunction. Intraoperatively, the liver has abnormal color and turgor with coagulopathy, and it may require immediate hepatectomy with a diverting portal caval shunt. The only option is retransplantation, and patients should be listed status 1a. While waiting for a liver, support with continuous dialysis, coagulation factors, plasma, and vasopressors is necessary. The mortality while waiting for retransplantation is over 50%.

Feng *et al.* [2] have developed a Donor Risk Index (DRI) scoring system that utilizes easily identifiable donor and recipient factors to assist transplant surgeons in selecting appropriate donor–recipient pairs with optimal outcomes. Both donor and recipient factors can lead to severe early graft dysfunction or PNF. Many times, it is best to choose a donor graft with high risk factors, such as long ischemia time, advanced age, or significant macrosteatosis, to implant into a recipient with a more stable hemodynamic profile and more normal renal function, such as a patient with advanced HCC but no physiologic decompensation, who may better tolerate the insult imparted by the transplant.

Small graft-for-size syndrome (SFSS) is defined as early graft dysfunction, in particular the triad of hyperbilirubinemia, coagulopathy, and ascites, in donors with less than 30% functional hepatic mass or a graft-to-recipient body weight ratio of less than 0.8. It is most common in adult-to-adult LDLT and adult split-liver transplantation, and is thought to be related to portal hyperperfusion. Many patients recover function with time, but splenic artery ligation/embolization is also used to decrease portal flow. Some surgeons advocate a temporary partial portosystemic shunt to alleviate this syndrome. Some patients may require retransplantation. Livers from donors with prolonged ischemic time, particularly from donation after cardiac death, can develop ischemic biliary structuring, which may require retransplantation.

Living Donor Liver Transplantation

The topic of LDLT is covered in Chapter 92, but the same major principles described for deceased donor liver transplantation apply. The additional special considerations to be aware of for LDLT recipients center around the much more complex and highly technically challenging operation of engraftment, as well as the postoperative management. Due to the much smaller diameter and multiplicity of blood vessels and bile ducts, surgical complications are far more common, especially the biliary anastomotic issues. As with deceased donors, HAT and HAS, PVT and PVS all occur, but at higher rates (up to 20% incidence in some reports). The bile ducts have become the Achilles' heel of the LDLT, with complication rates of stenosis or leak of up to 50%. Reoperations for biliary complications seem to be less advantageous, while endoscopic or percutaneous management has a high success rate in over 80% of patients. Overall, the advantage for recipients of these life-saving grafts is a higher long-term survival: beyond 3 years according to the A2ALL study group reports and the experience at these authors' center. This is despite a higher early complication rate, which is predominant in the first 30 days post LDLT.

Conclusion

Liver transplantation remains the only treatment for end-stage liver disease. Though surgical techniques have improved significantly over the last 20 years, it remains a complex operation, with multiple potential complications. Transplant recipients are more ill and donors less optimal than in the past. Transplant hepatologists need a thorough knowledge of the liver transplant operation in order to diagnose and treat these complications. A high index of suspicion will lead to early identification of complications, producing improved patient outcomes.

Take Home Points

- Liver transplantation remains the only life-saving therapy for patients with end-stage liver disease and certain malignancies.
- There is a persistent shortage of livers for transplantation, exacerbated by a growing demand of patients on the waitlist.
- The process of organ allocation aims to distribute life-saving liver allografts in a fair, useful, and just manner. As such, new modifications to allocation schemes are expected.
- Donor and recipient selection and pairing are key to a successful outcome.
- Knowledge of hepatic anatomy is vital to understanding surgical outcomes.
- A liver transplant is undertaken in three major phases: total hepatectomy, anhepatic, and implantation/reperfusion. There are a variety of technical approaches to each of these steps, each with its own merits and flaws.
- The most common early postoperative complication is hemorrhage, which usually requires surgical intervention.
- Hepatic artery thrombosis (HAT) can present subtly with devastating consequences, so a high index of suspicion for this entity must always exist.
- The most common complication overall is biliary stenosis or leak. Endoscopic or percutaneous therapies are usually successful, but there should be a low threshold for surgical revision, especially in the early postoperative period.
- Living donor liver transplants (LDLTs) are available to approximately 20% of potential recipients. Despite having a higher rate of early complications, especially of the biliary anastomoses, LDLT recipients enjoy a higher long-term survival than those receiving a deceased donor graft.

References

1 Kamath PS, Wiesner RH, Malinchoc M, *et al.* A model to predict survival in patients with end-stage liver disease. *Hepatology* 2001; **33**(2): 464–70.

2 Feng S, Goodrich NP, Bragg-Gresham JL, *et al.* Characteristics associated with liver graft failure: the concept of a donor risk index. *Am J Transplant* 2006; **6**(4): 783–90.

3 Anon. A definition of irreversible coma. Report of the Ad Hoc Committee of the Harvard Medical School to Examine the Definition of Brain Death. *JAMA* 1968; **205**(6): 337–40.

4 Ethics Committee, American College of Critical Care Medicine; Society of Critical Care Medicine. Recommendations for nonheartbeating organ donation. A position paper by the Ethics Committee, American College of Critical Care Medicine, Society of Critical Care Medicine. *Crit Care Med* 2001; **29**(9): 1826–31.

5 Potts JT, Herdman R; Institute of Medicine. *Non-Heart-Beating Organ Transplantation: Medical and Ethical Issues in Procurement*. Washington, DC: National Academy Press, 1997.

6 Jay C, Ladner D, Wang E, *et al.* A comprehensive risk assessment of mortality following donation after cardiac death liver transplant – an analysis of the national registry. *J Hepatol* 2011; **55**(4): 808–13.

7 Jay CL, Lyuksemburg V, Ladner DP, *et al.* Ischemic cholangiopathy after controlled donation after cardiac death liver transplantation: a meta-analysis. *Ann Surg* 2011; **253**(2): 259–64.

8 Callaghan CJ, Charman SC, Muiesan P, *et al.* Outcomes of transplantation of livers from donation after circulatory death donors in the UK: a cohort study. *BMJ Open* 2013; **3**(9): e003287.

9 Reich DJ, Mulligan DC, Abt PL, *et al.* ASTS recommended practice guidelines for controlled donation after cardiac death organ procurement and transplantation. *Am J Transplant* 2009; **9**(9): 2004–11.

10 Hiatt JR, Gabbay J, Busuttil RW. Surgical anatomy of the hepatic arteries in 1000 cases. *Ann Surg* 1994; **220**(1): 50–2.

11 Moreno C, Sabate A, Figueras J, *et al.* Hemodynamic profile and tissular oxygenation in orthotopic liver transplantation: Influence of hepatic artery or portal vein revascularization of the graft. *Liver Transpl* 2006; **12**(11): 1607–14.

CHAPTER 93

12 Hoffmann K, Weigand MA, Hillebrand N, *et al.* Is veno-venous bypass still needed during liver transplantation? A review of the literature. *Clin Transplant* 2009; **23**(1): 1–8.

13 Tzakis A, Todo S, Starzl TE. Orthotopic liver transplantation with preservation of the inferior vena cava. *Ann Surg* 1989; **210**(5): 649–52.

14 Belghiti J, Panis Y, Sauvanet A, *et al.* A new technique of side to side caval anastomosis during orthotopic hepatic transplantation without inferior vena caval occlusion. *Surg Gynecol Obstet* 1992; **175**(3): 270–2.

15 Chari RS, Gan TJ, Robertson KM, *et al.* Venovenous bypass in adult orthotopic liver transplantation: routine or selective use? *J Am Coll Surg* 1998; **186**(6): 683–90.

16 Shaw BW Jr. Auxiliary liver transplantation for acute liver failure. *Liver Transpl Surg* 1995; **1**(3): 194–200.

17 Margarit C, Lazaro JL, Hidalgo E, *et al.* Cross-clamping of the three hepatic veins in the piggyback technique is a safe and well tolerated procedure. *Transpl Int* 1998; **11**(Suppl. 1): S248–50.

18 Borchert DH. Cavoportal hemitransposition for the simultaneous thrombosis of the caval and portal systems – a review of the literature. *Ann Hepatol* 2008; **7**(3): 200–11.

19 Schumann R, Mandell MS, Mercaldo N, *et al.* Anesthesia for liver transplantation in United States academic centers: intraoperative practice. *J Clin Anesth* 2013; **25**(7): 542–50.

20 Sueyoshi E, Hayashida T, Sakamoto I, Uetani M. Vascular complications of hepatic artery after transcatheter arterial chemoembolization in patients with hepatocellular carcinoma. *Am J Roentgenol* 2010; **195**(1): 245–51.

21 Shimizu S, Onoe T, Ide K, *et al.* Complex vascular reconstruction using donor's vessel grafts in orthotopic liver transplantation. *Transplant Proc* 2012; **44**(2): 574–8.

22 Muralidharan V, Imber C, Leelaudomlipi S, *et al.* Arterial conduits for hepatic artery revascularisation in adult liver transplantation. *Transpl Int* 2004; **17**(4): 163–8.

23 Nikitin D, Jennings LW, Khan T, *et al.* Twenty years' follow-up of portal vein conduits in liver transplantation. *Liver Transpl* 2009; **15**(4): 400–6.

24 Scatton O, Meunier B, Cherqui D, *et al.* Randomized trial of choledochocholedochostomy with or without a T tube in orthotopic liver transplantation. *Ann Surg* 2001; **233**(3): 432–7.

25 Vallera RA, Cotton PB, Clavien PA. Biliary reconstruction for liver transplantation and management of biliary complications: overview and survey of current practices in the United States. *Liver Transpl Surg* 1995; **1**(3): 143–52.

26 Castaldo ET, Pinson CW, Feurer ID, *et al.* Continuous versus interrupted suture for end-to-end biliary anastomosis during liver transplantation gives equal results. *Liver Transpl* 2007; **13**(2): 234–8.

27 Haberal M, Sevmis S, Karakayali H, *et al.* Bile duct reconstruction without a stent in liver transplantation: early results of a single center. *Transplant Proc* 2008; **40**(1): 240–4.

28 Neuhaus P, Blumhardt G, Bechstein WO, *et al.* Technique and results of biliary reconstruction using side-to-side choledochocholedochostomy in 300 orthotopic liver transplants. *Ann Surg* 1994; **219**(4): 426–34.

29 Razonable RR, Findlay JY, O'Riordan A, *et al.* Critical care issues in patients after liver transplantation. *Liver Transpl* 2011; **17**(5): 511–27.

30 Mehrabi A, Fonouni H, Muller SA, Schmidt J. Current concepts in transplant surgery: liver transplantation today. *Langenbecks Arch Surg* 2008; **393**(3): 245–60.

31 Mueller AR, Platz KP, Kremer B. Early postoperative complications following liver transplantation. *Best Pract Res Clin Gastroenterol* 2004; **18**(5): 881–900.

32 Sanchez-Bueno F, Robles R, Ramirez P, *et al.* Hepatic artery complications after liver transplantation. *Clin Transplant* 1994; **8**(4): 399–404.

33 Tzakis AG, Gordon RD, Shaw BW Jr., *et al.* Clinical presentation of hepatic artery thrombosis after liver transplantation in the cyclosporine era. *Transplantation* 1985; **40**(6): 667–71.

34 Freise CE, Gillespie BW, Koffron AJ, *et al.* Recipient morbidity after living and deceased donor liver transplantation: findings from the A2ALL Retrospective Cohort Study. *Am J Transplant* 2008; **8**(12): 2569–79.

35 Parrilla P, Sanchez-Bueno F, Figueras J, *et al.* Analysis of the complications of the piggy-back technique in 1112 liver transplants. *Transplantation* 1999; **67**(9): 1214–17.

36 Krok KL, Cardenas A, Thuluvath PJ. Endoscopic management of biliary complications after liver transplantation. *Clin Liver Dis* 2010; **14**(2): 359–71.

37 Kohler S, Pascher A, Mittler J, *et al.* Management of biliary complications following living donor liver transplantation – a single center experience. *Langenbecks Arch Surg* 2009; **394**(6): 1025–31.

38 Poley JW, Lekkerkerker MN, Metselaar HJ, *et al.* Clinical outcome of progressive stenting in patients with anastomotic strictures after orthotopic liver transplantation. *Endoscopy* 2013; **45**(7): 567–70.

39 Lock JF, Schwabauer E, Martus P, *et al.* Early diagnosis of primary nonfunction and indication for reoperation after liver transplantation. *Liver Transpl* 2010; **16**(2): 172–80.

CHAPTER 94

Immunosuppression Used in Liver Transplantation

Rebecca L. Corey[1] and David D. Douglas[2]

[1] Transplant Center, Mayo Clinic Hospital, Phoenix, AZ, USA
[2] Division of Gastroenterology and Hepatology, Mayo Clinic, Scottsdale, AZ, USA

Summary

Once considered an "experimental procedure," liver transplantation is now an accepted and successful solution for patients with end-stage liver disease and/or hepatocellular carcinoma (HCC). Since the first successful liver transplant, performed by Dr. Thomas E. Starzl in 1967, all aspects of liver transplantation have experienced tremendous progress. Not only have surgical techniques improved during the last 4–5 decades, but clinical experience and scientific research have continued to advance our knowledge and understanding of the immune system and of the mechanisms of organ rejection. Rates of acute rejection and graft loss from rejection have decreased dramatically with current immunosuppression combinations. However, a key therapeutic challenge that still remains is to determine an optimal approach for preventing the renal, metabolic, and infectious complications that may result from long-term immunosuppression.

Case

A 53-year-old male with past medical history significant for chronic hepatitis C, HCC, and deceased donor liver transplantation presents to the outpatient liver transplant clinic for a routine follow-up. Prior to his clinic visit, he was seen by his local gastroenterologist for dyspepsia, diagnosed with *H. pylori*, and started on treatment. At his visit, he presents with a headache and hand tremors.
Medications:
- tacrolimus (TAC) 2 mg twice daily;
- mycophenolate 500 mg twice daily;
- prednisone 2.5 mg daily;
- amlodipine 5 mg daily;
- clarithromycin 500mg twice daily (started recently);
- amoxicillin 1000mg twice daily (started recently);
- metronidazole 500mg twice daily (started recently);
- omeprazole 20mg twice daily (dose increased recently).
Lab tests:
Hemoglobin 10.7 g/dL, hematocrit 31%, white blood cells (WBCs) 9.1×10^9/L, platelet 130×10^9/L, total bilirubin 1.1 mg/dL, aspartate aminotransferase (AST) 17 U/L, alanine aminotransferase (ALT) 25 U/L, potassium 5.8 mmol/L (previously 4.5 mmol/L), magnesium 1.8 mg/dL, blood urea nitrogen (BUN) 49 mg/dL, serum creatinine 2.5 mg/dL (previously 1.1 mg/dL), TAC trough 27 ng/mL (previously 6.3 ng/mL).

Immunosuppressive Drugs

General Principles

Transplanted liver allografts are generally less susceptible to rejection than other organ transplants. A very small number of liver transplant recipients may develop tolerance, but until tolerance can be routinely achieved in clinical practice, effective chemical immunosuppression will remain an essential prerequisite for preventing rejection and achieving successful outcomes. In the absence of tolerance, immunosuppression is required as long as the transplanted liver is functioning. More intense immunosuppression is typically used in the early post-transplant period, when the risk of rejection is highest. Thereafter, immunosuppression can be gradually reduced, provided that allograft function remains stable without rejection episodes. Importantly, the level and type of immunosuppression must always be balanced with the short- and long-term risks, including infectious, renal, and metabolic complications.

"Induction immunosuppression" refers to the use of intense immunosuppression during the early post-transplant period to prevent early rejection. Specialized induction antibodies may be used during the perioperative period to not only prevent early rejection but also avoid or delay calcineurin inhibitor (CNI) therapy and thereby prevent further exacerbation of renal dysfunction. "Maintenance immunosuppression" refers to the long-term use of immunosuppressive drug(s) to prevent rejection. Maintenance immunosuppressive drugs used in liver transplantation are either primary or adjunct immunosuppressive drugs and can be divided into various classes based on mechanism of action: CNIs, antiproliferative/antimetabolite agents, mammalian target of rapamycin (mTOR) inhibitors, and corticosteroids.

Immunosuppressive strategies vary widely among transplant centers and may be tailored for individual patients. Initial immunosuppressive regimens used in liver transplantation often combine drugs with different mechanisms and adverse effects in order to use lower doses of each individual drug, thereby maximizing efficacy and minimizing short- and long-term toxicities. Choice of immunosuppression can be influenced by multiple factors, including transplant center experience/protocols, indication for transplantation, comorbidities, toxicity/adverse effects, likelihood of pregnancy, risk of rejection, history of severe or recurrent rejection, and history or risk of malignancy and/or infections.

Practical Gastroenterology and Hepatology Board Review Toolkit, Second Edition. Edited by Nicholas J. Talley, Kenneth R. DeVault, Michael B. Wallace, Bashar A. Aqel and Keith D. Lindor.
© 2016 John Wiley & Sons, Ltd. Published 2016 by John Wiley & Sons, Ltd. Companion website: www.practicalgastrohep.com

Table 94.1 Immunosuppression in adult and pediatric liver transplant recipients. Source: OPTN 2014.

Immunosuppression	Adult	Pediatric
No induction	69.3%	70%
Induction	30.7%	30%
T cell-depleting	10.3%	10.8%
IL2-RA	20.4%	19.2%
CNIs	96.1%	96.3%
TAC	91.1%	95.5%
Cyclosporine	5%	0.8%
Antiproliferative/antimetabolite	84.3%	47.3%
Mycophenolate[a]	82.1%	46.5%
AZA	2.2%	0.8%
Corticosteroids (2011 data)		
At transplant	80.2%	87.7%
At 1 year after transplant	42.4%	53.8%
mTOR inhibitors (2011 data)		
At transplant	3.4%	1.6%
At 1 year after transplant	9.0%	5.6%

[a]Includes MMF and mycophenolate sodium.
CNI, calcineurin inhibitor; TAC, tacrolimus; AZA, azathioprine; mTOR, mammalian target of rapamycin; MMF, mycophenolate mofetil.

Clinical trends in the use of immunosuppressive drugs in liver transplantation in the United States were recently reported by the Scientific Registry of Transplant Recipients (SRTR) (Table 94.1).

Calcineurin Inhibitors (Cyclosporine, Tacrolimus)

CNIs represent one of the most important breakthroughs in immunosuppression for organ transplantation. Despite their potential short- and long-term toxicities, CNIs have proven to substantially reduce the risk of acute rejection and thus continue to be the cornerstone of many maintenance immunosuppressive drug regimens today.

Cyclosporine A (CSA) was first isolated by Jean F. Borel from a soil fungus, *Tolypocladium inflatum,* in the early 1970s. The introduction of CSA into clinical use in the early 1980s revolutionized immunosuppression for organ transplantation. CSA was initially approved in 1983 for use in kidney transplantation, but its use quickly expanded to liver transplantation and other types of organ transplantation, as well as various autoimmune diseases. The initial oil-based CSA formulation was characterized by significant inter- and intrapatient pharmacokinetic variability and poor oral bioavailability (mean bioavailability 30%, range 1–89%). This formulation required emulsification by bile acids for absorption, and the extent of oral absorption varied significantly with the presence of food, bile flow, and gastrointestinal (GI) motility. The development and approval of a "modified" CSA microemulsion formulation in 1995 led to improved oral bioavailability and greater independence from bile secretion. Modified CSA formulations contain CSA in a microemulsion, which creates micelles in the stomach that are then absorbed in the small intestine with less need for the presence of bile, thereby enhancing bioavailability and reducing variability. Due to differences in bioavailability, CSA and modified CSA formulations are not interchangeable, and patients should take the same product/formulation consistently. Currently, CSA is typically used as an alternative primary immunosuppressive drug in liver transplant recipients who do not tolerate TAC.

TAC, also known as FK506, was initially isolated from the fermentation broth of *Streptomyces tsukubaensis*, a bacterium found in the soil near Mt. Tsukuba in Japan. The results of initial research demonstrated that the *in vitro* and *in vivo* immunosuppressive

activity of TAC was approximately 100 times more potent than that of CSA. TAC absorption is independent of bile, but as with CSA, the oral bioavailability of TAC is quite variable (mean 29%, range 5–93%). TAC received initial Food and Drug Administration (FDA) approval in April 1994 for prevention of rejection in liver transplant recipients, and later was also approved for use in kidney and heart transplantation. Like CSA, TAC is available as brand name or generic, and patients should take the same product consistently. Currently, TAC is the primary drug used for prevention of rejection in liver, kidney, and heart transplant recipients, as well as other types of organ transplantation and various autoimmune disorders. A once-daily extended-release TAC formulation was FDA approved in 2013, but currently only for use in kidney transplant recipients.

TAC and CSA exert their primary immunosuppressive effects by inhibiting calcineurin and thereby preventing interleukin (IL)-2 transcription and T-lymphocyte activation. CSA and TAC have the same overall mechanism of action but bind to different cytoplasmic immunophilins within T lymphocytes: CSA binds to cyclophilin and TAC to FK-binding protein 12 (FKBP12). Once CSA or TAC binds to its respective immunophilin, a pentameric complex is formed with calcineurin, calmodulin, and calcium. Formation of this complex inhibits the phosphatase activity of calcineurin, thereby preventing dephosphorylation of nuclear factor of activated T cells (NF-AT) in the cytoplasm by calcineurin. As a result, NF-AT is unable to translocate into the nucleus, where it would be responsible for initiating transcription of lymphokines such as IL-2 that are involved in T-cell activation

Dosing of CSA and TAC varies widely; details regarding the usual dosing and administration of CSA and TAC are included in Table 94.2. Both CNIs are critical drugs characterized by a narrow therapeutic index, significant inter- and intrapatient pharmacokinetic variability, and numerous drug interactions; therefore, close therapeutic drug monitoring (TDM) is essential to ensure adequate efficacy and safety. Routine measurement of whole blood trough concentrations has traditionally been the accepted standard TDM for both CNIs. Some data suggest that overall exposure of CSA is better correlated with concentrations drawn 2 hours after administration (C2 level). However, in order for C2 monitoring to be clinically useful, levels must be drawn 2 hours (±15 minutes) after administration; due to this logistical difficulty, many centers continue to use trough (C0) concentrations for TDM of CSA. Ideally, CNI concentrations should be obtained after the drug has reached a steady-state concentration, which typically occurs 2–4 days after CNI initiation or a dose change. In addition, if patients switch to a different CSA or TAC formulation, levels should be monitored closely until stable. Target trough concentrations vary, and depend upon multiple factors, including but not limited to (i) institution protocols, (ii) type of organ transplant, (iii) time since transplant, (iv) risk or history of rejection, (v) adverse effects/tolerability, (vi) other comorbidities, (vii) concomitant immunosuppression, (viii) infection/malignancy risk, and (ix) the methodology (assay) used to measure concentrations. General TDM ranges are described in Table 94.2.

Both TAC and CSA are extensively metabolized to multiple metabolites, predominantly by hepatic and intestinal cytochrome P450 3A enzyme systems – primarily CYP450 3A4 and 3A5 – with less than 1% of parent drugs appearing in urine. Notably, genetic polymorphisms have been shown to influence TAC dosing. Indeed, individuals with one or more CYP3A5*1 alleles often require higher TAC doses to achieve therapeutic levels. Individuals with the homozygous CYP3A5*1/*1 genotype require the highest tacrolimus dose compared to heterozygotes CYP3A5*1/*3 or

Table 94.2 Maintenance immunosuppressive drugs.

Immunosuppressive drug	Class	Usual dosing and administration	Therapeutic drug monitoring	Key information
Tacrolimus (TAC) 0.5, 1.0, 5.0 mg capsules Suspension may be extemporaneously compounded by selected pharmacies Injectable for IV infusion	CNI	Varies; dose adjusted based on blood concentration Oral: • Generally given in two divided doses; if once-daily, administer in the morning • Typical starting dose 1–3 mg twice daily • Administer consistently ± food IV: • Rarely used • Continuous 24-hour infusion • Dose is only one-quarter of total daily oral dose	Whole blood trough level Target level varies General range: 5–15 ng/mL	Key adverse effects: • Nephrotoxicity • Hyperglycemia • Hypomagnesemia • Hyperkalemia Neurotoxicity (tremor, headache, neuropathy, rarely seizure) • Hypertension (less than CSA) • Hyperlipidemia (less than CSA) • Alopecia CYP3A4/3A5 and P-gp substrate Many drug–drug interactions
Cyclosporine (CSA) 25, 100 mg gelcaps 100 mg/mL oral solution Injectable for IV infusion	CNI	Varies; dose adjusted based on blood concentration Oral: • Generally given in two divided doses; if once-daily, administer in the morning • Typical starting dose 100–300 mg twice daily • Administer consistently ± food IV: • Rarely used • Continuous 24-hour infusion • Dose is only one-third of total daily oral dose	Whole blood trough level Target level varies General range: 100–400 ng/mL	Key adverse effects: • Nephrotoxicity • Hyperglycemia (less than TAC) • Hypomagnesemia • Hyperkalemia • Neurotoxicity (tremor, headache, neuropathy, rarely seizure; less than TAC) • Hypertension • Hyperlipidemia • Hirsutism CSA modified formulation is not interchangeable with standard CSA CYP3A4/3A5 and P-glycoprotein substrate Many drug–drug interactions
Mycophenolate mofetil (MMF) 250 mg capsules 500mg tablets 200 mg/mL oral suspension Injectable for IV infusion	Antiproliferative (prodrug: active metabolite MPA)	Varies Oral: • Usual starting dose 1000 mg twice daily • Empty stomach preferred, but may administer with food in case of GI upset IV: • Same as oral dose (1 : 1 conversion) • Administer over at least 2 hours	Routine TDM not necessary General range for MPA level: 1.0–3.5 μg/mL	Key adverse effects (dose-related): • Diarrhea • Nausea/vomiting • Myelosuppression
Enteric coated mycophenolate sodium (EC-MPS) 180 mg enteric coated tablet 360 mg enteric coated tablet	Antiproliferative (active moiety: MPA)	Varies Oral: • Approximate equivalent doses: • MMF 1000 mg ≈ 720 mg MPS • MMF 750 mg ≈ 540 mg MPS • MMF 500 mg ≈360 mg MPS • MMF 250 mg ≈180 mg MPS • Empty stomach preferred, but may take with food in case of GI upset	Routine TDM not necessary General range for MPA level: 1.0–3.5 μg/mL	Key adverse effects (dose-related): • Diarrhea • Nausea/vomiting • Myelosuppression
Azathioprine (AZA) 50, 100 mg tablet	Antiproliferative	Varies Oral: • 1–3 mg/kg/day in one or two divided doses • Administer with food to decrease nausea	Routine TDM not performed Evaluate for TPMT deficiency prior to initiation	Key adverse effects (dose-related): • Nausea • Myelosuppression Patients with TMPT deficiency or reduced activity are at increased risk of myelotoxicity • Avoid or decrease dose by 75% if used with allopurinol or febuxostat
Sirolimus (SRL) 0.5, 1.0, 2.0 mg tablet 1 mg/mL oral solution	mTOR inhibitor	Varies • Usual oral dose: 0.5 mg to 4 mg once daily • May administer initial/single loading dose (3× maintenance dose) • Administer consistently ± food • If used with CSA, administer 4 hours *after* morning CSA dose	Trough concentration • Target level varies • General range: 5–15 ng/mL	Key adverse effects: • Hypertriglyceridemia • Hypercholesterolemia • Myelosuppression • Mouth ulcers • Rash • Interstitial pneumonitis • Hepatic artery thrombosis • Delayed wound healing • Hyperglycemia • Fluid accumulation/swelling • Nephrotoxicity, if used with full-dose CNI • Proteinuria CYP3A4/3A5 and P-glycoprotein substrate Many drug–drug interactions

(continued)

CHAPTER 94

Table 94.2 *(Continued)*

Immunosuppressive drug	Class	Usual dosing and administration	Therapeutic drug monitoring	Key information
Everolimus (EVL) 0.25, 0.5, 0.75 mg tablet	mTOR inhibitor	Varies • Usual oral dose: 0.25–1.5 mg twice daily • Administer consistently ± food	Trough concentration • Target level varies • General range: 3–8 ng/mL	Key adverse effects: • Hypertriglyceridemia • Hypercholesterolemia • Myelosuppression • Mouth ulcers • Rash • Interstitial pneumonitis • Hepatic artery thrombosis • Delayed wound healing • Hyperglycemia • Fluid accumulation/swelling • Nephrotoxicity, if used with full-dose CNI • Proteinuria CYP3A4/3A5 and P-glycoprotein substrate Many drug–drug interactions
Prednisone 1.0, 2.5, 5.0, 10.0, 20.0, 50.0 mg tablet Oral solution 5 mg/5 mL Oral concentrate solution 5 mg/mL	Corticosteroid	Varies • Tapered dosing schedule • Usual maintenance dose 5–10 mg daily • Administer with food	Not necessary	Key adverse effects: • Hyperglycemia • Edema • Hypertension • Weight gain • Cataracts, glaucoma • Cosmetic changes • Adrenal suppression • Impaired wound healing

CNI, calcineurin inhibitor; IV, intravenous; P-gp, P-glycoprotein; CSA, cyclosporine; TAC, tacrolimus; GI, gastrointestinal; MPA, mycophenolic acid; TDM, therapeutic drug monitoring; MMF, mycophenolate mofetil; MPS, mycophenolate sodium; TPMT, thiopurine methyltransferase; mTOR, mammalian target of rapamycin.

homozygous CYP3A5*3/*3. Though the CYP3A5*1 allele is relatively uncommon in European Caucasians, approximately 40% of African ethnic groups and African Americans and 25% of Asian ethnic groups possess the allele. The majority of the published data regarding CYP3A genetic polymorphisms focus on TAC. It is not entirely clear why the CYP3A5 genotype is less predictive for CSA compared to TAC, but one possible explanation is that TAC may be a better substrate for CYP3A5 than is CSA. Both CSA and TAC are major substrates for CYP450 3A4. Additionally, TAC and CSA are also substrates for P-glycoprotein (P-gp), a membrane-bound transporter found throughout the body, including in the renal proximal tubule, the blood–brain barrier (BBB), and the intestinal epithelium. Drugs, foods, and other substances that inhibit or induce CYP450 metabolism will increase or decrease blood concentrations of TAC/CSA, respectively. Similarly, drugs or other substances that inhibit or induce P-gp transport will also increase or decrease absorption/blood concentrations of TAC/CSA, respectively. Examples of medications, foods, and substances that will increase or decrease TAC/CSA levels through varying mechanisms are given in Table 94.3. Importantly, CNIs may also affect other drugs. Additive nephrotoxicity can occur when CNIs are combined with other potentially nephrotoxic drugs, such as non-steroidal anti-inflammatory drugs (NSAIDs), aminoglycosides, amphotericin B, and other nephrotoxic drugs. Additive hyperkalemia can also occur when CNIs, especially TAC, are combined with other drugs that may increase potassium, such as potassium supplements, potassium-sparing diuretics (e.g., spironolactone, triamterene, etc.), angiotensin-converting enzyme (ACE) inhibitors, or angiotensin receptor antagonists. Finally, due to its ability to inhibit P-gp, CYP450 3A4, and the organic anion transport pump (OATP), CSA may increase the effects of other drugs, such as HMG-CoA reductase inhibitors. The majority of the HMG-CoA reductase inhibitors used for hypercholesterolemia are OATP and/or CYP3A4 substrates, and therefore coadministration with CSA may increase

overall exposure to the statin and risk of toxicity. Clinicians should start with the lowest dose when initiating statin therapy in patients taking CSA and refer to specific prescribing information in order to determine the maximum statin dose when combining with CSA. Some statins (e.g., lovastatin, simvastatin, atorvastatin, pitavastatin) are not recommended for use with CSA, due to the drug interaction and the increased risk of rhabdomyolysis. TAC does not appear to affect HMG-CoA reductase inhibitors to the same degree as CSA.

Though CSA and TAC have the same mechanism of action, there are a few key differences in their adverse effects. Adverse effects of CSA include nephrotoxicity, hypertension, hyperlipidemia, hypomagnesemia, hyperkalemia, gingival hyperplasia, gout,

Table 94.3 Selected drug interactions with immunosuppressive drugs.

Selected substances that INCREASE TAC, CSA, SRL, and EVL levels	
Calcium channel blockers	Verapamil, diltiazem, nicardipine
Antibiotics	Erythromycin, clarithromycin, quinupristin/dalfopristin
Antifungal agents	Ketoconazole, fluconazole,[a] voriconazole, itraconazole, posaconazole, isavuconazole
Amiodarone	
Protease inhibitors	Nelfinavir, ritonavir, boceprevir, telaprevir, indinavir, saquinavir, fosamprenavir
Grapefruit, grapefruit juice	
Cimetidine	
Metoclopramide[b]	
Selected substances that DECREASE TAC, cyclosporine, SRL, and EVL levels	
Anticonvulsants	Phenytoin, phenobarbital, carbamazepine
Antibiotics	Rifampin, rifabutin, nafcillin
Antifungals	Caspofungin
Efavirenz	
St. John's wort	

[a]Dose-dependent.
[b]Due to increased gastric emptying.
Note: List of interacting drugs is not all-inclusive.
TAC, tacrolimus; SRL, sirolimus; EVL, everolimus.

and hirsutism. In addition, CSA can occasionally cause neurologic adverse effects (neuropathy, tremors, and rarely seizures) and hyperglycemia, but at lower rates than TAC. Adverse effects of TAC include nephrotoxicity, hyperkalemia, hypomagnesemia, alopecia, hypertension, pruritus, hyperlipidemia, and hyperglycemia, as well as neurologic adverse effects. Neurologic toxicity due to TAC can manifest as a mild tremor, headache, or peripheral neuropathy, or as more severe but less common toxicities such as seizures and posterior reversible encephalopathy syndrome (PRES). Both TAC and CSA appear to have a similar risk of nephrotoxicity, but TAC is more diabetogenic, with a higher rate of new-onset diabetes after transplantation (NODAT) compared to CSA. In contrast, CSA is more likely than TAC to cause hypertension and hyperlipidemia. Finally, TAC may cause hair thinning or alopecia in some patients, whereas CSA may cause hirsutism.

Overall, TAC use in liver transplantation is associated with reduced mortality, graft loss, and lower rates of acute rejection and steroid-resistant acute rejection, but a higher incidence of diabetes, compared to use of CSA. Though TAC is used more commonly in liver transplantation recipients, CSA remains an effective alternative in patients who do not tolerate TAC.

Antiproliferative/Antimetabolite Agents (Azathioprine, Mycophenolate Mofetil/Mycophenolate Sodium)

Antiproliferative agents and antimetabolites exert their immunosuppressive effects by inhibiting *de novo* purine nucleotide synthesis and thereby preventing T- and B-lymphocyte proliferation. Unlike other cells, which can use alternative salvage pathways, T- and B lymphocytes are critically dependent on the *de novo* pathway of purine synthesis for proliferation. Azathioprine (AZA) in combination with prednisone was initially used in the 1960s for prevention of rejection in kidney and liver transplant recipients. However, its use in this area has now been largely supplanted by mycophenolate. In clinical trials involving liver transplant recipients, mycophenolate mofetil (MMF) in combination with corticosteroids and cyclosporine resulted in a lower rate of acute rejection at 6 months and a similar rate of death or retransplantation at 1 year compared to AZA in combination with cyclosporine and corticosteroids. Currently, the combination of mycophenolate and TAC ($\pm$ steroids) is used as the initial immunosuppression regimen in the majority of liver transplant recipients.

Azathioprine

AZA, an imidazolyl derivative of 6-mercaptopurine, is a prodrug that acts as an antimetabolite and exerts its immunosuppressive effects by inhibiting the *de novo* pathway of purine nucleotide synthesis and thereby suppressing T- and B-lymphocyte proliferation. After administration, AZA undergoes hepatic metabolism to an active metabolite, 6-mercaptopurine, which then undergoes further metabolism to form 6-thioguanine nucleotides, the major active metabolites that are incorporated into DNA and thus block the *de novo* pathway for purine synthesis in lymphocytes. Importantly, 6-mercaptopurine is metabolized to inactive compounds via two major pathways mediated by the enzymes thiopurine methyltransferase (TPMT) and xanthine oxidase. Genetic polymorphisms of TPMT can result in reduced or deficient TPMT activity. Approximately 11% of the population has reduced TPMT activity and 0.3% has a true deficiency of TPMT. Though true TPMT deficiency is rare, it has important implications for patient safety. Patients with intermediate TPMT activity are at higher risk for myelosuppression

and those with absent or low TPMT activity are at even greater risk for severe, life-threatening myelotoxicity. In patients with reduced TPMT activity, the addition of medications that inhibit TPMT activity (e.g., sulfasalazine, olsalazine) can further increase the risk of myelotoxicity. In addition, concomitant use of medications that inhibit xanthine oxidase activity (e.g., allopurinol, febuxostat) also increases the risk of myelotoxicity. If AZA is used concurrently with allopurinol or febuxostat, the AZA dose should be reduced by 75% and the patient should be monitored closely for myelosupression. Screening for TPMT deficiency or reduced activity prior to starting AZA therapy may help identify patients who are at higher risk for severe myelosuppression and thus prevent or minimize this toxicity.

Key adverse effects of AZA include nausea, myelosuppression, and hepatotoxicity (including hepatic sinusoidal obstruction syndrome). Recently, cases of hepatosplenic T-cell lymphoma have been reported in patients with inflammatory bowel disease (IBD) treated with AZA or mercaptopurine. Details regarding usual dosing and administration are included in Table 94.2.

Mycophenolic Acid

Two mycophenolate formulations are currently available: (i) MMF and (ii) enteric coated mycophenolate sodium (EC-MPS). MMF is FDA approved for prevention of rejection in kidney (1995), heart (1998), and liver (2000) transplant recipients, whereas EC-MPS is only approved for use in kidney transplantation (2004). After administration, MMF, a prodrug, is rapidly hydrolyzed to its active metabolite, mycophenolic acid (MPA). EC-MPS contains the same active moiety (MPA) as MMF, but in an enteric coated delayed-release formulation. MPA, the active moiety of both mycophenolate formulations, selectively inhibits T- and B-lymphocyte proliferation via non-competitive, reversible inhibition of inosine monophosphate dehydrogenase (IMPDH). Inhibition of IMPDH prevents production of guanosine and deoxyguanosine nucleotides, which are necessary for *de novo* purine synthesis in T and B lymphocytes. Though MPA has a similar mechanism of action to AZA, it is more selective for lymphocytes. MPA is fivefold more potent at inhibiting the type II isoform of IMPDH expressed in activated lymphocytes than the type I IMPDH isoform expressed in most other cell types.

After administration, oral absorption of MMF is rapid and essentially complete, and MMF is hydrolyzed within minutes to MPA (active metabolite) by plasma esterases. MPA is then glucuronidated in the liver to an inactive mycophenolic acid glucuronide (MPAG) metabolite. Gut bacteria glucuronidases reconvert MPAG to MPA, which then undergoes enterohepatic recirculation, resulting in a secondary peak plasma concentration 6–12 hours after the dose. MMF is well absorbed, and absolute bioavailablity is approximately 94%. EC-MPS contains the same active drug moiety as MMF, but in a different formulation designed for improved GI tolerability. After administration of EC-MPS, MPA is not released from the enteric coated tablet until it reaches the small intestine; the mean absolute bioavailability of EC-MPS is approximately 71%. MPA and MPAG are highly protein-bound to albumin (97 and 82%, respectively), and approximately 90% of the orally administered dose is excreted in the urine as MPAG. Multiple factors, including hypoalbuminemia and accumulation of MPAG in renal failure (which can displace MPA from albumin), can alter protein binding of MPA. Information regarding dosing and administration can be found in Table 94.2.

The most common adverse effects observed with MMF/EC-MPS are GI toxicity (nausea, diarrhea) and myelosuppression, both of which appear to be dose-related. Due to the enteric coated delayed-release formulation, EC-MPS may potentially have fewer GI adverse effects in some patients. Other rare but serious potential adverse effects of MMF/EC-MPS include JC virus-associated progressive multifocal leukoencephalopathy (PML) and pure red cell aplasia. Importantly, MMF/EC-MPS can cause fetal harm if administered to a pregnant female. Females of reproductive potential must be made aware of the increased risk of first trimester pregnancy loss and congenital malformations, and must be counseled regarding pregnancy prevention and planning.

Trough plasma levels of MPA are not routinely monitored in clinical practice, but may occasionally be ordered (therapeutic range: 1.0–3.5 µg/mL) when there is concern regarding reduced efficacy or toxicity. Key drug interactions with MMF/EC-MPS include (i) additive myelotoxicity when combined with other drugs that can cause bone marrow suppression, (ii) decreased absorption when taken simultaneously with magnesium or aluminum salts, and (iii) reduced enterohepatic recirculation in patients taking cholestyramine. Proton pump inhibitors (PPIs) may reduce MPA concentrations when administered with MMF, but the EC-MPS formulation doesn't appear to be affected.

Antiproliferative agents are adjunct immunosuppressive drugs, and are primarily used in combination with CNIs. In liver transplant recipients, MMF is most commonly used in combination with TAC to prevent rejection, but EC-MPS and AZA may be used as alternatives in patients who do not tolerate MMF.

Corticosteroids (Methylprednisolone, Prednisone, Prednisolone)

Corticosteroids have been used for the prevention and treatment of rejection in transplant recipients since the 1960s. Before the introduction of CSA, in the 1960s and 70s, corticosteroids in combination with AZA were the primary immunosuppression regimen. Though corticosteroids continue to be an important component of many immunosuppressive regimens today, steroid minimization or avoidance strategies are growing trends at many transplant centers, due to their numerous undesirable long-term effects. Effects of chronic corticosteroid use include new-onset diabetes mellitus after transplantation, hypertension, and hyperlipidemia, all of which may lead to cardiovascular complications and increased risk of infections, *de novo* malignancies, and bone disease.

Methylprednisolone sodium succinate is often administered as a single high dose followed by tapering doses in the early perioperative period. High doses of intravenous (IV) methylprednisolone (500–1000 mg/day for several days) may also be used for the treatment of acute cellular rejection after liver transplantation. Importantly, in hepatitis C virus (HCV)-positive transplant recipients, high-dose steroid therapy increases viral replication and may contribute to more rapid progression of recurrent HCV and allograft failure after liver transplantation. Therefore, HCV-positive liver transplant recipients with mild to moderate acute cellular rejection are sometimes initially treated with increasing doses of maintenance immunosuppression (TAC, mycophenolate), with steroid boluses used only in patients who do not respond. Oral corticosteroids used as adjunct maintenance immunosuppression include prednisone and prednisolone. After administration, oral prednisone is metabolized in the liver to prednisolone. Oral prednisone (or prednisolone) in a tapering dose is often included as part of the initial maintenance regimen after transplantation, but then gradually discontinued over a period of months. Indeed, approximately half of liver transplant recipients discontinue corticosteroid therapy by the end of the first year. However, patients with autoimmune liver disease or a history of acute rejection may continue low-dose prednisone indefinitely.

The immunosuppressive effects of corticosteroids are multifactorial. Corticosteroids act primarily on T-cell activation by inhibiting the production of T-cell cytokines such as IL-2, IL-6, and interferon gamma (IFN-γ), which are required to enhance the response of lymphocytes and macrophages to allograft antigens.

Common adverse effects of steroids include sodium and fluid retention, hypertension, hyperglycemia, psychosis/altered mental status (high doses), cataracts, glaucoma, osteoporosis, myopathy, hyperlipidemia, growth retardation (pediatric patients), cosmetic changes (buffalo hump, moon face, acne), suppression of the pituitary–adrenal axis (chronic use), obesity/weight gain, impaired wound healing, and infection. Details regarding usual dosing and administration are included in Table 94.2

Mammalian Target of Rapamycin Inhibitors (Sirolimus, Everolimus)

Sirolimus (SRL, rapamycin), a macrocyclic lactone derived from *Streptomyces hydroscopicus*, was first discovered on Easter Island (Rapa Nui). SRL is FDA approved for use in kidney transplantation (1999), but has also been used off-label in liver transplantation despite a black box warning for hepatic artery thrombosis in liver transplant recipients. Everolimus (EVL), a rapamycin derivative, is currently FDA approved for use in both kidney (2010) and liver (2013) transplantation. Notably, EVL is also approved and marketed under a different brand name in higher doses to treat various oncologic indications (e.g., neuroendocrine tumors, breast cancer, etc.).

After binding to FKBP12, SRL and EVL block the function of mTOR and thereby inhibit growth factor-stimulated cellular proliferation, leading to cell cycle arrest at the G1 stage. Thus, by inhibiting mTOR activity, EVL and SRL block IL-2-mediated proliferation and clonal expansion of activated T lymphocytes. The mTOR inhibitor/FKBP12 complex does not affect calcineurin activity. Also, compared to CNIs, which act early (G0–G1 phase), mTOR inhibitors act later in the cell cycle (G1 stage) and consequently are not as robust as CNIs in terms of immunosuppressive effects and ability to prevent rejection. Notably, the antiproliferative effects of mTOR inhibitors are not limited to lymphoid cells: they can also impair the normal fibroblast response to fibroblast growth factor, thus interfering with the wound-healing process. In contrast, the antifibrotic effects of mTOR inhibitors may also have beneficial effects in certain patients. In one study, long-term use of SRL in liver transplant recipients with recurrent HCV infection was associated with a reduction in hepatic fibrosis progression. In addition to their immunosuppressive effects, mTOR inhibitors have also demonstrated antitumor effects through antiproliferation and antiangiogenesis; there is thus growing interest in their use for transplant recipients with or at risk for malignancies.

One notable difference between SRL and EVL is in their respective elimination half-lives. SRL has a mean elimination half-life of 60 hours in adults, compared to approximately 30 hours for EVL. Thus, SRL is typically administered once daily and EVL twice daily. Details regarding usual dosing and administration of SRL and EVL are included in Table 94.2. Like CNIs, SRL and EVL are critical drugs characterized by significant pharmacokinetic variability, a narrow therapeutic index, and numerous drug interactions. As with all critical drugs, TDM is essential to ensure safe and effective use. Due to its long elimination half-life, daily levels are generally not necessary for SRL. Trough concentrations should be measured once steady-state concentration has been reached after initiation or a dose change (~1 week for SRL and 3–5 days for EVL).

Adverse effects of mTOR inhibitors include leukopenia, thrombocytopenia, anemia, hypercholesterolemia, hypertriglyceridemia, rash, mouth ulcers, delayed wound healing, lymphocele formation, interstitial pneumonitis, proteinuria, fluid accumulation/swelling, hyperglycemia, infection, nephrotoxicity if used with full-dose CNI, and thrombotic microangiopathy, thrombotic thrombocytopenia purpura, or hemolytic uremic syndrome when used with CNIs. In addition, mTOR inhibitors have also been associated with an increased risk of hepatic artery thrombosis, particularly when used within the first 30 days after liver transplantation. Importantly, though mTOR inhibitors are often used in renal-sparing protocols, liver transplant recipients who develop massive proteinuria after conversion from a CNI to an mTOR inhibitor may experience deterioration in renal function. Finally, due to impaired wound healing, in transplant recipients undergoing elective surgical procedures, discontinuation of mTOR inhibitor therapy (e.g., conversion to CNI) should be strongly considered several weeks before surgery. Post-surgery mTOR inhibitor should be not be restarted until the surgical wound has completely healed.

Like CNIs, both SRL and EVL undergo extensive metabolism by the CYP450 3A4 enzyme system and are P-gp substrates. Thus, any substances (food, drug, etc.) that inhibit or induce CYP450 3A4 metabolism/P-gp transport will increase or decrease SRL/EVL levels, respectively. CSA inhibits CYP3A4 and P-gp, and thereby increases SRL and EVL; prescribing information for EVL indicates that CSA and EVL may be administered at the same time, but when SRL is used in combination with CSA, it is recommended that SRL be administered 4 hours after the morning CSA dose. Examples of key substances that may interact with mTOR inhibitors through varying mechanisms are included in Table 94.3.

The role of mTOR inhibitors in the early post-transplant period is limited by wound-healing complications and a black box warning for hepatic artery thrombosis. In liver transplantation, mTOR inhibitors are primarily used as an alternative to CNIs or as adjunct immunosuppressive drugs in combination with low-dose CNI therapy for their renal-sparing effects. Despite this, it is essential to monitor for proteinuria during mTOR inhibitor use in order to prevent deterioration of renal function. In addition, due to their antitumor effects, there is growing interest in using mTOR inhibitors to prevent recurrent HCC and other malignancies. Additional scientific studies are needed to confirm whether mTOR inhibitor therapy can indeed impact HCC recurrence rates or the development of other malignancies, and if so, what dosage/level is required to achieve antitumor benefits.

Induction Antibodies

"Induction immunosuppression" refers to the use of intense immunosuppression during the early postoperative period to prevent rejection. Specialized antibodies that may be used for induction during the early post-transplant/perioperative period include lymphocyte-depleting (alemtuzumab or rabbit antithymocyte globulin (rATG)) and non-lymphocyte-depleting (basiliximab) antibody preparations. Induction agents have not received FDA approval for use in liver transplantation and are therefore considered "off-label." The primary purposes of induction therapy are (i) to provide potent immunosuppression and thereby prevent early rejection and (ii) to delay or minimize maintenance immunosuppressive agents and thus their associated toxicities (e.g., nephrotoxicity due to CNIs). In contrast to other types of solid organ transplantation, induction therapy is used infrequently in liver transplant

recipients. The majority of liver transplant recipients (70%) receive no induction, and among the remaining 30%, approximately 20 and 10% receive induction with an IL-2 receptor antagonist or a T cell-depleting agent, respectively. Lymphocyte-depleting agents such as rATG may also be used off-label in liver transplant recipients for treatment of severe and/or steroid-resistant acute cellular rejection.

Lymphocyte-Depleting Antibodies (Antithymocyte Globulin, Alemtuzumab)

rATG is a purified, pasteurized polyclonal antibody obtained through immunization of rabbits with human thymocytes. The final rATG product contains cytotoxic antibodies directed at multiple receptors (e.g., CD2, CD3, CD4, CD8, CD11a, CD18, etc.) expressed on the surface of human T lymphocytes. Administration of rATG results in rapid, profound, and long-lasting T-lymphocyte depletion followed by immune reconstitution. The extent and duration of T-cell depletion correlates with cumulative dose, and can persist for a period of months to years. Though a range of doses have reportedly been used, the most common is 1.5 mg/kg daily, administered as an IV infusion over 4–6 hours for several days (typical cumulative dose is 6 mg/kg). Duration of therapy varies with indication and patient tolerability. An equine-derived antithymocyte globulin is also available, but is rarely used in solid organ transplant recipients. If it is used, the dose is higher than that of the rabbit-derived ATG product. rATG is FDA approved for treatment of rejection in kidney transplant recipients; its use for induction or treatment of rejection in liver transplantation is off-label.

Alemtuzumab, a humanized monoclonal antibody, targets the CD52 receptor on the surface of T and B lymphocytes, as well as monocytes, macrophages, natural killer cells (NKCs), and a subpopulation of granulocytes. After administration, alemtuzumab binds to CD52-positive cells, resulting in a rapid and profound antibody-dependent lysis of lymphocytes and other cells. Like rATG, it may take several months for B lymphocyte to recover, and even longer for T lymphocytes. Use of alemtuzumab in any solid organ transplant recipient, including liver transplant recipients, is off-label.

The most common adverse effects associated with lymphocyte-depleting antibodies are related to myelosuppression (leukopenia, neutropenia, thrombocytopenia) and cytokine release following rapid lymphocyte destruction. Premedications (e.g., acetaminophen, diphenhydramine, and steroids) are recommended prior to administration to prevent or minimize infusion reactions. In addition, due to their potent immunosuppressive effects, lymphocyte-depleting antibodies may increase the risk of any infection, particularly viral infections, as well as post-transplant lymphoproliferative disease. When used in hepatitis C-positive transplant recipients, alemtuzumab was associated with hepatitis C recurrence and progressive liver failure after transplantation.

Non-Lymphocyte-Depleting Antibodies (Basiliximab)

Basiliximab, a chimeric (mouse/human) monoclonal antibody and IL-2 receptor antagonist (IL-2-RA), binds to CD25 on the alpha chain of the IL-2 receptor expressed on activated T lymphocytes. Basiliximab inhibits but does not deplete T lymphocytes. It is well tolerated, and its adverse effects were similar to placebo in clinical trials. Rarely, hypersensitivity reactions can occur. Basiliximab induction typically consists of 2 intravenous doses (20 mg in adults, 10 mg for pediatric patients <35 kg) on postoperative days 0 & 4. Basiliximab is FDA approved for prevention of rejection in kidney

CHAPTER 94

transplant recipients; use as an induction agent in liver transplantation is off-label. Basiliximab is not used to treat rejection.

Rescue Treatment for Episodes of Acute Rejection

Once a histologic diagnosis of acute cellular rejection is made, the most common initial treatment consists of high-dose IV corticosteroid therapy. Severe acute cellular rejection or rejection that is unresponsive to high-dose corticosteroid therapy may be treated with a lymphocyte-depleting antibody. Transplant recipients with mild rejection may be treated with increasing doses of maintenance immunosuppression or by addition of a new maintenance immunosuppressive drug. Additionally, in patients with HCV, increased maintenance immunosuppression may be tried before high-dose steroid therapy, due to the deleterious effects of high-dose steroid therapy on hepatitis C progression.

Immunosuppressive Strategies to Minimize Long-Term Adverse Effects

As patients continue to live longer with functioning grafts after liver transplantation, minimizing the long-term adverse effects of immunosuppression has become increasingly important. Indeed, cardiovascular disease (CVD) and renal failure are the leading nonhepatic causes of morbidity and mortality late after liver transplantation. The majority of liver transplant recipients who survive more than 6 months develop chronic kidney disease. In a longitudinal analysis that included 36 849 liver transplant recipients during the pre-Model for End-Stage Liver Disease (MELD) era, the risk of renal failure (glomerular filtration rate (GFR) < 30 mL/min) 5 and 10 years after liver transplantation was 18 and 25%, respectively. In transplant recipients who developed chronic kidney disease, the risk of death was increased fourfold. In another, more recent study, the majority (59%) of the 4904 non-renal adult transplant recipients placed on the kidney transplant waiting list between 1995 and 2008 were liver transplant recipients. Though long term use of CNIs plays a key role in the etiology of chronic kidney disease, other factors such as hypertension, diabetes mellitus, chronic HCV infection, and perioperative acute kidney injury also contribute. Chronic kidney disease, hypertension, and diabetes mellitus each confer a twofold increased risk of mortality after liver transplantation. The prevalence of hypertension in liver transplant recipients ranges from 60 to 70%, hyperlipidemia from 50 to 70%, and new-onset diabetes mellitus after transplantation (NODAT) from approximately 5 to 30%, with an even higher prevalence (40–60%) in HCV-infected patients. CNIs (CSA more than TAC) and corticosteroids contribute to hypertension. CNIs (CSA more than TAC), mTOR inhibitors, and corticosteroids contribute to hyperlipidemia. CNIs (TAC more than CSA), corticosteroids, and mTOR inhibitors can all contribute to NODAT. Finally, obesity can occur in up to 20% of liver transplant recipients during the first 3 years after transplant, further increasing the risk of cardiovascular morbidity and mortality.

Due to the long-term risk of chronic kidney disease, newer immunosuppressive strategies focusing on CNI minimization or avoidance are being evaluated, including (i) induction and delayed CNI introduction, (ii) CNI avoidance, and (iii) CNI minimization combined with the use of adjunct agents (mTOR inhibitors or antiproliferative/antimetabolite). Importantly, the benefits of CNI minimization or avoidance must be carefully balanced with the potential increased risk of rejection. Data suggest that complete

CNI avoidance is associated with higher rejection rates and that late conversion to mTOR inhibitors in patients with established chronic kidney disease may have a diminished benefit compared to earlier conversion. In a prospective, randomized, multicenter study, patients receiving MMF/CNI were randomized at 4–12 weeks post-transplant to continue MMF/CNI or switch to MMF/SRL. MMF/SRL was associated with significantly improved renal function (mean change in GFR 19.0 vs 1.2% for the MMF/CNI group) at 12 months, but biopsy-proven acute rejection (BPAR) was significantly greater in the MMF/SRL group than in the MMF/CNI group (12.2 vs. 4.1%, p = 0.02). Notably, malignancy-related deaths were lower in the MMF/SRL group, but more patients in this group discontinued therapy due to adverse effects (34.2 vs. 24.1%). In another large, prospective, randomized study, patients who were between 6 and 144 months post transplant were randomized to abrupt conversion from CNI to SRL. Abrupt CNI discontinuation/SRL conversion was associated with higher rates of BPAR and no demonstrable benefit 1 year after conversion from CNI to SRL. In a third study, conversion from CNI to EVL 4 weeks after liver transplantation was associated with a similar risk of BPAR and improved GFR. Finally, in a 24-month prospective, randomized, multicenter, open-label study, liver transplant recipients were randomized at 4 weeks after transplant to discontinue TAC/switch to EVL, continue TAC alone, or add EVL combined with reduced TAC. Early introduction of EVL to low-dose TAC at 1 month post transplant resulted in an improvement in renal function at 2 years without an increased risk of rejection. The arm randomized to TAC elimination at 4 weeks was stopped early due to significantly higher rates of BPAR. Use of induction to delay CNI introduction or to produce CNI minimization has been attempted in several centers, with varying results. As with all immunosuppression, the potential benefits of induction antibodies must be weighed carefully against the risks. Similarly, various steroid minimization/withdrawal strategies have been used, with varying results. In general, most liver transplant recipients who are beyond the first 90 days and are not at high risk for rejection can gradually discontinue steroids with close monitoring, but whether early steroid avoidance is feasible still remains to be determined.

Take Home Points

- Despite long-term adverse effects, calcineurin inhibitors (CNIs) are still the cornerstone of immunosuppression following liver transplantation.
- Long-term renal, metabolic, and infectious complications from immunosuppression are associated with increased morbidity and mortality after liver transplantation.
- Strategies to minimize the long-term consequences of immunosuppression continue to evolve.

References

1 US Department of Health and Human Services Health Resources and Services Administration. OPTN/SRTR 2012 Annual Data Report. Available from: http://srtr.transplant.hrsa.gov/annual_reports/2012/pdf/2012_SRTR_ADR.pdf (last accessed February 15, 2016).

2 Anon. A comparison of tacrolimus (FK506) and cyclosporine for immunosuppression in liver transplant. The US Multicenter FK506 Liver Study Group. *N Engl J Med* 1994; **331**: 1110–15.

3 McAlister VC, Haddad E, Renouf E, *et al.* Cyclosporin versus tacrolimus as primary immunosuppressant after liver transplantation: a meta-analysis. *Am J Transplant* 2006; **6**: 1578–85.

4 Ojo AO, Held PJ, Port FK, *et al.* Chronic renal failure after transplantation of a nonrenal organ. *N Engl J Med* 2003; **349**: 931–40.

5 Srinivas TR, Stephany BR, Budev M, *et al.* An emerging population: kidney transplant candidates who are placed on the waiting list after liver, heart, and lung transplantation. *Clin J Am Soc Nephrol* 2010; **5**: 1881–6.

6 Saliba F, De Simone P, Nevens F, *et al.* Renal function at two years in liver transplant patients receiving everolimus: results of a randomized, multicenter study. *Am J Transplant* 2013; **13**: 1734–45.

7 Fischer L, Klempnauer J, Beckebaum S, *et al.* A randomized, controlled study to assess the conversion from calcineurin-inhibitors to everolimus after liver transplantation – PROTECT. *Am J Transplant* 2012; **12**: 1855–65.

8 Abdelmalek MF, Humar A, Stickel F, *et al.* Sirolimus conversion regimen versus continued calcineurin inhibitors in liver allograft recipients: a randomized trial. *Am J Transplant* 2012; **12**: 694–705.

9 Teperman L, Moonka D, Sebastian A, *et al.* Calcineurin inhibitor-free mycophenolate mofetil/sirolimus maintenance in liver transplantation: the randomized spare-the-nephron trial. *Liver Transpl* 2013; **19**: 675–89.

10 Londono M-C, Rimola A, O'Grady JO, Sanchez-Fueyo A. Immunosuppression minimization vs. complete drug withdrawal in liver transplantation. *J Hepatol* 2013; **59**: 872–9.

11 Bishop AG, Bertolino PD, Bowen DG, *et al.* Tolerance in liver transplantation. *Best Pract Res Clin Gastro* 2012; **26**: 73–84.

12 Thervet E, Anglicheau D, Legendre C, Beaune P. Role of pharmacogenetics of immunosuppressive drugs in organ transplantation. *Ther Drug Monit* 2008; **30**: 143–50.

13 Chan AJ, Lake JR. Immunosuppression in HCV-positive liver-transplant recipients. *Curr Opin Organ Transplant* 2012; **17**: 648–54.

14 McKenna GJ, Trotter JF, Klintmalm E, *et al.* Limiting hepatitis C virus progression in liver transplant recipients using sirolimus-based immunosuppression. *Am J Transplant* 2011; **11**: 2379–87.

15 Wadei HM, Zaky ZS, Keaveny AP, *et al.* Proteinuria following sirolimus conversion is associated with deterioration of kidney function in liver transplant recipients. *Transplantation* 2010; **93**: 1006–12.

16 Bhat M, Sonenberg N, Gores GJ. The mTOR pathway in hepatic malignancies. *Hepatology* 2013; **58**: 810–18.

17 Yamanaka K, Petrulionis M, Lin S, *et al.* Therapeutic potential and adverse effects of everolimus for treatment of hepatocellular carcinoma – systemic review and meta-analysis. *Cancer Med* 2013; **2**: 862–71.

18 Weisner RH, Fung JJ. Present state of immunosuppressive therapy in liver transplant recipients. *Liver Transpl* 2011; **17**: S1–9.

19 Watt KD, Charlton MR. Metabolic syndrome and liver transplantation: a review and guide to management. *J Hepatol* 2010; **53**: 199–206.

20 Lucey MR, Terrault N, Ojo L, *et al.* Long-term management of the successful adult liver transplant: 2012 practice guidelines by the American Association for the Study of Liver Diseases and the American Society of Transplantation. *Liver Transpl* 2013; **19**(1): 3–26.

21 Beckbaum S, Cicinnati VR, Radtke A, Kabar I. Calcineurin inhibitors in liver transplantation – still champions or threatened by serious competitors? *Liver Int* 2013; **33**: 656–65.

22 Turner AP, Knechtle SJ. Induction immunosuppression in liver transplantation: a review. *Transpl Int* 2013; **26**: 673–83.

23 Knight SR, Morris PJ. Steroid sparing protocols following nonrenal transplants: the evidence is not there. A systemic review and meta-analysis. *Transpl Int* 2011; **24**: 1198–207.

CHAPTER 95

Medical Management of the Liver Transplant Patient

William C. Palmer and Denise M. Harnois

Division of Transplantation, Mayo Clinic, Jacksonville, FL, USA

Summary

Liver transplantation represents the definitive treatment for decompensated cirrhosis, acute fulminant liver failure, and certain primary hepatic malignancies. Post-liver transplant medical management starts with monitoring of immunosuppression and graft function, but also requires regular monitoring for complications of multiple organ systems, which are influenced by both donor and recipient factors. Primary disease or malignancy recurrences can take months or years to manifest, but medical complications can appear in any post-transplant stage. Improved immunosuppression and updated infectious disease prophylaxis and treatment have improved liver transplantation outcomes, but this has led to cardiovascular disease (CVD) and *de novo* malignancies increasingly impacting long-term survival. A multidisciplinary approach to management immediately after liver transplantation supports improvement in short- and long-term outcomes.

Immunosuppression

Advances in immunosuppression induction and maintenance therapies have reduced both acute and chronic organ rejection. Standard induction regimens combines agents, with each agent influencing different rejection cascade elements. The most commonly used regimens include calcineurin inhibitors (CNIs), mycophenolate mofetil (MMF), and tapered corticosteroids.

Induction, or initiation of immune suppression immediately after transplant, commonly employs intravenous methylprednisolone intraoperatively, with transition to oral prednisone. The schedule varies with center-specific protocols. Basiliximab and daclizumab (monoclonal anti-CD25 antibodies) represent alternative induction options. Thymoglobulin (a polyclonal lymphocyte-depleting antibody) is a viable substitute for steroids in certain cases. Sirolimus and everolimus, which inhibits mechanistic target of rapamycin (mTOR) and interleukin (IL)-2, may be an option where there is a risk of cancer or in patients intolerant to CNI therapy [1]. However, they are contraindicated initially post-liver transplantation secondary to concerns of impaired wound healing and possible hepatic artery thrombosis [2, 3]. CNIs, such as cyclosporine or tacrolimus, are the most common maintenance therapies; they inhibit calcineurin and reduce transcription of certain genes, including IL-2, which promotes T-cell activation. CNIs are metabolized by cytochrome P450, predisposing to drug–drug interaction and necessitating frequent level monitoring. Though they produce similar 1-year survival outcomes, tacrolimus appears less nephrotoxic than cyclosporin, with lower incidence of acute rejection and steroid-refractory rejection. However, neurogenic and diabetic complications are increased [4]. MMF (a T- and B-cell inhibitor) and sirolimus are not nephrotoxic, and are ideal for renal insufficiency. Azathioprine, a plasma cell inhibitor previously used frequently in maintenance immunosuppression, is uncommonly used today.

Medical Complications

Biliary Complications

Biliary complications post liver transplantation include leaks, strictures, and sludge/stone formation. One-third of biliary complications occur in the first month after liver transplantation, and 80% within 6 months [5]. Biliary strictures occur over time, while bile leaks usually present in the first 3 months. Biliary complications can present with right upper quadrant abdominal discomfort, but hepatic denervation and immunosuppression may reduce or eliminate pain. Biliary assessment requires imaging with ultrasound, magnetic resonance cholangiopancreatography (MRCP), cholangiogram via biliary tube, percutaneous tube cholangiography (PTC), or endoscopic retrograde cholangiopancreatography (ERCP). Combined routine ultrasonography and Doppler ultrasonography can accurately assess both the biliary system and vascular patency, which are important in the investigation of biliary complications. Most biliary leaks are managed via ERCP with stent placement and subsequent exchange over 2–3 months. Persistent leaks may require surgical revision [6]. Advanced cases require retransplantation. Organs donated after cardiac death produce higher rates of biliary complications, with up to 60% reported [7].

Rejection

Liver allograft rejection enjoys some tolerance compared to that of other transplanted organs, secondary to a high percentage of unconventional lymphoid cells. Pharmacological advances in immunosuppression have decreased the occurrence of acute cellular rejection (ACR) from near 75% to less than 30%. Chronic rejection leading to graft loss occurs in less than 4% of cases [8]. Liver biopsy classified according to the Banff criteria is necessary to confirm rejection [9]. ACR presents with histopathological changes of lymphocytic portal tract infiltration, bile duct damage, and

Practical Gastroenterology and Hepatology Board Review Toolkit, Second Edition. Edited by Nicholas J. Talley, Kenneth R. DeVault, Michael B. Wallace, Bashar A. Aqel and Keith D. Lindor.
© 2016 John Wiley & Sons, Ltd. Published 2016 by John Wiley & Sons, Ltd. Companion website: www.practicalgastrohep.com

venular inflammation, which usually responds to increased immunosuppression and pulse-dosed intravenous corticosteroids. Severe cases or steroid-resistant episodes (incidence: 5%) require alternative therapies, such as thymoglobulin [10], MMF [11], or basiliximab [12]. Long-term allograft function is not affected in those effectively treated, except in hepatitis C patients, who are noted to have worse outcomes after corticosteroid boluses [13]. Chronic rejection, ductopenic rejection, and vanishing bile duct syndrome occur less commonly but can lead to graft failure and the need for retransplantation. Syndrome hallmarks include graft dysfunction and progressive cholestasis, along with histopathologic changes such as foam cell arteriopathy, loss of bile ducts, and pruning of distal portal venous branches from persistent inflammation.

Infectious Complications

Infection following liver transplantation is the leading cause of mortality, with one series reporting 64% of 321 deaths from infection [14]. High-risk patients include those with poor graft function, who require increased immunosuppression [15]. Liver transplant patients with fever and even common infections require immediate assessment. Drug interactions in antimicrobial therapy combined with immunosuppression require special attention, as certain antimicrobials can alter immunosuppressant serum levels [9].

Bacterial

Early (30 days post liver transplantation) bacterial complications stem primarily from nosocomial causes, such as surgical-site infections, catheter-related bacteremia, pneumonia, urinary tract infections (UTIs), and *Clostridium difficile* colitis. Perioperative antibiotic prophylaxis targeted against gastrointestinal (GI) flora and *Staphlococcus aureus* combined with specific regimens against colonization by resistant pathogens (methicillin-resistant *S. aureus*, vancomycin-resistant *Enterococi*, extended-spectrum beta-lactamase-producing *Escherichia coli* and *Klebsiella pneumoniae*) are administered for the first 24–48 hours following liver transplantation. Trimethoprim-sulfamethoxazole prophylaxis against *Pneumocystis carinii* pneumonia has become standard, with dapsone or inhaled pentamidine as alternatives.

Bilomas are fluid collections inside or near the allograft resulting from biliary complications in approximately 10% of patients, primarily occurring in the first year after liver transplantation. Clinical presentation includes fever, abdominal pain, transaminitis, and/or leukocytosis. Percutaneous drainage provides diagnostic and therapeutic management, and may prevent progression to peritonitis or bacteremia. *Enterococci*, coagulase-negative *Staphylococci*, and *Candida* are the most commonly cultured pathogens. Most are managed without surgery, except for persistent or large ductal defects.

Post-liver transplantation peritonitis secondary to wound infections, surgical complications, intra-abdominal bleeding, strictures, bowel leaks, or perforations can be catastrophic. Risk factors include higher pretransplant MELD score, long surgical times, Roux-en-Y biliary anastomosis, and post-transplantation dialysis. Management includes correction of the underlying problem, broad-spectrum antimicrobial therapies, and supportive care [16].

Fungal

Candida and *Aspergillus* constitute the predominant post-liver transplantation fungal infections, with less common pathogens including *Cryptococcus*, *Histoplasmosis*, and *Coccidiomycosis*.

Antibiotic prophylaxis, fulminant hepatic failure, retransplantation, large intraoperative transfusion needs, longer operative times, renal failure, and post-liver transplantation dialysis are known risk factors for invasive candidiasis. Oral thrush is commonly managed prophylactically with oral nystatin. Systemic fungal prophylaxis in high-risk recipients is given for 6–12 weeks post liver transplantation with amphotericin B, voriconazole, or an echinocandin. Manifestations include intravascular catheters with candidemia, intra-abdominal abscess/peritonitis, and surgical-site infections. First-line treatment for *Candida albicans*, *C. tropicalis*, and *C. parapsilosis* is fluconazole, with alternative therapies, including echinocandin, amphotericin B, and voriconazole, reserved for resistant strains, such as *Candida glabrata*. Removal of any intravascular catheters and drainage of any abscess with wound debridement are required, along with retinal examination for endophthalmitis.

Cryptococcal cerebrospinal fluid (CSF) or serum antigen is most advantageous for diagnosis, while urinary histoplasmosis and Blastomyces antigens assist [9]. Invasive aspergillosis occurs rarely (less than 10% patients), but carries a mortality as high as 60%, with half of cases occurring after 6 months and one-third after 1 year [17]. The majority of cases present with pneumonia, diagnosed with respiratory cultures from induced sputum or bronchoscopy. Voriconazole is the treatment of choice, with amphotericin B a second-line agent.

Viral

Viral infections in the liver transplantation patient can occur from primary infection or from reactivation of a donor or recipient virus. Though cytomegalovirus (CMV) is the most common pathogen, herpes simplex virus (HSV), varicella zoster virus (VZV), and Epstein–Barr virus (EBV) are frequently encountered.

CMV-seropositive recipients (+CMV immunoglobulin G (IgG) antibodies) carry a risk of CMV reactivation regardless of donor status, but primary infection risk is increased when a seronegative recipient receives a seropositive allograft liver. CMV is the most common cause of fever post liver transplantation and independently increases the risk for bacteremia, invasive fungal infections, and EBV-related post-transplant lymphoproliferative disorders (PTLDs), while also causing primary acute and chronic allograft injury. ACR increases risk secondary to treatment with high-dose corticosteroids and antilymphocyte antibodies. CMV infections range from identification in body fluid or tissue specimens in asymptomatic recipients to end-organ disease. GI or hepatic tissue invasion occurs commonly, with pulmonary and central nervous system (CNS) infections also possible. CMV-seropositive recipients undergo periodic serum surveillance via pp65 antigenemia markers and quantitative CMV polymerase chain reaction (PCR) assays. CMV prophylaxis at 3 months is standard, with symptomatic or tissue-invasive CMV treated with oral valganciclovir or intravenous ganciclovir. Resistant CMV infection occurs in patients with prolonged ganciclovir or valganciclovir exposure with progressive CMV infection despite appropriate treatment. Genotypic assays should be performed and foscarnet therapy considered [9]. EBV infections associated with PTLDs can develop in CMV-infected patients after liver transplantation [18].

Vaccinations

All patients should receive vaccination against pneumococcus, hepatitis (A and B), varicella, zoster, influenza, and tetanus diphtheria prior to transplant if they are not already immune. Inactivated polio vaccine, cholera, plague, inactivated typhoid, rabies, and anthrax

CHAPTER 95

can be used safely if indicated. Live or attenuated vaccines such as measles, mumps, rubella, oral polio, bacille Calmette–Guérin (BCG), yellow fever, TY21a typhoid, and vaccinia are contraindicated secondary to concern for reactivation. Inactivated vaccinations post liver transplantation should be delayed at least 6 months, and live vaccines should not be given.

Renal Complications

Kidney disease commonly impacts liver transplantation recipients in terms of both short- and long-term outcomes. Acute renal failure (ARF) post liver transplantation carries a significantly increased mortality, extends hospitalization length, and increases cost [19]. ARF usually derives from acute tubular necrosis (earlier) or CNI toxicity (later). Hemodialysis pre or post liver transplantation is needed in up to 20% of patients [20]. Risk factors predicting need for dialysis post liver transplantation are preoperative serum creatine >1.9 mg/dL, preoperative blood urea nitrogen (BUN) >27mg/dL, intensive care stay longer than 3 days, and a Model for End-Stage Liver Disease (MELD) score >21. Continuous hemodialysis appears to be the preferred modality. Recovery from hepatorenal syndrome (HRS) post liver transplantation is 58.0–77.4%, with type 1 HRS and transplant MELD >20 known risk factors for worse outcomes after liver transplantation [21]. Chronic kidney disease (CKD) post liver transplantation is primarily a function of CNI toxicity, with rates of 14% at 3 years and 18% at 5 years [22]. Screening with urinalysis, microalbumin, and serum glomerular filtration rate (GFR) every 2–3 months initially and then every 6 months has been suggested [9]. Risk factors for CKD post liver transplantation include high preoperative serum creatine, high serum creatine 1 year postoperatively, intraoperative dialysis, previous HRS, and repeat transplantation. A long-term study showed that 9.5% of liver transplantation patients develop end-stage renal disease (ESRD) within 13 years, with 28.2% surviving (54.6% in the control group) and 3% requiring kidney transplantation [23]. Reduction of CNI doses or transition to an alternate CNI does not typically reverse renal impairment, but can slow progression [24]. Substitution with less nephrotoxic regimens, such as everolimus or sirolimus, is a reasonable option [25].

Cardiovascular Complications

Cardiovascular complications after liver transplantation vary from 9.4% at 5 years to 25% at 10 years [26], accounting for 21% of deaths surviving more than 3 years after liver transplantation [27]. Liver transplantation and the necessary sequelae independently increase the prevalence of hypertension, diabetes mellitus, dyslipidemia, and obesity. Cardiovascular events are independently increased in older transplant patients, males, and patients receiving MMF. Blood pressure screening should occur at least every 6 months following liver transplantation, with targets (<130/80) and lifestyle modification goals similar to the general population [9]. Hypertension post-liver transplantation derives primarily from immunosuppression and renal disease. Early post-liver transplantation hypertension is worsened by glucocorticoids and CNI medications like cyclosporine and tacrolimus. Initial studies demonstrated no difference in hypertension with cyclosporine and tacrolimus [24], but further trials suggest a lower incidence of late-onset hypertension with tacrolimus [28]. Thus, switching from cyclosporine to tacrolimus for hypertension management only is not recommended. Some patients lose normal circadian blood pressure patterns, developing nocturnal hypertension [29]. Up to 30% require more than one agent to control blood pressures [30]. Calcium channel blockers are preferred in liver transplantation patients, as they counter the effect of CNI-induced

afferent arteriolar vasoconstriction. Liver transplantation patients with proteinuria should receive an angiotensin-converting enzyme (ACE) inhibitor, angiotensin receptor blocker (ARB), or direct renin inhibitor [9].

Metabolic Complications

Dyslipidemia

Liver transplantation patients commonly (up to 70%) develop increased plasma cholesterol as well as hypertriglyceridemia after liver transplantation secondary to genetics, medications, body weight, and dietary habits [31]. Tacrolimus appears to have less effect than cyclosporine, with some evidence that transition to tacrolimus can improve dyslipidemia [32]. Corticosteroids cause weight gain and increase insulin resistance, acetyl-CoA carboxylase, free fatty acid synthetase, and HMG CoA reductase activity, and reduce lipoprotein lipase and low-density lipoprotein (LDL) receptor activity. Sirolimus causes dyslipidemia in up to 44% of patients. Lipid management takes a stepwise approach (Table 95.1). Pravastatin, the statin with the least potential for interaction with CNIs, should be started at the lowest dose and titrated up. Calcium channel blockers may elevate statin levels as well, and should be initiated with caution. Cholestyramine should be avoided due to absorption concerns with CI medications. Screening should occur at least annually [9].

Obesity

Obesity is a common issue following liver transplantation, with up to 20% of lean patients becoming obese within 2–3 years [33]. Genetic factors, decreased physical activity, immunosuppression (tacrolimus causes less weight gain than cyclosporine [34]), diabetes, and dietary habits, along with pre-existing obesity, combine to create a challenge for patients and providers. Though prednisone dosing is an independent risk factor for obesity post liver transplantation [35], prednisone tapering may not lead to weight loss [36]. Management includes dietary intervention, counseling, structured weight-loss programs, and exercise. Bariatric surgery can also be considered [9].

Diabetes Mellitus

The incidence of diabetes mellitus in liver transplantation patients is approximately 15%, with up to 40% of cases occurring within the first year post liver transplantation. Risk factors include older

Table 95.1 Management of dyslipidemia post liver transplant.

Low-density lipoprotein treatment thresholds	<100 mg/dL in very high–risk patients
	≤130 mg/dL in moderate–high-risk patients
	≤160 mg/dL in low-risk patients
Treatment options	Reduced cholesterol intake
	Reduced total fat intake
	Saturated fat <7%
	Decreased dietary transfats
	Increased soluble fiber intake
	Exercise
	Statins (HMG-CoA reductase inhibitors)
	Ezetimibe
Hypertriglyceridemia treatment	Omega-2 fatty acids 1000 mg twice daily, up to 4 g daily as tolerated
	Fibric acid derivatives
Refractory dyslipidemia	Conversion of cyclosporine to tacrolimus
	CNI reduction
	Removal of sirolimus

HMG-CoA, 3-hydroxy-3-methylglutaryl-coenzyme A; CNI, calcineurin inhibitor.

age, family history, Afro-Caribbean ethnicity, obesity, pre-existing impaired glucose tolerance, hepatitis C virus (HCV) infection [37], corticosteroid use, and tacrolimus therapy. Corticosteroid use is the single greatest risk factor, with dosing reductions demonstrating significant reduction in blood sugars [38]. Tacrolimus is more diabetogenic than cyclosporine [4]. Screening should occur at least every 6 months, as decreased survival in post-liver transplantation diabetics is noted at 10 years' follow-up [9]. Increased mortality from infection is noted in post-liver transplantation new-onset diabetics at 10 years' follow-up compared to controls [39]. Immediate post-transplant hyperglycemia is usually managed with insulin. Oral agents can subsequently be considered, with insulin monotherapy preferred in patients with ketosis or symptomatic hyperglycemia. Fasting plasma levels should be checked regularly after liver transplantation, with a goal HgbA1c <7%. Sulfonylureas and metformin are first-line therapy, but should be avoided in severe renal disease. Thiazoidinediones have been found to be effective in liver transplantation patients, but may cause weight gain and are contraindicated in heart failure.

Bone Health

Bone loss and fractures after liver transplantation have multiple predisposing factors, including immunosuppression, nutrition, lifestyle, parathyroid-calcium-vitamin D derangements, and preceding bone disease. The primary factor in osteoporosis after liver transplantation is corticosteroids, with the majority of bone loss and spinal fractures occuring in the first 6 months [40]. In animal models, CNIs have been demonstrated to cause high osteoclast and osteoblast activity, with a net loss of bone mass. MMF, sirolimus, and azathioprine show no effect on bone volume. Treatments are similar to those in the general population. Limited data exist on replacement of sex steroids in liver transplantation patients with osteoporosis. The evaluation and management of metabolic bone loss is outlined in Table 95.2.

Neurological Complications

Cerebral and systemic hemodynamic alterations during transplantation, graft dysfunction, embolic and hemorrhagic cerebrovascular accidents, opportunistic CNS infectious, and immunosuppressant neurotoxicity are all responsible for post-liver transplantation neurological complications. Immunosuppressant neurotoxicity, particularly from supratherapeutic CNIs [41], can produce cerebellar syndromes, posterior leukoencephalopathy, focal neurologic deficits, and even vegetative states. Seizures are also known complications [42].

Headaches, intention tremors, vivid nightmares, peripheral neuropathy, polyneuropathy, sleep disorders, restless leg syndrome, and hearing loss [43] can occur. Meningitis or meningoencephalitis

should be ruled out in headache patients post liver transplantation. Beta-blockers can treat tremors, and minor complications rarely necessitate immunosuppression substitutions.

Malignancy Complications

Malignancy in patients after liver transplantation increases with recipient age, age at transplantation, and time since transplantation [44]. Alcoholic cirrhosis patients are at an increased risk for malignancy. Skin, colon, oropharyngeal, esophageal, and lung cancers in tobacco smokers are more common in liver transplantation patients than in the general population [45]. Lymphomas, primarily PTLDs, are B-cell malignancies associated with EBV and occur most commonly in EBV-seropositive patients receiving aggressive immunosuppression [18]. Standardized intensive cancer screenings have been demonstrated to improve long-term survival in liver transplantation patients [46]. Table 95.3 outlines the surveillance of malignancies following liver transplantation.

Primary Disease Recurrence

Hepatitis C

Hepatitis C recurrence begins with serum HCV RNA levels increasing rapidly after the second postoperative week and peaking at month 4. HCV RNA levels tend to average 10–20 times higher than pretransplant levels. Approximately 2–5% of patients develop severe cholestatic hepatitis, leading to early graft failure. Cirrhosis can occur in 6–30% within 5 years, with approximately 30% of cases showing no fibrosis at 5 years [47]. Progression of fibrosis is influenced by high pretransplant viral loads, living donor transplants, donors over the age of 50, long warm ischemic times, graft steatosis, CMV infections, initial immunosuppression, and multiple episodes of rejection. CNI has an unclear impact on HCV infection, while MMF appears neutral or possibly beneficial in the long term. Data on IL-2 receptor antibodies (sirolimus and everolimus) are mixed.

Diagnosis of HCV recurrence is made initially on elevated liver enzymes, leading to liver biopsy. Histological features include prominent lobular inflammation, focal necrosis, acidophilic bodies, and macrovesicular steatosis. Lymphoid portal tract aggregates, interlobular bile duct damage, macrovesicular steatosis, and lobular infiltrates with apoptotic bodies indicate chronic changes. Differentiation from ACR is difficult, but relies on observed endothelialitis. Prophylactic HCV treatment prior to liver transplantation or in the initial postoperative period is limited by renal function. Liver biopsy demonstrating Metavir fibrosis grade 1 or higher with ongoing necroinflammatory activity suggests the need for therapy. Current therapy includes pegylated interferon and ribavirin for 48 weeks, except in genotype 2 and 3 patients achieving rapid viral clearance. The current wave of new drug therapies for hepatitis C makes the appropriate therapy a moving target, and trials to identify optimal treatments are ongoing. Despite standard therapies, worsened fibrosis and graft failure can occur, requiring retransplantation.

Hepatitis B

Recurrent hepatitis B infection can occur either on initial reperfusion or with delayed exposure from persistent viral replication at extrahepatic sites. Risk factors include high DBV DNA titers and insufficient post-liver transplantation prophylaxis, acquired prophylaxis resistance, and the presence of hepatitis B-e antigen. Mutations in hepatitis B surface antigen or YMDD motif can rarely cause reinfection. When viral loads are detectable at the time of transplant, post-liver transplantation prophylaxis with hepatitis B

Table 95.2 Management of bone loss post liver transplant.

Regular assessment	Serum calcium, phosphorus, thyroid, parathyroid, 25-hydroxyvitamin D levels
	Dietary calcium intake
	Urine calcium (200–300 mg/24 hours)
	Free testosterone (males), menopausal status (females)
	Bone mineral density (T scores)
	Lumbar spine radiographs
Possible treatments	Calcium and vitamin D supplements
	Weight-bearing exercise
	Bisphosphonates (oral or intravenous)
	Calcitonin

Table 95.3 Malignancies and suggested surveillance strategies post liver transplant.

Cancer	Type	Risk factors	Relative risk	Surveillance strategy
Skin (most common)	SCC BCC Melanoma	Fair skin Sun exposure Alcoholic liver disease History of skin cancers	20–70% (carcinomas) 2–5% (melanomas)	Annual dermatological examinations
Oropharynx (opx) Esophagus Lung	SCC Adenocarcinoma	Tobacco use Alcoholic liver disease Barrett's esophagus	3–14% (opx/esophagus) 1.7–2.5% (lung)	1–3 years with appropriate physical exam and imaging
Colon	Adenocarcinoma	UC History of neoplasm	25–30% (UC patients)	Yearly for UC patients Population guidelines for others
Lymphoma	PTLDs, B cell	EBV Thymoglobulin Immunosuppression	10–30%	Periodic follow-up as clinically indicated

SCC, squamous cell carcinoma; BCC, basal cell carcinoma; UC, ulcerative colitis; PTLD, post-transplant lymphoproliferative disorder; EBV, Epstein–Barr virus.

immune globulin (HBIG) and treatment with oral nucleos/tide analogues greatly decrease HBV recurrence. Initial data showed approximately 20% recurrence over 1–2 years using standard therapy [48]. With the availability of newer therapies, including those effective against lamivudine (LAM)-resistant HBV, recurrence rates have improved further. Nucleos/tide analogues, including entecavir and tenofovir, are selected post-transplant for continued remission.

Cholestatic and Autoimmune Liver Disease

Primary biliary cirrhosis (PBC) can recur on average 3–7 years post-liver transplantation, without correlated antimitochondrial antibody titers. Histological granulomatous bile duct destruction is the hallmark. Optimal immunosuppression is controversial. Ursodeoxycholic acid (UDCA) may be considered for histological recurrence [9]. Primary sclerosing cholangitis (PSC) recurs at 9–47%, with the need for endoscopic biliary stenting or dilation as initial treatment options. Retransplantation is required in 15% of cases. Autoimmune hepatitis recurs at 16–46%, with limited data on recurrence times. Risk factors include HLA-DR3-positive recipients of HLA-DR3-negative allografts. Increased immunosuppression is the treatment of choice.

Hepatocellular Carcinoma

Liver transplantation for hepatocellular carcinoma (HCC) can be achieved using defined selection criteria based on certain lesion size and absence of vascular invasion, with recurrence rates of 15–20% [49]. Recurrence risk factors include explant findings of poorly differentiated tumors, satellite lesions, portal vein invasion, tumor rupture, and lymph node involvement. Sirolimus may inhibit tumor recurrence by acting on the mTOR pathway [1]. Sorafenib, a multi-tyrosine kinase and angiogenesis inhibitor, has been shown to improve 3-month survival in post-liver transplantation recurrence [50], and has been demonstrated to be efficacious when combined with sirolimus immunosuppression [51].

Take Home Points

- Appropriate medical management of liver transplantation patients requires multidisciplinary care to produce acceptable outcomes.
- Immunosuppression selection necessitates estimation of expected complications and tolerance.
- Biliary complication management can be percutaneous, endoscopic, or surgical.
- Allograft rejection requires biopsy for diagnosis.

- Infection treatment entails monitoring for drug interactions with antimicrobial therapy and immunosuppression.
- Primary activation or reactivation of a donor or recipient virus can occur, especially Epstein–Barr virus (EBV) and cytomegalovirus (CMV).
- Live or attenuated vaccinations are contraindicated post liver transplantation, with other vaccinations delayed at least 6 months post transplantation.
- Acute and chronic kidney disease (CKD) both impact short- and long-term outcomes.
- Liver transplantation and sequelae independently increase the prevalence of hypertension, diabetes mellitus, dyslipidemia, and obesity.
- Bone loss and fractures should be monitored and treated aggressively.
- Malignancy surveillance is especially important in ulcerative colitis (UC) and alcoholic liver disease.
- Hepatitis C RNA levels tend to average 10–20 times higher than pretransplant levels.
- Cholestatic liver disease can recur without correlated serum titers.
- Liver transplantation for hepatocellular carcinoma (HCC) can be achieved with acceptable recurrence rates.

References

1 Toso C, Merani S, Bigam DL, *et al.* Sirolimus-based immunosuppression is associated with increased survival after liver transplantation for hepatocellular carcinoma. *Hepatology* 2010; **51**: 1237–43.

2 Cutler C, Stevenson K, Kim HT, *et al.* Sirolimus is associated with veno-occlusive disease of the liver after myeloablative allogeneic stem cell transplantation. *Blood* 2008; **112**: 4425–31.

3 Schäffer M, Schier R, Napirei M, *et al.* Sirolimus impairs wound healing. *Langenbecks Arch Surg* 2007; **392**: 297–303.

4 Haddad EM, McAlister VC, Renouf E, *et al.* Cyclosporin versus tacrolimus for liver transplanted patients. *Cochrane Database Syst Rev* 2006(4):CD005161.

5 Scanga AE, Kowdley KV. Management of biliary complications following orthotopic liver transplantation. *Curr Gastroenterol Rep* 2007; **9**: 31–8.

6 Londoño MC, Balderramo D, Cárdenas A. Management of biliary complications after orthotopic liver transplantation: the role of endoscopy. *World J Gastroenterol* 2008; **14**: 493–7.

7 Ayoub WS, Esquivel CO, Martin P. Biliary complications following liver transplantation. *Dig Dis Sci* 2010; **55**: 1540–6.

8 Wiesner RH, Menon KV. Late hepatic allograft dysfunction. *Liver Transpl* 2001; 7: S60–73.

9 Lucey MR, Terrault N, Ojo L, *et al.* Long-term management of the successful adult liver transplant: 2012 practice guideline by the American Association for the Study of Liver Diseases and the American Society of Transplantation. *Liver Transpl* 2013; **19**: 3–26.

10 Schmitt TM, Phillips M, Sawyer RG, *et al.* Anti-thymocyte globulin for the treatment of acute cellular rejection following liver transplantation. *Dig Dis Sci* 2010; **55**: 3224–34.

11 Akamatsu N, Sugawara Y, Tamura S, *et al.* Efficacy of mycofenolate mofetil for steroid-resistant acute rejection after living donor liver transplantation. *World J Gastroenterol* 2006; **12**: 4870–2.

12 Fernandes ML, Lee YM, Sutedja D, *et al.* Treatment of steroid-resistant acute liver transplant rejection with basiliximab. *Transpl Proc* 2005; **37**: 2179–80.

13 Samonakis DN, Germani G, Burroughs AK. Immunosuppression and HCV recurrence after liver transplantation. *J Hepatol* 2012; **56**: 973–83.

14 Torbenson M, Wang J, Nichols L, *et al.* Causes of death in autopsied liver transplantation patients. *Mod Pathol* 1998; **11**: 37–46.

15 Fishman JA, Rubin RH. Infection in organ-transplant recipients. *N Engl J Med* 1998; **338**: 1741–51.

16 Pungpapong S, Alvarez S, Hellinger WC, *et al.* Peritonitis after liver transplantation: incidence, risk factors, microbiology profiles, and outcome. *Liver Transpl* 2006; **12**: 1244–52.

17 Patel R, Portela D, Badley AD, *et al.* Risk factors of invasive *Candida* and non-*Candida* fungal infections after liver transplantation. *Transplantation* 1996; **62**: 926–34.

18 Gottschalk S, Rooney CM, Heslop HE. Post-transplant lymphoproliferative disorders. *Ann Rev Med* 2005; **56**: 29–44.

19 Bilbao I, Charco R, Balsells J, *et al.* Risk factors for acute renal failure requiring dialysis after liver transplantation. *Clin Transpl* 1998; **12**: 123–9.

20 Zand MS, Orloff MS, Abt P, *et al.* High mortality in orthotopic liver transplant recipients who require hemodialysis. *Clin Transpl* 2011; **25**: 213–21.

21 Alessandria C, Ozdogan O, Guevara M, *et al.* MELD score and clinical type predict prognosis in hepatorenal syndrome: relevance to liver transplantation. *Hepatology* 2005; **41**: 1282–9.

22 Ojo AO, Held PJ, Port FK, *et al.* Chronic renal failure after transplantation of a nonrenal organ. *N Engl J Med* 2003; **349**: 931–40.

23 Gonwa TA, Mai ML, Melton LB, *et al.* End-stage renal disease (ESRD) after orthotopic liver transplantation (OLTX) using calcineurin-based immunotherapy: risk of development and treatment. *Transplantation* 2001; **72**: 1934–9.

24 A comparison of tacrolimus (FK 506) and cyclosporine for immunosuppression in liver transplantation. The US Multicenter FK506 Liver Study Group. *N Engl J Med* 1994; **331**: 1110–15.

25 Neff GW, Montalbano M, Slapak-Green G, *et al.* Sirolimus therapy in orthotopic liver transplant recipients with calcineurin inhibitor related chronic renal insufficiency. *Transpl Proc* 2003; **35**: 3029–31.

26 Ciccarelli O, Kaczmarek B, Roggen F, *et al.* Long-term medical complications and quality of life in adult recipients surviving 10 years or more after liver transplantation. *Acta Gastroenterol Belg* 2005; **68**: 323–30.

27 Pruthi J, Medkiff KA, Esrason KT, *et al.* Analysis of causes of death in liver transplant recipients who survived more than 3 years. *Liver Transpl* 2001; **7**: 811–15.

28 Canzanello VJ, Textor SC, Taler SJ, *et al.* Late hypertension after liver transplantation: a comparison of cyclosporine and tacrolimus (FK 506). *Liver Transpl Surg* 1998; **4**: 328–34.

29 Taler SJ, Textor SC, Canzanello VJ, *et al.* Loss of nocturnal blood pressure fall after liver transplantation during immunosuppressive therapy. *Am J Hypertens* 1995; **8**: 598–605.

30 Neal DA, Tom BD, Luan J, *et al.* Is there disparity between risk and incidence of cardiovascular disease after liver transplant? *Transplantation* 2004; **77**: 93–9.

31 Laish I, Braun M, Mor E, *et al.* Metabolic syndrome in liver transplant recipients: prevalence, risk factors, and association with cardiovascular events. *Liver Transpl* 2011; **17**: 15–22.

32 Roy A, Kneteman N, Lilly L, *et al.* Tacrolimus as intervention in the treatment of hyperlipidemia after liver transplant. *Transplantation* 2006; **82**: 494–500.

33 Bianchi G, Marchesini G, Marzocchi R, *et al.* Metabolic syndrome in liver transplantation: relation to etiology and immunosuppression. *Liver Transpl* 2008; **14**: 1648–54.

34 Canzanello VJ, Schwartz L, Taler SJ, *et al.* Evolution of cardiovascular risk after liver transplantation: a comparison of cyclosporine A and tacrolimus (FK506). *Liver Transpl Surg* 1997; **3**: 1–9.

35 Everhart JE, Lombardero M, Lake JR, *et al.* Weight change and obesity after liver transplantation: incidence and risk factors. *Liver Transpl Surg* 1998; **4**: 285–96.

36 Stegall MD, Everson G, Schroter G, *et al.* Metabolic complications after liver transplantation. Diabetes, hypercholesterolemia, hypertension, and obesity. *Transplantation* 1995; **60**: 1057–60.

37 Bigam DL, Pennington JJ, Carpentier A, *et al.* Hepatitis C-related cirrhosis: a predictor of diabetes after liver transplantation. *Hepatology* 2000; **32**: 87–90.

38 Stegall MD, Everson GT, Schroter G, *et al.* Prednisone withdrawal late after adult liver transplantation reduces diabetes, hypertension, and hypercholesterolemia without causing graft loss. *Hepatology* 1997; **25**: 173–7.

39 Moon JI, Barbeito R, Faradji RN, *et al.* Negative impact of new-onset diabetes mellitus on patient and graft survival after liver transplantation: long-term follow up. *Transplantation* 2006; **82**: 1625–8.

40 Haagsma EB, Thijn CJ, Post JG, *et al.* Bone disease after orthotopic liver transplantation. *J Hepatol* 1988; **6**: 94–100.

41 Vizzini G, Asaro M, Miraglia R, *et al.* Changing picture of central nervous system complications in liver transplant recipients. *Liver Transpl* 2011; **17**: 1279–85.

42 Sancr FH, Sotiropoulos GC, Gu Y, *et al.* Severe neurological events following liver transplantation. *Arch Med Res* 2007; **38**: 75–9.

43 Rifai K, Kirchner GI, Bahr MJ, *et al.* A new side effect of immunosuppression: high incidence of hearing impairment after liver transplantation. *Liver Transpl* 2006; **12**: 411–15.

44 Sethi A, Stravitz RT. Review article: medical management of the liver transplant recipient – a primer for non-transplant doctors. *Aliment Pharmacol Ther* 2007; **25**: 229–45.

45 Chak E, Saab S. Risk factors and incidence of de novo malignancy in liver transplant recipients: a systematic review. *Liver Int* 2010; **30**: 1247–58.

46 Finkenstedt A, Graziadei IW, Oberaigner W, *et al.* Extensive surveillance promotes early diagnosis and improved survival of de novo malignancies in liver transplant recipients. *Am J Transpl* 2009; **9**: 2355–61.

47 Charlton M. Approach to recurrent hepatitis C following liver transplantation. *Curr Gastroenterol Rep* 2007; **9**: 23–30.

48 Mohanty SR, Cotler SJ. Management of hepatitis B in liver transplant patients. *J Clin Gastroenterol* 2005; **39**: 58–63.

49 Welker MW, Bechstein WO, Zeuzem S, Trojan J. Recurrent hepatocellular carcinoma after liver transplantation – an emerging clinical challenge. *Transpl Int* 2013; **26**: 109–18.

50 Llovet JM, Ricci S, Mazzaferro V, *et al.* Sorafenib in advanced hepatocellular carcinoma. *N Engl J Med* 2008; **359**: 378–90.

51 Gomez-Martin C, Bustamante J, Castroagudin JF, *et al.* Efficacy and safety of sorafenib in combination with mammalian target of rapamycin inhibitors for recurrent hepatocellular carcinoma after liver transplantation. *Liver Transpl* 2012; **18**: 45–52.

CHAPTER 95

Organ Allocation Policy: Practical Issues and Challenges to the Gastroenterologist

Jessica Yu[1] and Pratima Sharma[2]

[1] Division of Gastroenterology, Stanford University, Palo Alto, CA
[2] Division of Gastroenterology, University of Michigan, Ann Arbor, MI, USA

Summary

Current liver allocation policy is based upon urgency. The Model for End-stage Liver Disease (MELD) score measures the waitlist mortality risk among candidates with decompensated cirrhosis. Though the MELD score is a very well validated index of mortality, however, it is not suitable for allocation among certain subgroups of patients. This chapter highlights the liver allocation in those subgroups, as well as the common challenges faced by gastroenterologists in day-to-day clinical practice.

Introduction

Liver transplantation has evolved from a high-risk experimental procedure to life-saving standard of care for patients with decompensated cirrhosis, with a 1- and 5-year post-transplant patient survival of 90 and 75%, respectively [1].

Allocation

In the United States, the MELD score was adopted as an allocation tool for deceased donor liver allografts in February of 2002 [2]. The MELD score was originally developed from a cohort of 231 patients receiving transjugular intrahepatic portosystemic shunts (TIPS) for variceal bleeding or refractory ascites in order to predict 3-month mortality. It was subsequently validated in independent datasets of patients with excellent performance characteristics, including hospitalized (C-statistic 0.87) and ambulatory patients and those with cholestatic (C-statistic 0.80) and non-cholestatic (C-statistic 0.87) liver disease. Among the waitlisted patients, MELD score was better than Child–Turcotte–Pugh score in predicting 3-month mortality risk [3–5].

Based upon the readily available, objective laboratory values of serum creatinine, serum bilirubin, and International Normalized Ratio (INR) of prothrombin time, MELD score can be calculated as follows:

$$MELD = 10 \times (0.957 \text{ loge creatinine} + 0.378 \text{ loge bilirubin} + 1.12 \text{ loge INR} + 0.643)$$

The MELD score runs from 6 to 40. Candidates with calculated MELD score >40 are assigned a MELD score of 40. The lower bounds of serum bilirubin and serum creatinine are set at 1 mg/dL to avoid the non-negative integer. The upper bound of MELD is kept at 4 mg/dL to avoid giving undue advantage to patients with renal insufficiency. Candidates who have received renal replacement therapy in the previous week are given a creatinine of 4 mg/dL [6].

The Organ Procurement and Transplantation Network (OPTN), the governing body overseeing organ transplantation, requires that a patient's MELD score be reassessed and recertified at the transplant center. MELD scores must be submitted periodically for recertification, with updates at more frequent intervals required at higher MELDs [6] (Table 96.1). Recertification must be based on the most recent clinical information (e.g., laboratory test results and diagnosis), and the dates of laboratory tests must be given. Laboratory values must not be older than the value specified in Table 96.1. Failure to recertify a patient's MELD score in accordance with the schedule may result in reassignment to their previous lower MELD score. The candidate may remain at that previous lower score for the period allowed based upon the recertification schedule for the previous lower score, minus the time spent in the uncertified score. If the candidate remains uncertified past the recertification due date for the previous lower score, they will be assigned a MELD score of 6 [6].

Distribution

The United Network for Organ Sharing (UNOS) divides the United States into eleven geographic regions (see Chapter 93, Figure 93.1), each of which is fed by several local Donor Service Areas (DSAs). A DSA is a distinct, non-overlapping geographic area served by each of the 58 federally certified organ procurement organizations (OPOs). DSAs may include one or more transplant programs for a given organ and one or more donor hospitals. Organs are offered locally (in the specific DSA) and regionally, initially to those designated status 1A, which includes acute liver failure (ALF) with expected life expectancy of less than 1 week without a liver transplantation. Primary non-function of a transplant liver, an anhepatic candidate, and hepatic artery thrombosis within 7 days of transplant or acute decompensated Wilson's disease also qualifies as status 1A. After this, organs are offered to status 1B patients, who are pediatric patients (<17 years old). Adults and pediatric candidates with chronic liver disease are then offered organs in

Practical Gastroenterology and Hepatology Board Review Toolkit, Second Edition. Edited by Nicholas J. Talley, Kenneth R. DeVault, Michael B. Wallace, Bashar A. Aqel and Keith D. Lindor.
© 2016 John Wiley & Sons, Ltd. Published 2016 by John Wiley & Sons, Ltd. Companion website: www.practicalgastrohep.com

Table 96.1   MELD recertification schedule.

MELD score or status	Recertification	Laboratory values must be no older than
Status 1A	Every 7 days	48 hours
MELD ≥25	Every 7 days	48 hours
MELD 24–18	Every 1 month	7 days
MELD 17–11	Every 3 months	14 days
MELD 10–6	Every 12 months	30 days

Table 96.3   Evolution of the HCC MELD exception score since 2002.

	Feb 2002– Apr 2003	Apr 2003– Jan 2004	Jan 2004– Jan 2005	Jan 2005– Sept 2015
Stage I (T1) (one tumor of <2 cm)	15% risk MELD 24	8% risk MELD 20	Lab MELD	Lab MELD
Stage II (T2) (one tumor of 2–5 cm OR two or three tumors, the largest <3 cm)	30% risk MELD 29	15% risk MELD 24	15% risk MELD 24	15% risk MELD 22

descending MELD/Pediatric End-stage Liver Disease (PELD) order [6].

Modifications in Distribution Scheme

Survival benefit is defined as the risk ratio of post-transplant mortality to waitlist mortality. A risk ratio <1 represents survival benefit, whereas a risk ratio ≥1 represents harm from liver transplantation. Merion *et al.* [7] demonstrated that patients with MELD ≥18 with 1 year of post-transplant follow-up derived survival benefit from liver transplantation, whereas patients with MELD scores <15 had significant harm from liver transplantation, because their post-transplant mortality risk was higher than the waitlist mortality risk. This observation led to the implementation of the "Share 15" rule to improve access to deceased donor allograft for sicker patients in a given region.

More recently, in June 2013, to further improve the access to deceased donor organs among the sickest group of patients (MELD score ≥35) [8, 9], the "Share 35" rule was implemented in the distribution sequence. In this scheme, organs are offered locally and regionally to those with MELD ≥35, then locally to those with MELD 34–15, then regionally to those with MELD 34–15, then nationally to status 1A/1B candidates and to those with MELD ≥15, and finally to those with MELD <15. Table 96.2 summarizes the current allocation scheme for adult liver transplantation candidates.

MELD Exceptions

Despite the ability of the MELD score to objectively estimate mortality risk among candidates awaiting liver transplantation, there are several conditions for which waitlist mortality risk cannot be estimated based upon their intrinsic liver disease or MELD score alone. Waitlist mortality risk is deemed to be highest among candidates with fulminant hepatic failure. These candidates get the highest

priority, above MELD score. Candidates with hepatocellular carcinoma (HCC), hepatopulmonary syndrome (HPS), portopulmonary syndrome, familial amyloid polyneuropathy (FAP), cystic fibrosis, hilar cholangiocarincoma, or primary hyperoxaluria are prioritized through the MELD exception mechanism [10, 11].

Hepatocellular Carcinoma

Candidates who meet the Milan criteria (single lesion 2–5 cm in diameter or three lesions <3 cm diameter) without evidence of extrahepatic spread are eligible for MELD exception. These patients are assigned a MELD score of 22 and are eligible for an increase of 10% mortality risk every 3 months. Table 96.3 shows the evolution of the MELD exception score for HCC. Locoregional therapies should be considered for patients listed with MELD exception scores, to prevent progression of HCC [6].

HCC candidates exceeding the Milan criteria are not eligible for exception and are listed with their lab MELD score. These candidates may be considered for downstaging based upon their tumor burden. Once the tumor is downstaged, they may qualify for exception points based on review by the regional review board (RRB). Living donor liver transplantation is another option for these candidates.

Since October 8th, 2015, the allocation for HCC is revised. Under current HCC policy amendment, eligible candidates with decompensated cirrhosis and HCC who meet Milan criteria get listed with their calculated MELD score for 6 months. After six months they are assigned a MELD score of 28. The maximum value of exception scores for these candidates are capped at 34.

Hepatopulmonary Syndrome

Portal hypertension with evidence of an intrapulmonary shunt resulting in hypoxemia is associated with increased mortality. Candidates with evidence of intrapulmonary shunting and a documented PaO_2 <60 mmHg on room air may qualify for a MELD score of 22. The score will increase by 10% mortality equivalent every 3 months if PaO_2 remains <60 mmHg [6]. HPS is reversible after liver transplantation.

Cholangiocarcinoma

Candidates may qualify for exception points for an unresectable hilar cholangiocarcinoma smaller than 3 cm without intra- or extrahepatic spread. The diagnosis must be verified by cholangiogram and/or CA 19-9 of 100, with biopsy or cytology results confirming diagnosis. The center caring for these candidates must submit a written protocol of patient care, including selection criteria, neoadjuvant therapy before transplantation, and operative staging, to the OPTN committee [6].

Table 96.2   Evolution of the allocation scheme for adult liver transplantation candidates.

Feb 2002–Jul 2005	Jul 2005–Jun 2013 Share 15	Jun 2013–Present Share 35
Local: Status 1	Local: Status 1a/1b	Local: Status 1a/1b
Regional: Status 1	Regional: Status 1a/1b	Regional: Status 1a/1b
Local: MELD	Local: MELD ≥15	Local: MELD ≥35
Regional: MELD	Regional: MELD ≥15	Regional: MELD ≥35
National: Status 1	Local: MELD <15	Local: MELD 34–15
National: MELD	Regional: MELD <15	Regional: MELD 34–15
	National: Status 1	Local: MELD <15
	National: All others, in descending order	Regional: MELD <15
		National: Status 1
		National: All others, in descending order

Cystic Fibrosis

Cystic fibrosis leads to the development of cholestatic disease, much like primary biliary cirrhosis. Patients with cystic fibrosis with both liver and pulmonary disease have greater mortality than can be estimated by the progression of the liver disease alone. Therefore, if they have signs of reduced pulmonary function and a forced expiratory volume in 1 second (FEV1) <40%, they may qualify for exception points.

Familial Amyloid Polyneuropathy

FAP results from a mutation of a hepatic enzyme, which can lead to amyloid deposition in cardiac, neurologic, and ophthalmologic tissue. Those affected may thus benefit from liver transplantation regardless of their MELD score. Candidates must have a diagnosis that includes an echocardiogram (ECG) showing ejection fraction >40%, identification of the trans-thyretin (TTR) gene mutation, and biopsy-proven amyloid of the involved organ in order to be eligible for MELD exception [6]. Liver transplantation is the only curative option for FAP, and prevents the progression of symptoms.

Primary Hyperoxaluria

The liver plays a vital role in the metabolism of oxalate. Primary hyperoxaluria can result from genetic mutations leading to abnormal production of the enzymes responsible for oxalate metabolism. It can lead to renal failure. Candidates with alanine : glyoxylate aminotransferase (AGT) enzyme deficiency proven by liver biopsy (sample analysis and/or genetic analysis) and listed for liver–kidney transplant can qualify for a MELD exception [6]. Unlike those with other conditions, primary hyperoxaluria candidates receive a MELD exception score of 28.

Portal Pulmonary Syndrome

Pulmonary hypertension in the setting of liver disease is associated with worse outcomes. Candidates must have documented elevated mean pulmonary arterial pressure (MPAP) and pulmonary vascular resistance (PVR) prior to treatment, with a subsequent fall in MPAP <35 mmHG and PVR <400 dynes/s/cm^2. As persistently elevated MPAP is associated with poor outcome after liver transplantation, MELD exception is given only if MPAP remains <35 mmHG with treatment [6, 10].

Other Exceptions

Though many conditions qualify for standard MELD exceptions, the current exceptions are not all-inclusive. An illustrative example is provided by recurrent cholangitis. Structural biliary disease, such as primary sclerosing cholangitis (PSC), can lead to recurrent episodes of cholangitis prior to progression to cirrhosis. As cholangitis and bacteremia can lead to ineligibility for liver transplant, recurrent cholangitis can be considered for MELD exception by an RRB. Unfortunately, there are no standard exception criteria between RRBs. Consensus guidelines recommend exception points be awarded for patients with two or more episodes of cholangitis within a 6-month period or with septic complication of cholangitis. Cholangitis should not be related to iatrogenic etiology or biliary stent and should occur in patients who have been on antibiotics. This should be supported with evidence of the structural biliary disease not amenable to other therapy and with culture results confirming bacteremia and antibiotic failure [12].

Recurrent hepatic encephalopathy, pruritus, and gastrointestinal (GI) bleed associated with portal hypertension have been debated as criteria for MELD exception. A request for exception can be made with some of these conditions. Such requests are handled by RRBs on a case-by-case basis.

Practical Challenges

Allocation and Renal Dysfunction

Pre-liver transplantation renal failure has been an important predictor of waitlist mortality and of post-liver transplantation morbidity and mortality. Though policymakers bound the upper limit of creatinine to 4 mg/dL to curtail the undue advantage given to patients with renal insufficiency or on renal replacement therapy, serum creatinine is still the overweighted MELD component [13]. Pre-renal etiologies, including hepatorenal syndrome and acute tubular necrosis, are the most common causes of pre-liver transplantation renal dysfunction. GI bleed, infection, dehydration, and hypotension are among the major precipitating causes of acute kidney injury (AKI). The management of AKI and hepatorenal syndrome is discussed in Chapter 87.

Simple measures can be taken to prevent AKI among patients with decompensated cirrhosis. Renal functions should be frequently and closely monitored while on diuretics, especially after a dose change. Use of intravenous (IV) albumin on day 1 (1.5 mg/kg body weight) and day 3 (1 g/kg body weight), along with appropriate use of antibiotics, prevents AKI and decreases mortality from 29 to 10% among patients with spontaneous bacterial peritonitis (SBP). A more recent study has shown that albumin should be given when the serum creatinine is >1 mg/dL, blood urea nitrogen (BUN) >30 mg/dL, or total bilirubin >4 mg/dL but is not necessary in patients who do not meet these criteria [14]. A 5-day course of antibiotics among patients with decompensated cirrhosis and GI bleed prevents SBP and, therefore, decreases AKI. Albumin infusion of 6–8 g per liter of fluid removed after a large-volume paracentesis (≥5 L) appears to improve survival and is recommended in American Association for the Study of Liver Diseases (AASLD) practice guidelines [14, 15]. Non-steroidal anti-inflammatory drugs (NSAIDs), angiotensin-converting enzyme (ACE) inhibitors, and angiotensin receptor blockers (ARBs) should be avoided in patients with refractory ascites. Systemic hypotension and hyperkalemia often complicate ACE and ARB use [15].

Allocation and Hyponatremia

Splanchnic vasodilation, a hallmark of portal hypertension, leads to activation of endogenous vasoconstrictors, including antidiuretic hormones, and promotes water retention and hyponatremia. The prevalence of hyponatremia in patients with cirrhosis and ascites is high. Many studies have shown that pre-transplant hyponatremia, defined as serum sodium ≤134 mMol/L, is associated with high waitlist mortality among liver transplantation candidates. Kim et al. [16] showed that the effect of hyponatremia on waitlist mortality gradually diminishes as the MELD score increases, and concluded that adding serum sodium to the MELD score could reduce waitlist mortality by as much as 7%.

Data regarding short- and long-term mortality following liver transplantation among patients with pre-liver transplantation hyponatremia are conflicting. Many single-center studies suggest that the presence of pre-liver transplantation hyponatremia is associated with a high rate of post-liver transplantation neurologic disorders, infectious complications, prolonged hospitalization, and renal failure [17, 18]. Management of hyponatremia is discussed in the management of ascites.

Addition of serum sodium to MELD, as proposed recently by the OPTN Liver and Intestine Committee, might increase access to liver transplantation for low-MELD patients with hyponatremia. It would provide 1–13 additional MELD points, depending on the serum sodium value at a given MELD score. For example, a candidate with MELD 12 and serum sodium 125 mMol/L would receive 11 additional points for a total MELD score of 23. Though the addition of serum sodium points to the MELD score might improve waitlist mortality among low-MELD patients by providing them with enhanced access to donor organs, the effect of hyponatremia on the survival benefit of liver transplantation has not been studied.

Infections

A thorough infection workup should be performed if a candidate develops decompensation in terms of worsening synthetic function, mental status changes, fevers, GI bleed, or renal dysfunction, or if there is a rapid increase in their MELD score. Infected candidates are usually put on hold for transplant; they can be reactivated after completion of treatment. Candidates with PSC and recurrent cholangitis should be put on suppressive antibiotics. Magnetic resonance imaging (MRI)/ magnetic resonance cholangiopancreatography (MRCP) should be performed to assess for dominant strictures or cholangiocarcinoma in these patients. As already discussed, they may qualify for a MELD exception score.

Portal Vein Thrombosis

Portal vein thrombosis (PVT) is common, with a prevalence of 8–25% among liver transplantation recipients. It is associated with the severity of the patient's liver disease, and can lead to complications such as intestinal ischemia, worsening of portal hypertension, and ascites. PVT on ultrasound Doppler study should be confirmed by a dynamic study such as magnetic resonance venogram or computed tomographic (CT) venogram. Patients may be deemed untransplantable for technical reasons if the clot is extensive and extends to the superior mesenteric vein and splenic vein. Anticoagulation may be considered if patients with PVT have evidence of intestinal ischemia. Candidates with HCC and evidence of tumor thrombus of the portal vein are deemed not to be transplant candidates. PVT is also an independent risk factor for post-transplant mortality [19].

Conclusion

MELD-based allocation in the United States has contributed to transparency of the allocation system and the use of objective elements. It is important to understand that there are other factors beyond the components of MELD that contribute to waitlist mortality. Evidence-based incremental refinements in the current allocation process may improve waitlist and post-transplant outcomes.

Take Home Points

- Liver allocation in United States is prioritized based upon "urgency" and measured by Model for End-Stage Liver Disease (MELD) score.
- The MELD score consists of serum creatinine, serum bilirubin, and International Normalization Ratio (INR) of prothrombin time.
- MELD scores must be reassessed and recertified on a frequency determined by the Organ Procurement and Transplantation Network (OPTN).

- The goal of the "Share 35" distribution scheme is to enhance organ availability to the sickest candidates (MELD ≥35) by promoting regional sharing of deceased donor livers.
- Candidates with hepatocellular carcinoma (HCC), hepatopulmonary syndrome (HPS), cholangiocarcinoma, cystic fibrosis, familial amyloid polyneuropathy (FAP), primary hyperoxaluria, and portopulmonary syndrome are considered for MELD exception if they meet the OPTN criteria.
- Renal failure is associated with high waitlist and post-liver transplantation mortality.
- Measures should be taken to prevent acute kidney injury (AKI) in pre-transplant candidates.
- Hyponatremia is also associated with increased waitlist mortality.
- Portal vein thrombosis (PVT) should be confirmed by computed tomographic (CT) or magnetic resonance venogram, as extensive PVT may preclude patients from transplant.

Acknowledgement

Dr. Sharma is supported by National Institutes of Health (NIH) grant KO8 DK-088946.

Videos of interest to readers of this chapter can be found by visiting the companion website at:

http://www.practicalgastrohep.com/

96.1 Pancreatic cancer fine needle injection of antitumor necrosis factor (TNF) drug.
96.2 Pancreatic cancer endoscopic ultrasound fine needle aspiration.
96.3 Pancreatic cyst fine needle aspiration.
96.4 Pancreatic cyst fine needle aspiration.
96.5 Rectal cancer endoscopic ultrasound Stage T3, N1.

References

1 Kim WR, Stock PG, Smith JM, *et al*. OPTN/SRTR 2011 Annual Data Report: liver. *Am J Transplant* 2013; **13**(Suppl. 1): 73–102.

2 Wiesner RH, McDiarmid SV, Kamath PS, *et al*. MELD and PELD: application of survival models to liver allocation. *Liver Transpl* 2001; **7**(7): 567–80.

3 Malinchoc M, Kamath PS, Gordon FD, *et al*. A model to predict poor survival in patients undergoing transjugular intrahepatic portosystemic shunts. *Hepatology* 2000; **31**(4): 864–71.

4 Kamath PS, Wiesner RH, Malinchoc M, *et al*. A model to predict survival in patients with end-stage liver disease. *Hepatology* 2001; **33**(2): 464–70.

5 Wiesner R, Edwards E, Freeman R, *et al*. Model for end-stage liver disease (MELD) and allocation of donor livers. *Gastroenterology* 2003; **124**(1): 91–6.

6 Organ Procurement and Transplantation Network (OPTN) Policies. Policy 9: Allocation of Livers and Liver-Intestines. Available from: https://optn.transplant.hrsa.gov/media/1200/optn_policies.pdf#nameddest=Policy_09 (last accessed February 15, 2016).

7 Merion RM, Schaubel DE, Dykstra DM, *et al*. The survival benefit of liver transplantation. *Am J Transpl* 2005; **5**(2): 307–13.

8 Sharma P, Schaubel DE, Gong Q, *et al*. End-stage liver disease candidates at the highest model for end-stage liver disease scores have higher wait-list mortality than status-1A candidates. *Hepatology* 2012; **55**(1): 192–8.

9 Washburn K, Pomfret E, Roberts J. Liver allocation and distribution: possible next steps. *Liver Transpl* 2011; **17**(9): 1005–12.

10 Freeman RB Jr., Gish RG, Harper A, *et al.* Model for end-stage liver disease (MELD) exception guidelines: results and recommendations from the MELD Exception Study Group and Conference (MESSAGE) for the approval of patients who need liver transplantation with diseases not considered by the standard MELD formula. *Liver Transpl* 2006; **12**(12 Suppl. 3): S128–36.

11 Wiesner R, Lake JR, Freeman RB, Gish RG. Model for end-stage liver disease (MELD) exception guidelines. *Liver Transpl* 2006; **12**(12 Suppl. 3): S85–7.

12 Gores GJ, Gish RG, Shrestha R, Wiesner RH. Model for end-stage liver disease (MELD) exception for bacterial cholangitis. *Liver Transpl* 2006; **12**(12 Suppl. 3): S91–2.

13 Sharma P, Schaubel DE, Sima CS, *et al.* Re-weighting the model for end-stage liver disease score components. *Gastroenterology* 2008; **135**(5): 1575–81.

14 Sigal SH, Stanca CM, Fernandez J, *et al.* Restricted use of albumin for spontaneous bacterial peritonitis. *Gut* 2007; **56**(4): 597–9.

15 Runyon BA. Introduction to the revised American Association for the Study of Liver Diseases Practice Guideline management of adult patients with ascites due to cirrhosis 2012. *Hepatology* 2013; **57**(4): 1651–3.

16 Kim WR, Biggins SW, Kremers WK, *et al.* Hyponatremia and mortality among patients on the liver-transplant waiting list. *N Engl J Med* 2008; **359**(10): 1018–26.

17 Heuman DM, Abou-Assi SG, Habib A, *et al.* Persistent ascites and low serum sodium identify patients with cirrhosis and low MELD scores who are at high risk for early death. *Hepatology* 2004; **40**(4): 802–10.

18 Londono MC, Guevara M, Rimola A, *et al.* Hyponatremia impairs early posttransplantation outcome in patients with cirrhosis undergoing liver transplantation. *Gastroenterology* 2006; **130**(4): 1135–43.

19 Englesbe MJ, Schaubel DE, Cai S, *et al.* Portal vein thrombosis and liver transplant survival benefit. *Liver Transpl* 2010; **16**(8): 999–1005.

CHAPTER 97

Endoscopic Ultrasound

Thomas J. Savides

Division of Gastroenterology, University of California, San Diego, CA, USA

Summary

Endoscopic ultrasound (EUS) has become critically important in evaluating a variety of pancreatic, small-bowel, and colorectal diseases. In the absence of distant metastatic disease, locoregional EUS staging of pancreatic, ampullary, and rectal cancer can impact management. EUS is excellent in the evaluation of benign pancreatic lesions such as pancreatic cysts, chronic pancreatitis, and autoimmune pancreatitis. EUS with fine-needle aspiration (FNA) is especially accurate in obtaining diagnostic cytologic material for pancreatic lesions. Anal EUS is one of the best modalities for evaluating prior obstetrical trauma as a cause of fecal incontinence. Interventional EUS techniques are increasingly being used for therapies such as pancreatic pseudocyst drainage, injection therapy to assist pancreatic cancer treatment, and transcolonic drainage of perirectal fluid collections.

Case

A 65-year-old woman presents with a 1-month history of diarrhea with floating oil droplets. The referring gastroenterologist found she had a normal colonoscopy and a normal esophagogastroduodenoscopy (EGD) with duodenal biopsies. In the 2 weeks since the initial evaluation, she has developed dark urine and unintentionally lost 6.8 kg (15 pounds). Pancreatic EUS reveals a 3 cm mass in the pancreatic head, causing upstream dilation of both the bile duct and pancreas and abutment of the superior mesenteric vein (SMV). EUS-guided transduodenal FNA reveals pancreatic adenocarcinoma. In addition to being referred to a pancreatic surgeon, she is started on oral pancreatic enzymes before meals, which resolves her diarrhea and fecal incontinence.

Introduction

EUS incorporates an ultrasound transducer on the tip of an endoscope. It can be performed with a radial echoendoscope, which provide images perpendicular to the axis of the scope and corresponds to the axial computed tomography (CT) or magnetic resonance imaging (MRI) slices in the rectum, esophagus, and stomach, or with a linear-array EUS scope, which provides an image parallel to the shaft of the endoscope and allows real-time visualization of needle aspiration or therapeutic maneuvers. This chapter will focus on pancreatic, small-bowel, and colorectal EUS.

Pancreatic EUS

Pancreatic Cancer

EUS can detect pancreatic masses in patients with abnormal CT scans or unexplained biliary obstructions (Figure 97.1). When a solid pancreatic mass is identified, EUS FNA has a sensitivity and specificity of 85 and 95%, respectively, for diagnosing malignancy [1]. A large multicenter study found that when solid pancreatic masses undergo EUS FNA, the overall cancer diagnosis yield is 72%, with variation among endosonographers possibly related to the underlying rates of chronic pancreatitis in the population and to technical, cytopathology, and operator issues [2].

Once pancreatic cancer is diagnosed or highly suspected, the next important step is to dertmine resectability. CT or MRI scan should first be obtained to exclude distant metastases. Though traditionally invasion of the superior mesenteric artery (SMA), SMV, or portal vein has been considered unresectable for cure, recently some expert pancreatic surgeons have attempted resection with vascular reconstruction in select patients [3]. The accuracy of EUS for determining the resectability of pancreatic cancers ranges from 62 to 93%, and recent studies comparing EUS to CT and MRI have not yielded a clearly superior test for determining respectability [4].

Interventional EUS can play a role in the palliation of unresectable pancreatic cancer patients. EUS fine-needle injection can implant metal radiopaque fiducials to assist stereotactic radiation therapy, and can inject experimental chemotherapy directly into the lesion for localized treatment [5,6].

Pancreatic Cysts

Pancreatic cysts are an increasingly common problem, being frequently found as incidental lesions. Approximately 13.5% of abdominal MRI scans will incidentally detect small pancreatic cysts (average size 7 mm) [7]. Serial CT scan studies usually show no change in these lesions over a several-year period, suggesting the natural history of most small, incidentally found cysts is benign. The challenge is to determine which cysts are actually cancer or could turn into cancer.

Pancreatic cystic lesions are described in detail in Chapter 64, but briefly, they can be separated into three categories: those that are benign (simple cysts, pseudocysts, serous cystadenomas), those that are cancerous (adenocarcinomas, endocrine tumors), and those that have malignant potential (cystadenomas, branch-type intraductal papillary mucinous neoplasms (IPMNs), main-duct IPMNs). The

Practical Gastroenterology and Hepatology Board Review Toolkit, Second Edition. Edited by Nicholas J. Talley, Kenneth R. DeVault, Michael B. Wallace, Bashar A. Aqel and Keith D. Lindor.

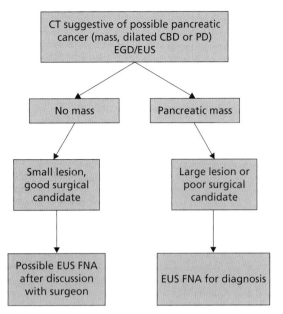

Figure 97.1 Algorithm for an EUS-guided approach to a suspected pancreatic mass. CT, computed tomography; CBD, common bile duct; PD, pancreatic duct; EGD, esophagogastroduodenoscopy; EUS, endoscopic ultrasound; FNA, fine-needle aspiration.

natural history of lesions with malignant potential is unknown, and it is quite likely that for many patients the risk of developing a life-threatening cancer is less than the risk of surgical cyst resection.

EUS is extremely useful in the initial evaluation of pancreatic cysts, as it can determine whether there is an associated mass that is likely to represent cancer. EUS FNA can aspirate cysts to obtain fluid for carcinoembryonic antigen (CEA), amylase, and cytology, which can help distinguish between mucinous and non-mucinous lesions. However, the actual utility of pancreatic cyst aspiration is uncertain as the results are often confusing to interpret and cannot indicate which patient will go on to develop cancer. Pancreatic cyst aspiration is associated with rare risks of bleeding, pancreatitis, and cyst infection. If a pancreatic cyst is aspirated, it is common practice to aspirate it completely and provide the patient with intravenous (IV) and/or oral antibiotics for 3–7 days in order to reduce complications. Benign-appearing cysts can generally be observed with serial imaging studies.

Large and/or symptomatic pancreatic pseudocysts can be safely and effectively drained with EUS-guided transgastric stent placement to form a cystgastrostomy [8].

Chronic Pancreatitis
The use of EUS in the evaluation of chronic pancreatitis is debated, and true accuracy estimates are hampered by the lack of a gold standard. EUS findings suggestive of chronic pancreatitis include stones/calcifications, echogenic foci, echogenic stranding, hyperechoic main pancreatic duct, dilated pancreatic duct, irregular pancreatic duct, visible pancreatic size branches, lobular echotexture, and cysts. Agreement among expert endosonographers is moderate for diagnosis of "early" chronic pancreatitis [9], except in the presence of obvious pancreatic stones/calcifications, which can generally be diagnosed with other, less invasive imaging studies. Due to its high sensitivity, the main role of EUS is likely to exclude chronic pancreatitis in patients with chronic, pancreatic-type, epigastric pain.

Autoimmune Pancreatitis
Autoimmune pancreatitis is an infrequent, but increasingly recognized, cause of biliary obstruction. It is important to consider, because it is treated with steroids rather than surgery. Most patients are males over the age of 55. The most commonly described CT finding is a diffusely swollen, sausage-shaped pancreas with a narrowed pancreatic duct, but the CT can also find pancreatic masses and isolated biliary strictures. EUS is very helpful in identifying possible autoimmune pancreatitis, because the pancreas will appear diffusely hypoechoic and enlarged. EUS FNA with core biopsy and serum immunoglobulin G (IgG) subtype 4 levels support the diagnosis of autoimmune pancreatitis [10, 11].

Pancreatic Endocrine Tumors
Pancreatic endocrine tumors are classified as either functional or non-functional, depending upon their production of symptomatic hormones (insulin, gastrin, glucagon, vasoactive intestinal peptide, somatostatin). The majority of pancreatic endocrine tumors do not cause endocrine symptoms, but are found either due to pain or on an incidental imaging study. EUS is extremely useful for detecting small, symptomatic, hormone-producing pancreatic endocrine tumors, such as insulinomas or gastrinomas; confirmation is by EUS FNA cytology.

Small-Bowel EUS

Ampullary Adenomas and Cancers
EUS can accurately assess ampullary adenomas or superficial ampullary adenocarcinomas that are being considered for possible endoscopic resection. If EUS shows extension into the bile duct, pancreatic duct, or peripancreatic lymph nodes, then invasive cancer should be suspected and surgical resection should be considered, rather than endoscopic ampullectomy.

Duodenal Polyps and Cancers
EUS can evaluate mucosal/submucosal lesions of the duodenum prior to endoscopic resection. These lesions can include carcinoid tumors, cysts, adenomas, and paraganglionomas, among others. EUS has a more limited role in the evaluation of duodenal adenocarcinoma, as this is usually treated surgically.

Colorectal EUS

Colon Cancer
There is no role for EUS in the staging of colon cancer. This is because colon cancer can easily and safely be resected with wide margins, which allows complete removal and locoregional staging in one step.

Rectal Cancer
Compared to colon cancer surgery, rectal cancer surgery is limited by the inability to obtain sufficient radial and proximal/distal resection margins, due to limitations imposed by the pelvic bones and the anus. Because of the risk of local recurrence after rectal cancer resection, preoperative chemoradiation is generally recommended for locally advanced rectal cancers. EUS is ideally suited for evaluating rectal cancer (Figure 97.2), because it can find tumors extending into the perirectal fat (T3) or with adjacent lymph nodes (N1), prompting preoperative chemoradiation. If a tumor is found to be

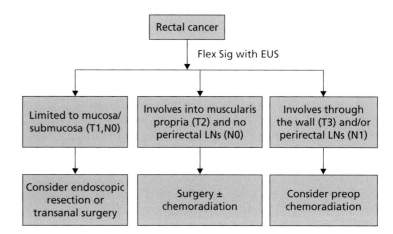

Figure 97.2 Algorithm for EUS-guided management of rectal cancer. Flex Sig, flexible sigmoidoscopy; EUS, endoscopic ultrasound; LN, lymph node.

limited to the mucosa/submucosal layer (T1), then it is amenable to transanal resection or endoscopic mucosal resection. EUS has an overall accuracy for the T- and N-staging of rectal cancers of approximately 85 and 75%, respectively [12]. EUS has greatly diminished staging accuracy following radiation therapy.

Anal Cancer

EUS has limited utility in anorectal cancer evaluation, because staging is based on tumor length and more distant lymph node metastases (iliac and femoral nodes), rather than local extension.

Fecal Incontinence

Fecal incontinence is usually caused by prior obstetrical trauma, which can result in either trauma to the anal sphincters or pudendal nerve damage. Fecal incontinence becomes more common in women over the age of 60; this is believed to be due to age-related weakening of already damaged anal sphincters and nerves. Postobstetrical damage to the anal sphincters is seen after 40% of vaginal deliveries based on EUS studies [13]. Patients with a significant defect of the anal sphincters on EUS may be considered for overlapping surgical sphincteroplasty.

Anal Fistulas

EUS can also detect such perianal findings as fistulas, abscesses, and fissures in patients with perirectal pain or a history of Crohn's disease. Examination is challenging, given the complexity of the fistulas, and might better be done with endoanal coil MRI or complete examination under anesthesia by an experienced colorectal surgeon.

Complications of EUS

Complications associated with EUS are similar to those for standard EGD, except that the rigid long tip of the echoendoscope can lead to a higher rate of esophageal or duodenal perforation. The risks of pancreatic EUS FNA are approximately 1%; they include bleeding, infection, perforation, and pancreatitis [14].

- EUS with fine-needle aspiration (FNA) has a high accuracy rate in obtaining tissue diagnosis of pancreatic cancer.
- Pancreatic cysts can be evaluated by EUS to help stratify the risk of malignancy.
- EUS is a sensitive method of excluding chronic pancreatitis in patients with epigastric pain.
- Therapeutic interventional EUS is a growing field that includes pseudocyst drainage, celiac plexus block, and fine-needle injection to aid in targeted chemotherapy and radiation.
- EUS is accurate for the staging of rectal cancer but plays no significant role in the staging of colon cancer.
- Anal EUS can detect post-obstetric anal sphincter damage, which may contribute to fecal incontinence.

Videos of interest to readers of this chapter can be found by visiting the companion website at:

http://www.practicalgastrohep.com/

97.1 Animated video of how to perform an antegrade double balloon enteroscopy.

Take Home Points

- Endoscopic ultrasound (EUS) can detect small pancreatic masses that may not be visualized well with computed tomography (CT) or magnetic resonance imaging (MRI).
- EUS is complimentary to CT and MRI for the staging of pancreatic cancer.

References

1 Eloubeidi MA, Chen VK, Eltoum IA, *et al.* Endoscopic ultrasound-guided fine needle aspiration biopsy of patients with suspected pancreatic cancer: diagnostic accuracy and acute and 30-day complications. *Am J Gastroenterol* 2003; **98**: 2663–8.

2 Gress F, Savides T, Cummings O, *et al.* Radial scanning and linear array endosonography for staging pancreatic cancer: a prospective randomized comparison. *Gastrointest Endosc* 1997; **45**: 138–42.

3 Al-Haddad M, Martin JK, Nguyen J, *et al.* Vascular resection and reconstruction for pancreatic malignancy: a single center survival study. *J Gastrointest Surg* 2007; **11**: 1168–74.

4 Dewitt J, Devereaux B, Chriswell M, *et al.* Comparison of endoscopic ultrasonography and multidetector computed tomography for detecting and staging pancreatic cancer. *Ann Intern Med* 2004; **141**: 753–63.

5 Chang KJ, Lee JG, Holcombe RF, *et al.* Endoscopic ultrasound delivery of an antitumor agent to treat a case of pancreatic cancer. *Nat Clin Pract Gastroenterol Hepatol* 2008; **5**: 107–11.

6 Pishvaian AC, Collins B, Gagnon G, *et al.* EUS-guided fiducial placement for CyberKnife radiotherapy of mediastinal and abdominal malignancies. *Gastrointest Endosc* 2006; **64**: 412–7.

7 Lee KS, Sehkar A, Rofsky NM, Pedrosa I. Prevalence of incidental pancreatic cysts in the adult population on MR imaging. *Am J Gastroenterol* 2010; **105**: 2079–84.

8 Varadarajulu S, Tamhane A, Blakely J. Graded dilation technique for EUS-guided drainage of peripancreatic fluid collections: an assessment of outcomes and complications and technical proficiency (with video). *Gastrointest Endosc* 2008; **68**: 656–66.

9 Catalano, MF, Sahai A, Levy M, *et al.* EUS-based criteria for the diagnosis of chronic pancreatitis: the Rosemont classification. *Gastrointest Endosc* 2008; **69**: 1251–61.

10 Kamisawa T, Chari ST, Lerch MM, *et al.* Recent advances in autoimmune pancreatitis: type 1 and type 2. *Gut* 2013; **62**; 1373–80.

11 Levy MJ, Reddy RP, Wiersema MJ, *et al.* EUS-guided trucut biopsy in establishing autoimmune pancreatitis as the cause of obstructive jaundice. *Gastrointest Endosc* 2005; **61**: 467–72.

12 Savides TJ, Master SS. EUS in rectal cancer. *Gastrointest Endosc* 2002; **56**(4 Suppl.): S12–18.

13 Sultan AH, Kamm MA, Hudson CN, *et al.* Anal-sphincter disruption during vaginal delivery. *N Engl J Med* 1993; **329**: 1905–11.

14 Early DA, Acosta RD, Chandrasekhara V, *et al.* Adverse events associated with EUS and EUS with FNA. *Gastrointest Endosc* 2013; **77**: 839–43.

CHAPTER 97

Index

Page numbers in *italics* refer to figures and those in **bold** to tables, but note that figures and tables are only indicated when they are separated from their text references. Index entries are filed in letter-by-letter alphabetical order.

ABCB4 gene   582–583, 591
ABCB11 gene   583, 591
abdominal aortic aneurysm screening   **210**
abdominal bloating/distension   412–415
  acute colonic pseudo-obstruction   343
  aerophagia   57
  differential diagnosis   **413**
  treatment   413–415
abdominal examination   208, 432–433
abdominal pain
  acute, in pregnancy   360–361
  acute pancreatitis   374
  chronic functional *see* functional abdominal pain
      syndrome
  chronic pancreatitis   378, 379
  diffuse   **205**
  diverticulitis   338–339
  drug therapy in pregnancy for   **358**, 359
  four-quadrants approach   203, *204*
  gastroparesis   133
  history and physical exam   44, 203, **204**
  intestinal obstruction   313
  location-based differentiation   **205**
  mesenteric ischemia   309
  nine-regions approach   203, *204*
  pancreatic pseudocyst   380
abdominal paracentesis   557, 558, 569
abdominal radiographs
  acute colonic pseudo-obstruction   344
  intestinal obstruction   313, *314, 316*
abdominal wall congenital anomalies   177–178
abuse, history of   207, 408
acanthosis nigricans   **165**
acarbose   562
acetaldehyde   499
acetaminophen (APAP)
  therapy, hepatitis A   468
  toxicity   435, 503
    clinical features   504
    diagnosis   436, 505
    liver transplant criteria   440, **604**
    management   437, **438**, 506–507
    prognosis   506
    risk factors   505
achalasia   28–31
  diagnosis   29, *30*
  treatment   30–31, 55
acid reflux, role in heartburn   47
acid-suppressive therapy
  peptic ulcer bleeding   118, 141
  short-bowel syndrome   300, **302**
  see also histamine type 2 receptor antagonists; proton
      pump inhibitors

acotiamide   72
acoustic radiation force impulse (ARFI) imaging   **452**,
    453
acrokeratosis paraneoplastica   **165**
Actinomyces spp.   **492**
acupuncture   64, 397
acute abdominal pain, in pregnancy   360–361
acute cellular rejection, liver allografts   624,
    626–627
acute colonic pseudo-obstruction (ACPO)   319,
    343–348
  clinical features   343–344
  diagnosis   344
  pathophysiology   343
  prognosis   348
  treatment   344–348
acute fatty liver of pregnancy (AFLP)   582
  clinical features   583–584
  diagnosis   584
  pathophysiology   583, 592–593
  prognosis and recurrence   585
  treatment   585
acute kidney injury (AKI)   634
  see also hepatorenal syndrome
acute liver failure (ALF)   435–440
  diagnostic evaluation   436, **437**
  drug-induced   435, **438**, 504, 506
  etiology   435
  hepatic encephalopathy   **436**, 439, 562
  hepatitis A   466–467
  hepatitis E   469
  liver transplantation   440, 603, **604**
  management   437–440
  pathophysiology   436
  prognostic scoring systems   440
Acute Liver Failure Study Group Index
    440
acute mesenteric ischemia (AMI)   308–312
  clinical features   309
  diagnosis   309–310
  non-occlusive   309, 312
  treatment   310–312
adalimumab
  Crohn's disease   **276**, 277
  perianal Crohn's disease   253–254
  in pregnancy   **358**
adaptive immune system   188–189
Addison's disease   540
adefovir, hepatitis B   476, 477
adenomas
  ampullary   459
  colonic *see* colonic adenomas
  gallbladder   546

  gastric   145–146
  hepatic   444–445
  small bowel   279, 282
adenoma-to-carcinoma sequence, colon   199–200,
    349, *350*
adenomyomatosis, gallbladder   447–448, 546
adherence, pediatric liver transplant recipients
    595
adverse drug reactions (ADR)
  liver injury *see* drug-induced liver injury
  transplant recipients   422
adverse reactions to food   227–230
  diagnosis   229–230
  immune-mediated   228
  management   230
  non-immune-mediated   228–229
aerophagia   56–58
aflatoxins   575
AIDS   363, 364
  see also HIV infection
AIDS cholangiopathy   489
Alagille syndrome (AGS)   591–592
alanine aminotransferase (ALT), serum   433
albumin
  extracorporeal dialysis   562
  intravenous therapy   558, 559, 560
  serum   433–434
  serum ascites gradient (SAAG)   557, **558**
alcohol (ethanol)
  abstinence   500, 501–502
  consumption   498
  induced hiccups   62
  metabolism   498, 499
  percutaneous injection (PEI), liver cancer
    578
alcohol dehydrogenase (ADH)   498, 499
alcoholic fatty liver (steatosis)   498, 499
alcoholic hepatitis   498, 499, 500
  ascites   558
  management   501
  prognostic scoring   500
alcoholic liver disease (ALD)   498–502
  clinical features   430–431, 499
  diagnosis   499–500
  differential diagnosis   500
  liver transplantation   501–502, 603–604
  management   500–501
  pathophysiology   498–499
  prognosis   500
alcoholic liver disease/non-alcoholic fatty liver disease
    (ALD/NAFLD) index (ANI)   500
alemtuzumab   623
alkaline phosphatase, serum   433

Practical Gastroenterology and Hepatology Board Review Toolkit, Second Edition. Edited by Nicholas J. Talley, Kenneth R. DeVault, Michael B. Wallace, Bashar A. Aqel
and Keith D. Lindor.
© 2016 John Wiley & Sons, Ltd. Published 2016 by John Wiley & Sons, Ltd. Companion website: www.practicalgastrohep.com

alosetron
    colonic ischemia   335
    fecal incontinence   258
    irritable bowel syndrome   395
Alper's syndrome   **593**
alpha-1-antitrypsin (A1AT)   590
    clearance test   305–306
    deficiency
        liver disease   536, 539, 590–591
        liver transplantation   536, 605
alpha-fetoprotein (AFP)   576
alverine citrate + simethicone   **396**
Amanita mushroom poisoning   437, **438**
amantadine   64
amebic liver abscess   488–489
American Association for the Study of Liver Diseases
        (AASLD)
    alcoholic liver disease   501
    hepatitis B   475–476, 477
    hepatitis C   480
    hepatocellular carcinoma screening   576
    Wilson's disease diagnosis   534
American Board of Internal Medicine (ABIM)   3, 4
American College of Gastroenterology (ACG),
        colorectal cancer screening   263, **264**
American trypanosomiasis see Chagas' disease
amiloride   558
aminosalicylates
    Crohn's disease   275, **276**
    in pregnancy   **358**
    ulcerative colitis   326
aminotransferases, serum   433
amitriptyline   258, **410**
ammonia excess   560–561, 592
ammonium tetrathiomolybdate   535
amoxicillin-clavulanate, hepatotoxicity   503, 504
ampullary tumors   459, 638
amyloidosis
    liver   541–542
    upper GI involvement   **161**, 162, *163*
anal cancer   **199**
    endoscopic ultrasound   639
    transplant recipients   421
anal fistulas see perianal fistulas
anal manometry see anorectal manometry
anal sphincteroplasty   258–259
anal sphincters   195, 256
    weakness   257
anal wink reflex   208
Ancylostoma duodenale   364–365
angioectasia, small bowel   243
angiography
    acute mesenteric ischemia   311
    hematochezia   238, *239*
    obscure GI bleeding   242–243
angiomas, upper GI bleeding   144
angiomyolipoma (AML), hepatic   446
angioplasty
    Budd–Chiari syndrome   515
    percutaneous mesenteric (PTMA)   312
anhepatic phase, liver transplant surgery   611–612
annular pancreas   **178**
anoctamin 1 (ANO1)   192
anomalous pancreaticobiliary ductal union
        (APBDU)   180
anorectal cancer   **199**, 639
anorectal disorders, functional   400–405
anorectal manometry
    dyssynergic defecation   248, *401*, 403
    fecal incontinence   258
anorectal varices   555, 556
anorectum
    motor activity   195
    neuromuscular apparatus   191

anorexia   224
anosmia   224
antacids, in pregnancy   **358**
antibiotics
    abdominal bloating/distension   414
    acute cholangitis   489
    acute diarrhea   216
    acute diverticulitis   341
    acute liver failure   437–438
    acute pancreatitis   376
    -associated osmotic diarrhea   330
    C. difficile infection   330
    chronic intestinal pseudo-obstruction   318
    Crohn's disease   276
    hepatic encephalopathy   562
    hepatotoxic   505
    HIV infection   365
    irritable bowel syndrome   395
    liver transplant recipients   627
    perianal fistulas   252–253
    protein-losing gastroenteropathy   307
    pyogenic liver abscess   487–488
    small-intestinal bacterial overgrowth   287–288
    spontaneous bacterial peritonitis   559
    tropical sprue   294–295
    variceal bleeding   80, 555
    Whipple's disease   297–298
anticoagulation
    acute mesenteric ischemia   311–312
    Budd–Chiari syndrome   515
    liver biopsy and   451
anticonvulsants
    acute liver failure   439–440
    hiccups   64
antidepressants
    functional abdominal pain syndrome   409, **410**
    functional dyspepsia   72
    irritable bowel syndrome   396
    see also tricyclic antidepressants
antidiarrheal agents
    acute diarrhea   216
    chronic diarrhea   220, **222**
    HIV infection   365
    irritable bowel syndrome   395
    pregnancy   **358**
    short-bowel syndrome   300, **302**
antiemetic agents
    gastroparesis   **135**, 136
    nausea and vomiting   77–78
    in pregnancy   **358**
antigen uptake, intestinal   187–188
antigliadin antibodies   291–292
anti-hepatitis B core antigen (HBc) antibodies   474
anti-hepatitis B e antigen (HBe) antibodies   474–475
anti-hepatitis B surface antigen (HBs) antibodies
        474
anti-hepatitis C virus (HCV) antibody   480
antimetabolites   **619**, 621–622
antimitochondrial antibodies (AMA)   510
antinuclear antibodies (ANA)   509, 524
antiobesity drugs   232
antioxidants, alcoholic hepatitis   501
antiphospholipid syndrome   540
antiplatelet therapy, high-ulcer risk patients   117
antiproliferative agents   **619**, 621–622
antireflux surgery   89
    Barrett's esophagus   94
    gastroparesis after   133
    imaging after   23–26
antiretroviral therapy, combination (cART)   364, 365
antispasmodics
    irritable bowel syndrome   395–396
    in pregnancy   359
antithrombin III (ATIII)   519

antithymocyte globulin (ATG)   623, 626
antituberculous drugs, hepatotoxicity   505, 506
anti-tumor necrosis factor-α (TNF-α) agents
    alcoholic hepatitis   501
    Crohn's disease   **276**, 277
    perianal Crohn's disease   253–254
    ulcerative colitis   326
antiviral therapy
    hepatitis B   475–477, 478
    hepatitis C   481–486
    hepatitis delta virus infection   478
antroduodenal manometry   38
    rumination syndrome   66, *67*
aortoenteric fistula   143–144
aortoiliac reconstruction, colonic ischemia   333
APACHE (Acute Physiology and Chronic Health
        Evaluation) II score   374, 440, 570
APC gene mutations   349, 351
appendicitis, in pregnancy   360
appetite, loss of   224, 226
appetite stimulants   226
arc of Riolan   308, *309*
argon plasma coagulation (APC)
    esophageal strictures   108–109
    malignant obstruction   266
arthritis
    inflammatory bowel disease   324
    Whipple's disease   297
Ascaris lumbricoides   496
ascites   557–559
    clinical features   432, 557
    complications   558–559
    culture-negative neutrocytic (CNNA)   559
    diagnosis   557, **558**
    refractory   225, 558, 569
    treatment   558
Asian Pacific Association for the Study of the Liver
        (APASL), hepatitis B recommendations   475–477
aspartate aminotransferase (AST), serum   433
Aspergillus infections   494, 627
aspiration therapy, for obesity   235
aspirin
    Barrett's esophagus   94
    high-cardiovascular risk patients   117
    high-ulcer risk patients   117
    peptic ulcer disease   115–116
asterixis   561
asthma, GERD   86, 87
atopy patch test   229
ATP7B gene mutations   533, 534
Auerbach's (myenteric) plexus   192
autism spectrum disorders (ASD)   184
autoimmune gastritis   130
autoimmune hepatitis (AIH)   508–510
    acute liver failure   435, 437, **438**
    diagnostic criteria   508–509
    drug-induced   506, 507
    liver transplantation   510, 605
    overlap syndrome   511
autoimmune liver diseases   508–512
autoimmune pancreatitis   638
autonomic nervous system (ANS)   192–193
azathioprine (AZA)
    autoimmune hepatitis   509, 510
    Crohn's disease   **276**, 277
    hepatotoxicity   503
    liver transplant recipients   **619**, 621
    perianal Crohn's disease   253, 254
    in pregnancy   **358**
    ulcerative colitis   326

Bacillus cereus food poisoning   214
baclofen   64, 66
bacterascites   559

bacterial infections
    acute diarrhea   214–216
    HIV infection   364, 365, **366**
    liver   487–491, **492–493**
    transplant recipients   421, 627
balsalazide   275, **276**
barbiturates   439
Barcelona Clinic Liver Cancer (BCLC) staging
    system   576
bariatric surgery   233–234
    endoscopic   234–235
    imaging after   25, 26
barium enema, double-contrast (DCBE), colorectal
    cancer screening   262
barium esophagram (swallow)   23, 28
    esophageal strictures, rings and webs   107
    modified   23
Barrett's dysplasia   94–95
    high-grade (HGD)   93, 94–95
    HPV association   91, *92*
    low-grade (LGD)   92, 93, 94
Barrett's esophagus   87, 91–96
    endoscopic evaluation   93
    epidemiology   91–92
    management   93–94
    non-dysplastic (NDBE)   92, 93, 94
    predictors of progression   92–93
    screening and surveillance   93
Barrett's metaplasia–dysplasia–adenocarcinoma
    sequence   91, 92–93
barrier function, intestinal mucosa and
    epithelium   187
Bartonella henselae   **492**
basiliximab   623–624, 626
Bazex syndrome   **165**
BCG infection   **492**
behavioral therapy, rumination syndrome   66
Behçet's disease   160, 540
belching   56–58, 72
    gastric   56
    supragastric   56–57, 58
benign recurrent intrahepatic cholestasis (BRIC)
    591
β-blockers, variceal bleeding prophylaxis   555, 556
bevacizumab   **353**
Bianchi procedure   302
Bifidobacterium infantis   396, 414
bile acid metabolism, inborn errors   **593**
bile duct hamartomas   446
bile duct stones *see* choledocholithiasis
bile leaks
    endoscopic management   459
    liver transplant recipients   614, 626
bile reflux, role in heartburn   47
bile salt replacement, short-bowel syndrome   301
biliary anastomosis, liver transplantation   612–613
biliary atresia   587–589
    liver transplantation   589, 593
    pathophysiology and types   587
biliary atresia splenic malformation (BASM)   587
biliary colic   543–544
biliary complications, liver transplant
    recipients   457–458, 614, 615, 626
biliary cystadenoma   442, *443*
biliary obstruction   457–459
    acute cholangitis   489, 546
    benign   457–458
    indeterminate   459
    malignant   458–459
biliary stents
    biliary obstructions   457–459, 546
    liver transplant surgery   612
    malignant gastric outlet obstruction   267–268
    primary sclerosing cholangitis   459, 551

biliary strictures/stenosis
    benign   457–458
    indeterminate   459
    liver transplant recipients   457–458, 614, 626
    malignant   458–459
    primary sclerosing cholangitis   459, 551
biliary tract disease   543–552
    endoscopic techniques   455–460
    history and physical exam   429–434
    transplant recipients   422
biliary tree
    cancer   547–550
    imaging   442–448
biliary tumors, malignant   446–447
biliopancreatic diversion   233
    with duodenal switch   233, 234
bilirubin, serum   433
bilomas, liver transplant recipients   627
biofeedback therapy
    dyssynergic defecation   249, 405
    fecal incontinence   258
biomarkers
    GI neoplasms   200
    liver fibrosis   452–453, *453*
biostatistics   5
bird-beak appearance, achalasia   29
bisacodyl   **249, 404**
    in pregnancy   358
Bismuth–Corlette classification,
    cholangiocarcinoma   549
bismuth subsalicylate
    acute diarrhea   216
    in pregnancy   358, 359
bleeding
    acute liver failure   438
    complicating liver biopsy   451
    complicating liver transplantation   613
    complicating TIPS   570–571
    GI *see* gastrointestinal bleeding
blood pressure screening   **210**
Board Examination, Gastroenterology   3–5
board review courses   4
body mass index (BMI)   224, 231
Borchardt triad   13
Borrelia spp.   **492**
bosentan   564
botulinum toxin injection
    esophageal motility disorders   30, 31, 55
    gastroparesis   136
bougie dilation, esophageal strictures, rings and
    webs   108, 110–111
bowel complaints   204–205, **206**
bowel resection
    extensive, short-bowel syndrome   299–300,
    302
    protein-losing enteropathy   307
bowel sounds   208
brachytherapy, endoscopic   266, 267
breath tests   413
    gastric emptying   36–37, 134
    small-intestinal bacterial overgrowth   287, *288*
Bristol Stool Form Scale   204–205
Brucella spp.   **492**
bruits, abdominal   432
Brunner gland hyperplasia   280
Budd–Chiari syndrome (BCS)   513–516, 539
    clinical features   514
    diagnosis   515
    etiology   513–514
    treatment   515–516, 570
budesonide
    Crohn's disease   **276**, 277
    eosinophilic esophagitis   100, 101
    in pregnancy   358

bulking agents, dietary   **249**
    irritable bowel syndrome   394
    pregnancy   359
bumetanide   558
Burkholderia pseudomallei   **492**
Burkitt-type lymphoma of small intestine   280–281
buspirone   409, **410**
busulfan   518
Byler's disease   591

CA19-9, serum   551, 579
CAGE questions   430–431
calcineurin inhibitors (CNIs)   618–621, 624, 626
    see also cyclosporine; tacrolimus
calcium (Ca^{2+}), intestinal motility   191, 192
calories
    decreased utilization   224–225
    reduced intake   224
Cameron erosions   143
Campylobacter infections   **214**, 216
candidiasis
    liver   494
    transplant recipients   421, 627
cannabis use, cyclic vomiting syndrome   72
Cantlie's line   609, *610*
capecitabine   **353**
Capillaria hepatica   496
capsule endoscopy *see* video-capsule endoscopy
caput medusae   555
carbohydrate metabolism, inherited disorders   592,
    593
carbon dioxide portography   567, *568*
carcinoembryonic antigen (CEA)   352, 380, 386
carcinoids   185
    gastric   128, 130, 149, *150*
    small bowel   280
    see also neuroendocrine tumors
carcinoid syndrome   185
CARD15/NOD2   187, 273
cardiac surgery, protein-losing gastroenteropathy   307
cardiovascular disease (CVD)
    hepatic involvement   538–539
    liver transplant recipients   624, 628
    NSAIDs and   117
Carnett's sign   44, 408
carvedilol   555
castor oil, in pregnancy   **358**
caudate lobe, liver transplant surgery   609, 611
$CD4^+$ T cells
    HIV infection   363, 364
    Th1 and Th2 subsets   188–189
cecal volvulus   315
cecostomy, percutaneous   347
cefotaxime   559
ceftriaxone
    HIV-associated proctitis   365
    variceal bleeding   555
    Whipple's disease   297
celiac-associated T-cell high-grade lymphoma, small
    bowel   280
celiac axis   308
celiac disease   291–294
    clinical features   291
    diagnosis   291–293
    dyspepsia   71
    epidemiology   291
    extraintestinal manifestations   **209**
    liver disease   512, 540
    pathogenesis   189
    pregnancy and   360
    treatment   293–294
    tropical sprue vs.   **294**
cerebral edema, acute liver failure   436, 439–440
certification examination   3–4

certolizumab
   Crohn's disease **276**, 277
   perianal Crohn's disease **253**, 254
   in pregnancy **358**
ceruloplasmin, serum 533, 534
cetuximab **353**, 354
Chagas' disease, esophageal involvement 30, 161–162
Charcot's triad 431, 489, **544**, 545
chemical gastritis/gastropathies 129–130
chemotherapy
   cholangiocarcinoma 549, 580
   colorectal cancer 353–354
   hepatocellular carcinoma 578
chest pain 48–50
   functional (FCP) 49–50, 169, 170, 171
   non-cardiac (NCCP) 48–49
   psychological evaluation 50
Chicago classification, esophageal motility disorders 28
Child–Turcotte–Pugh scoring system 601, **602**
Chlamydia trachomatis proctitis, HIV infection 365
chloride channel (ClC-2) activator *see* lubiprostone
chlorpromazine
   hepatotoxicity 503
   for hiccups 64
cholangiocarcinoma (CCA) 548–550, 578–580
   classification 578, *579*
   imaging 446–447, 548–549, 579
   liver transplantation 549–550, 580, 606, 633
   management 549–550, 579–580
   risk factors 547, 548, 551, 578–579
   staging **548**, 549
cholangiography, primary sclerosing cholangitis 550
cholangioscopy 459
cholangitis
   acute/ascending 489, **544**, 545–546
     diagnosis 431, 489, 545
     treatment 489, 545–546
   Oriental recurrent 489
   primary sclerosing *see* primary sclerosing cholangitis
   recurrent, biliary atresia 588
cholecystectomy
   biliary strictures after 457–458
   gallbladder cancer 548
   gallbladder polyps 547
   gallstone disease 544, 545
cholecystitis, acute 544
   in pregnancy 360
cholecystokinin (CCK) **182**, 183
cholecystostomy, percutaneous 544
choledocholithiasis **544**, 545
   diagnosis 447–448, 545
   primary sclerosing cholangitis 551
   treatment 456–457, 545
cholelithiasis *see* gallstones
cholestatic liver diseases, liver transplantation 605, 630
cholesterol abnormalities
   screening **210**
   see also dyslipidemia
cholesterol ester storage disease **593**
cholesterol polyps, gallbladder 546
cholestyramine
   primary biliary cholangitis 511
   short-bowel syndrome 301–302
cholinergic nerves, esophageal motor function 15, 16
chronic intestinal pseudo-obstruction (CIPO) 315–318
   causes 316, **318**
   clinical features 225, 315–316
   diagnosis 316–317
   management 317–318

chronic kidney disease (CKD), liver transplant recipients 624, 628
chronic mesenteric ischemia/insufficiency (CMI) 308, 312
   clinical features 225, 312
ciprofloxacin
   perianal fistulas 252–253
   spontaneous bacterial peritonitis prophylaxis 559–560
   variceal hemorrhage 80, 555
cirrhosis
   alcoholic 499, 500
   ascites 557
   cardiac 539
   cryptogenic 526–527
   decompensated 602, 634
   drug-induced 506
   hepatic encephalopathy 560–561
   hepatitis B 475, **476**
   hepatitis C 481
   hepatocellular carcinoma 574–575, 576
   hereditary hemochromatosis 533
   portal hypertension 554
   screening, chronic liver disease *482*
   variceal bleeding 555–556
   see also liver fibrosis
cisapride 318
citalopram **410**
clonidine 220, **222**
Clonorchis sinensis 495–496, 547
clopidogrel 117, 451
closed-eyes sign, during examination 408
Clostridium difficile infection (CDI) 328–331
   clinical features 329
   diagnosis 329
   differential diagnosis 330, 334, 344
   epidemiology 328
   HIV infection 364
   pathophysiology 328–329
   prognosis 331
   transplant recipients 421
   treatment 330, *331*
Clostridium perfringens 214
clubbing, digital 431
coagulation abnormalities, acute liver failure 438
Coccidioides 494
codeine
   chronic diarrhea **222**
   short-bowel syndrome 300, **302**
cognitive behavioral therapy (CBT)
   functional abdominal pain syndrome 410
   irritable bowel syndrome 396–397
colectomy, slow-transit constipation 249, 403, 405
colitis
   drug-induced 334–335
   indeterminate 323, 324
   inflammatory bowel disease 323–327
   ischemic *see* colonic ischemia
   pseudomembranous 328, 329
   ulcerative *see* ulcerative colitis
colon
   blood supply 177
   motility 194–195, *196*
   neuromuscular apparatus 191–193
colonic adenomas 198, 349
   cancer risk 350
   hereditary syndromes 351
   serrated 349
colonic adenoma-to-carcinoma sequence 199–200, 349, *350*
colonic decompression tubes 347
colonic diseases 321–367
   in pregnancy 359–361
colonic inertia *see* constipation, slow transit

colonic ischemia 333–336
   acute colonic pseudo-obstruction 344, 347–348
   clinical features 335–336
   diagnosis 336, *337*
   pathophysiology 333–335
   treatment 336
   see also mesenteric ischemia
colonic manometry 194–195, 403
colonic obstruction 314–315, *317*
   endoscopic palliation 268
colonic perforation
   acute colonic pseudo-obstruction 344, 347–348
   acute diverticulitis 339, 341
   transplant recipients 422
colonic polyps 349
   adenomatous *see* colonic adenomas
   hereditary syndromes 351
   hyperplastic (HPPs) 349
colonic pseudo-obstruction, acute *see* acute colonic pseudo-obstruction
colonic stents, malignant obstruction 268
colonic transit studies 248, 402
colonic volvulus 315
colonoscopy
   acute colonic pseudo-obstruction 346–347, **348**
   colorectal cancer 352
   colorectal cancer screening 262
   colorectal cancer surveillance 263, **264**
   Crohn's disease 274
   hematochezia 238, 239
   inflammatory bowel disease 325
   irritable bowel syndrome 393
   obscure GI bleeding 241
colorectal adenocarcinoma 349
colorectal adenomas *see* colonic adenomas
colorectal cancer (CRC) 349–354
   clinical features 352
   diagnosis 352
   differential diagnosis 352–353
   endoscopic palliation of obstruction 268
   endoscopic ultrasound 638–639
   epidemiology **199**, 349
   familial risks 350–351
   inflammatory bowel disease 324, 350
   pathophysiology 349–352
   prevention 352
   primary sclerosing cholangitis 551
   prognosis 354
   screening 261–264, 352
     guidelines **210**, 261, 263
     methods 261–263
   surveillance 261
     guidelines 263, **264**
     inflammatory bowel disease 325
   transplant recipients 421
   treatment 353–354
   young onset 351–352
colovaginal fistula 339
colovesical fistula 339
combined antegrade and retrograde dilation (CARD), esophageal strictures 108
commensal flora 189
   see also microbiota, gut
common bile duct stones *see* choledocholithiasis
complementary and alternative medicine 397, 414
computed tomography (CT)
   acute pancreatitis *372*
   esophagus 23
   intestinal obstruction 313, *317*
   pancreatic cancer 383, *384*
   pancreatic pseudocysts 379–380
   portal hypertension 554
   small bowel tumors 281
   stomach 26

computed tomography (CT) colonography
  colorectal cancer 352
  double-contrast (DCBE) 262–263
computed tomography (CT) enteroclysis, small bowel
    tumors 281
computed tomography enterography (CTE)
  Crohn's disease 275
  intestinal obstruction 313, 314, *317*
  nausea and vomiting 75
  obscure GI bleeding 242, **243**
congenital anomalies 177–178
  upper GI tract 12–13, **178**
congestive hepatopathy 538–539
connective-tissue diseases, esophageal and gastric
    involvement 156–157
constipation 246–250
  alarm signs 205
  chronic functional 400–405
    clinical features 401–402
    diagnosis 402–403
    management 403–405
    pathophysiology 400, *402*
    Rome III criteria **247, 401**
  clinical features 204–205, **206**, 247–248
  diagnosis 248
  differential diagnosis 248, **403**
  history and physical exam **206**
  irritable bowel syndrome 248, 392, **393**,
      394–395
  pathophysiology 246
  in pregnancy **358**, 359
  prognosis 249
  slow transit (colonic inertia) 246
    diagnosis 248, 403
    management 249, 405
    pathophysiology 246, 400
  therapy 248–249
constitutional DNA mismatch repair deficiency
    (CMMRD) 351
continuous positive airways pressure (CPAP),
    aerophagia 56, 57
contractile deceleration point (CDP) 28
contractile front velocity (CFV) 28
copper
  hepatic concentration 534
  overload 533, 534
  urinary excretion 534, 535
coronary artery disease, non-cardiac chest pain
    49
corrected sinusoidal pressure (CSP) 567–568
corticosteroids
  acute liver failure 437
  alcoholic liver disease 501
  autoimmune hepatitis 509, 510
  chronic intestinal pseudo-obstruction 318
  Crohn's disease 276–277
  drug-induced liver injury 506–507
  eosinophilic esophagitis 100, 101
  eosinophilic gastroenteritis 154
  HELLP syndrome 585
  intralesional, benign esophageal strictures 108,
      110–111
  liver transplant recipients **620**, 622
  in pregnancy **358**
  protein-losing gastroenteropathy 306
  ulcerative colitis 326
co-trimoxazole 559–560
cough, chronic, GERD 86, 87, 89
Cowden syndrome
  extraintestinal manifestations **209**
  GI manifestations **165**, 351
COX-2-selective NSAIDs 115–116, 117
Coxiella burnetii **493**
crepe paper esophagus 99

CREST syndrome 540
cricopharyngeal myotomy 54
Crigler–Najjar syndrome 592
Crohn's disease 273–278
  cancer risk 280, 350
  clinical features 273
  colitis 323
  diagnosis 274–275
  differential diagnosis 275
  epidemiology 273
  esophageal and gastric 159, **160**, *160*
  extraintestinal manifestations **209**, 273, 540
  grading of severity 273–274
  pathophysiology 187, 188, 273, *274*, 323
  perianal 251–254
  prognosis 278
  small-intestinal bacterial overgrowth 285
  treatment 275–277
Crohn's Disease Activity Index (CDAI) 273–274
Cronkhite–Canada syndrome **209**
cryptococcosis 494, 627
Cryptosporidium diarrhea 214, 364, 421
CT *see* computed tomography
culture-negative neutrocytic ascites (CNNA) 559
Cushing's disease 540
cutaneous diseases
  gastroenterological disease 5
  inflammatory bowel disease 324
  upper GI involvement 163–164, **165**
cutaneous hyperkeratosis syndromes 164, **165**
cyclic vomiting syndrome (CVS) 72, 133
  coalescent 133
cyclophosphamide (CY), hepatotoxicity 518
Cyclospora infections 214
cyclosporine (CSA)
  drug interactions 620
  GI side effects 422
  hepatitis C therapy interactions 485
  liver transplant recipients 618–621, 624, 626
  in pregnancy **358**
  ulcerative colitis 326
CYP3A gene polymorphisms 618–620
cystadenomas
  biliary 442, *443*
  pancreatic 385, **386**
cystic fibrosis
  liver disease 539, 589–590
  liver transplantation 634
cystic fibrosis transmembrane conductance regulator
    (CFTR) 589
cytokeratin (CK)-18 526
cytokines 188–189
cytomegalovirus (CMV) infection
  hepatitis 471
  HIV infection 364
  Ménétrier's disease 147
  transplant recipients 420, 594, 627

daclatasvir (DCV) 481, **482, 483**, 485
daclizumab 626
dasabuvir *see* ombitasvir/paritaprevir/ritonavir plus
    dasabuvir
deaminated gliadin antibodies 291–292
decompensated end-stage liver disease 602, 634
defecation, normal 256–257, 400, *402*
defecation disorders 246
  diagnosis 248
  fecal incontinence 257
  treatment 249
  see also dyssynergic defecation
defecography 248, 258
defensins 187
deferasirox 533
defibrotide 519

deglutitive inhibition 16
dental problems, halitosis 59
depression, unintentional weight loss 224
dermatologic diseases *see* cutaneous diseases
dermatomyositis 156, **157**, *159*
desipramine **410**
device-assisted enteroscopy (DAE), obscure GI
    bleeding 242, **243**, 244
diabetes mellitus
  gastroparesis 132, 133, 135, 157–158
  hepatic manifestations 540
  new onset, after transplantation (NODAT) 624,
      628–629
  screening **210**
  type 2 (T2DM)
    colorectal cancer risk 350
    NAFLD 524
  upper GI involvement 157–158, **159**
diarrhea
  acute 213–217
    clinical features 213–214
    common pathogens causing **214**
    diagnosis 214
    differential diagnosis 214–216
    treatment *215*, 216–217
  antibiotic-associated 330
  C. difficile-associated *see Clostridium difficile*
    infection
  chronic 218–222
    clinical features 218
    diagnosis 219–220, *221*
    prognosis 222
    treatment 220–222
  drug-induced 216
  fatty **220**, *221*
  fecal incontinence 258
  history taking 44, 204–205, **206**
  HIV infection 364–365
  hospitalized patients 330
  infectious 213–216, 330
    HIV infection 364
    transplant recipients **420**, 421
  inflammatory 215–216, **220**, *221*
    HIV infection 364
  irritable bowel syndrome 218, 392, **393**, 395
  osmotic 220, *221*
    antibiotic-associated 330
  pathophysiology 213, 218
  in pregnancy **358**, 359
  secretory 220, *221*
  short-bowel syndrome 301–302
  small-intestinal bacterial overgrowth 288
  transplant recipients **420**, 422, 423
  watery 214, 220
    HIV infection 364
  VIPoma syndrome 185
dicyclomine, in pregnancy **358**, 359
dietary factors, abdominal bloating/distension 412
dietary modification
  abdominal bloating/distension 414
  chronic nausea and vomiting 76–77
  eosinophilic esophagitis 100–101
  fecal incontinence 258
  gastroparesis 135
  irritable bowel syndrome 393
  NAFLD 527–528
  nausea and vomiting of pregnancy 359
  protein-losing gastroenteropathy 307
  short-bowel syndrome 300–301
  small-intestinal bacterial overgrowth 288
diethylpropion 232
Dieulafoy lesions, bleeding 142
digital rectal examination 208–209
dilated intercellular spaces (DISs) 47

diphenoxylate (with atropine) 220, **222**
    fecal incontinence 258
    in pregnancy **358**
    short-bowel syndrome 300, **302**
dipivoxil **477**
direct-acting antiviral (DAA) agents, hepatitis
    C 481–486, 604–605
disconnected pancreatic tail syndrome 381
distal contractile integral (DCI) 28
distal esophageal spasm (DES) 31–32, 55
distal latency (DL) 28
diuretics, for ascites 558
diverticular abscesses 340, 341
diverticular disease of colon 338, *339*
diverticulitis, acute 338–342
    clinical features 338–339
    complicated 339, 341
    diagnosis 340
    management 340–342
    uncomplicated 338–339, 340–341
DNA mismatch repair (MMR) gene mutations 349,
    351
docusate **249**
domperidone
    chronic intestinal pseudo-obstruction 318
    functional dyspepsia 72
    gastroparesis 136
donation after brain death (DBD) 603, 609
donation after cardiac death (DCD) 603, 609
Donor Risk Index (DRI) scoring system 615
Donor Service Areas (DSAs) 608, 632
double-balloon enteroscopy (DBE)
    obscure GI bleeding 242, **243**
    small bowel tumors 282
double-contrast barium enema (DCBE), colorectal
    cancer screening 262
double-duct sign, pancreatic cancer 383, *384*
doxylamine/vitamin B$_6$ **358**
drug-induced colon injury 334–335
drug-induced diarrhea 216
drug-induced GI events, transplant recipients 422
drug-induced liver injury (DILI) 503–507
    acute liver failure 435, **438**, 504
    causative drugs 505
    clinical features 430, 504
    diagnostic evaluation 504–505
    hematopoietic stem cell transplantation 516, **517**,
        517
    idiosyncratic 503, 504–505, 506
    management 506–507
    prognosis 506
    risk factors 505–506
Dubin–Johnson syndrome 592
duloxetine 409, **410**
duodenal adenomas 279
duodenal atresia **178**
duodenal cancer
    endoscopic ultrasound 638
    upper GI bleeding 143
duodenal duplication **178**
duodenal polyps 638
duodenal stenosis **178**
duodenal ulcers 115–119
    H. pylori 116, 122
    see also peptic ulcers
duodenal varices 556
duodenoscope 455, 456
duplications
    esophageal **12**, 13
    gastric 13
Dupuytren contracture 431
dyschezia 205
dysentery 215–216
    HIV infection 364

dysguesia 224
dyskeratosis congenita **165**
dyslipidemia
    liver transplant recipients 624, 628
    NAFLD 524
    screening guidelines **210**
dyspepsia 70–72
    alarm symptoms 70–71
    functional (FD) 70, 71–72, 122
    peptic ulcer disease 116
dysphagia 52–55, 85
    after antireflux surgery 25
    clinical features 52–53
    diagnosis 53
    eosinophilic esophagitis 99
    esophageal 44, 53, 54–55, **106**
    esophageal motility disorders 29, 33–34
    esophageal strictures, rings and webs 105, 106
    functional 169, 170, 171
    history and physical exam 44, **53**
    malignant, endoscopic palliation 266–267
    oropharyngeal 44, 52–53, 54
    pathophysiology 52
    prognosis 55
    radiology 23, *24*
    solid foods 44, 53, **100**, 106
    solids and liquids 44, 53
    therapeutics 53–55
dysphagia lusoria 13
dysplastic nodules (DNs), hepatic 446
dyspnea, hepatopulmonary syndrome 563
dyssynergic defecation 246, 400–405
    clinical features 402
    diagnosis 248, **401**, *401*, 403
    management 249, *404*, 405
    pathophysiology 400, *402*

echinococcosis 442, 495
echocardiography 563
echoendoscopes 455
edema
    liver disease 431–432
    protein-losing gastroenteropathy 305
EGD *see* esophagogastroduodenoscopy
egg allergy 228, 230
ehrlichiosis **492**
elastography, liver **452**, 453–454, 526
elbasvir (EBV) 481, **482, 483**
elderly patients
    acute diarrhea 216–217
    esophageal dysmotility 34
    liver transplantation 603
    reduced caloric intake 224
electrogastrography (EGG) 37–38
    nausea and vomiting 76
electromyography (EMG), anal sphincter 258
elemental diets, eosinophilic esophagitis 100
elimination diets
    abdominal bloating/distension 414
    eosinophilic esophagitis 100, 101
embolectomy, superior mesenteric artery 311
emphysema, alpha-1-antitrypsin deficiency 590
endoanal ultrasound, fecal incontinence 258
EndoBarrier GI liner 235
endocrine cell hyperplasia, stomach 128, 130
endocrine diseases
    hepatic manifestations 539–540
    upper GI involvement 157–159
endocrinology, gastrointestinal 181–186
endomysic band ligation
    non-variceal upper GI bleeding 139
    variceal bleeding 142, 556
endoscopic clips 139

endoscopic hemostasis
    hematochezia 239
    modalities 139
    peptic ulcer bleeding 118, 140–141
    upper GI bleeding 81, 139
    variceal bleeding 141–142, 556
endoscopic mucosal resection (EMR), Barrett's
    esophagus 94–95
endoscopic retrograde cholangiopancreatography
    (ERCP) 455–460
    acute cholangitis 546
    biliary obstructions 457–459
    cholangiocarcinoma 549, 579
    choledocholithiasis 456–457, 545
    complications 459–460
    pancreatic cancer 383, *384*
    pancreatic cystic neoplasms 386, 387
    pancreatic pseudocysts 381, 382
    procedure 456
endoscopic sclerotherapy
    non-variceal upper GI bleeding 139
    variceal bleeding 142, 556
endoscopic screening tests, colorectal cancer 262
endoscopic-sleeve gastroplasty 235
endoscopic (biliary) sphincterotomy
    acute pancreatitis 376
    bleeding after 143
    choledocholithiasis 456–457, 545
endoscopic therapy
    acute colonic pseudo-obstruction 346–347, **348**
    Barrett's esophagus 94–95
    esophageal strictures, rings and webs 108–109
    hemostatic *see* endoscopic hemostasis
    malignant GI obstruction 266–268
    obesity 234–235
    pancreatic pseudocyst drainage *379*, 381
endoscopic thermal contact probes 139
endoscopic ultrasound (EUS) 637–639
    Barrett's esophagus 94
    choledocholithiasis 545
    complications 459–460, 639
    gallbladder cancer 547, 548
    gastric tumors 146, 147, 148, 149, *150*
    large bowel 638–639
    liver and biliary tree disease 455–459
    pancreas 637–638
    pancreatic pseudocysts 381
    perianal fistulas 252
    procedure 456
    small bowel 638
endoscopic ultrasound-guided fine needle aspiration
    (EUS-FNA)
    gastric submucosal tumors 149–150
    liver lesions 459
    malignant biliary obstructions 458
    pancreatic masses 383, *384*, 386, 637
endoscopic variceal ligation (EVL) 555, 556
endoscopy
    C. difficile infection 329
    Crohn's disease 274–275
    fecal incontinence 258
    inflammatory bowel disease 325
    see also colonoscopy; esophagogastroduodenoscopy
endothelin receptor antagonists 564
endotracheal intubation, hematemesis 79, 139
end-stage liver disease, decompensated 602, 634
energy expenditure, increased 225
Entamoeba histolytica **214**, 488–489
entecavir, hepatitis B 476, 477
enteral nutrition 226
    acute liver failure 437
    acute pancreatitis 376
    chronic intestinal pseudo-obstruction 318
    short-bowel syndrome 300

enteral tubes, palliation of malignant obstruction   268
enteric dysmotility syndromes, without visceral
　　dilation   318–319
enteric nervous system (ENS)   192, 193
　　congenital anomalies   178
enteroclysis
　　intestinal obstruction   313, 314
　　small bowel tumors   281
enterocolitis, HIV-related   365, **366**
entero-endocrine cells   181
enteropathy-associated T-cell lymphoma, small
　　bowel   280
eosinophilic esophageal infiltration (EEI)   98
eosinophilic esophagitis (EoE)   98–102
　　clinical features   99
　　diagnosis   *24*, 99, 107
　　differential diagnosis   100
　　epidemiology   98
　　pathophysiology   98–99
　　prognosis   102
　　treatment   54, 100–101, *102*
eosinophilic gastroenteritis (EG)   152–154, 228
　　clinical features   153
　　diagnosis   153–154
　　pathophysiology   152–153
　　treatment   154
eosinophilic gastrointestinal (GI) disease   228
eotaxin 3   99
epidermolysis bullosa   163, **164**
epigastric pain   **205**
epigastric pain syndrome (EPS)   71
epinephrine, endoscopic injection   118, 139
eponyms, medical   5
epoprostenol   564
Epstein–Barr virus (EBV)
　　hepatitis   471
　　transplant recipients   420, 421–422, 594
ERCP *see* endoscopic retrograde
　　cholangiopancreatography
erosive esophagitis   86–87
eructation *see* belching
erythrocytapheresis   533
erythromycin   80, 136, 318
Escherichia coli
　　enterohemorrhagic   **214**
　　enteroinvasive   **214**
　　enteropathogenic   214
　　enterotoxigenic   214
　　Shiga toxin-producing   216
escitalopram   **410**
esophageal adenocarcinoma (EAC)
　　Barrett's esophagus related   91, 92
　　biomarkers of risk   92–93
　　HPV-related risk   91, 92, 93
　　intramucosal Barrett's   94–95
　　prevention, Barrett's esophagus   94
esophageal atresia   12–13
esophageal body   11
　　motor function   16
esophageal cancer
　　dysphagia   54
　　endoscopic palliation   266–267
　　epidemiology   **199**
　　upper GI bleeding   143
esophageal dilation
　　achalasia   31, 55
　　dysphagia   54, 55
　　eosinophilic esophagitis   99, 101
　　strictures, rings and webs   108, 110–111
esophageal disorders   83–111
　　functional   169–171
　　in pregnancy   357–359
　　in systemic and cutaneous diseases   156–165
esophageal duplications   **12**, 13, **178**

esophageal impedance–pH monitoring
　　belching and aerophagia   56–57, 58
　　chest pain   49
　　GERD   88
　　heartburn   47
esophageal manometry   *17*, 28
　　achalasia   29, *30*
　　belching   56–57
　　eosinophilic esophagitis   99
　　esophageal strictures, rings and webs   107
　　non-cardiac chest pain   49
esophageal motility   15–16, *17*
esophageal motility disorders   5, 28–34
　　diagnostics   28
　　hypotensive   32–34
　　non-achalasia   31–32
　　non-cardiac chest pain   49
　　treatment   54–55
　　see also achalasia
esophageal pH monitoring
　　GERD   87–88
　　non-cardiac chest pain   49
esophageal pressure topography (EPT)   28
esophageal rings   *12*, 13, 105–111
　　clinical features   106
　　diagnosis   107
　　treatment   107–108
　　see also Schatzki rings
esophageal spasm, distal (DES)   31–32, 55
esophageal stenosis, congenital   **12**, 13, **178**
esophageal stents
　　benign strictures, rings and webs   109–110,
　　　111
　　malignant dysphagia   266–267
esophageal strictures   105–111
　　anastomotic   108–109, *110*
　　clinical features   106
　　complex   105, 107
　　diagnosis   107
　　eosinophilic esophagitis   99, 101
　　pathophysiology   106
　　recurrent   105
　　refractory   105, 110–111
　　simple   105, 107
　　treatment   54, 107–111
esophageal varices   555–556
　　see also variceal bleeding
esophageal webs   *12*, 13, 105–111
　　clinical features   106
　　diagnosis   107
　　treatment   107–108
esophagectomy
　　anastomotic strictures after   108–109, *110*
　　esophageal intramucosal cancer   95
esophagitis
　　eosinophilic *see* eosinophilic esophagitis
　　erosive   86–87
　　infectious   52, 54
　　Los Angeles (LA) classification   87, *88*
　　pill-induced   422
　　reflux   85, 87
　　upper GI bleeding   142
esophagogastric junction (EGJ) outflow
　　obstruction   31
esophagogastroduodenoscopy (EGD)
　　Barrett's esophagus   93
　　dyspepsia   71
　　esophageal strictures, rings and webs   107
　　GERD   87
　　hematemesis   80, 81
　　nausea and vomiting   76
　　non-cardiac chest pain   48
　　obscure GI bleeding   241
　　varices   555

esophagus
　　anatomy   11–12
　　congenital malformations   12–13, **178**
　　embryology   12
　　hypercontractile   32
　　jackhammer   32
　　motor function   15–16, *17*
　　muscle innervation   15
　　nutcracker   32, *33*, 55
　　radiologic approach   23–26
　　vascular anomalies   **12**, 13
essential thrombocytosis   516
ethanol *see* alcohol
ethics   5
European Association for the Study of the Liver
　　(EASL)
　　alcoholic liver disease guidelines   501
　　hepatitis B recommendations   475–476
　　Wilson's disease diagnosis   534
EUS *see* endoscopic ultrasound
everolimus (EVL)
　　drug interactions   **620**
　　liver transplant recipients   **620**, 622–623, 624, 626
　　pancreatic neuroendocrine tumors   186
excitation–contraction coupling, gut smooth
　　muscle   191
exercise-induced colonic ischemia   335
exercise/physical activity
　　constipation   404
　　irritable bowel syndrome   393–394
external anal sphincter   195, 256
　　needle EMG   258
　　sphincteroplasty   258–259
　　weakness   257
extrapancreatic fluid collections   371–372

factor V Leiden   309, 514, 583
familial adenomatous polyposis (FAP)   199, 351
　　extraintestinal manifestations   **209**
　　gastric polyps   145
familial amyloid polyneuropathy (FAP)   606, 634
Fasciola hepatica   495, 496
fatty acid oxidation, inborn errors of
　　mitochondrial   592–593
fatty liver *see* hepatic steatosis
fecal continence, mechanisms   256–257
fecal immunochemical test (FIT)   261–262
fecal impaction   315
fecal incontinence (FI)   256–260
　　clinical features   205, 257–258
　　diagnostic testing   258
　　endoscopic ultrasound   633
　　etiology   256, **257**
　　management   258–259
　　pathophysiology   257
fecal microbiota transplant (FMT), *C. difficile*
　　infection   330
fecal occult blood test, guaiac-based (gFOBT)   261
fecal osmotic gap (FOG)   220
Felty's syndrome   540
fermentable oligo-di-monosaccharides and polyols
　　(FODMAPs)   229, 393, 414
fermentation, microbial   413
ferritin, serum   524, 532, 533
fertility, in GI diseases   359–360
fiber, dietary   404
FIC1 gene mutations   591
fidaxomicin, *C. difficile* infection   330
Finkelstein tonsil-smelling test   60
fish-mouth deformity, pancreatic intraductal papillary
　　mucinous neoplasms (IPMNs)   *386*, 387
fish-odor syndrome   59
Fistula Drainage Assessment Measure
　　(FDAM)   251–252

fistulas, gastrointestinal
  diverticulitis 339
  perianal 251–254, 639
  unintentional weight loss 225
FK506 *see* tacrolimus
fluid intake, constipation 404
fluid replacement
  acute diarrhea 216
  acute pancreatitis 375
  upper GI bleeding 79, 138
  variceal bleeding 555
flukes, hepatobiliary 495–496, 547
flumazenil 562
fluoroquinolones, in pregnancy **358**
5-fluorouracil (5-FU) **353**
fluoxetine **410**
fluticasone, eosinophilic esophagitis 100
focal nodular hyperplasia (FNH) 443–444
FODMAPs (fermentable oligo-di-monosaccharides and
      polyols) 229, 393, 414
folate deficiency, short-bowel syndrome 302
FOLFOX/FOLFIRI chemotherapy 353–354
Fontan procedure 304, 306, 307
food allergies 227–230
  diagnosis 229–230
  IgE-mediated 228
  management 230
  non-IgE-mediated (NFA) 228
  predisposing factors 227–228
Food Allergy Research and Education (FARE)
      230
food aversion 229
food challenge testing 229
food intolerances 227–230
food poisoning 214, 216, 228
food protein-induced enterocolitis syndrome
      (FPIES) 228
foregut 177
Forrest classification, peptic ulcers 117, **118**
foveolar hyperplasia, gastric 127
Francisella tularensis **493**
free fatty acids (FFAs) 499, 523
fructosemia, hereditary **593**
fulminant hepatic failure *see* acute liver failure
functional abdominal pain syndrome (FAPS)
      407–411
  clinical features 408
  diagnosis 408
  differential diagnosis 409
  pathophysiology 407–408
  treatment 409–411
functional chest pain (FCP) 49–50, 169, 170, 171
functional dyspepsia (FD) 70, 71–72, 122
functional esophageal disorders (FEDs) 169–171
functional gastrointestinal disorders (FGIDs) 70
  history of abuse 207
  small and large bowel 389–415
fundoplication, imaging after 23–26
fungal infections
  HIV infection 364, **366**
  liver 494
  transplant recipients 421, 627
furosemide 558

gabapentin 64, 409
galactosemia **593**
gallbladder
  adenomyomatosis 447–448, 546
  strawberry 546
gallbladder adenomas 546
gallbladder cancer **199**, 547–548
  imaging 447, 547–548
  staging 548
gallbladder disease 543–552

gallbladder polyps 546–547
  carcinomatous 546
  cholesterol 546
  malignancy risk 546–547
gallstones (cholelithiasis) 543–546
  after bariatric surgery 234
  complications 544–546
  endoscopic diagnosis 459
  imaging 447–448
  pregnancy 360
  short-bowel syndrome 300
  uncomplicated 543–544
  see also choledocholithiasis
Gardner syndrome **209**
gas, intestinal
  abdominal bloating/distension 413
  aerophagia 57
gastrectomy, Ménétrier's disease 307
gastric accommodation 16, 17
  testing 38–39
gastric adenocarcinoma *see* gastric cancer
gastric adenomas 145–146
gastric antral vascular ectasia (GAVE) 143,
      556–557
gastric atresia 13, **178**
gastric barostat 38
gastric biopsies
  eosinophilic gastroenteritis 154
  gastric submucosal tumors 149–150
  gastritis 126, *127*
  H. pylori 123
  peptic ulcers 116
gastric cancer (adenocarcinoma)
  epidemiology **199**
  H. pylori association 122
  prevention 124
  upper GI bleeding 143
  see also gastric tumors
gastric disorders 113–165
  in pregnancy 357–359
  in systemic and cutaneous diseases 156–165
gastric duplications 13, **178**
gastric dysplasia 128
gastric electrical rhythm 16–17
  testing 37–38
gastric electrical stimulation, gastroparesis 136–137
gastric emptying 17–18
  factors affecting 18
  GERD and 85–86
gastric emptying scintigraphy 36, *37*, 133–134
gastric emptying testing 36–37
  clinical utility 37
  gastroparesis 133–134
  nausea and vomiting 76
  techniques 36–37
gastric intraepithelial neoplasia 128
gastric lymphoma 147
gastric MALT lymphoma 122, 147
gastric motility 15, 16–18
  distal stomach 17–18
  electrophysiology 16–17
  fasting 18
  proximal stomach 17
  testing 36–39, 76
gastric motility disorders **37**
gastric mucosa 11–12
  heterotopic 13
gastric outlet obstruction (GOO), endoscopic palliation
      of malignant 267-268
gastric pacemaker 16–17, *18*
gastric polyps 145–147
  adenomatous 145–146
  fundic gland (FGP) 145, **146**, *146*
  hamartomatous 146

hyperplastic 145, **146**, *146*
  inflammatory fibroid 146
gastric tumors 145–150
  mucosal 145–148
  submucosal **146**, 148–150
  see also gastric cancer
gastric ulcers 115–119
  H. pylori 116, 122
  see also peptic ulcers
gastric varices 555, 556
  isolated (IGV) 556
  management 556, 569
gastric volvulus 13, **178**
gastrin 181–183
gastrin 17 levels, gastritis 127
gastrinoma 147–148, 182
gastrin receptor antagonists 183
gastritis 126–130
  active 127
  assessment 126–127
  atrophic 128, 129
  autoimmune 130
  chemical 129–130
  definition 126
  etiological classification 128–130
  H. pylori 128–129
  lymphocytic 127
  morphology 127–128
  OLGA/OLGIM staging systems 126–127
gastrocolonic response 194, *196*
gastroduodenal stents, malignant gastric outlet
      obstruction 267, *268*
Gastroenterology Board Examination 3–5
gastroesophageal reflux 16
gastroesophageal reflux disease (GERD) 85–90
  after *H. pylori* eradication 124
  Barrett's esophagus 87, 92
  belching and aerophagia 56
  clinical features 43, 86–87
  diagnosis 87–88
  distal esophageal spasm 32
  esophageal eosinophilia 99, 100
  esophageal strictures 105
  extraesophageal manifestations 85, 86, 87, 89
  heartburn symptoms predicting 46
  hypotensive esophageal dysmotility 32, 33
  non-cardiac chest pain 48, 87
  pathophysiology 85–86
  pregnancy 357, **358**
  transplant recipients 422
  treatment 54, 88–89, 94
gastroesophageal varices 555
  type 1 (GOV1) 556
  type 2 (GOV2) 556
gastrointestinal (GI) bleeding
  hematochezia 237–239
  history and physical exam 206–207
  obscure *see* obscure gastrointestinal bleeding
  variceal *see* variceal bleeding
  see also lower gastrointestinal bleeding; upper
      gastrointestinal bleeding
gastrointestinal (GI) cancer 198–200
gastrointestinal (GI) disorders
  common complaints/diagnoses **204**
  diagnosis and differential diagnosis 213–260
  with extraintestinal complaints **209**
  history and physical exam 203–211
  HIV infection 363–367
  liver disease 540
  obesity-associated 231–232
  pregnancy 357–361
gastrointestinal manometry 38
  rumination syndrome 66, *67*
gastrointestinal (GI) neoplasia 198–200

gastrointestinal stromal tumors (GIST)
  small bowel 280, 283
  stomach 148
gastrointestinal (GI) tract
  anatomy and embryology 177
  congenital anomalies 177–178
  hormones and neurotransmitters 181–186
  sensory pathways 193
gastroparesis 71, 132–137
  clinical presentation 133
  diabetic 132, 133, 135, 157–158
  etiology 132–133
  evaluation 133–134
  idiopathic 133
  postsurgical 133
  treatment 134–137
  unintentional weight loss 225
gastropathy 126
  chemical 129–130
  reactive 127
gastroplasty techniques, endoscopic 235
gastroschisis 177–178
GERD see gastroesophageal reflux disease
ghrelin family **182**
Giardia infections **214**
ginger 359
Glasgow Alcoholic Hepatitis Score (GAHS) 500
Glasgow–Blatchford score (GBS), peptic ulcer
    bleeding 117–118
gliadin antibodies 291–292
glial cells, enteric 192
globus sensation 85, 169, 170, 171
glucagon **182**
glucagon-like peptide 2 (GLP2), short-bowel
    syndrome 302
glucagonoma 185
glucose breath test (GBT) 287, **288**
glutaraldehyde colitis 335
gluten challenge testing 292–293
gluten-free diet (GFD) 293–294, 414, 512
gluten sensitivity, non-celiac (NCGS) 228
glycemic control, diabetic gastroparesis 135
glycogen storage diseases 592
gonorrhea **492**
Gottren's signs 156, 159
graciloplasty, dynamic 259
graft rejection, liver 624, 626–627
graft-versus-host disease (GVHD) 423
  hepatic (HGVHD) 516, 517
grandfather board certification 4
granular cell tumors (GCT), gastric 149
granulomatous hepatitis 490, **491**
grazoprevir (GR7) 471, **482**, 483, 484, 485
growth hormone, short-bowel syndrome 302
guanylate cyclase C agonist see linaclotide
guidelines, evidence-based societal 4–5
gut-associated lymphoid tissue (GALT), HIV
    infection 363–364

halitophobia 59
halitosis 58–61
  diagnosis 59–60
  etiology and pathophysiology 59
  therapeutics 60
hamartomas
  bile duct 446
  small bowel 280, 282
healthy diet counseling **210**
heartburn 46–48
  functional (FH) 169, 170–171
  history and physical exam 43
  mechanisms 47–48
  predicting GERD 46
  pregnancy 357

Helicobacter pylori 121–124
  bacteriology 121
  controversies in management 123–124
  diagnosis 116, 122–123, 141
  disease associations 122, **123**
  dyspepsia 71, 72
  epidemiology and transmission 121–122
  gastric MALT lymphoma 122, 147
  gastric polyps 145
  gastritis 128–129
  halitosis 59, 60
  histology 123, 124, 126
  pathogenesis 122
  peptic ulcer disease 115, 116, 122
  transplant recipients 422
  treatment 116, 123
Heller myotomy, modified 31, 55
HELLP syndrome 582
  clinical features 583
  diagnosis 584
  pathophysiology 583, 592–593
  prognosis and recurrence 585
  treatment 584–585
helminth infections
  HIV infection 364–365
  liver 495–496
hemangioma, liver 442–443, 444
hematemesis 79–81, 206
  causes 79, **80**
  initial assessment and management 79–80,
      138–139
  see also upper gastrointestinal (GI) bleeding
hematochezia 138, 206, 237–239
  clinical features 237
  diagnosis 238, **239**
  differential diagnosis 238–239
  prognosis 239
  treatment 239
hematologic disorders
  Budd–Chiari syndrome 514
  liver disease 541
hematopoietic cell transplantation (HCT)
  GI complications 419–424
  liver complications 516–520
hemobilia 143
hemochromatosis
  hereditary 530–533
    clinical features 530–532
    diagnosis 532–533
    liver transplantation 605
    treatment 533
  neonatal **593**
hemolytic anemia, liver disease 541
hemorrhage see bleeding
hemorrhagic colitis, penicillin-associated
    334
hemosuccus pancreaticus 143
Henoch–Schönlein purpura **209**, 540
heparin
  acute mesenteric ischemia 311–312
  protein-losing gastroenteropathy 306
  sinusoidal obstruction syndrome 519
hepatectomy, total 611
hepatic adenoma (HA) 444–445
hepatic adenomatosis 445
hepatic artery
  anastomosis, liver grafting 612
  anatomic variations 610
  liver transplant complications 613–614
hepatic artery–portal vein fistulas 539
hepatic artery stenosis (HAS), liver transplant
    recipients 613, 614
hepatic artery thrombosis (HAT) 539
  liver transplant recipients 422, 613–614

hepatic encephalopathy 560–562
  acute liver failure **436**, 439, 562
  chronic 561–562
  classification **561**
  post-TIPS 561, 571
hepatic hemangioma 442–443, 444
hepatic infarction 539
hepatic iron concentration (HIC) 532, 533
hepatic metastases 446
hepatic steatosis (fatty liver) 514, 522
  alcoholic 498, 499
  diagnosis 524–525, 526
  epidemiology 522–523
  pathophysiology 523
  prognosis 527
  see also acute fatty liver of pregnancy
hepatic vein
  complications of liver transplant 614
  piggyback liver transplant technique 611
hepatic vein pressure gradient (HVPG) 554,
      567–568
hepatic veno-occlusive disease (VOD) see sinusoidal
      obstruction syndrome
hepatitis
  acute, differential diagnosis **467**
  alcoholic see alcoholic hepatitis
  autoimmune see autoimmune hepatitis
  chronic, staging systems **452**
  granulomatous 490, **491**
  interface 509
  ischemic 538, 539
  viral see viral hepatitis
hepatitis A 465–469
  clinical features 430, 466–467
  diagnosis 467
  pathophysiology 465–466
  prevention 468
  treatment 467–468
  vaccination **210**, 468
hepatitis A virus (HAV) 465–466
hepatitis B
  acute liver failure 435, **438**
  chronic 473–479
    HBeAg-negative 475–476, 477
    HBeAg-positive 474–475, **476**, 477
    hepatitis delta virus infection 478
    liver cancer risk 475, 574
    natural history 474–475
    predictors of progression 475
    treatment 475–477, 478
  extraintestinal manifestations **209**
  hepatitis C co-infection 100
  history taking 430
  liver transplantation 605, 629–630
  screening **210**
  transplant recipients 420–421
  vaccination **210**
hepatitis B e antigen (HBeAg) 473–474, 477
hepatitis B immune globulin (HBIG) 605
hepatitis B surface antigen (HBsAg) 473–474, 477
hepatitis B virus (HBV) 473–474
  antibodies 474
  DNA, serum levels 474, 475, **476**
  genotypes 473
hepatitis C 480–486
  clinical features **209**, 430
  diagnosis and evaluation 480–481
  liver cancer risk 574–575
  liver transplantation 604–605
    antiviral therapy and 483–484, 485–486
    corticosteroid therapy 622
    disease recurrence 629
  screening **210**
  sustained virological response (SVR) 481

hepatitis C (*Continued*)
  transplant recipients 420–421
  treatment 481–486
hepatitis C virus (HCV) 480
  genotype 1, therapy 481–485
  genotype 2, therapy **482**, 485
  genotype 3, therapy **482**, 485
  genotype 4, therapy **482**, 485
  genotypes 5 and 6, therapy **482**, 485–486
  resistance associated variant (RAV) **482, 483**
  RNA testing 480
hepatitis delta virus (HDV) 478
hepatitis E **466**, 469–470
hepatitis E virus (HEV) 469
hepatocellular carcinoma (HCC) 574–578
  alpha-1-antitrypsin deficiency 536
  chronic hepatitis B 475, 574
  clinical features 575–576
  diagnosis and screening 446, 576, *577*
  hereditary hemochromatosis 533
  liver transplantation 576–578, 606, 630, 633
  pathogenesis 575
  risk factors 574–575
  treatment 576–578
hepatomegaly, physical examination 432–433
hepatoportoenterostomy (HPE) (Kasai) 588–589
hepatopulmonary syndrome (HPS) 562–563
  biliary atresia 588
  clinical features 431, 563
  liver transplantation 606, 633
hepatorenal syndrome (HRS) 560, 569–570, 628
hepcidin 530, *531*
herbal medicine, irritable bowel syndrome 397
hereditary mixed polyposis syndrome 351
hereditary non-polyposis colorectal cancer (HNPCC)
    see Lynch syndrome
herpes simplex virus (HSV)
  anogenital infection 365
  hepatitis 437, **438**, 470
  transplant recipients 420
herpesvirus infections
  acute hepatitis 470–471
  transplant recipients 420
heterotopic gastric mucosa 13
HFE gene mutations 524, 530, 532
hiatal hernia 25–26, 85
hiccups 61–64
  benign transient 61–62
  persistent or intractable 62–64
high-amplitude propagating contractions
    (HAPCs) 194, *196*
hindgut 177
Hirschsprung (HSCR) disease 178, 248
histamine 182, 229
histamine type 2 receptor antagonists (H2RAs)
  functional dyspepsia 72
  GERD 88–89
  peptic ulcer disease 117
  in pregnancy **358**
histidine–ketoglutarate–tryptophan (HTK)
    solution 612
histopathology 5
Histoplasma capsulatum 364, *490*, 494
history-taking, clinical 203–207, **208**
HIV infection
  enterocolitis 364–365, **366**
  GI consequences 363–367
    clinical features 364–365
    diagnosis 365, **366**
    differential diagnosis 365
    epidemiology 363
    pathogenesis 363–364
    treatment 365, *367*
  hepatitis C co-infection 480

leishmaniasis 494
  liver transplantation 603
  proctitis 365, **366**
HIV Organ Policy Equity (HOPE) Act 609
HLA haplotypes, celiac disease 292
Hodgkin's disease 541
hookworms, dog 153
hormones, gastrointestinal 181–186
HSV *see* herpes simplex virus
5-HT₃ antagonists 335, 395
5-HT₄ agonists
  colonic ischemia 335
  constipation 395, 405
human chorionic gonadotrophin (hCG) 357
human granulocytic anaplasmosis (HGA) **492**
human immunodeficiency virus *see* HIV
human monocytic ehrlichiosis (HME) **492**
human papillomavirus (HPV)
  esophageal adenocarcinoma risk 91, *92*, 93
  vaccination recommendations **210**
humoral immune response 189
hydatid disease (echinococcosis) 442, 495
hydrogen breath tests 287, *288*, 413
hydrothorax, hepatic 558–559, 569
hygiene hypothesis 227
hyoscyamine
  irritable bowel syndrome 395–396
  in pregnancy **358**, 359
hyperbilirubinemia 433
hypercontractile esophagus 32
hyperemesis gravidarum (HG) 357–359, 582
  clinical features 583
  diagnosis 584
  pathophysiology 582
  prognosis and recurrence 585
  treatment 584
hypergastrinemia 182–183
hyperglycemia, gastric emptying and 132, 134, 135
hyperkalemia, liver transplant surgery 612
hyperkeratosis plantaris and palmaris (tylosis) 44, **165**
hyperkeratosis syndromes, cutaneous 164, **165**
hyperlipidemia *see* dyslipidemia
hyperoxaluria 605–606, 634
hyperplastic polyps
  colon 349
  stomach 145, **146**, *146*
hypertension
  liver transplant recipients 624, 628
  NAFLD 524
hyperthyroidism 159, 539–540
hypertonic saline 439
hyperventilation 439
hypnotherapy 397, 410
hypoalbuminemia, protein-losing
    gastroenteropathy 304, 305
hypogastric pain **205**
hyponatremia
  ascites management 558
  liver transplant candidates 601, 634–635
hypoproteinemia, protein-losing
    gastroenteropathy 304, 305
hypothermia, induced 439
hypothyroidism 158–159, 540
Hy's rule, drug-induced liver injury 506

IBS *see* irritable bowel syndrome
icterus *see* jaundice
idiopathic thrombocytopenic purpura (ITP) 122
IgA
  deficiency, celiac disease 292
  secretory 189
IgE 189
  blood levels 229
  mediated food allergy 228

ileus, postoperative 319
imaging *see* radiology
imatinib mesylate, gastrointestinal stromal
    tumors 283
imipramine **410**
immunoproliferative small intestinal disease 281
immunosuppressive therapy
  autoimmune hepatitis 509–510
  drug interactions **620**
  hepatitis C 605
  liver transplantation 617–624, 626
    acute rejection episodes 624
    clinical trends **618**
    drugs used 618–623
    induction 617, 623–624
    long-term adverse effects 624, 628–629
    maintenance 617, **619–620**
  see also azathioprine; corticosteroids
impedance, multichannel
  esophageal *see* esophageal impedance–pH
      monitoring
  small intestine 193
inclusion-body myositis 156, **157**
incontinence products 258
indeterminate colitis 323, 324
infections
  acute liver failure 437–438
  causing dysphagia/odynophagia 52
  liver (non-viral) 487–496
  liver dysfunction 542
  liver transplant candidates 635
  transplant recipients 419–421, 627
  see also diarrhea, infectious; *specific infections*
Infectious Diseases Society of America (IDSA) 480
inferior mesenteric artery (IMA) 308, 334
inferior vena cava (IVC)
  complications of liver transplant 614
  liver transplant surgery 610, 611–612
infertility, in GI diseases 359–360
inflammatory bowel disease (IBD)
  C. difficile infection 328, 330
  colitis 323–327
  colorectal cancer risk 324, 350
  complications 324
  differential diagnosis **325**, 330
  extraintestinal manifestations 324, 540, 550
  pathophysiology 187, 188–189, 323
  pregnancy **358**, 359–360
  treatment 325–327
  unclassified (IBD-U) 323, 324
  see also Crohn's disease; ulcerative colitis
inflammatory diseases, upper GI
    involvement 159–161
inflammatory myopathies, upper GI involvement 156,
    157
inflammatory pseudotumor (IPT), hepatic 446
infliximab
  Crohn's disease **276**, 277
  perianal Crohn's disease 253
  in pregnancy **358**
influenza vaccination **210**
inlet patches 13
innate immune system 187
insulin **182**
insulinoma 185
insulin resistance 523
integrated relaxation pressure (IRP) 28
interferon (IFN)
  hepatitis B 476–477
  hepatitis delta virus infection 478
  see also pegylated interferon
internal anal sphincter 195, 256
  weakness 257
International Antiviral Society (IAS) 480

International Autoimmune Hepatitis Group
    (IAIHG) 508–509
interstitial Cajal cells (ICCs)
    esophagus 15
    intestinal 191–192
    stomach 17
intestinal angina *see* chronic mesenteric
    ischemia/insufficiency
intestinal epithelial cells
    antigen uptake 188
    barrier function 187
intestinal failure 299
intestinal ischemia *see* mesenteric ischemia
intestinal lymphangiectasia
    primary 304, 307
    secondary 304
intestinal metaplasia
    Barrett's esophagus 91, 93
    stomach 122, 128, 129
intestinal obstruction 313–315
    causes 313, **314**
    complications and recurrence 314
    diagnosis 313–314, **315**, *316, 317*
    management 313–315, **318**
    in pregnancy 361
intestinal pseudo-obstruction 315–319
    chronic *see* chronic intestinal pseudo-obstruction
    enteric dysmotility without visceral
        dilation 318–319
intestinal transplantation 302, 318
intestine
    history and physical exam 203–211
    motor and sensory function 191–197
    mucosal immunology 187–189
    pathobiology 175–200
intracranial pressure (ICP), raised
    acute liver failure *436, 439,* 562
    management 436
intraductal papillary mucinous neoplasms (IPMNs),
        pancreas 385–386, 387
intragastric balloons (IGBs), endoscopically
        placed 234–235
intrahepatic cholestasis
    benign recurrent (BRIC) 591
    progressive familial (PFIC) 591
intrahepatic cholestasis of pregnancy (ICP) 582
    clinical features 583
    diagnosis 584
    pathophysiology 582–583
    prognosis and recurrence 585
    treatment 584
intraoperative enteroscopy
    obscure GI bleeding 243, 244
    small bowel tumors 282
irinotecan **353**
iron
    hepatic concentration (HIC) 532, 533
    overload 530, 532–533
    serum 524
iron deficiency (anemia)
    H. pylori-related 122
    inflammatory bowel disease 324
    pathophysiology **531**
irritable bowel syndrome (IBS) 391–397
    abdominal bloating/distension 412, 413
    clinical features 392
    constipation-predominant (IBS-C) 248, 392, **393**,
        394–395
    diagnosis 392–393
    diarrhea-predominant (IBS-D) 218, 392, **393**, 395
    drug-induced colonic ischemia 335
    epidemiology 391
    pathophysiology 391–392, 407–408
    in pregnancy **358**, 359

prognosis 397
small-intestinal bacterial overgrowth and 285, 413
subtypes 392, **393**
treatment 393–397, 410
ischemic colitis *see* colonic ischemia
ischemic hepatitis 538, 539
isoniazid, hepatotoxicity 505

jackhammer esophagus 32
JAK2 gene mutations 514
Jarisch–Herxheimer reaction 297–298
jaundice
    cholangiocarcinoma 548
    drug-induced 504, 506
    history taking 207, **208**, 429
    pancreatic cancer 383
    physical exam 431
jejunostomy, proximal 299
Joint Guidelines
    colonoscopy surveillance **264**
    colorectal cancer screening 263
juvenile polyposis syndrome (JPS) 351

kala-azar 494
Kasai portoenterostomy 588–589
Kayser–Fleischer (KF) rings 534
keratoconjunctivitis sicca 511
King's College criteria, acute liver failure 440, 603, **604**
Klebsiella pneumoniae, liver abscess 487

lactitol, hepatic encephalopathy 561–562
lactose intolerance 228–229, 230
lactulose **249, 404**
    hepatic encephalopathy 561–562
    in pregnancy 358
lactulose breath test (LBT) 287, **288**
lamina propria
    esophagus 11
    fibrosis, gastric 127
lamivudine, hepatitis B 476, 477
laparoscopic adjustable gastric banding (LAGB) 26,
        233, 234
laparoscopic cholecystectomy 544, 545, 547
laparoscopic Roux-en-Y gastric bypass
        (LRYGB) 233–234
laparoscopic-sleeve gastrectomy (LSG) 234
large-bowel disorders 321–367
    functional 321–367
    HIV infection 364–365
    see also colonic diseases
large-bowel obstruction 314–315, *317*
    endoscopic palliation of malignant 268
large intestine
    anatomy and embryology 177
    motor function 194–196
    neuromuscular apparatus 191–193
    sensation 193, 195–196
large-volume paracentesis (LVP), for ascites 558, 569
laryngopharyngeal reflux 87, 88, 89
laryngoscopy, GERD 88
laxatives 248–249, 404–405
    irritable bowel syndrome **394**, 395
    in pregnancy 358, *359*
ledipasvir (LDV) 481, **482**, 483–484, 485
left lower quadrant (LLQ) pain **205, 340**
left-sided colitis 323
left upper quadrant (LUQ) pain **205**
Legionella spp. **492**
leiomyoma
    gastric 148
    small bowel 280, 282
leishmaniasis 494
leprosy **492**
leptospirosis **492**

leukemia, liver involvement 541
levofloxacin 555
lichen planus 163–164
lifestyle modification
    alcoholic liver disease 500–501
    GERD 88, 94
    obesity 232
Lille score 500
linaclotide
    constipation 249, **404**, 405
    irritable bowel syndrome **394**, 395
lipoma, gastric 149
lipopolysaccharide (LPS) 364
Listeria monocytogenes **492**
lithotripsy, endoscopic 456
liver
    imaging 442–448
    surgical anatomy 609–610
liver abscess
    amebic 488–489
    pyogenic 487–488
liver biopsy 436, 444
    alcoholic liver disease 500
    Budd–Chiari syndrome 515
    complications and risks 450–451
    drug-induced liver injury 505
    EUS-guided 459
    hepatitis C 481
    liver fibrosis 450–452
    monitoring after 451–452
    NAFLD **523**, 525–526
    preprocedure assessment 451
    primary sclerosing cholangitis 550
    safety 450
    sinusoidal obstruction syndrome *518*, 519
    technique 451
liver cancer **199**, 446–447, 574–580
    see also cholangiocarcinoma; hepatocellular
        carcinoma
liver cysts
    echinococcal 442, 495
    imaging 442, *443*
liver disease 463–595
    alcoholic *see* alcoholic liver disease
    autoimmune 508–512
    diagnostic approaches 427–460
    drug-induced *see* drug-induced liver injury
    endoscopic techniques 455–460
    history and physical exam 429–434
    pediatric 587–595
    pregnancy and 582–586
    short bowel syndrome 300
    in systemic diseases 538–542
    vascular 513–520
liver elastography **452**, 453–454, 526
liver fibrosis
    assessment 450–454
    hepatitis B 475
    hepatitis C 481
    liver biopsy 450–452
    NAFLD 525, 526
    non-invasive markers 452–454
    Schistosoma infections 496
    staging systems **452**
    see also cirrhosis
liver function tests 433–434
liver–kidney transplantation, simultaneous
        (SLKT) 603
liver rupture, HELLP syndrome 585
liver support devices 440
liver transplantation 599–639
    acute graft rejection 624, 626–627
    acute liver failure 440, 603, **604**
    Alagille syndrome 592

liver transplantation (*Continued*)
  alcoholic liver disease   501–502, 603–604
  alpha-1-antitrypsin deficiency   536, 605
  assessment of patients for   602–603
  autoimmune hepatitis   510, 605
  biliary atresia   589, 593
  Budd–Chiari syndrome   516
  cholangiocarcinoma   549–550, 580, 606, 633
  cholestatic liver diseases   605, 630
  complications
    biliary   457–458, 614, 615, 626
    gastrointestinal   422
    medical   626–630
    surgical   613–615
  contraindications   602–603
  deceased donor   603, 609
  donor selection   603, 609
  drug-induced liver injury   506, 507
  extended criteria donors (ECDs)   603
  graft rejection   626–627
  HELLP syndrome   585
  hepatitis B   605, 629–630
  hepatitis C *see under* hepatitis C
  hepatocellular carcinoma   576–578, 606, 630,
      633
  hepatopulmonary syndrome   606, 633
  hepatorenal syndrome   560
  immunosuppression   617–624, 626
  indications   602
  living donor *see* living donor liver transplantation
  medical management   626–630
  metabolic diseases   **602**, 605–606
  non-alcoholic steatohepatitis   604
  organ allocation   608–609, 632–635
    distribution scheme   608, 632–633
    future trends   608–609
    hyponatremia and   634–635
    infections and   635
    MELD exceptions   633–634
    portal vein thrombosis and   635
    prognosis and   601–602
    renal dysfunction and   634
  pediatric   593–595
  piggyback (Barcelona) technique   610, 611
  portopulmonary hypertension   564, 606, 634
  primary biliary cirrhosis   511, 605, 630
  primary non-function (PNF)   614–615
  primary sclerosing cholangitis   551, 605, 630
  progressive familial intrahepatic cholestasis   591
  selection of patients   601–607
  surgery   609–615
    complications   613–615
    phases   611–613
    relevant anatomy   609–610
    techniques   610–611
  timing of evaluation for   602
  Wilson's disease   535–536, 605
liver tumors
  benign   442–446
  malignant   **199**, 446–447, 574–580
living donor liver transplantation (LDLT)   603
  pediatric   594
  surgical complications   613, 614, 615
  surgical technique   611
long-chain 3-hydroxyacyl CoA dehydrogenase
    (LCHAD) deficiency   583
loperamide   220, **222**
  acute diarrhea   216
  fecal incontinence   258
  irritable bowel syndrome   395
  in pregnancy   **358**
  short-bowel syndrome   300, **302**
lorcaserin   232
L-ornithine-L-aspartate (LOLA)   562

lower esophageal sphincter (LES)   11
  mechanical disruption, achalasia   30–31
  motor function   16, *17*
  myotomy   31, 55
  transient relaxations (TLESR)   16, 56, 85
lower gastrointestinal (GI) bleeding
  diverticular disease   339
  hematochezia   237–239
  history taking   206–207
lubiprostone
  constipation   249, **404**, 405
  irritable bowel syndrome   **394**, 395
lymphocyte-depleting antibodies   623
lymphocytes, mucosal   188
lymphogranuloma venereum, HIV infection   365
lymphoma
  gastric   147
  liver   541
  small bowel   280–281, 283
Lynch syndrome   199–200, 351

Maddrey Discriminant Function (MDF)   500
magnesium salts, laxative   248–249
magnetic resonance cholangiopancreatography
    (MRCP)
  choledocholithiasis   456
  primary sclerosing cholangitis   550
magnetic resonance elastography (MRE)   **452**, 454
magnetic resonance enteroclysis, small bowel
    tumors   281–282
magnetic resonance enterography   75
  Crohn's disease   275
  intestinal obstruction   313, 314
magnetic resonance imaging (MRI)
  cholangiocarcinoma   549, *579*
  fecal incontinence   258
  perianal fistulas   252
  portal hypertension   554
  small bowel tumors   281–282
  small intestinal motility   193
Maintenance of Certification (MOC) examination   3, 4
malabsorption, intestinal
  chronic pancreatitis   378
  short-bowel syndrome   299, 300
  small-intestinal bacterial overgrowth   286
  unintentional weight loss   224–225
malaria   491
malignant obstruction
  biliary, endoscopic management   458–459
  endoscopic palliation   266–268
malignant tumors
  GI, transplant recipients   421–422
  post-liver transplantation   629, **630**
Mallory–Weiss tears   142–143
malrotation and midgut volvulus   **178**
MALT lymphoma (maltoma)
  gastric   122, 147
  small bowel   281
mammalian target of rapamycin (mTOR)
    inhibitors   **619–620**, 622–623
mannitol   439, 562
manometry   5
  anorectal *see* anorectal manometry
  colonic   194–195, 403
  esophageal *see* esophageal manometry
  gastrointestinal *see* gastrointestinal manometry
  small intestinal   193, 317
marginal artery of Drummond   308, *309*
MDR3 gene   582–583, 591
Meckel diverticulum   178
Mediterranean lymphoma, small bowel   281
medium-chain fatty acid disorder (MCAD)   592
megacolon   248
megarectum   248

Meissner's (submucosal) plexus   192
MELD (Model for End-Stage Liver Disease)
  score   601–602, 608, 632
  acute liver failure   440
  alcoholic liver disease   500
  exceptions   **602**, 608, 633–634
  hepatitis C   604–605
  hepatocellular carcinoma   576, 606
  pediatric liver transplantation   594
  plus serum sodium (MELD-Na)   570, 601, 634–635
  post-TIPS mortality   570
  primary sclerosing cholangitis   605
  recertification   632, **633**
  Share 35 rule   608, 633
melena   138, 206
melioidosis   **492**
Ménétrier's disease   147, 307
men who have sex with men (MSM), amebic liver
    abscess   488
6-mercaptopurine (6-MP)   621
  Crohn's disease   **276**, 277
  perianal Crohn's disease   253, 254
  in pregnancy   **358**
  ulcerative colitis   326
meropenem, Whipple's disease   297
mesalamine (5-ASA)   275, **276**, 326
mesenteric angiography   311
mesenteric ischemia   308–312
  non-occlusive   309, 312, 333
  see also acute mesenteric ischemia; chronic
      mesenteric ischemia/insufficiency; colonic
      ischemia
mesenteric lymph nodes   187–188
mesenteric vasculature   308–309, 334
mesenteric venous thrombosis (MVT)
  colonic ischemia   335, 336
  small-bowel ischemia   309, 311–312
metabolic bone disease
  inflammatory bowel disease   324
  liver transplant recipients   629
  primary biliary cholangitis   511
metabolic diseases
  inherited, causing liver disease   592–593
  liver transplantation   **602**, 605–606
  upper GI involvement   157–159
metabolic syndrome   524
metaplasia, gastric gland   128
metastases, liver   446
methane   413
methotrexate
  Crohn's disease   **276**, 277
  male fertility and   360
  in pregnancy   **358**
methylcellulose   **249**, **404**
methylmalonic acidemia   **593**
methylprednisolone   **276**, 622
methynatrexone   346
metoclopramide
  chronic intestinal pseudo-obstruction   317–318
  functional dyspepsia   72
  gastroparesis   135
  GERD   89
  hematemesis   80
  hiccups   64
  in pregnancy   **358**
Metorchis bilis   495–496
metronidazole
  C. difficile infection   330, **331**
  hepatic encephalopathy   562
  perianal fistulas   252
  in pregnancy   **358**
  spontaneous bacterial peritonitis   559
Meyenburg complexes   446
microaspiration   85, 86

microbiota, gut   189
  food allergy risk and   227–228
  gas production   413
  influence on motility and sensation   195–196
  mechanisms maintaining normal   285–286
microfold (M) cells   188
microgastria   **178**
microlithiasis, endoscopic diagnosis   459
microsomal ethanol-oxidizing system (MEOS)   498, 499
midgut   177
  congenital anomalies   177, **178**
midodrine   560
migrating motor complexes (MMCs)   193–194, *195*
Milan criteria, hepatocellular carcinoma   576, 606, 633
milk allergy   228, 230
mineral oil, in pregnancy   **358**
mismatch repair (MMR) gene mutations   349, 351
misoprostol, slow-transit constipation   249
mitochondrial fatty acid oxidation, inborn errors of   592–593
mitochondrial neurogastrointestinal encephalopathy   319
mixed connective-tissue disease (MCTD)   156–157
Model for End-Stage Liver Disease score *see* MELD score
molecular adsorbent recirculating system (MARS)   562
montelukast, eosinophilic esophagitis   101
morphine, chronic diarrhea   **222**
motilin   18, **182**, 185
mouth, chewing and swallowing   15
MRI *see* magnetic resonance imaging
mTOR inhibitors   **619–620**, 622–623
mucinous cystadenoma, pancreatic   385, **386**
mucosa-associated lymphoid tissue *see* MALT
mucosal immune system   187–189
  adaptive immunity   188–189
  antigen uptake/induction of immune response   187–188
  humoral immunity   189
  innate immunity   187
  mucosal and epithelial barrier   187
  tolerance   189
mucositis, transplant recipients   422
mucus layer, barrier function   187
Muir–Torre syndrome   351
multiple hamartoma syndrome *see* Cowden syndrome
Murphy's sign   544
muscle, smooth *see* smooth muscle
muscularis mucosae hyperplasia, gastric   127
mycobacteria, non-tuberculous   **493**
Mycobacterium avium complex (MAC) infection   297, 364, **493**
Mycobacterium leprae   **492**
Mycobacterium tuberculosis   364, **493**
mycophenolate mofetil (MMF)
  GI side effects   422, 621–622
  liver transplant recipients   **619**, 621–622, 624, 626
mycophenolate sodium, enteric coated (EC-MPS)   **619**, 621–622
mycophenolic acid (MPA)   621–622
myeloablative conditioning therapy   422
myeloma, multiple   541
myeloproliferative disorders (MPD)
  Budd–Chiari syndrome   514, 516
  liver involvement   541
myenteric ganglionitis, with intestinal dysmotility   318
myenteric (Auerbach's) plexus   192
MYH-associated polyposis (MAP)   351

N-acetylcysteine (NAC)
  acetaminophen toxicity   437, **438**, 506
acute liver failure   562
  alcoholic hepatitis   501
nadolol   555
NAFLD *see* non-alcoholic fatty liver disease
NAFLD Fibrosis Score   526
narcotic bowel syndrome   319, 409, **411**
nasal disease, halitosis   59
nasogastric aspiration, upper GI bleeding   80, 138
natalizumab
  Crohn's disease   **276**, 277
  in pregnancy   **358**
National Comprehensive Cancer Network (NCCN), colorectal cancer screening   263, **264**
National Guideline Clearinghouse   5
nausea and vomiting   74–78
  chronic   72, 75
  clinical features   75
  diagnosis   75–76
  differential diagnosis   76
  history and physical exam   44, 206, **207**
  intestinal obstruction   313
  non-GI causes   **206**
  pathophysiology   74–75
  of pregnancy (NVP)   357–359
  therapeutics   76–78
needle-knife electrocautery, esophageal strictures   108–109
Neisseria gonorrhoeae
  liver involvement   **492**
  proctitis, HIV infection   365
nematodes   496
neomycin   562
neoplasia, gastrointestinal   198–200
neostigmine, acute colonic pseudo-obstruction   319, 345–346
netazepide   183
neuroendocrine tumors (NETs), gastropancreatic   185–186
  endoscopic ultrasound   638
  extraintestinal manifestations   **209**
  functioning   185
  non-functioning   185
  small bowel   280, 282–283
  treatment   185, 186
  see also carcinoids
neurofibromatosis, small bowel   280, 282
neurological disorders
  liver transplant recipients   629
  Whipple's disease   297
neuromodulation therapy, chronic constipation   405
neuromuscular diseases   161–163
neuropeptide Y (NPY)   184
neurotransmitters   181–186, 192
new onset diabetes mellitus after transplantation (NODAT)   624, 628–629
Nissen fundoplication, imaging after   23, *24, 25*
nitric oxide (NO)
  esophageal motor function   15, 16
  portal hypertension   554, 563
NOD2/CARD15   187, 273
nodular regenerative hyperplasia (NRH), liver   445–446, 542
non-alcoholic fatty liver disease (NAFLD)   522–528
  assessment of severity   526
  clinical/diagnostic features   430, 523–526
  diagnosis   526
  differential diagnosis   500, 526–527
  epidemiology   522–523
  liver cancer risk   575
  obesity and   231, 523, 524
  pathophysiology   523
  prognosis   527
  staging systems   **452**
  treatment   527–528
non-alcoholic steatohepatitis (NASH)   231, 522
  diagnosis   525–526
  differential diagnosis   500
  liver transplantation   604
  prognosis   527
  treatment   528
non-cardiac chest pain (NCCP)   48–49, 85
  diagnostic evaluation   48–49
  esophageal vs. non-esophageal causes   49
  functional   49–50
  GERD-related   48, 87
non-celiac gluten sensitivity (NCGS)   228
non-celiac wheat sensitivity (NCWS)   228
non-dysplastic Barrett's esophagus (NDBE)   92, 93, 94
non-erosive reflux disease (NERD)   85, 87
non-steroidal anti-inflammatory drugs (NSAIDs)
  ascites   558
  Barrett's esophagus   94
  colonic ischemia   335
  COX-2-selective   115–116, 117
  gastritis/gastropathy   130
  hepatotoxicity   505
  high cardiovascular risk patients   117
  liver biopsy and   451
  peptic ulcer disease   115–116, 117
  prevention of ulcers   117
norfloxacin   80, 555, 559–560
norovirus infection   214
nortriptyline   **410**
nucleotide/nucleoside analogues, hepatitis B   477
nucleus tractus solitarius (NST)   74
nutcracker esophagus   32, *33*, 55
nutritional deficiencies
  alcoholic liver disease   500–501
  protein-losing gastroenteropathy   305, 307
  short-bowel syndrome   299–300, 302
  small-intestinal bacterial overgrowth   286
nutritional disease   5
nutritional supplements
  alcoholic liver disease   501
  oral   226
nutritional support
  acute liver failure   437
  acute pancreatitis   376
  chronic intestinal pseudo-obstruction   318
  protein-losing gastroenteropathy   307
  short-bowel syndrome   299, 300, 302

obesity   231–235
  central   524
  comorbidities   231–232
  definitions   231
  epidemiology   231
  hepatitis C   480
  liver transplant surgery risks   603, 604
  management options   232–235
  NAFLD   231, 523, 524
  post-liver transplantation   624, 628
  screening and counseling   **210**
  surgery *see* bariatric surgery
obscure gastrointestinal bleeding (OGIB)   241–244
  clinical features   241
  diagnosis   241–243
  differential diagnosis   243
  management   243–244
obstetric injury, fecal incontinence   256, **257**
octanoate breath test   134
octreotide   184–185
  chronic diarrhea   220, **222**
  chronic intestinal pseudo-obstruction   318
  hematemesis   80
  pancreatic pseudocysts   380
  protein-losing gastroenteropathy   306

octreotide (*Continued*)
  short-bowel syndrome 300, **302**
  variceal bleeding 141, 555
odynophagia 52, 106
Ogilvie syndrome *see* acute colonic pseudo-obstruction
OLGA/OLGIM gastritis staging systems 126–127
olsalazine 275, **276**
omalizumab 230
ombitasvir (OBV) 481, 484
ombitasvir/paritaprevir/ritonavir **483**
ombitasvir/paritaprevir/ritonavir plus dasabuvir
      (3D) 481, **482, 483**
    drugs contraindicated with **483**
    genotype 1 HCV 484
    genotype 4 HCV 485
omeprazole, short-bowel syndrome **302**
omphalocele 177–178
omphalomesenteric band 178
omphalomesenteric cyst 178
omphalomesenteric duct *see* Meckel diverticulum
ondansetron, in pregnancy **358**
opiate antidiarrheal agents 220, **222**
Opisthorchis flukes 495–496, 547
oral allergy syndrome (OAS) 228
oral contraceptive pill (OCP) 443, 444, 445
oral disease, halitosis 59, 60
oral hygiene 60
oral rehydration solutions (ORS)
    diarrhea 216, 220, **222**
    short-bowel syndrome 300
oral tolerance 189
organ failure, acute pancreatitis 374
Organ Procurement and Transplantation Network
      (OPTN) 594, 608, 632
orlistat 232
L-ornithine-L-aspartate (LOLA) 562
Osler–Weber–Rendu syndrome 539
osteoporosis
    inflammatory bowel disease 324
    liver transplant recipients 629
    primary biliary cholangitis 511
otilonium bromide **396**
oxalate kidney stones, short-bowel syndrome 300
oxaliplatin **353**
oxidative stress, alcoholic liver disease 499

P53 immunohistochemistry, Barrett's dysplasia
      92
pain, complicating liver biopsy 450–451
pancolitis 323
pancreas
    anatomy and embryology 178–179
    congenital anomalies **178**, 179–180
    ectopic 179
    pathobiology 175–200
pancreas divisum (PD) 179
pancreatic agenesis 179
pancreatic and peripancreatic necrosis, walled-off
      373
pancreatic cancer 383–385
    diagnosis 383, *384*, 458
    endoscopic ultrasound 637
    epidemiology **199**, 383
    management 384, **385**, *385*, 458
    risk factors 379, 383
pancreatic cystic lesions 383–387
    clinical features 386
    congenital 179–180
    diagnosis 386–387
    differential diagnosis 379–380, **386**
    endoscopic ultrasound 637–638
    pathophysiology 385–386
    treatment 387
pancreatic ductal adenocarcinoma 383

pancreatic enzymes 379
pancreatic masses
    diagnostic evaluation 383, *384*
    differential diagnosis **384**
    endoscopic ultrasound 637–638, *638*
pancreatic necrosis 371, *372*
    acute 374
    management 375–376
    prognosis 376
    walled-off (WOPN) 373, 374, 380
pancreatic neoplasms, cystic *see* pancreatic cystic
      lesions
pancreatic neuroendocrine tumors (NETs) 185,
      638
pancreatic polypeptide (PP) family **182**, 184
pancreatic pseudocysts 379–382, **386**
    acute pancreatitis 371, 372–373, 374
    diagnosis 379–380
    drainage *379*, 380 381
    natural history 379
    recurrence 381–382
    symptoms 380
pancreatic rest 149, *150*
pancreatitis
    acute 371–376
      clinical features 374
      diagnosis 374–375
      differential diagnosis 375
      epidemiology 373
      pathophysiology 373–374
      prognosis 376
      treatment 375–376
    autoimmune 638
    chronic 224, 378–382
      biliary strictures 458
      clinical features 376
      diagnosis 376–377
      endoscopic ultrasound 638
      pancreatic pseudocysts 379, 380
      treatment 377
    interstitial 371, *372*, 375
    necrotizing 371, *372*
      management 375–376
      prognosis 376
      see also pancreatic necrosis
    post-ERCP 459–460
    in pregnancy 360–361
Paneth cells 187
panitumumab **353**
paracentesis, abdominal 557, 558, 569
paraneoplastic syndromes, upper GI involvement **161**,
      162–163
parasitic infections
    acute diarrhea 214
    HIV infection 364–365
    liver 491–494, 495–496
    transplant recipients 421
parasympathetic nervous system 192–193
parenteral nutrition (PN) 226
    acute pancreatitis 376
    chronic intestinal pseudo-obstruction 318
    short-bowel syndrome 299, 300, 302
parietal pain 203
paritaprevir *see* ombitasvir/paritaprevir/ritonavir
paroxetine 359, **410**
paroxysmal nocturnal hemoglobinuria 514, 541
pasireotide 184
Paterson–Brown–Kelly syndrome 13, 105, 107
pathogen recognition receptors (PRRs) 187
PDR5 inhibitors 564
peanut allergy 228
Pearson's syndrome **593**
Pediatric End-Stage Liver Disease (PELD) 594
pediatric liver disease 587–595

pediatric liver transplantation 593–595
pegylated interferon (PEG-IFN)
    hepatitis B 476–477
    hepatitis C 485
    hepatitis delta virus infection 478
    hepatitis E 470
pelvic floor dyssynergia *see* defecation disorders
pelvic floor exercises, fecal incontinence 258
pemphigoid 163, **164**
pemphigus 163, **164**
pemphigus vulgaris 163, **164**, *164*
D-penicillamine 535
penicillin G, Whipple's disease 297
pentagastrin 183
pentoxifylline 501
peppermint oil **396**
pepsinogen testing, gastritis 127
peptic ulcers 115–119, **358**
    bleeding 117–118, 140–141
      acid-suppressive therapy 118, 141
      endoscopic hemostasis 118, 140–141
      H. pylori testing 141
      management algorithm *119*
      rebleeding 118, 140, 141
      scoring systems 117–118
    clinical features 116
    diagnosis 116
    etiologies 115–116
    H. pylori 115, 116, 122
    non-NSAID, non-*H. pylori* idiopathic 116, 117
    NSAID 115–116, 117
    perforation 116
    pregnancy 357
    therapeutics 116–118, *119*
    transplant recipients 422
peptide histidine isoleucine (PHI) 185
peptide hormones 181–185
peptide YY (PYY) 184
percutaneous endoscopic cecostomy 347
percutaneous ethanol injection (PEI), hepatocellular
      carcinoma 578
percutaneous mesenteric angioplasty (PTMA) 312
perforations
    colonic *see* colonic perforation
    complicating ERCP 460
    peptic ulcer 116
perianal disease
    Crohn's disease 251–254
    HIV infection 365
    transplant recipients 422–423
Perianal Disease Activity Index (PDAI) 252
perianal fistulas 251–254
    complex and simple 251, *252*
    diagnosis 251–252
    endoscopic ultrasound 639
    pathophysiology 251, *252*
    treatment 252–254
perianal injectable bulking agents 259
peripancreatic fluid collections 371–376
    acute 374
    definitions 371–373
peripancreatic necrosis
    acute 374
    walled-off 372, 373, 374
peristalsis
    esophageal 16, *17*
    gastric 17
peritoneal friction rubs 432
peritonitis
    perforated diverticulitis 339, 341
    post-liver transplantation 627
    secondary bacterial 559
    spontaneous bacterial (SBP) 559–560
per-oral endoscopic myotomy (POEM) 31, 55

Peutz–Jeghers syndrome (PJS)
  colorectal cancer 351
  extraintestinal manifestations **209**
  small bowel hamartomas 280, 282
Peyer patches 187–188
pharyngeal motor function 15–16
phentermine 232
phenytoin 439–440
phlebotomy, hereditary hemochromatosis 533
photodynamic therapy (PDT), malignant
    obstruction 266, 267
physical activity see exercise/physical activity
physical examination 208–209
pioglitazine 528
Plasmodium infections 491
platelet-derived growth factor alpha (PDGFα)
    cells 192
platelets 434
platypnea, hepatopulmonary syndrome 563
pleural effusion, portal hypertension 558–559
Plummer–Vinson syndrome 13, 105, 107
pneumatic dilation, achalasia 31, 55
POLG mutation **593**
pollen-food allergy syndrome 228
polyarteritis nodosa 540
polycystic kidney disease 539
polycystic liver disease 442
polycythemia vera 516
polyethylene glycol (PEG)
  acute colonic pseudo-obstruction 346
  constipation 248, **249**, 404
  hematochezia 238
  irritable bowel syndrome **394**, 395
  in pregnancy **358**
Polyflex stents, esophageal strictures 109–110
polymyalgia rheumatica 540
polymyositis 156, **157**
porphyria 5
portal hypertension 554–565, 567–568
  Budd–Chiari syndrome 515–516
  diagnosis 554, 567–568
  elastographic evaluation 454
  nodular regenerative hyperplasia 446
portal hypertensive gastropathy (PHG) 143, 556–557
portal vein 609–610
  liver transplant complications 614
  liver transplant surgery 612
  septic thrombophlebitis 488
  stenosis (PVS) 614
portal vein thrombosis (PVT)
  liver transplant candidate 625
  liver transplant surgery and 609–610, 612
  post-liver transplantation 614
  systemic diseases 539
portography 567, 568
portopulmonary hypertension (PPH) 562, 563–564
  biliary atresia 588
  liver transplantation 564, 606, 634
portosystemic shunts 142
positron emission tomography (PET), small bowel
    tumors 282
postoperative ileus 319
postprandial distress syndrome (PDS) 71, 72
post-transplant lymphoproliferative disorder
    (PTLD) 421–422
practice questions 5
prebiotics, small-intestinal bacterial overgrowth 289
prednisone (or prednisolone)
  autoimmune hepatitis 509, 510
  Crohn's disease 276–277
  eosinophilic gastroenteritis 154
  liver transplant recipients **620**, 622
pre-eclampsia 582, 583, 584
pregabalin 409

pregnancy 5
  acute liver failure 435, **438**
  acute viral hepatitis 470
  drugs for GI disease **358**
  H. pylori management 124
  liver disease 582–586
  luminal GI disease 357–361
preventative services, national guidelines **210**, 211
primary afferent neurons 193
primary biliary cholangitis/cirrhosis (PBC) 510–512
  liver transplantation 511, 605, 630
primary non-function (PNF), liver grafts 614–615
primary obesity surgery endoluminal (POSE)
    procedures 235
primary sclerosing cholangitis (PSC) 489, 550–551
  cholangiocarcinoma risk 548, 551, 579
  complications 551
  diagnosis 448, 550
  gallbladder polyps 546
  inflammatory bowel disease association 324, 550
  liver transplantation 551, 605, 630
  management 459, 551
probiotics
  abdominal bloating 414
  C. difficile infection 330
  hepatic encephalopathy 562
  irritable bowel syndrome 396
prochlorperazine, in pregnancy **358**
proctitis
  HIV infection 365, **366**
  ulcerative 323
proctography, dynamic 258
proctosigmoiditis 323
progressive familial intrahepatic cholestasis
    (PFIC) 591
prokinetic agents
  abdominal bloating/distension 414
  chronic intestinal pseudo-obstruction 317–318
  functional constipation 405
  functional dyspepsia 72
  gastroparesis **134**, 135–136
  GERD 89
  nausea and vomiting 77, 78
  small-intestinal bacterial overgrowth 289
promethazine, in pregnancy **358**
propionic acidemia **593**
propranolol 555
prostacyclin 564
protein–energy malnutrition 223
protein-losing gastroenteropathy (PLGE) 304–307
  clinical features 305
  diagnosis 305, 306
  etiology 304–305, **306**
  pathophysiology 304, 305
  treatment 306, 307
protein-restricted diet, hepatic encephalopathy 561
prothrombin time 434
proton pump inhibitors (PPI)
  eosinophilic esophagitis 100
  functional dyspepsia 72
  functional esophageal disorders 170
  GERD 89, 94
  hematemesis 80
  hepatitis C therapy and 484
  hypergastrinemia due to 182
  peptic ulcer bleeding 118, 141
  peptic ulcer disease 116, 117
  in pregnancy **358**
  small-intestinal bacterial overgrowth and 285
  test, non-cardiac chest pain 48–49
protozoal infections
  HIV infection 364, **366**
  liver 491–494
  transplant recipients 421

prucalopride
  chronic intestinal pseudo-obstruction 318
  constipation 395, **404**, 405
pruritus
  intrahepatic cholestasis of pregnancy 583
  primary biliary cholangitis 511, 605
  progressive familial intrahepatic cholestasis 591
pseudomembranous colitis 328, 329
pseudopancreatic metaplasia, stomach 128
pseudopyloric metaplasia, stomach 128
psychiatric illness, unintentional weight loss 224
psychological assessment
  chest pain 50
  functional abdominal pain syndrome 408, **409**
  nausea and vomiting 76
psychological therapies
  functional abdominal pain syndrome 410
  irritable bowel syndrome 396–397
  rumination syndrome 66
psyllium **249**, 394, **404**
pulmonary disorders, hepatic manifestations 539
push enteroscopy (PE)
  obscure GI bleeding 242, **243**, 244
  small bowel tumors 282
pyelphlebitis 488
pyloric stenosis **178**
pylorospasm, diabetic gastroparesis 136
pylorus 17, 18
pyogenic liver abscess 487–488
pyrosis see heartburn

Q-fever **493**
quality of life
  biliary atresia 589
  pediatric liver transplant recipients 594–595
quetiapine 409–410

radiation enteritis 225
radiation therapy
  colorectal cancer 354
  liver complications 518
radiofrequency ablation (RFA)
  Barrett's esophagus 94, 95
  hepatocellular carcinoma 578
radiology 5
  colorectal cancer screening 262–263
  esophagus and stomach 23–26
  liver and bile ducts 442–448
radionuclide scintigraphy
  gastric emptying measurement 26, 27, 130, 131
  hematochezia 238, **239**
  obscure GI bleeding 242–243
radiopaque markers, colonic transit studies 248,
    402
ramosetron 395
ranitidine, short-bowel syndrome **302**
rapamycin see sirolimus
rectal cancer
  endoscopic ultrasound 638–639
  treatment **353**, 354
  see also colorectal cancer
rectal compliance, assessment 258
rectal diseases 321–367
  HIV infection 364–365
rectal examination, digital 208–209
rectal sensation
  assessment 258, 403
  dysfunctional 257
rectal stents, malignant obstruction 268
rectal varices 555, 556
referred pain 203
reflux esophagitis 85, 87
regenerative nodules (RNs), hepatic 446
regulatory T cells 189

regurgitation 46–48
  esophageal strictures 106
  GERD 85
  predicting GERD 46
  vomiting vs. 74
renal disorders, hepatic manifestations 539
renal dysfunction/failure
  acute liver failure 436
  advanced liver disease 560
  liver transplant candidates 634
  post-liver transplantation 624, 628
  see also hepatorenal syndrome
renal support, acute liver failure 439
renal transplantation
  colonic ischemia 333–334
  GI complications 422
  simultaneous liver transplant (SLKT) 603
reperfusion, transplanted liver 612
respiratory chain defects **593**
retching 74
Reynold's pentad 489, **544**, 545
rheumatoid arthritis (RA) 540
rheumatological disorders, liver disease 540
ribavirin (RBV)
  hepatitis C **482**, 483–484, 485
  hepatitis E 470
Rickettsia rickettsii **493**
rifampin 511
rifaximin
  abdominal bloating/distension 414
  hepatic encephalopathy 562
  irritable bowel syndrome 395
  in pregnancy **358**
  small-intestinal bacterial overgrowth 288, 289
  tropical sprue 295
right lower quadrant (RLQ) pain **205**
right upper quadrant (RUQ) pain **205**, 431
ritonavir *see* ombitasvir/paritaprevir/ritonavir
rituximab 421–422
Rockall score, upper GI bleeding 117–118, 139
Rocky Mountain spotted fever **493**
Rome criteria
  dyssynergic defecation **401**
  functional abdominal pain syndrome **408**
  functional chest pain 49–50
  functional constipation **247, 401**
  irritable bowel syndrome 392, **393**
  rumination syndrome 65
rosiglitazone 528
roundworms 496
Roux-en-Y gastric bypass (RYGBP) 25, 26, 233–234
Roux-en-Y stasis syndrome 133
rumination 64–67, 72
  clinical features 65
  differential diagnosis 66, 74
  pathophysiology and diagnosis 65–66, *67*
  treatment 66–67
rumination (R) waves 66

sacral nerve stimulation (SNS) 259, 405
Salmonella infections
  diarrhea **214**, 216
  hepatitis **493**
  HIV infection 364
sarcoidosis
  esophagus and stomach **160**, 161
  liver *490*, 541
Schatzki rings 23, *24*, 105
  treatment 109, 111
Schistosoma spp. 496
scintigraphy *see* radionuclide scintigraphy
scleroderma *see* systemic sclerosis
sclerotherapy, endoscopic *see* endoscopic sclerotherapy
scombroid fish poisoning 229

secretagogues, intestinal 405, 414–415
secretin **182**, 183–184
secretory IgA 189
seizures, acute liver failure 439–440
selective serotonin reuptake inhibitors (SSRIs)
  functional abdominal pain syndrome 409, **410**
  irritable bowel syndrome 396
  in pregnancy **358**, 359
selenium deficiency, short-bowel syndrome 302
self-expanding biodegradable stents (SEBS) 110, 111
self-expanding metal stents (SEMS)
  biliary obstructions 457–459
  complications 267
  esophageal strictures 109, 111
  palliation of malignant obstruction 266, 267
self-expanding plastic stents (SEPS)
  esophageal strictures 109–110, 111
  malignant dysphagia 267
self-help therapies 397, 414
senna 248, **249, 404**
  in pregnancy **358**
sensation, gut 193
serial transverse enteroplasty procedure (STEP) 302
serotonin modular therapy, colonic ischemia 335
serotonin-norepinephrine reuptake inhibitors
  (SNRIs) 409, **410**
serous cystadenoma, pancreatic 385, **386**
serrated polyposis syndrome 351
sertraline 511
serum ascites–albumin gradient (SAAG) 557, **558**
sexual abuse, history of 408
Share 35 rule, donor liver allocation 608, 633
shellfish allergy 228
Shiga toxin-producing *Escherichia coli* 216
Shigella infections **214**, 215–216
short-bowel syndrome (SBS) 299–303
  clinical features 224–225, 300
  pathophysiology 299–300
  prognosis 302
  treatment 300–302
short-chain fatty acids (SCFAs) 301
sicca syndrome 511
sickle cell anemia 541
sigmoidoscopy, flexible, colorectal cancer
  screening 262
sigmoid volvulus 315
sildenafil 55
simeprevir 481, 484–485
simulation, medical 209–211
simultaneous liver–kidney transplantation
  (SLKT) 603
single-balloon enteroscopy (SBE), obscure GI
  bleeding 242, **243**
singultus *see* hiccups
sinusoidal obstruction syndrome (SOS) 423, 516–520
  clinical features 518
  diagnosis 518–519
  pathophysiology 516–517
  prognosis 520
  treatment 519
sirolimus (SRL)
  drug interactions **620**
  GI side effects 422
  liver transplant recipients **619**, 622–623, 624, 626
Sitzmarks 402
Sjögren's syndrome 157, 540
skin prick testing 229
sleeve gastrectomy **233**, 234
sleeve gastroplasty, endoscopic 235
slow waves, electrical
  gastric smooth muscle 16–17
  intestinal smooth muscle 191–192
small-bowel adenocarcinoma 280, 282
small-bowel adenomas 279, 282

small-bowel biopsy
  celiac disease 292
  Whipple's disease 297, 298
small-bowel cancer 280–281
  epidemiology **199**, 279
  staging **281**
  treatment 282–283
small bowel–colon anastomosis, short-bowel
  syndrome 302
small-bowel culture 286–287, **288**
small-bowel diseases 271–319
  endoscopic ultrasound 638
  functional 389–415
  obscure GI bleeding 243
  in pregnancy 359–361
small bowel follow-through 281
small-bowel ischemia 308–312
  see also acute mesenteric ischemia; chronic
      mesenteric ischemia/insufficiency
small-bowel lymphoma 280–281, 283
small-bowel manometry 193, 317
small-bowel obstruction 313–314, *316*
small-bowel tumors 279–283
  benign 279–280, 282
  clinical features 281
  diagnosis 281–282
  malignant 280–281
  therapy 282–283
small-(liver) graft-for-size syndrome (SFSS) 615
small-intestinal bacterial overgrowth (SIBO) 224,
      285–289
  chronic intestinal pseudo-obstruction 318
  clinical features 286
  diagnosis 286–287, **288**, *288*
  pathophysiology 285–286, *287*, 413
  treatment 287–289
small intestine
  anatomy and embryology 177
  hormones and neurotransmitters 181–186
  motility 193–194
  neuromuscular apparatus 191–193
  sensory function 193
Smartpill wireless motility capsule (WMC) 37, 134,
      402
smoking, cigarette 323, 352, 590
smooth muscle
  esophageal 11, 15, 16
  intestinal 191
smooth-muscle antibodies (SMA) 509, 524
smooth-muscle cells (SMCs), small intestine 191
smooth-muscle hyperplasia, gastric 127
sodium benzoate 562
sodium restriction, ascites 558
sofosbuvir (SOF) 481, **482**, 483–484, 485
solid organ transplantation (SOT)
  GI complications 419–424
  hepatitis E after 469, 470
somatostatin **182**, 184–185
  variceal bleeding 555
somatostatin analogues 184–185
  variceal bleeding 555
  see also octreotide
somatostatinoma 184
somatostatin receptor scintigraphy (SRS) 185, 186
sorafenib 578
soy allergy 228
spasmolytic polypeptide-expressing metaplasia
      (SPAM), gastric 128
sphincter of Oddi dysfunction (SOD) 459
spider angiomas 431
spiral enteroscopy, obscure GI bleeding **243**
spironolactone 558
splenomegaly, physical examination 432, 433
spontaneous bacterial empyema (SBE) 559

spontaneous bacterial peritonitis (SBP) 559–560
spontaneous portosystemic shunts (SPSS) 562
squamocolumnar junction (SCJ), esophageal 93
staphylococcal toxic shock syndrome **493**
Staphylococcus aureus food poisoning 214
statins
    Barrett's esophagus 94
    hepatotoxicity 505–506
steatosis, hepatic *see* hepatic steatosis
stents
    malignant obstructions 266, 267–268
    TIPS 567, 571
    see also biliary stents; esophageal stents;
        self-expanding metal stents
Still's disease 540
stomach
    anatomy 11–12
    congenital malformations 13, **178**
    embryology 12
    motor function *see* gastric motility
    radiologic approach 26
stool-based tests, colorectal cancer screening 261–262
stool cultures 214
streptococcal toxic shock syndrome **493**
streptomycin, Whipple's disease 297
stress ulcers, bleeding 142
Strongyloides stercoralis 364–365, 496
submucosal (Meissner's) plexus 192
sucralfate, in pregnancy **358**
sulfasalazine 275, **276**
    hepatotoxicity 503
    male fertility and 360
sunitinib 186
superior mesenteric artery (SMA) 308, 334
    embolism 309, 311
    thrombosis 309, 311
superior mesenteric vein (SMV), interposition
        graft 610
swallowing 15–16, *17*
    difficulty *see* dysphagia
    radiologic evaluation 23
    rehabilitation 54
Symmers fibrosis 496
sympathetic nervous system 192
syphilis 365, **493**
systemic diseases
    esophageal and gastric involvement 156–165
    hepatic manifestations 538–542
systemic inflammatory response syndrome
        (SIRS) 374, 436
systemic lupus erythematosus (SLE) 157, 540
systemic sclerosis (scleroderma)
    esophageal disease 32, 33, 156, **157**, *158*
    gastric disease 156, **157**
    liver disease 540

tachykinins **182**
tacrolimus (TAC)
    drug interactions 620
    GI side effects 422
    liver transplant recipients 618–621, 624, 626
    perianal Crohn's disease 253
taste abnormalities 224
T cells 188–189
tegaserod 249, 395, 405
telbivudine, hepatitis B 476, 477
tenia coli 191
tenofovir, hepatitis B 476, 477
terlipressin 555, 560
Test Center, ABIM examination 3
Th1/Th2 cells 188
thalidomide, in pregnancy **358**
thermal contact probes, endoscopic hemostasis 139
thiopurine methyltransferase (TPMT) 621

thiopurines 277, 326
3D regimen *see* ombitasvir/paritaprevir/ritonavir plus
        dasabuvir
thrombocytopenic purpura, idiopathic (ITP) 122
thrombolytic therapy, Budd–Chiari syndrome 515
TIPS *see* transjugular intrahepatic portosystemic shunt
tissue plasminogen activator (tPA) 519
tissue transglutaminase antibodies (tTGA) 292, 512
toll-like receptors (TLRs) 187
tonsilloliths, halitosis 59
toxic reactions to food 229
Toxocara canis 496
toxoplasmosis 494
tracheoesophageal fistula 12–13
transarterial chemoembolization (TACE),
        hepatocellular carcinoma 578
transarterial radioembolization (TARE), hepatocellular
        carcinoma 578
transferrin saturation 532
transient elastography, liver fibrosis **452**, 453–454
transient lower esophageal sphincter relaxations
        (TLESR) 16, 56, 85
transjugular intrahepatic portosystemic shunt
        (TIPS) 567–572
    Budd–Chiari syndrome 515–516, 570
    complications 570–571
    contraindications **570**
    diagnostic methods 567–569
    equipment 567
    hepatic encephalopathy complicating 561, 571
    hepatorenal syndrome 560, 569–570
    indications 569–570
    procedure 567, *568*
    prognostic scoring 570
    refractory ascites 558
    variceal bleeding 142, 556, 569
transplantation
    GI complications 419–424
    see also intestinal transplantation; liver
        transplantation
travelers, hepatitis A 465, 468
traveler's diarrhea 214, 216
trefoil factors 187
trematodes (flukes) 495–496, 547
Treponema pallidum 365, **493**
tricyclic antidepressants (TCAs)
    chronic nausea and vomiting 78
    functional abdominal pain syndrome 409, **410**
    gastroparesis 136
    irritable bowel syndrome 396
    in pregnancy **358**, 359
trientine 555
trimethoprim-sulfamethoxazole (TMP-SMX),
        Whipple's disease 297
trimethylaminuria 59
trituration, gastric 16, 17
troglitazone 504
Tropheryma whipplei 296, **493**
tropical enteropathy 294
tropical sprue 291, 294–295
trypanosomiasis, American *see* Chagas' disease
tuberculosis **493**
tularemia **493**
tumor necrosis factor-α (TNF-α)-inhibiting agents *see*
        anti-tumor necrosis factor-α agents
Turcot syndrome **209**, 351
Twinrix vaccine 468
tylosis 44, **165**
tyramine reactions 229
tyrosinemia **593**

ulcerative colitis (UC) 323–327
    clinical features 323–324
    colorectal cancer risk 324, 350

diagnosis 324–325
differential diagnosis **325**
epidemiology 323
extraintestinal manifestations **209**, 324, 540
pathophysiology 188–189, 323
small-intestinal bacterial overgrowth 285
treatment 325–327
ulcerative proctitis 323
ultrasonography
    endoscopic *see* endoscopic ultrasound
    gallbladder cancer 547
    gallstone disease 544, 545
    gastric emptying measurement 37
    hepatocellular carcinoma 576, *577*
    liver biopsy guidance 450
    nausea and vomiting 75–76
    physical examination and 209
    portal hypertension 554
    small intestinal motility 193
    TIPS surveillance 568–569
ultrasound-based liver elastography **452**, 453–454
umbilical-intestinal fistula 178
umbilical pain **205**
United Network for Organ Sharing (UNOS) 608, 609,
        632–633
University of Wisconsin (UW) solution 612
upper esophageal sphincter (UES) 11
    motor function 15–16, *17*
upper gastrointestinal (GI) bleeding 138–144
    causes 79, 80, 138, 141
    endoscopy 81, 139
    hematemesis 79–81
    hematochezia 237
    history 79, 206
    initial assessment and management 79–80,
        138–139
    medical therapy 80–81
    non-variceal 138–144
    peptic ulcers *see* peptic ulcers, bleeding
    variceal 80, 141–142
upper gastrointestinal endoscopy *see*
        esophagogastroduodenoscopy
upper gastrointestinal series (UGI) 23, 26
upper gastrointestinal (GI) tract
    anatomy and embryology 11–12
    congenital malformations 12–13, **178**
    diagnostic modalities 21–39
    history and physical exam (H&P) 43–45
    pathobiology 9–18
    problem-based approach to 43–81
urea breath test (UBT) 123
urea cycle defects 592
urease test, rapid 123
ursodeoxycholic acid (UDCA)
    intrahepatic cholestasis of pregnancy 584
    NAFLD 528
    primary biliary cholangitis 511
    primary sclerosing cholangitis 551
    progressive familial intrahepatic cholestasis
        591
    sinusoidal obstruction syndrome 519
US Preventive Services Task Force (USPSTF)
        guidelines **210**, 211, 263

vaccinations **210**, 627–628
VACTERL association 12
vagotomy, gastroparesis after 133
vagus nerve
    esophageal motor function 15, 16
    gastric motility 17
vancomycin, *C. difficile* infection 330, *331*
variceal bleeding 555–557
    acute, management 80, 141–142, 555–556
    peristomal 551

variceal bleeding (*Continued*)
  primary prophylaxis   555
  secondary prophylaxis   556, 569
varicella zoster virus (VZV), hepatitis   471
varices   554–557
  bleeding *see* variceal bleeding
  detection   555
  ectopic   556
  management   555–556
  pathophysiology   555
  peristomal   551, 556
vascular anomalies, esophagus   **12**, 13
vascular diseases of liver   513–520
vasculitis   540
vasoactive intestinal polypeptide (VIP)   16, **182**, 185
vasoconstrictors, hepatorenal syndrome   560
vasodilators, portopulmonary hypertension   564
vasopressin   555
vedolizumab
  Crohn's disease   **276**, 277
  in pregnancy   **358**
velpatasvir   481, 484, 485
venlafaxine   **410**
veno-occlusive disease (VOD), hepatic *see* sinusoidal
    obstruction syndrome
veno-venous bypass, liver transplantation   610, 611
Verner–Morrison syndrome   185
vertical-banded gastroplasty (VBG)   234
Viatorr stent graft, TIPS   567, 571
Vibrio parahemolyticus   **214**, 215
video capsule endoscopy (VCE)
  Crohn's disease   274
  obscure GI bleeding   241–242, **243**

small bowel tumors   282
small intestinal motility   193
VIPoma   185
viral hepatitis   5
  acute   465–471
  acute liver failure   435
  chronic   473–479
  history taking   429–430
viral infections
  acute diarrhea   214
  HIV infection   364, 365, **366**
  transplant recipients   420–421, 627
visceral pain   203
vitamin B$_6$ **358**
vitamin deficiencies
  primary biliary cholangitis   511
  protein-losing gastroenteropathy   307
  short-bowel syndrome   302
vitamin E   528
vitelline cyst   178
vitelline duct congenital anomalies   178
volvulus
  colonic   315
  gastric   13, **178**
vomiting *see* nausea and vomiting
vomiting center   74–75
Von Gierke's disease   592

Waldenström's macroglobulinemia   541
waterbrash   46
watermelon stomach   143, 557
watery diarrhea, hypokalemia and hypochlorhydria or
    achlorhydria (WDHA) syndrome   185

weight loss, intentional
  bariatric surgery   233
  NAFLD   527–528
  obesity management   232
weight loss, unintentional   223–226
  causes   224–225
  evaluation   225–226
  history and physical exam   223–224
  nutrition management   226
West Haven classification, hepatic
    encephalopathy   **561**
Whipple's disease   296–298
  clinical features   296–297
  diagnosis   297
  extraintestinal manifestations   **209**, 297, **493**, 540
  pathophysiology   296
  treatment   297–298
Wilson's disease   **438**, 533–536
  clinical features   533–534
  diagnosis   534, **535**
  liver transplantation   535–536, 605
  treatment   534–536
wireless motility capsule (WMC; Smartpill)   37, 134,
    402
Wolman's disease   **593**

Yersinia infections   **214**, 216

zinc
  deficiency, short-bowel syndrome   302
  therapy   535, 562
Zollinger–Ellison syndrome (ZES)   147–148, 182,
    184